Cancer Cytogenetics

Cancer Cytogenetics

Chromosomal and Molecular Genetic Aberrations of Tumor Cells

Fourth Edition

EDITED BY

Sverre Heim

Section for Cancer Cytogenetics
Institute for Cancer Genetics and Informatics
Oslo University Hospital
Oslo, Norway

Felix Mitelman

Department of Clinical Genetics
University of Lund
Lund, Sweden

WILEY Blackwell

This edition first published 2015 © 2015 by John Wiley & Sons, Ltd.
Third edition published 2009 © 2009 by John Wiley & Sons, Inc.

Registered Office
John Wiley & Sons, Ltd, The Atrium, Southern Gate, Chichester, West Sussex, PO19 8SQ, UK

Editorial Offices
9600 Garsington Road, Oxford, OX4 2DQ, UK
The Atrium, Southern Gate, Chichester, West Sussex, PO19 8SQ, UK
111 River Street, Hoboken, NJ 07030-5774, USA

For details of our global editorial offices, for customer services and for information about how to apply for permission to reuse the copyright material in this book please see our website at www.wiley.com/wiley-blackwell

Library of Congress Cataloging-in-Publication Data

Cancer cytogenetics (Heim)
  Cancer cytogenetics : chromosomal and molecular genetic aberrations of tumor cells / edited by Sverre Heim,
Felix Mitelman. – Fourth edition.
       p. ; cm.
  Includes bibliographical references and index.
  ISBN 978-1-118-79553-8 (cloth)
I. Heim, Sverre, editor.   II. Mitelman, Felix, editor.   III. Title.
[DNLM: 1. Neoplasms–genetics.   2. Chromosome Disorders–genetics.   3. Cytogenetics–methods.   QZ 202]
  RC268.4
  616.99′4042–dc23
                                        2015015465
A catalogue record for this book is available from the British Library.

Wiley also publishes its books in a variety of electronic formats. Some content that appears in print may not be available in electronic books.

Set in 9.5/12pt Minion by SPi Global, Pondicherry, India
Printed and bound in Singapore by Markono Print Media Pte Ltd

1   2015

Contents

Contributors

Sietse M. Aukema
Institute of Human Genetics
University Hospital Schleswig-
Holstein Campus Kiel
Christian-Albrechts University Kiel
Germany

Georgia Bardi
BioAnalytica-GenoType SA
Molecular Cytogenetic Research
and Applications
Athens, Greece

Petter Brandal
Section for Cancer Cytogenetics
Institute for Cancer Genetics and
Informatics
Olso University Hospital
Oslo, Norway

Jörn Bullerdiek
Center for Human Genetics
University of Bremen
Bremen, Germany

Paola Dal Cin
Department of Pathology
Brigham and Women's Hospital
Boston, MA, USA

Thoas Fioretos
Department of Clinical Genetics
University of Lund
Lund, Sweden

David Gisselsson
Department of Clinical Genetics
University of Lund
Lund, Sweden

Susanne M. Gollin
Department of Human Genetics
University of Pittsburgh Graduate
School of Public Health
University of Pittsburgh Cancer
Institute
Pittsburgh, PA, USA

Christine J. Harrison
Leukaemia Research Cytogenetics
Group
Northern Institute for Cancer
Research
Newcastle University
Newcastle upon Tyne, UK

Sverre Heim
Section for Cancer Cytogenetics
Institute for Cancer Genetics and
Informatics
Olso University Hospital
Oslo, Norway

Bertil Johansson
Department of Clinical Genetics
University of Lund
Lund, Sweden

Eeva Kettunen
Health and Work Ability
Systems Toxicology
Finnish Institute of Occupational
Health
Helsinki, Finland

Sakari Knuutila
Department of Pathology
Haartman Institute and HUSLAB
University of Helsinki and Helsinki
University Central Hospital
Helsinki, Finland

Michelle M. Le Beau
Section of Hematology/Oncology
University of Chicago
Chicago, IL, USA

Nils Mandahl
Department of Clinical Genetics
University of Lund
Lund, Sweden

Fredrik Mertens
Department of Clinical Genetics
University of Lund
Lund, Sweden

Francesca Micci
Section for Cancer Cytogenetics
Institute for Cancer Genetics and
Informatics
Olso University Hospital
Oslo, Norway

Lucienne Michaux
Centre for Human Genetics
University Hospitals Leuven
University of Leuven
Leuven, Belgium

Felix Mitelman
Department of Clinical
Genetics
University of Lund
Lund, Sweden

Penny Nymark
Department of Toxicogenomics
Maastricht University
Maastricht, The Netherlands;
Institute of Environmental
Medicine
Karolinska Institute
Stockholm, Sweden

Harold J. Olney
Centre Hospitalier de l'Universitié
de Montréal (CHUM)
Université de Montréal
Montréal, Quebec, Canada

Ioannis Panagopoulos
Section for Cancer Cytogenetics
Institute for Cancer Genetics and
Informatics
Olso University Hospital
Oslo, Norway

Nikos Pandis
Department of Genetics
Saint Savas Hospital
Athens, Greece

Reiner Siebert
Institute of Human Genetics
University Hospital Schleswig-
Holstein Campus Kiel
Christian-Albrechts University Kiel
Germany

Karen Sisley
Academic Unit of Ophthalmology
and Orthoptics
Department of Oncology
The Medical School
University of Sheffield
Sheffield, UK

Manuel R. Teixeira
Department of Genetics
Portuguese Oncology Institute
Porto, Portugal

Peter Vandenberghe
Centre for Human Genetics
University Hospitals Leuven
University of Leuven
Leuven, Belgium

Preface to the Fourth Edition

Although only six years have passed since the publication of the third edition of *Cancer Cytogenetics*, the field has undergone marked changes. New information about many tumor types has been gathered using chromosome banding and various molecular cytogenetic techniques, but first and foremost it is the increasing addition of state-of-the-art genomic analyses to the chromosome-level studies of neoplastic cells that has now brought about a more detailed and better understanding of how neoplastic transformation occurs in different disease entities. Inevitably, therefore, this fourth edition contains a wider coverage of the molecular genetic changes that neoplastic cells have acquired than was possible in previous editions. The main focus nevertheless remains unaltered: the genomic aberrations of neoplastic cells as they appear at the chromosomal level of organization. To put the molecular knowledge and studies—especially those involving various ways to search for pathogenetic fusion genes by means of whole genome sequencing—into an integrated molecular genetic–cytogenetic perspective, an entire new chapter was added. Otherwise the overall structure of the book remains the same as it was in the previous edition: the first five chapters, Chapters 1–5, are more generic in nature, Chapters 6–11 deal with hematologic malignancies and lymphomas, and Chapters 12–24 review existing cytogenetic and molecular genetic knowledge on solid tumors.

In all the chapters of this edition, we have strived to emphasize the clinical impact of the various acquired rearrangements, be it diagnostic or prognostic, as much as possible. Cancer cytogenetics has come of age as one of the several means whereby different neoplastic diseases could and should be diagnosed—especially hematologic disorders, malignant lymphomas, and tumors of bone and soft tissue but also increasingly other solid tumors—and it is imperative that cancer cytogeneticists communicate these aspects of their work to the pathologists and clinicians who are in direct charge of the patients. The closer the dialogue with other diagnosticians and clinicians, the more useful the karyotype and other cytogenetic and molecular findings will be in the risk assessment and choice of therapy for individual patients.

At the same time, cancer cytogenetics remains pivotal in the examination of neoplastic cells for research purposes. Chromosome banding analysis is a robust and unbiased method whereby global genetic information can be obtained at the cytogenetic level. All molecular examinations of tumor cells should ideally be viewed against the background of knowledge about the tumor karyotype.

A large number of experts have helped us write the various chapters of *Cancer Cytogenetics*, Fourth Edition. They have done a better job than we ever could even if we had had unlimited time on our hands, and we are profoundly grateful to all of them. The heterogeneity inevitable resulting from multiple authorship reflects reality within the scientific community and we choose to see it as an advantage rather than a disadvantage. We have nevertheless strived to impart a recognizable common format on the various organ-specific chapters so as to comply with the overall plan of the book. It is our hope that those who read and use this book will agree with us that the final result does the field of cancer cytogenetics the credit that is its due.

Sverre Heim
Felix Mitelman
Oslo and Lund, December 2014

CHAPTER 1

How it all began: cancer cytogenetics before sequencing

Felix Mitelman[1] and Sverre Heim[2]

[1] Department of Clinical Genetics, University of Lund, Lund, Sweden
[2] Section for Cancer Cytogenetics, Institute for Cancer Genetics and Informatics,
Oslo University Hospital, Oslo, Norway

The role of genetic changes in neoplasia has been a matter of debate for more than 100 years. The earliest systematic study of cell division in malignant tumors was made in 1890 by the German pathologist David von Hansemann. He drew attention to the frequent occurrence of aberrant mitoses in carcinoma biopsies and suggested that this phenomenon could be used as a criterion for diagnosing the malignant state. His investigations as well as other studies associating nuclear abnormalities with neoplastic growth were, a quarter of a century later, forged into a systematic somatic mutation theory of cancer, which was presented in 1914 by Theodor Boveri in his famous book *Zur Frage der Entstehung maligner Tumoren*. According to Boveri's hypothesis, chromosome abnormalities were the cellular changes causing the transition from normal to malignant proliferation.

For a long time, Boveri's remarkably prescient idea, the concept that neoplasia is brought about by an acquired genetic change, could not be tested. The study of sectioned material yielded only inconclusive results and was clearly insufficient for the examination of chromosome morphology. Technical difficulties thus prevented reliable visualization of mammalian chromosomes, in both normal and neoplastic cells, throughout the entire first half of the 20th century.

During these "dark ages" of mammalian cytogenetics (Hsu, 1979), plant cytogeneticists made spectacular progress, very much through their use of squash and smear preparations. These techniques had from 1920 onward greatly facilitated studies of the genetic material in plants and insects, disclosing chromosome structures more reliably and with greater clarity than had been possible in tissue sections. Around 1950, it was discovered that some experimental tumors in mammals, in particular the Ehrlich ascites tumor of the mouse, could also be examined using the same squash and smear approach. These methods were then rapidly tried with other tissues as well, and in general, mammalian chromosomes were found to be just as amenable to detailed analysis as the most suitable plant materials.

Simultaneously, tissue culturing became more widespread and successful, one effect of which was that the cytogeneticists now had at their disposal a stable source of *in vitro* grown cells. Of crucial importance in this context was also the discovery that colchicine pretreatment resulted in mitotic arrest and dissolution of the spindle apparatus and that treatment of arrested cells with a hypotonic salt solution greatly improved the quality of metaphase spreads. Individual chromosomes could now be counted and analyzed. The many

Cancer Cytogenetics: Chromosomal and Molecular Genetic Aberrations of Tumor Cells, Fourth Edition.
Edited by Sverre Heim and Felix Mitelman.
© 2015 John Wiley & Sons, Ltd. Published 2015 by John Wiley & Sons, Ltd.

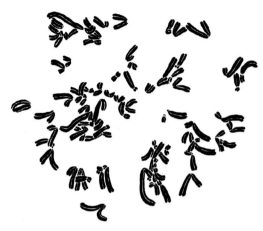

Figure 1.1 Camera lucida drawing of tumor cell mitosis from one of the first (early 1950s) human cancerous effusions submitted to detailed chromosome analysis. The modal number was 75. The stemline also contained numerous abnormal chromosome shapes (Courtesy of Prof. Albert Levan).

methodological improvements ushered in a period of vivid expansion in mammalian cytogenetics, culminating in the description of the correct chromosome number of man by Tjio and Levan (1956) and, shortly afterward, the discovery of the major constitutional human chromosomal syndromes. Two technical breakthroughs around the turn of the decade were of particular importance: the finding that phytohemagglutinin (PHA) has a mitogenic effect on lymphocytes (Nowell, 1960) and the development of a reliable method for short-term culturing of peripheral blood cells (Moorhead et al., 1960).

Cytogenetic studies of animal ascites tumors during the early 1950s, followed soon by investigations of malignant exudates in humans (Figure 1.1), uncovered many of the general principles of karyotypic patterns in highly advanced, malignant cell populations: the apparently ubiquitous chromosomal variability within the tumor, surmised by pathologists since the 1890s; the stemline concept, first defined by Winge (1930); and the competition between stemlines resulting in labile chromosomal equilibria responsive to environmental alterations. The behavior of malignant cell populations could now be described in Darwinian terms: by selective pressures, a dynamic equilibrium is maintained, but any environmental change may upset the balance, causing shifts of the stemline karyotype. Evolution

thus occurs in tumor cell populations in much the same manner as in populations of organisms: chromosomal aberrations generate genetic diversity, and the relative "fitness" imparted by the various changes decides which subclones will prevail.

The elucidation of these evolutionary principles in numerous studies by a number of investigators, for example, Hauschka (1953), Levan (1956), and Makino (1956), paved the way for the new and growing understanding of the role of karyotypic changes in neoplasia and laid the foundation of modern cancer cytogenetics. In humans as well as in other mammals, the results strongly indicated that the chromosomal abnormalities observed were an integral part of tumor development and evolution (see, e.g., Levan, 1967; Koller, 1972; Hsu, 1979; Sandberg, 1980, for review of the early data). It should be kept in mind, however, that the object of these early investigations was always metastatic tumors, often effusions, that is, highly malignant cell populations. Hence, few, if any, conclusions could be drawn from them as to the role of chromosomal abnormalities in early tumor stages.

Interest in cancer cytogenetics influenced human cytogenetics much more profoundly than is currently appreciated. For example, the main goal behind the study that eventually led to the description of the correct chromosome number in man (Tjio and Levan, 1956) was to identify what distinguished a cancer cell. The motivation was not primarily an interest in the normal chromosome constitution, which at that time had no obvious implications, but the hope that such knowledge would help answer the basic question of whether chromosome changes lay behind the transformation of a normal to a cancer cell.

The first spectacular success in cancer cytogenetics came when Nowell and Hungerford (1960) discovered that a small karyotypic marker (Figure 1.2), the Philadelphia (Ph) chromosome, replaced one of the four smallest autosomes (the G-group chromosomes according to the nomenclature at the time) in the bone marrow cells of seven patients with chronic myeloid leukemia (CML). This was the first consistent chromosome abnormality in a human cancer, and its detection seemed to provide conclusive verification of Boveri's idea. It was reasonable to assume that the acquired chromosomal abnormality—a perfect example of a somatic

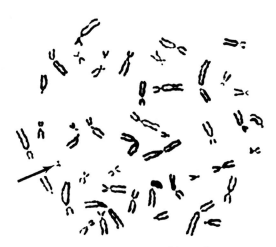

Figure 1.2 Unbanded metaphase cell from a bone marrow culture established from a patient with chronic myeloid leukemia. The arrow indicates the Ph chromosome (previously called Ph[1]); the superscript indicated that this was the first cancer-specific aberration detected in Philadelphia. This naming practice was later abandoned, but the abbreviation Ph has for sentimental reasons been retained, since it was the first consistent chromosome abnormality detected in a human malignancy.

mutation in a hematopoietic stem cell—was the direct cause of the neoplastic state.

Nowell and Hungerford's discovery greatly stimulated interest in cancer cytogenetics in the early 1960s, but for several reasons, the Ph chromosome long remained an exceptional finding. The confusing plethora of karyotypic aberrations encountered in other malignancies suggested that the changes were epiphenomena incurred during tumor progression rather than essential early pathogenetic factors. The enthusiasm for tumor cytogenetics as a result gradually faded. With this change of mood, the perceived significance of the Ph chromosome also changed, and the very uniqueness of the marker came to be regarded as a perplexing oddity. Why should there be such a simple association between a chromosomal trait and one particular malignant disease, when more and more data from other neoplasms showed either no chromosome aberrations at all or a confusing mixture of apparently meaningless abnormalities?

That an orderly pattern existed in what had hitherto been seen as chaos was suggested independently in the mid-1960s by Levan (1966) and van Steenis (1966). Surveying chromosomal data available in the literature, mainly on ascitic forms of gastric, mammary, uterine, and ovarian carcinomas, they found clear evidence that certain chromosome types tended to increase and others to decrease in number in the tumors. Soon afterward, the nonrandomness of karyotypic changes was also demonstrated beyond doubt in specific types of human hematologic disorders and solid tumors; for example, trisomy of a C chromosome in acute myeloid leukemia (Hungerford and Nowell, 1962), deletion of an F-group chromosome in polycythemia vera (Kay et al., 1966), loss of a G chromosome in meningioma (Zang and Singer, 1967), and a C–G translocation in acute myeloid leukemia (Kamada et al., 1968). The results of comprehensive cytogenetic studies of experimental tumors, including more than 200 primary sarcomas induced by the Rous sarcoma virus in mice, rats, and the Chinese hamster, supported the same conclusion (Mitelman, 1974). In both humans and animals, the karyotypic abnormalities seemed to be of two essentially different kinds: nonrandom changes preferentially involving particular chromosomes and a frequently more massive random or background variation affecting all chromosomes. To differentiate between the two could be exceedingly difficult, however. As a consequence, in spite of painstaking efforts, little progress was made in cancer cytogenetics during this period.

The situation changed dramatically in 1970 with the introduction by Caspersson and Zech of chromosome banding techniques (Caspersson et al., 1970a). The new methodology completely revolutionized cytogenetic analyses. Each chromosome could now be precisely identified on the basis of its unique banding pattern; whereas formerly identification was restricted to chromosome groups, all descriptions of chromosome deviations immediately became more precise and the conclusions based on them more stringent. As a consequence, a steadily increasing number of cancer cases, initially predominantly malignant hematologic disorders, were investigated with the new techniques, and a number of characteristic, specific, sometimes even pathognomonic changes were soon discovered (Table 1.1). Caspersson et al. (1970b) first used banding in this context and identified the Ph chromosome as a deleted chromosome 22, and in 1972, three of the nonrandom aberrations described in the 1960s were clarified: the additional C-group

Table 1.1 Characteristic neoplasia-associated cytogenetic aberrations detected by banding analyses 1970–1979

Year	Disease	Aberration	References
1970	Chronic myeloid leukemia	del(22q)	Caspersson et al. (1970b)
1972	Acute myeloid leukemia	+8	de la Chapelle et al. (1972)
	Burkitt lymphoma	14q+	Manolov and Manolova (1972)
	Meningioma	−22	Mark et al. (1972) and Zankl and Zang (1972)
	Polycythemia vera	del(20q)	Reeves et al. (1972)
1973	Acute myeloid leukemia	t(8;21)(q22;q22)	Rowley (1973a)
	Acute myeloid leukemia	i(17)(q10)	Mitelman et al. (1973)
	Acute myeloid leukemia	−7/del(7q)	Petit et al. (1973) and Rowley (1973c)
	Chronic myeloid leukemia	t(9;22)(q34;q11)	Rowley (1973b)
	Acute myeloid leukemia/	+9	Davidson and Knight (1973), Rowley (1973d),
	Myeloproliferative disorders		and Rutten et al. (1973)
1974	Acute myeloid leukemia	+21	Mitelman and Brandt (1974)
	Refractory anemia	del (5q)	van den Berghe et al. (1974)
1975	Myeloproliferative disease	t(11;20)(p15;q11)	Berger (1975)
1976	Acute myeloid leukemia	t(6;9)(p23;q34)	Rowley and Potter (1976)
	Burkitt lymphoma	t(8;14)(q24;q32)	Zech et al. (1976)
1977	Acute lymphoblastic leukemia	t(4;11)(q21;q23)	Oshimura et al. (1977)
	Acute promyelocytic leukemia	t(15;17)(q22;q21)	Rowley et al. (1977)
	Neuroblastoma	del(1p)	Brodeur et al. (1977)
1978	Acute monocytic leukemia	t(8;16)(p11;p13)	Mitelman et al. (1978)
	Acute myeloid leukemia	ins(3;3)(q21;q21q26)	Golomb et al. (1978)
1979	Acute lymphoblastic leukemia	t(8;14)(q24;q32)	Berger et al. (1979a) and Mitelman et al. (1979)
	Burkitt lymphoma	t(2;8)(p12;q24)	Miyoshi et al. (1979) and van den Berghe et al. (1979)
	Burkitt lymphoma	t(8;22)(q24;q11)	Berger et al. (1979b)
	Chronic lymphocytic leukemia	+12	Autio et al. (1979)
	Follicular lymphoma	t(14;18)(q32;q21)	Fukuhara et al. (1979)
	Mouse plasmacytoma	t(6;15), t(12;15)	Ohno et al. (1979)

chromosome in acute myeloid leukemia was identified as trisomy 8 (de la Chapelle et al., 1972), the lost G-group chromosome in meningioma corresponded to monosomy 22 (Mark et al., 1972; Zankl and Zang, 1972), and the deleted F-group chromosome in polycythemia vera was a del(20q) (Reeves et al., 1972). A previously unrecognized recurrent abnormality, a 14q + marker chromosome in Burkitt lymphoma (BL), was also described the very same year (Manolov and Manolova, 1972). The first recurrent balanced rearrangements were reported shortly afterward: a reciprocal translocation between chromosomes 8 and 21, that is, t(8;21)(q22;q22), was found in the bone marrow cells of some patients with acute myeloid leukemia (Rowley, 1973a), and the Ph chromosome of CML was demonstrated to stem from a t(9;22)(q34;q11), not a deletion of chromosome 22 as was previously

thought (Rowley, 1973b). Among other important translocations also soon identified were t(8;14) (q24;q32), t(2;8)(p12;q24), and t(8;22)(q24;q11) in BL (Zech et al., 1976; Berger et al., 1979b; Miyoshi et al., 1979; van den Berghe et al., 1979), t(15;17) (q22;q21) in acute promyelocytic leukemia (Rowley et al., 1977), t(4;11)(q21;q23) in acute lymphoblastic leukemia (Oshimura et al., 1977), and t(14;18)(q32;q21) in follicular lymphoma (Fukuhara et al., 1979). Ohno et al. (1979) identified two characteristic translocations—t(6;15) and t(12;15)—in mouse plasmacytomas (MPC), the first specific rearrangements in experimental neoplasms and, as it turned out (see below), the perfect equivalents of the characteristic translocations in human BL. In total, more than 1200 neoplasms with clonal abnormalities were reported during this first decade of banding cytogenetics,

Table 1.2 Characteristic cytogenetic aberrations detected by banding analyses of solid tumors 1980–1989

Year	Tumor type	Aberration	References
1980	Salivary gland adenoma	t(3;8)(p21;q12)	Mark et al. (1980)
1982	Germ cell tumors	i(12)(p10)	Atkin and Baker (1982)
	Lung cancer	del(3)(p14p23)	Whang-Peng et al. (1982)
	Retinoblastoma	i(6)(p10)/del(13q)	Balaban et al. (1982) and Kusnetsova et al. (1982)
	Rhabdomyosarcoma (alveolar)	t(2;13)(q36;q14)	Seidal et al. (1982)
1983	Ewing sarcoma	t(11;22)(q24;q12)	Aurias et al. (1983) and Turc-Carel et al. (1983)
	Salivary gland adenoma	der(12)(q13–15)	Stenman and Mark (1983)
	Wilms' tumor	der(16)t(1;16)(q21;q13)	Kaneko et al. (1983)
1985	Chondrosarcoma (myxoid)	t(9;22)(q31;q12)	Hinrichs et al. (1985)
1986	Kidney cancer	t(X;1)(p11;q21)	de Jong et al. (1986)
	Lipoma	t(3;12)(q27;q13)	Heim et al. (1986) and Turc-Carel et al. (1986)
	Liposarcoma (myxoid)	t(12;16)(q13;p11)	Limon et al. (1986a)
	Salivary gland carcinoma	t(6;9)(q23;p23)	Stenman et al. (1986)
	Synovial sarcoma	t(X;18)(p11;q11)	Limon et al. (1986b)
1987	Kidney cancer	del(3p)/der(3)t(3;5)(p13;q22)	Kovacs et al. (1987)
	Lipoma	Ring chromosome(s)	Heim et al. (1987)
	Lipoma	der(12)(q13–15)	Mandahl et al. (1987)
1988	Primitive neuroectodermal tumor	i(17)(q10)	Griffin et al. (1988)
	Salivary gland cystadenolymphoma	t(11;19)(q21;p13)	Bullerdiek et al. (1988)
	Uterine leiomyoma	del(7)(q22q31)	Boghosian et al. (1988)
	Uterine leiomyoma	t(12;14)(q14;q24)	Heim et al. (1988), Mark et al. (1988), and Turc-Carel et al. (1988)
1989	Infantile fibrosarcoma	+8,+11,+20	Mandahl et al. (1989) and Speleman et al. (1989)
	Lipoma	der(6)(p21)	Sait et al. (1989)
	Ovarian cancer	add(19)(p13)	Pejovic et al. (1989)

and more than 60 recurrent chromosomal aberrations were identified.

The following decade saw a rush of data coming from studies of solid tumors, initially in particular mesenchymal neoplasms. The chromosome abnormalities of more than 2000 solid tumors were reported between 1980 and 1989, and almost 200 recurrent structural changes were identified. Several of them were no less specific than those previously found among hematologic disorders (Table 1.2), for example, t(2;13)(q36;q14) in alveolar rhabdomyosarcoma (Seidal et al., 1982), t(11;22)(q24;q12) in Ewing sarcoma (Aurias et al., 1983; Turc-Carel et al., 1983), and t(12;16) (q13;p11) in myxoid liposarcoma (Limon et al., 1986a). At this time, it also became clear that many benign tumors carried characteristic aberrations, including reciprocal translocations, for example,

t(3;8)(p21;q12) in salivary gland adenoma (Mark et al., 1980), t(3;12)(q27;q13) in lipoma (Heim et al., 1986; Turc-Carel et al., 1986), and t(12;14) (q14;q24) in uterine leiomyoma (Heim et al., 1988; Mark et al., 1988; Turc-Carel et al., 1988).

The identification of specific cytogenetic aberrations enabled meaningful clinical–cytogenetic association studies, the most important of which were the International Workshops on Chromosomes in Leukemia established in the late 1970s. The workshops provided an arena for a fruitful and at the time unique collaboration among cytogeneticists, clinicians, and pathologists who shared their data and insights in order to find diagnostically and prognostically interesting associations between cytogenetic aberrations and clinical characteristics in various hematologic disorders. The results obtained by this collaborative study group over a 10-year period showed that cytogenetics could subdivide phenotypically identical leukemias and lymphomas into distinct subgroups on the basis of specific abnormalities and that this classification had important clinical implications. For example, the workshop collaborators demonstrated that the diagnostic karyotype in childhood acute lymphoblastic leukemia was of greater prognostic importance than any hitherto known risk factor, such as patient age, white blood cell count, or immunophenotype (Bloomfield et al., 1986). The studies performed by the Workshops on well-characterized patient materials from different parts of the world were thus instrumental in consolidating cytogenetics as clinically well-nigh indispensable in hematology. A similar collaborative study group dedicated to the genetic analysis of mesenchymal tumors—the Chromosomes and Morphology (CHAMP) study group—was formed a decade later and has identified several important clinical–cytogenetic associations among different bone and soft tissue tumors (e.g., Mertens et al., 1998).

Technological advances at the same time made it possible to supplement cytogenetic investigations by molecular genetic studies of the same tumor types. Analyses in the early 1980s of the specific translocations in MPC, BL, and CML proved particularly pivotal for our understanding of how chromosome aberrations contribute to neoplastic transformation not only in these specific disorders but also generally (Mitelman et al., 2007). The picture to emerge was that reciprocal translocations exert their effects by one of two main alternative mechanisms: deregulation, usually resulting in overexpression, of a seemingly normal gene in one of the breakpoints (the BL scenario) or the creation of a hybrid, chimeric gene through fusion of parts of two genes, one in each breakpoint (the CML scenario). Deregulation of an oncogene by juxtaposition to a constitutively active gene region was predicted by Klein already in 1981, and the principle was soon demonstrated in MPC (Adams et al., 1982; Harris et al., 1982; Kirsch et al., 1982) and human BL (Dalla Favera et al, 1982; Taub et al., 1982; Croce et al., 1983; Erikson et al., 1983). The breakpoints of the characteristic translocations in mice and humans were found to be located within or close to the MYC oncogene and one of

the immunoglobulin heavy- or light-chain genes (IGH, IGK, or IGL). As a consequence of the translocations, the entire coding part of MYC is juxtaposed to one of the immunoglobulin genes, resulting in deregulation of MYC because the gene is now driven by regulatory elements of the immunoglobulin genes. The alternative mechanism—the creation of a fusion gene—was documented at the same time in CML with the demonstration that the Ph chromosome, that is, the der(22)t(9;22)(q34;q11), contains a fusion in which the 3′ part of the ABL oncogene from 9q34 has become juxtaposed with the 5′ part of a gene from 22q11 called the BCR gene, resulting in the creation of an in-frame BCR–ABL fusion transcript (de Klein et al., 1982; Heisterkamp et al., 1983; Groffen et al., 1984; Shtivelman et al., 1985).

These and similar molecular insights into how cancer-specific chromosomal abnormalities act pathogenetically sparked an enormous interest in cytogenetics as a powerful means to pinpoint the locations of genes important in tumorigenesis (Heim and Mitelman, 1987). An impressive amount of information has been accumulated through these efforts. More than 65 000 neoplasms with at least one clonal cytogenetic change have been identified, and more than 700 gene fusions have been found by genomic characterization of breakpoints in cytogenetically identified aberrations in various leukemias, lymphomas, and solid tumors (Mitelman et al., 2015). We now know that practically all acquired balanced rearrangements lead to in principle the same consequences as the ones originally elucidated in BL and CML, that is, deregulation of a seemingly normal gene or the creation of a hybrid gene. In addition to oncogene activation via translocations and other balanced rearrangements (inversions, insertions), gene fusions may also be produced by unbalanced changes such as deletions leading to fusion of genes in the deletion edges.

The advent of molecular genetics in the 1980s and the development of a range of powerful molecular cytogenetic technologies during the last three decades, such as fluorescence *in situ* hybridization (FISH), multicolor FISH, comparative genomic hybridization (CGH), various array-based genotyping technologies, and DNA and RNA sequencing (Lander, 2011; Ozsolak and Milos, 2011;

Le Scouarnac and Gribble, 2012; Mwenifumbo and Marra, 2013; Mertens and Tayebwa, 2014), have dramatically widened our knowledge and understanding of the molecular mechanisms that are operative in neoplastic initiation and progression. The new techniques have enabled researchers to investigate tumor cells at the level of individual genes, even at the level of single base pairs, and the molecular consequences of an ever increasing number of cancer-associated genomic aberrations have thus been laid bare (Vogelstein et al., 2013).

It is obvious that the cross-fertilization between cytogenetics and molecular genetics has led to conceptually new advances and insights into the fundamental cell biology mechanisms that are disrupted when neoplastic transformation occurs. At the same time, the clinical usefulness of cytogenetic abnormalities as diagnostic and prognostic aids in cancer medicine has been increasingly appreciated. The ultimate goal is to arrive at specific therapies individualized to counter those molecular mechanisms that have gone awry in each patient's cancerous disease. The development of imatinib (Druker, 2008) as a therapeutic agent for CML—the first example of a targeted therapy against a specific fusion gene in cancer—is a wonderful example of how progress in cytogenetics and molecular biology has led to a qualitatively new treatment approach: the discovery of the Ph chromosome, the finding that the Ph chromosome results from a reciprocal translocation, the identification of the two genes in the breakpoints of the translocation, and the subsequent characterization of the fusion gene and its protein product. Similar targeted therapies are presently being developed against a number of fusion genes, and some have already turned out to be successful, for example, crizotinib targeting the *EML4–ALK* fusion gene generated by an inversion on the short arm of chromosome 2 in a subset of patients with non-small cell lung cancer (Shaw and Engelman, 2013). While it took 40 years from the discovery of the Ph chromosome to the development of imatinib, it only took a few years from the description of the *EML4–ALK* fusion in lung cancer to the development of crizotinib. We are convinced that many similar success stories are unfolding as we write; cancer genetic research helps obtain more effective and less toxic treatments for malignant diseases. Thus, in the 100 years since Boveri first

postulated that chromosome change may initiate the carcinogenic process, cancer cytogenetics has come of age. It is no longer a purely descriptive discipline but one that attempts to synthesize information from several investigative approaches. Cancer cytogenetics has become both a central methodology in basic cancer research and an important clinical tool in oncology.

References

Adams JM, Gerondakis S, Webb E, Mitchell J, Bernard O, Cory S (1982): Transcriptionally active DNA region that rearranges frequently in murine lymphoid tumors. *Proc Natl Acad Sci USA* 22:6966–6970.

Atkin NB, Baker MC (1982): Specific chromosome change, i(12p), in testicular tumors? *Lancet* 2:1349.

Aurias A, Rimbaut C, Buffe D, Dubousset J, Mazabraud A (1983): Chromosomal translocations in Ewing's sarcoma. *N Engl J Med* 309:496–497.

Autio K, Turunen O, Penttila O, Eramaa E, de la Chapelle A, Schröder J (1979): Human chronic lymphocytic leukemia: Karyotypes in different lymphocyte populations. *Cancer Genet Cytogenet* 1:147–155.

Balaban G, Gilbert F, Nicholas W, Meadows AT, Shields J (1982): Abnormalities of chromosome #13 in retinoblastomas from individuals with normal constitutional karyotypes. *Cancer Genet Cytogenet* 6:213–221.

Berger R (1975): Translocation t(11;20) et polyglobulie primitive. *Nouv Presse Med* 4:1972.

Berger R, Bernheim A, Brouet JC, Daniel MT, Flandrin G (1979a): t(8;14) translocation in a Burkitt's type of lymphoblastic leukaemia (L3). *Br J Haematol* 43:87–90.

Berger R, Bernheim A, Weh H-J, Flandrin G, Daniel MT, Brouet J-C, et al. (1979b): A new translocation in Burkitt's tumor cells. *Hum Genet* 53:111–112.

van den Berghe H, Cassiman JJ, David G, Fryns JP, Michaux JL, Sokal G (1974): Distinct haematological disorder with deletion of long arm of no. 5 chromosome. *Nature* 251:437–438.

van den Berghe H, Parloir C, Gosseye S, Englebienne V, Cornu G, Sokal G (1979): Variant translocation in Burkitt lymphoma. *Cancer Genet Cytogenet* 1:9–14.

Bloomfield CD, Goldman AI, Alimena G, Berger R, Borgström GH, Brandt L, et al. (1986): Chromosomal abnormalities identify high-risk and low-risk patients with acute lymphoblastic leukemia. *Blood* 67:415–420.

Boghosian L, Dal Cin P, Sandberg AA (1988): An interstitial deletion of chromosome 7 may characterize a subgroup of uterine leiomyoma. *Cancer Genet Cytogenet* 34:207–208.

Boveri T (1914): *Zur Frage der Entstehung maligner Tumoren*. Jena: Gustav Fischer.

Brodeur GM, Sekhon GS, Goldstein MN (1977): Chromosomal aberrations in human neuroblastomas. *Cancer* 40:2256–2263.

Bullerdiek J, Haubrich J, Meyer K, Bartnitzke S (1988): Translocation t(11;19)(q21;p13.1) as the sole chromosome abnormality in a cystadenolymphoma (Warthin's tumor) of the parotid gland. *Cancer Genet Cytogenet* 35:129–132.

Caspersson T, Zech L, Johansson C (1970a): Differential binding of alkylating fluorochromes in human chromosomes. *Exp Cell Res* 60:315–319.

Caspersson T, Gahrton G, Lindsten J, Zech L (1970b): Identification of the Philadelphia chromosome as a number 22 by quinacrine mustard fluorescence analysis. *Exp Cell Res* 63:238–240.

de la Chapelle A, Schröder J, Vuopio P (1972): 8-Trisomy in the bone marrow. Report of two cases. *Clin Genet* 3:470–476.

Croce CM, Thierfelder W, Erikson J, Nishikura K, Finan J, Lenoir GM, et al. (1983): Transcriptional activation of an unrearranged and untranslocated c-myc oncogene by translocation of a C lambda locus in Burkitt. *Proc Natl Acad Sci USA* 80:6922–6926.

Dalla-Favera R, Bregni M, Erikson J, Patterson D, Gallo RC, Croce CM (1982): Human c-myc onc gene is located on the region of chromosome 8 that is translocated in Burkitt lymphoma cells. *Proc Natl Acad Sci USA* 79:7824–7827.

Davidson WM, Knight LA (1973): Acquired trisomy 9. *Lancet* 1:1510.

Druker BJ (2008): Translation of the Philadelphia chromosome into therapy for CML. *Blood* 112:4808–4817.

Erikson J, Nishikura K, ar-Rushdi A, Finan J, Emanuel B, Lenoir G, et al. (1983): Translocation of an immunoglobulin kappa locus to a region 3′ of an unrearranged c-myc oncogene enhances c-myc transcription. *Proc Natl Acad Sci USA* 80:7581–7585.

Fukuhara S, Rowley JD, Variakojis D, Golomb HM (1979): Chromosome abnormalities in poorly differentiated lymphocytic lymphoma. *Cancer Res* 39:3119–3128.

Golomb HM, Vardiman JW, Rowley JD, Testa JR, Mintz U (1978): Correlation of clinical findings with quinacrine-banded chromosomes in 90 adults with acute nonlymphocytic leukemia. An eight-year study (1970–1977). *N Engl J Med* 299:613–619.

Griffin CA, Hawkins AL, Packer RJ, Rorke LB, Emanuel BS (1988): Chromosome abnormalities in pediatric brain tumors. *Cancer Res* 48:175–180.

Groffen J, Stephenson JR, Heisterkamp N, de Klein A, Bartram CR, Grosveld G (1984): Philadelphia chromosomal breakpoints are clustered within a limited region, bcr, on chromosome 22. *Cell* 36:93–99.

von Hansemann D (1890): Ueber asymmetrische Zelltheilung in Epithelkrebsen und deren biologische Bedeutung. *Virchows Arch Anat* 119:299–326.

Harris LJ, Lang RB, Marcu KB (1982): Non-immunoglobulin-associated DNA rearrangements in mouse plasmacytomas. *Proc Natl Acad Sci USA* 79:4175–4179.

Hauschka TS (1953): Cell population studies on mouse ascites tumors. *Ann N Y Acad Sci* 16:64–73.

Heim S, Mitelman F (1987): *Cancer Cytogenetics*. New York: Alan R. Liss, Inc.

Heim S, Mandahl N, Kristoffersson U, Mitelman F, Rööser B, Rydholm A, Willén H (1986): Reciprocal translocation t(3;12)(q27;q13) in lipoma. *Cancer Genet Cytogenet* 23:301–304.

Heim S, Mandahl N, Kristoffersson U, Mitelman F, Rööser B, Rydholm A, Willén H (1987): Marker ring chromosome—a new cytogenetic abnormality characterizing lipogenic tumors? *Cancer Genet Cytogenet* 24:319–326.

Heim S, Nilbert M, Vanni R, Floderus U-M, Mandahl N, Liedgren S, Lecca U, Mitelman F (1988): A specific translocation, t(12;14)(q14–15;q23–24), characterizes a subgroup of uterine leiomyomas. *Cancer Genet Cytogenet* 32:13–17.

Heisterkamp N, Stephenson JR, Groffen J, Hansen PF, de Klein A, Bartram CR, Grosveld G (1983): Localization of the c-abl oncogene adjacent to a translocation break point in chronic myelocytic leukaemia. *Nature* 306:239–242.

Hinrichs SH, Jaramillo MA, Gumerlock PH, Gardner MB, Lewis JP, Freeman AE (1985): Myxoid chondrosarcoma with a translocation involving chromosomes 9 and 22. *Cancer Genet Cytogenet* 14:219–226.

Hsu TC (1979): *Human and Mammalian Cytogenetics*. An Historical Perspective. New York: Springer Verlag.

Hungerford DA, Nowell PC (1962): Chromosome studies in human leukemia III. Acute granulocytic leukemia. *J Natl Cancer Inst* 29:545–565.

de Jong B, Molenaar IM, Leeuw JA, Idenberg VJS, Oosterhuis JW (1986): Cytogenetics of a renal adenocarcinoma in a 2-year-old child. *Cancer Genet Cytogenet* 21:165–169.

Kamada N, Okada K, Ito T, Nakatsui T, Uchino H (1968): Chromosomes 21–22 and neutrophil alkaline phosphatase in leukaemia. *Lancet* 1: 364.

Kaneko Y, Kondo K, Rowley JD, Moohr JW, Maurer HS (1983): Further chromosome studies on Wilms' tumor cells of patients without aniridia. *Cancer Genet Cytogenet* 10:191–197.

Kay HEM, Lawler SD, Millard RE (1966): The chromosomes in polycythemia vera. *Br J Haematol* 12: 507–527.

Kirsch IR, Morton CC, Nakahara K, Leder P (1982): Human immunoglobulin heavy chain genes map to a region of translocations in malignant B lymphocytes. *Science* 216:301–303.

Klein G (1981): The role of gene dosage and genetic transpositions in carcinogenesis. *Nature* 294:313–318.

de Klein A, van Kessel AG, Grosveld G, Bartram CR, Hagemeijer A, Bootsma D, et al. (1982): A cellular oncogene is translocated to the Philadelphia chromosome in chronic myelocytic leukaemia. *Nature* 300:765–767.

Koller PC (1972): *The Role of Chromosomes in Cancer Biology. Recent Results in Cancer Research.* Vol 38. Berlin: Springer Verlag.

Kovacs G, Szücs S, de Riese W, Baumgärtel H (1987): Specific chromosome aberration in human renal cell carcinoma. *Int J Cancer* 40:171–178.

Kusnetsova LE, Prigogina EL, Pogosianz HE, Belkina BM (1982): Similar chromosomal abnormalities in several retinoblastomas. *Hum Genet* 61:201–204.

Lander ES (2011): Initial impact of the sequencing of the human genome. *Nature* 470:187–197.

Le Scouarnac S, Gribble SM (2012): Characterising chromosome rearrangements: Recent technical advances in molecular cytogenetics. *Heredity* 108:75–85.

Levan A (1956): Chromosomal studies on some human tumors and tissues of normal origin, grown in vivo and in vitro at the Sloan-Kettering Institute. *Cancer* 9:648–663.

Levan A (1966): Non-random representation of chromosome types in human tumor stemlines. *Hereditas* 55:28–38.

Levan A (1967): Some current problems of cancer cytogenetics. *Hereditas* 57:343–355.

Limon J, Turc-Carel C, Dal Cin P, Rao U, Sandberg AA (1986a): Recurrent chromosome translocations in liposarcoma. *Cancer Genet Cytogenet* 22:93–94.

Limon J, Dal Cin P, Sandberg AA (1986b): Translocations involving the X chromosome in solid tumors: Presentation of two sarcomas with t(X;18)(q13;p11). *Cancer Genet Cytogenet* 23:87–91.

Makino S (1956): Further evidence favoring the concept of the stem cell in ascites tumors of rats. *Ann N Y Acad Sci* 63:818–830.

Mandahl N, Heim S, Johansson B, Bennet K, Mertens F, Olsson G, et al. (1987): Lipomas have characteristic structural chromosomal rearrangements of 12q13–q14. *Int J Cancer* 39:685–688.

Mandahl N, Heim S, Rydholm A, Willén H, Mitelman F (1989): Nonrandom numerical chromosome aberrations (+8, +11, +17, +20) in infantile fibrosarcoma. *Cancer Genet Cytogenet* 40:137–139.

Manolov G, Manolova Y (1972): Marker band in one chromosome 14 from Burkitt lymphomas. *Nature* 237:33–34.

Mark J, Levan G, Mitelman F (1972): Identification by fluorescence of the G chromosome lost in human meningomas. *Hereditas* 71:163–168.

Mark J, Dahlenfors R, Ekedahl C, Stenman G (1980): The mixed salivary gland tumor—a normally benign human neoplasm frequently showing specific chromosomal abnormalities. *Cancer Genet Cytogenet* 2:231–241.

Mark J, Havel G, Grepp C, Dahlenfors R, Wedell B (1988): Cytogenetical observations in human benign uterine leiomyomas. *Anticancer Res* 8:621–626.

Mertens F, Tayebwa J (2014): Evolving techniques for gene fusion detection in soft tissue tumours. *Histopathology* 64:151–162.

Mertens F, Fletcher CDM, Dal Cin P, De Wever I, Mandahl N, Mitelman F, et al. (1998): Cytogenetic analysis of 46 pleomorphic soft tissue sarcomas and correlation with morphologic and clinical features: A report of the CHAMP Study Group. *Genes Chromosomes Cancer* 22:16–25.

Mitelman F (1974): The Rous sarcoma virus story: Cytogenetics of tumors induced by RSV. In German J (ed): *Chromosomes and Cancer.* New York: John Wiley & Sons, pp. 675–693.

Mitelman F, Brandt L (1974): Chromosome banding pattern in acute myeloid leukemia. *Scand J Haematol* 13:321–330.

Mitelman F, Brandt L, Levan G (1973): Identification of iso-chromosome 17 in acute myeloid leukaemia. *Lancet* 2:972.

Mitelman F, Brandt L, Nilsson PG (1978): Relation among occupational exposure to potential mutagenic/carcinogenic agents, clinical findings, and bone marrow chromosomes in acute nonlymphocytic leukemia. *Blood* 52:1229–1237.

Mitelman F, Andersson-Anvret M, Brandt L, Catovsky D, Klein G, Manolov G, et al. (1979): Reciprocal 8;14 translocation in EBV-negative B-cell acute lymphocytic leukemia with Burkitt-type cells. *Int J Cancer* 24:27–33.

Mitelman F, Johansson B, Mertens F (2007): The impact of translocations and gene fusions on cancer causation. *Nat Rev Cancer* 7:233–245.

Mitelman F, Johansson B, Mertens F (Eds.) (2015): Mitelman Database of Chromosome Aberrations and Gene Fusions in Cancer. http://cgap.nci.nih.gov/Chromosomes/Mitelman.

Miyoshi I, Hiraki S, Kimura I, Miyamoto K, Sato J (1979): 2/8 translocation in a Japanese Burkitt's lymphoma. *Experientia* 35:742–743.

Moorhead PS, Nowell PC, Mellman WJ, Battips DM, Hungerford DA (1960): Chromosome preparations of leukocytes cultured from human peripheral blood. *Exp Cell Res* 20:613–616.

Mwenifumbo JC, Marra MA (2013): Cancer genome-sequencing study design. *Nat Rev Genet* 14:321–332.

Nowell PC (1960): Phytohemagglutinin: An initiator of mitosis in cultures of normal human leukocytes. *Cancer Res* 20:462–466.

Nowell PC, Hungerford DA (1960): A minute chromosome in human chronic granulocytic leukemia. *Science* 132:1497.

Ohno S, Babonits M, Wiener F, Spira J, Klein G, Potter M (1979): Nonrandom chromosome changes involving the Ig gene-carrying chromosomes 12 and 6 in pristane-induced mouse plasmacytomas. *Cell* 18:1001–1007.

Oshimura M, Freeman AI, Sandberg AA (1977): Chromosomes and causation of human cancer and leukemia. XXVI. Banding studies in acute lymphoblastic leukemia (ALL). *Cancer* 40:1161–1172.

Ozsolak F, Milos PM (2011): RNA sequencing: Advances, challenges and opportunities. *Nat Rev Genet* 12:87–98.

Pejovic T, Heim S, Mandahl N, Elmfors B, Flodérus U-M, Furgyik S, et al. (1989): Consistent occurrence of a 19p + marker chromosome and loss of 11p material in ovarian seropapillary cystadenocarcinomas. *Genes Chromosomes Cancer* 1:167–171.

Petit P, Alexander M, Fondu P (1973): Monosomy 7 in erythroleukaemia. *Lancet* 2:1326–1327.

Reeves BR, Lobb DS, Lawler SD (1972): Identity of the abnormal F-group chromosome associated with polycythaemia vera. *Humangenetik* 14:159–161.

Rowley JD (1973a): Identification of a translocation with quinacrine fluorescence in a patient with acute leukemia. *Ann Genet* 16:109–112.

Rowley JD (1973b): A new consistent chromosomal abnormality in chronic myelogenous leukaemia identified by quinacrine fluorescence and Giemsa staining. *Nature* 243:290–293.

Rowley JD (1973c): Deletions of chromosome 7 in haematological disorders. *Lancet* 2:1385–1386.

Rowley JD (1973d): Acquired trisomy 9. *Lancet* 2:390.

Rowley JD, Potter D (1976): Chromosomal banding patterns in acute nonlymphocytic leukemia. *Blood* 47: 705–721.

Rowley JD, Golomb HM, Dougherty C (1977): 15/17 translocation, a consistent chromosomal change in acute promyelocytic leukaemia. *Lancet* 1:549–550.

Rutten FJ, Hustinx TW, Scheres MJ, Wagener DJ (1973): Acquired trisomy 9. *Lancet* 2:455.

Sait SNJ, Dal Cin P, Sandberg AA, Leong S, Karakousis C, Rao U, et al. (1989): Involvement of 6p in benign lipomas. A new cytogenetic entity? *Cancer Genet Cytogenet* 37:281–283.

Sandberg AA (1980): *The Chromosomes in Human Cancer and Leukemia*. New York: Elsevier/North-Holland.

Seidal T, Mark J, Hagmar B, Angervall L (1982): Alveolar rhabdomyosarcoma: A cytogenetic and correlated cytological and histological study. *APMIS* 90:345–354.

Shaw AT, Engelman JA (2013): ALK in lung cancer: Past, present, and future. *J Clin Oncol* 31:1105–1111.

Shtivelman E, Lifshitz B, Gale RP, Canaani E (1985): Fused transcript of abl and bcr genes in chronic myelogenous leukaemia. *Nature* 315:550–554.

Speleman F, Dal Cin P, De Potter K, Laureys G, Roels HJ, Leroy J, et al. (1989): Cytogenetic investigation of a case of congenital fibrosarcoma. *Cancer Genet Cytogenet* 39:21–24.

van Steenis H (1966): Chromosomes and cancer. *Nature* 209:819–821.

Stenman G, Mark J (1983): Specificity of the involvement of chromosomes 8 and 12 in human mixed salivary-gland tumours. *J Oral Pathol* 12:446–457.

Stenman G, Sandros J, Dahlenfors R, Juberg-Ode M, Mark J (1986): 6q- and loss of the Y chromosome – two common deviations in malignant human salivary gland tumors. *Cancer Genet Cytogenet* 22:283–293.

Taub R, Kirsch I, Morton C, Lenoir G, Swan D, Tronick S, et al. (1982): Translocation of the c-myc gene into the immunoglobulin heavy chain locus in human Burkitt lymphoma and murine plasmacytoma cells. *Proc Natl Acad Sci USA* 79:7837–7841.

Tjio JH, Levan A (1956): The chromosome number of man. *Hereditas* 42:1–6.

Turc-Carel C, Philip I, Berger M-P, Philip T, Lenoir GM (1983): Chromosomal translocations in Ewing's sarcoma. *N Engl J Med* 309:497–498.

Turc-Carel C, Dal Cin P, Rao U, Karakousis C, Sandberg AA (1986): Cytogenetic studies of adipose tissue tumors. I. A benign lipoma with reciprocal translocation t(3;12) (q28;q14). *Cancer Genet Cytogenet* 23:283–289.

Turc-Carel C, Dal Cin P, Boghosian L, Terk-Zakarian J, Sandberg AA (1988): Consistent breakpoints in region 14q22–q24 in uterine leiomyoma. *Cancer Genet Cytogenet* 32:25–31.

Vogelstein B, Papadopoulos N, Velculescu VE, Zhou S, Diaz LA Jr, Kinzler KW (2013): Cancer genome landscapes. *Science* 339:1546–1558.

Whang-Peng J, Bunn PA, Kao-Shan CS, Lee EC, Carney DN, Gazdar A, Minna JO (1982) A nonrandom chromosomal abnormality, del 3p(14–23),in human small lung cancer. *Cancer Genet Cytogenet* 6:119–134.

Winge Ö (1930): Zytologische Untersuchungen über die Natur maligner Tumoren. II. Teerkarzinome bei Mäusen. *Z Zellforsch Mikrosk Anat* 10:683–735.

Zang KD, Singer H (1967): Chromosomal constitution of meningiomas. *Nature* 216: 84–85.

Zankl K, Zang KD (1972): Cytological and cytogenetical studies on brain tumors. 4. Identification of the missing G chromosome in human meningiomas as no. 22 by fluorescence technique. *Humangenetik* 14:167–169.

Zech L, Haglund U, Nilsson K, Klein G (1976): Characteristic chromosomal abnormalities in biopsies and lymphoid-cell lines from patients with Burkitt and non-Burkitt lymphomas. *Int J Cancer* 17:47–56.

CHAPTER 2

Cytogenetic methods

David Gisselsson

Department of Clinical Genetics, University of Lund, Lund, Sweden

The human chromosome complement consists of 22 pairs of autosomes and one pair of sex chromosomes, XX in females and XY in males. The autosomes are numbered after their relative lengths, with the exception of chromosomes 21 and 22. For stable function of a chromosome, a *centromere* somewhere along its length and a *telomere* at each terminus are required. The centromere is associated with the kinetochore protein complex necessary for anchoring of the spindle fibers and for separation of sister chromatids at the metaphase–anaphase transition. Centromeric regions contain large areas of repetitive DNA sequences, some of which contribute to the segments of *constitutive heterochromatin* found around the centromeres of all chromosomes, though most prominently in 1, 9, 16, and Y. Another type of repetitive DNA element is located at the telomeres. These tandemly repeated TTAGGG hexamer units maintain the structural integrity of chromosome termini and ensure complete replication of the most terminal nonrepetitive sequences.

Since the correct chromosome number of man was reported more than half a century ago (Tjio and Levan, 1956), our possibilities to analyze the human chromosome complement have improved steadily. This chapter is an attempt to outline the methods currently employed in cancer cytogenetics, spanning from chromosome banding to array- and sequencing-based techniques. Cytogenetic methods have traditionally been based on microscopic examination of individual cells, and it can be argued that next-generation sequencing (NGS) and genomic arrays are not cytogenetics. However, also these techniques can be used to obtain significant data on overall genome architecture in cells and could therefore with all rights be considered high-resolution cytogenetics. The practical details and protocols of the specific methods will only be touched upon, and the reader is referred to the individual articles cited in this and later chapters for more detailed information.

Sampling for cytogenetic analysis

A correct sampling procedure is the basis for correct scientific and diagnostic conclusions. A first issue to consider is whether the sample is sufficient for the planned analyses. Chromosome preparation requires live cells, whereas *in situ* hybridization at least requires intact nuclei, and genome arrays as well as sequencing rely on DNA that has not been extensively degraded. Another issue to consider is whether the sample is representative of the lesion to be investigated. Cytogeneticists rarely know precisely which cells they study. Exceptions to this are when *in situ* hybridization is combined with immunohistochemical staining of intact cells or when DNA is extracted for analysis

Cancer Cytogenetics: Chromosomal and Molecular Genetic Aberrations of Tumor Cells, Fourth Edition.
Edited by Sverre Heim and Felix Mitelman.

from fixed microdissected solid tumor components, from reviewed cryosections, or from flow-sorted cells. When analysis is performed on cultured cells, it is further important to consider whether the results are representative of the *in vivo* situation. Two main types of heterogeneity can be expected at cytogenetic analysis of a tumor sample: that between neoplastic and nonneoplastic cells and that among various neoplastic cells (Pandis et al., 1994; Lindgren et al., 2011). *In vitro* overgrowth of normal cells or of neoplastic subclones can bias the cytogenetic results. This is a major reason why the use of established cell lines can have serious disadvantages. Pronounced selection may occur among clones that were present already *in vivo*, and chromosomal aberrations that emerge *in vitro* may be mistaken for *in vivo* changes (Gisselsson et al., 2010). Finally, many human tumor cell lines are contaminated by other human or animal cells (Lacroix, 2008). Direct preparations or short-term cultures are therefore usually preferred for chromosome banding analysis.

Chromosome banding

Chromosomes are typically studied at the metaphase stage of the cell cycle when the chromatin is highly condensed and the chromosome morphology is well defined. In most banding methods, individual chromosomes are identified by their relative size, the position of the centromere, and the patterns of transverse striations. Based on this, the short (p) and long (q) chromosome arms are divided into different morphological *regions*, which in turn can be subdivided into *bands* and *subbands*, their number depending on the resolution of the preparation technique. The first of these methods to be invented was *Q-banding* (Caspersson et al., 1970), for which metaphase chromosomes are stained with quinacrine mustard and examined through a fluorescence microscope. A partial explanation of the Q-banding pattern is that quinacrine stains AT-rich sequences brighter than GC-rich sequences (Weisblum and De Haseth, 1972). Most striking are the very bright Q-bands containing highly AT-rich satellite DNA, particularly in the distal part of the Y chromosome. *G-banding* (Figure 2.1A) is obtained when the chromosomes are pretreated with a salt solution or a proteolytic enzyme before staining with Giemsa or equivalent stains. G-banding yields approximately the same information as Q-banding;

bands that fluoresce intensely by Q-banding stain darkly by G-banding. *R-banding* is obtained by pretreatment with hot alkali and subsequent staining with Giemsa or acridine orange (Dutrillaux and Lejeune, 1971). As the name indicates, R-banding yields a pattern that is the reverse of that obtained by G-and Q-banding. However, since R-banding stains the chromosome ends intensely, this technique may be preferable to G- or Q-banding when it comes to detecting terminal chromosome rearrangements.

G-banding and other whole-genome banding methods are still used in routine cytogenetic diagnostic investigations and in research. In fact, chromosome banding remains the only truly low-cost genome screening technique allowing the identification of balanced as well as unbalanced genomic rearrangements in single cells (Table 2.1). Besides these whole-genome banding methods, there are several sequence-specific techniques, of which *C-banding* is most commonly used. This is produced by denaturing the chromosomes prior to Giemsa staining (Sumner, 1972). The method labels the constitutive heterochromatin, thus especially demarcating the variable heterochromatic blocks on chromosomes 1, 9, 16, and Y.

In situ hybridization

In situ hybridization techniques are based on the inherent organization of DNA into two antiparallel complementary strands. After denaturation of target DNA in metaphase spreads or interphase nuclei, single-stranded DNA probes are allowed to form hybrid double-stranded complexes with their complementary genomic sequences. Before hybridization, probes can be labeled by fluorophores to allow direct detection by fluorescence microscopy (Pinkel et al., 1986; Cremer et al., 1988). This fluorescence *in situ* hybridization (FISH) strategy allows simultaneous detection of several genomic sequence targets as fluorophores of different wavelengths can be combined in the same hybridization experiment and concurrently detected (Figure 2.1B–D). However, probes can also be labeled with nonfluorescent haptens, allowing secondary detection by enzymatic methods analogous to those used in immunohistochemistry. This chromogenic *in situ* hybridization (CISH) technique avoids the problem of tissue autofluorescence and can therefore be advantageous for direct analysis of fixed tissue sections (Tanner et al., 2000; Hsi et al., 2002).

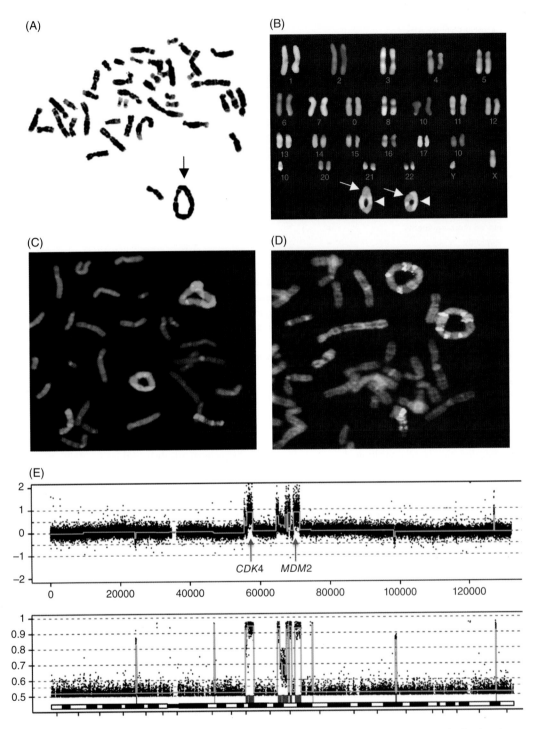

Figure 2.1 Examples of how different cytogenetic techniques can be used to delineate chromosome aberrations at different levels of resolution. A supernumerary ring chromosome (arrow) is identified by G-banding (A) in a soft tissue tumor and shown by multicolor FISH paint (B) to contain sequences from chromosomes 9 (arrowhead) and 12 (arrow). Whole-chromosome painting (C) of chromosomes 9 (red) and 12 (green) corroborates these findings, and multicolor chromosome 12 banding with single-copy probes (D) shows that sequences from the *MDM2* (yellow) and *CDK4* (violet) genes in 12q13–15 are amplified in the rings. Further analysis with SNP array (E) defines the boundaries of the 12q-amplified segments, which include *CDK4* and *MDM2*. The *y*-axis of the upper panel corresponds to relative gene copy number (log2 ratio). The *y*-axis of the lower panel shows the mirrored B-allele frequency (mBAF), which is shifted toward homozygosity (mBAF = 1) in the amplified regions. Array images are courtesy of Dr. K. Hansén Nord.

Table 2.1 Comparison of cytogenetic methodologies

	Chromosome banding	Metaphase FISH	Interphase FISH	Genomic array	Next-generation sequencing*
Approximate resolution level	>5 Mb	>1–5 Mb	>50 kb	>50 kb[†]	1 nt
Cell culture required	+	+	−	−	−
Preselected probes required	−	+	+	−	−
Direct link to sequence map	−	+/−[‡]	+/−[‡]	+	+
Intercellular heterogeneity detected	+	+	+	+/−[§]	+/−[§]
Type of aberration detected					
Balanced rearrangements	+	+	+	−	+
Aneuploidy	+	+	+	+	+[¶]
Structural imbalances	+	+	+	+	+
Copy number-neutral allelic imbalances	−	−	−	+/−[††]	+

*Applies to whole-genome sequencing with optimal coverage.
[†]Order of magnitude of maximal functional resolution according to Coe et al. (2007).
[‡]Library-based single-copy probes are typically defined on physical genome maps, but painting probes and satellite probes are not.
[§]Requires single cell preparation or specific bioinformatic interpretation.
[¶]Requires bioinformatic/statistical analysis of read numbers.
[††]Possible if SNPs are included in the array.

However, the number of colors available for chromogenic detection is still quite limited.

One great advantage of FISH is its versatility with respect to target sequences. Whole chromosomes or large parts of the chromosomes can be targeted by *painting probes*, whereas centromeres, telomeres, and polymorphic satellites can be detected by specific *repeat sequence probes*. Furthermore, *single-copy probes* can be manufactured by amplification of genomic DNA cloned into libraries of various vectors such as cosmids, fosmids, and bacterial artificial chromosomes. These probes can target unique sequences down to the gene level. Single-copy probes are highly useful to map chromosome breakpoints in metaphase preparations or to search for copy number changes in metaphase or interphase cells. All these FISH applications require preexperimental selection of which sequences to examine; one only gets information about those sequences one probes for. Differential labeling of several probes may circumvent this problem and thus make whole-genome screening by FISH possible. In *multicolor karyotyping*, simultaneous hybridization of differently labeled painting probes allows chromosome identification by assigning each pair of homologous chromosomes a certain spectral signature (Schröck et al., 1996;

Speicher et al., 1996; Tanke et al., 1999). This application is particularly useful for resolving the composition of complex structural aberrations but may have limited resolution when very small chromosome fragments are involved (Lee et al., 2001). Similar combinatorial labeling of single-copy probes can also be used to create *color banding* along the length of one or several chromosomes. Some of these methods are based on cross-species hybridization or microdissection of chromosome segments (Müller et al., 1998; Chudoba et al., 2004), whereas others are based on smaller sequences that can be traced back directly to the human genome sequence map (Lengauer et al., 1993; Gisselsson et al., 2000). For routine cancer genetic purposes, FISH is typically used either to assess amplicon status of importance for risk stratification and/or treatment such as *ERBB2* amplification in breast cancer and *MYCN* amplification in neuroblastoma.

Genomic arrays

Genomic arrays are highly efficient tools for obtaining data on genomic imbalances present in a tumor sample. In its most original form, DNA was first extracted from a tumor specimen and a normal reference sample, respectively, differentially labeled with fluorophores, mixed, and allowed to hybridize competitively to complementary target sequences (Kallioniemi et al., 1992). Originally, the target sequences were normal chromosome spreads where the ratio of test-to-reference fluorescence along the chromosomes was quantified using digital image analysis. Defined DNA fragments fixed in a matrix system provide much higher resolution and have now largely replaced this approach. Currently available genomic array platforms are based on single-stranded oligonucleotides (*oligonucleotide arrays*), which may or may not include polymorphic probes to detect single nucleotide polymorphisms (*SNP arrays*). Apart from efficiently detecting gains and losses of genome sequences at a very high resolution, SNP arrays can be employed to assess genomic imbalances not reflected as copy number abnormalities, such as loss of heterozygosity by uniparental disomy (Bignell et al., 2004; Zhao et al., 2004).

The resolution of arrays primarily depends on their underlying design concept, for example, the total number of DNA target sequences, their individual lengths, and the distance between them (Aradhya and Cherry, 2007). Even within a specific array platform, the resolution is often different for different parts of the genome. Furthermore, the resolution for an individual tumor sample depends on unique experimental conditions such as the degree of contamination by DNA from nonneoplastic tissues, which often makes the practical resolution of genomic arrays lower than expected from theoretical calculations (Coe et al., 2007). Another disadvantage of the array methodology is that it reflects a theoretical average of a tumor sample so that intercellular variability is difficult to assess. Techniques have long been established for unbiased PCR amplification of small amounts of DNA, for instance, from microdissected tumor samples (Speicher et al., 1993, 1995; Wiltshire et al., 1995) or from single cells (Klein et al., 1999; Wells et al., 1999). This has made it possible to compare genomic profiles from different parts of a single tumor. These techniques are sensitive to differences in sample quality and are rarely used in a clinical setting. Through the use of relatively simple bioinformatic tools, it is now possible to determine the relative prevalence of different genomic aberrations in a single sample (Lindgren et al., 2011). This, in turn, enables indirect characterization of clonal

hierarchies in a tumor (Lundberg et al., 2013). However, a remaining disadvantage of genomic array techniques is their failure to detect completely balanced aberrations, such as inversions, insertions, and translocations. Nevertheless, the typically high resolution of genomic arrays, their potential for robotic streamlining, and the fact that they do not require living cells for analysis (Table 2.1) have quickly made them ubiquitous tools in cancer cytogenetics.

Large-scale sequencing

The advent of massive parallel/second-generation/ NGS technology has radically transformed the field of cancer cytogenetics. More than 800 genomes of more than 25 cancer types have now been sequenced (Mwenifumbo and Marra, 2013). This has provided a flood of novel cancer genetic data, including but not limited to the identification of novel driver mutations, somatic mutational signatures correlating with carcinogenic exposures, and further details on clonal evolution through ultra-deep sequencing or multisample/multiregion sequencing. NGS has also increased our possibilities to perform refined mapping of chromosomal rearrangements down to the single nucleotide level (Table 2.1). This has enabled the delineation of complex structural rearrangements such as combined deletion–inversion events, in particular through the methodology of whole-genome sequencing using paired-end reads (Inaki and Liu, 2012). Also, novel architectural features of the cancer genome have been described through NGS, such as the *tandem duplicator phenotype* (Stephens et al., 2009; Hillmer et al., 2011; McBride et al., 2012), *chromothripsis* (massive numbers of genomic rearrangements involving several chromosomes with minimal corresponding change in copy numbers; Stephens et al., 2011), and *kataegis* (clusters of somatic single nucleotide variants that often colocalize with structural rearrangements; Nik-Zainal et al., 2012).

From a methodological standpoint, NGS at its current state has higher requirements with respect to sample tissue than does genome arrays. This mainly stems from the need to separate constitutional variants from somatic events. Not only is a high (60–80%) content of neoplastic cells recommended but also nonneoplastic control tissue from each patient (Mwenifumbo and Marra, 2013).

Further requirements for robust ascertainment of somatic single nucleotide variations include a high number of redundant reads (high coverage), critical filtering against databases of constitutional variants, and some extent of confirmative resequencing. Taken together, this demands not only a robust infrastructure for material collection but also extensive bioinformatic skills and resources. NGS technology has thereby transformed cancer cytogenetics to a multidisciplinary field. Considering the continuously decreasing costs for NGS analysis together with its unprecedented level of resolution, it can be expected to largely replace older cytogenetic methods, not only as a research tool but also as a clinical instrument. However, NGS should not uncritically be regarded as a method that surpasses other whole-genome analysis technologies in all respects as it still faces significant limitations. For example, in contrast to banding and *in situ* hybridization, it does not on its own allow single cell resolution; even though the presence of multiple neoplastic clones can be ascertained by high-coverage sequencing, it provides no direct information about which genetic aberrations inhabit the same cells. Furthermore, compared to *in situ* methods, NGS provides limited topographical information, making it difficult to precisely locate significant aberrations, such as amplicons, in the genome. This in turn could make it hard to dissect precisely the mechanisms behind complex genomic changes by virtue of NGS alone.

Interpretation of cytogenetic data

Even though the technical possibilities to detect genomic rearrangements in neoplasms have increased tremendously in recent years, several principal issues regarding the interpretation of cytogenetic data remain unresolved. One example is the finding of a normal karyotype/flat genomic array profile in a neoplastic sample (Pandis et al., 1994). In many cases, particularly when the cells were cultured prior to analysis, this could be explained by the presence of nonneoplastic cells in the sample. Another explanation is that the studied cells were truly neoplastic but that their pathogenic mutations were below the resolution level of the method used for analysis. Finally, the possibility remains that no mutation was present in the neoplastic cells, leaving the

alternatives that pathogenic abnormalities exist at the epigenetic level or were caused by nonhuman DNA, for example, oncogenic viruses, not picked up by, for example, genomic arrays.

Another question is whether all abnormalities found upon analysis of a seemingly representative sample are actually significant. Considering the high resolution of array- and NGS-based approaches and the high degree of polymorphic variation in the human genome, both at the single nucleotide level and at the copy number level, it is of great importance to determine which changes are of pathogenic importance and which are part of the normal spectrum of interindividual genome variation (Rodriguez-Revenga et al., 2007). This is stressed by the fact that clonal chromosome changes have also been found in several reactive/inflammatory lesions that are classified as nonneoplastic by morphological and clinical criteria (Ray et al., 1991; Johansson et al., 1993; Broberg et al., 1999). Recent data have also indicated that genomic imbalances commonly accumulate with age in somatic nonneoplastic tissues (Forsberg et al., 2013), suggesting that such human somatic mosaicism may constitute a confounding factor in the cancer context. It is evident that delineation of the extent of somatic genetic variation in humans of different ages and with different nonneoplastic conditions is becoming increasingly important for the interpretation of cancer genetic data.

References

Aradhya S, Cherry AM (2007) Array-based comparative genomic hybridization: Clinical contexts for targeted and whole-genome designs. *Genet Med* 9:553–559.

Bignell GR, Huang J, Greshock J, Watt S, Butler A, West S, et al. (2004) High-resolution analysis of DNA copy number using oligonucleotide microarrays. *Genome Res* 14:287–295.

Broberg K, Höglund M, Limon J, Lindstrand A, Toksvig-Larsen S, Mandahl N, et al. (1999) Rearrangement of the neoplasia-associated gene HMGIC in synovia from patients with osteoarthritis. *Genes Chromosomes Cancer* 24:278–282.

Caspersson T, Zech L, Johansson C (1970) Differential binding of alkylating fluorochromes in human chromosomes. *Exp Cell Res* 60:315–319.

Chudoba I, Hickmann G, Friedrich T, Jauch A, Kozlowski P, Senger G (2004) mBAND: A high resolution multicolor banding technique for the detection of complex intrachromosomal aberrations. *Cytogenet Genome Res* 104:390–393.

Coe BP, Ylstra B, Carvalho B, Meijer GA, Macaulay C, Lam WL (2007) Resolving the resolution of array CGH. *Genomics* 89:647–653.

Cremer T, Lichter P, Borden J, Ward DC, Manuelidis L (1988) Detection of chromosome aberrations in metaphase and interphase tumor cells by in situ hybridization using chromosome-specific library probes. *Hum Genet* 80: 235–246.

Dutrillaux B, Lejeune J (1971) Sur une nouvelle technique d'analyse du caryotype humaine. *C R Acad Sci Paris D* 272:2638–2640.

Forsberg LA, Absher D, Dumanski JP (2013) Non-heritable genetics of human disease: Spotlight on post-zygotic genetic variation acquired during lifetime. *J Med Genet* 50:1–10.

Gisselsson D, Mandahl N, Pålsson E, Gorunova L, Höglund M (2000) Locus-specific multifluor FISH analysis allows physical characterization of complex chromosome abnormalities in neoplasia. *Genes Chromosomes Cancer* 28:347–352.

Gisselsson D, Lindgren D, Mengelbier LH, Øra I, Yeger H (2010) Genetic bottlenecks and the hazardous game of population reduction in cell line based research. *Exp Cell Res* 316:3379–3386.

Hillmer AM, Yao F, Inaki K, Lee WH, Ariyaratne PN, Teo AS, et al. (2011) Comprehensive long-span paired-end-tag mapping reveals characteristic patterns of structural variations in epithelial cancer genomes. *Genome Res* 21:665–675.

Hsi BL, Xiao S, Fletcher JA (2002) Chromogenic in situ hybridization and FISH in pathology. *Methods Mol Biol* 204:343–351.

Inaki K, Liu ET (2012) Structural mutations in cancer: Mechanistic and functional insights. *Trends Genet* 28:550–559.

Johansson B, Heim S, Mandahl N, Mertens F, Mitelman F (1993) Trisomy 7 in nonneoplastic cells. *Genes Chromosomes Cancer* 6:199–205.

Kallioniemi A, Kallioniemi OP, Sudar D, Rutovitz D, Gray JW, Waldman F, et al. (1992) Comparative genomic hybridization for molecular cytogenetic analysis of solid tumors. *Science* 258:818–821.

Klein CA, Schmidt-Kittler O, Schardt JA, Pantel K, Speicher MR, Riethmuller G (1999) Comparative genomic hybridization, loss of heterozygosity, and DNA sequence analysis of single cells. *Proc Natl Acad Sci USA* 96:4494–4499.

Lacroix M (2008) Persistent use of "false" cell lines. *Int J Cancer* 122:1–4.

Lee C, Gisselsson D, Jin C, Nordgren A, Ferguson DO, Blennow E, et al. (2001) Limitations of chromosome classification by multicolor karyotyping. *Am J Hum Genet* 68:1043–1047.

Lengauer C, Speicher MR, Popp S, Jauch A, Taniwaki M, Nagaraja R, et al. (1993) Chromosomal bar codes produced by multicolor fluorescence in situ hybridization with multiple YAC clones and whole chromosome painting probes. *Hum Mol Genet* 2:505–512.

Lindgren D, Höglund M, Vallon-Christersson J (2011) Genotyping techniques to address diversity in tumors. *Adv Cancer Res* 112:151–182.

Lundberg G, Jin Y, Sehic D, Øra I, Versteeg R, Gisselsson D (2013) Intratumour diversity of chromosome copy numbers in neuroblastoma mediated by on-going chromosome loss from a polyploid state. *PLoS One* 8:e59268.

McBride DJ, Etemadmoghadam D, Cooke SL, Alsop K, George J, Butler A, et al. (2012) Tandem duplication of chromosomal segments is common in ovarian and breast cancer genomes. *J Pathol* 227:446–455.

Müller S, O'Brien PC, Ferguson-Smith MA, Wienberg J (1998) Cross-species colour segmenting: A novel tool in human karyotype analysis. *Cytometry* 33:445–452.

Mwenifumbo JC, Marra MA (2013) Cancer genome-sequencing study design. *Nat Rev Genet* 14:321–332.

Nik-Zainal S, Alexandrov LB, Wedge DC, Van Loo P, Greenman CD, Raine K, et al. (2012) Mutational processes molding the genomes of 21 breast cancers. *Cell* 149:979–993.

Pandis N, Bardi G, Heim S (1994) Interrelationship between methodological choices and conceptual models in solid tumor cytogenetics. *Cancer Genet Cytogenet* 76:77–84.

Pinkel D, Straume T, Gray JW (1986) Cytogenetic analysis using quantitative, high-sensitivity, fluorescence hybridization. *Proc Natl Acad Sci USA* 83:2934–2938.

Ray RA, Morton CC, Lipinski KK, Corson JM, Fletcher JA (1991) Cytogenetic evidence of clonality in a case of pigmented villonodular synovitis. *Cancer* 67:121–125.

Rodriguez-Revenga L, Mila M, Rosenberg C, Lamb A, Lee C (2007) Structural variation in the human genome: the impact of copy number variants on clinical diagnosis. *Genet Med* 9:600–606.

Schröck E, du Manoir S, Veldman T, Schoell B, Wienberg J, Ferguson-Smith MA, et al. (1996) Multicolor spectral karyotyping of human chromosomes. *Science* 273:494–497.

Speicher MR, du Manoir S, Schröck E, Holtgreve-Grez H, Schoell B, Lengauer C, et al. (1993) Molecular cytogenetic analysis of formalin-fixed, paraffin-embedded solid tumors by comparative genomic hybridization after universal DNA-amplification. *Hum Mol Genet* 2:1907–1914.

Speicher MR, Jauch A, Walt H, du Manoir S, Ried T, Jochum W, et al. (1995) Correlation of microscopic phenotype with genotype in a formalin-fixed, paraffin-embedded testicular germ cell tumor with universal DNA amplification, comparative genomic hybridization, and interphase cytogenetics. *Am J Pathol* 146:1332–1340.

Speicher MR, Gwyn Ballard S, Ward DC (1996) Karyotyping human chromosomes by combinatorial multi-fluor FISH. *Nat Genet* 12:368–375.

Stephens PJ, McBride DJ, Lin ML, Varela I, Pleasance ED, Simpson JT, et al. (2009) Complex landscapes of somatic rearrangement in human breast cancer genomes. *Nature* 462:1005–1010.

Stephens PJ, Greenman CD, Fu B, Yang F, Bignell GR, Mudie LJ, et al. (2011) Massive genomic rearrangement acquired in a single catastrophic event during cancer development. *Cell* 144:27–40.

Sumner AT (1972) A simple technique for demonstrating centromeric heterochromatin. *Exp Cell Res* 75:304–306.

Tanke HJ, Wiegant J, vanGijlswijk RP, Bezrookove V, Pattenier H, Heetebrij RJ, et al. (1999) New strategy for multi-colour fluorescence in situ hybridisation: COBRA: COmbined Binary RAtio labelling. *Eur J Hum Genet* 7:2–11.

Tanner M, Gancberg D, DiLeo A, Larsimont D, Rouas G, Piccart MJ et al. (2000) Chromogenic *in situ* hybridization: a practical alternative for fluorescence in situ hybridization to detect HER-2/neu oncogene amplification in archival breast cancer samples. *Am J Pathol* 157:1467–1472.

Tjio JH, Levan A (1956) The chromosome number of man. *Hereditas* 42:1–6.

Weisblum B, De Haseth PL (1972) Quinacrine, a chromosome stain specific for deoxyadenylate–deoxythymidylate rich regions in DNA. *Proc Natl Acad Sci USA* 69:629–632.

Wells D, Sherlock JK, Handyside AH, Delhanty JD (1999) Detailed chromosomal and molecular genetic analysis of single cells by whole genome amplification and comparative genomic hybridisation. *Nucleic Acids Res* 27:1214–1218.

Wiltshire RN, Duray P, Bittner ML, Visakorpi T, Meltzer PS, Tuthill RJ et al. (1995) Direct visualization of the clonal progression of primary cutaneous melanoma: Application of tissue microdissection and comparative genomic hybridization. *Cancer Res* 55:3954–3957.

Zhao X, Li C, Paez JG, Chin K, Janne PA, Chen TH, et al. (2004) An integrated view of copy number and allelic alterations in the cancer genome using single nucleotide polymorphism arrays. *Cancer Res* 64:3060–3071.

3

CHAPTER 3

Cytogenetic nomenclature

Sverre Heim[1] and Felix Mitelman[2]

[1] Section for Cancer Cytogenetics, Institute for Cancer Genetics and Informatics, Oslo University Hospital, Oslo, Norway

[2] Department of Clinical Genetics, University of Lund, Lund, Sweden

Human chromosome nomenclature is based on a consensus reached at several international conferences, after each of which reports containing recommendations for a uniform system of karyotype description have been published. The most recent and authoritative document is "An International System for Human Cytogenetic Nomenclature (2013)," abbreviated ISCN (2013), and the reader is well advised to consult this text for detailed descriptions and definitions and as a daily working guide to how abnormal karyotypes should be interpreted and written. What follows is only a brief summary of the most essential cytogenetic terminology related to the description of chromosome aberrations in neoplastic cells.

Chromosomes are classified according to their size, the location of the centromere (that separates the chromosome into two arms), and the banding pattern along each arm. The autosomes are numbered from 1 to 22 in descending order of length; the sex chromosomes are referred to as X and Y. A schematic illustration, an idiogram, of the normal human male karyotype is presented in Figure 3.1.

Designation of regions and bands

Each chromosome arm—the short arm is called p, the long one q—may consist of one or more regions. Each region is delimited by specific landmarks, that is, consistent, distinct, morphologic features of importance in chromosome identification. Landmarks include the ends of chromosome arms (the telomeres), the centromere, and also certain characteristic bands. A region consists of one or more bands and is defined as the area that lies between two adjacent landmarks. A band is defined as a chromosomal area that is distinguishable from adjacent segments by appearing darker or lighter with one or more banding techniques. Since the chromosomes are visualized as consisting of a continuous series of light and dark transverse bands, no "interbands" exist.

Regions and bands are numbered consecutively from the centromere outward along each chromosome arm. Thus, the two regions adjacent to the centromere are number 1 in each arm; the next, more distal region is number 2, and so on. A band used as a landmark by definition belongs entirely to the region distal to the landmark and hence constitutes band number 1 of that region.

Cancer Cytogenetics: Chromosomal and Molecular Genetic Aberrations of Tumor Cells, Fourth Edition.
Edited by Sverre Heim and Felix Mitelman.

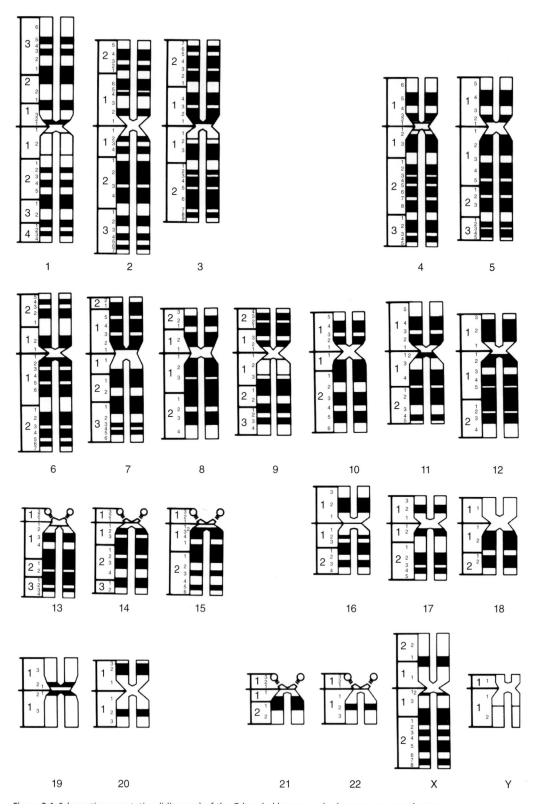

Figure 3.1 Schematic presentation (idiogram) of the G-banded human male chromosome complement.

In designating any particular band, four items are therefore required: the chromosome number, the arm symbol, the region number, and the band number within that region. These items are given in consecutive order without spacing or punctuation. For example, 9q34 means chromosome 9, the long arm, region 3, band 4.

The mitotic process is characterized by increasing chromosomal contraction, and chromosomes in prometaphase or early metaphase are therefore more elongated than midmetaphase chromosomes. The banding pattern of these earlier mitotic phases is more complex, as several of the conventional, midmetaphase bands are split into subbands. Thus, with high resolution or fine structure banding, smaller details of chromosome morphology may be visualized. Whenever a midmetaphase band is subdivided, a decimal point followed by the number assigned to each subband is placed after the original band designation. Like the midmetaphase bands, the subbands are numbered consecutively from the centromere outward. For example, the original band 1q42 may be subdivided into three subbands, labeled 1q42.1, 1q42.2, and 1q42.3. If subbands are subdivided, additional digits, but no further punctuation, are used. For example, subband 1q42.1 may be further subdivided into 1q42.11, 1q42.12, and so on.

Karyotypic nomenclature

In the karyotype description, the first item to be recorded is the total number of chromosomes, followed by a comma (,). The sex chromosome constitution is given next. Thus, a normal female karyotype is written as 46,XX, and the normal male karyotype as 46,XY.

To specify structurally altered chromosomes, single- and three-lettered abbreviations (given subsequently) are used. The number of the chromosome or chromosomes involved in the rearrangement is specified within parentheses immediately following the symbol indicating the type of rearrangement. If two or more chromosomes are altered, a semicolon (;) is used to separate their designations. If one of the rearranged chromosomes is a sex chromosome, this is listed first; otherwise, the rule is that the lowest chromosome number is mentioned first. The

breakpoints, given within parentheses, are specified in the same order as the chromosomes involved, and semicolon is again used to separate the breakpoints. Note that punctuation is never used in intrachromosomal rearrangements, that is, to separate breakpoints in the same chromosome.

The terms used to describe abnormal karyotypes are defined by the ISCN (2013). Below are given some of the more common abbreviations and examples of how they are used:

Translocation, abbreviated *t*: This means that a chromosomal segment moves from one chromosome to another (Figure 3.2). The translocation may or may not be reciprocal. 46,XX,t(9;22)(q34;q11) thus describes an otherwise normal female karyotype containing a translocation between chromosomes 9 and 22 with the breakpoint in chromosome 9 at band q34 and in chromosome 22 at band q11. Similarly, t(3;9;22)(q13;q34;q11) indicates a three-break rearrangement involving band q13 in chromosome 3, band q34 in chromosome 9, and band q11 in chromosome 22.

Insertion, abbreviated *ins*: This means that a chromosomal segment moves to a new, interstitial position in the same or another chromosome. The chromosome in which the segment is inserted is always specified first. For example, ins(5;2)(p14;q22q32) means that breakage and reunion have occurred at band 5p14 in the short arm of chromosome 5 and bands 2q22 and 2q32 in the long arm of chromosome 2. The segment from 2q22 to 2q32 has been inserted into 5p at band 5p14. The designation ins(2)(q13p13p23) describes an insertion of the segment between bands 2p13 and 2p23 into the long arm of chromosome 2 at 2q13.

Inversion, abbreviated *inv*: This designates a rotation 180° of a chromosome segment. In the karyotype 46,XY,inv(16)(p13q22), breakage and reunion have occurred at bands 16p13 and 16q22. The segment between these bands is still present but upside down (Figure 3.3).

Deletion, abbreviated *del*: This means loss of a chromosomal segment (Figure 3.4). Whether a deletion is interpreted as terminal or interstitial is apparent from the breakpoint designations. Thus, del(1)(q23) indicates a terminal deletion with the break at band 1q23 and loss of the distal long arm segment. The remaining chromosome consists of

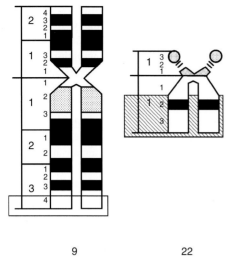
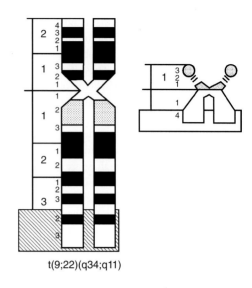

9   22   t(9;22)(q34;q11)

Figure 3.2 Translocation, illustrated as t(9;22)(q34;q11).

the entire short arm of chromosome 1 and the part of the long arm that is between the centromere and band 1q23. In contrast, del(1)(q21q31) indicates an interstitial deletion with breakage and reunion at bands 1q21 and 1q31.

Duplication, abbreviated *dup*: This indicates the presence of an extra copy of part of a chromosome (Figure 3.5). The breakpoints delineate the duplicated segment, for example, dup(1)(q21q31).

Isochromosome, abbreviated *i*: Isochromosomes consist of arms that are mirror images of one another. They result from misdivision of the centromere (transverse breakage). One example is i(12p), an isochromosome for the short arm of chromosome 12 (Figure 3.6). The designation i(12p) may be used in text, but the isochromosome should be written as i(12)(p10) in karyotype descriptions. The "band" 12p10 is a fictitious one; it is the side of the midcentromeric plane that faces toward the short arm. An isochromosome for the long arm of chromosome 12 would have been written as i(12)(q10).

Ring chromosome, abbreviated *r*: The essential feature of a ring chromosome is evident from the name. Breaks have occurred in both the short and the long arms with subsequent fusion to form a ring structure, for example, r(6)(p21q24).

Marker chromosomes, abbreviated *mar*: This is used to signify any structurally rearranged chromosome. When the banding pattern is recognizable, however,

the marker can be adequately described by the standard nomenclature, and so the term is better avoided for these situations. The precise current definition of a mar is a structurally abnormal chromosome in which no part can be identified. When *additional material of unknown origin* is attached to a chromosome region or band, this may be described by the term *add* before the breakpoint designation. For example, add(19)(p13) indicates that extra material has become attached to band 19p13, but neither the origin of the added segment nor the type of rearrangement is known. Such abnormalities have often been described using the symbols t and ?, for example, t(19;?)(p13;?), but since it is only rarely known that the rearranged chromosome actually results from a translocation, the use of the symbol *add* is recommended.

Derivative chromosomes, abbreviated *der*: This means not only any structurally rearranged chromosome generated by an abnormality involving two or more chromosomes but also the structural rearrangements generated by more than one aberration within a single chromosome. The term *der* always refers to the chromosome(s) that has an intact centromere. The derivative chromosome is specified in parentheses, followed by all aberrations involved in the generation of the derivative chromosome. For example, der(1)t(1;3) (p32;q21)t(1;11)(q25;q13) specifies a derivative chromosome 1 generated by two translocations,

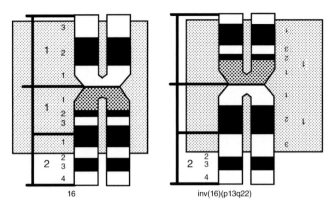

Figure 3.3 Inversion, illustrated as inv(16)(p13q22).

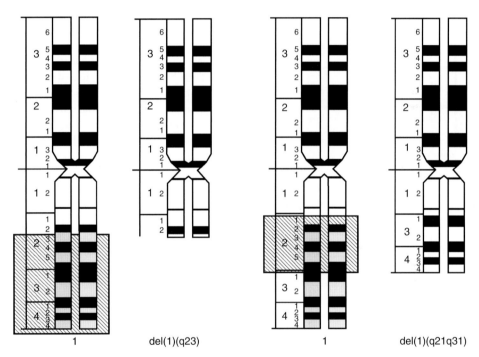

Figure 3.4 Deletions may be terminal or interstitial. The terminal deletion del(1)(q23) is illustrated to the left, and the interstitial del(1)(q21q31) to the right.

one involving the short arm with a breakpoint in 1p32 and the other involving the long arm with a breakpoint in 1q25.

Homogeneously staining regions and *double minute chromosomes*, cytogenetic signs of gene amplification, are abbreviated *hsr* and *dmin*, respectively.

Plus (+) and *minus* (−) *signs* are placed before a chromosome number to indicate an additional or missing whole chromosome. They are placed after a symbol to indicate an increase or decrease in the length of a chromosomal arm. Thus, 47,XY, +21 means a male karyotype with 47 chromosomes, including an additional chromosome 21, whereas 21q + indicates an increase in the length of the long arm of one chromosome 21. The latter terminology should be restricted to written text; in formal descriptions of karyotypes, a 21q + should be described using the add symbol, that is, add(21)(q?).

Nomenclature of tumor cell populations

A *clone* is defined as a cell population derived from a single progenitor. It is common practice to infer a clonal origin when a number of cells have the same or closely related abnormal chromosome complements. A clone is therefore not necessarily completely homogeneous, neither karyotypically nor phenotypically, since subclones may have evolved during the development of the tumor.

An internationally accepted operational definition (ISCN 1991, 2013) says that a clone exists if two or more cells are found with the same structural aberration or supernumerary chromosome. If the abnormality is a missing chromosome, the same change must be present in at least three mitoses. The general rule in tumor cytogenetics is that only clonal chromosomal abnormalities should be reported in the tumor karyotype.

The *stemline* indicates the most basic clone in a tumor cell population. All additional deviating clonal findings are termed *sidelines*. When more than one clone is present, the karyotype designations of each clone are separated by a *slant line* (/). Such multiple clones may be cytogenetically related or unrelated.

The *modal number* is the most common chromosome number in a tumor cell population. The modal number may be described as *near-diploid* when it is approximately diploid but without a sharp mode. The modal number is *hypodiploid* when the mode is less than 46 chromosomes, and *hyperdiploid* when it is more than 46. Modal numbers in tumor cell populations may also be described as haploid, triploid, tetraploid, hypotriploid, near-triploid, hypertriploid, hypotetraploid, near-tetraploid, hypertetraploid, and so on, depending on the predominant chromosome number. Karyotypes with a normal chromosome number but that nevertheless

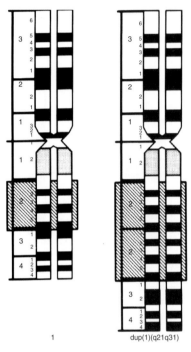

Figure 3.5 Duplication, illustrated as dup(1)(q21q31).

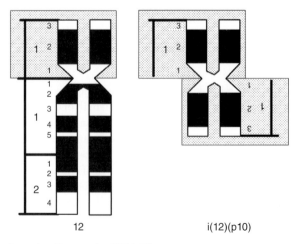

Figure 3.6 Isochromosome formation, illustrated as i(12)(p10).

contain numerical and/or structural aberrations, may be described as *pseudodiploid*.

In situ hybridization nomenclature

The introduction of various *in situ* hybridization technologies into the cytogenetic analysis of interphase and metaphase cells has led the International Standing Committee on Human Cytogenetic Nomenclature to propose an *in situ* hybridization (*ish*) nomenclature system that may be used to describe abnormalities at the molecular level by indicating, for example, the presence, absence, amplification, or separation of specific probe signals. The major aim of this ish nomenclature is to enable investigators to evaluate at a glance in a shorthand system how an individual chromosomal abnor-

mality has been identified and characterized. The information obtained by *in situ* hybridization studies or other techniques used to study chromosome aberrations, for example, comparative genomic hybridization, can always be transcribed into a karyotype description using the established cytogenetic nomenclature system. For a description of the special symbols and abbreviations used to report how ish results are obtained, the reader should consult ISCN (2013).

References

ISCN (1991) *Guidelines for Cancer Cytogenetics: Supplement to an International System for Human Cytogenetic Nomenclature*. Mitelman F, editor. Basel: S. Karger.

ISCN (2013) *An International System for Human Cytogenetic Nomenclature*. Shaffer LG, McGowen-Jordan J, Schmid M, editors. Basel: S. Karger.

CHAPTER 4

Nonrandom chromosome abnormalities in cancer: an overview

Sverre Heim[1] and Felix Mitelman[2]

[1] Section for Cancer Cytogenetics, Institute for Cancer Genetics and Informatics, Oslo University Hospital, Oslo, Norway

[2] Department of Clinical Genetics, University of Lund, Lund, Sweden

The main conclusion to emerge from modern cancer cytogenetics is that the karyotypic changes of tumor cells are unevenly distributed throughout the genome. Different chromosomes, regions, and bands are preferentially involved in rearrangements in different neoplasms. Furthermore, a steadily increasing number of specific abnormalities are found to be associated with particular diseases or disease subgroups, as is described in detail in Chapters 6–24. In this chapter, we discuss neoplastic karyotypes in more general terms. We shall emphasize the difference between primary and secondary changes; address the questions of why, how, when, and where chromosome abnormalities arise; compare numerical and structural aberrations in terms of how they contribute to tumor development; and also touch upon the issues of what causes cancer-associated chromosome abnormalities and whether they are necessary and/or sufficient to transform a normal cell into a cancer cell. Some of the more principal differences between the cytogenetic and molecular genetic approaches to the study of acquired somatic cell mutations will also be discussed, before we end by dwelling a bit on the relative virtues of pathogenetic versus phenotypic classifications of tumors.

At the very beginning, however, it may be worthwhile to get an overview of the totality of information available for assessment. The cancer cytogenetics database is undergoing rapid changes as numerous reports describing new karyotypic abnormalities in human neoplasia are continuously being added to the scientific literature (Figure 4.1). All published cytogenetic data are systematically recorded in the Mitelman Database of Chromosome Aberrations and Gene Fusions in Cancer (Mitelman et al., 2015) that catalogues detailed karyotypic descriptions and clinical and morphological features on all reported neoplastic cases with a clonal cytogenetic abnormality identified by banding analysis. The database also contains information on the molecular genetic consequences and the prognostic impact of acquired cytogenetic and/or molecular genetic rearrangements in neoplasia. The information is integrated into the "Cancer Genome Anatomy Project" (CGAP)—an interdisciplinary program with the aim to create an information infrastructure of the genes associated with carcinogenesis and to develop technological tools to support the analysis of the molecular profile of cancer cells (Strausberg, 2001; Wheeler et al., 2005; Sayers et al., 2010). The CGAP thus facilitates the integration of cytogenetic, mapping,

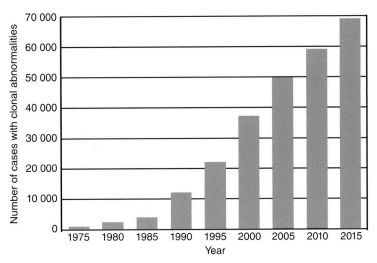

Figure 4.1 Overview of the cancer cytogenetics database as it has evolved since the first descriptions of acquired chromosome aberrations identified by banding techniques in the early 1970s.

and sequence data pertaining to cancer diseases from a variety of sources.

At the time of writing, clonal chromosome aberrations have been identified in more than 65 000 neoplasms, including malignant hematologic disorders, malignant lymphomas, and benign and malignant solid tumors. This is undoubtedly an impressive figure, and it might perhaps be tempting to conclude that sufficient data must now be at hand to deduct all information on cancer biology that may be gained through cytogenetic analysis. However, a closer look at the material reveals that for many important tumor types (e.g., carcinomas of the uterine cervix, prostate, pancreas, and skin), the knowledge is actually extremely limited. In general, the leukemias are by far the most thoroughly investigated. Of the present total, hematologic disorders comprise 60%, lymphomas comprise 15%, and solid tumors make up the remaining 25% of the cases. The number of cytogenetically characterized solid tumors is hence totally disproportionate to the relative impact of these diseases on human morbidity and mortality. One might even say that an inverse relationship exists between the number of studied cases and their clinical importance. The leukemias and malignant lymphomas make up three-fourths of all cases but cause only 10% of human cancer deaths, whereas the major cancer killer, the malignant epithelial tumors responsible for 90% of cancer mortality, is

represented by less than 10% of the cases in the database. In fact, we know less about the cytogenetics of all carcinomas today than we did about one leukemia subtype, acute myeloid leukemia, 20 years ago.

In addition, there are technical and analytical problems that limit the information value of the existing cytogenetic data on malignant epithelial tumors. First, the chromosome morphology is often poor or at least inferior to that in leukemias and lymphomas, which means that many of the published cases have been only partially karyotyped. Second, investigations of carcinomas have often been performed late in the disease, on samples from effusions or metastases, that is, at a time when the karyotype may be dominated by complex secondary karyotypic changes (see the following text) accrued during tumor progression. A further challenge is the presence of cytogenetically unrelated clones, which are found in less than 3% of leukemias, lymphomas, and mesenchymal tumors but have been reported in up to 50% of various carcinomas (Jin et al., 2001). All these circumstances compound the difficulties in pinpointing the essential genomic rearrangements in early tumor development. More cytogenetic data are therefore particularly badly needed for epithelial neoplasms. However, also in the most extensively investigated leukemias, new aberrations and new clinicocytogenetic correlations are still being discovered, illustrating the continuing necessity for cytogenetic research even in those disorders for which the database is most solid. It should also be noted that a substantial proportion of the cytogenetically abnormal leukemias published so far represent selected cases reported because they had a characteristic or unusual chromosome abnormality (Mitelman et al., 2015), giving a false impression of the actual frequencies of many recurrent cytogenetic aberrations. More data on consecutive series of unselected patient materials are needed in order to establish the true prevalence of all chromosome abnormalities also in leukemias and lymphomas.

Primary and secondary neoplasia-associated chromosome abnormalities

Numerous specific chromosomal abnormalities have been detected in almost all tumor types that have been examined, and the remainder of this book contains detailed discussions of these cytogenetic–pathologic relationships and the molecular consequences of the aberrations whenever such knowledge is available. In spite of the unquestionable karyotypic nonrandomness, the main impression gained from a cursory examination of the total database is its enormous heterogeneity. Practically all kinds of abnormalities have been reported; only the frequencies and the clinicomorphologic contexts vary. More often than not, several changes are present simultaneously. One is compelled to ask the following questions: are all the aberrations pathogenetically important, are only some aberrations important, or—in principle equally possible— do none of them reflect essential events in the neoplastic transformation of initially normal cells? That the latter query must be answered in the negative has now been established beyond doubt, inasmuch as the molecular consequences of several rearrangements (activation of oncogenes or inactivation of suppressor genes) have been clarified and shown to be causally important in the tumorigenic process (Chapters 6–24).

The best approximation to biological reality may be achieved by subdividing the various clonal aberrations into those that are primary and those that are secondary (Heim and Mitelman, 1989). The acquisition of microscopically visible mutations

by the tumor cells is, like tumorigenesis itself, in most instances a multistage process. *Primary aberrations* are frequently found as the sole karyotypic abnormalities in cancer and are often specifically associated with particular tumor types. The term primary not only refers to the fact that these are the first changes we see in neoplastic cells but also reflects their causal role in tumorigenesis; they are essential in establishing the neoplasm. In principle, of course, what we detect first need not necessarily be the first mutation, and one has to be open to the possibility that submicroscopic mutation(s) may in given instances precede the primary chromosomal abnormality (see also the following text). The issue remains unresolved, but at least it seems fair to say that a broad consensus has evolved that the tumor-specific primary chromosome abnormalities occur in the earliest stages of carcinogenesis, that they represent rate-limiting steps, and that they indeed are a *conditio sine qua non* for the whole process.

Secondary aberrations, on the contrary, are rarely or never found alone; as the name implies, they develop in cells already carrying a primary abnormality. In later disease stages, however, they may be so numerous as to completely dominate the karyotypic picture. Although less specific than primary changes, secondary aberrations nevertheless demonstrate nonrandom features with distribution patterns that appear to be dependent both on which primary abnormality is present and on the type of neoplasm. This is presumably achieved in the following manner (Nowell, 1976, 1986; Heim et al., 1988; Heim, 1993): chance disturbances of the mitotic process, in some cases presumably facilitated by a mutator phenotype effect of the primary abnormality, provide a random background of genetic variability in the tumor. The genetically rearranged cells that thus emerge are immediately and continuously tested for "evolutionary fitness" in a Darwinian manner, with proliferatively superior subclones gradually expanding at the expense of less fit cells. Depending on how the selection pressure changes, typically when infiltrating or metastatic cells find themselves in a new locale or after cytostatic treatment is instituted, the total tumor karyotype may evolve toward greater or less complexity (genetic divergence and convergence, respectively). We emphasize that this evolutionary scenario is not principally dependent on whether the neoplastic process starts out as monoclonal (as implied earlier) or begins with the more or less simultaneous transformation of many cells. If the latter, polyclonal pathway is the one followed by some neoplasms—and cytogenetic data on many carcinomas indicate that this may be the case— then oligo- or monoclonality may develop secondarily, for example, after the basal lamina is penetrated and the tumor begins to infiltrate (Heim et al., 1988; Heim, 1993; Teixeira and Heim, 2011).

The operational division between primary and secondary acquired chromosome aberrations outlined earlier has also been proposed to reflect a deeper genetic, and hence most likely functional, distinction (Johansson et al., 1996) in that primary aberrations consist of specific gene rearrangements, whereas secondary chromosomal changes result in large-scale genomic imbalances. According to this hypothesis, then, there are no unbalanced primary aberrations, only secondary imbalances masquerading as primary. This proposition, if correct, has a number of conceptual ramifications (Johansson et al., 1996). First, the genetic mechanisms underlying tumor initiation and progression would seem to be totally different. Second, the elucidation of the molecular consequences of the secondary aberrations will be an arduous task, even if one were to adhere to the, in our opinion overly simplistic, view that cytogenetically identified genomic imbalances may be reduced to simple gains or losses of single oncogenes or tumor suppressor genes (TSG). Third, the cytogenetic diagnosis of neoplasms will have to take into account that unbalanced "primary" abnormalities are secondary to submicroscopic, truly primary changes of major diagnostic and prognostic importance. Whether the suggested scheme is correct about submicroscopic mutations always preceding chromosomal ones is uncertain, but analyses by recently introduced methods that allow single-cell sequencing (Navin et al., 2011) may, at least in theory, go some way toward resolving the issue. At any rate, it is an observable fact that secondary changes do not always bring about large-scale chromosomal imbalances. For example, the Burkitt lymphoma/leukemia-specific 8;14-translocation sometimes occurs secondarily in follicular non-Hodgkin lymphomas with t(14;18) as the primary abnormality (Chapter 11; Gauwerky et al., 1988),

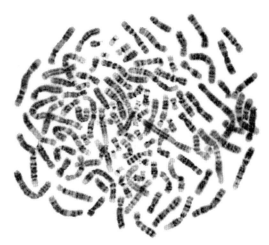

Figure 4.2 Metaphase from a cancer cell showing extreme karyotypic complexity. Among the massive numerical as well as structural chromosome abnormalities were also many that represented cytogenetic noise, changes that were found in this cell only.

which then alter their clinical behavior correspondingly, and if an inv(16) occurs during clonal evolution of chronic myeloid leukemia (CML) with the primary 9;22-translocation, an acute myelomonocytic leukemia results (Chapter 6; Heim et al., 1992; Ninomiya et al., 2011). Sometimes, primary chromosome rearrangements may occur secondarily, evidently, and it would be surprising if the opposite were not also the case, albeit possibly on rare occasions only.

In addition to the evolutionarily important primary and secondary chromosome aberrations that by definition must be found in clonal proportions, not only extreme cytogenetic complexity (Figure 4.2) but also variability with no two identical cells is sometimes seen, especially in solid tumors. The term *cytogenetic noise* has been used for these extensive but nonclonal abnormalities (Heim and Mitelman, 1989).

Why and how do chromosome aberrations arise?

Are primary and secondary chromosome abnormalities always the result of chance events? Are they only, as the secondary changes were depicted earlier, the products of stochastic alterations occurring more or less continuously throughout the genome, with selection for proliferative advantage determining which ones will give rise to tumors and, hence, can be detected? This is a thoroughly logical, simple, and attractive possibility, and it is probably the hypothesis shared by the majority of researchers in the field. However, a different scenario cannot be ruled out: certain genomic rearrangements, perhaps especially those which frequently occur as primary abnormalities, might be preferentially induced, for example, through direct interaction between a carcinogenic agent and specific genomic sites in the target cells. It has been convincingly shown that many external genotoxic agents induce chromosomal breaks (Obe et al., 2002), and epidemiological studies have shown an association between the extent of chromosomal damage and cancer risk (Bonassi et al., 2005, 2008). Some early evidence from cytogenetic investigations of experimental tumors also supports the view that more or less specific chromosomal aberration patterns may be dependent on the inducing agent (Mitelman et al., 1972; Mitelman, 1981). This proposition has also been substantiated in some human malignancies associated with occupational, environmental, and/or genotoxic exposures (Mitelman et al., 1978; Mauritzson et al., 2002; Irons et al., 2013), and several agents have been shown to increase the risk of particular translocations/gene fusions, deletions, as well as numerical abnormalities, for example, DNA topoisomerase II inhibitors (Zhang and Rowley, 2006), alkylating agents (Escobar et al., 2007), agricultural pesticides (Chiu et al., 2006), radiation (Rabes et al., 2000), and benzene (Zhang et al., 2012).

An important topic in this context is the observation of geographic heterogeneity of cancer chromosome abnormalities. It has long been known that cancer frequencies differ both geographically and among ethnic groups. Data have also come forth indicating that the aberration patterns of apparently identical malignancies may vary significantly among laboratories from different parts of the world (Johansson et al., 1991; Moorman et al., 2010; Marques et al., 2011; Chen et al., 2012). Partly, this probably reflects different ascertainment practices due to such factors as variable referral routines and differences in age composition among the patients investigated. The choice of technical procedures, including which media are used and whether direct preparations or short-term cultures are relied upon

(Jin et al., 1993; Pandis et al., 1994), may also be important. However, for several abnormalities, explanations along these lines seem insufficient to account for the observed variability. Population differences in the response to carcinogens, possibly reflecting polymorphic variability in DNA repair capacity, could perhaps explain some of the geographic variations. Another explanation, however, might be that specific etiologic factors directly or indirectly induce or influence the nonrandom aberration patterns.

In addition to external agents, host factors might also have a role in the origin of specific chromosome aberrations. One important host factor is chromosome instability. There are many inherited cancer-predisposing disorders, including the well-known chromosome breakage syndromes associated with instability at the chromosomal and/or DNA level (Taylor, 2001; Eyfjord and Bodvarsdottir, 2005; Bellacosa, 2013) and an increased incidence of translocations involving some chromosomal regions more than others (Aplan, 2006). For example, patients with ataxia-telangiectasia, caused by mutation of the ATM gene (11q22) that plays an important role in the recognition and repair of DNA double-strand breaks, are prone to develop translocations involving the T-cell or immunoglobulin antigen-receptor loci (Rotman and Shiloh, 1998). Also, patients with the Nijmegen breakage syndrome, caused by a mutation in the NBN gene (8q21) that, like ATM, is involved in the repair of DNA double-strand breaks, frequently display translocations affecting immunoglobulin and T-cell receptor genes (Chrzanowska et al., 2012). Another cause of chromosome instability is telomere dysfunction, which through breakage—fusion—bridge cycles may cause primarily structural chromosome aberrations (Murname, 2012). Aneuploidy, on the other hand, seems to be largely brought about by mitotic spindle defects (Ganem et al., 2009) or spindle multipolarity combined with cytokinetic failure (Gisselsson et al., 2010). It was recently shown that missegregating chromosomes can be damaged during cytokinesis, leading to DNA double-strand breaks and unbalanced translocations in the daughter cells, thus implying an overlap between the routes leading to numerical and structural aberrations (Janssen et al., 2011). Overall, a general tolerance to DNA breaks seems to be a common feature of tumor cells compared with non-neoplastic cells, allowing the driver mechanisms behind genomic recombination to become established in tumors and enhancing the probability of tumorigenic mutations (Lord and Ashworth, 2012).

Common chromosomal fragile sites (Durkin and Glover, 2007), which are known to contribute to the formation of DNA breaks, have long been discussed as a possible predisposing factor to chromosome rearrangements. Several reports in the 1980s pointed out that the breakpoints of consistently cancer-associated chromosome abnormalities and fragile sites clustered to the same bands, and it was widely speculated that the constitutional presence of certain fragile sites predisposed to these chromosomal rearrangements and, hence, to cancer. The statistical basis for the observed association was later subjected to criticism, and in some instances, cancer-associated breakpoints were shown to differ at the molecular level from those of constitutional fragile sites in the same chromosome bands. Much of the interest in the connection between fragile sites and cancer consequently cooled off (see Heim and Mitelman, 1995, for a review of the early data). Recent findings have again linked common fragile sites to chromosome rearrangements and tumorigenesis, however. An extensive study of 746 cancer cell lines revealed a strong association between fragile sites and regions of cancer-causing homozygous deletions (Bignell et al., 2010), and exposure of thyroid cells to chemicals that induce fragile sites has been found to result in formation of the *CCDC6–RET* and *NCOA4–RET* gene fusions (Chapter 19) frequently found in papillary thyroid carcinoma (Gandhi et al., 2010). The results provide evidence that the involvement of chromosomal fragile sites in the generation of cancer-specific chromosome abnormalities is not fortuitous. At present, the bulk of available evidence therefore again appears to indicate that inherited or acquired genomic instability generated by formation of DNA breaks and/or failure of cell cycle checkpoints facilitates the appearance of chromosome aberrations and predisposes individuals to develop various cancers.

It stands to reason that the three-dimensional chromosome architecture within the interphase nucleus, the organization of the genetic material into relatively well-defined spatial intranuclear domains (Cremer and Cremer, 2010; Cavalli and Misteli, 2013; Cremer et al., 2014), in some way must influence the likelihood with which various structural chromosome aberrations arise. Probably, DNA double-strand breaks are required for most, if not all, such aberrations. Therefore, at least some degree of physical proximity between breakpoint regions seems essential for the formation of any chromosome rearrangement. In fact, several loci recombined in specific translocations—*BCR–ABL1* in CML (Chapter 8), *PML–RARA* in acute promyelocytic leukemia (Chapter 6), *RET–CCDC6* in thyroid cancer (Chapter 19), and *IGH–MYC, IGH–CCND1*, and *IGH–BCL2* in B-cell malignancies (Chapter 11)—have been found to be close to each other in the corresponding normal cell types (references in Mitelman et al., 2007; Roukos et al., 2013). However, in view of the fact that more than 20 000 recurrent balanced aberrations involving every chromosome band have been reported in neoplasia (Mitelman et al., 2015) and the profound cell-to-cell variability of nuclear architecture in living cells during development and cell differentiation (Cremer et al., 2014), it seems unlikely that the interphase position of the breakpoints involved will be able to explain the origin of neoplasia-associated rearrangements any time soon. Another factor that might facilitate illegitimate recombination in a major way is shared sequence motifs at the chromosome breakpoints (Aplan, 2006; Povirk, 2006; Tsai et al., 2008; Roukos et al., 2013). Future sequencing efforts will no doubt shed light on this issue, including the relative contribution of chance to what might appear as specific aberration induction, as will also additional studies of the interphase nuclear anatomy of susceptible target cells.

We see, therefore, that many of the "whys" and "hows" interact, the distinction between them is sometimes blurred and anything but easy, and the main mechanisms are not mutually exclusive. Taken together, however, there is little evidence favoring any substantial impact of specific external or internal factors on the genesis of nonrandom chromosome abnormalities. For the time being and at our present level of understanding of the processes involved, we are compelled to believe that most of the primary and secondary cancer-associated cytogenetic aberrations arise as stochastic events.

When do chromosome aberrations arise?

It is clear that tumors with chromosome abnormalities may be diagnosed at any age. Structural and numerical aberrations have been recorded in newborns and patients up to the age of 100 years (Mitelman et al., 2015). When the aberrations arise, however, is a moot point. For childhood hematologic malignancies, there is ample evidence, based on twin studies and polymerase chain reaction (PCR) analyses of specific gene fusions in Guthrie spots, that they may be formed already in utero, several years prior to overt leukemia (Greaves and Wiemels, 2003; Greaves et al., 2011). To what extent leukemias in adults have a clonal origin that can be traced many years back, perhaps even to early childhood or prenatal life, is not known.

For solid tumors, lack of appropriate preneoplastic tissue samples collected before diagnosis has precluded similar investigations. It would undoubtedly be of great interest, for example, in cancer epidemiological studies, to identify more exactly when in life translocations and gene fusions arise in different cell types. It is difficult to envisage how such information could possibly be obtained, however; perhaps, as stated by Boveri already in 1914, it will never be possible to study a tumor "*in statu nascendi.*"

In which cells do chromosome aberrations arise?

Cancer stem cells have attracted much attention. It is now generally accepted that hematologic malignancies are sustained by leukemic stem cells, capable of both initiating and maintaining the disease. More recently, the cancer stem cell concept has been shown to be applicable also to some malignant solid tumors, for example, of the breast, colon, lung, and central nervous system (Valent et al., 2012; Visvader and Lindeman, 2012; Sugihara and Saya, 2013; Tirino et al., 2013). A fundamental question is whether the neoplasia-inducing primary chromosome abnormalities arise in normal stem cells or whether they occur at a later stage in differentiation. A paradigmatic example of a translocation originating in a stem cell is the t(9;22) giving rise to the Philadelphia chromosome in CML, as demonstrated already in the early 1960s

(references in Johansson et al., 2002). Also, a few other gene fusions have been shown to be present in the stem cell compartment or in early progenitors in acute leukemias (Castor et al., 2005; Hotfilder et al., 2005; Hong et al., 2008; Bueno et al., 2011), but most leukemia-associated gene fusions have not been subjected to this type of investigation. In addition, it is at present questionable which cell should be regarded as the most relevant one in this context. Convincing evidence for the presence of pre-leukemic hematopoietic stem cells ancestral to the dominant leukemia clone was recently presented (Shlush et al., 2014). In solid tumors, such studies are difficult to perform because so little is known about the differentiation hierarchy in the tissues from which they derive. Recent data indicate, however, that bone marrow-derived mesenchymal progenitor cells may be involved in sarcoma development (Riggi et al., 2005, 2006). It is undoubtedly going to be an arduous task to design and carry out experiments capable of identifying and characterizing the target cells, but only then will it be possible to understand why some chromosome aberrations, including gene fusions resulting from structural chromosomal rearrangements, such as *ETV6–NTRK3*, occur in a variety of morphologically and clinically distinct neoplasms, including soft tissue fibrosarcoma, mesoblastic nephroma, secretory breast and salivary gland carcinoma, colon cancer, acute myeloid leukemia, chronic eosinophilic leukemia, and astrocytoma (Mitelman et al., 2015), whereas most others seem to be restricted to very specific cell and tumor types.

Are acquired chromosome aberrations sufficient for neoplastic proliferation?

Several lines of evidence strongly indicate that the answer to this question is negative. The most compelling argument is that many similar aberrations have been found in nonneoplastic cells of healthy individuals. For example, trisomy 7 may be seen as the only change not only in both benign and malignant solid tumors but also in several unquestionably nonneoplastic disease lesions (e.g., osteoarthritis, Dupuytren's contracture, and focal steatosis of the liver) and even in apparently normal tissues of, for example, the brain, kidney, and lung (Johansson et al., 1993; Mertens et al., 1996; Broberg et al., 2001, Micci et al., 2007). Several typical leukemia- and lymphoma-associated structural rearrangements have also been detected in normal cells by both chromosome banding and molecular means, in particular using sensitive PCR assays (Bäsecke et al., 2002; Janz et al., 2003; Brassesco et al., 2009; Hirt et al., 2013). Among the gene fusions identified in healthy individuals are *RUNX1–RUNX1T1* corresponding to t(8;21)(q22;q22), *BCR–ABL1* corresponding to t(9;22)(q34;q11), *ETV6–RUNX1* corresponding to t(12;21)(p13;q22), and *IGH–BCL2* corresponding to t(14;18)(q32;q21). Cells carrying leukemia-associated gene fusions may occasionally be detectable several years after successful treatment, for example, when the patients are in long-term complete remission and there is little risk of relapse (Nucifora et al., 1993; Jurlander et al., 1996). Long and disparate latency periods before overt leukemia in twins born with the same gene fusion, transmitted in utero, have been well documented (Greaves and Wiemels, 2003). Finally, there is circumstantial as well as direct evidence from murine leukemia models that additional events are a prerequisite for malignant transformation (Kelly and Gilliland, 2002). Thus, besides the necessity that the leukemogenic or carcinogenic events take place in suitably primed, susceptible cells, something we do not know to be the case in the studies demonstrating low-level presence of leukemogenic gene products in healthy individuals, the available data indicate that secondary changes, most likely mutations, are necessary, at least in the context of hematologic malignancies. In contrast, there is some evidence that the expression of certain sarcoma-associated gene fusions is sufficient for transformation of bone marrow-derived mesenchymal progenitor cells in mice (Riggi et al., 2005, 2006). Also, conditional expression of *EWSR1–ATF1* human cDNA in mice has been found to generate clear cell sarcoma-like tumors with 100% penetrance (Straessler et al., 2013); the *EWSR1–ATF1* is generated by a t(12;22)(q13;q12) characterizing clear cell sarcoma in man (see Chapter 24). Whether the same holds true also for other solid tumors, including gene fusion-driven carcinogenesis in humans, remains to be clarified, and so does the spectrum of mutated genes associated with different gene fusions in both hematologic and solid neoplasms. It is clear

that our conceptual models of the pathogenetic impact of chromosome abnormalities need to take into account the surprisingly large number of other, submicroscopic somatic mutations recently identified by whole-genome sequencing in human malignancies (Stratton, 2011; Kandoth et al., 2013; Vogelstein et al., 2013; Weinstein et al., 2013); we still do not always know what is signal and what is noise in the vast amount of such data now being made available.

Do all tumors have chromosome abnormalities, and are such changes present only in neoplastic cells?

A negative answer to the first question seems obvious, since examples abound of tumors in which only normal metaphases were found. It should be made absolutely clear, however, that this in no way runs counter to the predictions of the somatic mutation theory of cancer. The haploid human genome contains roughly 3×10^9 base pairs (bp), and since structural rearrangements involving chromosomal segments much smaller than a band are not detected with present-day cytogenetic techniques, it follows that genetic changes of as much as 10^6–10^7 bp may occur without visible alteration of chromosomal morphology. So even if the somatic mutation theory were to show 100% concordance with reality, some of the acquired mutations would be expected to be too small to be seen microscopically. As recently shown in, for example, cancer of the prostate (Rubin et al., 2011), lung (Hammerman et al., 2012), colon (Seshagiri et al., 2012), and breast (Asmann et al., 2012), gene fusions do occur in important tumor types with the breakpoints so close to each other or involving so similar-looking chromosomal segments that their detection had to await the introduction of methodologies other than chromosome banding, including genome-wide expression and sequencing analyses.

An additional but partly related problem is that one cannot be certain whether cytogenetically normal cells isolated from tumor samples really are part of the tumor parenchyma. In the absence of any information about possible submicroscopic aberrations in these cells, is it not more likely that they in most instances belong to one of the stromal components ubiquitous to every tumor? Banding analysis alone evidently cannot provide a conclusive answer. Combined analyses of the cells' genotype and phenotype, something that has proved notoriously difficult to obtain, could provide more reliable knowledge about this problem and might also be expected to shed light on what at first glance seems to be the diametrically opposite issue, namely, the ontologic and pathogenetic status of the cytogenetically unrelated clones that are found so often in many solid epithelial tumors (see, e.g., Chapters 14 and 16). It is not clear whether these cells, which typically carry only relatively simple aberrations, belong to the tumor parenchyma (in which case one has to consider seriously the possibility of polyclonal carcinogenesis) or whether they are non-neoplastic. A quality grading of the chromosomal aberrations (simple or complex?) based on cytogenetic impressions alone is not always sufficient; many examples are known of balanced, solitary chromosomal rearrangements that have a most profound tumorigenic impact (Mitelman et al., 2007). The question has major implications for our reasoning about the pathogenesis of cancerous as well as other hyperproliferative disease processes and should, sooner rather than later, be addressed by means of appropriate combinations of cytogenetic and other techniques.

General effects of structural and numerical chromosome abnormalities

Two main classes of cancer-relevant genes, the oncogenes and the TSG, have been recognized as main pathogenetic targets for cancer-associated karyotypic abnormalities, and numerous examples of oncogene activation and suppressor gene inactivation are given in the further chapters. Here, we shall only outline in a very schematic fashion the principal genetic effects that different types of chromosomal rearrangements may have. Either they lead to loss of genetic material, gain of material, or balanced relocation of chromosomal segments (Figure 4.3).

Net loss of chromosomal material

This may be caused by deletions, unbalanced translocations, or loss of entire chromosomes (monosomy). Standard pathogenetic theory holds that such changes are carcinogenic by removing TSG. However, there are now numerous examples of fusion genes identified by whole-transcriptome sequencing that have been produced by juxtaposition of parts of two genes delineating, most often, cryptic deletions in hematologic disorders as well

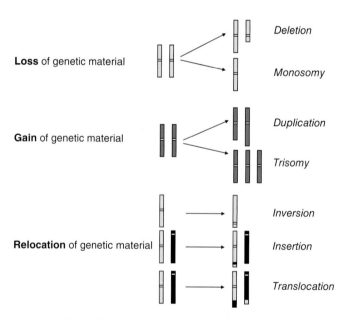

Figure 4.3 The chromosome aberrations of cancer may in principle exert their effect through gain or loss of genetic material or through structural or regulatory changes brought about by relocation of chromosomal segments.

as various solid tumors (Rubin et al., 2011; Asmann et al., 2012; Hammerman et al., 2012; Seshagiri et al., 2012; Mitelman et al., 2015). A major challenge will be to verify by functional studies which of the alleged gene fusions are pathogenetically important and which are either secondary progressional changes or nonconsequential noise abnormalities, either unimportant chance events or attributable to technical problems with cutoff levels, transsplicing, and read-through fusions across adjacent genes (Mertens and Tayebwa, 2014; Panagopoulos et al, 2014). It also remains to be established what role is played by epigenetic gene silencing, which is now more and more being appreciated as an alternative to mutations and deletions to disrupt TSG function in cancer cells (You and Jones, 2012; Goodell and Godley, 2013; Fabbri et al., 2013). Finally, even when deletions work by loss of TSG, we do not know how consistently this loss of function adheres to the two-hit model of Knudson (1971). Some recent evidence from, for example, the del(5q) of acute myeloid leukemia and myelodysplasia (Chapters 6 and 7) indicates that loss of a single allele (haploinsufficiency) is a crucial pathogenetic step but may not be sufficient for the defect to make itself felt phenotypically (Joslin et al., 2007; Ebert et al., 2008; Stoddart et al., 2014).

Net gain of chromosomal material

Malsegregation may give rise to trisomy or more extensive polysomies. Duplication and triplication of particular chromosomal regions or segments may also lead to an unbalanced gene product. In all cases, a simple dose effect could conceivably be the mechanism whereby the extra DNA is influential, for example, by adding one or more active oncogene alleles. It should be stressed that this explanation is still entirely speculative, however. Several studies have shown that the expression of a considerable fraction of genes located in regions of gains or losses of chromosomal material varies consistently with DNA copy number, but not all genes affected by copy number changes show an altered expression. In a study of acute myeloid leukemia (Schoch et al., 2006), gain of chromosome 8 was found to lead to a higher expression of genes located on chromosome 8, but no consistent pattern of over-expressed genes was identified that would have allowed a clear discrimination of trisomy 8 cases

from those with a normal karyotype. Also, as discussed in Chapter 14, Platzer et al. (2002) and Cardoso et al. (2007) found that the great majority of genes located in areas of chromosome amplification in colorectal cancer did not show upregulation of expression. The general conclusions from these and other recent correlative analyses of DNA copy number and mRNA expression data performed in several biological models (Wang et al., 2011; Mesquita et al., 2013) thus agree that gene copy number changes do not necessarily result in altered expression.

Relocation of sequences with no gain or loss of genetic material

Rearrangements leading to this result may be interchromosomal (translocations and insertions) or intrachromosomal (inversions). By recombining DNA sequences in this manner, genes may be destroyed, new fusion genes may be created, or the regulatory control of genes may be interfered with. Such position effects are the mechanism behind the chromosomal activation of oncogenes in several human neoplasms (Mitelman et al., 2007), and numerous examples to this effect will be presented in the following chapters. We also need to be cognizant of the fact that even in what seems cytogenetically to be balanced rearrangements, cryptic deletions or duplications in the breakpoint region(s) may occur (Sinclair et al., 2000; Kolomietz et al., 2001; Howarth et al., 2011). A mixture and blurring of the boundaries between the three major mechanisms by which cytogenetic alterations exert their effects may therefore be more common than was initially appreciated.

At what resolution level are neoplasia-associated mutations best studied?

The genetic profile of tumors can be assessed at many different levels of resolution, all of which depend on the utilization of particular methodologies that each has its own developmental history, advantages, and disadvantages. The techniques include classic cytology, whereby the size, shape, and staining characteristics of individual nuclei are determined; flow cytometry, which gives information about the total DNA content of the average tumor cell; cytogenetics, the main topic of this book; and molecular genetic studies at the level of genes or primary DNA structure.

It is the latter approach that in the last three decades has commanded the greatest interest, both in the scientific community and among the general public. At times, the focus on the molecular genetics of cancer has been so strong that all other and older means of gaining relevant information seem to have been forgotten; surely, the fascination with new things and toys is one of the most profound character traits in man. If it were so that the molecular genetic approach really helped answer all relevant questions about the acquired genetic changes of neoplastic cells better than can be done by, say, cytogenetic analysis, then the total and unconditional embracing of the new should not be lamented but welcomed. If, on the contrary, the suspicion arises that important aspects of cancer genetics are neglected by a one-sided molecular-level strategy, then one should try to readdress our current approaches to see if they really are optimally suited to what is the common goal of all cancer geneticists: to achieve the best possible understanding of the genetic processes that drive tumorigenesis. A clear appreciation of the ontological, methodological, and epistemological relationship between the cytogenetics and molecular genetics of tumor cells is vital to obtaining such a balanced attitude. We here want to emphasize only some of the factors that play a role. A fuller discussion of the topic may be found in Heim (1992).

On the face of it, the one important difference between the cytogenetic and DNA levels is that the objects under investigation differ in size. Point mutations, small deletions, and any other rearrangements involving stretches of DNA smaller than the minimum required for microscopic detection cannot be evaluated by morphologic methods but may be studied by molecular genetic techniques. That such small changes may be functionally important is beyond question; hence, in this regard, the molecular genetics of cancer is obviously superior to cytogenetic investigations.

The chemical nature of modern-day molecular genetic techniques and their enormous resolution power also lead to some inherent limitations, however, which sometimes tend to be overlooked when the genomic changes of tumors are discussed only from a molecular perspective. First and foremost, most molecular genetic methods are dependent on probing with DNA sequences that hybridize specifically at given sites. No information is obtained about those areas that are not probed, no matter how massive rearrangements they may contain. Alternatively, although the data generated by approaches such as whole-transcriptome sequencing is without bias, the shear amount of it is so immense as to make the analytical process ungainly at best: which of the hundreds of suggested fusion genes represent biologically and clinically important acquired mutations of tumorigenic significance, and which are noise of one or the other kind? Banding analysis, on the contrary, is a screening method that poses nonspecific, open-frame questions. All that can be seen cytogenetically is seen, within the boundaries set by the resolution achieved in that particular mitotic cell; the method is not dependent on any ability to "guess right" when the investigation is planned. In the last few years, important technological breakthroughs have been made that promise to bridge the epistemological gap between the molecular methods with their inherent specificity and the screening qualities of karyotyping techniques. Array-based techniques and sequencing not only can detect copy number imbalances whenever these are present but can also identify chromosomal breakpoints with unprecedented precision. New sequencing methods, among them parallel paired-end mapping (Mertens and Tayebwa, 2014), offer unique possibilities to screen the entire transcriptome for balanced rearrangements in a novel manner. The technology has already been applied to cancer studies and has led to the identification of previously unknown fusion genes (Chapter 5) in, for example, prostate, breast, ovarian, colon, and lung cancer; it is a fascinating new approach to look for cancer-associated rearrangements in an unbiased, genome-wide fashion. Whenever meaningful cytogenetic data exist on tumors that are examined by RNA sequencing, the karyotypic information can be put to good use as a means of selecting those candidate fusion genes that are likely to play a pathogenetic role; those fusions that correspond to the observed cytogenetic rearrangements are the ones of most interest, the ones whose involvement should first and foremost be looked for using verification by FISH, PCR, and Sanger sequencing (Panagopoulos et al., 2014).

Whereas molecular genetic analyses of a cancer begin with the isolation of DNA or RNA from a smaller or larger tumor sample, cytogenetic studies require that live, individual cells are removed from the tumor parenchyma. Almost all molecular genetic analyses in the cancer context have hitherto been performed on a mix of nucleic acids stemming from many cells, some of which belong to the tumor parenchyma and others to stromal elements. Next to nothing—FISH analyses excepted—has been done on single nuclei, something that would be a requirement if these techniques were to be used in the assessment of cell-to-cell genomic variability. Exciting new technical developments are now being made indicating that also molecular techniques may soon become cytological in nature. It was recently shown that whole-genome amplification and massive parallel sequencing of flow-sorted nuclei from breast cancers could accurately quantify genomic copy numbers within even an individual nucleus (Navin et al., 2011).

In normal molecular genetic practice, however, the DNA or RNA is obtained from all cell types within the sample, be they stromal or truly neoplastic, and after the extraction, there is no way to differentiate between the materials deriving from the different sources. The subsequent analysis therefore yields a picture of an idealized, average tumor cell that not only may incorporate features of nontumorous components but that will also fail to reveal genomic differences among different subsets of tumor parenchyma cells. The result is an inherent bias toward homogeneity; whatever heterogeneity there might have been among clones or subclones of neoplastic cells remains undetected.

It is our conviction that analyses should ideally proceed from the large to the small and that one should scrutinize the details only after one has a good idea as to which of them are likely to be the most important. If one can combine investigative techniques, this is almost always preferable for no one technique is capable alone to reveal all that is of interest in complex biological systems such as neoplasms. Likewise, the search for information about ever smaller entities of pathogenetic importance—be they isolated at the genic or DNA primary structure level—should be accompanied by parallel and no less consistent synthetic efforts, by attempts to see how the new data fit the knowledge obtained at higher levels of complexity. In short, cytogenetic and molecular genetic investigations of neoplastic cells must be balanced, and they must operate in concert. Only then can the partly overlapping, partly unique information yielded by the two approaches be synthesized into a picture of carcinogenesis that is at the same time both profound in understanding and comprehensive in scope.

Pathogenetic versus phenotypic tumor classification

In all the remaining chapters of this book, chromosomal aberration patterns are being correlated with diagnoses. Sometimes, remarkable concordance between the pathological diagnosis and one cytogenetic or molecular genetic rearrangement or a given aberration pattern will be noted; sometimes, a nonrandom relationship will be pointed out but not one that is completely specific; but on other occasions, no clear-cut cytogenetic—pathologic or cytogenetic–clinical relationship can be discerned. How are we to make sense of this variability if the acquired chromosomal aberrations are pathogenetically essential?

Current classification of neoplasias occurs according to several mostly morphological schemes—gross anatomical, histological, and cytological—to which modifying information from other fields, often histochemistry and immunology, may be added. Pathogenetic considerations traditionally play no or only a negligible role in the diagnostic grouping of cancers, and as long as the therapeutic measures are not specifically directed against the molecular mechanisms that have gone awry, there is not much impetus for this to change; adequate surgical removal of a macroscopic tumor is not dependent on an understanding of what made the tumor grow. Once treatment targets the molecular defects of the cells making up the neoplastic parenchyma, however, accurate pathogenetic classification, including cytogenetic classification, becomes essential. This was first seen for CML (Chapter 8). Formerly, it was accepted that some CML cases did not have t(9;22) or the corresponding gene fusion, BCR–ABL1, just as it was accepted that some cases of polycythemia vera and other chronic myeloproliferative disorders did. The introduction of imatinib mesylate (Druker, 2008), a drug that specifically counteracts the abnormal tyrosine kinase activity of the protein product of the fusion gene, served as a great stimulus to trim the borderlines of the disease category: cases displaying the *BCR–ABL1* fusion were accepted as CML even if some phenotypic features were at odds with the usual mode of presentation, whereas cases without this genotypic marker were now referred to other diagnoses (Swerdlow et al., 2008).

The increased understanding of leukemogenesis, especially, but also carcinogenesis and other types of tumorigenesis resulting from cytogenetic and other studies in the last few decades has paved the way for the introduction of many new biologically active drugs that target specifically the defining molecular details of different neoplastic processes. Once many such drugs become available, and this is going to happen in the next few years, it becomes adamant to determine whether any given tumor has the genetic feature in question, that is, a pathogenetic (cytogenetic, genomic) tumor classification will be of the essence (Brandal et al., 2010). Eventually, the goal is that the increased pathogenetic knowledge will be translated into specific and efficient therapies tailor-made to each individual cancer case. The treatment can then become both rational and individualized, the latter term now meaning that it is specifically directed against the genetic individuality of the cancer cells as well as administered in a manner that is best adapted to the genetic individuality of the host organism, the patient.

References

Aplan PD (2006): Causes of oncogenic chromosomal translocation. *Trends Genet* 22:46–55.

Asmann YW, Necela BM, Kalari KR, Hossain A, Baker TR, Carr JM, et al. (2012): Detection of redundant fusion transcripts as biomarkers or disease-specific therapeutic targets in breast cancer. *Cancer Res* 72:1921–1928.

Bäsecke J, Griesinger F, Trümper L, Brittinger G (2002): Leukemia-and lymphoma-associated genetic aberrations in healthy individuals. *Ann Hematol* 81:64–75.

Bellacosa A (2013): Developmental disease and cancer: Biological and clinical overlaps. *Am J Med Genet* 161: 2788–2796.

Bignell GR, Greenman CD, Davies H, Butler AP, Edkins S, Andrews JM, et al. (2010): Signatures of mutation and selection in the cancer genome. *Nature* 463:893–898.

Bonassi S, Ugolini D, Kirsch-Volders M, Strömberg U, Vermeulen R,, Tucker JD (2005): Human population studies

with cytogenetic biomarkers: Review of the literature and future prospectives. *Environ Mol Mutagen* 45:258–270.

Bonassi S, Norppa H, Ceppi M, Strömberg U, Vermeulen R, Znaor A, et al. (2008): Chromosomal aberration frequency in lymphocytes predicts the risk of cancer: Results from a pooled cohort study of 22 358 subjects in 11 countries. *Carcinogenesis* 29:1178–1183.

Boveri T (1914): *Zur Frage der Entstehung maligner Tumoren.* Jena: Gustav Fisher.

Brandal P, Teixeira MR, Heim S (2010): Genotypic and phenotypic classification of cancer: How should the impact of the two diagnostic approaches best be balanced? *Genes Chromosomes Cancer* 49:763–774.

Brassesco MS, Montaldi AP, Gras DE, de Paula Queiroz RG, Martinez-Rossi NM, Tone LG,et al. (2009): MLL leukemia-associated rearrangements in peripheral blood lymphocytes from healthy individuals. *Genet Mol Biol* 32:234–241.

Broberg K, Toksvig-Larsen S, Lindstrand A, Mertens F (2001): Trisomy 7 accumulates with age in solid tumors and non-neoplastic synovia. *Genes Chromosomes Cancer* 30:310–315.

Bueno C, Montes R, Catalina P, Rodríguez R, Menendez P (2011): Insights into the cellular origin and etiology of the infant pro-B acute lymphoblastic leukemia with MLL-AF4 rearrangement. *Leukemia* 25:400–410.

Cardoso J, Boer J, Morreau H, Fodde R (2007): Expression and genomic profiling of colorectal cancer. *Biochim Biophys Acta Rev Cancer* 1775:103–137.

Castor A, Nilsson L, Åstrand-Grundström I, Buitenhuis M, Ramirez C, Anderson K, Strömbeck B, et al. (2005): Distinct patterns of hematopoietic stem cell involvement in acute lymphoblastic leukemia. *Nat Med* 11:630–637.

Cavalli G, Misteli T (2013): Functional implications of genome topology. *Nat Struct Mol Biol* 20:290–299.

Chen B, Wang YY, Shen Y, Zhang WN, He HY, Zhu YM et al. (2012): Newly diagnosed acute lymphoblastic leukemia in China (I): abnormal genetic patterns in 1346 childhood and adult cases and their comparison with the reports from Western countries. *Leukemia* 26:1608–1616.

Chiu BC, Dave BJ, Blair A, Gapstur SM, Zahm SH, Weisenburger DD (2006): Agricultural pesticide use and risk of t(14;18)-defined subtypes of non-Hodgkin lymphoma. *Blood* 108:1363–1369.

Chrzanowska KH, Gregorek H, Dembowska-Bagińska B, Kalina MA, Digweed M (2012): Nijmegen breakage syndrome (NBS). *Orphanet J Rare Dis.* 7:13.

Cremer T, Cremer M (2010): Chromosome territories. *Cold Spring Harb Perspect Biol.* 12:a003889.

Cremer T, Cremer C, Lichter P (2014): Recollections of a scientific journey published in human genetics: From chromosome territories to interphase cytogenetics and comparative genome hybridization. *Hum Genet* 133:403–416.

Druker BJ (2008): Translation of the Philadelphia chromosome into therapy for CML. *Blood* 112:4808–4812.

Durkin SG, Glover TW (2007): Chromosome fragile sites. *Annu Rev Genet* 41:169–192.

Ebert BL, Pretz J, Bosco J, Chang CY, Tamayo P, Galili N, et al. (2008): Identification of RPS14 as a 5q–syndrome gene by RNA interference screen. *Nature* 451:335–339.

Escobar PA, Smith MT, Vasishta A, Hubbard AE, Zhang L (2007): Leukaemia-specific chromosome damage detected by comet with fluorescence in situ hybridization (comet-FISH). *Mutagenesis* 22:321–327.

Eyfjord JE, Bodvarsdottir SK (2005): Genomic instability and cancer: Networks involved in response to DNA damage. *Mutat Res* 592:18–28.

Fabbri M, Calore F, Paone A, Galli R, Calin GA (2013): Epigenetic regulation of miRNAs in cancer. *Adv Exp Med Biol* 754:137–148.

Gandhi M, Dillon LW, Pramanik S, Nikiforov YE, Wang YH (2010): DNA breaks at fragile sites generate oncogenic RET/PTC rearrangements in human thyroid cells. *Oncogene* 29:2272–2280.

Ganem NJ, Godinho SA, Pellman D (2009): A mechanism linking extra centrosomes to chromosomal instability. *Nature* 460:278–282.

Gauwerky CE, Hoxie J, Nowell PC, Croce CM (1988): Pre-B-cell leukemia with a t(8;14) and a t(14;18) translocation is preceded by follicular lymphoma. *Oncogene* 2:431–435.

Gisselsson D, Jin Y, Lindgren D, Persson J, Gisselsson L, Hanks S, et al. (2010): Generation of trisomies in cancer cells by multipolar mitosis and incomplete cytokinesis. *Proc Natl Acad Sci USA* 107:20489–20493.

Goodell MA, Godley LA (2013): Perspectives and future directions for epigenetics in hematology. *Blood* 121:5131–5137.

Greaves MF, Wiemels J (2003): Origins of chromosome translocations in childhood leukaemia. *Nat Rev Cancer* 3:639–649.

Greaves M, Colman SM, Kearney L, Ford AM (2011): Fusion genes in cord blood. *Blood* 117:369–370.

Hammerman PS, Hayes DN, Wilkerson MD, Schultz N, Bose R, Chu A, et al. (2012): Comprehensive genomic characterization of squamous cell lung cancers. *Nature* 489:519–525.

Heim S (1992): Is cytogenetics reducible to the molecular genetics of cancer cells? *Genes Chromosomes Cancer* 5:188–196.

Heim S (1993): Tumor progression—karyotypic keys to multistage pathogenesis. In Iversen OH (ed.): *New Frontiers in Cancer Causation: Exploring New Frontiers.* Washington, DC: Hemisphere Publishing Corporation, pp. 247–259.

Heim S, Mitelman F (1989): Primary chromosome abnormalities in human neoplasia. *Adv Cancer Res* 52:1–44.

Heim S, Mitelman F (1995): *Cancer Cytogenetics. Chromosomal and Molecular Genetic Aberrations of Tumor Cells,* Second Edition. New York: Wiley-Liss.

Heim S, Mandahl N, Mitelman F (1988): Genetic convergence and divergence in tumor progression. *Cancer Res* 48: 5911–5916.

Heim S, Christensen BE, Fioretos T, Sørensen AG, Pedersen NT (1992): Acute myelomonocytic leukemia with inv(16) (p13q22) complicating Philadelphia chromosome positive chronic myeloid leukemia. *Cancer Genet Cytogenet* 59:35–38.

Hirt C, Weitmann K, Schüler F, Kiefer T, Rabkin CS, Hoffmann W, et al. (2013): Circulating t(14;18)-positive cells in healthy individuals: Association with age and sex but not with smoking. *Leuk Lymphoma* 54:2678–2684.

Hong D, Gupta R, Ancliff P, Atzberger A, Brown J, Soneji S, et al. (2008): Initiating and cancer-propagating cells in TEL-AML1-associated childhood leukemia. *Science* 319:336–339.

Hotfilder M, Röttgers S, Rosemann A, Schrauder A, Schrappe M, Pieters R, et al. (2005): Leukemic stem cells in childhood high-risk ALL/t(9;22) and t(4;11) are present in primitive lymphoid-restricted CD34+CD19– cells. *Cancer Res* 65:1442–1449.

Howarth KD, Pole JC, Beavis JC, Batty EM, Newman S, Bignell GR, et al. (2011): Large duplications at reciprocal translocation breakpoints that might be the counterpart of large deletions and could arise from stalled replication bubbles. *Genome Res* 21:525–534.

Irons RD, Chen Y, Wang X, Ryder J, Kerzic PJ (2013): Acute myeloid leukemia following exposure to benzene more closely resembles de novo than therapy related-disease. *Genes Chromosomes Cancer* 52:887–894.

Janssen A, van der Burg M, Szuhai K, Kops GJ, Medema RH (2011): Chromosome segregation errors as a cause of DNA damage and structural chromosome aberrations. *Science* 333:1895–1898.

Janz S, Potter M, Rabkin CS (2003): Lymphoma-and leukemia-associated chromosomal translocations in healthy individuals. *Genes Chromosomes Cancer* 36:211–223.

Jin Y, Mertens F, Mandahl N, Heim S, Olegård C, Wennerberg J, Biörklund A, et al. (1993): Chromosome abnormalities in eighty-three head and neck squamous cell carcinomas: Influence of culture conditions on karyotypic pattern. *Cancer Res* 53:2140–2146.

Jin Y, Martins C, Salemark L, Persson B, Jin C, Miranda J, et al. (2001): Nonrandom karyotypic features in basal cell carcinomas of the skin. *Cancer Genet Cytogenet* 131:109–119.

Johansson B, Mertens F, Mitelman F (1991): Geographic heterogeneity of neoplasia-associated chromosome aberrations. *Genes Chromosomes Cancer* 3:1–7.

Johansson B, Heim S, Mandahl N, Mertens F, Mitelman F (1993): Trisomy 7 in nonneoplastic cells. *Genes Chromosomes Cancer* 6:199–205.

Johansson B, Mertens F, Mitelman F (1996): Primary vs. secondary neoplasia-associated chromosomal abnormalities—balanced rearrangements vs. genomic imbalances? *Genes Chromosomes Cancer* 16:155–163.

Johansson B, Fioretos T, Mitelman F (2002): Cytogenetic and molecular genetic evolution of chronic myeloid leukemia. *Acta Haematol* 107:76–94.

Joslin JM, Fernald AA, Tennant TR, Davis EM, Kogan S C, Anastasi J, et al. (2007): Haploinsufficiency of EGR1, a candidate gene in the del(5q), leads to the development of myeloid disorders. *Blood* 110:719–726.

Jurlander J, Caligiuri MA, Ruutu T, Baer MR, Strout MP, Oberkircher AR, et al. (1996): Persistence of the AML1/ETO fusion transcript in patients treated with allogeneic bone marrow transplantation for t(8;21) leukemia. *Blood* 88:2183–2191.

Kandoth C, McLellan MD, Vandin F, Ye K, Niu B, Lu C, Xie M, et al. (2013): Mutational landscape and significance across 12 major cancer types. *Nature* 502:333–339.

Kelly LM, Gilliland DG (2002): Genetics of myeloid leukemias. *Annu Rev Genomics Hum Genet* 3:179–198.

Knudson AG (1971): Mutation and cancer: Statistical study of retinoblastoma. *Proc Natl Acad Sci USA* 68:820–823.

Kolomietz E, Al-Maghrabi J, Brennan S, Karaskova J, Minkin S, Lipton J, et al. (2001): Primary chromosomal rearrangements of leukemia are frequently accompanied by extensive submicroscopic deletions and may lead to altered prognosis. *Blood* 97:3581–3588.

Lord CJ, Ashworth A (2012): The DNA damage response and cancer therapy. *Nature* 481:287–294.

Marques EA, Neves L, Fonseca TC, Lins MM, Pedrosa F, Lucena-Silva N (2011): Molecular findings in childhood leukemia in Brazil: High frequency of MLL-ENL Fusion/t(11;19) in infant leukemia. *J Pediatr Hematol Oncol* 33:470–474.

Mauritzson N, Albin M, Rylander L, Billström R, Ahlgren T, Mikoczy Z, Björk J, et al. (2002): Pooled analysis of clinical and cytogenetic features in treatment-related and de novo adult acute myeloid leukemia and myelodysplastic syndromes based on a consecutive series of 761 patients analyzed 1976–1993 and on 5098 unselected cases reported in the literature 1974–2001. *Leukemia* 16:2366–2378.

Mertens F, Tayebwa J (2014): Evolving techniques for gene fusion detection in soft tissue tumours. *Histopathology* 64:151–162).

Mertens F, Pålsson E, Lindstrand A, Toksvig-Larsen S, Knuutila S, Larramendy ML, et al. (1996): Evidence of somatic mutations in osteoarthritis. *Hum Genet* 98:651–656.

Mesquita B, Lopes P, Rodrigues A, Pereira D, Afonso M, Leal C, et al. (2013): Frequent copy number gains at 1q21 and 1q32 are associated with overexpression of the ETS transcription factors ETV3 and ELF3 in breast cancer irrespective of molecular subtypes. *Breast Cancer Res Treat* 138:37–45.

Micci F, Micci F, Haugom L, Abeler VM, Bjerkehagen B, Heim S (2007): Trisomy 7 in postoperative spindle cell nodules. *Cancer Genet Cytogenet* 174:147–150.

Mitelman F (1981): Tumor etiology and chromosome pattern—evidence from human and experimental neoplasms.

In Arrighi FE, Rao PN, Stubblefield E (eds.): *Genes, Chromosomes, and Neoplasia*. New York: Raven Press, pp. 335–350.

Mitelman F, Mark J, Levan G, Levan A (1972): Tumor etiology and chromosome pattern. *Science* 176:1340–1341.

Mitelman F, Brandt L, Nilsson PG (1978): Relation among occupational exposure to potential mutagenic/carcinogenic agents, clinical findings, and bone marrow chromosomes in acute nonlymphocytic leukemia. *Blood* 52:1229–1237.

Mitelman F, Johansson B, Mertens F (2007): The impact of translocations and gene fusions on cancer causation. *Nat Rev Cancer* 7:233–245.

Mitelman F, Johansson B, Mertens F, editors (2015): Mitelman Database of Chromosome Aberrations and Gene Fusions in Cancer. http://cgap.nci.nih.gov/Chromosomes/Mitelman.

Moorman AV, Chilton L, Wilkinson J, Ensor HM, Bown N, Proctor SJ (2010): A population-based cytogenetic study of adults with acute lymphoblastic leukemia. *Blood* 115:206–214.

Murname JP (2012): Telomere dysfunction and chromosome instability. *Mutation Res* 730:28–36.

Navin N, Kendall J, Troge J, Andrews P, Rodgers L, McIndoo J, et al. (2011): Tumour evolution inferred by single-cell sequencing. *Nature* 472:90–94.

Ninomiya S, Kanemura N, Tsurumi H, Kasahara S, Hara T, Yamada T, et al. (2011): Coexistence of inversion 16 and the Philadelphia chromosome comprising P. 190 BCR/ABL in chronic myeloid leukemia blast crisis. *Int J Hematol* 93:806–810.

Nowell PC (1976): The clonal evolution of tumor cell populations. Acquired genetic lability permits stepwise selection of variant sublines and underlies tumor progression. *Science* 194:23–28.

Nowell PC (1986): Mechanisms of tumor progression. *Cancer Res* 46:2203–2207.

Nucifora G, Larson RA, Rowley JD (1993): Persistence of the 8;21 translocation in patients with acute myeloid leukemia type M2 in long-term remission. *Blood* 82:712–715.

Obe G, Pfeiffer P, Savage JR, Johannes C, Goedecke W, Jeppesen P, et al. (2002): Chromosomal aberrations: Formation, identification and distribution. *Mutat Res* 504:17–36.

Panagopoulos I, Thorsen J, Gorunova L, Micci F, Heim S (2014): Sequential combination of karyotyping and RNA-sequencing in the search for cancer-specific fusion genes. *Int J Biochem Cell Biol* 53:462–465.

Pandis N, Bardi G, Heim S (1994): Interrelationship between methodological choices and conceptual models in solid tumor cytogenetics. *Cancer Genet Cytogenet* 76:77–84.

Platzer Upender MB, Wilson K, Willis J, Lutterbaugh J, Norratti A, Willson JKV, et al. (2002): Silence of chromosomal amplifications in colon cancer. *Cancer Res* 62:1134–1138.

Povirk LF (2006): Biochemical mechanisms of chromosomal translocations resulting from DNA double-strand breaks. *DNA Repair* 5:1199–1212.

Rabes HM, Demidchik EP, Sidorow JD, Lengfelder E, Beimfohr C, Hoelzel D, et al. (2000): Pattern of radiation-induced RET and NTRK1 rearrangements in 191 post-Chernobyl papillary thyroid carcinomas: Biological, phenotypic, and clinical implications. *Clin Cancer Res* 6:1093–1103.

Riggi N, Cironi L, Provero P, Suvà ML, Kaloulis K, Garcia-Echeverria C, et al. (2005): Development of Ewing's sarcoma from primary bone marrow-derived mesenchymal progenitor cells. *Cancer Res* 65:11459–11468.

Riggi N, Cironi L, Provero P, Suvà ML, Stehle JC, Baumer K, et al. (2006): Expression of the FUS-CHOP fusion protein in primary mesenchymal progenitor cells gives rise to a model of myxoid liposarcoma. *Cancer Res* 66:7016–7023.

Rotman G, Shiloh Y (1998): ATM: From gene to function. *Hum Mol Genet* 7:1555–1563.

Roukos V, Burman B, Misteli T (2013): The cellular etiology of chromosome translocations. *Curr Opin Cell Biol* 25:357–364.

Rubin MA, Maher CA, Chinnaiyan AM (2011): Common gene rearrangements in prostate cancer. *J Clin Oncol* 29:3659–3668.

Sayers EW, Barrett T, Benson DA, Bolton E, Bryant SH, Canese K, et al. (2010): Database resources of the National Center for Biotechnology Information. *Nucleic Acids Res* 38:D5–D16.

Schoch C, Kohlmann A, Dugas M, Kern W, Schnittger S, Haferlach T (2006): Impact of trisomy 8 on expression of genes located on chromosome 8 in different AML subgroups. *Genes Chromosomes Cancer* 45:1164–1168.

Seshagiri S, Stawiski EW, Durinck S, Modrusan Z, Storm EE, Conboy CB, et al. (2012): Recurrent R-spondin fusions in colon cancer. *Nature* 488:660–664.

Shlush LI, Zandi S, Mitchell A, Chen WC, Brandwein JM, Gupta V, et al. (2014): Identification of pre-leukaemic haematopoietic stem cells in acute leukaemia. *Nature* 506:328–333.

Sinclair PB, Nacheva EP, Leversha M, Telford N, Chang J, Reid A, et al. (2000): Large deletions at the t(9;22) breakpoint are common and may identify a poor-prognosis subgroup of patients with chronic myeloid leukemia. *Blood* 95:738–743.

Stoddart A, Fernald AA, Wang J, Davis EM, Karrison T, Anastasi J, et al. (2014): Haploinsufficiency of del(5q) genes, Egr1 and Apc, cooperate with Tp53 loss to induce acute myeloid leukemia in mice. *Blood* 123:1069–1078.

Straessler KM, Jones KB, Hu H, Jin H, van de Rijn M, et al. (2013): Modeling clear cell sarcomagenesis in the mouse: Cell of origin differentiation state impacts tumor characteristics. *Cancer Cell* 23:215–227.

Stratton M (2011): Exploring the genomes of cancer cells: Progress and promise. *Science* 331:1553–1558.

Strausberg RL (2001): The cancer genome anatomy project: New resources for reading the molecular signatures of cancer. *J Pathol* 195:31–40.

Sugihara E, Saya H (2013): Complexity of cancer stem cells. *Int J Cancer* 132:1249–1259.

Swerdlow SH, Campo E, Harris NL, Jaffe ES, Pileri SA, Stein H et al. (2008): *WHO Classification of Tumours of Haematopoietic and Lymphoid Tissues.* Lyon: IARC Press.

Taylor AM (2001): Chromosome instability syndromes. *Best Pract Res Clin Haematol* 14:631–644.

Teixeira MR, Heim S (2011): Cytogenetic analysis of tumor clonality. *Adv Cancer Res* 112:127–149.

Tirino V, Desiderio V, Paino F, De Rosa A, Papaccio F, et al. (2013): Cancer stem cells in solid tumors: An overview and new approaches for their isolation and characterization. *FASEB J* 27:13–24.

Tsai AG, Lu H, Raghavan SC, Muschen M, Hsieh CL, Lieber MR (2008): Human chromosomal translocations at CpG sites and a theoretical basis for their lineage and stage specificity. *Cell* 135:1130–1142.

Valent P, Bonnet D, De Maria R, Lapidot T, Copland M, Melo JV, et al. (2012): Cancer stem cell definitions and terminology: The devil is in the details. *Nat Rev Cancer* 12:767–775.

Visvader JE, Lindeman GJ (2012): Cancer stem cells: Current status and evolving complexities. *Cell Stem Cell* 10: 717–728.

Vogelstein B, Papadopoulos N, Velculescu VE, Zhou S, Diaz LA Jr, Kinzler KW (2013): Cancer genome landscapes. *Science* 339:1546–1558.

Wang RT, Ahn S, Park CC, Khan AH, Lange K, Smith DJ (2011): Effects of genome-wide copy number variation on expression in mammalian cells. *BMC Genomics* 12:562–576.

Weinstein JN, Collisson EA, Mills GB, Shaw KR, Ozenberger BA, Ellrott K, et al. (2013): The cancer genome atlas pan-cancer analysis project. *Nat Genet* 10:1113–1120.

Wheeler DL, Barrett T, Benson DA, Bryant SH, Canese K, Church DM, et al. (2005): Database resources of the National Center for Biotechnology Information. *Nucleic Acids Res* 33:D39–D45.

You JS, Jones PA (2012): Cancer genetics and epigenetics: Two sides of the same coin? *Cancer Cell* 22:9–20.

Zhang Y, Rowley JD (2006): Chromatin structural elements and chromosomal translocations in leukemia. *DNA Repair* 5:1282–1297.

Zhang L, Lan Q, Ji Z, Li G, Shen M, Vermeulen R, et al. (2012): Leukemia-related chromosomal loss detected in hematopoietic progenitor cells of benzene-exposed workers. *Leukemia* 26:2494–2498.

CHAPTER 5

From chromosomes to genes: searching for pathogenetic fusions in cancer

Ioannis Panagopoulos

Section for Cancer Cytogenetics, Institute for Cancer Genetics and Informatics, Olso University Hospital, Oslo, Norway

Fusion genes constitute a class of mutations in cancer that have attracted much attention as an important biomarker of neoplasia. They often exhibit distinctive covariation with histopathology and other phenotypic features, but first and foremost, they encode pathogenetic mutations that can serve as therapeutic targets for antioncogenic medicines that interact directly with the molecular change responsible for neoplastic transformation. Fusion genes also play a key role for the accurate diagnosis and subclassification of neoplasms. For example, *FUS–DDIT3* and *SS18–SSX* are pathognomonic for myxoid liposarcoma and synovial sarcoma, respectively (Fletcher et al., 2013). In acute myeloid leukemia (AML), t(8;16)(p11;p13) leading to the *KAT6A–CREBBP* fusion gene characterizes a distinct disease entity (Gervais et al., 2008; Haferlach et al., 2009). Furthermore, fusion genes have prognostic significance. In AML, *RUNX1–RUNX1T1*, *CBFB–MYH11*, and *MLL–ARHGAP26* define disease entities that have a relatively favorable prognosis, whereas *KAT6A–CREBBP*, *DEK–NUP214*, and *MLL–AFF1* correspondingly signify a poor prognosis (Chapter 6). In children with alveolar rhabdomyosarcoma, the presence of the *PAX3–FOXO1A* fusion gene is an independent predictor of poor outcome (Sorensen et al., 2002). In synovial sarcoma, the *SS18–SSX* fusion is a significant prognostic factor for overall survival, and the *SS18–SSX1* fusion type is associated with a high rate of tumor cell proliferation and poor clinical outcome (Kawai et al., 1998; Nilsson et al., 1999; Inagaki et al., 2000; Ladanyi et al., 2002). Because of their pathogenetically essential role – only the cells of the neoplastic parenchyma harbor them—fusion genes are ideal targets of molecular therapy, the paradigmatic examples being (i) the treatment for chronic myeloid leukemia (CML) carrying *BCR–ABL1*, which was dramatically improved by the introduction of an ABL-specific tyrosine kinase (TK) inhibitor, imatinib mesylate, into the clinic (Druker, 2008), and (ii) the use of *all-trans* retinoic acid (ATRA)/arsenic trioxide (ATO) in the treatment of acute promyelocytic leukemia (APL) carrying the *PML–RARA* fusion, which is the key player in APL leukemogenesis generated by t(15;17). Both ATRA and ATO trigger catabolism of the PML–RARA fusion protein, targeting the retinoic acid receptor α (RARA) and promyelocytic leukemia (PML) moieties, respectively (Zhou et al., 2007).

Cancer-specific fusion genes have been found in hematologic malignancies, mesenchymal tumors, and carcinomas in steadily increasing numbers. During 1982–1988, 10 such fusion genes were

---

Cancer Cytogenetics: Chromosomal and Molecular Genetic Aberrations of Tumor Cells, Fourth Edition.
Edited by Sverre Heim and Felix Mitelman.

identified, followed by 162 during 1990–1999, 420 during 2000–2009, and 1792 during 2010–2013 (http://cgap.nci.nih.gov/Chromosomes/Mitelman; updated on January 10, 2014). The list of fusion genes important in tumorigenesis is certain to increase further as more samples become available for testing and new methodologies are brought to bear (Mitelman et al., 2014).

Types of fusion genes

Fusion genes involving regulatory elements of the immunoglobulin and T-cell receptor genes

These fusions are found in lymphoid leukemias and lymphomas of the B- and T-cell lineages and lead to the quantitative deregulation of a gene in the breakpoint region of a tumor-specific chromosomal rearrangement, often a translocation. A good example is the activation of *MYC* in Burkitt lymphoma by the translocations t(8;14)(q24;q32), t(2;8)(p11;q24), or t(8;22)(q24;q11). The breakpoint in chromosome 8 is within or adjacent to the *MYC* gene. The other breakpoint is always within an immunoglobulin gene encoding either the heavy chain (*IGH* on 14q32) or the kappa (*IGK* on 2p11) or lambda (*IGL* on 22q11) light chains. As a consequence of the translocations, *MYC* becomes constitutively expressed owing to the influence of regulatory elements from the immunoglobulin genes (Klein, 2009).

Promoter swapping

The breakpoint in this situation is located in the 5′ untranslated region (UTR) of the gene, resulting in ectopic overexpression of a wild-type, full-length, downstream gene product.

Gene fusion resulting in promoter swapping was first observed as a consequence of the reciprocal t(3;8)(p21;q12) in pleomorphic adenomas of the salivary gland (Kas et al., 1997). The breakpoint of this translocation occurs in the 5′ noncoding regions of both *PLAG1* (8q12) and *CTNNB1* (3p21) so that regulatory control elements of both genes are swapped while preserving the coding sequences. Consequently, *PLAG1* is activated while expression levels of *CTNNB1* are reduced (Kas et al., 1997) in what was subsequently shown to be the most common mechanism of *PLAG1* activation (Van

Dyck et al., 2007). Upregulation of *SOX5* by promoter swapping with the *P2RY8* gene was demonstrated in follicular lymphoma (Storlazzi et al., 2007). In aneurysmal bone cysts, five chromosomal aberrations have been reported rearranging the *USP6/TRE17* gene and fusing it with one of five different partners, namely *CDH11*, *ZNF9*, *COL1A1*, *TRAP150*, and *OMD* (Oliveira et al., 2004, 2005). The translocation always results in promoter swapping leading to the highly active promoter of the translocation partner gene being fused to the first coding exon of *USP6/TRE17* resulting in its transcriptional upregulation.

Fusion genes coding for fusion proteins

As a result of a chromosomal aberration (often translocation), in this scenario, two protein-coding regions (or portions thereof) are fused in-frame, producing a chimeric protein. It is generally accepted that fusion proteins resulting from chromosome aberrations are oncogenic and their generation represents important and early steps in carcinogenesis (Boxer and Dang, 2001; Xia and Barr, 2005; Mitelman et al., 2007).

Often, at least one of the two rearranged genes encodes a transcription factor, and the hybrid gene functions as an abnormal transcription factor (Sorensen and Triche, 1996; Boxer and Dang, 2001; Xia and Barr, 2005). When expressed, the fusion product retains the DNA-binding specificity of one gene partner while activating transcription inappropriately through transactivating domains contributed by the second gene moiety. The result is abnormal regulation of downstream genes.

Another important type of fusion genes encodes chimeric TK (Medves and Demoulin, 2012). These fusions are produced by translocations and other chromosomal rearrangements targeting a subset of TK genes that includes *ABL1*, *PDGFRA*, *PDGFRB*, *FGFR1*, *SYK*, *RET*, *JAK2*, and *ALK*. In most TK proteins, the TK domain is located in the C-terminus, while inhibitory domains are in the N-terminal. In the chimeric protein, the moiety encoded by the partner gene always replaces the N-terminal part (thus, inhibitory domains are deleted), whereas the C-terminal TK domain is retained (Medves and Demoulin, 2012). The N-terminal moiety of the partner protein, which often includes a coiled-coil or a helix–loop–helix domain, plays an important role by controlling the oligomerization required for TK activation, cytoskeletal localization, neoplastic transformation, and the expression level of the fusion oncoprotein (since the fusion product is driven by the promoter of the partner gene).

"Out-of-frame" fusion transcripts

Rearrangements involving chromosome bands 12q13-15 in lipomas and other benign connective tissue tumors often result in out-of-frame fusions of the *HMGA2* gene with a variety of partners (Cleynen and Van de Ven, 2008). A stop codon is encountered quickly so that only few amino acids are added to the AT-hooks of HMGA2. The fusion transcript codes for a truncated form of HMGA2, called HMGA2Tr, mainly consisting of the three DNA-binding domains. An example is the fusion of *HMGA2* with *RDC1* in lipomas as a result of chromosomal rearrangements involving chromosome bands 2q35 and 12q13-15 (Broberg et al., 2002). Out-of-frame fusion transcripts have also been found for *ETV6* in leukemias. They usually involve the first two *ETV6* exons, generating a truncated ETV6 protein containing no functional domains. A loss of function of *ETV6* and the partner gene has been suggested (De Braekeleer et al., 2012).

Generation of fusion genes

The initial event in the creation of a fusion gene by chromosomal aberrations is the formation of a DNA double-strand break (DSB), which can be induced both physiologically, such as during the maturation of the immune system, or by exogenous DNA-damaging agents (Nambiar and Raghavan, 2011). Proper repair of all these DSB is essential for genome stability. Mechanisms to repair DSB involve two principal pathways: nonhomologous end joining (NHEJ) and homologous recombination (HR). NHEJ joins two free DNA ends after a break by direct religation, whereas HR uses a homologous template for repair, most typically a sister chromatid. In some instances, these pathways function inappropriately and rejoin ends incorrectly to produce genomic rearrangements, including chromosomal aberrations (Nambiar and Raghavan, 2011).

Sequence analysis of individual DNA breakpoints reveals different DNA recombination and repair mechanisms involved in chromosomal translocations, depending on the differentiation stage of the target cell at initiation. For example, chromosomal fusion sites of lymphoid malignancies are often linked to aberrant recombination activating gene (RAG)-mediated V(D)J recombination (Raghavan et al., 2001). Activation-induced deaminase (AID) is required for the chromosome breaks in *MYC* that lead to *IGH–MYC* fusion (Robbiani et al., 2008). Chromosomal breakpoints in therapy-related acute lymphoblastic leukemia are clustered close to topoisomerase II binding sites in the *MLL* gene (Domer et al., 1995).

Many breakpoint junctions (from chromosomal rearrangements) contain a few base pairs (2–20 bp) of overlapping sequences between joining chromosomal ends, a phenomenon broadly referred to as "microhomology" (Lawson et al., 2011; Villarreal et al., 2012; Berger et al., 2013). The frequent presence of microhomology at breakpoints of chromosomal translocations could provide insights into the repair mechanisms used to form these chromosomal aberrations (Villarreal et al., 2012 and references therein). The precise mechanisms of microhomology-mediated DSB repair and its role in chromosomal aberration, and consequently in fusion gene formation, are not yet unraveled, but multiple microhomology-mediated repair (MHMR) pathways have been proposed to explain the use of microhomology to repair DNA breaks (Villarreal et al., 2012). Moreover, a more general "illegitimate recombination mechanism" was also suggested in the generation of the *EWSR1–FLI1* fusion gene to explain the duplications, deletions, and inversions found on the der(11)t(11;22)(q23;q12) and der(22) t(11;22)(q23;q12) of Ewing sarcoma (Zucman-Rossi et al., 1998). The mechanism is based on the independent generation of single-strand DNA ends that are processed individually before interchromosomal joining.

In recent years, evidence for the existence of fusion transcripts that span two adjacent, independent genes has emerged (Akiva et al., 2006; Parra et al., 2006). Typically, such chimeric transcripts begin at the promoter of the upstream gene and end at the termination point of the downstream gene. The intergenic region is spliced out of the transcript as an intron so that the resulting fused transcripts possess exons from both genes. The RNA products are called transcription-induced chimeras (TIC), read-through fusions, or conjoined genes, since run-off transcription is the most likely mechanism involved in their generation (Akiva et al., 2006; Parra et al., 2006; Prakash et al., 2010). In the latter study of 800 TIC, a database was developed that contains detailed information about the TIC identified in the human genome (http://metasystems.riken.jp/conjoing/index). TIC are not restricted to humans but have been identified in mouse and drosophila as well (Prakash et al., 2010), in all three species showing tight regulation and unique expression patterns (Akiva et al., 2006; Parra et al., 2006; Nacu et al., 2011). For example, the two adjacent genes *HHLA1* and *OC90*, both located in 8q24, generate the *HHLA1–OC90* fusion transcript that is restricted to teratocarcinoma cell lines (Kowalski et al., 1999). The *LY75–CD302* chimera is restricted to the Reed–Sternberg cells of Hodgkin disease (Kato et al., 2003). The two genes are located in band 2q24 and are separated by only 5.4 kb. TIC fusion can change the properties of the participating proteins or change their localization. The *TMEM189–UEV* mRNA is a naturally occurring read-through transcript of the neighboring *TMEM189* and *UBE2V1* genes located in 20q13 (Thomson et al., 2000). The chimeric protein clusters to the cytoplasm, whereas UBE2Vl is a nuclear protein. The best characterized human TIC fusion transcript involves two members of the TNF ligand family, *TNFSF12* (previously known as *TWEAK*) and *TNFSF13* (*APRIL*), which encode a type II transmembrane and a secreted protein, respectively (Pradet-Balade et al., 2002). The chimeric TNFSF12–TNFSF13 protein, which is composed of TNFSF12 cytoplasmic and transmembrane domains fused to the TNFSF13 C-terminal domain, is expressed and translated endogenously in human primary T cells and monocytes. The chimeric protein is membrane anchored and presents the TNFSF13 receptor-binding domain at the cell surface. It is a biologically active ligand that stimulates cycling in T- and B-lymphoma cell lines (Pradet-Balade et al., 2002).

Transsplicing, that is, fusion of transcripts from nonadjacent genes without a corresponding fusion at the DNA level, is a common phenomenon in certain organisms such as trypanosomes and nematodes (Michaeli, 2011; Blumenthal, 2012) and has also been suggested as a mechanism for the generation of fusion transcripts (Li et al., 2008). Two neoplasia-associated fusion transcripts have been suggested that could be the products of a transsplicing mechanism: *JAZF1–SUZ12* in endometrial stromal sarcomas and *SLC45A3–ELK4* in prostate cancer (Li et al., 2008; Rickman et al., 2009). However, the importance of this mechanism for the generation of fusion transcripts has been questioned (Panagopoulos, 2010; Zhang et al., 2012). A *JAZF1–SUZ12* transcript was found in the immortalized T HESCs cell line (Li et al., 2008) that was derived from stromal cells obtained from an adult female with myomas and immortalized by transfection of the human telomerase gene (Krikun et al., 2004). Since this cell line has a normal karyotype and there is no fusion of the two genes at the genomic level, the authors proposed that the *JAZF1–SUZ12* transcript of T HESCs cells is generated from regulated transsplicing between precursor RNAs for *JAZF1* and *SUZ12* (Li et al., 2008). However, a *JAZF1–SUZ12* chimeric transcript was not found in the same human normal endometrial stromal cell line, at least not in a constant, reproducible manner (Panagopoulos, 2010).

The *SLC45A3–ELK4* chimera was shown to be formed by *cis*-splicing of adjacent genes/read-through and does not involve DNA rearrangements (Zhang et al., 2012). The expression of the chimera is induced by androgen treatment probably by overcoming the read-through block imposed by intergenic CCCTC insulators bound by CTCF repressor protein (Zhang et al., 2012). The *SLC45A3–ELK4* chimera is not restricted to prostate cancer but has also been found in normal prostate tissue (Nacu et al., 2011).

Methods to identify fusion genes

Methodologies based on cytogenetics

During the 1980s and in the beginning of the 1990s, the methodologies relied on for the identification and characterization of fusion genes included somatic cell hybrids and extensive restriction endonucleases/Southern blot and Northern blot analyses with utilization of radioactive material. The detection of a fusion gene was not a "one-step" process (not only because of the methods used but also because of the limited knowledge of the human genome at the time); nevertheless, its ability to elicit important new findings is exemplified by the discovery of *BCR–ABL1*, the fusion gene of CML. In 1982, de Klein and coworkers showed that *ABL1* is moved from chromosome 9 to chromosome 22 by the translocation. Heisterkamp et al. (1983) molecularly cloned a DNA fragment from a CML case that was shown to be a chimeric DNA fragment that contained sequences from chromosome 22 and chromosome 9. The following year, Groffen et al. (1984) showed in 17 CML patients that the breakpoint always occurred in a region of 5.8 kb, which was named the "breakpoint cluster region." The same year, an 8 kb *ABL1* RNA was found to be present in leukemic cells from CML patients with t(9;22) but not in normal cells, suggesting that it was a consequence of the translocation (Gale and Canaani, 1984). Heisterkamp et al. (1985) then showed that the "breakpoint cluster region" was part of a gene that was named *BCR*. Finally, sequence analysis of cDNA clones demonstrated that the result of t(9;22)(q34;q11) in CML was the generation of a *BCR1–ABL1* chimeric gene (Heisterkamp et al., 1985; Shtivelman et al., 1985).

The introduction of the polymerase chain reaction (PCR) and fluorescence *in situ* hybridization (FISH) techniques facilitated the identification of a plethora of fusion genes in various neoplasias. PCR is an *in vitro* method to amplify specific segments of DNA, using two oligonucleotide primers that hybridize to opposite strands and flank the region of interest in the target DNA (Saiki et al., 1985). A repetitive series of cycles involving template denaturation, primer annealing, and the extension of the annealed primers by DNA polymerase results in the exponential accumulation of a specific DNA fragment whose termini are defined by the 5′ ends of the primers (Saiki et al., 1985). If the two primers flank a chromosomal translocation junction, exponential amplification is contingent upon the presence of the translocation (Lee et al., 1987). Two independent research groups modified this approach to include RNA as the initial template in the amplification scheme. The RNA was first converted to single-stranded cDNA (by reverse transcriptase), which could then be used for enzymatic amplification of sequences between specific primers using a thermostable DNA polymerase (Dobrovic et al., 1988; Kawasaki et al., 1988). In both studies, this new approach, which nowadays is named reverse transcription PCR (RT-PCR), was used to identify chimeric *BCR–ABL1* transcripts in RNA from patients with CML or ALL carrying a Philadelphia chromosome. The method had high sensitivity (it detected the transcript in a 1:10^5 dilution of 1 μg RNA from the *BCR–ABL1*-positive K562 cell line) and overcame the difficulties related to variable genomic breakpoints within the *BCR* and *ABL1* genes. While the breakpoints within *BCR* and *ABL1* are variable, RNA splicing results in precise joining of *BCR* and *ABL1* exons so that the hybrid mRNA has one of two sequences that differ only in whether or not they contain the 75 base pair (bp) *BCR*. Thus, the *BCR–ABL1* fusion transcripts can be detected by synthesizing the corresponding cDNA and amplifying it by PCR using primers flanking the translocation junction (Dobrovic et al., 1988; Kawasaki et al., 1988). Frohman et al. (1988) devised a PCR-based technique, termed "rapid amplification of cDNA ends" (RACE), that achieved amplification and cloning of the region between a single short sequence in a cDNA molecule and its unknown 3′ or 5′ end. RACE can be used to identify the partner gene whenever one of the genes of the fusion transcript is known. Both RT-PCR and RACE shift the "hunting of fusion genes" from the DNA to the RNA level.

In 1986, Pinkel et al. described the use of FISH for chromosome classification and the detection of chromosome aberrations. Biotin-labeled DNA was hybridized to target chromosomes and subsequently rendered fluorescent by successive treatments with fluorescein-labeled avidin and biotinylated antiavidin antibody (Pinkel et al., 1986). As a spin-off of the Human Genome Project (HUGO), more and more probes from cloned and mapped segments of the human genome (cosmids, fosmids, PACs, BACs, and YACs) became available for FISH (e.g., BAC Resource Consortium; Cheung et al., 2001). The steadily increasing number of available probes, the high sensitivity and specificity of FISH, and the speed with which the assays can be performed made FISH a powerful technique for fusion gene detection.

The combination of cytogenetics (G-, Q- or R-banding), FISH, and molecular analyses (PCR, RT-PCR, RACE) has proved consistently effective in the identification of pathogenetic fusions in cancer, and many such chimeric genes have been detected using this sequential approach (Figure 5.1). The working flow starts with cytogenetic analysis of tumor cells to identify a characteristic chromosomal rearrangement, including mapping of the genomic breakpoints to a distinct band on each chromosome. The second step is the utilization of FISH techniques on abnormal metaphase plates using various probes such as YACs, BACs, PACs, cosmids, and fosmids to find the smallest probe that spans the chromosomal breakpoint (the signal for this probe will be split between the two derivative chromosomes). The third step involves molecular cloning often using various techniques such as PCR,

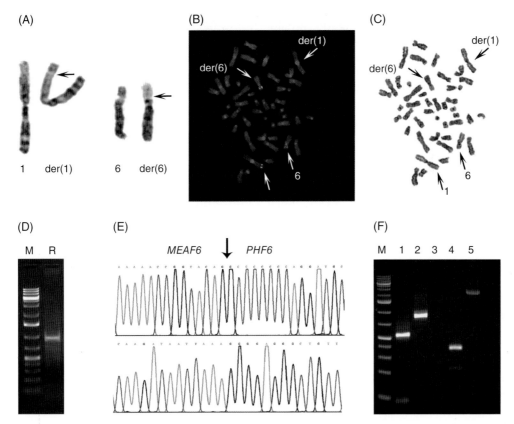

Figure 5.1 Cytogenetics-based approach for the detection of fusion genes exemplified by the detection of *MEAF6–PHF1* in low-grade endometrial stromal sarcoma. (A) Partial karyotype showing chromosome aberrations der(1) t(1;6)(p34;p21) and der(6)t(1;6)(p34;p21) together with the corresponding normal chromosomes; breakpoint positions are indicated by arrows. (B) FISH using BAC RP11-508 M23 (green signal) from 1p34 containing the *MEAF6* gene and pool of the RP11-600P03 and RP11-436 J22 BACs (red signal) from 6p21 containing the *PHF1* gene. A part of the probe from 6p21 (red signal) has moved to the derivative chromosome 1, while the entire probe containing *MEAF6* has moved to the derivative chromosome 6. The data suggest that the functional fusion gene is generated on the der(6). (C) G-banding of the metaphase spread shown in (B).

(D) Amplification of a 1 kb cDNA in the 5′-RACE analysis (R) using reverse *PHF1* primers and the universal forward primers. (E) Partial sequence chromatograms of the 1 kb cDNA fragment showing the junctions (arrow) of the *MEAF6–PHF1* chimeric transcript (upper) and genomic hybrid DNA fragment (lower). (F) RT-PCR and genomic PCR using specific *MEAF6* and *PHF1* primers. Lane 1, amplification of *MEAF6–PHF1* cDNA fragment; lane 2: amplification of *MEAF6* transcript; lane 3, reciprocal *PHF1–MEAF6* cDNA not amplified; lane 4, amplification of *PHF1* transcript; lane 5, amplification of *MEAF6–PHF1* genomic hybrid DNA fragment. M, 1 kb DNA ladder. *Source*: Panagopoulos et al. (2012) Novel fusion of *MYST/Esa1*-associated factor 6 and PHF1 in endometrial stromal sarcoma. Plos ONE 7, e39354.

RT-PCR, and RACE to localize the breakpoint more precisely and to identify the genes fused by the chromosomal rearrangement. The aforementioned sequential procedure is very robust and reliable, and a plethora of fusion genes have been cloned by such means in various types of malignancies (Heim and Mitelman, 2009; Mitelman et al., 2014).

A "shortcut" to the aforementioned methodology has been the candidate gene approach. de Thé et al. (1990) used it to identify the molecular consequences of the t(15;17)(q22;q21) chromosomal translocation, the hallmark of APL. Because (i) retinoic acid was known to induce *in vivo* differentiation of APL cells to mature granulocytes leading to morphological complete, albeit temporary, remission, (ii) the retinoic acid receptor alpha gene (*RARA*) was located in chromosomal band 17q21, and (iii) the t(15;17)(q22;q21) is specifically associated with APL, de Thé et al. (1990) decided to find out whether *RARA* was rearranged by the translocation. They showed that t(15;17)(q22;q21) fuses *RARA* to *PML* (myl in their publication), resulting in a chimeric *PML–RARA* fusion transcript.

The candidate gene approach has been extensively used to find fusion genes. For example, Åman et al. (1992) showed that *DDIT3* is rearranged in myxoid liposarcoma with t(12;16) (q13;p11). *DDIT3* maps to 12q13 and belongs to the C/EBP family of transcription factors. Members of the C/EBP family are expressed at high levels in fat and are involved in adipocyte differentiation of fibroblasts. *DDIT3* is induced during the differentiation of 3 T3-Ll cells to adipocytes and may play a role in the regulation of fat-specific gene expression. The t(12;16)(q13;p11) translocation was assumed to rearrange one or two genes in 12q13 and/or 16p11, loci that should be important in the normal control of fat cell differentiation and proliferation. Using a cDNA probe that spans the *DDIT3* coding region, *DDIT3* was found to be consistently rearranged in liposarcomas carrying t(12;16)(q13;p11) but not in other tumors with rearrangements of 12q13–15 (Åman et al., 1992). Among other neoplasia-associated fusion genes found by this approach, *FUS–ERG* in AML with t(16;21(p11;q22) and *EWSR1–DDIT3* in myxoid liposarcoma may be mentioned (Ichikawa et al., 1994; Panagopoulos et al., 1994, 1996).

A gene that has been found involved in one fusion gene is considered to be a candidate gene also for other rearrangements involving a break of the same chromosomal band. An example is the *EWSR1* gene in 22q12 (Fisher, 2014). *EWSR1* is a "promiscuous" gene that can fuse as the 5′ partner with many different genes in a wide range of clinically and pathologically diverse tumors (Fisher, 2014). In mesenchymal tumors with a chromosomal aberration involving chromosome band 22q12, *EWSR1* is immediately considered a candidate rearranged gene, and one searches first for its possible involvement before more time-consuming and complicated investigations are undertaken.

The cytogenetics-based methods are used for identification of fusion genes in cases with simple structural aberrations or in cases with recurrent chromosome abnormalities; they cannot be used in cases where banding analysis showed either a normal or complex karyotype.

"Omics" and gene expression-based methodologies

Wachtel et al. (2004) used gene expression signatures to identify a novel *PAX3–NCOA1* fusion in an alveolar rhabdomyosarcoma. Hierarchical clustering analysis showed that the tumor segregated with the branch of *PAX3–FKHR*, *PAX3–AFX*, and *PAX7–FKHR* fusion-positive alveolar rhabdomyosarcomas although RT-PCR analysis demonstrated that none of the earlier transcripts were expressed by the tumor. The authors calculated the probability of a translocation involving *PAX3* being present based on 100 genes of the translocation-specific signature and concluded that an alternative translocation involving the DNA-binding domains of *PAX3* or *PAX7* must be responsible for the translocation-specific expression signature. Using RACE experiments, they verified the *PAX3–NCOA1* fusion and thus described, using gene expression and molecular methodology, the gene-level equivalent of a translocation t(2;2)(q35;p23) or an inversion inv(2)(p23q35) (Wachtel et al., 2004).

Tomlins et al. (2005) reported a recurrent fusion of *TMPRSS2* with the *ERG* or *ETV1* genes in prostate cancer based on outlier gene expression analysis. They developed a method called cancer outlier profile analysis (COPA) to find genes with high expression in a subset of the samples and applied it on the Oncomine cancer microarray database (www.oncomine.org) (Rhodes et al., 2004). The principle of COPA is described by MacDonald and Ghosh (2006). In some prostate cancers, the *ERG* gene (21q22.3) was strongly expressed, while in some others, the *ETV1* gene (7p21.2) showed strong expression. Since both *ERG* and *ETV1* were known to be 3′-end partners in the *EWSR1–ERG* and *EWSR1–ETV1* fusion genes found in Ewing sarcomas and since they maintained DNA-binding domains in the aforementioned chimeras, Tomlins and coworkers (2005) hypothesized that *ERG* and *ETV1* might be involved in prostate cancer in a similar way, and subsequently, applying 5′-RACE methodology, they found the *TMPRSS2–ERG* and *TMPRSS2–ETV1* fusions.

A similar approach was used to identify the *HEY1–NCOA2* as a recurrent fusion gene in mesenchymal chondrosarcoma (Wang et al., 2012). In these experiments, the Affymetrix GeneChip® Human Exon 1.0 ST Array was used. This array consists of 1.4 million probe sets targeting more than one million exon clusters across the entire genome. It enables two complementary levels of analysis: "gene-level" expression analysis and "exon-level" expression analysis. The "exon-level" analysis can distinguish between different isoforms of gene transcripts. The fundamental rationale for exon-level expression profiling in the detection of fusion genes is based on the observation that most gene fusions leading to the formation of a chimeric protein cause an intragenic discontinuity in the RNA expression level of the exons that are 5′ or 3′ to the fusion point in one or both fusion partners. This is attributable to the differences in the strength or activity of the promoters of the two translocation partner genes. Additionally, in some cases, the nononcogenic, reciprocal fusion gene may be lost due to an unbalanced translocation event. Wang et al. (2012) therefore developed a genome-wide screen for gene fusions using Affymetrix Exon array expression data to study a variety of tumor samples with poorly understood genetics, of which the majority were mesenchymal or embryonal tumors. They demonstrated the successful application of this approach to detect gene fusions without prior knowledge of the genetic background of a given case and described the

identification of a novel, recurrent *HEY1–NCOA2* fusion in mesenchymal chondrosarcoma. Both genes are located on the long arm of chromosome 8, *HEY1* in 8q21.13 and *NCOA2* in 8q13.3, and are approximately 10 Mb apart. Wang et al. (2012) showed that, at least in one case, the *HEY1–NCOA2* fusion resulted from a small deletion of the 5′ portion of *NCOA2* spanning from the 5′ UTR to exon 12 of *NCOA2*. Suehara et al. (2012) applied a similar approach, that is, differential expression of 5′ and 3′ ends using NanoString Technology (Geiss et al., 2008) (http://www.nanostring.com/), and found *GOPS–ROS1* and *KIF5B–RET* fusions in lung adenocarcinomas.

Comparative genomic hybridization-based methodology

Array-based comparative genomic hybridization (aCGH) data can be used to identify novel fusion genes. The rationale is that sometimes gene fusions arising from inter- or intrachromosomal rearrangements are associated with an alteration in intragenic copy numbers that can be identified in a general screen. High-resolution aCGH analysis of salivary gland tumors revealed fusion (and amplification) of the *FGFR1* and *PLAG1* genes in ring chromosomes (Persson et al., 2008).

Ozawa et al. (2010) described a *KDR–PDGFRA* fusion in glioblastoma based on aCGH data. They used high-resolution aCGH to screen for potential rearrangements involving TK genes in glioma samples and identified a complex amplicon within 4q12 spanning the *PDGFRA* and *KDR* genes. The profile suggested amplification of chromosomal regions preserving the 5′ end of *KDR* and the kinase domain and 3′ portion of *PDGFRA*. Based on the pattern of copy number changes across this region, the authors hypothesized that an intrachromosomal rearrangement may have resulted in a gene fusion between *KDR* and *PDGFRA*. Indeed, RT-PCR confirmed a *KDR–PDGFRA* fusion transcript in the tumor.

Such et al. (2011) used aCGH to identify a novel *NUP98–RARG* fusion in an AML carrying a t(11;12)(p15;q13) chromosome translocation. To search for minor or cryptic genomic imbalances flanking the translocation breakpoint, they performed aCGH and found a 1.0 Mb microdeletion in 11p15 and a 2.5 Mb microdeletion in 12q13 involving the *NUP98* and *RARG* genes, respectively. They hypothesized that the genomic deletions would result in the formation of a *NUP98–RARG* fusion gene, which was confirmed by subsequent RT-PCR (Such et al., 2011). aCGH was also used to identify a *STAT5B–RARA* fusion in an APL (Chen et al., 2012) and a recurrent *STRN–ALK* fusion in thyroid carcinomas (Pérot et al., 2014).

Protein-based methodologies

A phosphoproteomic approach was used to study TK signaling in non-small cell lung cancer (Rikova et al., 2007). In some of the samples, high-level phosphorylation of ALK or ROS was found. Western blot analysis showed that ALK and ROS fragments had smaller molecular weight than predicted for wild-type proteins. Performing RACE, RT-PCR, and sequencing analyses, the authors showed that the fusion genes *TFG–ALK*, *SLC34A2–ROS*, and *CD75–ROS* were present.

Recently, *FGFR3* fusion genes were found in bladder cancer using Western blot as initial methodology. Williams et al. (2013) screened 43 bladder tumor cells lines by Western blot and found three cell lines that had abnormally high molecular weight forms of FGFR3 in addition to the expected normal FGFR protein. Further experiments with immunoprecipitation and deglycosylation suggested that these high molecular weight forms of FGFR3 might be fusion proteins. Subsequent RT-PCR studies showed the presence of *FGFR3–BAIAP2L1* in one cell line and the *FGFR3–TACC3* fusion gene in two others. Interestingly, the same fusion gene, *FGFR3–TACC3*, was also found in a subset of glioblastomas using high-throughput paired-end RNA sequencing (RNA-Seq) (Singh et al., 2012).

DNA-mediated transformation methodology

DNA-mediated transformation technique (also called gene transfer or transfection assay) is another approach to find fusion genes. The method is based on the ability of donor DNA from a tumor to induce oncogenetic transformation of the NIH 3 T3 immortalized mouse cell line in a single step (Krontiris and Cooper, 1981; Cooper, 1982). A number of oncogenes have been found using this approach, among them members of the *RAS* family

(Der et al., 1982; Fasano et al., 1984). In some cases, however, oncogenes identified by gene transfer were shown to be activated by rearrangements occurring during the experimental procedure, meaning that they were not present in the human tumors that served as the source of donor DNA, as in the case of *RET* that was subsequently found genuinely rearranged and activated in papillary thyroid carcinomas (Takahashi et al., 1985; Fusco et al., 1987; Grieco et al., 1990).

Soda et al. (2007) used an improved DNA-mediated transformation technique looking for oncogenes in non-small cell lung carcinoma. They generated a retroviral cDNA expression library, prepared recombinant retrovirus, and infected the mouse 3 T3 cell line with them. Subsequently, they isolated genomic DNA from the 3 T3-transformed loci and used it as template in PCR to amplify the inserted retroviral cDNA clones. One of the clones contained the *EML4–ALK* fusion transcript. RT-PCR on tumor material verified the presence of the chimeric *EML4–ALK* gene in the tumor.

Clinic-based methodology

Schaller and Burkland (2001) treated a patient with idiopathic hypereosinophilia with imatinib mesylate. The attempt was undertaken because both idiopathic hypereosinophilia and CML were hypothesized to have a common regulatory association (Malbrain et al., 1996). The following year, two more reports described the successful treatment of hypereosinophilia patients with imatinib (Ault et al., 2002; Gleich et al., 2002). The results implicated a kinase, similar to BCR–ABL1, KIT, and PDGFR, in the pathogenesis of eosinophilia in these patients. Analysis for KIT activation loop mutation (D816V) in four responding patients was negative, suggesting that KIT was not the target of imatinib (Gleich et al., 2002). Cools et al. (2003) reported that 9 of 11 patients treated with imatinib had responses lasting more than three months in which the eosinophil count returned to normal. None of the patients had mutations in exons encoding the activation loops or juxtamembrane domains of PDGFRA, PDGFRB, and KIT, which were known targets of imatinib. One of the patients who responded carried a t(1;4) (q44;q12) in his bone marrow cells. Since both *PDGFRA* and *KIT* are located in chromosome band 4q12, they were further investigated for possible involvement. FISH experiments showed that the translocation was associated with a deletion in 4q12 with a breakpoint near *PDGFRA*. The subsequent 5′-RACE experiments revealed a novel *FIP1L1–PDGFRA* chimeric transcript that arose from an interstitial hemizygous deletion linking together two genes that were normally located 900 kb apart on 4q12, a deletion not detectable by standard cytogenetics (Cools et al., 2003).

Next-generation sequencing-based methodologies

Next-generation sequencing (NGS, also called second-generation sequencing, high-throughput sequencing, deep sequencing, massively parallel sequencing, etc.) involves sequencing of short stretches of DNA and alignment to a reference genome. Alignments with unexpected position, orientation, or separation distance often reflect genomic rearrangements such as translocations, inversions, or deletions. Thus, NGS can detect previously unknown fusions in neoplasms with highly complex karyotypes or without any cytogenetic information (Meyerson et al., 2010).

Whole-genome sequencing (WGS), exome sequencing (also known as targeted exome capture), and whole-transcriptome sequencing (RNA-Seq) are the three major NGS technologies. WGS determines the complete DNA sequence of a sample in a single experiment. Exome sequencing selectively sequences the coding regions of the genome. RNA-Seq provides a picture of the RNA present at a given moment in time, enabling a search for alternative gene spliced transcripts, posttranscriptional changes, gene fusions, mutations/single-nucleotide polymorphisms (SNPs), and changes in gene expression (Chu and Corey, 2012). WGS and RNA-Seq are the two major NGS technologies for fusion gene detection, while exome sequencing is mostly used to identify somatic point mutations (Liu et al., 2013).

A variety of fusion genes have been discovered using WGS technology (e.g., Bass et al., 2011; Totoki et al., 2011; Welch et al., 2011). WGS of colorectal adenocarcinomas identified 11 rearrangements encoding predicted in-frame fusion proteins, including a recurrent *VTI1A–TCF7L2* fusion found in three out of 97 large bowel cancers (Bass et al., 2011). In a primary hepatitis C virus-positive

hepatocellular carcinoma, WGS revealed 33 somatic chromosomal rearrangements, most of them intrachromosomal (Totoki et al., 2011). Additional RT-PCR and Sanger sequencing confirmed four fusion transcripts generated by the rearrangements: the *BCORL1–ELF4* and *CTNND1–STX5* fusion genes created by intrachromosomal inversions of Xq25 and 11q12, respectively; the *VCL–ADK* fusion gene predicted to be generated by an interstitial deletion in 10q22; and the *CABP2–LOC645332* fusion gene generated by a tandem duplication in 11q13. WGS was also used to diagnose a cryptic fusion oncogene in an APL with no pathogenic *RARA* fusion identified by routine metaphase cytogenetics or interphase FISH (Welch et al., 2011). A cytogenetically cryptic event was found: a 77 kb segment from chromosome 15 had been inserted into the second intron of the *RARA* gene on chromosome 17 resulting in a classic *PML–RARA* fusion gene. In a recent study, WGS was carried out on 41 ependymomas, and a novel fusion gene between *RELA* and *C11orf95* was found in eight of nine analyzed supratentorial tumors (Parker et al., 2014). The *C11orf95–RELA* fusion was further verified with RNA-Seq, RT-PCR, Sanger sequencing, and FISH.

WGS has not been extensively used for the detection of fusion genes because it requires a great deal of sequencing and intensive computational analysis; the whole process of WGS, from sample preparation to fusion identification and verification, may take months to complete (Welch et al., 2011). In addition, the significance of a fusion gene discovered using WGS relies on its effects on expression and on whether it produces fusion transcripts.

In 2009, two reports were published showing that RNA-Seq is an efficient tool to detect fusion genes in cancer (Maher et al., 2009a, 2009b). The initial reports were followed by a cascade of studies exploring the presence of fusion genes in various cancers using high-throughput sequencing. The great interest in this topic has led to the development of multiple open-source software tools and pipelines that simplify the computational task of identifying novel fusion genes among millions of sequencing reads (Annala et al., 2013; Wang et al., 2013).

In a typical RNA-Seq experiment, RNA is first extracted, DNA contamination is removed using DNase, and the remaining RNA is broken up into short fragments. The RNA fragments are then reverse transcribed into cDNA, sequencing adaptors are ligated, and fragment size selection is undertaken. Finally, the ends of the cDNAs are sequenced using NGS technology to produce many short reads. If both ends of the cDNAs are sequenced, then paired-end reads are generated. Downstream data analysis consists of quality control such as trimming of sequencing adapters and removal of reads with poor-quality scores followed by mapping reads, analysis of differential expression, identification of novel transcripts, and pathway analysis. For the discovery of fusion transcripts, various programs have been developed such as FusionSeq, FusionMap, deFuse, nFuse, FusionFinder, and others (Sboner et al., 2010; Ge et al., 2011; Francis et al., 2012; McPherson et al., 2011, 2012). All of them follow a three-step procedure to detect gene fusions: (i) mapping and filtering, (ii) fusion junction detection, and (iii) fusion gene assembly and selection (Annala et al., 2013; Wang et al., 2013).

RNA-Seq is currently very popular in cancer-related fusion gene studies. The technique allows the detection of multiple alternative splice variants resulting from a fusion event and has low cost, and the turnaround time is quick. A limitation of RNA-Seq is that it cannot detect fusion events involving nontranscribed regions (Kim and Salzberg, 2011). Tissue specificity and the broad dynamic range of expression in the human transcriptome may also complicate the detection of gene fusions, especially when transcript expression is low (Taylor and Ladanyi, 2011).

Even in the early days of NGS, a puzzling finding was that the detected fusion genes were so many and definitely more than one (Ruan et al., 2007). In the initial reports of RNA-Seq as a tool for fusion gene detection, Maher et al. (2009a, 2009b) detected 111 chimeras in the K562 CML cell line, among them the BCR–ABL1 fusion, and 118 fusion transcripts in the VcaP prostate cancer cell line. Today, it is well established that RNA-Seq and analysis of the data with software specific for the detection of fusion genes result in long lists of fusion genes. Some of them are artifacts produced during the RNA library preparation stage (Quail et al., 2008; Annala et al., 2013). Others could be read-through transcripts generated when the RNA polymerase continues beyond the normal termination sequence into an adjacent gene (Nacu et al., 2011), while others still could be cancer-related fusion genes found in normal cells (individuals) such as BCR–ABL1 (Bose et al., 1998), TFG–GRP128 (Chase et al., 2010), and NPM–ALK (Trumper et al., 1998). Intratumor heterogeneity and clonal evolution shown at both cytogenetic and molecular level (Teixeira and Heim, 2011; Gerlinger et al., 2012) might also contribute to the multiplicity of detected fusion genes. Some fusion genes are tumor-causing drivers, while others could be the tumor-maintaining passengers (Vogelstein et al., 2013). The challenge is to identify the driver fusion gene(s) from the long list of fusion transcripts generated by the programs for fusion gene detection. Two computational approaches were recently described with the aim to identify driver fusion genes (Shugay et al., 2013; Wu et al., 2013).

Because the chromosomal rearrangement leading to a fusion gene is often seen as the sole aberration at cytogenetic analysis, it is assumed to be a primary tumorigenic event. Thus, a combination of banding cytogenetics and RNA-Seq would be uniquely well suited to identify the "primary" driver fusion genes in neoplasms carrying only one or a few chromosomal rearrangements (Figure 5.2). By using two completely distinct screening techniques operating at different levels of genomic organization (karyotyping and RNA-Seq) and laying the results on top of each other, one detects only one or very few points of correspondence (i.e., a fusion gene located in a chromosomal breakpoint), thus omitting the necessity to examine equally vigorously all the hundreds of fusion candidates identified by sequencing alone.

The combination of banding cytogenetics and RNA-Seq was used first to identify the recurrent WWTR1–CAMTA chimeric gene in epithelioid hemangioendothelioma (Tanas et al., 2011). RNA-Seq was performed on a tumor carrying the t(1;3)(p33;q25) translocation, and the data were analyzed using the FusionSeq algorithm (Sboner et al., 2010; Tanas et al., 2011). Because CAMTA1 and WWTR1 are located in chromosomal bands 1p36 and 3q25, respectively, the 26th in rank order WWTR1–CAMTA1 chimera was assumed to be the driver fusion gene (Tanas et al., 2011). Subsequent RT-PCR on this and four additional

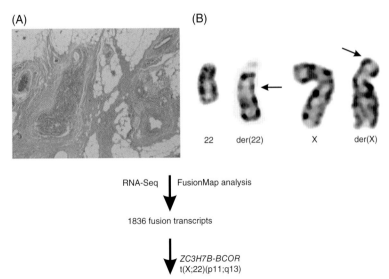

(A)   (B)

22   der(22)   X   der(X)

RNA-Seq   FusionMap analysis

1836 fusion transcripts

ZC3H7B-BCOR
t(X;22)(p11;q13)

(C)
GCCGTACTCGGAGACCCGGCTGGATGCACTCGACAGCTTTGGGTCGACACGAGGCTCNCTGGACAAACCTGACTCCTTCATGGGCGAGTATAGTGTTGGA
CGAGGCTCCCTGGACAAACCTGACTCCTTCATGGGCGAGTATAGTGTTTCCAACACTATACTCGCCCATGAAGGAGTCAGGCTCCCTGGACAAACCTGAC
CGGCTGGATGCACTCGACAGCTTTGGGTCGACACGAGGCTCCCTGGACAAACCTGACTCCTTCATGGGCGAGTATAGTGTTGGAAACAAGCACCGTGATC
GCTGGATGCACTCGACAGCTTTGGGTCGACACGAGGCTCCCTGGACAAACCTGACTCCTTCATGGGCGAGTATAGTGTTGGAAACAAGCACCGTGATCCC
CCTGGACAAACCTGACTCCTTCATGGGCGAGTATAGTGTTGGAAACAAGCACCGTGATCCCTTTGAAGCCCCAGAGGACAAAGATCTTCCTGTGGAGAAG
AACCTGACTCCTTCATGGGCGAGTATAGTGTTGGAAACAAGCACCGTGATCCCTTTGAAGCCCCAGAGGACAAAGATCTTCCTGTGGAGAAGTACTTTGT
CTCGACAGCTTTGGGTCGACACGAGGCTCCCTGGACAAACCTGACTCCTTCATGGGCGAGTATAGGGTTGGAAACAAGCACCGTGATCCCTTTGAAGCCC
GCTGGATGCACTCGACAGCTTTGGGTCGACACGAGGCTCCCTGGACAAACCTGACTCCTTCATGGGCGAGTATAGTGTTGGAAACAAGCACCGTGATCCC
ACGAGGCTCCCTGGACAAACCTGACTCCTTCATGGGCGAGTATAGTGTTGGAAACAAGCACCGTGATACCTTTGAAGCCCCAGAGGACAAAGATCTTCCT
CTCGGAGACCCGGCTGGATGCACTCGACAGCTTTGGGTCGACACCAGGCTCCGTGGACAAACCTGACTCCTTCATGGGCGAGTATAGTGTTGGAAACAAG
AACCTGACTCCTTCATGGGCGAGTATAGTGTTGGAAACAAGCACCGTGATCCCTTTGAAGCCCCAGAGGACAAAGATCTTCCTGTGGAGAAGTACTTTGT
GGAGACCCGGCTGGATGCACTCGACAGCTTTGGGTCGACACGAGGCTCCCTGGACAAACCTGACTCCTTCATGGGCGAGTATAGTGTTGGAAACAAGCAC
CGACAGCTTTGGGTCGACACGAGGCTCCCTGGACAAACCTGACTCCTTCATGGGCGAGTATAGTGTTGGAAACAAGCACCGTGATCCCTTTGAAGCCCCA
GCTGGATGCACTCGACAGCTTTGGGTCGACACGAGGCTCCCTGGACAAACCTGACTCCTTCATGGGCGAGTATAGTGTTGGAAACAAGCACCGTGATCCC

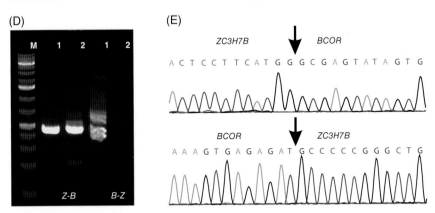

(D)

M   1   2   1   2

Z-B   B-Z

(E)

ZC3H7B   BCOR

A C T C C T T C A T G G G C G A G T A T A G T G

BCOR   ZC3H7B

A A A G T G A G A G A T G C C C C C G G G C T G

Figure 5.2 Combination of banding cytogenetics and RNA-Seq for the detection of the *ZC3H7–BCOR* fusion gene in low-grade endometrial stromal sarcoma. (A) H&E stained section of the endometrial stromal sarcoma. (B) Chromosomal aberrations der(22)t(X;22)(p11;q13) and der(X)t(X;22)(p11;q13) together with the corresponding normal chromosome homologs. RNA was extracted and sequenced. The data were analyzed with FusionMap and 1836 potential fusion transcripts were found, among them the *ZC3H7–BCOR* fusion transcript. *ZC3H7–BCOR* was investigated further because *ZC3H7B* and *BCOR* map to chromosome bands 22q13 and Xp11, respectively. (C) Chimeric *ZC3H7–BCOR* cDNA sequences identified with RNA-Seq. The junction "TCCTTCATGGGCGAGTTATAGT" is in yellow. (D) Verification of *ZC3H7–BCOR* (*Z-B*) and the reciprocal *BCOR–ZC3H7* (*B-Z*) using RT-PCR in two endometrial stromal sarcomas carrying a der(22)t(X;22)(p11;q13). A *ZC3H7B–BCOR* cDNA fragment was found in both cases, whereas the reciprocal *BCOR–ZC3H7B* fusion was detected only in case 1 that was used for RNA-Seq. (E) Sanger sequencing confirmed the *ZC3H7B–BCOR* and *BCOR–ZC3H7B* fusion transcripts.

epithelioid hemangioendotheliomas demonstrated that all carried the *WWTR1–CAMTA1* fusion (Tanas et al., 2011). Using the same approach, Lee et al. (2012) identified the *YWHAE–FAM22A/B* chimeric genes in high-grade endometrial stromal sarcomas carrying the translocation t(10;17) (q22;p13). FISH experiments revealed rearrangement of the *YWHAE* gene and the localization of the breakpoint in two close but different bands on chromosome 10 (10q22.3 and 10q23.2) separated by only 7.8 Mb. However, 3′-RACE experiments were unsuccessful because of the abundant expression of the wild-type *YWHAE*. RNA-Seq of a cell line carrying the t(10;17)(q22;p13) and analysis of the sequence reads with the deFuse program (McPherson et al., 2011) identified an in-frame *YWHAE–FAM22A* fusion transcript, which came out first in the rank order of the detected fusion genes (Lee et al., 2012). RT-PCR testing with forward *YWHAE* primers and consensus reverse primers for *FAM22A/B* identified the presence of *YWHAE–FAM22A* or *YWHAE–FAM22B* in all examined tumors.

A similar sequential combination of methods—banding cytogenetics and RNA-Seq—was used to demonstrate that *ZC3H7–BCOR* is a recurrent chimera in a subset of endometrial stromal sarcomas characterized cytogenetically by an X;22 translocation (Figure 5.2). RNA-Seq was performed on a tumor whose karyotype was 46,X,t(X;22) (p11;q13),t(3;4)(p23;q27) (Panagopoulos et al., 2013c), and the sequence reads were analyzed using the FusionMap software (Ge et al., 2011). A *ZC3H7–BCOR* chimeric transcript corresponding to the t(X;22)(p11;q13) was found ranked in the ninth place. RT-PCR and Sanger sequencing of the same tumor as well as another one carrying a der(22)t(X;22)(p11;q13) confirmed the presence of the *ZC3H7–BCOR* chimeric transcript in both. The cytogenetic guidance was a necessity to identify the fusion gene of interest (Panagopoulos et al., 2013c). The same sequential approach comparing karyotypic and sequencing data was also used to identify recurrent *EWSR1–YY1* fusions in a subset of mesotheliomas (Panagopoulos et al., 2013d). RNA-Seq was performed on a mesothelioma carrying a t(14;22)(q32;q12) as the sole chromosomal aberration, and the sequence reads were analyzed using the FusionMap software. The *YY1–EWSR1*

fusion transcript was ranked first, while the reciprocal *EWSR1–YY1* was ranked 15th. Taking into consideration that *YY1* and *EWSR1* map to chromosome bands 14q32 and 22q12, respectively, the same chromosomal bands involved in the rearrangement, the presence of *EWSR1–YY1* and *YY1–EWSR1* fusion transcripts in the tumor was further investigated and confirmed with molecular techniques. When screening additional cases of mesothelioma, one more tumor was identified carrying an *EWSR1–YY1* fusion gene but not the reciprocal *YY1–EWSR1* transcript (Panagopoulos et al., 2013d).

RNA-Seq and the FusionMap software were also used to examine in detail an acute erythroid leukemia with the translocation t(1;16)(p31;q24) and a FISH-detected split of *CBFA2T3* in 16q24 (Micci et al., 2011). An *NFIA–CBFA2T3* (the former gene is located in 1p31) chimeric transcript ranked 10th in a list of over 500 possible fusion genes was found to correspond to the translocation (Micci et al., 2013). The same sequential approach was also used to identify the *ZMYND8–RELA* fusion in a congenital acute erythroid leukemia carrying a t(11;20)(p11;q13) translocation (Panagopoulos et al., 2013b) and the *IRF2BP2–CDX1* fusion in a mesenchymal chondrosarcoma with t(1;5)(q42;q32) as the sole karyotypic aberration (Nyquist et al., 2012).

RNA-Seq of an AML with the karyotype 46,XX,add(1)(p36),der(2)t(2;3)(q21;q21),del(3) (q21),der(10)t(1;10)(q32;q24),der(16)(2qter-->2q 21::16p11-->16q24::16p11-->16pter) identified a cryptic *FUS–ERG* fusion transcript (Panagopoulos et al., 2013a). All the structural chromosome aberrations could have generated fusion genes. Screening with FISH for all possibly rearranged genes within the abnormal karyotype would have been laborious and an almost impossibly time-consuming procedure. It was therefore decided to perform RNA-Seq to compare karyotyping and sequencing data and concentrate exclusively on those suggested fusion genes that were found in chromosomal breakpoints. From the 500 fusion genes indicated by the RNA-Seq data using the FusionMap algorithm, only *FUS–ERG* showed correspondence with karyotype features (*FUS* maps to 16p11, a chromosome band that was rearranged in the karyotype) (Panagopoulos et al., 2013a).

RNA-Seq combined with FISH and banding cytogenetics was also used for the identification of the recurrent *MBTD1–CXorf67* fusion transcript in a subgroup of low-grade endometrial stromal sarcomas carrying a reciprocal t(X;17)(p11.2;q21.33) translocation (Dewaele et al., 2014) and for the identification of the *SERPINE1–FOSB* fusion in pseudomyogenic hemangioendothelioma with a balanced translocation t(7;19)(q22;q13) (Walther et al., 2014).

The aforementioned studies show that RNA-Seq used together with algorithms specifically designed to discover fusion genes is a particularly powerful approach when the grid of information thus obtained is laid on top of the grid of information obtained by karyotyping. The algorithms alone gave many fusion genes, and their ranking order was not necessarily in accordance with their biological or clinical importance; at the very least, one can say that the fusions corresponding to the cytogenetically visible rearrangement did not always come out on top.

Fusion detection programs are many (Wang et al., 2013), and each of them has specific biases as regards sensitivity and specificity that, however, have not been extensively compared or investigated. In a recent study, eight fusion detection softwares were tested (FusionHunter, FusionMap, FusionFinder, MapSplice, deFuse, Bellerophontes, ChimeraScan, and TopHat-Fusion) to detect fusion events using synthetic and real datasets that included chimeras (Carrara et al., 2013). The study showed that analysis of synthetic data could generate misleading results with most fusion detection programs generating a very high number of false-positive chimeras, leading the investigators to conclude that "there is space for further improvement in the fusion-finder algorithms" (Carrara et al., 2013).

In two cases, fusion detection programs failed to detect the biologically important fusion genes. The first was an AML that was suspected of having a t(8;16)(p11;p13) resulting in a *KAT6A–CREBBP* fusion because the bone marrow was packed with monoblasts showing marked erythrophagocytosis (Panagopoulos et al., 2014b). Since the diagnostic karyotype contained the chromosomal aberrations add(1)(p13), t(8;21)(p11;q22), and der(16)t(1;16) (p13;p13) but no t(8;16), no direct confirmation of the suspicion could be given although both 8p11

and 16p13 seemed to be rearranged. The leukemic cells were examined in two ways to find out whether a cryptic *KAT6A–CREBBP* was present. The first was the "conventional" approach: G-banding was followed by FISH and RT-PCR. The second was RNA-Seq followed by data analysis using the FusionMap and FusionFinder programs with special emphasis on candidates located in the 1p13, 8p11, 16p13, and 21q22 breakpoints. The "conventional" approach showed that a chimeric *KAT6A–CREBBP* transcript was present in the patient's bone marrow. Surprisingly, *KATA6A–CREBBP* was not among the 874 and 35 fusion transcripts identified by the FusionMap and FusionFinder programs, respectively, although 11 sequences of the raw RNA-sequencing data were *KATA6A–CREBBP* fragments (Panagopoulos et al., 2014b). Instead, three other *KAT6A* (referred to as *MYST3* in the FusionMap output) fusions were found: *DTX3L–MYST3* ranking 91, *MYST3–SLK* ranking 193, and *MYST–DNAJC14* ranking 606. Based on the map information on the genes, these fusions would have corresponded to the translocations t(3;8)(q21;p11), t(8;10)(p11;q24), and t(8;12) (p11;q13), respectively, none of which was seen by karyotyping. One *CREBBP* fusion transcript was found, *CREBBP–TTc58*, that was ranked 401st in the list of fusion transcripts. The transcript would have corresponded to a t(16;22)(p13;q12), which was not found by G-banding.

The second case was a small round cell tumor in which a t(4;19)(q35;q13) was found in a complex karyotype but where the initial reverse transcriptase PCR (RT-PCR) examination did not detect the *CIC–DUX4* fusion transcript previously described as the crucial gene-level outcome of this specific translocation (Panagopoulos et al., 2014a). The RNA-Seq data were analyzed using the FusionMap, FusionFinder, and ChimeraScan programs that identified 1024, 103, and 101 fusion transcripts, respectively, but *CIC–DUX4* was not among them. This notwithstanding, the "grep" command-line utility captured 15 chimeric *CIC–DUX4* cDNA sequences, and the fusion between the *CIC* and *DUX4* genes was mapped precisely (Panagopoulos et al., 2014a).

The two studies showed that at least some fusion detection programs (FusionMap, FusionFinder, and ChimeraScan) generate a plethora of fusion transcripts but do not always detect the biologically important chimeric transcripts, *KAT6A–CREBBP* in the AML and *CIC–DUX4* in the small round cell sarcoma. These programs are useful but suffer from imperfections with regard to both sensitivity and specificity. The "grep" command is an excellent tool to capture chimeric transcript from RNA-Seq data when the pathological and/or cytogenetic information strongly indicates the presence of a specific fusion gene that the bioinformatic programs fail to identify.

Conclusion

During the last three decades, identification of fusion genes has become an important part of cancer research. Many approaches have been used, of which the cytogenetics–FISH–PCR–Sanger sequencing methodology emerged as the gold standard. As NGS becomes cheaper and more NGS platforms become available, one can assume that this approach will become increasingly widespread and lead to the detection of ever more fusion genes in different types of cancer. However, the algorithms used to find the fusion genes typically give hundreds of alleged fusions that cannot all be equally important and many of which are almost certainly unimportant. The algorithms may furthermore fail to list the driver fusion genes among the candidates they identify; both their sensitivity and specificity are incomplete. To perform all the verification/falsification work necessary on this high number of alleged fusion genes in almost each tumor is hardly doable for a normal-sized lab, but a combination of G-banding (or other chromosome banding techniques) and RNA-Seq (or any other type of NGS) helps us detect the fusion gene(s) associated with a visible chromosome aberration. At the same time, this circumvents the highly laborious FISH stage at which one formerly had to try out ever new FISH probes looking for the one split by the rearrangement; most FISH studies can now be performed later as part of the confirmation of the sequencing findings. Sequencing of many tumors of the same type in order to find one or more fusion genes common to several of them is another approach. Either way, the continuous improvement of the bioinformatics methodology is of the essence to reduce the number of false positives while simultaneously ensuring that no actual fusion gene is missed (Kangaspeska et al., 2012; Carrara et al., 2013).

References

Akiva P, Toporik A, Edelheit S, Peretz Y, Diber A, Shemesh R, et al. (2006): Transcription-mediated gene fusion in the human genome. *Genome Res* 16:30–36.

Åman P, Ron D, Mandahl N, Fioretos T, Heim S, Arheden K, et al. (1992): Rearrangement of the transcription factor gene CHOP in myxoid liposarcomas with t(12;16)(q13;p11). *Genes Chromosomes Cancer* 5:278–285.

Annala MJ, Parker BC, Zhang W, Nykter M (2013): Fusion genes and their discovery using high throughput sequencing. *Cancer Lett* 340:192–200.

Ault P, Cortes J, Koller C, Kaled ES, Kantarjian H (2002): Response of idiopathic hypereosinophilic syndrome to treatment with imatinib mesylate. *Leuk Res* 26:881–884.

Bass AJ, Lawrence MS, Brace LE, Ramos AH, Drier Y, Cibulskis K, et al. (2011): Genomic sequencing of colorectal adenocarcinomas identifies a recurrent VTI1A-TCF7L2 fusion. *Nat Genet* 43:964–968.

Berger M, Dirksen U, Braeuninger A, Koehler G, Juergens H, Krumbholz M, et al. (2013): Genomic EWS-FLI1 fusion sequences in Ewing sarcoma resemble breakpoint characteristics of immature lymphoid malignancies. *PLoS One* 8: e56408.

Blumenthal T (2012): Trans-splicing and operons in *C. elegans*. *WormBook*, 1–11.

Bose S, Deininger M, Gora-Tybor J, Goldman JM, Melo JV (1998): The presence of typical and atypical BCR-ABL fusion genes in leukocytes of normal individuals: Biologic significance and implications for the assessment of minimal residual disease. *Blood* 92:3362–3367.

Boxer LM, Dang CV (2001): Translocations involving c-myc and c-myc function. *Oncogene* 20:5595–5610.

Broberg K, Zhang M, Strombeck B, Isaksson M, Nilsson M, Mertens F, et al. (2002): Fusion of RDC1 with HMGA2 in lipomas as the result of chromosome aberrations involving 2q35-37 and 12q13-15. *Int J Oncol* 21:321–326.

Carrara M, Beccuti M, Lazzarato F, Cavallo F, Cordero F, Donatelli S, et al. (2013): State-of-the-art fusion-finder algorithms sensitivity and specificity. *Biomed Res Int* 2013:340620.

Chase A, Ernst T, Fiebig A, Collins A, Grand F, Erben P, et al. (2010): TFG, a target of chromosome translocations in lymphoma and soft tissue tumors, fuses to GPR128 in healthy individuals. *Haematologica* 95:20–26.

Chen H, Pan J, Yao L, Wu L, Zhu J, Wang W, et al. (2012): Acute promyelocytic leukemia with a STAT5b-RARalpha fusion transcript defined by array-CGH, FISH, and RT-PCR. *Cancer Genet* 205:327–331.

Cheung VG, Nowak N, Jang W, Kirsch IR, Zhao S, Chen XN, et al. (2001): Integration of cytogenetic landmarks into the draft sequence of the human genome. *Nature* 409:953–958.

Chu Y, Corey DR (2012): RNA sequencing: Platform selection, experimental design, and data interpretation. *Nucleic Acid Ther* 22:271–274.

Cleynen I, Van de Ven WJ (2008): The HMGA proteins: A myriad of functions (Review). *Int J Oncol* 32:289–305.

Cools J, DeAngelo DJ, Gotlib J, Stover EH, Legare RD, Cortes J, et al. (2003): A tyrosine kinase created by fusion of the PDGFRA and FIP1L1 genes as a therapeutic target of imatinib in idiopathic hypereosinophilic syndrome. *N Engl J Med* 348:1201–1214.

Cooper GM (1982): Cellular transforming genes. *Science* 217:801–806.

De Braekeleer E, Douet-Guilbert N, Morel F, Le Bris MJ, Basinko A, De Braekeleer M (2012): ETV6 fusion genes in hematological malignancies: A review. *Leuk Res* 36:945–961.

De Klein A, van Kessel AG, Grosveld G, Bartram CR, Hagemeijer A, Bootsma D, et al. (1982): A cellular oncogene is translocated to the Philadelphia chromosome in chronic myelocytic leukaemia. *Nature* 300:765–767.

De Thé H, Chomienne C, Lanotte M, Degos L, Dejean A (1990): The t(15;17) translocation of acute promyelocytic leukaemia fuses the retinoic acid receptor alpha gene to a novel transcribed locus. *Nature* 347:558–561.

Der CJ, Krontiris TG, Cooper GM (1982): Transforming genes of human bladder and lung carcinoma cell lines are homologous to the ras genes of Harvey and Kirsten sarcoma viruses. *Proc Natl Acad Sci USA* 79:3637–3640.

Dewaele B, Przybyl J, Quattrone A, Finalet Ferreiro J, Vanspauwen V, Geerdens E, et al. (2014): Identification of a novel, recurrent MBTD1-CXorf67 fusion in low-grade endometrial stromal sarcoma. *Int J Cancer* 134:1112–1122.

Dobrovic A, Trainor KJ, Morley AA (1988): Detection of the molecular abnormality in chronic myeloid leukemia by use of the polymerase chain reaction. *Blood* 72:2063–2065.

Domer PH, Head DR, Renganathan N, Raimondi SC, Yang E, Atlas M (1995): Molecular analysis of 13 cases of MLL/11q23 secondary acute leukemia and identification of topoisomerase II consensus-binding sequences near the chromosomal breakpoint of a secondary leukemia with the t(4;11). *Leukemia* 9:1305–1312.

Druker BJ (2008): Translocation of the Philadelphia chromosome into therapy for CML. *Blood* 112:4804–4817.

Fasano O, Birnbaum D, Edlund L, Fogh J, Wigler M (1984): New human transforming genes detected by a tumorigenicity assay. *Mol Cell Biol* 4:1695–1705.

Fisher C (2014): The diversity of soft tissue tumours with EWSR1 gene rearrangements: A review. *Histopathology* 64:134–150.

Fletcher CDM, Bridge JA, Hogendoorn PCW, Mertens F (2013) *WHO Classification of Tumours of Soft Tissue and Bone.* Lyon: IARC.

Francis RW, Thompson-Wicking K, Carter KW, Anderson D, Kees UR, Beesley AH (2012): FusionFinder: A software tool to identify expressed gene fusion candidates from RNA-Seq data. *PLoS One* 7: e39987.

Frohman MA, Dush MK, Martin GR (1988): Rapid production of full-length cDNAs from rare transcripts: Amplification using a single gene-specific oligonucleotide primer. *Proc Natl Acad Sci USA* 85:8998–9002.

Fusco A, Grieco M, Santoro M, Berlingieri MT, Pilotti S, Pierotti MA, et al. (1987): A new oncogene in human thyroid papillary carcinomas and their lymph-nodal metastases. *Nature* 328:170–172.

Gale RP, Canaani E (1984): An 8-kilobase abl RNA transcript in chronic myelogenous leukemia. *Proc Natl Acad Sci USA* 81:5648–5652.

Ge H, Liu K, Juan T, Fang F, Newman M, Hoeck W (2011): FusionMap: Detecting fusion genes from next-generation sequencing data at base-pair resolution. *Bioinformatics* 27:1922–1928.

Geiss GK, Bumgarner RE, Birditt B, Dahl T, Dowidar N, Dunaway DL, et al. (2008): Direct multiplexed measurement of gene expression with color-coded probe pairs. *Nat Biotechnol* 26:317–325.

Gerlinger M, Rowan AJ, Horswell S, Larkin J, Endesfelder D, Gronroos E, et al. (2012): Intratumor heterogeneity and branched evolution revealed by multiregion sequencing. *N Engl J Med* 366:883–892.

Gervais C, Murati A, Helias C, Struski S, Eischen A, Lippert E, et al. (2008): Acute myeloid leukaemia with 8p11 (MYST3) rearrangement: an integrated cytologic, cytogenetic and molecular study by the Groupe Francophone de Cytogenetique Hematologique. *Leukemia* 22:1567–1575.

Gleich GJ, Leiferman KM, Pardanani A, Tefferi A, Butterfield JH (2002): Treatment of hypereosinophilic syndrome with imatinib mesilate. *Lancet* 359:1577–1578.

Grieco M, Santoro M, Berlingieri MT, Melillo RM, Donghi R, Bongarzone I, et al. (1990): PTC is a novel rearranged form of the ret proto-oncogene and is frequently detected in vivo in human thyroid papillary carcinomas. *Cell* 60:557–563.

Groffen J, Stephenson JR, Heisterkamp N, de Klein A, Bartram CR, Grosveld G (1984): Philadelphia chromosomal breakpoints are clustered within a limited region, bcr, on chromosome 22. *Cell* 36:93–99.

Haferlach T, Kohlmann A, Klein HU, Ruckert C, Dugas M, Williams PM, et al. (2009): AML with translocation t(8;16) (p11;p13) demonstrates unique cytomorphological, cytogenetic, molecular and prognostic features. *Leukemia* 23:934–943.

Heim S, Mitelman F (2009): *Cancer Cytogenetics. Chromosomal and Molecular Genetic Aberrations of Tumor Cells.* Third Edition. New York: Wiley-Blackwell.

Heisterkamp N, Stephenson JR, Groffen J, Hansen PF, de Klein A, Bartram CR, et al. (1983): Localization of the c-abl oncogene adjacent to a translocation break point in chronic myelocytic leukaemia. *Nature* 306:239–242.

Heisterkamp N, Stam K, Groffen J, de Klein A, Grosveld G (1985): Structural organization of the bcr gene and its role in the Ph' translocation. *Nature* 315:758–761.

Ichikawa H, Shimizu K, Hayashi Y, Ohki M (1994): An RNA-binding protein gene, TLS/FUS, is fused to ERG in human myeloid leukemia with t(16;21) chromosomal translocation. *Cancer Res* 54:2865–2868.

Inagaki H, Nagasaka T, Otsuka T, Sugiura E, Nakashima N, Eimoto T (2000): Association of SYT-SSX fusion types with proliferative activity and prognosis in synovial sarcoma. *Mod Pathol* 13:482–488.

Kangaspeska S, Hultsch S, Edgren H, Nicorici D, Murumagi A, Kallioniemi O (2012): Reanalysis of RNA-sequencing data reveals several additional fusion genes with multiple isoforms. *PLoS One* 7: e48745.

Kas K, Voz ML, Roijer E, Astrom AK, Meyen E, Stenman G, et al. (1997): Promoter swapping between the genes for a novel zinc finger protein and beta-catenin in pleiomorphic adenomas with t(3;8)(p21;q12) translocations. *Nat Genet* 15:170–174.

Kato M, Khan S, Gonzalez N, O'Neill BP, McDonald KJ, Cooper BJ, et al. (2003): Hodgkin's lymphoma cell lines express a fusion protein encoded by intergenically spliced mRNA for the multilectin receptor DEC-205 (CD205) and a novel C-type lectin receptor DCL-1. *J Biol Chem* 278:34035–34041.

Kawai A, Woodruff J, Healey JH, Brennan MF, Antonescu CR, Ladanyi M (1998): SYT-SSX gene fusion as a determinant of morphology and prognosis in synovial sarcoma. *N Engl J Med* 338:153–160.

Kawasaki ES, Clark SS, Coyne MY, Smith SD, Champlin R, Witte ON, et al. (1988): Diagnosis of chronic myeloid and acute lymphocytic leukemias by detection of leukemia-specific mRNA sequences amplified in vitro. *Proc Natl Acad Sci USA* 85:5698–5702.

Kim D, Salzberg SL (2011): TopHat-Fusion: An algorithm for discovery of novel fusion transcripts. *Genome Biol* 12: R72.

Klein G (2009): Burkitt lymphoma – a stalking horse for cancer research? *Semin Cancer Biol* 19:347–350.

Kowalski PE, Freeman JD, Mager DL (1999): Intergenic splicing between a HERV-H endogenous retrovirus and two adjacent human genes. *Genomics* 57:371–379.

Krikun G, Mor G, Alvero A, Guller S, Schatz F, Sapi E, et al. (2004): A novel immortalized human endometrial stromal cell line with normal progestational response. *Endocrinology* 145:2291–2296.

Krontiris TG, Cooper GM (1981): Transforming activity of human tumor DNAs. *Proc Natl Acad Sci USA* 78:1181–1184.

Ladanyi M, Antonescu CR, Leung DH, Woodruff JM, Kawai A, Healey JH, et al. (2002): Impact of SYT-SSX fusion type on the clinical behavior of synovial sarcoma: A multi-institutional retrospective study of 243 patients. *Cancer Res* 62:135–140.

Lawson AR, Hindley GF, Forshew T, Tatevossian RG, Jamie GA, Kelly GP, et al. (2011): RAF gene fusion breakpoints in pediatric brain tumors are characterized by significant enrichment of sequence microhomology. *Genome Res* 21:505–514.

Lee MS, Chang KS, Cabanillas F, Freireich EJ, Trujillo JM, Stass SA (1987): Detection of minimal residual cells carrying the t(14;18) by DNA sequence amplification. *Science* 237:175–178.

Lee CH, Ou WB, Marino-Enriquez A, Zhu M, Mayeda M, Wang Y, et al. (2012): 14–3–3 fusion oncogenes in high-grade endometrial stromal sarcoma. *Proc Natl Acad Sci USA* 109:929–934.

Li H, Wang J, Mor G, Sklar J (2008): A neoplastic gene fusion mimics trans-splicing of RNAs in normal human cells. *Science* 321:1357–1361.

Liu X, Wang J, Chen L (2013): Whole-exome sequencing reveals recurrent somatic mutation networks in cancer. *Cancer Lett* 340:270–276.

MacDonald JW, Ghosh D (2006): COPA—cancer outlier profile analysis. *Bioinformatics* 22:2950–2951.

Maher CA, Kumar-Sinha C, Cao X, Kalyana-Sundaram S, Han B, Jing X, et al. (2009a): Transcriptome sequencing to detect gene fusions in cancer. *Nature* 458:97–101.

Maher CA, Palanisamy N, Brenner JC, Cao X, Kalyana-Sundaram S, Luo S, et al. (2009b): Chimeric transcript discovery by paired-end transcriptome sequencing. *Proc Natl Acad Sci USA* 106:12353–12358.

Malbrain ML, Van den Bergh H, Zachee P (1996): Further evidence for the clonal nature of the idiopathic hypereosinophilic syndrome: Complete haematological and cytogenetic remission induced by interferon-alpha in a case with a unique chromosomal abnormality. *Br J Haematol* 92:176–183.

McPherson A, Hormozdiari F, Zayed A, Giuliany R, Ha G, Sun MG, et al. (2011): deFuse: An algorithm for gene fusion discovery in tumor RNA-Seq data. *PLoS Comput Biol* 7: e1001138.

McPherson A, Wu C, Wyatt AW, Shah S, Collins C, Sahinalp SC (2012): nFuse: Discovery of complex genomic rearrangements in cancer using high-throughput sequencing. *Genome Res* 22:2250–2261.

Medves S, Demoulin JB (2012): Tyrosine kinase gene fusions in cancer: Translating mechanisms into targeted therapies. *J Cell Mol Med* 16:237–248.

Meyerson M, Gabriel S, Getz G (2010): Advances in understanding cancer genomes through second-generation sequencing. *Nat Rev Genet* 11:685–696.

Micci F, Thorsen J, Haugom L, Zeller B, Tierens A, Heim S (2011): Translocation t(1;16)(p31;q24) rearranging CBFA2T3 is specific for acute erythroid leukemia. *Leukemia* 25:1510–1512.

Micci F, Thorsen J, Panagopoulos I, Nyquist KB, Zeller B, Tierens A, et al. (2013): High-throughput sequencing identifies an NFIA/CBFA2T3 fusion gene in acute erythroid leukemia with t(1;16)(p31;q24). *Leukemia* 27:980–982.

Michaeli S (2011): Trans-splicing in trypanosomes: Machinery and its impact on the parasite transcriptome. *Future Microbiol* 6:459–474.

Mitelman F, Johansson B, Mertens F (2007): The impact of translocations and gene fusions on cancer causation. *Nat Rev Cancer* 7:233–245.

Mitelman F, Johansson B, Mertens F (2014): Mitelman Database of Chromosome Aberrations and Gene Fusions in Cancer. http://cgap.nci.nih.gov/Chromosomes/Mitelman.

Nacu S, Yuan W, Kan Z, Bhatt D, Rivers CS, Stinson J, et al. (2011): Deep RNA sequencing analysis of readthrough gene fusions in human prostate adenocarcinoma and reference samples. *BMC Med Genomics* 4:11.

Nambiar M, Raghavan SC (2011): How does DNA break during chromosomal translocations? *Nucleic Acids Res* 39:5813–5825.

Nilsson G, Skytting B, Xie Y, Brodin B, Perfekt R, Mandahl N, et al. (1999): The SYT-SSX1 variant of synovial sarcoma is associated with a high rate of tumor cell proliferation and poor clinical outcome. *Cancer Res* 59:3180–3184.

Nyquist KB, Panagopoulos I, Thorsen J, Haugom L, Gorunova L, Bjerkehagen B, et al. (2012): Whole-transcriptome sequencing identifies novel IRF2BP2-CDX1 fusion gene brought about by translocation t(1;5)(q42;q32) in mesenchymal chondrosarcoma. *PLoS One* 7: e49705.

Oliveira AM, Hsi BL, Weremowicz S, Rosenberg AE, Dal Cin P, Joseph N, et al. (2004): USP6 (Tre2) fusion oncogenes in aneurysmal bone cyst. *Cancer Res* 64:1920–1923.

Oliveira AM, Perez-Atayde AR, Dal Cin P, Gebhardt MC, Chen CJ, Neff JR, et al. (2005): Aneurysmal bone cyst variant translocations upregulate USP6 transcription by promoter swapping with the ZNF9, COL1A1, TRAP150, and OMD genes. *Oncogene* 24:3419–3426.

Ozawa T, Brennan CW, Wang L, Squatrito M, Sasayama T, Nakada M, et al. (2010): PDGFRA gene rearrangements are frequent genetic events in PDGFRA-amplified glioblastomas. *Genes Dev* 24:2205–2218.

Panagopoulos I (2010): Absence of the JAZF1/SUZ12 chimeric transcript in the immortalized non-neoplastic endometrial stromal cell line T HESCs. *Oncol Lett* 1:947–950.

Panagopoulos I, Åman P, Fioretos T, Höglund M, Johansson B, Mandahl N, et al. (1994): Fusion of the FUS gene with ERG in acute myeloid leukemia with t(16;21)(p11;q22). *Genes Chromosomes Cancer* 11:256–262.

Panagopoulos I, Höglund M, Mertens F, Mandahl N, Mitelman F, Åman P (1996): Fusion of the EWS and CHOP genes in myxoid liposarcoma. *Oncogene* 12:489–494.

Panagopoulos I, Micci F, Thorsen J, Gorunova L, Eibak AM, Bjerkehagen B Davidson B Heim S (2012): Novel fusion of MYST/Esal-associated factor 6 and PHF1 in endometrial stromal sarcoma. *Plos One* 7:e39354.

Panagopoulos I, Gorunova L, Zeller B, Tierens A, Heim S (2013a): Cryptic FUS-ERG fusion identified by RNA-sequencing in childhood acute myeloid leukemia. *Oncol Rep* 30:2587–2592.

Panagopoulos I, Micci F, Thorsen J, Haugom L, Buechner J, Kerndrup G, et al. (2013b): Fusion of ZMYND8 and RELA genes in acute erythroid leukemia. *PLoS One* 8: e63663.

Panagopoulos I, Thorsen J, Gorunova L, Haugom L, Bjerkehagen B, Davidson B, et al. (2013c): Fusion of the ZC3H7B and BCOR genes in endometrial stromal sarcomas carrying an X;22-translocation. *Genes Chromosomes Cancer* 52:610–618.

Panagopoulos I, Thorsen J, Gorunova L, Micci F, Haugom L, Davidson B, et al. (2013d): RNA sequencing identifies fusion of the EWSR1 and YY1 genes in mesothelioma with t(14;22)(q32;q12). *Genes Chromosomes Cancer* 52:733–740.

Panagopoulos I, Gorunova L, Bjerkehagen B, Heim S (2014a): The "grep" command but not FusionMap, FusionFinder or ChimeraScan captures the CIC-DUX4 fusion gene from whole transcriptome sequencing data on a small round cell tumor with t(4;19)(q35;q13). *Plos One* 9: e99439.

Panagopoulos I, Torkildsen S, Gorunova L, Tierens A, Tjønnfjord GE, Heim S (2014b): Comparison between karyotyping-FISH-reverse transcription PCR and RNA-sequencing-fusion gene identification programs in the detection of KAT6A-CREBBP in acute myeloid leukemia. *Plos One* 9: e96570.

Parker M, Mohankumar KM, Punchihewa C, Weinlich R, Dalton JD, Li Y, et al. (2014): C11orf95-RELA fusions drive oncogenic NF-kappaB signalling in ependymoma. *Nature* 506:451–455.

Parra G, Reymond A, Dabbouseh N, Dermitzakis ET, Castelo R, Thomson TM, et al. (2006): Tandem chimerism as a means to increase protein complexity in the human genome. *Genome Res* 16:37–44.

Pérot G, Soubeyran I, Ribeiro A, Bonhomme B, Savagner F, Boutet-Bouzamondo N, et al. (2014): Identification of a recurrent STRN/ALK fusion in thyroid carcinomas. *PLoS One* 9: e87170.

Persson F, Winnes M, Andren Y, Wedell B, Dahlenfors R, Asp J, et al. (2008): High-resolution array CGH analysis of salivary gland tumors reveals fusion and amplification of the FGFR1 and PLAG1 genes in ring chromosomes. *Oncogene* 27:3072–3080.

Pinkel D, Straume T, Gray JW (1986): Cytogenetic analysis using quantitative, high-sensitivity, fluorescence hybridization. *Proc Natl Acad Sci USA* 83:2934–2938.

Pradet-Balade B, Medema JP, Lopez-Fraga M, Lozano JC, Kolfschoten GM, Picard A, et al. (2002): An endogenous hybrid mRNA encodes TWE-PRIL, a functional cell surface TWEAK-APRIL fusion protein. *EMBO J* 21:5711–5720.

Prakash T, Sharma VK, Adati N, Ozawa R, Kumar N, Nishida Y, et al. (2010): Expression of conjoined genes: Another mechanism for gene regulation in eukaryotes. *PLoS One* 5: e13284.

Quail MA, Kozarewa I, Smith F, Scally A, Stephens PJ, Durbin R, et al. (2008): A large genome center's improvements to the Illumina sequencing system. *Nat Methods* 5:1005–1010.

Raghavan SC, Kirsch IR, Lieber MR (2001): Analysis of the V(D)J recombination efficiency at lymphoid chromosomal translocation breakpoints. *J Biol Chem* 276:29126–29133.

Rhodes DR, Yu J, Shanker K, Deshpande N, Varambally R, Ghosh D, et al. (2004): ONCOMINE: A cancer microarray database and integrated data-mining platform. *Neoplasia* 6:1–6.

Rickman DS, Pflueger D, Moss B, VanDoren VE, Chen CX, de la Taille A, et al. (2009): SLC45A3-ELK4 is a novel and frequent erythroblast transformation-specific fusion transcript in prostate cancer. *Cancer Res* 69:2734–2738.

Rikova K, Guo A, Zeng Q, Possemato A, Yu J, Haack H, et al. (2007): Global survey of phosphotyrosine signaling identifies oncogenic kinases in lung cancer. *Cell* 131: 1190–1203.

Robbiani DF, Bothmer A, Callen E, Reina-San-Martin B, Dorsett Y, Difilippantonio S, et al. (2008): AID is required for the chromosomal breaks in c-myc that lead to c-myc/IgH translocations. *Cell* 135:1028–1038.

Ruan Y, Ooi HS, Choo SW, Chiu KP, Zhao XD, Srinivasan KG, et al. (2007): Fusion transcripts and transcribed retrotransposed loci discovered through comprehensive transcriptome analysis using Paired-End diTags (PETs). *Genome Res* 17:828–838.

Saiki RK, Scharf S, Faloona F, Mullis KB, Horn GT, Erlich HA, et al. (1985): Enzymatic amplification of beta-globin genomic sequences and restriction site analysis for diagnosis of sickle cell anemia. *Science* 230:1350–1354.

Sboner A, Habegger L, Pflueger D, Terry S, Chen DZ, Rozowsky JS, et al. (2010): FusionSeq: A modular framework for finding gene fusions by analyzing paired-end RNA-sequencing data. *Genome Biol* 11:R104.

Schaller JL, Burkland GA (2001) Case report: Rapid and complete control of idiopathic hypereosinophilia with imatinib mesylate. *MedGenMed* 3:9.

Shtivelman E, Lifshitz B, Gale RP, Canaani E (1985): Fused transcript of abl and bcr genes in chronic myelogenous leukaemia. *Nature* 315:550–554.

Shugay M, Ortiz de Mendibil I, Vizmanos JL, Novo FJ (2013): Oncofuse: a computational framework for the prediction of the oncogenic potential of gene fusions. *Bioinformatics* 29:2539–2546.

Singh D, Chan JM, Zoppoli P, Niola F, Sullivan R, Castano A, et al. (2012): Transforming fusions of FGFR and TACC genes in human glioblastoma. *Science* 337:1231–1235.

Soda M, Choi YL, Enomoto M, Takada S, Yamashita Y, Ishikawa S, et al. (2007): Identification of the transforming EML4-ALK fusion gene in non-small-cell lung cancer. *Nature* 448:561–566.

Sorensen PH, Triche TJ (1996): Gene fusions encoding chimaeric transcription factors in solid tumours. *Semin Cancer Biol* 7:3–14.

Sorensen PH, Lynch JC, Qualman SJ, Tirabosco R, Lim JF, Maurer HM, et al. (2002): PAX3-FKHR and PAX7-FKHR gene fusions are prognostic indicators in alveolar rhabdomyosarcoma: A report from the children's oncology group. *J Clin Oncol* 20:2672–2679.

Storlazzi CT, Albano F, Lo Cunsolo C, Doglioni C, Guastadisegni MC, Impera L, et al. (2007): Upregulation of the SOX5 by promoter swapping with the P2RY8 gene in primary splenic follicular lymphoma. *Leukemia* 21:2221–2225.

Such E, Cervera J, Valencia A, Barragan E, Ibanez M, Luna I, et al. (2011): A novel NUP98/RARG gene fusion in acute myeloid leukemia resembling acute promyelocytic leukemia. *Blood* 117:242–245.

Suehara Y, Arcila M, Wang L, Hasanovic A, Ang D, Ito T, et al. (2012): Identification of KIF5B-RET and GOPC-ROS1 fusions in lung adenocarcinomas through a comprehensive mRNA-based screen for tyrosine kinase fusions. *Clin Cancer Res* 18:6599–6608.

Takahashi M, Ritz J, Cooper GM (1985): Activation of a novel human transforming gene, ret, by DNA rearrangement. *Cell* 42:581–588.

Tanas MR, Sboner A, Oliveira AM, Erickson-Johnson MR, Hespelt J, Hanwright PJ, et al. (2011): Identification of a disease-defining gene fusion in epithelioid hemangioendothelioma. *Sci Transl Med* 3:98ra82.

Taylor BS, Ladanyi M (2011): Clinical cancer genomics: How soon is now? *J Pathol* 223:318–326.

Teixeira MR, Heim S (2011): Cytogenetic analysis of tumor clonality. *Adv Cancer Res* 112:127–149.

Thomson TM, Lozano JJ, Loukili N, Carrio R, Serras F, Cormand B, et al. (2000): Fusion of the human gene for the polyubiquitination coeffector UEV1 with Kua, a newly identified gene. *Genome Res* 10:1743–1756.

Tomlins SA, Rhodes DR, Perner S, Dhanasekaran SM, Mehra R, Sun XW, et al. (2005): Recurrent fusion of TMPRSS2 and ETS transcription factor genes in prostate cancer. *Science* 310:644–648.

Totoki Y, Tatsuno K, Yamamoto S, Arai Y, Hosoda F, Ishikawa S, et al. (2011): High-resolution characterization of a hepatocellular carcinoma genome. *Nat Genet* 43:464–469.

Trumper L, Pfreundschuh M, Bonin FV, Daus H (1998): Detection of the t(2;5)-associated NPM/ALK fusion cDNA in peripheral blood cells of healthy individuals. *Br J Haematol* 103:1138–1144.

Van Dyck F, Declercq J, Braem CV, Van de Ven WJ (2007): PLAG1, the prototype of the PLAG gene family: Versatility in tumour development (review). *Int J Oncol* 30:765–774.

Villarreal DD, Lee K, Deem A, Shim EY, Malkova A, Lee SE (2012): Microhomology directs diverse DNA break repair pathways and chromosomal translocations. *PLoS Genet* 8:e1003026.

Vogelstein B, Papadopoulos N, Velculescu VE, Zhou S, Diaz LA, Jr., Kinzler KW (2013): Cancer genome landscapes. *Science* 339:1546–1558.

Wachtel M, Dettling M, Koscielniak E, Stegmaier S, Treuner J, Simon-Klingenstein K, et al. (2004): Gene expression signatures identify rhabdomyosarcoma subtypes and detect a novel t(2;2)(q35;p23) translocation fusing PAX3 to NCOA1. *Cancer Res* 64:5539–5545.

Walther C, Tayebwa J, Lilljebjörn H, Magnusson L, Nilsson J, Vult von Steyern F, et al. (2014): A novel SERPINE1-FOSB fusion gene results in transcriptional up-regulation of FOSB in pseudomyogenic haemangioendothelioma. *J Pathol* 232:534–540

Wang L, Motoi T, Khanin R, Olshen A, Mertens F, Bridge J, et al. (2012): Identification of a novel, recurrent HEY1-NCOA2 fusion in mesenchymal chondrosarcoma based on a genome-wide screen of exon-level expression data. *Genes Chromosomes Cancer* 51:127–139.

Wang Q, Xia J, Jia P, Pao W, Zhao Z (2013): Application of next generation sequencing to human gene fusion detection: computational tools, features and perspectives. *Brief Bioinform* 14:506–519.

Welch JS, Westervelt P, Ding L, Larson DE, Klco JM, Kulkarni S, et al. (2011): Use of whole-genome sequencing to diagnose a cryptic fusion oncogene. *JAMA* 305:1577–1584.

Williams SV, Hurst CD, Knowles MA (2013): Oncogenic FGFR3 gene fusions in bladder cancer. *Hum Mol Genet* 22:795–803.

Wu CC, Kannan K, Lin S, Yen L, Milosavljevic A (2013): Identification of cancer fusion drivers using network fusion centrality. *Bioinformatics* 29:1174–1181.

Xia SJ, Barr FG (2005): Chromosome translocations in sarcomas and the emergence of oncogenic transcription factors. *Eur J Cancer* 41:2513–2527.

Zhang Y, Gong M, Yuan H, Park HG, Frierson HF, Li H (2012): Chimeric transcript generated by cis-splicing of adjacent genes regulates prostate cancer cell proliferation. *Cancer Discov* 2:598–607.

Zhou GB, Zhang J, Wang ZY, Chen SJ, Chen Z (2007): Treatment of acute promyelocytic leukaemia with all-trans retinoic acid and arsenic trioxide: a paradigm of synergistic molecular targeting therapy. *Philos Trans R Soc Lond B Biol Sci* 362:959–971.

Zucman-Rossi J, Legoix P, Victor JM, Lopez B, Thomas G (1998): Chromosome translocation based on illegitimate recombination in human tumors. *Proc Natl Acad Sci USA* 95:11786–11791.

CHAPTER 6

Acute myeloid leukemia

Bertil Johansson[1] and Christine J. Harrison[2]

[1]Department of Clinical Genetics, University of Lund, Lund, Sweden
[2]Leukaemia Research Cytogenetics Group, Northern Institute for Cancer Research, Newcastle University, Newcastle upon Tyne, UK

Acute leukemia is a worldwide disease with an incidence of approximately 4/100 000 per year; 70% of the cases are acute myeloid leukemia (AML). Although acute lymphoblastic leukemia (ALL) predominates in childhood, AML is by far the most common type among adults. The incidence rises steeply after the age of 50 years with a median age of roughly 70 years (Juliusson et al., 2012). Men are slightly more often affected than women, and a male preponderance (55%) is also apparent in published AML with an aberrant karyotype. However, the median age of cytogenetically abnormal cases reported in the literature is only 45 years (Mitelman et al., 2014). Thus, there is definitely an age bias of the cytogenetic data on AML, with a clear under-reporting of karyotyped cases in elderly patients.

The salient pathologic feature of AML is the excessive accumulation of immature myeloid blasts in the bone marrow (BM). This maturation arrest, a characteristic of acute leukemias, prevents normal hematopoiesis and leads, directly or indirectly, to a lack of differentiated granulocytes (neutrophils, eosinophils, and basophils), monocytes, thrombocytes, and erythrocytes. Over the years, several attempts have been made to classify AML into entities that are reproducible, that contribute to a more profound understanding of the disease biology, and that are of prognostic and therapeutic importance. A major initiative and a step forward in this respect was taken by the cooperative French–American–British (FAB) study group who, in the mid-1970s, proposed a classification in which ALL and AML were separated and subdivided into three and six groups, respectively (Bennett et al., 1976). Initially, the FAB classification relied almost exclusively on morphologic criteria, but subsequent revisions also included information gained from other investigations, mainly cytochemical and immunophenotypic analyses (Bennett et al., 1985a, 1985b, 1991). Ultimately, the FAB classification recognized the following subgroups: minimally differentiated AML, AML without maturation, AML with maturation, acute promyelocytic leukemia (APL), acute myelomonocytic leukemia (including the subtype with BM eosinophilia), acute monoblastic and monocytic leukemia, acute erythroleukemia, and acute megakaryoblastic leukemia (AMKL).

Although the FAB classification was of utmost importance in bringing order out of "nosologic chaos," it has essentially been superseded by the World Health Organization (WHO) Classification of Tumours of the Haematopoietic and Lymphoid Tissues. The underlying principle is the incorporation of all available information—morphologic, cytochemical, immunophenotypic, genetic, and clinical features—into an effort to define subgroups that are

Cancer Cytogenetics: Chromosomal and Molecular Genetic Aberrations of Tumor Cells, Fourth Edition.
Edited by Sverre Heim and Felix Mitelman.
© 2015 John Wiley & Sons, Ltd. Published 2015 by John Wiley & Sons, Ltd.

Table 6.1 WHO classification of acute myeloid leukemia and related precursor neoplasms

*Acute myeloid leukemia (AML) with recurrent genetic abnormalities**
AML with t(8;21)(q22;q22) [*RUNX1–RUNX1T1*]
AML with inv(16)(p13q22)
or t(16;16)(p13;q22) [*CBFB–MYH11*]
APL with t(15;17)(q22;q21) [*PML–RARA*]
AML with t(9;11)(p21;q23) [*MLL–MLLT3*]
AML with t(6;9)(p22;q34) [*DEK–NUP214*]
AML with inv(3)(q21q26)
or t(3;3)(q21;q26) [*RPN1–MECOM*]
Acute megakaryoblastic leukemia with t(1;22) (p13;q13) [*RBM15–MKL1*]
AML with mutated *NPM1* (provisional entity)
AML with mutated *CEBPA* (provisional entity)
AML with myelodysplasia-related changes
Therapy-related myeloid neoplasms
AML, not otherwise specified
AML with minimal differentiation
AML without maturation
AML with maturation
Acute myelomonocytic leukemia
Acute monoblastic and monocytic leukemia
Acute erythroid leukemia
Erythroleukemia (erythroid/myeloid)
Pure erythroid leukemia
Acute megakaryoblastic leukemia
Acute basophilic leukemia
Acute panmyelosis with myelofibrosis
Myeloid sarcoma
Myeloid proliferations related to Down syndrome
Transient abnormal myelopoiesis
Myeloid leukemia associated with Down syndrome
Blastic plasmacytoid dendritic cell neoplasm

*Some gene names/breakpoints are different from the ones given in the WHO classification because of changes in gene nomenclature/localization.

Table 6.2 Frequencies of abnormal karyotypes in pediatric and adult AML

Pediatric AML		Adult AML	
Frequency (%)	References	Frequency (%)	References
75	Harrison et al. (2010)	48	Büchner et al. (2009)
76	Imamura et al. (2012)	51	Haferlach et al. (2012a)
76	Sandahl et al. 2014b	52	Röllig et al. (2011)
77	Rubnitz et al. (2010)	55	Yang et al. (2012)
78	Gibson et al. (2011)	58	Cheng et al. (2009b)
78	Tsukimoto et al. (2009)	59	Grimwade et al. (2010)
78	von Neuhoff et al. (2010)	59	Medeiros et al. (2010b)

such as age, previous treatment/genotoxic exposure, gender, geographic/ethnic origin, and constitutional genetics, as exemplified in the following.

Impact of age

Numerous studies have shown that pediatric AMLs are more often karyotypically abnormal than adult AML. In general, clonal changes are found in 75–80% of childhood cases, whereas the corresponding frequency in adult AML is 50–60% (Table 6.2).

Approximately 55 and 45% of cytogenetically abnormal AML cases in children and adults, respectively, are pseudodiploid (Mitelman et al., 2014). Hypodiploidy is more common in adult AML (~25%) than in pediatric AML (~15%), whereas hyperdiploidy is slightly more frequent in childhood AML (30% vs. ~25%).

Several chromosomal changes/karyotypic patterns are more common in pediatric than in adult AML and vice versa (Table 6.3). For example, t(1;22) (p13;q13), t(7;12)(q36p13), and t(X;6)(p11;q23) are almost exclusively seen in infant AML; t(5;11) (q35;p15), t(5;17)(q35;q21), t(6;9)(p22;q34), and t(7;11)(p15;p15) mainly occur in AML in children/ adolescents/younger adults; whereas t(1;3)(p36;q21), der(1;7)(q10;p10), t(4;12)(q12;p13), and monosomal karyotypes (MK) are primarily seen in AML in middle-aged or elderly patients. The reasons for

biologically homogeneous and have clinical relevance (Vardiman et al., 2009). At present (Swerdlow et al., 2008), seven subgroups are recognized, some of which comprise several entities (Table 6.1).

Most AML harbor clonal chromosomal abnormalities

Chromosome banding analyses reveal acquired, clonal chromosomal abnormalities in the majority of AML cases, with the frequencies and types of aberrations to some extent being influenced by factors

Table 6.3 Cytogenetic, molecular genetic, and clinical features of AML-associated chromosomal aberrations

Aberrations	Molecular genetic features	Gender	Median age	Characteristic features	Prognosis
t(1;3)(p36;q21)	PRDM16 deregulation	F = M	60	Dysmegakaryocytopoiesis, prior MDS	Poor
t(1;21)(p36;q22)	PRDM16 deregulation	F = M	60	t-AML	Poor
t(1;16)(p31;q24)	NFIA–CBFA2T3	M > F	1	Erythroleukemia	Poor
t(1;11)(p32;q23)	MLL–EPS15	F = M	7	De novo, myelomonocytic/ monoblastic/monocytic	Unclear
t(1;22)(p13;q13)	RBM15–MKL1	F > M	<1	AMKL, not Down syndrome	Intermediate
der(1;7)(q10;p10)		M > F	60	t-AML, prior MDS	Poor
t(1;11)(q21;q23)	MLL–MLLT11	F = M	2	De novo, myelomonocytic/ monoblastic/monocytic	Favorable
t(2;3) (p21~23;q26)	MECOM deregulation	F = M	55	De novo AML, dysmegakaryocytopoiesis	Poor
t(2;11)(p21;q23)	MLL rearrangement	M > F	60	Multilineage dysplasia, prior MDS	Unclear
t(2;11)(q31;p15)	NUP98–HOXD11(13)	F = M	30	De novo, myelomonocytic	Unclear
t(2;11)(q37;q23)	MLL–SEPT2	F = M	60	t-AML	Poor
inv(3)(q21q26)	MECOM deregulation	F = M	50	Dysmegakaryocytopoiesis, fibrosis, prior MDS	Poor
t(3;5)(q25;q35)	NPM1–MLF1	M > F	30	Dysmegakaryocytopoiesis, prior MDS	Intermediate
t(3;12)(q26;p13)	MECOM deregulation	F = M	50	Dysmegakaryocytopoiesis, prior MDS	Poor
t(3;21)(q26;q22)	MECOM deregulation	F = M	60	t-AML, multilineage dysplasia, prior MDS	Poor
+4 sole		F > M	55	De novo, minimal differentiation/ without maturation	Intermediate/ poor
t(4;12)(q12;p13)	CHIC2–ETV6	M > F	60	Minimal differentiation/without maturation, dysplasia	Poor
t(4;11)(q21;q23)	MLL–AFF1	F > M	<1	Myelomonocytic/monoblastic/ monocytic	Poor
–5/del(5q)		F = M	60–65	t-AML, dysplasia, prior MDS	Poor
t(5;11)(q31;q23)	MLL–ARHGAP26	M > F	<1	De novo, myelomonocytic/ monoblastic/monocytic	Unclear
t(5;11)(q35;p15)	NUP98–NSD1	M > F	<15	De novo, myelomonocytic/ monoblastic/monocytic	Poor
t(5;17)(q35;q21)	NPM1–RARA	F = M	<15	Atypical APL, no Auer rods	Favorable
t(6;9)(p22;q34)	DEK–NUP214	F = M	30	De novo AML with maturation, dysplasia, Auer rods	Poor
t(6;11)(q27;q23)	MLL–MLLT4	F = M	40	De novo, myelomonocytic/ monoblastic/monocytic	Poor
–7/del(7q)		M > F	45–55	t-AML, variable morphology	Poor
t(7;21)(p22;q22)	RUNX1–USP42	M > F	35	Myelomonocytic/monoblastic/ monocytic	Unclear
t(7;11)(p15;p15)	NUP98–HOXA9(11,13)	F > M	35	De novo AML with maturation, dysplasia, Auer rods	Poor
t(7;12)(q36;p13)	MNX1 deregulation	F = M	<1	Minimal differentiation/without maturation	Poor
+8 sole		F = M	50	De novo, variable morphology	Intermediate/ poor
inv(8)(p11q13)	KAT6A–NCOA2	F > M	15	Monoblastic, erythrophagocytosis	Poor
t(8;16)(p11;p13)	KAT6A–CREBBP	F > M	45	t-AML, monoblastic, erythrophagocytosis	Poor
t(8;22)(p11;q13)	KAT6A–EP300	M > F	35	De novo, monoblastic, erythrophagocytosis	Poor

Table 6.3 (Continued)

Aberrations	Molecular genetic features	Gender	Median age	Characteristic features	Prognosis
t(8;21)(q22;q22)	RUNX1–RUNX1T1	M > F	30	De novo AML with maturation, dysplasia, Auer rods	Favorable
t(9;11)(p22;p15)	NUP98–PSIP1	F > M	50	De novo AML with maturation	Poor
t(9;11)(p21;q23)	MLL–MLLT3	F = M	20	t-AML, monoblastic/monocytic	Intermediate
del(9q) sole		M > F	45	De novo AML with maturation, dysplasia, Auer rods	Intermediate
t(9;22)(q34;q11)	BCR–ABL1	M > F	40	De novo AML with/without maturation	Poor
+10 sole		M > F	50	De novo, minimal differentiation/ without maturation	Intermediate/ poor
t(10;11)(p12;q14)	PICALM–MLLT10	F = M	20	De novo, minimal differentiation/ without maturation	Intermediate/ poor
10p12/11q23 rear.	MLL–MLLT10	M > F	2	De novo, monoblastic	Poor
t(10;11)(q21;q23)	MLL–TET1	F = M	40	De novo, myelomonocytic/ monoblastic/monocytic	Poor
t(10;16)(q22;p13)	KAT6B–CREBBP	F > M	30	Myelomonocytic/monoblastic/ monocytic	Poor
+11 sole		F = M	60	De novo AML with/without maturation, Auer rods	Poor
inv(11)(p15q22)	NUP98–DDX10	M > F	40	t-AML, variable morphology	Unclear
t(11;12)(p15;p13)	NUP98–KDM5A	F = M	2	AMKL, not Down syndrome	Poor
t(11;12)(p15;q13)	NUP98–HOXC11(C13)	F > M	40	De novo AML with maturation	Poor
t(11;20)(p15;q12)	NUP98–TOP1	F > M	25	AML with maturation, t-AML	Poor
11q gain	MLL amplification	M > F	>60	Minimal differentiation or with/ without maturation	Poor
t(11;16)(q23;p13)	MLL–CREBBP	F = M	40	t-AML, myelomonocytic/monoblastic/ monocytic	Poor
t(11;17)(q23;q12)	MLL–MLLT6	F = M	15	De novo, myelomonocytic/ monoblastic/monocytic	Poor
t(11;17)(q23;q21)	ZBTB1–RARA	M > F	55	Atypical APL, Pelger–Huët-like cells, coagulopathy	Intermediate/ poor
t(11;17)(q23;q25)	MLL–SEPT9	M > F	25	Myelomonocytic/monoblastic/ monocytic	Poor
t(11;19) (q23;p13.1)	MLL–ELL	F = M	50	t-AML, myelomonocytic/monoblastic/ monocytic	Poor
t(11;19) (q23;p13.3)	MLL–MLLT1	F = M	7	t-AML, myelomonocytic/monoblastic/ monocytic	Poor
t(11;22)(q23;q11)	MLL–SEPT5	F = M	30	De novo, myelomonocytic	Unclear
del(12p)		F = M	50	Variable morphology, t-AML	Intermediate/ poor
t(12;22)(p13;q12)	MN1–ETV6	F = M	50	Variable morphology, often unclassified	Poor
+13 sole		M > F	65	De novo AML with minimal differentiation, dysplasia	Poor
t(15;17)(q22;q21)	PML–RARA	F = M	40	APL, Auer rods, coagulopathy	Favorable
inv(16)(p13q22)	CBFB–MYH11	M > F	40	Myelomonocytic, eosinophilia	Favorable
inv(16)(p13q24)	CBFA2T3–GLIS2	F > M	1	AMKL, not Down syndrome	Intermediate/ poor

(Continued)

Table 6.3 (Continued)

Aberrations	Molecular genetic features	Gender	Median age	Characteristic features	Prognosis
t(16;21)(p11;q22)	FUS–ERG	M > F	25	AML with/without maturation, erythrophagocytosis	Poor
t(16;21)(q24;q22)	RUNX1–CBFA2T3	F > M	40	t-AML, with maturation	Poor
del(17p)	TP53	M > F	60	Dysgranulocytopoiesis, Pelger–Huët anomaly	Poor
i(17q) sole		M > F	>65	Dysgranulocytopoiesis, dysmegakaryocytopoiesis	Poor
del(20q) sole		M > F	>60	De novo AML, variable morphology	Intermediate/poor
+21 sole		M > F	35	De novo AML, variable morphology	Intermediate/poor
+22 sole		M > F	30	De novo AML, variable morphology	Intermediate
t(X;6)(p11;q23)	MYB–GATA1	M > F	<1	Acute basophilic leukemia, hyperhistaminemia	Unclear
Xq24/11q23 rear.	MLL–SEPT6	F = M	<1	De novo AML with maturation, myelomonocytic	Unclear
–Y sole		M only	60	Variable morphology, Auer rods	Intermediate

this age-related frequency variation are unknown, but most likely, differences in exposures to "leukemogenic factors" underlie some of the variability.

Impact of previous treatment/genotoxic exposure

That prior treatment with chemo- and/or radiotherapy influences the karyotypic features seen in the ensuing therapy-related AML (t-AML) has been known since the late 1970s. In the WHO classification, two main t-AML types are recognized (Vardiman et al., 2008), one following exposure to alkylating agents and/or ionizing radiation and one after treatment with DNA topoisomerase II inhibitors; these differ clinically as well as genetically. Briefly, previous treatment with alkylators is strongly associated with t-AML occurring 5–10 years after the exposure, often with a prior myelodysplastic syndrome (MDS) and signs of BM failure with cytopenia. These t-AML cases are usually cytogenetically complex and hypodiploid, primarily harboring genomically unbalanced anomalies such as deletions of 5q, 7q, and 17p. In contrast, t-AML arising after treatment with drugs targeting DNA topoisomerase II develops 1–5 years after exposure, usually without an antecedent MDS. These t-AML cases are cytogenetically characterized by balanced translocations that frequently involve MLL at 11q23, NUP98 at 11p15, RARA at 17q21 or RUNX1 at 21q22 (Mauritzson et al., 2002; Pedersen-Bjergaard et al., 2008; Joannides and Grimwade, 2010; Churpek and Larson, 2013). It should, however, be emphasized that this dichotomy between alkylator- and DNA topoisomerase-related t-AML is a simplification, not least considering that many patients have received a combination of such agents.

Other therapeutic agents have also been linked to certain chromosomal changes. For example, AML following granulocyte colony-stimulating factor treatment of pediatric patients with aplastic anemia or Kostmann syndrome (severe congenital granulocytopenia) and AML occurring after immunosuppressive therapy with azathioprine have been associated with monosomy 7 (Freedman and Alter, 2002; Kwong, 2010).

Surprisingly little is known about the impact of prior occupational, environmental, or lifestyle exposures on AML-associated karyotypic features, although this important question has been addressed in numerous studies. In the early 1980s, it was suggested that AML occurring in individuals occupationally exposed to potential mutagenic/carcinogenic agents were more often karyotypically abnormal, frequently showing whole or partial losses of chromosomes 5 and 7 (Mitelman et al., 1981). However, this correlation has, with a few exceptions, not been confirmed in later studies (Crane et al., 1996; Albin et al., 2000). Similarly, even though significant associations between certain types of exposure and chromosomal abnormalities have been reported, such as smoking and −5, del(5q), −7, del(7q), +8, t(8;21)(q22;q22), and inv(16)(p13q22); alcohol and −5, del(5q), −7, and del(7q); paints and t(8;21)(q22;q22); pesticides and herbicides and −5 and del(5q); and organic solvents and +8 (Sandler et al., 1993; Crane et al., 1996; Davico et al., 1998; Albin et al., 2000; Moorman et al., 2002; Björk et al., 2009; Irons et al., 2013), these associations have often been inconclusive, with imprecise estimates and rarely verified in subsequent independent patient cohorts. Thus, caution is definitely required before concluding that a particular environmental exposure is the cause of an AML with a certain chromosomal change.

Impact of gender

Several AML-associated abnormalities display an unequal sex distribution (Table 6.3). For example, t(1;22)(p13;q13), t(4;11)(q21;q23), t(8;16)(p11;p13), and t(16;21)(q24;q22) are more common in AML in females, whereas the opposite is true for der(1;7)(q10;p10), t(5;11)(q31;q23), t(11;17)(q23;q21), and +13. Whether such gender-related differences in frequency reflect constitutional heterogeneity or different iatrogenic/environmental exposure is unknown.

Impact of geographic/ethnic origin

Mitelman and Levan (1978) were the first to describe differences in the incidence of chromosomal aberrations in hematologic malignancies diagnosed in different parts of the world. In a later review by Johansson et al. (1991), who ascertained close to 1500 AML cases, a significant frequency variation was identified for −5, del(5q), +8, t(8;21)(q22;q22), and t(15;17)(q22;q21) among patients from Asia, Europe, and the USA. Although some of the observed differences were most likely fortuitous, the overall findings strongly suggested heterogeneity in geographic frequency of AML-associated abnormalities. Since then, a few translocations have been shown to be particularly common in some geographic/ethnic groups, such as t(7;11)(p15;p15) in patients from Asia (Wei et al., 2013)

and t(6;11)(q27;q23) in African Americans in the USA (Blum et al., 2004).

Impact of constitutional genetics

Some constitutional genetic abnormalities not only increase the risk of AML but also influence the type and frequency of acquired aberrations seen in the leukemic cells. For example, children with Down syndrome (DS) have a pronounced risk of developing AML, in particular AMKL (Hasle, 2001). The genetic features of myeloid leukemia associated with DS differ from those seen in non-DS-AML: *GATA1* mutations, dup(1q), del(6q), del(7p), dup(7q), +8, +11, del(16q), and acquired +21 are significantly more common in DS-AML, whereas t(1;22)(p13;q13), t(8;21)(q22;q22), 11q23 rearrangements, t(15;17)(q22;q21), and inv(16)(p13q22) are much more frequent in non-DS-AML (Forestier et al., 2008; Khan et al., 2011; Blink et al., 2014). Thus, DS-AML is clearly a distinct entity, as also recognized by the present WHO classification (Table 6.1).

Certain Mendelian disorders are also known to increase the risk of AML with characteristic chromosomal abnormalities. For example, AML in patients with the autosomal recessive chromosome breakage syndrome Fanconi anemia often harbors gains of 1q, 3q, and 11q, monosomy 7 or del(7q), del(11q), del(20q), and *RUNX1* abnormalities (Mehta et al., 2010; Quentin et al., 2011; Rochowski et al., 2012). Monosomy 7 is also common in AML occurring in other inherited conditions predisposing to leukemia, such as "familial platelet disorder with propensity to acute myelogenous leukemia" and neurofibromatosis type 1 (Shannon et al., 1992; Minelli et al., 2004).

Characteristic chromosomal abnormalities in AML

The cytogenetic, molecular genetic, and clinical features of AML-associated numerical and structural abnormalities, reported in a sufficient number to allow comments on clinicogenetic associations, are summarized in the following in order of chromosome number; aberrations involving the same chromosome are listed from pter to qter. For each anomaly, the Mitelman Database of Chromosome Aberrations and Gene Fusions in Cancer (Mitelman et al., 2014) has been searched to identify the number of cases reported, the frequency and type of secondary changes, age and sex distribution, and morphologic subtypes. For the sake of brevity, this database is not referred to in the following. As the Mitelman database contains all cytogenetic references to the various abnormalities, and in order to minimize the number of references in the text, only the most pertinent studies, mainly initial reports and larger series, are referred to.

Throughout, we have emphasized the cytogenetic features and the clinical implications of the aberrations, whereas the descriptions of the molecular genetic/biologic consequences of the changes are only briefly mentioned, partly because they lie outside the main scope of this book and partly because the lifetime of such data is quite short. However, the genes rearranged as a result of an abnormality are always mentioned to allow more information to be retrieved from various databases on the Internet. The molecular genetic findings as well as some pertinent clinical and prognostic features associated with the various abnormalities are also briefly summarized in Table 6.3.

t(1;3)(p36;q21) [RPN1–PRDM16]

Approximately 50 AML cases with t(1;3) (Figure 6.1) have been reported, with the translocation being the sole chromosomal aberration in two-thirds of cases. The most frequent additional change is del(5q), found in 15%.

The t(1;3) results in transcriptional upregulation of the PRDM16 gene through promoter swapping with the housekeeping gene RPN1. Thus,

overexpression of PRDM16 is the functionally important outcome of the translocation, as in other 1p36/PRDM16 rearrangements (Mochizuki et al., 2000; Duhoux et al., 2012).

The t(1;3) is equally common in females and males and mainly occurs in adults; the median age among published cases is 60 years. The majority of t(1;3)-positive myeloid malignancies are AML, but many, including those in the first published series (Moir et al., 1984), are diagnosed during an often short MDS phase characterized by trilineage dysplasia, in particular dyserythropoiesis and dysmegakaryocytopoiesis (Secker-Walker et al., 1995). Welborn et al. (1987) described patients with t(1;3)-positive AML/MDS as typically middle-aged and severely anemic, with macrocytosis and a relatively high platelet count; thrombocytosis was, however, not confirmed in a recent large series of t(1;3)-positive myeloid malignancies (Duhoux et al., 2012). The dysmegakaryocytopoietic features and the involvement of 3q21 led to the suggestion that the t(1;3) is a variant of inv(3)(q21q26)/t(3;3)(q21;q26), and indeed, it is now known that also the molecular genetic consequences of t(1;3) and inv(3)/t(3;3) are similar, with the promoter of RPN1 driving the expression of the structurally and functionally related PRDM16 and MECOM genes, respectively.

Prior genotoxic exposure has been reported in 15–20% of t(1;3)-positive AML, but in contrast to most other balanced translocations in t-AML, the t(1;3) is not strongly associated with topoisomerase II inhibitors but rather with irradiation and alkylating agents (Welborn et al., 1987; Block et al., 2002; Charrin et al., 2002; Mauritzson et al., 2002). A dismal outcome of t(1;3)-positive AML, with most cases being virtually nonresponsive to conventional chemotherapy, has been emphasized (Lugthart et al., 2010; Duhoux et al., 2012).

t(1;21)(p36;q22) [RUNX1–PRDM16]

The t(1;21) rearranges the RUNX1 and PRDM16 genes, leading to deregulated PRDM16 expression, akin to the aforementioned t(1;3)(p36;q21) (Roulston et al., 1998; Sakai et al., 2005; Duhoux et al., 2012).

Only a few AML cases with t(1;21) have been reported, but some characteristic clinical features of t(1;21)-positive AML have nevertheless emerged (Roulston et al., 1998; Hromas et al., 2000; Stevens-Kroef et al., 2006): most cases are t-AML, often

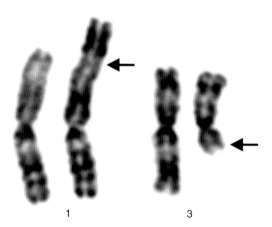

1   3

Figure 6.1 The t(1;3)(p36;q21) is strongly associated with dysmegakaryocytopoiesis. Arrows indicate breakpoints.

after previous exposure to irradiation, including a nuclear explosion (sic) and/or topoisomerase II inhibitors. The outcome is dismal.

t(1;16)(p31;q24) [*NFIA–CBFA2T3*]

The t(1;16), which results in an *NFIA–CBFA2T3* fusion, has so far only been described in a handful of AML cases (Micci et al., 2013). However, all patients reported to date have been young boys with erythroleukemia and with a poor outcome.

t(1;11)(p32;q23) [*MLL–EPS15*]

This translocation, leading to an *MLL–EPS15* chimera (Bernard et al., 1994), has been reported in approximately 10 AML cases. It is most often the sole abnormality, but monosomy 7 and trisomy 8 are recurrent secondary changes. There is no gender-related frequency difference, and the t(1;11) is found both in infant/childhood and, albeit rarely, adult AML; the median age is 7 years. Most cases are acute myelomonocytic or monoblastic/monocytic leukemia and the vast majority are de novo AML. The prognostic impact is unclear, but considering the involvement of the *MLL* gene, a t(1;11)-positive AML will, by default, be grouped as "adverse" in most treatment protocols.

t(1;22)(p13;q13) [*RBM15–MKL1*]

The t(1;22), which results in a fusion between the *RBM15* and *MKL1* genes (Ma et al., 2001; Mercher et al., 2001), has been described in approximately 40 AMLs and has been the sole change in the majority (80%) of cases. Those with secondary aberrations are often high hyperdiploid or hypotriploid, with chromosome numbers ranging from 51 to 61.

The first reported t(1;22)-positive AML was classified as an infant acute erythroid leukemia (FIWCL, 1984a), but this diagnosis was made several years before criteria for AMKL were published. In fact, all ensuing cases have been AMKL, and since the early 1990s, it has become apparent that the t(1;22) is pathognomonic for AMKL in young children, most often infants without DS, prior MDS, and a transient leukemoid reaction (Baruchel et al., 1991; Carroll et al., 1991; Bernstein et al., 2000; Dastugue et al., 2002). In contrast to AMKL in children with DS, t(1;22)-positive cases rarely harbor *GATA1* mutations (Hama et al., 2008). The patients typically present with hepatosplenomegaly,

BM myelofibrosis, and a clear female predominance, with a sex ratio (SR) of 2.4. Early reports suggested that the t(1;22) conferred a poor prognosis but the change has since been associated with a superior outcome compared with AMKL without this translocation (Rubnitz et al., 2010; de Rooij et al., 2013).

der(1;7)(q10;p10)

This unbalanced whole-arm translocation between chromosomes 1 and 7 (Figure 6.2), leading to gain and loss of the entire 1q and 7q, respectively, is present in roughly 0.5% of cytogenetically abnormal AML. However, some cases may go undetected if the chromosome morphology is poor because the der(1;7) may be misinterpreted as a "+del(1p),−7." It is the sole change in 60%; among the remainder, the most frequent secondary change is +8. In addition, t-MDS/t-AML cases with der(1;7) often harbor *IDH1* and *IDH2* mutations (Westman et al., 2013).

The initial studies of this translocation reported that the breakpoints were located very close to the centromeres of both chromosomes, with the centromere most likely belonging to chromosome 1. It was therefore initially described as "+der(1)t(1;7)(p11;p11),−7" (Geraedts et al., 1980). However, it was later shown that the t(1;7) translocation contains α satellite DNA from both chromosomes (Wang et al., 2003). Thus, it is a true whole-arm translocation that should be designated der(1;7)(q10;p10).

The der(1;7) is mainly seen in elderly AML patients (median age ~60 years) and is exceedingly rare in childhood AML. It is more common in males (SR 1.8). Most der(1;7)-positive myeloid

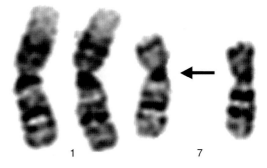

Figure 6.2 The whole-arm der(1;7)(q10;p10), leading to gain of 1q and loss of 7q, is associated with t-AML. The arrow indicates the centromeric breakpoints.

malignancies are initially diagnosed as MDS, but 25% present as full-fledged AML and 10% as myeloproliferative neoplasms. The der(1;7) is strongly associated with prior iatrogenic exposure (Scheres et al., 1985); in fact, 30–60% of der(1;7)-positive myeloid malignancies are diagnosed in patients previously treated with chemo- and/or radiotherapy (Mauritzson et al., 2002; Hsiao et al., 2006; Sanada et al., 2007). Several investigators have reported that der(1;7) confers a poor prognosis (Hsiao et al., 2006). Although the dismal survival often has been attributed to the del(7q) generated through the der(1;7), this may not be the correct explanation. Sanada et al. (2007) compared MDS with der(1;7) with those with −7/del(7q) and showed that the der(1;7)-positive cases had lower blast counts, higher hemoglobin concentrations, slower progression to AML, and significantly better outcome than MDS with −7/del(7q). However, this has not been confirmed in other studies (Hsiao et al., 2006; Slovak et al., 2009).

t(1;11)(q21;q23) [*MLL–MLLT11*]

The rare t(1;11), generating an *MLL–MLLT11* fusion (Tse et al., 1995), is the sole abnormality in most instances; the only recurrent secondary changes to date have been +6 and +19. It is equally common in girls and boys and mainly occurs in infant/childhood AML (median age 2 years). Morphologically, most cases are acute myelomonocytic or monoblastic/monocytic leukemia, as is usual for *MLL*-positive AML, but in contrast to many other *MLL* translocations, the t(1;11) is not associated with prior genotoxic therapy (Harrison et al., 1998; Busson-Le Coniat et al., 1999). Based on the study by Busson-Le Coniat et al. (1999), who reported that five out of six patients relapsed, it was initially concluded that the t(1;11) was associated with a poor outcome. However, a later retrospective study of 25 pediatric t(1;11)-positive ALL cases (Balgobind et al., 2009) reported a 5-year overall survival rate of 100%, hence associating this 11q23/*MLL* subgroup with an excellent prognosis.

t(2;3)(p11~23;q23~28) [*MECOM* deregulation]

Close to 70 AML cases with t(2;3) (Figure 6.3) have been published. As seen from the designation earlier, the breakpoints have been variable, although

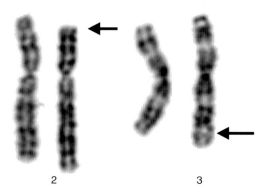

Figure 6.3 The t(2;3)(p21~23;q26) is associated with dysmegakaryocytopoiesis. Arrows indicate breakpoints.

most have been reported to involve 2p21~23 and 3q26~28. Considering that the translocation has been shown to rearrange the *MECOM* locus at 3q26.2, resulting in increased expression of this gene (Stevens-Kroef et al., 2004; Trubia et al., 2006), it should perhaps rather be written as "t(2;3) (p21~23;q26)." The t(2;3) is the sole chromosomal aberration in almost 50% of cases, with the most common secondary change, monosomy 7, being seen in one-third; in fact, −7 is a frequent additional aberration in AML cases with various types of 3q26/*MECOM* rearrangement.

To date, only a few t(2;3)-positive AML cases have been reported in children and adolescents; most patients are adults (median age 55 years) and there is no clear gender-related difference (Stevens-Kroef et al., 2004; Trubia et al., 2006; Lugthart et al., 2010). The vast majority are de novo AML associated with dysmegakaryocytopoiesis, near-normal platelet counts or even thrombocytosis, and a dismal outcome.

t(2;11)(p21;q23) [*MLL* rearrangement (?)]

This translocation was first identified in a few cases of MDS (Feder et al., 1985) but is now known to be present also in AML. It is the sole change in 50%; del(5q) and monosomy 7 are common secondary changes. The t(2;11) has, in a few cases, been shown to rearrange the *MLL* gene (Thirman et al., 1993; Meyer et al., 2013). However, in a larger series of MDS and AML with t(2;11), Bousquet et al. (2008) could not confirm involvement of *MLL*. The partner gene at 2p21 has not yet been identified.

There is a clear overrepresentation of males (SR 4.5), and t(2;11)-positive AML is most often seen in adults (median age 60 years). In most instances, the BM displays multilineage dysplasia, and there are several examples of AML evolving from MDS with t(2;11). Thus, many—if not all—AMLs with t(2;11) are secondary to MDS (Bousquet et al., 2008). The prognostic impact is unclear, but considering the relatively high age of the patients and the strong association with prior MDS, it would seem likely that t(2;11) is associated with a poor outcome.

t(2;11)(q31;p15) [*NUP98–HOXD11(13)*]

This rare translocation, which is the sole chromosomal change in most cases, results in a fusion between *NUP98* and different members of the *HOXD* family (Raza-Egilmez et al., 1998; Taketani et al., 2002b), thus representing one of several *NUP98-HOX* rearrangements in AML (see the following). The t(2;11) occurs both in children and adults (median age 30 years), mainly in de novo AML, and is equally common in males and females. The morphology varies, but acute myelomonocytic leukemia is quite common. Due to the rarity of t(2;11), its prognostic implication is unknown.

t(2;11)(q37;q23) [*MLL–SEPT2*]

The t(2;11) has so far been reported only in a few cases, most often as the sole aberration. As it may escape detection, in particular if the chromosome morphology is suboptimal, masquerading as a "del(11)(q23)," its true prevalence remains to be determined. Molecularly, the t(2;11) rearranges the *MLL* gene with *SEPT2* (Cerveira et al., 2006), and it is hence an example of the growing number of translocations fusing *MLL* with different members of the septin family, coding for GTPases involved in several key steps of mitosis (Cerveira et al., 2011). Most t(2;11)-positive cases have been described in adults, with the majority being t-AML after previous exposure to DNA topoisomerase II poisons (van Binsbergen et al., 2007; Bielorai et al., 2010). Albeit based on few cases, the t(2;11) seems to be associated with a poor outcome.

inv(3)(q21q26)/t(3;3)(q21;q26) [*RPN1–MECOM*]

The inv(3) or t(3;3) (Figure 6.4) is found in approximately 1% of AML, with the inversion being twice as common as the translocation. The inv(3) may be

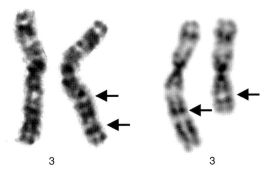

Figure 6.4 The inv(3)(q21q26) (left) and t(3;3)(q21;q26) (right) are strongly associated with prominent dysmegakaryocytopoiesis. Arrows indicate breakpoints.

even more frequent considering that it easily escapes detection if the chromosome morphology is poor. The inv(3)/t(3;3) is the sole cytogenetic change in approximately 40% of cases. The only secondary change found in a large proportion of inv(3)/t(3;3)-positive AML is monosomy 7 (40%). Furthermore, deletions of the *NF1* gene and mutations of the *KRAS*, *NRAS*, and *RUNX1* genes are found in 20–30% (Haferlach et al., 2011a). The inv(3) and t(3;3) both result in deregulated expression of the *MECOM* gene at 3q26 through juxtaposition with *RPN1* enhancer elements (Fichelson et al., 1992; Morishita et al., 1992; Suzukawa et al., 1994).

The inv(3) and t(3;3) are extremely rare in pediatric AML (Harrison et al., 2010). Instead, they are characteristic of adult AML with a median age of 50 years (Grimwade et al., 2010; Rogers et al., 2014), and they are seen equally often in males and females. The first 3q21q26 aberrations, initially described as ins(3;3)(q21;q21q26) or ins(3;3)(q26;q21q26) although later reinterpreted as t(3;3), were published by Rowley and Potter (1976) and Golomb et al. (1978). Soon afterward, this translocation was associated with dysplastic megakaryocytes and increased platelets (Sweet et al., 1979). A few years later, the more common inv(3) was identified and also shown to correlate with dysmegakaryocytopoiesis (Bernstein et al., 1982). Studies of several larger patient series subsequently confirmed the existence of a characteristic "3q21q26 syndrome" (Secker-Walker et al., 1995; Charrin et al., 2002; Lugthart et al., 2010; Medeiros et al., 2010a; Sun et al., 2011; Rogers et al., 2014): AML with inv(3)/t(3;3) is associated with normal or, less frequently, elevated platelets, an increased number of (micro)megakaryocytes, frequently an antecedent MDS phase, trilineage dysplasia, often fibrosis or increased reticulin in the BM, and an immunophenotype characterized by expression of CD7, CD13, CD33, CD34, CD38, CD56, CD117, and HLA-DR.

The prognosis of inv(3)/t(3;3)-positive AML is universally poor, with minimal or no response to chemotherapy, with complex and monosomal karyotypes, often with −7, and dysgranulocytopoiesis seemingly conferring an even worse outcome (Weisser et al., 2007; Lugthart et al., 2010; Rogers et al., 2014). However, emerging data suggest that allogeneic stem cell transplantation (alloSCT) is beneficial (Weisser et al., 2007; Sun et al., 2011; Rogers et al., 2014).

t(3;5)(q25;q35) [*NPM1–MLF1*]

More than 70 AML cases with t(3;5)(q25;q35), which results in the *NPM1–MLF1* fusion gene (Yoneda-Kato et al., 1996), have been reported, with the t(3;5) as the sole change in approximately 80%. The only relatively common secondary change is trisomy 8.

AML with t(3;5) is more common in males (SR 2.0) and mainly occurs in younger patients (median age 30 years). None of the reported cases has been associated with previous radio- or chemotherapy; hence, t(3;5)-positive cases are typically de novo AML. However, a prior MDS phase is not uncommon (Lim et al., 2010; Dumézy et al., 2013). A general morphologic feature of t(3;5)-positive cases, shared with many other AML with aberrations involving 3q, is trilineage dysplasia, in particular dysmegakaryocytopoiesis with an increased number of (micro)megakaryocytes. Based on the limited immunophenotypic data available, most cases are positive for CD13, CD33, and CD117 but negative for CD34 (Dumézy et al., 2013). Initially, the prognosis was considered poor, but several long-term survivors have since been reported and t(3;5)-positive cases are now often grouped as intermediate-risk AML (Raimondi et al., 1989a; Secker-Walker et al., 1995; Arber et al., 2003; Grimwade et al., 2010; Dumézy et al., 2013).

t(3;12)(q26;p13) [*ETV6–MECOM*]

Close to 40 AML cases with t(3;12) have been published, with the translocation being the sole change in 60%. Though clearly a primary AML-associated abnormality, the translocation is also found, albeit rarely, in CML during blast crisis (BC). The only recurrent secondary changes in t(3;12)-positive AML identified so far are del(5q) and monosomy 7; these aberrations have not been described in CML BC with t(3;12).

Raynaud et al. (1996) showed that all the 12p13 breakpoints occurred within *ETV6* and Peeters et al. (1997) reported that the t(3;12) resulted in a fusion between *ETV6* and *MECOM*. As the *ETV6* gene did not contribute any functional domains to the chimera, it was suggested that the pathogenetically important consequence might be deregulated expression of *MECOM*. In fact, subsequent studies have confirmed the presence of *ETV6–MECOM* transcripts and/or increased expression of *MECOM* in t(3;12)-positive AML (Poppe et al., 2006).

Despite the fact that the first reported case with t(3;12) was an infant AML (Massaad et al., 1990), this translocation is very rare in children. Most patients are adults (median age 50 years), without any clear gender difference. The clinical features include prior MDS that often rapidly progresses to AML with a variable—often unclassifiable—morphology, dysplastic megakaryocytes, normal or decreased platelet counts, and a dismal outcome (Secker-Walker et al., 1995; Raynaud et al., 1996; Voutsadakis and Maillard, 2003).

t(3;21)(q26;q22) [*RUNX1–MECOM*]

To date, approximately 60 AML cases with t(3;21) (Figure 6.5) have been reported, with the translocation being the sole change in 50%. Relatively frequent additional changes include monosomy 7, trisomies 8 and 12, as well as gain of the der(21)t(3;21). Nucifora and Rowley (1995) showed that the promoter region

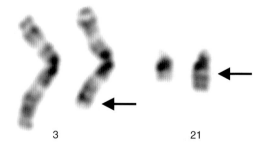

3   21

Figure 6.5 The t(3;21)(q26;q22) is associated with t-AML. Arrows indicate breakpoints.

of *RUNX1* moves to the der(3)t(3;21), rearranging with several genes in 3q26, but mainly *MECOM*.

The t(3;21), which is equally common in males and females, is mainly found in adult AML; the median age is approximately 60 years. Initial reports of t(3;21) emphasized its association with acute transformation of MDS/myeloproliferative neoplasms and/or prior chemotherapy (Akahoshi et al., 1987; Rubin et al., 1987), and subsequent studies confirmed that t(3;21) is a recurring abnormality in t-AML strongly correlated with previous treatment with DNA topoisomerase II poisons and/or alkylating agents. In fact, the majority of t(3;21)-positive cases are t-AML (Rubin et al., 1990; Pedersen-Bjergaard et al., 1994; Mauritzon et al., 2002; Slovak et al., 2002; Li et al., 2012). Morphologically, most cases are unclassifiable, as expected of t-AML, with multilineage dysplasia and megakaryocytic hypoplasia. The t(3;21) has been associated with a poor prognosis by most investigators.

Trisomy 4

Trisomy 4 as the sole aberration is found in approximately 1% of AML. Interestingly, there is an association between +4 and the presence of double minutes (dmin); approximately 10% of AML cases with +4 as the "sole" abnormality also harbor dmin, sometimes with +4 in the stemline and dmin only in a subclone but occasionally vice versa. The dmin are known to carry the *MYC* gene (Govberg et al., 2000), and it was initially surmised that this gene was the target of the amplification, based mainly on its importance in other hematologic malignancies such as ALL, lymphomas, and multiple myeloma (Chapters 10 and 11). However, detailed mapping and expression analyses of *MYC*-containing dmin have revealed that they harbor several 8q24-linked genes in addition to *MYC* and that the latter gene is not overexpressed, in effect excluding *MYC* as the likely target gene (Storlazzi et al., 2006).

The molecular genetic consequences of +4 are, as for numerical chromosomal changes in general, unknown. Possible mechanisms include gene dosage effects and/or duplication of rearranged or mutated genes on chromosome 4. Beghini et al. (2004) found evidence in support of the latter, identifying duplications of a mutated *KIT* gene at 4q12 in two of six AML cases with +4 as the sole

change, and Schnittger et al. (2006) subsequently reported *KIT* mutations in two cases with +4 as the sole change. However, only one of 10 AMLs with isolated trisomy 4 was shown to harbor a *KIT* mutation in a later study by Bains et al. (2012), who instead observed internal tandem duplications of *FLT3* (*FLT3*-ITD) and *NPM1* mutations in 40–50% of cases. Thus, the jury is still out on the possible association between the presence of a mutated *KIT* gene and trisomy 4.

Trisomy 4 as the sole change is somewhat more common in women than in men (SR 1.4) and is primarily seen in adult AML (median age 55 years). The morphology varies, but several cases have been classified as AML with minimal differentiation or without maturation. In the initial report of +4 as a single anomaly, Mecucci et al. (1986) suggested that it characterized a novel subgroup of AML not associated with prior genotoxic exposure. Indeed, several studies have since confirmed that trisomy 4-positive cases mainly are de novo AML and have also suggested that +4 is associated with marked leukocytosis, high BM blast counts, extramedullary leukemia, and hand-mirror appearance of the blasts (Weber et al., 1990; UKCCG, 1992a; Suenaga et al., 1993; Bains et al., 2012). Based on a review of 30 cases, Gupta et al. (2003) concluded that the outcome appeared to be poor compared with other cytogenetic entities in the intermediate-risk group. The dismal outcome of several of the patients reported by Bains et al. (2012) agrees well with this conclusion. In fact, and as will be mentioned in the relevant sections in the following, several AML-associated trisomies are associated with an intermediate to poor prognosis when found as single anomalies; apart from +4, this is the case for +8, +11, and +13.

t(4;12)(q12;p13) [*CHIC2–ETV6*]

Approximately 25 AML cases with t(4;12) (Figure 6.6) have been published. It has been the sole change in 70% of them; the only recurrent secondary changes reported are del(5q), −7, −11, i(17q), and +21.

Cools et al. (1999) showed that the t(4;12) leads to a fusion between *CHIC2* and *ETV6*. However, the molecular genetic consequence of this translocation is more complex. Not only is there breakpoint heterogeneity at 4q12, but also some t(4;12)-positive cases that do not express the *CHIC2–ETV6* fusion (Cools et al., 2002).

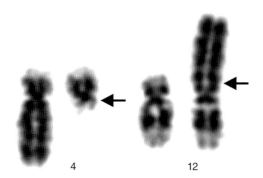

Figure 6.6 The t(4;12)(q12;p13) is associated with AML with minimal differentiation or without maturation, trilineage dysplasia, and basophilia. Arrows indicate breakpoints.

AML with t(4;12) is more common in men (SR 1.6) and most patients are adults (median age 60 years). The first t(4;12)-positive AML was a "myelo-megakaryocytic" leukemia (Ohyashiki, 1984), but subsequent reports have shown that most are AML with minimal differentiation/without maturation or unclassifiable (Harada et al., 1995; Ma et al., 1997; Cools et al., 1999; Chauffaille et al., 2003). It has gradually become apparent that AML with t(4;12) represents a specific subgroup characterized by trilineage dysplasia, lymphoid-like morphology of the blasts, absent or low myeloperoxidase activity, basophilia, a myeloid immunophenotype with frequent aberrant expression of the T-cell antigen CD7, and a dismal outcome.

t(4;11)(q21;q23) [MLL–AFF1]
The t(4;11) is strongly associated with ALL (Chapter 10); however, it also occurs, albeit more rarely, in AML, in which it is the sole change in 60%. Recurrent secondary changes include +6, –7, +8, and +19. As in ALL, the t(4;11) in AML results in the MLL–AFF1 chimera (Corral et al., 1993).

AML cases with t(4;11) are more common in females (SR 1.9) and most patients are children, often infants. Among the few adult patients, the median age is approximately 40 years. The leukemic blasts of the first reported AML cases with t(4;11) had a monocytic morphology (Parkin et al., 1982), and most published cases since have been myelo-monocytic or monoblastic/monocytic leukemias (Johansson et al., 1998; Bloomfield et al., 2002; Balgobind et al., 2009). Other characteristic features

include leukocytosis, hepatosplenomegaly, previous chemotherapy with DNA topoisomerase II inhibitors (mainly in adults), and a poor prognosis.

Monosomy 5/del(5q)
Monosomy 5 is one of the most common numerical changes in AML, seen in 2–3% of all cases, almost exclusively together with other abnormalities such as –7, del(7q), –17, del(17p), and –18. In fact, only 10 AMLs with –5 as the single aberration have been reported. Deletion of 5q is more common than –5, occurring in 5% of AML. As for mono-somy 5, del(5q) is most often present together with other changes, again in particular whole or partial losses of chromosomes 7, 17, and 18. However, del(5q) is, in contrast to monosomy 5, relatively often the sole anomaly; more than 200 such AML cases have been reported. Of these, approximately one-third had subclones containing other aberrations, most frequently +8 and +21.

The pathogenetic consequences of monosomy 5 remain elusive, as indeed they do for all mono-somies. It may seem obvious that –5 results in a hemizygous loss of all genes located on chromosome 5. However, several FISH- and array-based studies have shown that –5 in AML, at least in cases with complex karyotypes (CK), frequently is not a true monosomy. Instead, such analyses have revealed chromosome 5 material elsewhere in the genome, as deletions or as part of unbalanced translocations or insertions, resulting in net loss of 5q material only (Mrózek et al., 2002; Schoch et al., 2002; Van Limbergen et al., 2002; Bram et al., 2003; Galván et al., 2010; Jerez et al., 2012a). Thus, one really has to question, as Bram et al. (2003) and Galván et al. (2010) did, whether monosomy 5 is a common change in AML—it actually seems to be rare once data from all types of investigations are assessed. As regards del(5q), its functionally important outcome is probably loss of genes rather than creation of a fusion gene, considering the variable proximal and distal breakpoints (Douet-Guilbert et al., 2012; Jerez et al., 2012a). Initially, deletion of one or several tumor suppressor genes, coupled with inactivating mutations of the remaining allele(s) on the normal homologue, was believed to be the patho-genetically essential mechanism. However, despite numerous efforts to identify such genes, the results were meager. Instead, haploinsufficiency of one or several genes has become the focus of attention, with recent data suggesting that haploinsufficiency of the *EGR1* and *APC* genes in 5q plays a crucial role (Stoddart et al., 2014).

Monosomy 5 is more common in men (SR 1.5) and is most often found in adult AML (median age 60 years). In contrast, deletion of 5q as the sole change shows a female preponderance with an SR of 1.6. However, together with other changes, del(5q) does not display any gender difference. Similar to monosomy 5, del(5q) is mainly found in elderly people (median age 60–65 years) with several studies having shown that the percentage of AML cases with −5/del(5q) increases with age (Schoch et al., 2005a; Appelbaum et al., 2006a; Sanderson et al., 2006; Cheng et al., 2009b; Lazarevic et al., 2014). Correspondingly, these changes are very rare in pediatric AML (Harrison et al., 2010; von Neuhoff et al., 2010; Johnston et al., 2013; Sandahl et al., 2014b).

Monosomy 5 and del(5q) were first identified in AML in the mid-1970s (Oshimura et al., 1976; Rowley, 1976; Van Den Berghe et al., 1976). A close association between whole or partial losses of chromosome 5, often as part of hypodiploid CK, and AML was soon established. It was later shown that −5/del(5q) is significantly more common in t-AML than in de novo AML and that these abnormalities are strongly associated with prior exposure to alkylating agents, irradiation, or both (Mauritzson et al., 2002; Smith et al., 2003; Pedersen-Bjergaard et al., 2006). The AML blasts with −5/del(5q) typically express CD2, CD7, CD13, CD14, CD15, CD18, CD33, and CD34, and CK with −5/del(5q) are particularly common in AML with myelodysplasia-related changes, with minimal differentiation and acute erythroid leukemia (Cuneo et al., 1990, 1995; Olopade et al., 1992; Casasnovas et al., 1998; Béné et al., 2001; Hrušák and Porwit-MacDonald, 2002).

Soon after the identification of −5 and del(5q) in AML, it became apparent that they were associated with resistance to chemotherapy and, hence, with an adverse prognosis (Larson et al., 1983; FIWCL, 1984b; Keating et al., 1987). As a result, cases with 5q loss are stratified as high-risk AML, with several studies reporting a dismal outcome even after alloSCT (Gale et al., 1995; Ferrant et al., 1997; Schoch et al., 2001; Burnett et al., 2002; van der Straaten et al., 2005; Middeke et al., 2012). New and

innovative therapeutic strategies are therefore urgently needed for this common AML group. Some recent preliminary data suggest that treatment with lenalidomide may be beneficial; however, the results have been conflicting (Möllgård et al., 2011; Sekeres et al., 2011; Dennis et al., 2013).

t(5;11)(q31;q23) [*MLL–ARHGAP26*]

The t(5;11), which results in a fusion between *MLL* and *ARHGAP26* (Borkhardt et al., 2000), has so far been reported in only a few AML cases, being the sole change in all of them. The first reported t(5;11)-positive case was an elderly woman with a previous history of chemotherapy and with AML without maturation (Hoyle et al., 1989). However, all subsequent cases have been boys with de novo acute myelomonocytic or monoblastic/monocytic leukemia and, with one exception, infants (Itoh et al., 1999; Borkhardt et al., 2000; Panagopoulos et al., 2004; Wilda et al., 2005). The patients have responded well to conventional chemotherapy or alloSCT; thus, the t(5;11) may actually characterize a small subgroup of infant *MLL*-positive AML with a favorable prognosis.

t(5;11)(q35;p15) [*NUP98–NSD1*]

This translocation, leading to *NUP98–NSD1* (Jaju et al., 2001), has been described in close to 40 AML cases. However, as it is cytogenetically cryptic, this number is undoubtedly an underreporting. The t(5;11) is the sole abnormality in the majority of cases. The most common secondary aberrations are del(5q) and trisomy 8.

The t(5;11) was first identified by Jaju et al. (1999) by FISH screening of a series of pediatric and adult MDS and AML with del(5q) as the "sole" aberration. Subsequent investigations have identified the *NUP98–NSD1* fusion in 4–7% and 1–2% of pediatric and adult AML, respectively (Hollink et al., 2011; Akiki et al., 2013; Fasan et al., 2013; Shiba et al., 2013; Thol et al., 2013), with the prevalence in cytogenetically normal childhood AML being approximately 15%. The median age in children is 10 years and in adults 45 years; to date, no patient below the age of 2 years has been reported. Based on the aforementioned studies, it has become clear that *NUP98–NSD1*-positive AMLs characteristically are de novo AML (with a seemingly normal karyotype [NK]) with a male predominance

(SR 1.7), myelomonocytic or monoblastic/monocytic morphology, high incidence of *FLT3*-ITD and *WT1* mutations, hyperleukocytosis, and a poor response to treatment. Although the t(5;11) is associated with a dismal outcome, alloSCT has been suggested to improve survival (Akiki et al., 2013).

t(5;17)(q35;q21) [*NPM1–RARA*]

Roughly 10 AML cases with t(5;17) have been published. Although the translocation rarely is the sole anomaly, no secondary changes have been recurrent. The t(5;17) leads to a fusion between the *NPM1* and *RARA* genes (Redner et al., 1996); it is thus one of several rare variant translocations involving *RARA*.

The t(5;17) is equally common in men and women but is clearly associated with young age; most reported patients have been children below the age of 15 years. The first t(5;17)-positive AML published was a pediatric APL displaying an atypical morphology without Auer rods and responding poorly to all-*trans* retinoic acid (ATRA) treatment (Corey et al., 1994), and subsequent reports (Grimwade et al., 2000; Sainty et al., 2000; Otsubo et al., 2012) confirmed a strong association with childhood APL, mainly of the hypogranular type and without Auer rods. These studies have also shown that the t(5;17) is very rare in APL, comprising less than 1% of such cases, and that, in contrast to the initial report, the response to ATRA is usually good.

t(6;9)(p22;q34) [*DEK–NUP214*]

The t(6;9), which fuses the *DEK* gene from 6p with the *NUP214* gene from 9q (von Lindern et al., 1992), is seen in approximately 1% of AML, with a median age of 10 years in children and 45 years in adults (Grimwade et al., 2010; Gupta et al., 2010; Harrison et al., 2010; Sandahl et al., 2014a). t(6;9)-positive AML has generally not been reported to display any gender-related frequency difference, but there was a clear overrepresentation of boys in a recent international compilation of more than 60 pediatric patients (Sandahl et al., 2014a). It is the sole aberration in 80%; the most common secondary changes are +8 and +13. In addition, *FLT3*-ITD is present in approximately 70%, a frequency much higher than usually seen in translocation-positive AML (Oyarzo et al., 2004; Garçon et al., 2005; Slovak et al., 2006; Sandahl et al., 2014a).

The first AML with t(6;9) was reported by Rowley and Potter (1976), and with the description of several additional cases in the early 1980s, this translocation was firmly established as a primary AML-associated abnormality. Since then, several investigators have identified morphologic and clinical features that characterize t(6;9)-positive AML (Oyarzo et al., 2004; Garçon et al., 2005; Slovak et al., 2006; Chi et al., 2008; Grimwade et al., 2010; Gupta et al., 2010; Harrison et al., 2010; Sandahl et al., 2014a). The majority are de novo AML, most often AML with maturation or myelomonocytic leukemia, although some cases are secondary AML after a prior MDS phase. Auer rods are present in a substantial proportion of cases, and the blasts are typically positive for CD9, CD13, CD15, CD33, CD34, CD38, CD45, CD117, and HLA-DR. Trilineage dysplasia is common, and so is BM basophilia. The response to chemotherapy is often poor, and survival has been reported to be dismal. Thus, t(6;9) is now included in the high-risk group in most treatment protocols. Encouraging results have, however, been obtained after alloSCT (Garçon et al., 2005; Slovak et al., 2006; Gupta et al., 2010; Ishiyama et al., 2012; Sandahl et al., 2014a).

t(6;11)(q27;q23) [*MLL–MLLT4*]

The t(6;11), resulting in an *MLL–MLLT4* gene fusion (Prasad et al., 1993), is seen in 0.5% of AML and is the sole change in close to 90%; the most frequent secondary aberrations are gain of the der(6)t(6;11) and trisomy for chromosomes 8, 19, and 21. In addition, *RAS* mutations are present in 45% of cases (Coenen et al., 2014).

The t(6;11) is equally common in women and men and is mainly found in adults (median age 40 years). Although the aberration was first described in the early 1980s (Hagemeijer et al., 1981; Yunis et al., 1981), only a few additional t(6;11)-positive cases were reported during that decade, probably because of difficulties in identifying it. In fact, AML with del(11)(q23) as the sole change may well harbor the t(6;11), as shown by FISH analyses of "terminal" deletions of 11q23 (Kobayashi et al., 1993).

Several studies have delineated morphologic and clinical features typical of t(6;11)-positive AML (Martineau et al., 1998; Bloomfield et al., 2002; Blum et al., 2004; Balgobind et al., 2009; Grimwade et al., 2010; Chen et al., 2013). The vast majority are morphologically characterized as acute myelomonocytic or monoblastic/monocytic leukemia, and leukocytosis and hepatosplenomegaly are common. In contrast to many other *MLL* translocations, t(6;11)-positive cases are most often de novo AML. A poor response to chemotherapy and a dismal prognosis have been stressed by most investigators, and there are conflicting reports as to whether alloSCT improves the outcome (Blum et al., 2004; Balgobind et al., 2009; Krauter et al., 2009; Chen et al., 2013). Thus, novel treatment strategies need to be developed. Interestingly, recent *in vitro* experiments suggested that agents targeting aberrant histone methylation may be beneficial.

Monosomy 7/del(7q)

Next to trisomy 8, monosomy 7 is the most common numerical chromosomal abnormality in AML. It is found together with other changes, mainly −5, del(5q), and −17, in 10% of all cytogenetically abnormal AML. However, −7 is frequently (5%) the sole change. Deletions of 7q are also common (5%) and most often present with additional aberrations, again in particular losses of chromosomes 5 and 17. In contrast to −7, only 1% of karyotypically aberrant AML cases have del(7q) as the sole anomaly. Another cytogenetic difference between −7 and del(7q) is the fact that cases with monosomy 7 as an isolated change rarely harbor subclones with other aberrations, whereas AMLs with del(7q) as the sole aberration display subclones, or occasionally unrelated clones, in almost one-third of cases; +8 is often the other change.

The pathogenetically important molecular genetic consequence of monosomy 7 is unknown. As for monosomy 5, it has been shown that −7 in AML with CK often is not a true whole chromosome loss, but rather a del(7q) in disguise (Mrózek et al., 2002; Schoch et al., 2002; Van Limbergen et al., 2002). Most molecular genetic studies of del(7q) have focused on identifying mutated tumor suppressor genes on the remaining normal homologue, but despite numerous efforts, no target genes have been identified. Instead, haploinsufficient expression of genes on 7q has been proposed to be the pathogenetically important outcome, with emerging data indicating that the *CUX1* and *SAMD9L* genes contribute to the myeloid transformation (Jerez et al., 2012b; McNerney et al., 2013; Nagamachi et al., 2013).

AML cases with −7 or del(7q) were reported already in the early 1970s (Petit et al., 1973; Rowley, 1973a), and whole or partial losses of chromosome 7 were quickly established as nonrandom AML-associated abnormalities. Monosomy 7 is more common in men (SR 1.9) when seen as the sole change, whereas del(7q) is equally common in males and females. The median age of AML patients with −7/del(7q) is higher (55 years) when other aberrations are present than when found alone (45 years), with the frequencies of AML with −7/del(7q) in CK increasing with age, similar to chromosome 5 losses (Schoch et al., 2005a; Appelbaum et al., 2006a; Sanderson et al., 2006; Cheng et al., 2009b; Lazarevic et al., 2014). In contrast to −5/del(5q), chromosome 7 loss is also common in pediatric AML, occurring in 5% of cases (Harrison et al., 2010; von Neuhoff et al., 2010; Sandahl et al., 2014b).

There is a clear association between AML with −7/del(7q) and previous genotoxic treatment, in particular with alkylators and/or radiotherapy (Mauritzson et al., 2002; Smith et al., 2003; Pedersen-Bjergaard et al., 2006). Both t-AML and de novo cases are often morphologically unclassifiable; the most common morphologic types among those that can be classified are AML with minimal differentiation or without maturation, acute erythroid leukemia, and AMKL (Cuneo et al., 1990, 1995; Olopade et al., 1992; Béné et al., 2001; Dastugue et al., 2002). The blasts are typically positive for CD7, CD13, CD15, CD18, CD33, and CD34 (Casasnovas et al., 1998; Hrušák and Porwit-MacDonald, 2002).

That −7/del(7q) has an adverse prognostic impact was realized already in the early 1980s (Borgström et al., 1980; Larson et al., 1983), and it is today well recognized that AMLs with these changes display a poor response to chemotherapy and, hence, have a dismal outcome (Hasle et al., 2007; Grimwade et al., 2010; Harrison et al., 2010). It is questionable whether more intensive chemotherapy or alloSCT improves survival (Gale et al., 1995; Schoch et al., 2001; Burnett et al., 2002; van der Straaten et al., 2005).

t(7;21)(p22;q22) [*RUNX1–USP42*]

Although this cytogenetically semicryptic translocation, resulting in a *RUNX1–USP42* fusion (Paulsson et al., 2006a), has been reported in only a handful of AML cases, certain characteristic features have nevertheless emerged (Jeandidier et al., 2012). Most patients are relatively young males (median age 35 years) with myelomonocytic or monoblastic/monocytic leukemia and frequent aberrant expression of CD7 and CD56. Furthermore, rearrangements of 5q, leading to loss of this chromosome arm, are common secondary changes. The clinical outcome has been variable, so the prognostic impact remains to be elucidated.

t(7;11)(p15;p15) [*NUP98–HOXA9(11,13)*]

Almost 70 AML cases with t(7;11) (Figure 6.7) have been published making this the most common translocation involving 11p15/*NUP98*. The translocation is the sole change in approximately 85%; trisomy 8 is the only recurrent secondary change observed to date. *FLT3*, *RAS*, and *WT1* mutations are present in 20–40% (Chou et al., 2009).

Borrow et al. (1996a) and Nakamura et al. (1996) showed that the t(7;11) results in a fusion between the *NUP98* gene at 11p15 and the *HOXA9* gene at 7p15. Subsequent studies not only confirmed this chimera in t(7;11)-positive AML but also identified fusions with other *HOXA* members, that is, *HOXA11* and *HOXA13* (Fujino et al., 2002; Taketani et al., 2002a).

The t(7;11), which is slightly more common in women (Chou et al. 2009, Wei et al., 2013), occurs mainly in young adults (median age 35 years). The t(7;11) was first identified in an AML in a Japanese patient (Ohyashiki, 1984), and it has since become apparent that this translocation is more common in patients of Oriental origin, being seen in 0.5–2% of adult Chinese AML patients (Kwong and Pang, 1999; Chou et al., 2009; Wei et al., 2013). With only few exceptions, all published t(7;11)-positive cases have been de novo AML, and most have been AML

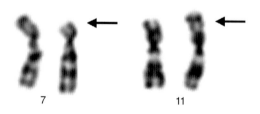

Figure 6.7 The t(7;11)(p15;p15) is associated with AML with maturation or myelomonocytic leukemia, trilineage dysplasia, and Auer rods. Arrows indicate breakpoints.

with maturation or myelomonocytic leukemia, often with Auer rods and trilineage dysplasia. The immunophenotype is usually positive for CD13, CD33, CD34, CD117, and HLA-DR but negative for lymphoid-associated antigens (Sato et al., 1987; Kwong and Pang, 1999; Chou et al. 2009; Wei et al., 2013). A poor survival has been emphasized.

t(7;12)(q36;p13) [*MNX1–ETV6*]

Many, if not most, t(7;12)-positive cases escape detection in conventional chromosome banding analysis because this translocation is very difficult to identify, almost cytogenetically cryptic (Hagemeijer et al., 1981; Heim et al., 1987b; Raimondi et al., 1999). The t(7;12) is rarely the sole change; with a few exceptions, also trisomy 19 is usually present. Another relatively common secondary aberration is trisomy 8. Therefore, infant AML (see the following) with +19 and/or +8 should definitely be tested for the presence of t(7;12).

Tosi et al. (1998) and Wlodarska et al. (1998) reported that the t(7;12) rearranges the *ETV6* gene at 12p13, and Beverloo et al. (2001) identified a fusion between the *MNX1* gene at 7q36 and *ETV6*. However, several t(7;12)-positive cases have 7q breakpoints that do not map within the *MNX1* gene and do not result in *MNX1–ETV6*. It was therefore questioned whether a fusion gene is the important result of the translocation (Tosi et al., 2000, 2003; Simmons et al., 2002). Additional *MNX1–ETV6*-positive cases were subsequently reported by von Bergh et al. (2006), who also identified ectopic expression of the *MNX1* gene in all t(7;12)-positive cases, with or without the *MNX1–ETV6* fusion. Thus, aberrant expression of *MNX1* appears to be the functionally important outcome.

Approximately 20 AML and a few ALL cases with t(7;12)(q36;p13) have been published, all below the age of 2 years (Tosi et al., 2000, 2003; Slater et al., 2001; von Bergh et al., 2006; Park et al., 2009; Wildenhain et al., 2010). The t(7;12) is present in 20% of infant AML making it the second most common rearrangement after 11q23/*MLL* changes in this age group. The morphology of t(7;12)-positive cases is variable, but a significant proportion is AML with minimal differentiation or without maturation, with expression of both myeloid and T-cell-associated antigens such as CD4, CD7, CD13, CD15, CD33, CD34, CD56, and

CD117. The outcome, at least after conventional chemotherapy, has been very poor.

Trisomy 8

Trisomy 8—the most common chromosomal change in AML—is the sole change in 5% of all cytogenetically abnormal cases and occurs together with other aberrations in an additional 10%. The functional consequences of +8 are unknown but may include global gene expression changes, deregulation of imprinted loci, and duplication of rearranged or mutated genes on chromosome 8. However, as reviewed by Paulsson and Johansson (2007), investigations addressing these issues have so far been unfruitful. Genes on chromosome 8 are often overexpressed, but different genes have been shown to be up- or downregulated in different studies. Also, and in contrast to what is seen in AML with well-known primary translocations and inversions, there does not seem to be a strong gene expression signature associated with +8. Furthermore, the origin of the additional chromosome 8 may be maternal as well as paternal, arguing against imprinting being of pathogenetic importance. Finally, and to the best of our knowledge, no gene on chromosome 8 has been shown to be mutated or rearranged and duplicated in AML with +8.

There is ample evidence that trisomy 8 is not sufficient for leukemogenesis. First, although individuals with a constitutional +8 mosaicism have an increased risk of AML, only a minority develops this disease, and then after a long latency period (Welborn, 2004). Second, there does not seem to be an increased risk of AML in CML patients with trisomy 8-positive/t(9;22)-negative clones emerging after treatment with imatinib (Baccarani et al., 2013). Third, Schoch et al. (2005b) reported that the discriminating gene expression pattern of AML with isolated +8 did not depend on the upregulation of chromosome 8 genes alone, concluding that additional genetic changes may be present. In fact, array-based analyses have revealed several cryptic chromosomal changes in AML with +8 as the seemingly sole change (Paulsson et al., 2006b; Hahm et al., 2013), and mutations of the *ASXL1*, *JAK2*, and *TET2* genes have been shown to be common (Schnittger et al., 2007, 2013; Chou et al., 2010, 2011).

Trisomy 8 does not display any gender-related frequency difference and occurs in all age groups but with the incidence increasing with age; the median age is 50 years. Although +8 may be found in all morphologic subtypes of AML, it is particularly frequent in AML with or without maturation, myelomonocytic leukemia, and monoblastic leukemia (Schoch et al., 1997; Byrd et al., 1998; Elliott et al., 2002; Farag et al., 2002; Haferlach et al., 2002; Wolman et al., 2002). Trisomy 8-positive AML do not have any specific immunophenotypic features (Hrušák and Porwit-MacDonald, 2002) but may differ from cytogenetically abnormal AML by having a lower expression of CD34 and a higher expression of CD36 (Casasnovas et al., 1998; Perea et al., 2005).

Trisomy 8 as an isolated change is rarely associated with previous genotoxic exposure; instead, it is significantly more common in de novo AML than in t-AML (Mauritzson et al., 2002). Regarding the prognostic impact of +8, several studies have reported that it is associated with an intermediate prognosis (Dastugue et al., 1995; Schoch et al., 1997; Wolman et al., 2002; Jaff et al., 2007; Grimwade et al., 2010). However, some investigators have identified a poorer outcome than is usually seen in the intermediate group, suggesting that alloSCT should be considered (Byrd et al., 1998; Elliott et al., 2002; Farag et al., 2002; Schaich et al., 2007; Chevallier et al., 2009).

inv(8)(p11q13) [*KAT6A–NCOA2*]

This inversion, which results in a *KAT6A–NCOA2* fusion (Carapeti et al., 1998), is a rare abnormality in AML but mostly occurs as the sole change. Despite its rarity, several clinical characteristics have emerged: the vast majority are females (SR 6.0) and young (median age 15 years), most cases are myelomonocytic or monoblastic leukemia, erythrophagocytosis is common, and the outcome is usually dismal (Coulthard et al., 1998; Panagopoulos et al., 2000; Billio et al., 2002). These features are indistinguishable from those seen in cases with t(8;16)(p11;p13), the more common *KATA6A* rearrangement in AML.

t(8;16)(p11;p13) [*KAT6A–CREBBP*]

Although more than 100 AML cases with t(8;16) (Figure 6.8) leading to the *KAT6A–CREBBP* chimera (Borrow et al., 1996b) have been reported, this translocation is nevertheless rare; less than 0.5% of all cytogenetically aberrant AML carry this abnormality.

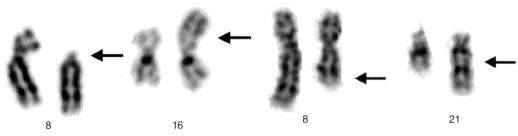

8   16

Figure 6.8 The t(8;16)(p11;p13) is strongly associated with acute myelomonocytic or monoblastic/monocytic leukemia and erythrophagocytosis. Arrows indicate breakpoints.

8   21

Figure 6.9 The t(8;21)(q22;q22) is strongly associated with AML with maturation, granulocytic dysplasia, and Auer rods. Arrows indicate breakpoints.

The t(8;16) is the sole change in 60%; the most common secondary aberrations are +8 and +21. Based on array analyses, gain of the *MYB* gene has also been shown to be frequent (Murati et al., 2009).

The t(8;16), which is more common in females (SR 1.9), occurs in infants, children, and, mainly younger, adults (median age 45 years). An association between t(8;16) and monocytic/monoblastic differentiation, often with extensive erythrophagocytosis, was stressed already in the initial reports of this translocation (Bernstein et al., 1987; Heim et al., 1987a). Subsequent larger series of t(8;16)-positive cases have clearly shown that they are most often acute monoblastic/monocytic leukemia, occasionally myelomonocytic leukemia. Erythrophagocytosis is present in 75% of cases, leukemia cutis in 30%, and disseminated intravascular coagulation in 40%. The latter coagulopathy, together with the presence of promyeloblast-like cells, may mimic APL. A large proportion of the patients received previous chemotherapy, such as anthracyclines, alkylating agents, topoisomerase II inhibitors, and/or radiotherapy (Hanslip et al., 1992; Quesnel et al., 1993; Block et al., 2002; Gervais et al., 2008; Haferlach et al., 2009; Brown et al., 2012; Diab et al., 2013). A very poor prognosis, at least after conventional chemotherapy, has been emphasized by all investigators. Interestingly, spontaneous remission of congenital AML with t(8;16) has been reported in several instances (Coenen et al., 2013).

t(8;22)(p11;q13) [*KAT6A–EP300*]

This rare t(8;22) may be considered a variant of the t(8;16) as it also rearranges the *KAT6A* gene (Chaffanet et al., 2000) and is associated with acute monoblastic/monocytic leukemia, erythrophagocytosis, and

a dismal outcome (Lai et al., 1992; Kitabayashi et al., 2001). However, in contrast to t(8;16), t(8;22)-positive cases have, until now, most often been males and all but one were de novo AML.

t(8;21)(q22;q22) [*RUNX1–RUNX1T1*]

The t(8;21) (Figure 6.9), leading to a *RUNX1–RUNX1T1* fusion (Miyoshi et al., 1991; Erickson et al., 1992), is found in 15% and 5% of childhood and adult AML, respectively (Grimwade et al., 2010; Harrison et al., 2010), making it the most frequent translocation in this disease. It is the sole change in 45%; common secondary aberrations include, in decreasing frequency order, –Y, –X (females only), del(9q), +8, del(7q), and + der(21)t(8;21). In addition, mutations of the *ASXL1*, *KIT*, and *NRAS* genes are present in 10–15% of cases (Radtke et al., 2009; Pollard et al., 2010; Krauth et al., 2014).

Although the t(8;21) is easy to recognize cytogenetically, rearrangements between 8q22 and 21q22 may be masked within CK or may even be the result of cryptic insertions. Complex translocations involving 8q22, 21q22, and another chromosome band comprise almost 5% of the cases (GFCH, 1990)—some of these may not be interpreted as variants of t(8;21)—and almost 10% of *RUNX1–RUNX1T1*-positive cases harbor hidden insertions (Gamerdinger et al., 2003). Thus, an AML with morphologic, immunophenotypic, or clinical features (see the following) strongly suggesting the presence of a t(8;21) not observed by chromosome banding analysis should definitely be screened by targeted FISH or RT-PCR analyses.

The t(8;21) was first reported by Rowley (1973b) and was soon confirmed to be a specific AML-associated abnormality. There is a slight overrepresentation of males (SR 1.5), and the t(8;21) is seen in all age groups, although it is particularly common in children and young adults; the median age is only 30 years. Morphologically, the vast majority of t(8;21)-positive cases are AML with maturation—only occasional cases are classified as AML without maturation or myelomonocytic leukemia. In some instances, the blast percentage is quite low, something that prior to the present WHO classification would have resulted in a diagnosis of MDS. Typically, the BM displays Auer rods and dysplastic features of the granulocytes. Occasionally, dyserythropoiesis and/or dysmegakaryocytopoiesis are also seen, but trilineage dysplasia is rare. A certain degree of eosinophilia and an increased number of mast cells are common. Taken together, the t(8;21) subgroup has distinct morphologic features that set it apart from other types of AML (Swirsky et al., 1984; Haferlach et al., 1996; Billström et al., 1997; Nakamura et al., 1997; Pullarkat et al., 2013). The immunophenotype is also characteristic, with positivity for CD13, CD15, CD18, CD34, CD117, HLA-DR, and MPO but negativity for CD2, CD4, CD7, CD11, CD14, and CD33. Aberrant expression of the B-cell antigen CD19 and the NK-cell antigen CD56 is common (Hurwitz et al., 1992; Kita et al., 1992; Casasnovas et al., 1998; Ferrara et al., 1998; Hrušák and Porwit-MacDonald, 2002). In fact, the immunophenotypic features are so typical that they often predict the presence of t(8;21). From a clinical point of view, it is important to be aware of the fact that extramedullary leukemia, principally in the mastoid and orbital cavities or paraspinally, is seen in 10–25% of patients, either at the time of diagnosis or at relapse (Tallman et al., 1993; Billström et al., 1997).

Most t(8;21)-positive cases are de novo AML; only 5% are t-AML, arising mainly after treatment with topoisomerase II poisons—anthracyclines as well as epipodophyllotoxins (Quesnel et al., 1993; Mauritzson et al., 2002; Slovak et al., 2002; Gustafson et al., 2009). Patients with t(8;21)-positive AML usually achieve complete remission after conventional chemotherapy and have been shown to respond particularly well to high-dose cytarabine treatment (Bloomfield et al., 1998). The t(8;21) is therefore associated with a favorable prognosis (Haferlach et al., 1996; Byrd et al., 1999; Grimwade et al., 2010; Harrison et al., 2010). However, some features have repeatedly, albeit not

consistently, been associated with a worse outcome, namely, leukocytosis, extramedullary leukemia, and *KIT* mutations (Byrd et al., 1997; Schlenk et al., 2004; Paschka et al., 2006; Schnittger et al., 2006; Shimada et al., 2006; Prébet et al., 2009; Pollard et al., 2010; Kim et al., 2013).

t(9;11)(p22;p15) [*NUP98–PSIP1*]

This translocation, which leads to a fusion between the *NUP98* and *PSIP1* genes (Ahuja et al., 2000), has only been reported in a few cases, and then mostly as the sole aberration. This notwithstanding, the t(9;11) seems to be associated with certain characteristic features, such as predominance of females (SR 4.0); de novo AML with maturation; middle age (median age 50 years); expression of both mature and immature surface antigens, that is, CD11b, CD13, CD33, CD34, and HLA-DR; and a dismal outcome (Hussey et al., 2001; Lundin et al., 2011).

t(9;11)(p21;q23) [*MLL–MLLT3*]

The t(9;11) (Figure 6.10), which fuses the *MLL* gene with the *MLLT3* gene (Iida et al., 1993; Nakamura et al., 1993), is the most common *MLL* translocation in AML, comprising 20% of infant AML, 30–50% of pediatric AML, and 25% of adult AML with *MLL* rearrangements (Balgobind et al., 2009; Meyer et al., 2013).

In AML in general, the t(9;11) is seen in 1–2% of adult and in 5–10% of childhood cases (Raimondi et al., 1999; Forestier et al., 2003; Grimwade et al., 2010; Harrison et al., 2010; Lazarevic et al., 2014). It is most frequently found in infants, children, and

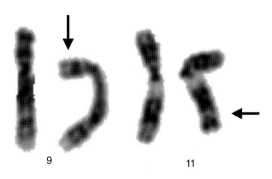

9   11

Figure 6.10 The t(9;11)(p21;q23) is strongly associated with monoblastic/monocytic leukemia and with t-AML. Arrows indicate breakpoints.

young adults (median age 20 years) and is equally common in females and males. It is the sole change in two-thirds of the cases. Trisomy 8, the most common secondary abnormality, is found in almost 20%; other relatively frequent additional changes include trisomies of chromosomes 6, 19, and 21 and *RAS* mutations (Chandra et al., 2010).

The t(9;11) is a relatively subtle translocation that may be overlooked in cases with inferior chromosome morphology. In addition, the *MLL–MLLT3* fusion may also arise through more complex mechanisms, such as three-way translocations and insertions; the latter may be difficult or even impossible to identify with chromosome banding analysis (Shago et al., 2004). Thus, the use of FISH or RT-PCR analysis is advisable in cases where the translocation is suspected for morphologic, immunophenotypic, or clinical reasons.

The t(9;11) was first reported as a characteristic translocation in AML by Hagemeijer et al. (1982) who emphasized its strong association with monoblastic leukemia. However, although t(9;11) predominantly occurs in monoblastic/monocytic leukemia, it is also seen in other subtypes such as myelomonocytic leukemia and AML without maturation. The t(9;11)-positive blasts are typically positive for CD11, CD13, CD15, and CD33 but less often express CD14, CD34, and lymphoid markers (Casasnovas et al., 1998; Swansbury et al., 1998). Extramedullary leukemia, mainly in the skin but also in the abdomen, orbit, and thorax, is common (Johansson et al., 2000; Park et al., 2001). Dewald et al. (1983) were the first to report a t-AML with t(9;11), and it was soon realized that this abnormality frequently is associated with prior chemotherapy, often including etoposide, a drug known to inhibit DNA topoisomerase II (Ratain et al., 1987; Pui et al., 1989; Pedersen-Bjergaard et al., 1990; Bloomfield et al., 2002). In fact, the prevalence of t(9;11) is significantly higher in t-AML than in de novo AML (Mauritzson et al., 2002).

In contrast to most translocations affecting the *MLL* gene, the t(9;11) does not seem to be associated with a particularly poor prognosis. Several studies of childhood t(9;11)-positive AML have instead reported a favorable outcome (Kalwinsky et al., 1990; Martinez-Climent et al., 1995; Rubnitz et al., 2002; Lie et al., 2003); however, this has not been seen in all pediatric series (Balgobind et al.,

2009; Harrison et al., 2010). In adult AML, the t(9;11) has also been correlated with superior survival, at least compared with other abnormalities involving 11q23 (Mrózek et al., 1997; Krauter et al., 2009; Grimwade et al., 2010; Chen et al., 2013). For this reason, 11q23 rearrangements in adult AML are often dichotomized into t(9;11) and non-t(9;11), with the former being included in the intermediate prognostic group and the latter in the high-risk group.

del(9q)

Deletions of the long arm of chromosome 9 are relatively common in AML, occurring in approximately 2 and 5% of adult and childhood cases, respectively (Grimwade et al., 2010; Harrison et al., 2010); among these, it is the sole abnormality in roughly one-third.

Mecucci et al. (1984), the first to investigate del(9q) in detail, concluded that the deletion was interstitial but that the breakpoints were variable. However, Sreekantaiah et al. (1989) subsequently reported a clustering of breaks in 9q21~22, suggesting that genes of importance in leukemogenesis were located within these bands, and further cytogenetic and molecular genetic characterization confirmed this position for the deletion (Peniket et al., 2005; Sweetser et al., 2005). The latter investigators identified a commonly deleted region within 9q21 with concomitant downregulation of several genes. As none of the genes was mutated, it was suggested that haploinsufficiency might be the essential leukemogenic outcome.

The first AML with del(9q) as the sole change was reported by Sasaki et al. (1976), with additional cases being described in the early 1980s. Due to the rarity of del(9q) as an isolated aberration, studies of its clinical implications have been few and far between. Based on all published cases, del(9q) is somewhat more common in men (SR 1.4) and is most often found in adult AML (median age 45 years). With one exception, all published cases have been de novo, most often AML with maturation, followed by AML without maturation and acute myelomonocytic leukemia. Many display a marked variation in size and nucleus-to-cell ratio of the blasts, Auer rods, erythroid dysplasia, and granulocytic lineage vacuolation (Hoyle et al., 1987; Peniket et al., 2005). The immunophenotypic features, admittedly based on only a few cases, include positivity for CD15, CD33, CD34, and HLA-DR, as well as aberrant expression of the T-cell antigen CD7 (Tien et al., 1995; Ferrara et al., 1996).

The few larger patient series in which the prognostic impact of del(9q) as the sole change has been investigated have all concluded that it belongs in the intermediate-risk group (Byrd et al., 2002; Peniket et al., 2005, Grimwade et al., 2010). Interestingly, *CEBPA* mutations, known to be associated with a favorable prognosis (Preudhomme et al., 2002), have been identified in close to 50% of del(9q)-positive AML (Fröhling et al., 2005); this is probably one reason for the relatively favorable outcome, at least within the intermediate group, of del(9q)-positive AML.

t(9;22)(q34;q11) [*BCR–ABL1*]

Apart from being characteristic of CML and also quite frequent in adult ALL, t(9;22) also occurs in 1% of AML. It is the sole anomaly in roughly 40% of these cases with the most common secondary changes being, in decreasing frequency order, +8, −7, +19, and +der(22) t(9;22). These aberrations are also frequent in CML BC, and the question therefore often arises whether a t(9;22)-positive AML represents CML in myeloid BC or whether it is a de novo Ph-positive AML.

There are some genetic and clinical differences between CML BC and de novo Ph-positive AML that may help discriminate between these two entities (Sasaki et al., 1983; Chen et al., 1988; Kantarjian et al., 1991; Tien et al., 1992; Cuneo et al., 1996; Soupir et al., 2007; Konoplev et al., 2013; Nacheva et al., 2013). First, although the *BCR* breakpoints in Ph-positive AML often map to the major breakpoint cluster region, leading to the P210 *BCR–ABL1* transcript as in CML, some are located upstream of this region, resulting in P190 *BCR–ABL1*; the latter may suggest (but certainly does not prove) de novo AML. Second, patients with Ph-positive AML often have a mixture of cytogenetically abnormal and normal cells at diagnosis; this is rare in CML BC. Third, *NPM1* mutations, although infrequent in de novo Ph-positive AML, may be specific for such cases. Fourth, Ph-positive AML may harbor distinct genomic imbalances as ascertained by array analyses. Finally, patients with de novo Ph-positive AML are less likely to have splenomegaly and peripheral basophilia.

Sasaki et al. (1975) were the first to describe the presence of t(9;22) in AML. Additional t(9;22)-positive AML cases were subsequently published during the late 1970s, clearly showing that this translocation was not restricted to CML or ALL. To date, more than 200 Ph-positive AML cases have been reported. Among these, the t(9;22) is more common in males (SR 1.6). It occurs in all age groups but is particularly frequent in younger and middle-aged adults; the median age is approximately 40 years.

Most t(9;22)-positive AML are morphologically classified as AML with or without maturation. The blasts often display both myeloid and lymphoid features that include rearrangements of the immunoglobulin heavy-chain and the T-cell receptor beta genes and expression of several lineage antigens, such as the stem cell antigen CD34, the myeloid markers CD13 and CD33, as well as the B-cell markers CD10 and CD19; this presumably reflects the immature nature of the hematopoietic cell in which the translocation arises (Chen et al., 1988; Tien et al., 1995; Cuneo et al., 1996; Casasnovas et al., 1998; Soupir et al., 2007). Only 1–2% of patients with t(9;22)-positive AML have a previous history of chemotherapy (Grimwade et al., 2010), and such t-AMLs are not specifically associated with any particular treatment modality—they may occur after radiotherapy alone or after chemotherapy with alkylating agents or DNA topoisomerase II inhibitors (Block et al., 2002; Mauritzson et al., 2002). That t(9;22)-positive AML responds poorly to chemotherapy, conferring a dismal prognosis, was shown already in the mid-1970s (Bloomfield et al., 1977), and subsequent studies confirmed that complete remission is rarely achieved with conventional chemotherapy alone (Cuneo et al., 1996; Soupir et al., 2007). However, treatment with imatinib seems to be beneficial (Cho et al., 2007; Shimizu et al., 2014).

Trisomy 10

Although trisomy 10 as the sole change is rare in AML, seen in approximately 0.5% of cases, it has nevertheless been associated with certain characteristic features (Morgan et al., 1996; Ohyashiki et al., 1996; Suzuki et al., 2000; Yuan et al., 2010). A relatively large proportion of the patients is of Asian descent, there is a male preponderance (SR 2.0), most patients are adults (median age 50 years), and most cases are de novo AML. Many display an immature morphology, that is, AML with minimal differentiation or without maturation, while the vast majority express the T-cell antigen CD7. The prognosis has been variably referred to as intermediate or poor.

t(10;11)(p12;q14) [*PICALM–MLLT10*]

More than 50 AML cases with t(10;11)(p12;q14), which fuses the *PICALM* and *MLLT10* genes (Dreyling et al., 1996; Kobayashi et al., 1997b), have been reported. It is, in this context, important to stress the presence of the *PICALM–MLLT10* fusion, because the t(10;11) may at the cytogenetic level easily be misinterpreted as a variant of the more common rearrangement between 10p12 and 11q23 that results in the *MLL–MLL10* fusion (see the following). The t(10;11) is the sole change in roughly half of the cases. Recurrent secondary changes include trisomies for chromosomes 4 and 19 and deletions of 17p (Borel et al., 2012).

The t(10;11), which is equally common in males and females, mainly occurs in children, adolescents, and young adults (median age 20 years). Extramedullary leukemia is present in the majority of patients. Although the t(10;11) may be found in most morphologic subtypes, many cases show a rather immature morphology, that is, AML with minimal differentiation or without maturation. Most cases are de novo AML, but approximately 20% are t-AML, in several instances after chemotherapy for diffuse large B-cell lymphoma. Immunophenotypically, t(10;11)-positive AML cases are often positive for CD13, CD33, CD34, CD65, CD117, HLA-DR, and MPO and the T-cell antigen CD7; in addition, rearrangements of the immunoglobulin heavy-chain and the T-cell receptor genes are common (Dreyling et al., 1998; La Starza et al., 2006; Caudell and Aplan, 2008: Borel et al., 2012). The prognosis has been reported to be intermediate or poor.

10p11.2–p12/11q23 rearrangements [*MLL–ABI1* or *MLL–MLLT10*]

Complex rearrangements involving 10p12 and 11q23, leading to an *MLL–MLLT10* chimera (Chaplin et al., 1995), occur in approximately 3% and 1% of childhood and adult AML, respectively

(Grimwade et al., 2010; Harrison et al., 2010), and comprise 20–25% of *MLL*-rearranged infant/pediatric AML and 5–10% of adult AML (Meyer et al., 2013). Additional abnormalities are found in two-thirds, with +8 and +19 as the most frequent.

The 10p12/11q23 abnormalities have been variably described as derivative chromosomes including t(10;11)(p12;q23), inv(11)(q13q23), and insertions of 10p into 11q or vice versa. The complexity of the various rearrangements, including more proximal 11q breakpoints, was investigated by Beverloo et al. (1995), who performed a detailed characterization of the changes and showed an opposite orientation of the two genes. Thus, two breaks as seen in a simple reciprocal translocation are not sufficient to create an in-frame fusion; at least three breaks are needed. Considering the cytogenetic heterogeneity of the various aberrations leading to *MLL–MLLT10*, acute myelomonocytic or monoblastic/monocytic leukemias (see the following) with abnormalities of 10p and 11q, almost irrespective of the bands involved, should be suspected to harbor this fusion. Hence, FISH or RT-PCR analyses should definitely be considered in such cases.

AML with 10p12/11q23 rearrangements are more common in males (SR 1.6) and are most often found in infants and children (median age 2 years). The first 10p12/11q23 rearrangement, an ins(10;11) (p11;q23q24) in an infant acute monoblastic/monocytic leukemia, was described by Kaneko et al. (1982), and soon afterward, several similar, often inverted, 11q insertions into 10p were identified in acute myelomonocytic or monoblastic/monocytic leukemias. Aberrations involving the same band at 10p but more proximal 11q bands were also reported (Carter et al., 1991); changes now known to represent der(10)t(10;11)(p12;q23) inv(11)(q13q23) based on the study by Beverloo et al. (1995). In the large series of 10p12/11q23-rearranged AML reported by Lillington et al. (1998) and Casillas et al. (2003), a close association with monoblastic and monocytic leukemias was confirmed. The vast majority are de novo leukemia. As for *MLL*-rearranged AML in general, hyperleukocytosis, central nervous system (CNS) involvement, and hepatosplenomegaly are common. Lillington et al. (1998) reported that children aged 1–14 years often achieved remission, whereas infants and elderly patients fared poorly. A dismal outcome in the latter age groups has subsequently been stressed in several studies (Dreyling et al., 1998; Casillas et al., 2003; Balgobind et al., 2009). In the international childhood study of Balgobind et al. (2009), another *MLL* partner, *ABI1*, was described at 10p11.2. Although the number of patients with this fusion was small, it was shown to have a dismal prognosis. From cytogenetic analysis alone, it is difficult to distinguish the *ABI1* fusion from *MLLT10*; therefore, molecular analysis is recommended.

t(10;11)(q21;q23) [*MLL–TET1*]

The 10q breakpoint in this rare *MLL* translocation is often designated as 10q22 but since the t(10;11) is known to involve the *TET1* gene (Ono et al., 2002b), mapping to 10q21.3, the latter chromosome band is used here. Among the approximately 10 AML cases with t(10;11) reported, it has been the sole change in most instances. The t(10;11) was first described in a monoblastic/monocytic leukemia by Thirman et al. (1993), and almost all subsequent cases have been de novo acute myelomonocytic or monoblastic/monocytic leukemia; BM dysplasia has been noted in several instances (Harrison et al., 1998; Lorsbach et al., 2003; Lee et al., 2013). Although t(10;11)-positive AML does occur in children, it is more common in adults (median age 40 years). There is no clear gender difference. Albeit based on few cases, most reported patients have succumbed to AML, indicating a poor prognostic impact of t(10;11).

t(10;16)(q22;p13) [*KAT6B–CREBBP*]

The t(10;16), which results in a *KAT6B–CREBBP* fusion (Panagopoulos et al., 2001), may be considered a rare variant of t(8;16) (see previous text) considering not only the molecular genetic similarities—both involve *CREBBP* and a member of the *KAT6* gene family—but also the clinical features (Panagopoulos et al., 2001; Vizmanos et al., 2003; Murati et al., 2004): most cases are myelomonocytic, monoblastic, or monocytic leukemias; there may be an overpresentation of females; it is found in infants, children, and, mainly younger, adults (median age 30 years); and the outcome has been dismal in most instances; however, in contrast to t(8;16)-positive AML, erythrophagocytosis seems to be rare.

Trisomy 11

Trisomy 11 is present in 2–3% of cytogenetically aberrant AML cases, as the single change in approximately 1% (Heinonen et al., 1998; Caramazza et al., 2010; Grimwade et al., 2010). Partial tandem duplication (PTD) of the *MLL* gene has been reported in a substantial proportion (25–90%) of cases, with the *MLL*-PTD being restricted to one of the three chromosomes 11 and relatively often associated with concomitant *FLT3*-ITD (Caligiuri et al., 1997; Slovak et al., 1995; Schnittger et al., 2000; Steudel et al., 2003; Rege-Cambrin et al., 2005; Alseraye et al., 2011). Although the *MLL*-PTD is most likely of importance, it may perhaps be too simplistic to ascribe the functionally essential consequence of +11 to the rearrangement of a single gene on that chromosome.

Trisomy 11-positive AML, which is equally common in men and women, mainly occurs in middle-aged and elderly patients (median age 60 years). Although trisomy 11 as a sole change in AML was reported already in the early 1980s (Hagemeijer et al., 1981; Yunis et al., 1981), it was not recognized as a nonrandom AML-associated aberration until Dang et al. (1985) reviewed a handful of such cases. Larger series have since been published identifying several clinical characteristics of AML with +11 (UKCCG, 1992a; Bilhou-Nabera et al., 1994; Slovak et al., 1995; Farag et al., 2002; Rege-Cambrin et al., 2005; Caramazza et al., 2010; Grimwade et al., 2010; Alseraye et al., 2011). The majority are de novo AML, at least in the sense that they are rarely associated with prior chemotherapy. However, many arise after a prior MDS phase and display trilineage dysplasia; hence, they are secondary AML. Most are AML with or without maturation or myelomonocytic leukemia with Auer rods and dysplastic features and express HLA-DR, CD13, CD15, CD33, CD34, and CD117. A poor response to chemotherapy and an unfavorable prognosis has been reported, with the outcome being particularly dismal for cases with *MLL*-PTD and/or *FLT3*-ITD.

inv(11)(p15q22) [*NUP98–DDX10*]

This inversion, generating a *NUP98–DDX10* fusion (Arai et al., 1997), has been described in more than 25 AML cases and been the sole anomaly in roughly 60%; the only recurrent secondary changes to date have been +8 and +21. The inv(11) is more common in males (SR 1.7) and occurs in all age groups (median age 40 years). The first AML cases with inv(11)—one de novo and one t-AML—were reported by Gibbons et al. (1987) and Pui et al. (1989), and subsequent studies have shown that almost half of all *NUP98–DDX10*-positive cases are t-AML, occurring after previous chemotherapy including DNA topoisomerase II inhibitors, with the prevalence of inv(11) being clearly higher in t-AML than in de novo AML (Kobayashi et al., 1997a; Nebral et al., 2005; Romana et al., 2006; Gorello et al., 2013). No specific morphologic subgroup has been associated with inv(11), and its prognostic implication remains unclear; however, the outcome has been reported to be dismal in some of the aforementioned studies.

t(11;12)(p15;p13) [*NUP98–KDM5A*]

This translocation, which is cytogenetically cryptic and leads to a *NUP98–KDM5*A fusion, was first reported in a 1-year-old child with AMKL (van Zutven et al., 2006). It has since been shown to be a recurrent abnormality in pediatric AMKL, occurring in approximately 10% of such cases (Gruber et al., 2012; de Rooij et al., 2013). In most instances, *NUP98–KDM5*A-positive cases are cytogenetically abnormal, often with hyperdiploid CK. The fusion gene is equally common in girls and boys and the median age is 2 years. Similar to the t(1;22) in AMKL (see previous text), the t(11;12) is not present in adult AMKL and none of the patients reported had DS. Clinically, t(11;12)-positive AMKL does not seem to differ from other pediatric AMKL, but the overall survival is dismal (de Rooij et al., 2013).

t(11;12)(p15;q13) [*NUP98–HOXC11(C13)*]

The t(11;12), resulting in a fusion between *NUP98* and *HOXC11* or *HOXC13* (Taketani et al., 2002c; Panagopoulos et al., 2003), has so far been reported in only 10 AML cases. This notwithstanding, certain genetic and clinical characteristics may be outlined (Wong et al., 1998; Gu et al., 2003; Tošić et al., 2009): it is almost always the sole chromosomal abnormality, is more common in females (SR 2.3), and is mostly detected in adult AML (median age 40 years). The majority are de novo AML with maturation, although some t-AML cases have been described. All reported patients have achieved complete remission after induction

therapy, but most have relapsed. Thus, the t(11;12) seems to be associated with a poor prognosis.

t(11;20)(p15;q12) [*NUP98–TOP1*]

Approximately 15 AML cases with t(11;20), leading to *NUP98–TOP1* (Ahuja et al., 1999), have been published, with the t(11;20) being the sole change in 80%; no recurrent secondary changes have been reported. The t(11;20) is clearly more common in women (SR 4.0) and is more frequent in younger patients; the median age is approximately 25 years. Although the first reported t(11;20)-positive case was a patient with polycythemia vera (Berger, 1975), subsequent cases have mainly been de novo AML or, in some instances, t-AML after multiagent chemotherapy including alkylators as well as DNA topoisomerase II poisons (Nebral et al., 2005; Romana et al., 2006). The morphology is variable, but most are AML with maturation or monoblastic/monocytic leukemias. The outcome is dismal.

11q gain [*MLL* amplification]

With the advent of FISH and locus-specific probes for the *MLL* gene in the 1990s, it was soon realized that approximately 1% of AML cases harbor intra- or extrachromosomal amplification of this gene, either in the form of double minutes, homogeneously staining regions, or ring chromosomes or as additional copies on other chromosomes (Tanaka et al., 1997; Allen et al., 1998; Andreasson et al., 1998; Ariyama et al., 1998; Felix et al., 1998; Avet-Loiseau et al., 1999). In most instances, the *MLL* gene is not rearranged. It should be emphasized that although the amplicons are not restricted to *MLL*, this gene has been shown to be differentially expressed in AML with 11q23 amplifications.

Most cases are cytogenetically complex, often hypodiploid with whole or partial losses of chromosomes 5 and 7 and *TP53* mutations. The morphology is variable, but AMLs with minimal differentiation or with/without maturation, often with BM dysplasia, are most common; in contrast to AML with *MLL* rearrangements, myelomonocytic, monoblastic, or monocytic leukemia is quite rare. The patients are mainly elderly (median age >60 years) with an overrepresentation of males (SR 1.6). There is relatively often a previous history of treatment with alkylating agents, and the prognosis has been reported to be extremely dismal, with minimal response to chemotherapy (Cuthbert et al., 2000; Michaux et al., 2000; Streubel et al., 2000; Andersen et al., 2001; Poppe et al., 2004; Zatkova et al., 2009).

t(11;16)(q23;p13) [*MLL–CREBBP*]

The t(11;16), leading to an *MLL–CREBBP* chimera (Sobulo et al., 1997; Taki et al., 1997), is a recurrent but relatively rare *MLL* translocation in AML, so far described in only approximately 15 cases, most often as the sole change. The first patient with t(11;16) reported had t-AML occurring after previous treatment with etoposide (Winick et al., 1993), and strikingly, all subsequent cases, with one exception, have been t-AML associated with prior therapy with topoisomerase II-targeting agents (Roulston et al., 1995; Rowley et al., 1997; Shali et al., 2006). The t(11;16) is equally common in females and males and has been described in both childhood and adult AML (median age 40 years). The morphologic subtypes have been acute myelo-monocytic or monoblastic/monocytic leukemia in most instances. The outcome has been variable, but many patients succumb to the disease, at least if treated with chemotherapy alone. Whether alloSCT improves the outcome remains to be elucidated.

t(11;17)(q23;q12) [*MLL–MLLT6*]

Approximately 50 AML cases with a translocation between 11q23 and 17q12~21 have been reported. Although almost identical at the cytogenetic level, cases with t(11;17) have been shown to differ molecularly as well as clinically. One group is characterized by various *MLL* fusions, all of them with genes mapping to 17q12 (Figure 6.11), whereas the other group involves the *RARA* gene at 17q21 and is associated with APL (see the following). Of the

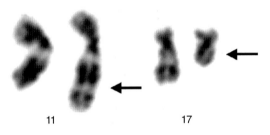

11   17

Figure 6.11 The t(11;17)(q23;q12) is associated with acute myelomonocytic and monoblastic/monocytic leukemia. Arrows indicate breakpoints.

approximately 35 non-APL cases reported with t(11;17), the translocation has been the sole change in 80%; the only recurrent secondary changes have been trisomy for chromosomes 5, 8, and 19. Three different genes on 17q12 have been shown to fuse to *MLL* as a consequence of t(11;17), namely *MLLT6*, *LASP1*, and *ACACA* (Prasad et al., 1994a; Strehl et al., 2003; Meyer et al., 2005). Involvement of the two latter genes is very rare; most t(11;17) result in *MLL–MLLT6* (Strehl et al., 2006; Meyer et al., 2013).

The t(11;17), which is equally common in males and females, almost exclusively occurs in AML in infants, children, adolescents, or young adults; the median age is 15 years. The first t(11;17)-positive AML published was a monoblastic leukemia (Zaccaria et al., 1982), and subsequent reports have confirmed a strong association with acute myelo-monocytic or monoblastic/monocytic leukemia, all of which, with one exception, were de novo AML (Harrison et al., 1998; Strehl et al., 2006). Little is known about the prognostic impact of t(11;17), but in the series compiled by Harrison et al. (1998), none of the patients was a long-term survivor, indicating a dismal outcome.

t(11;17)(q23;q21) [*ZBTB16–RARA*]

As mentioned earlier, the t(11;17) that rearranges the *RARA* gene, leading to a *ZBTB16–RARA* fusion (Chen et al., 1993), is cytogenetically almost indistinguishable from the one involving *MLL*. Among the roughly 15 APL cases with t(11;17) reported, the translocation has been the sole change in two-thirds. The only recurrent additional anomaly to date has been loss of the Y chromosome.

There is a pronounced male preponderance of t(11;17)-positive APL, with an SR of 10. Indeed, we know of no other abnormality in AML (except idic(X)(q13) in women and loss of the Y chromosome in males) that displays such a gender bias. As yet, t(11;17) has not been described in pediatric APL; instead, the patients have been young adults, middle aged, or elderly, with a median age of 55 years. The first patient had APL-like promyelocytes without Auer rods, and although treatment with ATRA resulted in myeloid maturation, no remission was achieved (Chen et al., 1993). Subsequent studies have shown that the t(11;17) is found in approximately 1% of all APL cases and that most patients present with a high percentage of promyelocytes in the BM and clinical and laboratory signs of disseminated intravascular coagulation. Notably, however, the BM morphology of t(11;17)-positive cases is not always easily classified as APL; instead, the blasts may have a regular round or oval nucleus, more suggestive of AML with maturation, and Pelger–Huët-like cells are common. However, similar to t(15;17)-positive APL, the blasts express CD13 and CD33 and are negative for HLA-DR and CD34, but in contrast to APL with t(15;17), aberrant CD56 expression is common in t(11;17)-positive APL (Scott et al., 1994; Licht et al., 1995; Koken et al., 1999; Grimwade et al., 2000; Sainty et al., 2000).

The initial reports of t(11;17) stressed the adverse prognostic impact of this abnormality, with poor response to conventional chemotherapy and/or ATRA. However, in the series published by Grimwade et al. (2000), complete remission was achieved in all patients treated with combination chemotherapy, half of whom also received ATRA, with the majority being alive at the time of reporting.

t(11;17)(q23;q25) [MLL–SEPT9]

More than 30 AML cases with t(11;17) leading to an MLL–SEPT9 fusion—the most common MLL–SEPT chimera in AML (Osaka et al., 1999; Taki et al., 1999; Cerveira et al., 2011)—have been published, with t(11;17) being the sole change in 65%. The most common secondary aberrations are trisomies 8 and 20.

The t(11;17) is somewhat more common in males (SR 1.4) and has been reported in all age groups but mainly in younger patients (median age 25 years). Although Yunis (1984) was the first to emphasize that t(11;17) was an AML-associated abnormality, single cases had already been reported in the late 1970s and early 1980s (Golomb et al., 1978; Mitelman et al., 1981). The translocation is particularly common in acute myelomonocytic and monoblastic/monocytic leukemia, but some are AML with or without maturation (Harrison et al., 1998; Santos et al., 2010; Lee et al., 2011). Roughly one-fifth of all cases are t-AML, mainly after chemotherapy that included DNA topoisomerase II inhibitors. The t(11;17) has been reported to confer a poor prognosis.

t(11;19)(q23;p13.1) [MLL–ELL]

Close to 200 AML cases with t(11;19)(q23;p13) have been reported. However, the t(11;19) is not a single entity, there are at least two different types of 11;19 translocation at the cytogenetic level (Huret et al., 1993; Moorman et al., 1998). The t(11;19)(q23;p13.1), that is, the one with a proximal 19p13 breakpoint, is identified cytogenetically as 11q+ and 19p− that are easier to detect by R-banding than by G-banding. In contrast, the t(11;19)(q23;p13.3) is seen as 11q− and 19p+ and is readily detected by G-banding but not by R-banding. The former is more often the sole aberration, whereas the latter is associated with additional changes in roughly half of the cases (Mrózek et al., 1997; Moorman et al., 1998; Bloomfield et al., 2002).

The t(11;19)(q23;p13.1), shown to fuse MLL with ELL by Thirman et al. (1994), is one of the most common 11q23 translocations in AML, constituting almost 20% of infant AML and 10% of pediatric and adult AML with MLL rearrangements (Balgobind et al., 2009; Meyer et al., 2013). However, it is nevertheless a relatively uncommon abnormality in AML in general, occurring in only 1% of cases (Byrd et al., 2002; Grimwade et al., 2010). It is equally common in males and females and found in all age groups, although most patients are adults with a median age of 50 years.

As is typical for MLL-rearranged AML, most MLL–ELL-positive cases are myelomonocytic or monoblastic/monocytic leukemias, and many are t-AML after previous therapy with DNA topoisomerase II inhibitors. Hepatosplenomegaly and massive leukocytosis are common, and the prognosis has been reported to be poor (Huret et al., 1993; Mrózek et al., 1997; Moorman et al., 1998; Secker-Walker et al., 1998; Bloomfield et al., 2002; Byrd et al., 2002; Chen et al., 2013).

t(11;19)(q23;p13.3) [MLL–MLLT1]

In contrast to the aforementioned t(11;19), the t(11;19)(q23;p13.3), resulting in the MLL–MLLT1 fusion (Tkachuk et al., 1992), is most often found in infant ALL. It is clearly less prevalent in AML (Meyer et al., 2013). Compared with MLL–ELL-positive cases, AML patients with MLL–MLLT1 are much younger (often infants); the median age was 7 years in the pediatric series reported by Balgobind et al. (2009). As for AML with MLL–ELL, cases with *MLL–MLLT1* do not display any gender-related frequency difference; most are myelomonocytic or monoblastic/monocytic leukemias expressing HLA-DR, CD13, CD14, CD15, CD33, and CD34; many are t-AML. Hepatosplenomegaly and leukocytosis are common and the outcome is dismal (Huret et al., 1993; Moorman et al., 1998; Balgobind et al., 2009).

t(11;22)(q23;q11) [*MLL–SEPT5*]

This is a rare *MLL* translocation that rearranges the *SEPT5* gene (Marukawa et al., 1996; Megonigal et al., 1998). To date, only approximately 10 AML cases with t(11;22) have been reported. It is the sole change in the majority of cases, occurs equally often in males and females, and is mainly found in young adults (median age 30 years). The translocation was first described in a de novo monoblastic leukemia by Kobayashi et al. (1990) and all t(11;22)-positive cases with this translocation described since have been de novo AML, often with maturation or myelomonocytic leukemia (Tatsumi et al., 2001; Cerveira et al., 2011). Due to the low number of cases reported, the clinical implications of t(11;22) remain to be elucidated.

del(12p)

Rearrangements resulting in loss of 12p, such as deletions, additions of unknown material, and unbalanced translocations, are seen in 1–2% of AML cases (Grimwade et al., 2010), most frequently (80%) in CK that often also harbor whole or partial losses of chromosomes 5 and 7. Several FISH studies have revealed that the 12p deletions are interstitial, with a minimal deleted region between the *ETV6* and the *CDKN1B* genes (Kobayashi et al., 1994; Sato et al., 1995; Höglund et al., 1996; Wlodarska et al., 1996; Andreasson et al., 1998). The target gene(s) has not been identified, but low expression of *CDKN1B* has been suggested to play a pathogenetic role (Haferlach et al., 2011b). Translocations involving 12p and usually *ETV6*, not always seen as part of a CK, are more frequent in children than in adults. Together with deletions, they comprise a newly defined subgroup of childhood AML (Harrison et al., 2010; von Neuhoff et al., 2010).

Deletions of 12p do not display any gender-related frequency difference, but mainly occur in adult AML (median age 50 years). Although the first AML cases, one de novo and one treatment related, with 12p loss were reported already in the mid-1970s (Yamada and Furusawa, 1976; Weinfeld et al., 1977), it took almost a decade before 12p deletions were clearly linked to AML. The morphology is quite variable and several cases are t-AML arising after treatment with alkylating agents or, less commonly, DNA topoisomerase II inhibitors (Wilmoth et al., 1985; Le Beau et al., 1986). AML with del(12p) is included either in the intermediate or poor prognosis risk groups by different study groups (Slovak et al., 2000; Byrd et al., 2002; Tallman et al., 2007; Grimwade et al., 2010). However, the subgroup of childhood AML with 12p abnormalities was confirmed to have a poor outcome in two independent studies (Harrison et al., 2010; von Neuhoff et al., 2010).

t(12;22)(p13;q12) [*MN1–ETV6*]

The t(12;22), generating an *MN1–ETV6* fusion (Buijs et al., 1995), is a rare translocation in AML, so far described in roughly 20 cases. It is seldom the only change; additional abnormalities are present in more than 80%, the most common being −7 and +21. AML with t(12;22) is equally common in men and women and mainly occurs in adults (median age 50 years). The t(12;22) was first described as a specific AML-related abnormality in two patients with de novo acute myelomonocytic leukemia by Callen et al. (1991), and it has since become apparent that this translocation is clearly associated with de novo AML; only one case to date has been t-AML (Haferlach et al., 2012b). The morphology is variable, with a majority being unclassifiable. Almost all patients reported have relapsed (Callen et al., 1991; Nakazato et al., 2001; Chen et al., 2007; Nofrini et al., 2011), strongly indicating a poor prognostic impact of this translocation.

Trisomy 13

Trisomy 13 is seen in 2–3% of karyotypically abnormal AML, being the sole change in 25% of these cases. When additional changes are present, trisomy 13 is generally not associated with any characteristic AML-related translocations or inversions; instead, it occurs together with other genomic imbalances, mainly numerical anomalies. However, +13 is fairly common in AML with t(6;9) (p22;q34). Little is known about the leukemogenic impact of +13. Because the *FLT3* gene is located in 13q12, *FLT3*-ITD was thought to be common in cases with trisomy 13, akin to *MLL*-PTD in AML with +11. However, this is clearly not the case (Powell et al., 2005). Instead, increased *FLT3* expression and *RUNX1* mutations have been shown to be present in almost all cases, indicating that these two changes cooperate in trisomy 13-associated leukemogenesis (Dicker et al., 2007; Silva et al., 2007).

Hsu et al. (1979) first associated +13, as the sole change, with myeloid malignancies. Since then, several larger series of trisomy 13-positive AML have been published (Döhner et al., 1990; Baer and Bloomfield, 1992; Soni et al., 1996; Mehta et al., 1998; Farag et al., 2002; Mesa et al., 2009), delineating characteristic features of this AML subgroup. Most patients are elderly males (SR 2.5 and median age 65 years) without any previous genotoxic treatment and presenting with leukocytosis. Although AML cases with +13 are morphologically heterogeneous, a substantial proportion has been classified as AML with minimal differentiation or without maturation, with the presence of +13 in the former subtype being associated with TdT expression (Patel et al., 2013). Transformation of an early hematopoietic cell has been implicated based on frequent expression of myeloid as well as lymphoid antigens. Other typical BM features include small blasts with few or no granules, hand-mirror blasts, lack of Auer rods, and trilineage dysplasia. All studies have emphasized a low complete remission rate and brief remission duration. Interestingly, morphologic and cytogenetic complete remission in a few cases treated with lenalidomide alone has been reported (Fehniger et al., 2009).

t(15;17)(q22;q21) [*PML–RARA*]

t(15;17) is the sole change in approximately 70% of cases, with +8 as the most common secondary change (10–15%). Other relatively frequent additional aberrations include del(7q); del(9q); ider(17)(q10)t(15;17), that is, an isochromosome of the derivative chromosome 17; and +21. Furthermore, *FLT3*-ITD and activating point mutations in *FLT3* have been shown to be present in 20–40% and 10–20% of cases, respectively (Kiyoi et al., 1997; Slack et al., 1997; Callens et al., 2005; Gale et al., 2005; Cervera et al., 2010; Grimwade et al., 2010; Barragán et al., 2011). The presence of secondary

changes has generally not been associated with a significantly worse outcome.

The t(15;17) (Figure 6.12), and its corresponding *PML–RARA* fusion (Borrow et al., 1990; de Thé et al., 1990; Longo et al., 1990), is considered pathognomonic for APL. Except for a few other *RARA* rearrangements in this disease entity (see the following), all APL cases harbor *PML–RARA*. Hence, the frequency of this gene fusion in AML almost equals that of APL.

Soon after the identification of *PML–RARA*, it was reported that this chimera also occasionally occurred in APL without the typical t(15;17), as a consequence of variant translocations or cytogenetically cryptic insertions, for example, ins(15;17)(q22;q21q21) and ins(17;15)(q21;q22q22) (Baranger et al., 1993; Hiorns et al., 1994; Grimwade et al., 1997). This finding highlighted the importance of combining cytogenetic and molecular genetic analyses in the accurate diagnosis of APL (Grimwade et al., 2000). Thus, if APL is suspected based on clinical, morphologic, or immunophenotypic grounds (see the following) but the t(15;17) is not seen cytogenetically, targeted analyses for the *PML–RARA* fusion should be considered mandatory, considering that the presence (or absence) of this abnormality is vital for proper treatment decision. Although FISH is a robust and quick method to detect *PML–RARA*, it should be stressed that some insertions resulting in this chimera are too small to be identified by FISH, at least if commercial probes are used (Kim et al., 2010; Campbell et al., 2013). Thus, it is definitely advisable to perform RT-PCR either at the time of diagnosis or when FISH results are negative if APL is suspected clinically.

As mentioned, although the *PML–RARA* fusion is by far the most common *RARA* rearrangement in APL, other genes have also been shown to fuse to *RARA* in APL, namely, *BCOR* [t(X;17)(p11;q21)],

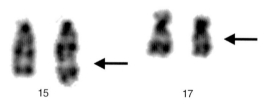

15   17

Figure 6.12 The t(15;17)(q22;q21) is pathognomonic for APL. Arrows indicate breakpoints.

FIP1L1 [t(4;17)(q12;q21)], *NABP1* [t(2;17)(q32;q21)], *NPM1* [t(5;17)(q35;q21); see previous text], *NUMA1* [t(11;17)(q13;q21)], *PRKAR1A* [t(17;17)(q21;q24)], *STAT5B* [rearrangement within 17q21], *TBLR1* [t(3;17)(q26;q21)], and *ZBTB16* [t(11;17)(q23;q21); see previous text]. Many of these display certain unique morphologic features, making them "APL-like," but most, although not all, are responsive to ATRA (Chen et al., 1993, 2014; Redner et al., 1996; Wells et al., 1997; Arnould et al., 1999; Catalano et al., 2007; Kondo et al., 2008; Yamamoto et al., 2010; Won et al., 2013).

In 1976, Rowley and Potter published a series of 50 cytogenetically analyzed AML cases, of which two were APL with a del(17)(q11q21) as the sole anomaly. These two cases were later presented separately by Golomb et al. (1976), who specifically associated the partial 17q deletions with APL. The same group (Rowley et al., 1977a) subsequently reported a third APL with "del(17q)." In that case, however, an abnormal 15q with a break in 15q22 was also observed. Based on these observations, and by reviewing the two former cases, they concluded that the karyotypic aberration in all three APL was an insertion of band 17q21 into 15q22. Kaneko and Sakurai (1977) and Okada et al. (1977), who had observed the same abnormality, suggested that it was a t(15;17)(q22;q21) rather than an insertion. Numerous subsequent studies soon confirmed their interpretation and firmly established t(15;17) as a remarkably specific APL-associated cytogenetic abnormality, occurring in close to 100% of pediatric as well as adult APL. The striking specificity of this clinicocytogenetic association is further underscored by the fact that when, albeit rarely, t(15;17) develops as a secondary change during CML BC, the ensuing AML exhibits disease characteristics indistinguishable from APL (Castaigne et al., 1984; Wiernik et al., 1991; Kashimura and Ohyashiki, 2010).

APL with t(15;17) is usually characterized by a predominance of abnormal promyelocytes with conspicuous granules and bundles of Auer rods, so-called faggot cells. In some instances, however, the cells are microgranular with an apparent paucity or absence of granules; these cells often have a bilobed nuclear shape. Rarely, a hyperbasophilic form is seen, with the leukemic cells typically having a strongly basophilic cytoplasm with no or only a few granules (Liso and Bennett, 2003). The blasts typically express CD13, CD33, CDw65, and CD117 but are most often negative for HLA-DR, CD4, CD7, CD10, CD11b, CD11c, CD14, CD16, CD34, and CD36; aberrant expression of CD2 is noteworthy (Ball et al., 1991; Marosi et al., 1992; Casasnovas et al., 1998; Guglielmi et al., 1998; Hrušák and Porwit-MacDonald, 2002; Dong et al., 2011). In fact, the immunophenotypic features are so characteristic that they alone strongly suggest a diagnosis of APL. Most APLs are de novo, but up to 20% of cases occur after previous chemotherapy, mainly with drugs targeting topoisomerase II, such as mitoxantrone and epirubicin (Detourmignies et al., 1992; Andersen et al., 2002; Joannides et al., 2011).

The outcome of APL is nowadays quite favorable, with the vast majority of patients achieving complete hematologic as well as molecular genetic remission when treated with chemotherapy combined with ATRA, arsenic trioxide or ATRA plus arsenic trioxide (Zhou et al., 2010; Lengfelder et al., 2012; Lo-Coco et al., 2013). However, the high tendency for disseminated intravascular coagulation still poses a serious threat at diagnosis—this is the main reason why rapid detection of *PML–RARA* using targeted analyses is important.

inv(16)(p13q22)/t(16;16)(p13;q22) [*CBFB–MYH11*]

The inv(16) (Figure 6.13) or t(16;16), which both result in a *CBFB–MYH11* fusion gene (Liu et al., 1993), is seen in 5% of pediatric and adult AML (Harrison et al., 2010; Grimwade et al., 2010), with the inversion being much more common (90–95%) than the translocation (5–10%); there are no clinical differences between inv(16)-positive and

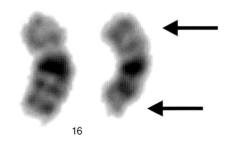

16

Figure 6.13 The inv(16)(p13q22) is characteristic for acute myelomonocytic leukemia with BM eosinophilia. Arrows indicate breakpoints.

t(16;16)-positive cases (Larson et al., 1986; Eghtedar et al., 2012). The inv(16)/t(16;16) is the sole anomaly in 70%. The most frequent secondary changes are, in decreasing frequency order, +22, +8, del(7q), and +21. In addition, *CBL*, *FLT3*, *KIT*, *KRAS*, and *NRAS* mutations and *NF1* deletions are present in 15–45% of cases (Haferlach et al., 2010; Paschka et al., 2013).

As the core-binding factor (CBF) transcription complex consists of the interacting proteins RUNX1, involved in t(8;21)(q22;q22) (see previous text), and CBFB, rearranged in inv(16)/t(16;16), cases with these changes are often referred to as "CBF AML." However, these two AML types should be seen as separate clinical entities with different prognostic implications, as emphasized by Marcucci et al. (2005) and shown in several studies (Appelbaum et al., 2006b; Kuwatsuka et al., 2009; Prébet et al., 2009).

Yunis et al. (1981) first described the inv(16) (p13q22) in a case of AML, and a few years later, a strong association between this inversion and acute myelomonocytic leukemia with abnormal BM eosinophils was reported by Le Beau et al. (1983). The variant t(16;16) was subsequently identified by Hogge et al. (1984). Based on these early studies as well as on numerous later investigations, inv(16)/t(16;16)-positive AML was recognized as a specific subgroup with typical morphologic, immunophenotypic, and clinical features. These characteristics are also important to take into account when performing cytogenetic analyses, as inv(16) is a subtle anomaly that may well escape detection in suboptimal chromosome preparations. Additional abnormalities of the inv(16), often translocations, are not uncommon and may mask the presence of this aberration (de la Chapelle and Lahtinen, 1983; Berger et al., 1995). Hence, if the inv(16) is not found by chromosome banding analysis but its presence is suspected based on clinical features, targeted analyses by FISH and/or RT-PCR should definitely be performed.

The inv(16)/t(16;16) is slightly more common in males (SR 1.3) and has been reported in all age groups, including infants as well as octogenarians. However, most patients are relatively young (median age 40 years). The majority of AML cases with inv(16)/t(16;16) are morphologically classified as acute myelomonocytic leukemia with a variable number of eosinophils at all stages of maturation,

often with nuclear blebs and Auer rods. The close association between these changes and BM eosinophilia is further supported by rare examples of inv(16)-positive CML BC displaying such features (Heim et al., 1992; Merzianu et al., 2005; Wu et al., 2006). This notwithstanding, a substantial proportion of cases belongs to other morphologic subgroups, mainly AML with maturation, and prior to the present WHO classification, some cases were diagnosed as MDS because the percentage of BM blasts was below the cutoff for AML (Campbell et al., 1991; Estey et al., 1992). The blasts typically express CD11, CD13, CD14, CD15, CD33, CD34, CD36, CDw65, CD117, and HLA-DR, with frequent aberrant expression of CD2 (Ball et al., 1991; Marosi et al., 1992; Adriaansen et al., 1993; Casasnovas et al., 1998; Hrušák and Porwit-MacDonald, 2002).

Several studies during the 1980s suggested that AML with inv(16)/t(16;16) had a propensity to relapse with CNS involvement, including leptomeningeal disease and intracerebral extramedullary leukemia (Holmes et al., 1985a; Glass et al., 1987; Ohyashiki et al., 1988), stressing the need for CNS prophylaxis. Although CNS leukemia nowadays is quite rare, possibly due to the protective effects of high-dose cytarabine therapy (Billström et al., 2002), it is still overrepresented in inv(16)/t(16;16)-positive AML cases (Shihadeh et al., 2012). Most patients present with marked leukocytosis (Grimwade et al., 1998; Delaunay et al., 2003), and the vast majority are de novo AML, with less than 5% occurring after previous chemotherapy (Mauritzson et al., 2002; Grimwade et al., 2010); these t-AML cases are characterized by prior exposure to DNA topoisomerase II inhibitors or radiotherapy, a short latency period, and absence of an antecedent MDS phase (Quesnel et al., 1993; Andersen et al., 2002).

Almost all studies have identified a favorable prognosis for patients with inv(16)/t(16;16)-positive AML; in fact, some investigators have reported that these patients have the best outcome of all cytogenetic AML subgroups, at least in adults. Additional chromosomal changes do not seem to confer a negative prognostic impact; in contrast, the presence of +22 has actually been reported to predict an improved outcome (Marlton et al., 1995; Schlenk et al., 2004; Marcucci et al., 2005; Prébet et al., 2009; Grimwade et al., 2010; Paschka et al., 2013). Treatment including high-dose cytarabine has been shown to be particularly effective, akin to the situation in t(8;21)-positive AML (Ghaddar et al., 1994; Bloomfield et al., 1998; Appelbaum et al., 2006b). However, some features have been associated, although not consistently, with an inferior outcome, namely, advanced age, leukocytosis, and *KIT* mutations (Delaunay et al., 2003; Appelbaum et al., 2006b; Paschka et al., 2006, 2013; Prébet et al., 2009; Pollard et al., 2010; Cairoli et al., 2013).

inv(16)(p13q24) [*CBFA2T3–GLIS2*]

The *CBFA2T3–GLIS2* fusion was identified in pediatric AMKL by the use of transcriptome sequencing (Gruber et al., 2012; Thiollier et al., 2012). This gene chimera, which is generated by a cryptic inv(16)(p13q24), was reported to be present in almost 30% of non-DS AMKL and to be associated with a significantly worse outcome compared with *CBFA2T3–GLIS2*-negative cases. Masetti et al. (2013) subsequently not only confirmed the poor prognostic impact of *CBFA2T3–GLIS2* but also identified this gene fusion in other morphologic subgroups of pediatric AML. However, de Rooij et al. (2013), who observed a lower frequency (12%) of *CBFA2T3–GLIS2* in childhood AMKL, did not find any evidence for a particularly poor outcome compared with other AMKL patients. Based on data extracted from the studies referred to in the previous text, the majority of *CBFA2T3–GLIS2*-positive cases are cytogenetically abnormal, most often with near-diploid karyotypes, the median age is 1 year, and there is an overrepresentation of girls (SR 1.9).

t(16;21)(p11;q22) [*FUS–ERG*]

Almost 60 AML cases with t(16;21) have been reported, with the translocation being the sole change in two-thirds; the most frequent secondary changes are +8, +10, and +12. The t(16;21) results in a *FUS–ERG* fusion (Ichikawa et al., 1994; Panagopoulos et al., 1994; Prasad et al., 1994b); interestingly, the same chimera has been identified also in a single case of ALL (Kanazawa et al., 2005) and in a few Ewing tumors (Shing et al., 2003). The t(16;21), which is somewhat more common in males (SR 1.3), occurs in most age groups, although most often in older children and younger adults (median age 25 years).

The t(16;21), albeit with a slightly different 16p breakpoint, was first described by Mecucci

et al. (1985), and shortly afterward, several additional patients, all from Japan, were reported (Minamihisamatsu and Ishihara, 1988; Yao et al., 1988). In fact, a substantial proportion of published t(16;21)-positive AML has been from Asia. Initially, the t(16;21) was thought to represent a variant of the more common t(8;21) because of the common 21q22 breakpoint, but the molecular genetic consequences are completely different and so are, to a large extent, the clinical features (Sadamori et al., 1990; Kong et al., 1997; Shikami et al., 1999; Imashuku et al., 2000; Kim et al., 2009; Jekarl et al., 2010). However, similar to AML with t(8;21), BM eosinophilia is common, often with dysplastic eosinophils, but in contrast to t(8;21)-positive AML, Auer rods are rare. The morphology is quite heterogeneous, but AML with or without maturation is most frequent and hemophagocytosis has been noted in several cases. The t(16;21)-positive blasts are often positive for CD11, CD13, CD18, CD33, CD34, CD117, and HLA-DR, with frequent expression of CD56, cytoplasmic myeloperoxidase, and the interleukin-2 receptor α chain. A dismal outcome has been stressed by most investigators.

t(16;21)(q24;q22) [*RUNX1–CBFA2T3*]

This translocation, generating a *RUNX1–CBFA2T3* fusion (Gamou et al., 1998), is a relatively rare abnormality, so far reported in slightly more than 20 AML cases. It is the sole change in 25%, with trisomy 8 as the only recurrent additional aberration, seen in 50%. Although the t(16;21) was initially described in a childhood AML (Raimondi et al., 1989b), most patients since have been adults, with a median age of 40 years and with an overrepresentation of women (SR 2.3). Morphologically, the vast majority have been AML with maturation. Traweek et al. (1994) first reported a t(16;21)-positive AML secondary to prior chemotherapy and an association between t(16;21) and t-AML, often after treatment with the topoisomerase II inhibitors etoposide and/or mitoxantrone, has subsequently been confirmed. In fact, 50% of cases are t-AML, with the initial tumor relatively often being breast cancer, something that may explain the predominance of females (Berger et al., 1996; Slovak et al., 2002; Boils and Mohamed, 2008). The outcome has been variable, but most published cases have succumbed to AML, indicating a poor prognosis.

del(17p)

Rearrangements leading to loss of 17p—deletions, additions, unbalanced translocations, and dicentric chromosomes—are seen in 2% of cytogenetically abnormal AML cases, in the vast majority (>98%) within CK that often also display losses of chromosomes 5, 7, and 18. Thus, a 17p deletion is seldom the sole change in AML. The 17p losses almost always include the *TP53* gene, and mutations of the remaining *TP53* allele are common (Lai et al., 1995; Wang et al., 1997; Soenen et al., 1998; Castro et al., 2000). Another abnormality that leads to deletion of 17p is i(17q), but as AML cases with this isochromosome seem to be genetically and clinically distinct from other 17p-deleted AMLs, they are discussed separately in the following.

Deletions of 17p are extremely rare in pediatric AML—they are mainly seen in elderly AML patients (median age 60 years), with a slight overrepresentation of men (SR 1.4). The morphology is quite variable, with many cases being unclassifiable. A characteristic feature, however, is the presence of dysgranulocytopoiesis and pseudo-Pelger–Huët cells (Lai et al., 1995). An association between 17p deletions, most often in complex, hypodiploid karyotypes also harboring chromosome 5 and 7 losses, and previous chemotherapy was noted already in the late 1970s and early 1980s (Rowley et al., 1977b; Sandberg et al., 1982). Such a correlation was subsequently confirmed in several studies, associating 17p loss with prior therapy with alkylating agents or hydroxyurea (Wang et al., 1997; Sterkers et al., 1998; Merlat et al., 1999; Mauritzson et al., 2002). A poor prognosis has been emphasized in all studies, and del(17p) is included as a high-risk abnormality in most treatment protocols; even after alloSCT, the outcome is dismal (Merlat et al., 1999; Slovak et al., 2000; Byrd et al., 2002; Farag et al., 2006; Seifert et al., 2009; Grimwade et al., 2010; Mohr et al., 2013; Lazarevic et al., 2014; Middeke et al., 2014).

i(17q)

Although most often referred to as an isochromosome—i(17)(q10)—this abnormality is in fact isodicentric, with breakpoints in 17p11, and should hence formally be designated idic(17)(p11) (Fioretos et al., 1999). However, for the sake of brevity, i(17q) is used in the following.

More than 150 AML cases with i(17q) have been published; the i(17q) has been the sole change in 40%. Thus, it is much more frequently a single change compared with other abnormalities resulting in 17p loss (see previous text). Common additional abnormalities include, in order of decreasing frequency, +8, −7, +13, and −5; in contrast to AML cases with del(17p), partial 5q and 7q deletions are rare. It should be stressed that i(17q) is not specific for AML; it is seen in several other hematologic malignancies, such as ALL, CML in BC, MDS, and myeloproliferative neoplasms as well as in a wide variety of solid tumors. In fact, i(17q) is by far the most frequent neoplasia-associated "isochromosome" overall (Mertens et al., 1994). The essential molecular genetic consequences of i(17q) are unknown. As it results in loss of the *TP53* gene, it was initially surmised that the functional outcome would be loss of one *TP53* allele with an inactivating mutation of the other allele. However, and in contrast to del(17p)-positive cases, *TP53* mutations are rare in AML with i(17q) (Schütte et al., 1993; Fioretos et al., 1999; Kanagal-Shamanna et al., 2012).

As a sole change, i(17q) is more common in males (SR 2.0) and is found almost exclusively in elderly patients (median age >65 years). The first AML with i(17q) was reported by Mitelman et al. (1973), and by the early 1980s, it had been firmly established as an AML-associated aberration (Borgström et al., 1982). As a single anomaly, i(17q) has been described in all morphologic subtypes, except acute erythroid leukemia and basophilic leukemia, with most cases being unclassifiable. Studies of (17q)-positive AML have delineated several characteristic features, such as male gender, advanced age, splenomegaly and/or hepatomegaly, prominent basophilia and eosinophilia, hypercellular BM, dysgranulocytopoiesis and dysmegakaryocytopoiesis, and positivity for CD13, CD33, CD34, CD38, CD117, HLA-DR, and myeloperoxidase (Weh et al., 1990; Kanagal-Shamanna et al., 2012). Whereas a substantial proportion of t-AML with del(17p) have been reported, as discussed earlier, cases with i(17q) as the sole change are almost always de novo AML, but like other 17p deletions, i(17q) is associated with a poor prognosis.

del(20q)

Deletions of the long arm of chromosome 20 are found in 1–2% of cytogenetically abnormal AML, and in one-third, the del(20q) is the sole anomaly. Abnormalities in addition to del(20q) include, in decreasing frequency order, –7, del(5q), +8, –18, –17, del(7q), and –5. Hence, it is not a common secondary change to AML-associated translocations/inversions.

Several lines of evidence indicate that del(20q) is not sufficient for overt leukemia. First, the proportion of mitoses with this abnormality, at least in MDS and myeloproliferative neoplasms, may decrease, occasionally even disappear, in subsequent cytogenetic analyses in the absence of treatment (Aatola et al., 1992; Matsuda et al., 2000). Second, there are a few examples of del(20q)-containing BM from patients with undiagnosed MDS being used successfully for transplantation, showing that such cells can home to the BM, proliferate, differentiate, and yield normal peripheral blood values (Redei et al., 1997; Mielcarek et al., 2006). Finally, and most important, del(20q) has been observed in patients with morphologically normal BM without cytopenia (Matsuda et al., 2000; Steensma et al., 2003).

Le Beau et al. (1985) showed that 20q deletions are interstitial and numerous subsequent studies have attempted to delineate minimally common deleted segments that might harbor pathogenetically important genes (Roulston et al., 1993; Bench et al., 2000; Huh et al., 2010; Okada et al., 2012). However, no confirmed target gene has been identified to date. Deletion of 20q as an isolated change is more common in men (SR 1.7). It is very rare in childhood AML, occurring mainly in elderly patients (median age >60 years). The morphology is highly variable, with no subtype being particularly common. The majority are de novo AML; only 10% are associated with previous chemotherapy, most often given for a prior myeloproliferative neoplasm (that may well have harbored 20q− before treatment). The prognostic impact of del(20q) is somewhat unclear. It is definitely not a favorable abnormality, as it is in MDS (Chapter 7); instead, it has variously been reported to be associated with either an intermediate or an unfavorable outcome (Campbell and Garson, 1994; Byrd et al., 2002; Farag et al., 2006).

Trisomy 21

Trisomy 21 is seen in 3–5% of pediatric and adult AML (Harrison et al., 2010; Grimwade et al., 2010), making it the third most common numerical anomaly, after +8 and –7, in this disease. It is most often (80%) present together with other aberrations, mainly other trisomies such as +6, +8, +19, and +22; monosomy 7 is also frequent (Harrison et al., 2010). It is also a relatively common secondary change to inv(16)/t(16;16). Among cases with trisomy 21 as the sole change, subclones with +8 are seen in 10%. The pathogenetically important consequence of trisomy 21 is unclear. However, mutations of the RUNX1 gene are found in approximately 50% of cases (Preudhomme et al., 2000; Snaddon et al., 2002; Taketani et al., 2003; Larsson et al., 2012).

Trisomy 21 as a sole change is somewhat more common in men (SR 1.4) and is seen in all age groups, although most often in younger patients (median age 40 years). It is not strongly associated with any specific morphologic subgroup, although it has been suggested to be particularly frequent in acute monoblastic/monocytic leukemia (Larsson et al., 2012). Little is known about the immunophenotypic features, but positivity for CD13, CD14, CD15, CD33, and MPO seems to be typical and aberrant CD7 expression has been noted in some cases (Cheng et al., 2009a; Yamamoto et al., 2002). The vast majority (95%) are de novo AML. The clinical impact of +21 is debatable; it has been associated with both intermediate and unfavorable prognosis (Cortes et al., 1995; Gale et al., 1995; Farag et al., 2002; Schaich et al., 2002; Grimwade et al., 2010).

Trisomy 22

Gain of chromosome 22 is found in 2–3% of cytogenetically abnormal AML, a frequency on par with +11 and +13. In the majority (90%) of cases, trisomy 22 occurs together with other changes, most often numerical anomalies such as +6, +8, +13, +19, and +21. Trisomy 22 is also the most common secondary chromosomal change to inv(16)/t(16;16). In fact, Grois et al. (1989) suggested that AML with +22 as the "sole" anomaly frequently, perhaps always, harbor this inversion. This has since been confirmed in several (Wong and Kwong, 1999; Litmanovich et al., 2000; Mitterbauer et al., 2000; Xu et al., 2008), but not all (Langabeer et al., 1998), studies addressing this issue. The molecular genetic consequences of +22 remain unknown. In contrast to +4, +8, +11, +13, and +21 in AML, trisomy 22 has, until now, not been associated with any specific gene mutations.

Isolated trisomy 22 is more frequent in men (SR 2.1). It is quite rare in children—no patient below the age of 10 has been described to date—occurring mainly in young adults (median age 30 years). All published cases have been de novo AML. Although +22 has been reported in several different morphologic subgroups, a substantial proportion has been acute myelomonocytic leukemia, many with pronounced BM eosinophilia (Najfeld et al., 1986; Niemeyer et al., 1986; UKCCG, 1992a); they may have had an undetected inv(16). The clinical impact of +22 has not been addressed in any large series, but AML cases with gain of this chromosome are usually included in the intermediate-risk group by default, that is, it is considered neither a favorable nor an adverse abnormality (Grimwade et al., 2010).

t(X;6)(p11;q23) [MYB–GATA1]

The t(X;11) is a rare abnormality resulting in a *MYB–GATA1* fusion (Quelen et al., 2011) that has only been described in a handful of AML cases, in all instances as the sole change. It is noteworthy that all patients have been male infants who, with one exception, were diagnosed with acute basophilic leukemia and had clinical signs of hyperhistaminemia, that is, urticarial rashes and gastrointestinal disorders (Dastugue et al., 1997; Chessells et al., 2002; Quelen et al., 2011). Despite the young age, all patients remain alive at the time of reporting, several of them in long-term complete remission, indicating a favorable prognosis.

Xq24/11q23
rearrangements [MLL–SEPT6]

Rearrangements involving Xq24 and 11q23, fusing *MLL* with *SEPT6* (Borkhardt et al., 2001), have been reported in approximately 15 AML cases, most often as the sole change. Occasionally, the abnormality is interpreted as a balanced reciprocal t(X;11)(q24;q23). However, akin to 10p12/11q23 rearrangements generating the *MLL–MLLT10* chimera, the opposite orientation of the *MLL* and *SEPT6* genes preludes an in-frame fusion unless at least three chromosome breaks take place. Thus, *MLL–SEPT6* fusions are the result of inverted insertions such as ins(X;11)

(q24;q23q23), ins(X;11)(q24;q23q13), and ins(11;X) (q23;q24q24) (Borkhardt et al., 2001; Ono et al., 2002a; Fu et al., 2003).

The first reported patient with an Xq24/11q23 rearrangement was an infant with acute monocytic leukemia (Köller et al., 1989), and all *MLL–SEPT6*-positive cases since, with one exception, have been pediatric, most often infant, de novo AML, without any clear gender-related frequency difference. AML with maturation has been the most common subtype, followed by acute myelomonocytic and monoblastic/monocytic leukemias (Harrison et al., 1998; Borkhardt et al., 2001; Ono et al., 2002a; Cerveira et al., 2008, 2011). The outcome has varied, but it should be noted that most cases treated with alloSCT were alive at the time of reporting.

Loss of the Y chromosome

Already in the prebanding era, Jacobs et al. (1963) reported that the frequency of Y chromosome loss in normal blood lymphocytes increases with age in healthy men. It was subsequently shown that loss of Y (LOY) in BM cells is fairly common in elderly males without hematologic malignancy (O'Riordan et al., 1970; Secker-Walker, 1971); thus, LOY should in most cases be accepted as a normal age-related phenomenon without any leukemogenic significance (Pierre and Hoagland, 1972; Sandberg and Sakurai, 1973; Abe et al., 1980; UKCCG, 1992b). However, Secker-Walker (1971) hypothesized that men with LOY could be predisposed to hematologic disease and, interestingly, mosaic LOY in peripheral blood was recently associated with shorter survival and increased risk of cancer (Forsberg et al., 2014).

Sometimes, however, LOY behaves like a bona fide AML-associated abnormality by disappearing in remission (Holmes et al., 1985b; Riske et al., 1994). Wiktor et al. (2000) reported that the percentages of BM metaphases with LOY differ between hematologically healthy controls and males with AML, with the latter generally displaying higher levels of LOY, suggesting that the presence of greater than 75% cells with LOY probably represents an AML-associated clone. However, as such a high frequency of LOY also can be seen in BM samples with no evidence of disease (Wong et al., 2008; Wiktor et al., 2011), this cutoff cannot be used in clinical decision making.

In AML, LOY is seen in almost 10% of cytogenetically abnormal cases, most often (85%) together with other changes, in particular t(8;21)(q22;q22). LOY as a sole change is, as expected, mainly found in middle-aged or elderly men (median age 60 years). Morphologically, AML with LOY is highly variable, with no subtype preference, although Auer rods have been reported to be common (Billström et al., 1987; Keating et al., 1987). AML with LOY is included in the intermediate-risk group (Holmes et al., 1985b; Keating et al., 1987; Schouten et al., 1991; Slovak et al., 2000; Byrd et al., 2002).

Characteristic karyotypic patterns in AML

During the early 1970s, several attempts were made to subgroup AML cases cytogenetically into prognostically relevant categories. For example, when cases were trichotomized into AA (only abnormal metaphases), AN (a mixture of abnormal and normal metaphases), and N (only normal metaphases), "N-patients" were shown to fare better than "AN-patients," with "AA-patients" having the worst outcome (Sakurai and Sandberg, 1973; FIWCL, 1978; Golomb et al., 1978). However, with the advent of chromosome banding techniques and the identification of several AML-associated translocations, inversions, deletions, and gains, the focus changed from clinical studies of general karyotypic patterns to analyses of the clinical features associated with specific chromosomal changes. Nevertheless, some karyotypic patterns in AML remain clinically important, either by conferring a poor prognostic impact, for example, CK or MK, or by necessitating further molecular genetic analyses for accurate risk stratification, for example, NK.

Complex Karyotype (CK)

That the number of chromosomal changes present in AML was associated with outcome was reported already in the mid-1970s by Trujillo et al. (1974) and Sakurai and Sandberg (1976), who compared cases harboring "minor karyotypic abnormalities," involving one or two chromosomes, with those having "major karyotypic abnormalities," that is, three or more changes, revealing that the latter group had an inferior prognosis. The term CK was

introduced in the 1980s to denote the presence of multiple aberrations, with several studies confirming a poor prognostic impact of CK (Yunis et al., 1984; Levin et al., 1986; Berger et al., 1987; Weh et al., 1988; Arthur et al., 1989; Fenaux et al., 1989). Furthermore, CK was associated with monosomies 5 and 7 and deletions of 5q, 7q, 12p, and 17p, high age, and t-AML. In fact, AML with CK is a distinct entity characterized by certain genomic imbalances and a specific gene expression pattern; in addition, *TP53* mutations are frequent and prognostically ominous (Schoch et al., 2005a; Bowen et al., 2009; Rücker et al., 2012; Volkert et al., 2014). However, it should be emphasized that CK does not always imply the same thing. First, it is variably defined as ≥3, ≥4, or ≥5 abnormalities by different investigators. Second, AML with favorable abnormalities, such as t(8;21), t(15;17), inv(16)/t(16;16), or t(9;11), may well be CK in the sense that they may harbor greater than or equal to 3 abnormalities but that does not "upgrade" them into the adverse group. Third, whereas it is clear that a hypodiploid karyotype with losses of 5q, 7q, and 17p should be considered high risk, the question of how to group hyperdiploid CK has rarely been addressed (Chilton et al., 2014).

AML with CK is less common in pediatric (10–15%) than in adult AML (15–40%), with the frequency generally increasing by age and with the prevalence clearly higher in t-AML (Raimondi et al., 1999; Slovak et al., 2000; Schoch et al., 2001, Mauritzson et al., 2002; Harrison et al., 2010; von Neuhoff et al., 2010; Lazarevic et al., 2014). The morphology is variable, but CK is particularly common in AML with minimal differentiation, acute erythroid leukemia, and AMKL. Today, AML cases with CK are included in the adverse risk group in most, if not all, treatment protocols. However, it should be stressed that CK is not always an independent risk factor when other parameters are taken into account, such as age, performance status, and presence of a chromosome change, such as monosomy 7, known to confer a poor prognostic impact. Reinforcing these exceptions, childhood AML with a CK in which those cases with good and adverse chromosomal abnormalities are removed is not considered high risk on current treatment trials (Harrison et al., 2010).

Monosomal Karyotype (MK)

The term monosomal karyotype (MK), coined by Breems et al. (2008), refers to two or more distinct autosomal monosomies or one single autosomal monosomy in the presence of structural abnormalities, excluding ring chromosomes and markers. As for CK, MK is not applicable for AML with t(8;21), t(15;17), or inv(16)/t(16;16). MK-AML constitutes 10–15% of all AML, with the percentage of MK-positive cases increasing with age. The morphology is, as for CK, variable.

Breems et al. (2008) presented evidence suggesting that MK provided better prognostic prediction than CK, although there was an overlap, as expected, between CK- and MK-positive cases. Similar findings were soon reported by other investigators; however, not all have confirmed an independent prognostic role of MK in multivariate analyses (Medeiros et al., 2010b; Perrot et al., 2011; Kayser et al., 2012; Haferlach et al., 2012a; Yanada et al., 2012; Lazarevic et al., 2014).

Normal Karyotype (NK)

As seen in Table 6.2, 20–25% of pediatric AML and 40–50% of adult AML do not harbor any cytogenetically identifiable abnormalities, that is, they have an NK. In some instances, the reasons are most likely technical, including division of only the nonneoplastic cells in culture or poor chromosome morphology precluding accurate analysis. Indeed, and as mentioned in the separate sections earlier, several translocations and inversions may go undetected in suboptimal preparations, such as inv(3)(q21q26), t(6;11)(q27;q23), t(11;19)(q23;p13), and inv(16)(p13q22). Furthermore, some abnormalities are cytogenetically cryptic, for example, t(5;11)(q35;p15), t(11;12)(p15;p13), and inv(16)(p13q24).

The aforementioned notwithstanding, most NK-AML cases are truly cytogenetically normal, at least in the sense that they do not harbor any known AML-associated translocations or inversions. However, they are definitely not genetically normal. For example, single-nucleotide polymorphism (SNP) array analyses have revealed partial uniparental isodisomies in 10–30% of NK-AML, and it has been shown that such regions frequently harbor mutated genes that through somatic recombination have become homozygous, such as CEBPA, FLT3, JAK2, NPM1, and RUNX1 mutations

(Fitzgibbon et al., 2005; Gorletta et al., 2005; Raghavan et al., 2005; Akagi et al., 2009; Bullinger et al., 2010). In addition, SNP array studies have disclosed cytogenetically cryptic copy number alterations in 25–50% of NK-AML cases (Akagi et al., 2009; Radtke et al., 2009; Tiu et al., 2009; Walter et al., 2009; Bullinger et al., 2010; Parkin et al., 2010; Yi et al., 2011). The heterogenous frequencies and patterns of such imbalances may possibly, at least partly, explain the clinical heterogeneity of NK-AML.

Furthermore, it is now well known that the presence of certain gene mutations provides important prognostic information, something that today is used in clinical practice: FLT3-ITDs are associated with a dismal outcome, whereas NPM1 and CEBPA mutations confer a favorable prognosis. More recently, numerous analyses, including next-generation sequencing, of NK-AML cases have identified several novel gene mutations, many of which were shown to be particularly common in NK-AML and often associated with an inferior outcome, involving, for example, ASXL1, BCOR, DNMT3A, IDH1, and IDH2 (Ley et al., 2008; Mardis et al., 2009; Metzeler et al., 2011; Grossmann et al., 2011; Walker and Marcucci, 2012; Estey, 2013; Martelli et al., 2013; The Cancer Genome Atlas Research, 2013).

Thus, from generally having been considered a rather uninteresting karyotypic AML subgroup, without any notable prognostic impact, NK-AML has emerged as an important subtype that, based on molecular events, can now be further divided into clinically relevant entities.

Acknowledgments

Financial support from the Swedish Cancer Society, the Swedish Childhood Cancer Foundation, the Swedish Research Council, Leukaemia and Lymphoma Research, UK, and Kay Kendall Leukaemia Fund is gratefully acknowledged.

References

Aatola M, Armstrong E, Teerenhovi L, Borgström GH (1992): Clinical significance of the del(20q) chromosome in hematologic disorders. *Cancer Genet Cytogenet* 62:75–80.

Abe S, Golomb HM, Rowley JD, Mitelman F, Sandberg AA (1980): Chromosomes and causation of human cancer and leukemia. XXXV. The missing Y in acute non-lymphocytic leukemia (ANLL). *Cancer* 45:84–90.

Adriaansen HJ, te Boekhorst PAW, Hagemeijer AM, Van Der Schoot CE, Delwel HR, Van Dongen JJM (1993): Acute myeloid leukemia M4 with bone marrow eosinophilia (M4Eo) and inv(16)(p13q22) exhibits a specific immuno-phenotype with CD2 expression. *Blood* 81:3043–3051.

Ahuja HG, Felix CA, Aplan PD (1999): The t(11;20) (p15;q11) chromosomal translocation associated with therapy-related myelodysplastic syndrome results in an NUP98-TOP1 fusion. *Blood* 94:3258–3261.

Ahuja HG, Hong J, Aplan PD, Tcheurekdjian L, Forman SJ, Slovak ML (2000): t(9;11)(p22;p15) in acute myeloid leukemia results in a fusion between NUP98 and the gene encoding transcriptional coactivators p52 and p75-lens epithelium-derived growth factor (LEDGF). *Cancer Res* 60:6227–6229.

Akagi T, Ogawa S, Dugas M, Kawamata N, Yamamoto G, Nannya Y, et al. (2009): Frequent genomic abnormalities in acute myeloid leukemia/myelodysplastic syndrome with normal karyotype. *Haematologica* 94:213–223.

Akahoshi M, Oshimi K, Mizoguchi H, Okada M, Enomoto Y, Watanabe Y (1987): Myeloproliferative disorders terminating in acute megakaryoblastic leukemia with chromosome 3q26 abnormality. *Cancer* 60:2654–2661.

Akiki S, Dyer SA, Grimwade D, Ivey A, Abou-Zeid N, Borrow J, et al. (2013): NUP98-NSD1 fusion in association with FLT3-ITD mutation identifies a prognostically relevant subgroup of pediatric acute myeloid leukemia patients suitable for monitoring by real time quantitative PCR. *Genes Chromosomes Cancer* 52:1053–1064.

Albin M, Björk J, Welinder H, Tinnerberg H, Mauritzson N, Johansson B, et al. (2000): Acute myeloid leukemia and clonal chromosome aberrations in relation to past exposure to organic solvents. *Scand J Work Environ Health* 26:482–491.

Allen RJ, Smith SD, Moldwin RL, Lu M-M, Giordano L, Vignon C, et al. (1998): Establishment and characterization of a megakaryoblast cell line with amplification of MLL. *Leukemia* 12:1119–1127.

Alseraye FM, Zuo Z, Bueso-Ramos C, Wang S, Medeiros LJ, Lu G (2011): Trisomy 11 as an isolated abnormality in acute myeloid leukemia is associated with unfavorable prognosis but not with an NPM1 or KIT mutation. *Int J Clin Exp Pathol* 4:371–377.

Andersen MK, Christiansen DH, Kirchhoff M, Pedersen-Bjergaard J (2001): Duplication or amplification of chromosome band 11q23, including the unrearranged MLL gene, is a recurrent abnormality in therapy-related MDS and AML, and is closely related to mutation of the TP53 gene and to previous therapy with alkylating agents. *Genes Chromosomes Cancer* 31:33–41.

Andersen MK, Larson RA, Mauritzson N, Schnittger S, Jhanwar SC, Pedersen-Bjergaard J (2002): Balanced chromosome abnormalities inv(16) and t(15;17) in therapy-related myelodysplastic syndromes and acute leukemia: report from an international workshop. *Genes Chromosomes Cancer* 33:395–400.

Andreasson P, Johansson B, Billström R, Garwicz S, Mitelman F, Höglund M (1998): Fluorescence in situ hybridization analyses of hematologic malignancies reveal frequent cytogenetically unrecognized 12p rearrangements. *Leukemia* 12:390–400.

Appelbaum FR, Gundacker H, Head DR, Slovak ML, Willman CL, Godwin JE, et al. (2006a): Age and acute myeloid leukemia. *Blood* 107:3481–3485.

Appelbaum FR, Kopecky KJ, Tallman MS, Slovak ML, Gundacker HM, Kim HT, et al. (2006b): The clinical spectrum of adult acute myeloid leukaemia associated with core binding factor translocations. *Br J Haematol* 135:165–173.

Arai Y, Hosoda F, Kobayashi H, Arai K, Hayashi Y, Kamada N, et al. (1997): The inv(11)(p15q22) chromosome translocation of de novo and therapy-related myeloid malignancies results in fusion of the nucleoporin gene, NUP98, with the putative RNA helicase gene, DDX10. *Blood* 89:3936–3944.

Arber DA, Chang KL, Lyda MH, Bedell V, Spielberger R, Slovak ML (2003): Detection of NPM/MLF1 fusion in t(3;5)-positive acute myeloid leukemia and myelodysplasia. *Hum Pathol* 34:809–813.

Ariyama Y, Fukuda Y, Okuno Y, Seto M, Date K, Abe T, et al. (1998): Amplification on double-minute chromosomes and partial-tandem duplication of the MLL gene in leukemic cells of a patient with acute myelogenous leukemia. *Genes Chromosomes Cancer* 23:267–272.

Arnould C, Philippe C, Bourdon V, Grégoire MJ, Berger R, Jonveaux P (1999): The signal transducer and activator of transcription STAT5b gene is a new partner of retinoic acid receptor α in acute promyelocytic-like leukaemia. *Hum Mol Genet* 8:1741–1749.

Arthur DC, Berger R, Golomb HM, Swansbury GJ, Reeves BR, Alimena G, et al. (1989): The clinical significance of karyotype in acute myelogenous leukemia. *Cancer Genet Cytogenet* 40:203–216.

Avet-Loiseau H, Godon C, Li J-Y, Daviet A, Mellerin M-P, Talmant P, et al. (1999): Amplification of the 11q23 region in acute myeloid leukemia. *Genes Chromosomes Cancer* 26:166–170.

Baccarani M, Deininger MW, Rosti G, Hochhaus A, Soverini S, Apperley JF, et al. (2013): European LeukemiaNet recommendations for the management of chronic myeloid leukemia: 2013. *Blood* 122:872–884.

Baer MR, Bloomfield CD (1992): Trisomy 13 in acute leukemia. *Leuk Lymphoma* 7:1–6.

Bains A, Lu G, Yao H, Luthra R, Medeiros LJ, Sargent RL (2012): Molecular and clinicopathologic characterization of AML with isolated trisomy 4. *Am J Clin Pathol* 137:387–394.

Balgobind BV, Raimondi SC, Harbott J, Zimmermann M, Alonzo TA, Auvrignon A, et al. (2009): Novel prognostic subgroups in childhood 11q23/MLL-rearranged acute myeloid leukemia: results of an international retrospective study. *Blood* 114:2489–2496.

Ball ED, Davis RB, Griffin JD, Mayer RJ, Davey FR, Arthur DC, et al. (1991): Prognostic value of lymphocyte surface markers in acute myeloid leukemia. *Blood* 77:2242–2250.

Baranger L, Gardembas M, Hillion J, Foussard C, Ifrah N, Boasson M, et al. (1993): Rearrangements of the RARA and PML genes in a cytogenetic variant of acute promyelocytic leukemia. *Genes Chromosomes Cancer* 6:118–120.

Barragán E, Montesinos P, Camos M, González M, Calasanz MJ, Román-Gómez J, et al. (2011): Prognostic value of FLT3 mutations in patients with acute promyelocytic leukemia treated with all-trans retinoic acid and anthracycline monochemotherapy. *Haematologica* 96:1470–1477.

Baruchel A, Daniel M-T, Schaison G, Berger R (1991): Nonrandom t(1;22)(p12-p13;q13) in acute megakaryocytic malignant proliferation. *Cancer Genet Cytogenet* 54:239–243.

Beghini A, Ripamonti CB, Cairoli R, Cazzaniga G, Colapietro P, Elice F, et al. (2004): KIT activating mutations: incidence in adult and pediatric acute myeloid leukemia, and identification of an internal tandem duplication. *Haematologica* 89:920–925.

Bench AJ, Nacheva EP, Hood TL, Holden JL, French L, Swanton S, et al. (2000): Chromosome 20 deletions in myeloid malignancies: reduction of the common deleted region, generation of a PAC/BAC contig and identification of candidate genes. *Oncogene* 19:3902–3913.

Béné MC, Bernier M, Casasnovas RO, Castoldi G, Doekharan D, van der Holt B, et al. (2001): Acute myeloid leukaemia M0: haematological, immunophenotypic and cytogenetic characteristics and their prognostic significance: an analysis in 241 patients. *Br J Haematol* 113:737–745.

Bennett JM, Catovsky D, Daniel MT, Flandrin G, Galton DAG, Gralnick HR, et al. (1976): Proposals for the classification of the acute leukaemias. French-American-British (FAB) co-operative group. *Br J Haematol* 33:451–458.

Bennett JM, Catovsky D, Daniel MT, Flandrin G, Galton DAG, Gralnick HR, et al. (1985a): Criteria for the diagnosis of acute leukaemia of megakaryocyte lineage (M7). A report of the French-American-British Cooperative Group. *Ann Intern Med* 103:460–462.

Bennett JM, Catovsky D, Daniel MT, Flandrin G, Galton DAG, Gralnick HR, et al. (1985b): Proposed revised criteria for the classification of acute myeloid leukemia. A report of the French-American-British Cooperative Group. *Ann Intern Med* 103:620–625.

Bennett JM, Catovsky D, Daniel MT, Flandrin G, Galton DAG, Gralnick HR, et al. (1991): Proposal for the recognition of minimally differentiated acute myeloid leukaemia (AML-M0). *Br J Haematol* 78:325–329.

Berger R (1975): Translocation t(11;20) et polyglobulie primitive. *Nouv Presse Med* 4:1972.

Berger R, Bernheim A, Ochoa-Noguera ME, Daniel M-T, Valensi F, Sigaux F, et al. (1987): Prognostic significance of chromosomal abnormalities in acute nonlymphocytic leukemia: a study of 343 patients. *Cancer Genet Cytogenet* 28:293–299.

Berger R, Derré J, Le Coniat M, Hébert J, Romana PS, Jonveaux P (1995): Inversion-associated translocations in acute myelomonocytic leukemia with eosinophilia. *Genes Chromosomes Cancer* 12:58–62.

Berger R, Le Coniat M, Romana SP, Jonveaux P (1996): Secondary acute myeloblastic leukemia with t(16;21) (q24;q22) involving the AML1 gene. *Hematol Cell Ther* 38:183–186.

von Bergh ARM, van Drunen E, van Wering ER, van Zutven LJCM, Hainmann I, Lönnerholm G, et al. (2006): High incidence of t(7;12)(q36;p13) in infant AML but not in infant ALL, with a dismal outcome and ectopic expression of HLXB9. *Genes Chromosomes Cancer* 45:731–739.

Bernard OA, Mauchauffe M, Mecucci C, Van Den Berghe H, Berger R (1994): A novel gene, AF-1p, fused to HRX in t(1;11)(p32;q23), is not related to AF-4, AF-9 nor ENL. *Oncogene* 9:1039–1045.

Bernstein R, Pinto MR, Behr A, Mendelow B (1982): Chromosome 3 abnormalities in acute nonlymphocytic leukemia (ANLL) with abnormal thrombopoiesis: report of three patients with a "new" inversion anomaly and a further case of homologous translocation. *Blood* 60:613–617.

Bernstein R, Pinto MR, Spector I, Macdougall LG (1987): A unique 8;16 translocation in two infants with poorly differentiated monoblastic leukemia. *Cancer Genet Cytogenet* 24:213–220.

Bernstein J, Dastugue N, Haas OA, Harbott J, Heerema NA, Huret JL, et al. (2000): Nineteen cases of the t(1;22)(p13;q13) acute megakaryoblastic leukaemia of infants/children and a review of 39 cases: report from a t(1;22) study group. *Leukemia* 14:216–218.

Beverloo HB, Le Coniat M, Wijsman J, Lillington DM, Bernard O, de Klein A, et al. (1995): Breakpoint heterogeneity in t(10;11) translocation in AML-M4/M5 resulting in fusion of AF10 and MLL is resolved by fluorescent in situ hybridization analysis. *Cancer Res* 55:4220–4224.

Beverloo HB, Panagopoulos I, Isaksson M, van Wering E, van Drunen E, de Klein A, et al. (2001): Fusion of the homeobox gene HLXB9 and the ETV6 gene in infant acute myeloid leukemias with the t(7;12)(q36;p13). *Cancer Res* 61:5374–5377.

Bielorai B, Meyer C, Trakhtenbrot L, Golan H, Rozner E, Amariglio N, et al. (2010): Therapy-related acute myeloid leukemia with t(2;11)(q37;q23) after treatment for osteosarcoma. *Cancer Genet Cytogenet* 203:288–291.

Bilhou-Nabera C, Lesesve J-F, Marit G, Lafage M, Dastugue N, Goullin B, et al. (1994): Trisomy 11 in acute myeloid leukemia: ten cases. *Leukemia* 8:2240–2241.

Billio A, Steer EJ, Pianezze G, Svaldi M, Casin M, Amato B, et al. (2002): A further case of acute myeloid leukaemia with inv(8)(p11q13) and MOZ-TIF2 fusion. *Haematologica* 87:ECR15.

Billström R, Nilsson P-G, Mitelman F (1987): Characteristic patterns of chromosome abnormalities in acute myeloid leukemia with Auer rods. *Cancer Genet Cytogenet* 28:191–199.

Billström R, Johansson B, Fioretos T, Garwicz S, Malm C, Zettervall O, et al. (1997): Poor survival in t(8;21)(q22;q22)-associated acute myeloid leukaemia with leukocytosis. *Eur J Haematol* 59:47–52.

Billström R, Ahlgren T, Békássy AN, Malm C, Olofsson T, Höglund M, et al. (2002): Acute myeloid leukemia with inv(16)(p13q22): involvement of cervical lymph nodes and tonsils is common and may be a negative prognostic sign. *Am J Hematol* 71:15–19.

van Binsbergen E, de Weerdt O, Buijs A (2007): A new subtype of MLL-SEPT2 fusion transcript in therapy-related acute myeloid leukemia with t(2;11)(q37;q23): a case report and literature review. *Cancer Genet Cytogenet* 176:72–75.

Björk J, Johansson B, Broberg K, Albin M (2009): Smoking as a risk factor for myelodysplastic syndromes and acute myeloid leukemia and its relation to cytogenetic findings: a case-control study. *Leuk Res* 33:788–791.

Blink M, Zimmermann M, von Neuhoff C, Reinhardt D, de Haas V, Hasle H, et al. (2014): Normal karyotype is a poor prognostic factor in myeloid leukemia of Down syndrome: a retrospective international study. *Haematologica* 99:299–307.

Block AW, Carroll AJ, Hagemeijer A, Michaux L, van Lom K, Olney HJ, et al. (2002): Rare recurring balanced chromosome abnormalities in therapy-related myelodysplastic syndromes and acute leukemia: report from an international workshop. *Genes Chromosomes Cancer* 33:401–412.

Bloomfield CD, Peterson LC, Yunis JJ, Brunning RD (1977): The Philadelphia chromosome (Ph1) in adults presenting with acute leukaemia: a comparison of Ph1+ and Ph1- patients. *Br J Haematol* 36:347–358.

Bloomfield CD, Lawrence D, Byrd JC, Carroll A, Pettenati MJ, Tantravahi R, et al. (1998): Frequency of prolonged remission duration after high-dose cytarabine intensification in acute myeloid leukemia varies by cytogenetic subtype. *Cancer Res* 58:4173–4179.

Bloomfield CD, Archer KJ, Mrózek K, Lillington DM, Kaneko Y, Head DR, et al. (2002): 11q23 balanced chromosome aberrations in treatment-related myelodysplastic syndromes and acute leukemia: report from an international workshop. *Genes Chromosomes Cancer* 33:362–378.

Blum W, Mrózek K, Ruppert AS, Carroll AJ, Rao KW, Pettenati MJ, et al. (2004): Adult de novo acute myeloid leukemia with t(6;11)(q27;q23): results from Cancer and Leukemia Group B Study 8461 and review of the literature. *Cancer* 101:1420–1427.

Boils CL, Mohamed AN (2008): t(16;21)(q24;q22) in acute myeloid leukemia: case report and review of the literature. *Acta Haematol* 119:65–68.

Borel C, Dastugue N, Cances-Lauwers V, Mozziconacci M-J, Prebet T, Vey N, et al. (2012): PICALM-MLLT10 acute myeloid leukemia: a French cohort of 18 patients. *Leuk Res* 36:1365–1369.

Borgström GH, Teerenhovi L, Vuopio P, de la Chapelle A, Van Den Berghe H, Brandt L, et al. (1980): Clinical implications of monosomy 7 in acute nonlymphocytic leukemia. *Cancer Genet Cytogenet* 2:115–126.

Borgström GH, Vuopio P, de la Chapelle A (1982): Abnormalities of chromosome No. 17 in myeloproliferative disorders. *Cancer Genet Cytogenet* 5:123–135.

Borkhardt A, Bojesen S, Haas OA, Fuchs U, Bartelheimer D, Loncarevic IF, et al. (2000): The human GRAF gene is fused to MLL in a unique t(5;11)(q31;q23) and both alleles are disrupted in three cases of myelodysplastic syndrome/acute myeloid leukemia with a deletion 5q. *Proc Natl Acad Sci USA* 97:9168–9173.

Borkhardt A, Teigler-Schlegel A, Fuchs U, Keller C, König M, Harbott J, et al. (2001): An ins(X;11)(q24;q23) fuses the MLL and the Septin 6/KIAA0128 gene in an infant with AML-M2. *Genes Chromosomes Cancer* 32:82–88.

Borrow J, Goddard AD, Sheer D, Solomon E (1990): Molecular analysis of acute promyelocytic leukemia breakpoint cluster region on chromosome 17. *Science* 249:1577–1580.

Borrow J, Shearman AM, Stanton VP Jr, Becher R, Collins T, Williams AJ, et al. (1996a): The t(7;11)(p15;p15) translocation in acute myeloid leukaemia fuses the genes for nucleoporin NUP98 and class I homeoprotein HOXA9. *Nat Genet* 12:159–167.

Borrow J, Stanton VP Jr, Andresen JM, Becher R, Behm FG, Chaganti RSK, et al. (1996b): The translocation t(8;16)(p11;p13) of acute myeloid leukaemia fuses a putative acetyltransferase to the CREB-binding protein. *Nat Genet* 14:33–41.

Bousquet M, Quelen C, Rosati R, Mansat-De Mas V, La Starza R, Bastard C, et al. (2008): Myeloid cell differentiation arrest by miR-125b-1 in myelodysplastic syndrome and acute myeloid leukemia with the t(2;11)(p21;q23) translocation. *J Exp Med* 205:2499–2506.

Bowen D, Groves MJ, Burnett AK, Patel Y, Allen C, Green C, et al. (2009): TP53 gene mutation is frequent in patients with acute myeloid leukemia and complex karyotype, and is associated with very poor prognosis. *Leukemia* 23:203–206.

Bram S, Swolin B, Rödjer S, Stockelberg D, Ögård I, Bäck H (2003): Is monosomy 5 an uncommon aberration? Fluorescence in situ hybridization reveals translocations and deletions in myelodysplastic syndromes or acute myelocytic leukemia. *Cancer Genet Cytogenet* 142:107–114.

Breems DA, Van Putten WLJ, De Greef GE, Van Zelderen-Bhola SL, Gerssen-Schoorl KBJ, Mellink CHM, et al. (2008): Monosomal karyotype in acute myeloid leukemia: a better indicator of poor prognosis than a complex karyotype. *J Clin Oncol* 26:4791–4797.

Brown T, Swansbury J, Taj MM (2012): Prognosis of patients with t(8;16)(p11;p13) acute myeloid leukemia. *Leuk Lymphoma* 53:338–341.

Büchner T, Berdel WE, Haferlach C, Haferlach T, Schnittger S, Müller-Tidow C, et al. (2009): Age-related risk profile and chemotherapy dose response in acute myeloid leukemia: a study by the German Acute Myeloid Leukemia Cooperative Group. *J Clin Oncol* 27:61–69.

Buijs A, Sherr S, van Baal S, van Bezouw S, van der Plas D, Geurts van Kessel A, et al. (1995): Translocation (12;22) (p13;q11) in myeloproliferative disorders results in fusion of the ETS-like TEL gene on 12p13 to the MN1 gene on 22q11. *Oncogene* 10:1511–1519.

Bullinger L 1, Krönke J, Schön C, Radtke I, Urlbauer K, Botzenhardt U, et al. (2010): Identification of acquired copy number alterations and uniparental disomies in cytogenetically normal acute myeloid leukemia using high-resolution single-nucleotide polymorphism analysis. *Leukemia* 24:438–449.

Burnett AK, Wheatley K, Goldstone AH, Stevens RF, Hann IM, Rees JHK, et al. (2002): The value of allogeneic bone marrow transplant in patients with acute myeloid leukaemia at differing risk of relapse: results of the UK MRC AML 10 trial. *Br J Haematol* 118:385–400.

Busson-Le Coniat M, Salomon-Nguyen F, Hillion J, Bernard OA, Berger R (1999): MLL-AF1q fusion resulting from t(1;11) in acute leukemia. *Leukemia* 13:302–306.

Byrd JC, Weiss RB, Arthur DC, Lawrence D, Baer MR, Davey F, et al. (1997): Extramedullary leukemia adversely affects hematologic complete remission rate and overall survival in patients with t(8;21)(q22;q22): results from Cancer and Leukemia Group B 8461. *J Clin Oncol* 15:466–475.

Byrd JC, Lawrence D, Arthur DC, Pettenati MJ, Tantravahi R, Qumsiyeh M, et al. (1998): Patients with isolated trisomy 8 in acute myeloid leukemia are not cured with cytarabine-based chemotherapy: results from Cancer and Leukemia Group B 8461. *Clin Cancer Res* 4:1235–1241.

Byrd JC, Dodge RK, Carroll A, Baer MR, Edwards C, Stamberg J, et al. (1999): Patients with t(8;21)(q22;q22) and acute myeloid leukemia have superior failure-free and overall survival when repetitive cycles of high-dose cytarabine are administered. *J Clin Oncol* 17:3767–3775.

Byrd JC, Mrózek K, Dodge RK, Carroll AJ, Edwards CG, Arthur DC, et al. (2002): Pretreatment cytogenetic abnormalities are predictive of induction success, cumulative incidence of relapse, and overall survival in adult patients with de novo acute myeloid leukemia: results from Cancer and Leukemia Group B (CALGB 8461). *Blood* 100:4325–4336.

Cairoli R, Beghini A, Turrini M, Bertani G, Nadali G, Rodeghiero F, et al. (2013): Old and new prognostic factors in acute myeloid leukemia with deranged core-binding factor beta. *Am J Hematol* 88:594–600.

Caligiuri MA, Strout MP, Oberkircher AR, Yu F, de la Chapelle A, Bloomfield CD (1997): The partial tandem duplication of ALL1 in acute myeloid leukemia with normal cytogenetics or trisomy 11 is restricted to one chromosome. *Proc Natl Acad Sci USA* 94:3899–3902.

Callen DF, Hull YJ, Toogood IRG, Fioretos T, Heim S, Mandahl N, et al. (1991): New chromosomal rearrangement, t(12;22)(p13;q12), in acute nonlymphocytic leukemia. *Cancer Genet Cytogenet* 51:255–258.

Callens C, Chevret S, Cayuela J-M, Cassinat B, Raffoux E, de Botton S, et al. (2005): Prognostic implication of FLT3 and Ras gene mutations in patients with acute promyelocytic leukemia (APL): a retrospective study from the European APL group. *Leukemia* 19:1153–1160.

Campbell LJ, Garson OM (1994): The prognostic significance of deletion of the long arm of chromosome 20 in myeloid disorders. *Leukemia* 8:67–71.

Campbell LJ, Challis J, Fok T, Garson OM (1991): Chromosome 16 abnormalities associated with myeloid malignancies. *Genes Chromosomes Cancer* 3:55–61.

Campbell LJ, Oei P, Brookwell R, Shortt J, Eaddy N, Ng A, et al. (2013): FISH detection of PML-RARA fusion in ins(15;17) acute promyelocytic leukaemia depends on probe size. *Biomed Res Int* 2013:164501.

Caramazza D, Ketterling RP, Knudson RA, Hanson CA, Siragusa S, Pardanani A, et al. (2010): Trisomy 11: prevalence among 22 403 unique patient cytogenetic studies and clinical correlates. *Leukemia* 24:1092–1094.

Carapeti M, Aguiar RCT, Goldman JM, Cross NCP (1998): A novel fusion between MOZ and the nuclear receptor coactivator TIF2 in acute myeloid leukemia. *Blood* 91:3127–3133.

Carroll A, Civin C, Schneider N, Dahl G, Pappo A, Bowman P, et al. (1991): The t(1;22)(p13;q13) is nonrandom and restricted to infants with acute megakaryoblastic leukemia: a Pediatric Oncology Group study. *Blood* 78:748–752.

Carter M, Kalwinsky DK, Mirro J Jr, Behm FG, Head D, Huddleston TF, et al. (1991): The t(10;11)(p14;q21) translocation in three children with acute myeloblastic leukemia. *Leukemia* 5:561–565.

Casasnovas RO, Campos L, Mugneret F, Charrin C, Béné MC, Garand R, et al. (1998): Immunophenotypic patterns and cytogenetic anomalies in acute non-lymphoblastic leukemia subtypes: a prospective study of 432 patients. *Leukemia* 12:34–43.

Casillas JN, Woods WG, Hunger SP, McGavran L, Alonzo TA, Feig SA (2003): Prognostic implications of t(10;11) translocations in childhood acute myelogenous leukemia: a report from the Children's Cancer Group. *J Pediatr Hematol Oncol* 25:594–600.

Castaigne S, Berger R, Jolly V, Daniel MT, Bernheim A, Marty M, et al. (1984): Promyelocytic blast crisis of chronic myelocytic leukemia with both t(9;22) and t(15;17) in M3 cells. *Cancer* 54:2409–2413.

Castro PD, Liang JC, Nagarajan L (2000): Deletions of chromosome 5q13.3 and 17p loci cooperate in myeloid neoplasms. *Blood* 95:2138–2143.

Catalano A, Dawson MA, Somana K, Opat S, Schwarer A, Campbell LJ, et al. (2007): The PRKAR1A gene is fused to RARA in a new variant acute promyelocytic leukemia. *Blood* 110:4073–4076.

Caudell D, Aplan PD (2008): The role of CALM-AF10 gene fusion in acute leukemia. *Leukemia* 22:678–685.

Cerveira N, Correia C, Bizarro S, Pinto C, Lisboa S, Mariz JM, et al. (2006): SEPT2 is a new fusion partner of MLL in acute myeloid leukemia with t(2;11)(q37;q23). *Oncogene* 25:6147–6152.

Cerveira N, Micci F, Santos J, Pinheiro M, Correia C, Lisboa S, et al. (2008): Molecular characterization of the MLL-SEPT6 fusion gene in acute myeloid leukemia: identification of novel fusion transcripts and cloning of genomic breakpoint junctions. *Haematologica* 93:1076–1080.

Cerveira N, Bizarro S, Teixeira MR (2011): MLL-SEPTIN gene fusions in hematological malignancies. *Biol Chem* 392:713–724.

Cervera J, Montesinos P, Hernandez-Rivas JM, Calasanz MJ, Aventin A, Ferro MT, et al. (2010): Additional chromosome abnormalities in patients with acute promyelocytic leukemia treated with all-trans retinoic acid and chemotherapy. *Haematologica* 95:424–431.

Chaffanet M, Gressin L, Preudhomme C, Soenen-Cornu V, Birnbaum D, Pébusque M-J (2000): MOZ is fused to p300 in an acute monocytic leukemia with t(8;22). *Genes Chromosomes Cancer* 28:138–144.

Chandra P, Luthra R, Zuo Z, Yao H, Ravandi F, Reddy N, et al. (2010): Acute myeloid leukemia with t(9;11)(p21-22;q23): common properties of dysregulated ras pathway signaling and genomic progression characterize de novo and therapy-related cases. *Am J Clin Pathol* 133:686–693.

de la Chapelle A, Lahtinen R (1983): Chromosome 16 and bone-marrow eosinophilia. *N Engl J Med* 309:1394.

Chaplin T, Bernard O, Beverloo HB, Saha V, Hagemeijer A, Berger R, et al. (1995): The t(10;11) translocation in acute myeloid leukemia (M5) consistently fuses the leucine zipper motif of AF10 onto the HRX gene. *Blood* 86:2073–2076.

Charrin C, Belhabri A, Treille-Ritouet D, Theuil G, Magaud J-P, Fiere D, et al. (2002): Structural rearrangements of chromosome 3 in 57 patients with acute myeloid leukemia: clinical, hematological and cytogenetic features. *Hematol J* 3:21–31.

Chauffaille Mde LLF, Fermino FA, Pelloso LAF, Silva MRR, Bordin JO, Yamamoto M (2003): t(4;12)(q11;p13): a rare chromosomal translocation in acute myeloid leukemia. *Leuk Res* 27:363–366.

Chen SJ, Flandrin G, Daniel M-T, Valensi F, Baranger L, Grausz D, et al. (1988): Philadelphia-positive acute leukemia: lineage promiscuity and inconsistently rearranged breakpoint cluster region. *Leukemia* 2:261–273.

Chen Z, Brand NJ, Chen A, Chen S-J, Tong J-H, Wang Z-Y, et al. (1993): Fusion between a novel Krüppel-like zinc finger gene and the retinoic acid receptor-alpha locus due to a variant t(11;17) translocation associated with acute promyelocytic leukaemia. *EMBO J* 12:1161–1167.

Chen S, Xue Y, Zhu X, Wu Y, Pan J (2007): Minimally differentiated acute myeloid leukemia with t(12;22)(p13;q11) translocation showing primary multidrug resistance and expressing multiple multidrug-resistant proteins. *Acta Haematol* 118:38–41.

Chen Y, Kantarjian H, Pierce S, Faderl S, O'Brien S, Qiao W, et al. (2013): Prognostic significance of 11q23 aberrations in adult acute myeloid leukemia and the role of allogeneic stem cell transplantation. *Leukemia* 27:836–842.

Chen Y, Li S, Zhou C, Li C, Ru K, Rao Q, et al. (2014): TBLR1 fuses to retinoid acid receptor alpha in a variant t(3;17)(q26;q21) translocation of acute promyelocytic leukemia. *Blood* 124(6):936–945.

Cheng Y, Wang H, Wang H, Chen Z, Jin J (2009a): Trisomy 21 in patients with acute leukemia. *Am J Hematol* 84:193–194.

Cheng Y, Wang Y, Wang H, Chen Z, Lou J, Xu H, et al. (2009b): Cytogenetic profile of de novo acute myeloid leukemia: a study based on 1432 patients in a single institution of China. *Leukemia* 23:1801–1816.

Chessells JM, Harrison CJ, Kempski H, Webb DKH, Wheatley K, Hann IM, et al. (2002): Clinical features, cytogenetics and outcome in acute lymphoblastic and myeloid leukaemia of infancy: report from the MRC Childhood Leukaemia working party. *Leukemia* 16:776–784.

Chevallier P, Labopin M, Nagler A, Ljungman P, Verdonck LF, Volin L, et al. (2009): Outcome after allogeneic transplantation for adult acute myeloid leukemia patients exhibiting isolated or associated trisomy 8 chromosomal abnormality: a survey on behalf of the ALWP of the EBMT. *Bone Marrow Transplant* 44:589–594.

Chi Y, Lindgren V, Quigley S, Gaitonde S (2008): Acute myelogenous leukemia with t(6;9)(p23;q34) and marrow basophilia: an overview. *Arch Pathol Lab Med* 132:1835–1837.

Chilton L, Hills RK, Harrison CJ, Burnett AK, Grimwade D, Moorman AV (2014): Hyperdiploidy with 49–65 chromosomes represents a heterogeneous cytogenetic subgroup of acute myeloid leukemia with differential outcome. *Leukemia* 28:321–328.

Cho B-S, Kim H-J, Lee S, Eom K-S, Min W-S, Lee J-W, et al. (2007): Successful interim therapy with imatinib prior to allogeneic stem cell transplantation in Philadelphia chromosome-positive acute myeloid leukemia. *Eur J Haematol* 79:170–173.

Chou W-C, Chen C-Y, Hou H-A, Lin L-I, Tang J-L, Yao M, et al. (2009): Acute myeloid leukemia bearing t(7;11)(p15;p15) is a distinct cytogenetic entity with poor outcome and a distinct mutation profile: comparative analysis of 493 adult patients. *Leukemia* 23:1303–1310.

Chou W-C, Huang H-H, Hou H-A, Chen C-Y, Tang J-L, Yao M, et al. (2010): Distinct clinical and biological features of de novo acute myeloid leukemia with additional sex comblike 1 (ASXL1) mutations. *Blood* 116:4086–4094.

Chou W-C, Chou S-C, Liu C-Y, Chen C-Y, Hou H-A, Kuo Y-Y, et al. (2011): TET2 mutation is an unfavorable prognostic factor in acute myeloid leukemia patients with intermediate-risk cytogenetics. *Blood* 118:3803–3810.

Churpek JE, Larson RA (2013): The evolving challenge of therapy-related myeloid neoplasms. *Best Pract Res Clin Haematol* 26:309–317.

Coenen EA, Zwaan CM, Reinhardt D, Harrison CJ, Haas OA, de Haas V, et al. (2013): Pediatric acute myeloid leukemia with t(8;16)(p11;p13), a distinct clinical and biological entity: a collaborative study by the International-Berlin-Frankfurt-Munster AML-study group. *Blood* 122: 2704–2713.

Coenen EA, Zwaan CM, Stary J, Baruchel A, de Haas V, Stam RW, et al. (2014): Unique BHLHB3 overexpression in pediatric acute myeloid leukemia with t(6;11)(q27;q23). *Leukemia* 28(7):1564–1568.

Cools J, Bilhou-Nabera C, Wlodarska I, Cabrol C, Talmant P, Bernard P, et al. (1999): Fusion of a novel gene, BTL, to ETV6 in acute myeloid leukemias with a t(4;12)(q11-q12;p13). *Blood* 94:1820–1824.

Cools J, Mentens N, Odero MD, Peeters P, Wlodarska I, Delforge M, et al. (2002): Evidence for position effects as a variant ETV6-mediated leukemogenic mechanism in myeloid leukemias with a t(4;12)(q11-q12;p13) or t(5;12)(q31;p13). *Blood* 99:1776–1784.

Corey SJ, Locker J, Oliveri DR, Shekhter-Levin S, Redner RL, Penchansky L, et al. (1994): A non-classical translocation involving 17q12 (retinoic acid receptor alpha) in acute promyelocytic leukemia (APML) with atypical features. *Leukemia* 8:1350–1353.

Corral J, Forster A, Thompson S, Lampert F, Kaneko Y, Slater R, et al. (1993): Acute leukemias of different lineages have similar MLL gene fusions encoding related chimeric proteins resulting from chromosomal translocation. *Proc Natl Acad Sci USA* 90:8538–8542.

Cortes JE, Kantarjian H, O'Brien S, Keating M, Pierce S, Freireich EJ, et al. (1995): Clinical and prognostic significance of trisomy 21 in adult patients with acute myelogenous leukemia and myelodysplastic syndromes. *Leukemia* 9:115–117.

Coulthard S, Chase A, Orchard K, Watmore A, Vora A, Goldman JM, et al. (1998): Two cases of inv(8)(p11q13) in AML with erythrophagocytosis: a new cytogenetic variant. *Br J Haematol* 100:561–563.

Crane MM, Strom SS, Halabi S, Berman EL, Fueger JJ, Spitz MR, et al. (1996): Correlation between selected environmental exposures and karyotype in acute myelocytic leukemia. *Cancer Epidemiol Biomarkers Prev* 5:639–644.

Cuneo A, Van Orshoven A, Michaux JL, Boogaerts M, Louwagie A, Doyen C, et al. (1990): Morphologic, immunologic and cytogenetic studies in erythroleukaemia: evidence for multilineage involvement and identification of two distinct cytogenetic-clinicopathological types. *Br J Haematol* 75:346–354.

Cuneo A, Ferrant A, Michaux JL, Boogaerts M, Demuynck H, Van Orshoven A, et al. (1995): Cytogenetic profile of minimally differentiated (FAB M0) acute myeloid leukemia: correlation with clinicobiologic findings. *Blood* 85:3688–3694.

Cuneo A, Ferrant A, Michaux J-L, Demuynck H, Boogaerts M, Louwagie A, et al. (1996): Philadelphia chromosome-positive acute myeloid leukemia: cytoimmunologic and cytogenetic features. *Haematologica* 81:423–427.

Cuthbert G, Thompson K, McCullough S, Watmore A, Dickinson H, Telford N, et al. (2000): MLL amplification in acute leukaemia: a United Kingdom Cancer Cytogenetics Group (UKCCG) study. *Leukemia* 14:1885–1891.

Dang CV, Stein PH, Gress DR, Dallabetta GA, Bender WL (1985): A case of agnogenic myeloid metaplasia evolving into acute myelogenous leukemia associated with the development of trisomy 11 in bone marrow cells. *Am J Hematol* 19:285–288.

Dastugue N, Payen C, Lafage-Pochitaloff M, Bernard P, Leroux D, Huguet-Rigal F, et al. (1995): Prognostic significance of karyotype in de novo adult acute myeloid leukemia. *Leukemia* 9:1491–1498.

Dastugue N, Duchayne E, Kuhlein E, Rubie H, Demur C, Aurich J, et al. (1997): Acute basophilic leukaemia and translocation t(X;6)(p11;q23). *Br J Haematol* 98:170–176.

Dastugue N, Lafage-Pochitaloff M, Pagès MP, Radford I, Bastard C, Talmant P, et al. (2002): Cytogenetic profile of childhood and adult megakaryoblastic leukemia (M7): a study of the Groupe Francais de Cytogenetique Hematologique (GFCH). *Blood* 100:618–626.

Davico L, Sacerdote C, Ciccone G, Pegoraro L, Kerim S, Ponzio G, et al. (1998): Chromosome 8, occupational exposures, smoking, and acute nonlymphocytic leukemias: a population-based study. *Cancer Epidemiol Biomarkers Prev* 7:1123–1125.

Delaunay J, Vey N, Leblanc T, Fenaux P, Rigal-Huguet F, Witz F, et al. (2003): Prognosis of inv(16)/t(16;16) acute myeloid leukemia (AML): a survey of 110 cases from the French AML Intergroup. *Blood* 102:462–469.

Dennis M, Culligan D, Karamitros D, Vyas P, Johnson P, Russell NH, et al. (2013): Lenalidomide monotherapy and in combination with cytarabine, daunorubicin and etoposide for high-risk myelodysplasia and acute myeloid leukaemia with chromosome 5 abnormalities. *Leuk Res Rep* 2:70–74.

Detourmignies L, Castaigne S, Stoppa AM, Harousseau JL, Sadoun A, Janvier M, et al. (1992): Therapy-related acute promyelocytic leukemia: a report on 16 cases. *J Clin Oncol* 10:1430–1435.

Dewald GW, Morrison-DeLap SJ, Schuchard KA, Spurbeck JL, Pierre RV (1983): A possible specific chromosome marker for monocytic leukemia: three more patients with t(9;11)(p22;q24) and another with t(11;17)(q24;q21), each with acute monoblastic leukemia. *Cancer Genet Cytogenet* 8:203–212.

Diab A, Zickl L, Abdel-Wahab O, Jhanwar S, Gulam MA, Panageas KS, et al. (2013): Acute myeloid leukemia with translocation t(8;16) presents with features which mimic acute promyelocytic leukemia and is associated with poor prognosis. *Leuk Res* 37:32–36.

Dicker F, Haferlach C, Kern W, Haferlach T, Schnittger S (2007): Trisomy 13 is strongly associated with AML1/RUNX1 mutations and increased FLT3 expression in acute myeloid leukemia. *Blood* 110:1308–1316.

Döhner H, Arthur DC, Ball ED, Sobol RE, Davey FR, Lawrence D, et al. (1990): Trisomy 13: a new recurring chromosome abnormality in acute leukemia. *Blood* 76:1614–1621.

Dong HY, Kung JX, Bhardwaj V, McGill J (2011): Flow cytometry rapidly identifies all acute promyelocytic leukemias with high specificity independent of underlying cytogenetic abnormalities. *Am J Clin Pathol* 135:76–84.

Douet-Guilbert N, De Braekeleer E, Basinko A, Herry A, Gueganic N, Bovo C, et al. (2012): Molecular characterization of deletions of the long arm of chromosome 5 (del(5q)) in 94 MDS/AML patients. *Leukemia* 26:1695–1697.

Dreyling MH, Martinez-Climent JA, Zheng M, Mao J, Rowley JD, Bohlander SK (1996): The t(10;11)(p13;q14) in the U937 cell line results in the fusion of the AF10 gene and CALM, encoding a new member of the AP-3 clathrin assembly protein family. *Proc Natl Acad Sci USA* 93:4804–4809.

Dreyling MH, Schrader K, Fonatsch C, Schlegelberger B, Haase D, Schoch C, et al. (1998): MLL and CALM are fused to AF10 in morphologically distinct subsets of acute leukemia with translocation t(10;11): both rearrangements are associated with a poor prognosis. *Blood* 91:4662–4667.

Duhoux FP, Ameye G, Montano-Almendras CP, Bahloula K, Mozziconacci MJ, Laibe S, et al. (2012): PRDM16 (1p36) translocations define a distinct entity of myeloid malignancies with poor prognosis but may also occur in lymphoid malignancies. *Br J Haematol* 156:76–88.

Dumézy F, Renneville A, Mayeur-Rousse C, Nibourel O, Labis E, Preudhomme C (2013): Acute myeloid leukemia with translocation t(3;5): new molecular insights. *Haematologica* 98:e52–e54.

Eghtedar A, Borthakur G, Ravandi F, Jabbour E, Cortes J, Pierce S, et al. (2012): Characteristics of translocation (16;16)(p13;q22) acute myeloid leukemia. *Am J Hematol* 87:317–318.

Elliott MA, Letendre L, Hanson CA, Tefferi A, Dewald GW (2002): The prognostic significance of trisomy 8 in patients with acute myeloid leukemia. *Leuk Lymphoma* 43:583–586.

Erickson P, Gao J, Chang K-S, Look T, Whisenant E, Raimondi S, et al. (1992): Identification of breakpoints in t(8;21) acute myelogenous leukemia and isolation of a fusion transcript, AML1/ETO, with similarity to Drosophila segmentation gene, runt. *Blood* 80:1825–1831.

Estey EH (2013): Acute myeloid leukemia: 2013 update on risk-stratification and management. *Am J Hematol* 88:318–327.

Estey E, Trujillo JM, Cork A, O'Brien S, Beran M, Kantarjian H, et al. (1992): AML-associated cytogenetic abnormalities (inv(16), del(16), t(8;21)) in patients with myelodysplastic syndromes. *Hematol Pathol* 6:43–48.

Farag SS, Archer KJ, Mrózek K, Vardiman JW, Carroll AJ, Pettenati MJ, et al. (2002): Isolated trisomy of chromosomes 8, 11, 13 and 21 is an adverse prognostic factor in adults with de novo acute myeloid leukemia: results from Cancer and Leukemia Group B 8461. *Int J Oncol* 21:1041–1051.

Farag SS, Archer KJ, Mrozek K, Ruppert AS, Carroll AJ, Vardiman JW, et al. (2006): Pretreatment cytogenetics add to other prognostic factors predicting complete remission and long-term outcome in patients 60 years of age or older with acute myeloid leukemia: results from Cancer and Leukemia Group B 8461. *Blood* 108:63–73.

Fasan A, Haferlach C, Alpermann T, Kern W, Haferlach T, Schnittger S (2013): A rare but specific subset of adult AML patients can be defined by the cytogenetically cryptic NUP98-NSD1 fusion gene. *Leukemia* 27:245–248.

Feder M, Finan J, Besa E, Nowell P (1985): A 2p;11q chromosome translocation in dysmyelopoietic preleukemia. *Cancer Genet Cytogenet* 15:143–150.

Fehniger TA, Byrd JC, Marcucci G, Abboud CN, Kefauver C, Payton JE, et al. (2009): Single-agent lenalidomide induces complete remission of acute myeloid leukemia in patients with isolated trisomy 13. *Blood* 113:1002–1005.

Felix CA, Megonigal MD, Chervinsky DS, Leonard DGB, Tsuchida N, Kakati S, et al. (1998): Association of germline p53 mutation with MLL segmental jumping translocation in treatment-related leukemia. *Blood* 91:4451–4456.

Fenaux P, Preudhomme C, Lai JL, Morel P, Beuscart R, Bauters F (1989): Cytogenetics and their prognostic value in de novo acute myeloid leukaemia: a report on 283 cases. *Br J Haematol* 73:61–67.

Ferrant A, Labopin M, Frassoni F, Prentice HG, Cahn JY, Blaise D, et al. (1997): Karyotype in acute myeloblastic leukemia: prognostic significance for bone marrow transplantation in first remission: a European group for blood and marrow transplantation study. *Blood* 90:2931–2938.

Ferrara F, Scognamiglio M, Di Noto R, Schiavone EM, Poggi V, Fiorillo A, et al. (1996): Interstitial 9q deletion is associated with CD7+ acute leukemia of myeloid and T lymphoid lineage. *Leukemia* 10:1990–1992.

Ferrara F, Di Noto R, Annunziata M, Copia C, Lo Pardo C, Boccuni P, et al. (1998): Immunophenotypic analysis enables the correct prediction of t(8;21) in acute myeloid leukaemia. *Br J Haematol* 102:444–448.

Fichelson S, Dreyfus F, Berger R, Melle J, Bastard C, Miclea JM, et al. (1992): Evi-1 expression in leukemic patients with rearrangements of the 3q25-q28 chromosome region. *Leukemia* 6:93–99.

Fioretos T, Strömbeck B, Sandberg T, Johansson B, Billström R, Borg Å, et al. (1999): Isochromosome 17q in blast crisis of chronic myeloid leukemia and in other hematologic malignancies is the result of clustered breakpoints in 17p11 and is not associated with coding TP53 mutations. *Blood* 94:225–232.

Fitzgibbon J, Smith L-L, Raghavan M, Smith ML, Debernardi S, Skoulakis S, et al. (2005): Association between acquired uniparental disomy and homozygous gene mutation in acute myeloid leukemias. *Cancer Res* 65:9152–9154.

FIWCL (First International Workshop on Chromosomes in Leukemia) (1978): Chromosomes in acute non-lymphocytic leukaemia. *Br J Haematol* 39:311–316.

FIWCL (Fourth International Workshop on Chromosomes in Leukemia, 1982) (1984a): Abnormalities of chromosome 22. *Cancer Genet Cytogenet* 11:316–318.

FIWCL (Fourth International Workshop on Chromosomes in Leukemia, 1982) (1984b): Clinical significance of chromosomal abnormalities in acute nonlymphoblastic leukaemia. *Cancer Genet Cytogenet* 11:332–350.

Forestier E, Heim S, Blennow E, Borgström G, Holmgren G, Heinonen K, et al. (2003): Cytogenetic abnormalities in childhood acute myeloid leukaemia: a Nordic series comprising all children enrolled in the NOPHO-93-AML trial between 1993 and 2001. *Br J Haematol* 121:566–577.

Forestier E, Izraeli S, Beverloo B, Haas O, Pession A, Michalová K, et al. (2008): Cytogenetic features of acute lymphoblastic and myeloid leukemias in pediatric patients with Down syndrome: an iBFM-SG study. *Blood* 111:1575–1583.

Forsberg LA, Rasi C, Malmqvist N, Davies H, Pasupulati S, Pakalapati G, et al. (2014): Mosaic loss of chromosome Y in peripheral blood is associated with shorter survival and higher risk of cancer. *Nat Genet* 46(6):624–628.

Freedman MH, Alter BP (2002): Risk of myelodysplastic syndrome and acute myeloid leukemia in congenital neutropenias. *Semin Hematol* 39:128–133.

Fröhling S, Schlenk RF, Krauter J, Thiede C, Ehninger G, Haase D, et al. (2005): Acute myeloid leukemia with deletion 9q within a noncomplex karyotype is associated with CEBPA loss-of-function mutations. *Genes Chromosomes Cancer* 42:427–432.

Fu J-F, Liang D-C, Yang C-P, Hsu J-J, Shih L-Y (2003): Molecular analysis of t(X;11)(q24;q23) in an infant with AML-M4. *Genes Chromosomes Cancer* 38:253–259.

Fujino T, Suzuki A, Ito Y, Ohyashiki K, Hatano Y, Miura I, et al. (2002): Single-translocation and double-chimeric transcripts: detection of NUP98-HOXA9 in myeloid leukemias with HOXA11 or HOXA13 breaks of the chromosomal translocation t(7;11)(p15;p15). *Blood* 99:1428–1433.

Gale RP, Horowitz MM, Weiner RS, Ash RC, Atkinson K, Babu R, et al. (1995): Impact of cytogenetic abnormalities on outcome of bone marrow transplants in acute myelogenous leukemia in first remission. *Bone Marrow Transplant* 16:203–208.

Gale RE, Hills R, Pizzey AR, Kottaridis PD, Swirsky D, Gilkes AF, et al. (2005): Relationship between FLT3 mutation status, biologic characteristics, and response to targeted therapy in acute promyelocytic leukemia. *Blood* 106:3768–3776.

Galván AB, Mallo M, Arenillas L, Salido M, Espinet B, Pedro C, et al. (2010): Does monosomy 5 really exist in myelodysplastic syndromes and acute myeloid leukemia? *Leuk Res* 34:1242–1245.

Gamerdinger U, Teigler-Schlegel A, Pils S, Bruch J, Viehmann S, Keller M, et al. (2003): Cryptic chromosomal aberrations leading to an AML1/ETO rearrangement are frequently caused by small insertions. *Genes Chromosomes Cancer* 36:261–272.

Gamou T, Kitamura E, Hosoda F, Shimizu K, Shinohara K, Hayashi Y, et al. (1998): The partner gene of AML1 in t(16;21) myeloid malignancies is a novel member of the MTG8(ETO) family. *Blood* 91:4028–4037.

Garçon L, Libura M, Delabesse E, Valensi F, Asnafi V, Berger C, et al. (2005): DEK-CAN molecular monitoring of myeloid malignancies could aid therapeutic stratification. *Leukemia* 19:1338–1344.

Geraedts JPM, den Ottolander GJ, Ploem JE, Muntinghe OG (1980): An identical translocation between chromosome 1 and 7 in three patients with myelofibrosis and myeloid metaplasia. *Br J Haematol* 44:569–575.

Gervais C, Murati A, Helias C, Struski S, Eischen A, Lippert E, et al. (2008): Acute myeloid leukaemia with 8p11 (MYST3) rearrangement: an integrated cytologic, cytogenetic and molecular study by the groupe francophone de cytogénétique hématologique. *Leukemia* 22:1567–1575.

GFCH (Groupe Français de Cytogénétique Hématologique) (1990): Acute myelogenous leukemia with an 8;21 translocation. A report on 148 cases from the Groupe Français de Cytogénétique Hématologique. *Cancer Genet Cytogenet* 44:169–179.

Ghaddar HM, Plunkett W, Kantarjian HM, Pierce S, Freireich EJ, Keating MJ, et al. (1994): Long-term results following treatment of newly-diagnosed acute myelogenous leukemia with continuous-infusion high-dose cytosine arabinoside. *Leukemia* 8:1269–1274.

Gibbons B, Czepulkowski B, Tucker J, Simpson E, Amess JAL, Young BD, et al. (1987): Subtle abnormalities in the short arm of chromosome 11 in acute myeloid leukemia. *Cancer Genet Cytogenet* 28:287–297.

Gibson BE, Webb DKH, Howman AJ, De Graaf SSN, Harrison CJ, Wheatley K (2011): Results of a randomized trial in children with acute myeloid leukaemia: medical research council AML12 trial. *Br J Haematol* 155:366–376.

Glass JP, Van Tassel P, Keating MJ, Cork A, Trujillo J, Holmes R (1987): Central nervous system complications of a newly recognized subtype of leukemia: AMML with a pericentric inversion of chromosome 16. *Neurology* 37:639–644.

Golomb HM, Rowley J, Vardiman J, Baron J, Locker G, Krasnow S (1976): Partial deletion of long arm of chromosome 17. A specific abnormality in acute promyelocytic leukemia? *Arch Intern Med* 136:825–828.

Golomb HM, Vardiman JW, Rowley JD, Testa JR, Mintz U (1978): Correlation of clinical findings with quinacrine-banded chromosomes in 90 adults with acute nonlymphocytic leukemia. An eight-year study (1970–1977). *N Engl J Med* 299:613–619.

Gorello P, Nofrini V, Brandimarte L, Pierini V, Crescenzi B, Nozza F, et al. (2013): Inv(11)(p15q22)/NUP98-DDX10 fusion and isoforms in a new case of de novo acute myeloid leukemia. *Cancer Genet* 206:92–96.

Gorletta TA, Gasparini P, D'Elios MM, Trubia M, Pelicci PG, Di Fiore PP (2005): Frequent loss of heterozygosity without loss of genetic material in acute myeloid leukemia with a normal karyotype. *Genes Chromosomes Cancer* 44:334–337.

Govberg IJ, Wolf JL, Cotter PD (2000): Trisomy 4 and double minutes in acute myeloid leukemia: further evidence that double minutes can occur as the primary cytogenetic abnormality. *Cancer Genet Cytogenet* 121:212–215.

Grimwade D, Gorman P, Duprez E, Howe K, Langabeer S, Oliver F, et al. (1997): Characterization of cryptic rearrangements and variant translocations in acute promyelocytic leukemia. *Blood* 90:4876–4885.

Grimwade D, Walker H, Oliver F, Wheatley K, Harrison C, Harrison G, et al. (1998): The importance of diagnostic cytogenetics on outcome in AML: analysis of 1, 612 patients entered into the MRC AML 10 trial. *Blood* 92:2322–2333.

Grimwade D, Biondi A, Mozziconacci M-J, Hagemeijer A, Berger R, Neat M, et al. (2000): Characterization of acute promyelocytic leukemia cases lacking the classic t(15;17): results of the European Working Party. *Blood* 96:1297–1230.

Grimwade D, Hills RK, Moorman AV, Walker H, Chatters S, Goldstone AH, et al. (2010): Refinement of cytogenetic classification in acute myeloid leukemia: determination of prognostic significance of rare recurring chromosomal abnormalities among 5876 younger adult patients treated in the United Kingdom Medical Research Council trials. *Blood* 116:354–365.

Grois N, Nowotny H, Tyl E, Krieger O, Kier P, Haas OA (1989): Is trisomy 22 in acute myeloid leukemia a primary abnormality or only a secondary change associated with inversion 16? *Cancer Genet Cytogenet* 43:119–129.

Grossmann V, Tiacci E, Holmes AB, Kohlmann A, Martelli MP, Kern W, et al. (2011): Whole-exome sequencing identifies somatic mutations of BCOR in acute myeloid leukemia with normal karyotype. *Blood* 118:6153–6163.

Gruber TA, Larson Gedman A, Zhang J, Koss CS, Marada S, Ta HQ, et al. (2012): An inv(16)(p13.3q24.3)-encoded CBFA2T3-GLIS2 fusion protein defines an aggressive subtype of pediatric acute megakaryoblastic leukemia. *Cancer Cell* 22:683–697.

Gu B-W, Wang Q, Wang J-M, Xue Y-Q, Fang J, Wong KF, et al. (2003): Major form of NUP98/HOXC11 fusion in adult AML with t(11;12)(p15;q13) translocation exhibits aberrant trans-regulatory activity. *Leukemia* 17:1858–1864.

Guglielmi C, Martelli MP, Diverio D, Fenu S, Vegna ML, Cantu-Rajnoldi A, et al. (1998): Immunophenotype of adult and childhood acute promyelocytic leukaemia: correlation with morphology, type of PML gene breakpoint and clinical outcome. A cooperative Italian study on 196 cases. *Br J Haematol* 102:1035–1041.

Gupta V, Minden MD, Yi Q-L, Brandwein J, Chun K (2003): Prognostic significance of trisomy 4 as the sole cytogenetic abnormality in acute myeloid leukemia. *Leuk Res* 27:983–991.

Gupta M, Ashok Kumar J, Sitaram U, Neeraj S, Nancy A, Balasubramanian P, et al. (2010): The t(6;9)(p22;q34) in myeloid neoplasms: a retrospective study of 16 cases. *Cancer Genet Cytogenet* 203:297–302.

Gustafson SA, Lin P, Chen SS, Chen L, Abruzzo LV, Luthra R, et al. (2009): Therapy-related acute myeloid leukemia with t(8;21) (q22;q22) shares many features with de novo acute myeloid leukemia with t(8;21)(q22;q22) but does not have a favorable outcome. *Am J Clin Pathol* 131:647–655.

Haferlach T, Bennett JM, Löffler H, Gassmann W, Andersen JW, Tuzuner N, et al. (1996): Acute myeloid leukemia with translocation (8;21). Cytomorphology, dysplasia and prognostic factors in 41 cases. *Leuk Lymphoma* 23:227–234.

Haferlach T, Schoch C, Schnittger S, Kern W, Löffler H, Hiddemann W (2002): Distinct genetic patterns can be identified in acute monoblastic and acute monocytic leukaemia (FAB AML M5a and M5b): a study of 124 patients. *Br J Haematol* 118:426–431.

Haferlach T, Kohlmann A, Klein H-U, Ruckert C, Dugas M, Williams PM, et al. (2009): AML with translocation t(8;16)(p11;p13) demonstrates unique cytomorphological, cytogenetic, molecular and prognostic features. *Leukemia* 23:934–943.

Haferlach C, Dicker F, Kohlmann A, Schindela S, Weiss T, Kern W, et al. (2010): AML with CBFB-MYH11 rearrangement demonstrate RAS pathway alterations in 92% of all cases including a high frequency of NF1 deletions. *Leukemia* 24:1065–1069.

Haferlach C, Bacher U, Haferlach T, Dicker F, Alpermann T, Kern W, et al. (2011a): The inv(3)(q21q26)/t(3;3)(q21;q26) is frequently accompanied by alterations of the RUNX1, KRAS and NRAS and NF1 genes and mediates adverse prognosis both in MDS and in AML: a study in 39 cases of MDS or AML. *Leukemia* 25:874–877.

Haferlach C, Bacher U, Kohlmann A, Schindela S, Alpermann T, Kern W, et al. (2011b): CDKN1B, encoding the cyclin-dependent kinase inhibitor 1B (p27), is located in the minimally deleted region of 12p abnormalities in myeloid malignancies and its low expression is a favorable prognostic marker in acute myeloid leukemia. *Haematologica* 96:829–836.

Haferlach C, Alpermann T, Schnittger S, Kern W, Chromik J, Schmid C, et al. (2012a): Prognostic value of monosomal karyotype in comparison to complex aberrant karyotype in acute myeloid leukemia: a study on 824 cases with aberrant karyotype. *Blood* 119:2122–2125.

Haferlach C, Bacher U, Schnittger S, Alpermann T, Zenger M, Kern W, et al. (2012b): ETV6 rearrangements are recurrent in myeloid malignancies and are frequently associated with other genetic events. *Genes Chromosomes Cancer* 51:328–337.

Hagemeijer A, Hählen K, Abels J (1981): Cytogenetic follow-up of patients with nonlymphocytic leukemia. II. Acute nonlymphocytic leukemia. *Cancer Genet Cytogenet* 3:109–124.

Hagemeijer A, Hählen K, Sizoo W, Abels J (1982): Translocation (9;11)(p21;q23) in three cases of acute monoblastic leukemia. *Cancer Genet Cytogenet* 5:95–105.

Hahm C, Mun YC, Seong CM, Han S-H, Chung WS, Huh J (2013): Single nucleotide polymorphism array-based karyotyping in acute myeloid leukemia or myelodysplastic syndrome with trisomy 8 as the sole chromosomal abnormality. *Acta Haematol* 129:154–158.

Hama A, Yagasaki H, Takahashi Y, Nishio N, Muramatsu H, Yoshida N, et al. (2008): Acute megakaryoblastic leukaemia (AMKL) in children: a comparison of AMKL with and without Down syndrome. *Br J Haematol* 140:552–561.

Hanslip JI, Swansbury GJ, Pinkerton R, Catovsky D (1992): The translocation t(8;16)(p11;p13) defines an AML subtype with distinct cytology and clinical features. *Leuk Lymphoma* 6:479–486.

Harada H, Asou H, Kyo T, Asaoku H, Iwato K, Dohy H, et al. (1995): A specific chromosome abnormality of t(4;12) (q11-12;p13) in CD7+ acute leukaemia. *Br J Haematol* 90:850–854.

Harrison CJ, Cuneo A, Clark R, Johansson B, Lafage-Pochitaloff M, Mugneret F, et al. (1998): Ten novel 11q23 chromosomal partner sites. *Leukemia* 12:811–822.

Harrison CJ, Hills RK, Moorman AV, Grimwade DJ, Hann I, Webb DKH, et al. (2010): Cytogenetics of childhood acute myeloid leukemia: United Kingdom Medical Research Council Treatment trials AML 10 and 12. *J Clin Oncol* 28:2674–2681.

Hasle H (2001): Pattern of malignant disorders in individuals with Down's syndrome. *Lancet Oncol* 2:429–436.

Hasle H, Alonzo TA, Auvrignon A, Behar C, Chang M, Creutzig U, et al. (2007): Monosomy 7 and deletion 7q in children and adolescents with acute myeloid leukemia: an international retrospective study. *Blood* 109:4641–4647.

Heim S, Avanzi G-C, Billström R, Kristoffersson U, Mandahl N, Bekassy AN, et al. (1987a): A new specific chromosomal rearrangement, t(8;16)(p11;p13), in acute monocytic leukaemia. *Br J Haematol* 66:323–326.

Heim S, Békassy AN, Garwicz S, Heldrup J, Wiebe T, Kristoffersson U, et al. (1987b): New structural chromosomal rearrangements in congenital leukemia. *Leukemia* 1:16–23.

Heim S, Egelund Christensen B, Fioretos T, Sörensen A-G, Tinggaard Pedersen N (1992): Acute myelomonocytic leukemia with inv(16)(p13q22) complicating Philadelphia chromosome positive chronic myeloid leukemia. *Cancer Genet Cytogenet* 59:35–38.

Heinonen K, Mrózek K, Lawrence D, Arthur DC, Pettenati MJ, Stamberg J, et al. (1998): Clinical characteristics of patients with de novo acute myeloid leukaemia and isolated trisomy 11: a Cancer and Leukemia Group B study. *Br J Haematol* 101:513–520.

Hiorns LR, Min T, Swansbury GJ, Zelent A, Dyer MJS, Catovsky D (1994): Interstitial insertion of retinoic acid receptor-α gene in acute promyelocytic leukemia with normal chromosomes 15 and 17. *Blood* 83:2946–2951.

Hogge DE, Misawa S, Parsa NZ, Pollak A, Testa JR (1984): Abnormalities of chromosome 16 in association with acute myelomonocytic leukemia and dysplastic bone marrow eosinophils. *J Clin Oncol* 2:550–557.

Höglund M, Johansson B, Pedersen-Bjergaard J, Marynen P, Mitelman F (1996): Molecular characterization of 12p abnormalities in hematologic malignancies: deletion of KIP1, rearrangement of TEL, and amplification of CCND2. *Blood* 87:324–330.

Hollink IHIM, van den Heuvel-Eibrink MM, Arentsen-Peters STCJM, Pratcorona M, Abbas S, Kuipers JE, et al. (2011): NUP98/NSD1 characterizes a novel poor prognostic group in acute myeloid leukemia with a distinct HOX gene expression pattern. *Blood* 118:3645–3656.

Holmes R, Keating MJ, Cork A, Broach Y, Trujillo J, Dalton WT Jr, et al. (1985a): A unique pattern of central nervous system leukemia in acute myelomonocytic leukemia associated with inv(16)(p13q22). *Blood* 65:1071–1078.

Holmes RI, Keating MJ, Cork A, Trujillo JM, McCredie KB, Freireich EJ (1985b): Loss of the Y chromosome in acute myelogenous leukemia: a report of 13 patients. *Cancer Genet Cytogenet* 17:269–278.

Hoyle C, Sherrington PD, Hayhoe FGJ (1987): Cytological features of 9q- deletions in AML. *Br J Haematol* 66:277–278.

Hoyle CF, de Bastos M, Wheatley K, Sherrington PD, Fischer PJ, Rees JKH, et al. (1989): AML associated with previous cytotoxic therapy, MDS or myeloproliferative disorders: results from the MRC's 9th AML trial. *Br J Haematol* 72:45–53.

Hromas R, Shopnick R, Jumean HG, Bowers C, Varella-Garcia M, Richkind K (2000): A novel syndrome of radiation-associated acute myeloid leukemia involving AML1 gene translocations. *Blood* 95:4011–4013.

Hrušák O, Porwit-MacDonald A (2002): Antigen expression patterns reflecting genotype of acute leukemias. *Leukemia* 16:1233–1258.

Hsiao H-H, Sashida G, Ito Y, Kodama A, Fukutake K, Ohyashiki JH, et al. (2006): Additional cytogenetic changes and previous genotoxic exposure predict unfavorable prognosis in myelodysplastic syndromes and acute myeloid leukemia with der(1;7)(q10;p10). *Cancer Genet Cytogenet* 165:161–166.

Hsu LYF, Greenberg ML, Kohan S, Wittman R (1979): Trisomy 13 in bone marrow cells in acute myelocytic leukemia and myelofibrosis. *Clin Genet* 15:327–331.

Huh J, Tiu RV, Gondek LP, O'Keefe CL, Jasek M, Makishima H, et al. (2010): Characterization of chromosome arm 20q abnormalities in myeloid malignancies using genome-wide single nucleotide polymorphism array analysis. *Genes Chromosomes Cancer* 49:390–399.

Huret JL, Brizard A, Slater R, Charrin C, Bertheas MF, Guilhot F, et al. (1993): Cytogenetic heterogeneity in t(11;19) acute leukemia: clinical, hematological and cytogenetic analyses of 48 patients – updated published cases and 16 new observations. *Leukemia* 7:152–160.

Hurwitz CA, Raimondi SC, Head D, Krance R, Mirro J Jr, Kalwinsky DK, et al. (1992): Distinctive immunophenotypic features of t(8;21)(q22;q22) acute myeloblastic leukemia in children. *Blood* 80:3182–3188.

Hussey DJ, Moore S, Nicola M, Dobrovic A (2001): Fusion of the NUP98 gene with the LEDGF/p52 gene defines a recurrent acute myeloid leukemia translocation. *BMC Genet* 2:20.

Ichikawa H, Shimizu K, Hayashi Y, Ohki M (1994): An RNA-binding protein gene, TLS/FUS, is fused to ERG in human myeloid leukemia with t(16;21) chromosomal translocation. *Cancer Res* 54:2865–2868.

Iida S, Seto M, Yamamoto K, Komatsu H, Tojo A, Asano S, et al. (1993): MLLT3 gene on 9p22 involved in t(9;11) leukemia encodes a serine/proline rich protein homologous to MLLT1 on 19p13. *Oncogene* 8:3085–3092.

Imamura T, Iwamoto S, Kanai R, Shimada A, Terui K, Osugi Y, et al. (2012): Outcome in 146 patients with paediatric acute myeloid leukaemia treated according to the AML99 protocol in the period 2003–06 from the Japan Association of Childhood Leukaemia Study. *Br J Haematol* 159:204–210.

Imashuku S, Hibi S, Sako M, Lin YW, Ikuta K, Nakata Y, et al. (2000): Hemophagocytosis by leukemic blasts in 7 acute myeloid leukemia cases with t(16;21)(p11;q22). Common morphologic characteristics for this type of leukemia. *Cancer* 88:1970–1975.

Irons RD, Chen Y, Wang X, Ryder J, Kerzic PJ (2013): Acute myeloid leukemia following exposure to benzene more closely resembles de novo than therapy related-disease. *Genes Chromosomes Cancer* 52:887–894.

Ishiyama K, Takami A, Kanda Y, Nakao S, Hidaka M, Maeda T, et al. (2012): Allogeneic hematopoietic stem cell transplantation for acute myeloid leukemia with t(6;9) (p23;q34) dramatically improves the patient prognosis: a matched-pair analysis. *Leukemia* 26:461–464.

Itoh M, Okazaki T, Tashima M, Sawada H, Uchiyama T (1999): Acute myeloid leukemia with t(5;11): two case reports. *Leuk Res* 23:677–680.

Jacobs PA, Brunton M, Court Brown WM, Doll R, Goldstein H (1963): Change of human chromosome count distribution with age: evidence for a sex differences. *Nature* 197: 1080–1981.

Jaff N, Chelghoum Y, Elhamri M, Tigaud I, Michallet M, Thomas X (2007): Trisomy 8 as sole anomaly or with other clonal aberrations in acute myeloid leukemia: impact on clinical presentation and outcome. *Leuk Res* 31:67–73.

Jaju RJ, Haas OA, Neat M, Harbott J, Saha V, Boultwood J, et al. (1999): A new recurrent translocation, t(5;11) (q35;p15.5), associated with del(5q) in childhood acute myeloid leukemia. *Blood* 94:773–780.

Jaju RJ, Fidler C, Haas OA, Strickson AJ, Watkins F, Clark K, et al. (2001): A novel gene, NSD1, is fused to NUP98 in the t(5;11)(q35;p15.5) in de novo childhood acute myeloid leukemia. *Blood* 98:1264–1267.

Jeandidier E, Gervais C, Radford-Weiss I, Zink E, Gangneux C, Eischen A, et al. (2012): A cytogenetic study of 397 consecutive acute myeloid leukemia cases identified three with a t(7;21) associated with 5q abnormalities and exhibiting similar clinical and biological features, suggesting a new, rare acute myeloid leukemia entity. *Cancer Genet* 205:365–372.

Jekarl DW, Kim M, Lim J, Kim Y, Han K, Lee A-W, et al. (2010): CD56 antigen expression and hemophagocytosis of leukemic cells in acute myeloid leukemia with t(16;21)(p11;q22). *Int J Hematol* 92:306–313.

Jerez A, Gondek LP, Jankowska AM, Makishima H, Przychodzen B, Tiu RV, et al. (2012a): Topography, clinical, and genomic correlates of 5q myeloid malignancies revisited. *J Clin Oncol* 30:1343–1349.

Jerez A, Sugimoto Y, Makishima H, Verma A, Jankowska AM, Przychodzen B, et al. (2012b): Loss of heterozygosity in 7q myeloid disorders: clinical associations and genomic pathogenesis. *Blood* 119:6109–6117.

Joannides M, Grimwade D (2010): Molecular biology of therapy-related leukaemias. *Clin Transl Oncol* 12:8–14.

Joannides M, Mays AN, Mistry AR, Hasan SK, Reiter A, Wiemels JL, et al. (2011): Molecular pathogenesis of secondary acute promyelocytic leukemia. *Mediterr J Hematol Infect Dis* 3:e2011045.

Johansson B, Mertens F, Mitelman F (1991): Geographic heterogeneity of neoplasia-associated chromosome aberrations. *Genes Chromosomes Cancer* 3:1–7.

Johansson B, Moorman AV, Haas OA, Watmore AE, Cheung KL, Swanton S, et al. (1998): Hematologic malignancies with t(4;11)(q21;q23) – a cytogenetic, morphologic, immunophenotypic and clinical study of 183 cases. *Leukemia* 12:779–787.

Johansson B, Fioretos T, Kullendorff C-M, Wiebe T, Békassy AN, Garwicz S, et al. (2000): Granulocytic sarcomas in body cavities in childhood acute myeloid leukemias with 11q23/MLL rearrangements. *Genes Chromosomes Cancer* 27:136–142.

Johnston DL, Alonzo TA, Gerbing RB, Hirsch B, Heerema NA, Ravindranath Y, et al. (2013): Outcome of pediatric patients with acute myeloid leukemia (AML) and -5/5q-abnormalities from five pediatric AML treatment protocols: a report from the Children's Oncology Group. *Pediatr Blood Cancer* 60:2073–2078.

Juliusson G, Lazarevic V, Hörstedt A-S, Hagberg O, Höglund M (2012): Acute myeloid leukemia in the real world: why population-based registries are needed. *Blood* 119:3890–3899.

Kalwinsky DK, Raimondi SC, Schell MJ, Mirro J Jr, Santana VM, Behm F, et al. (1990): Prognostic importance of cytogenetic subgroups in de novo pediatric acute nonlymphocytic leukemia. *J Clin Oncol* 8:75–83.

Kanagal-Shamanna R, Bueso-Ramos CE, Barkoh B, Lu G, Wang S, Garcia-Manero G, et al. (2012): Myeloid neoplasms with isolated isochromosome 17q represent a clinicopathologic entity associated with myelodysplastic/myeloproliferative features, a high risk of leukemic transformation, and wild-type TP53. *Cancer* 118:2879–2888.

Kanazawa T, Ogawa C, Taketani T, Taki T, Hayashi Y, Morikawa A (2005): TLS/FUS-ERG fusion gene in acute lymphoblastic leukemia with t(16;21)(p11;q22) and monitoring of minimal residual disease. *Leuk Lymphoma* 46:1833–1835.

Kaneko Y, Sakurai M (1977): 15/17 translocation in acute promyelocytic leukaemia. *Lancet* 1:961.

Kaneko Y, Rowley JD, Maurer HS, Variakojis D, Moohr JW (1982): Chromosome pattern in childhood acute nonlymphocytic leukemia (ANLL). *Blood* 60:389–399.

Kantarjian HM, Talpaz M, Dhingra K, Estey E, Keating MJ, Ku S, et al. (1991): Significance of the P210 versus P190 molecular abnormalities in adults with Philadelphia chromosome-positive acute leukemia. *Blood* 78:2411–2418.

Kashimura M, Ohyashiki K (2010): Successful imatinib and arsenic trioxide combination therapy for sudden onset promyelocytic crisis with t(15;17) in chronic myeloid leukemia. *Leuk Res* 34:e213–e214.

Kayser S, Zucknick M, Döhner K, Krauter J, Köhne C-H, Horst HA, et al. (2012): Monosomal karyotype in adult acute myeloid leukemia: prognostic impact and outcome after different treatment strategies. *Blood* 119:551–558.

Keating MJ, Cork A, Broach Y, Smith T, Walters RS, McCredie KB, et al. (1987): Toward a clinically relevant cytogenetic classification of acute myelogenous leukemia. *Leuk Res* 11:119–133.

Khan I, Malinge S, Crispino J (2011): Myeloid leukemia in Down syndrome. *Crit Rev Oncog* 16:25–36.

Kim J, Park TS, Song J, Lee K-A, Hong DJ, Min YH, et al. (2009): Detection of FUS-ERG chimeric transcript in two cases of acute myeloid leukemia with t(16;21)(p11.2;q22) with unusual characteristics. *Cancer Genet Cytogenet* 194:111–118.

Kim MJ, Cho SY, Kim M-H, Lee JJ, Kang SY, Cho EH, et al. (2010): FISH-negative cryptic PML-RARA rearrangement detected by long-distance polymerase chain reaction and sequencing analyses: a case study and review of the literature. *Cancer Genet Cytogenet* 203:278–283.

Kim H-J, Ahn HK, Jung CW, Moon JH, Park C-H, Lee K-O, et al. (2013): KIT D816 mutation associates with adverse outcomes in core binding factor acute myeloid leukemia, especially in the subgroup with RUNX1/RUNX1T1 rearrangement. *Ann Hematol* 92:163–171.

Kita K, Nakase K, Miwa H, Masuya M, Nishii K, Morita N, et al. (1992): Phenotypical characteristics of acute myelocytic leukemia associated with the t(8;21)(q22;q22) chromosomal abnormality: frequent expression of immature B-cell antigen CD19 together with stem cell antigen CD34. *Blood* 80:470–477.

Kitabayashi I, Aikawa Y, Yokoyama A, Hosoda F, Nagai M, Kakazu N, et al. (2001): Fusion of MOZ and p300 histone acetyltransferases in acute monocytic leukemia with a t(8;22)(p11;q13) chromosome translocation. *Leukemia* 15:89–94.

Kiyoi H, Naoe T, Yokota S, Nakao M, Minami S, Kuriyama K, et al. (1997): Internal tandem duplication of FLT3 associated with leukocytosis in acute promyelocytic leukemia. *Leukemia* 11:1447–1452.

Kobayashi H, Miyachi H, Ogawa T, Jimbo M (1990): Translocation t(11;22)(q23;q11) in an adult with acute monoblastic leukemia. *Jpn J Med* 29:527–532.

Kobayashi H, Espinosa R III, Thirman MJ, Fernald AA, Shannon K, Diaz MO, et al. (1993): Do terminal deletions of 11q23 exist? Identification of undetected translocations with fluorescence in situ hybridization. *Genes Chromosomes Cancer* 7:204–208.

Kobayashi H, Montgomery KT, Bohlander SK, Adra CN, Lim BL, Kucherlapati RS, et al. (1994): Fluorescence in situ hybridization mapping of translocations and deletions involving the short arm of human chromosome 12 in malignant hematologic diseases. *Blood* 84:3473–3482.

Kobayashi H, Arai Y, Hosoda F, Maseki N, Hayashi Y, Eguchi H, et al. (1997a): Inversion of chromosome 11, inv(11) (p15q22), as a recurring chromosomal aberration associated with de novo and secondary myeloid malignancies: identification of a P1 clone spanning the 11q22 breakpoint. *Genes Chromosomes Cancer* 19:150–155.

Kobayashi H, Hosoda F, Maseki N, Sakurai M, Imashuku S, Ohki M, et al. (1997b): Hematologic malignancies with the t(10;11)(p13;q21) have the same molecular event and a variety of morphologic or immunologic phenotypes. *Genes Chromosomes Cancer* 20:253–259.

Koken MHM, Daniel M-T, Gianni M, Zelent A, Licht J, Buzyn A, et al. (1999): Retinoic acid, but not arsenic trioxide, degrades the PLZF/RARα fusion protein, without inducing terminal differentiation or apoptosis, in a RA-therapy resistant t(11;17)(q23;q21) APL patient. *Oncogene* 18:1113–1118.

Köller U, Haas OA, Ludwig W-D, Bartram CR, Harbott J, Panzer-Grümayer R, et al. (1989): Phenotypic and genotypic heterogeneity in infant acute leukemia. II. Acute nonlymphoblastic leukemia. *Leukemia* 3:708–714.

Kondo T, Mori A, Darmanin S, Hashino S, Tanaka J, Asaka M (2008): The seventh pathogenic fusion gene FIP1L1-RARA was isolated from a t(4;17)-positive acute promyelocytic leukemia. *Haematologica* 93:1414–1416.

Kong X-T, Ida K, Ichikawa H, Shimizu K, Ohki M, Maseki N, et al. (1997): Consistent detection of TLS/FUS-ERG chimeric transcripts in acute myeloid leukemia with t(16;21) (p11;q22) and identification of a novel transcript. *Blood* 90:1192–1199.

Konoplev S, Yin CC, Kornblau SM, Kantarjian HM, Konopleva M, Andreeff M, et al. (2013): Molecular characterization of de novo Philadelphia chromosome-positive acute myeloid leukemia. *Leuk Lymphoma* 54:138–144.

Krauter J, Wagner K, Schäfer I, Marschalek R, Meyer C, Heil G, et al. (2009): Prognostic factors in adult patients up to 60 years old with acute myeloid leukemia and translocations of chromosome band 11q23: individual patient data-based meta-analysis of the German Acute Myeloid Leukemia Intergroup. *J Clin Oncol* 27:3000–3006.

Krauth M-T, Eder C, Alpermann T, Bacher U, Nadarajah N, Kern W, et al. (2014): High number of additional genetic lesions in acute myeloid leukemia with t(8;21)/RUNX1-RUNX1T1: frequency and impact on clinical outcome. *Leukemia* 28(7):1449–1458.

Kuwatsuka Y, Miyamura K, Suzuki R, Kasai M, Maruta A, Ogawa H, et al. (2009): Hematopoietic stem cell transplantation for core binding factor acute myeloid leukemia: t(8;21) and inv(16) represent different clinical outcomes. *Blood* 113:2096–2103.

Kwong YL (2010): Azathioprine: association with therapy-related myelodysplastic syndrome and acute myeloid leukemia. *J Rheumatol* 37:485–490.

Kwong Y-L, Pang A (1999): Low frequency of rearrangements of the homeobox gene HOXA9/t(7;11) in adult acute myeloid leukemia. *Genes Chromosomes Cancer* 25:70–74.

La Starza R, Crescenzi B, Krause A, Pierini V, Specchia G, Bardi A, et al. (2006): Dual-color split signal fluorescence in situ hybridization assays for the detection of CALM/AF10 in t(10;11)(p13;q14-q21)-positive acute leukemia. *Haematologica* 91:1248–1251.

Lai JL, Zandecki M, Fenaux P, Preudhomme C, Facon T, Deminatti M (1992): Acute monocytic leukemia with (8;22) (p11;q13) translocation. Involvement of 8p11 as in classical t(8;16)(p11;p13). *Cancer Genet Cytogenet* 60:180–182.

Lai J-L, Preudhomme C, Zandecki M, Flactif M, Vanrumbeke M, Lepelley P, et al. (1995): Myelodysplastic syndromes and acute myeloid leukemia with 17p deletion. An entity characterized by specific dysgranulopoiesis and a high incidence of P53 mutations. *Leukemia* 9:370–381.

Langabeer SE, Grimwade D, Walker H, Rogers JR, Burnett AK, Goldstone AH, et al. (1998): A study to determine whether trisomy 8, deleted 9q and trisomy 22 are markers of cryptic rearrangements of PML/RARα, AML1/ETO and CBFB/MYH11 respectively in acute myeloid leukaemia. *Br J Haematol* 101:338–340.

Larson RA, Le Beau MM, Vardiman JW, Testa JR, Golomb HM, Rowley JD (1983): The predictive value of initial cytogenetic studies in 148 adults with acute nonlymphocytic leukemia: a 12-year study (1970-1982). *Cancer Genet Cytogenet* 10:219–236.

Larson RA, Williams SF, Le Beau MM, Bitter MA, Vardiman JW, Rowley JD (1986): Acute myelomonocytic leukemia with abnormal eosinophils and inv(16) or t(16;16) has a favorable prognosis. *Blood* 68:1242–1249.

Larsson N, Lilljebjörn H, Lassen C, Johansson B, Fioretos T (2012): Myeloid malignancies with acquired trisomy 21 as the sole cytogenetic change are clinically highly variable and display a heterogeneous pattern of copy number alterations and mutations. *Eur J Haematol* 88:136–143.

Lazarevic V, Hörstedt A-S, Johansson B, Antunovic P, Billström R, Derolf A, et al. (2014): Incidence and prognostic significance of karyotypic subgroups in older patients with acute myeloid leukemia: the Swedish population-based experience. *Blood Cancer J* 4:e188.

Le Beau MM, Larson RA, Bitter MA, Vardiman JW, Golomb HM, Rowley JD (1983): Association of an inversion of chromosome 16 with abnormal marrow eosinophils in acute myelomonocytic leukemia. *N Engl J Med* 309:630–636.

Le Beau MM, Westbrook CA, Diaz MO, Rowley JD (1985): c-src is consistently conserved in the chromosomal deletion (20q) observed in myeloid disorders. *Proc Natl Acad Sci USA* 82:6692–6696.

Le Beau MM, Albain KS, Larson RA, Vardiman JW, Davis EM, Blough RR, et al. (1986): Clinical and cytogenetic correlations in 63 patients with therapy-related myelodysplastic syndromes and acute nonlymphocytic leukemia: further evidence for characteristic abnormalities of chromosomes No. 5 and 7. *J Clin Oncol* 4:325–345.

Lee S-G, Park TS, Oh SH, Park JC, Yang YJ, Marschalek R, et al. (2011): De novo acute myeloid leukemia associated with t(11;17)(q23;q25) and MLL-SEPT9 rearrangement in an elderly patient: a case study and review of the literature. *Acta Haematol* 126:195–198.

Lee S-G, Cho SY, Kim MJ, Oh SH, Cho EH, Lee S, et al. (2013): Genomic breakpoints and clinical features of MLL-TET1 rearrangement in acute leukemias. *Haematologica* 98:e55–e57.

Lengfelder E, Hofmann WK, Nowak D (2012): Impact of arsenic trioxide in the treatment of acute promyelocytic leukemia. *Leukemia* 26:433–442.

Levin M, Le Coniat M, Bernheim A, Berger R (1986): Complex chromosomal abnormalities in acute nonlymphocytic leukemia. *Cancer Genet Cytogenet* 22:113–119.

Ley TJ, Mardis ER, Ding L, Fulton B, McLellan MD, Chen K, et al. (2008): DNA sequencing of a cytogenetically normal acute myeloid leukaemia genome. *Nature* 456:66–72.

Li S, Yin CC, Medeiros LJ, Bueso-Ramos C, Lu G, Lin P (2012): Myelodysplastic syndrome/acute myeloid leukemia with t(3;21)(q26.2;q22) is commonly a therapy-related disease associated with poor outcome. *Am J Clin Pathol* 138:146–152.

Licht JD, Chomienne C, Goy A, Chen A, Scott AA, Head DR, et al. (1995): Clinical and molecular characterization of a rare syndrome of acute promyelocytic leukemia associated with translocation (11;17). *Blood* 85:1083–1094.

Lie SO, Abrahamsson J, Clausen N, Forestier E, Hasle H, Hovi L, et al. (2003): Treatment stratification based on initial in vivo response in acute myeloid leukaemia in children without Down's syndrome: results of NOPHO-AML trials. *Br J Haematol* 122:217–225.

Lillington DM, Young BD, Berger R, Martineau M, Moorman AV, Secker-Walker LM (1998): The t(10;11)(p12;q23) translocation in acute leukaemia: a cytogenetic and clinical study of 20 patients. *Leukemia* 12:801–804.

Lim G, Choi JR, Kim MJ, Kim SY, Lee HJ, Suh J-T, et al. (2010): Detection of t(3;5) and NPM1/MLF1 rearrangement in an elderly patient with acute myeloid leukemia: clinical and laboratory study with review of the literature. *Cancer Genet Cytogenet* 199:101–109.

von Lindern M, Fornerod M, van Baal S, Jaegle M, de Wit T, et al. (1992): The translocation (6;9), associated with a specific subtype of acute myeloid leukemia, results in the fusion of two genes, dek and can, and the expression of a chimeric, leukemia-specific dek-can mRNA. *Mol Cell Biol* 12:1687–1697.

Liso V, Bennett J (2003): Morphological and cytochemical characteristics of leukaemic promyelocytes. *Best Pract Res Clin Haematol* 16:349–355.

Litmanovich D, Zamir-Brill R, Jeison M, Gershoni-Baruch R (2000): Is inversion 16 a prerequisite and is trisomy 22 invariably associated with inversion 16 in AML-M4eo? *Cancer Genet Cytogenet* 121:106.

Liu P, Tarlé SA, Hajra A, Claxton DF, Marlton P, Freedman M, et al. (1993): Fusion between transcription factor CBFβ/PEBP2β and a myosin heavy chain in acute myeloid leukemia. *Science* 261:1041–1044.

Lo-Coco F, Avvisati G, Vignetti M, Thiede C, Orlando SM, Iacobelli S, et al. (2013): Retinoic acid and arsenic trioxide for acute promyelocytic leukemia. *N Engl J Med* 369:111–121.

Longo L, Pandolfi PP, Biondi A, Rambaldi A, Mencarelli A, Lo Coco F, et al. (1990): Rearrangements and aberrant expression of the retinoic acid receptor α gene in acute promyelocytic leukemias. *J Exp Med* 172:1571–1575.

Lorsbach RB, Moore J, Mathew S, Raimondi SC, Mukatira ST, Downing JR (2003): TET1, a member of a novel protein family, is fused to MLL in acute myeloid leukemia containing the t(10;11)(q22;q23). *Leukemia* 17:637–641.

Lugthart S, Gröschel S, Beverloo HB, Kayser S, Valk PJM, van Zelderen-Bhola SL, et al. (2010): Clinical, molecular, and prognostic significance of WHO type inv(3)(q21q26.2)/t(3;3)(q21;q26.2) and various other 3q abnormalities in acute myeloid leukemia. *J Clin Oncol* 28:3890–3898.

Lundin C, Horvat A, Karlsson K, Olofsson T, Paulsson K, Johansson B (2011): t(9;11)(p22;p15) [NUP98/PSIP1] is a poor prognostic marker associated with de novo acute myeloid leukaemia expressing both mature and immature surface antigens. *Leuk Res* 35:e75–e76.

Ma SK, Lie AKW, Au WY, Wan TSK, Chan LC (1997): CD7+ acute myeloid leukaemia with 'mature lymphoid' blast morphology, marrow basophilia and t(4;12)(q12;p13). *Br J Haematol* 97:978–980.

Ma Z, Morris SW, Valentine V, Li M, Herbrick J-A, Cui X, et al. (2001): Fusion of two novel genes, RBM15 and MKL1, in the t(1;22)(p13;q13) of acute megakaryoblastic leukemia. *Nat Genet* 28:220–221.

Marcucci G, Mrózek K, Ruppert AS, Maharry K, Kolitz JE, Moore JO, et al. (2005): Prognostic factors and outcome of core binding factor acute myeloid leukemia patients with t(8;21) differ from those of patients with inv(16): a Cancer and Leukemia Group B study. *J Clin Oncol* 23:5705–5717.

Mardis ER, Ding L, Dooling DJ, Larson DE, McLellan MD, Chen K, et al. (2009): Recurring mutations found by sequencing an acute myeloid leukemia genome. *N Engl J Med* 361:1058–1066.

Marlton P, Keating M, Kantarjian H, Pierce S, O'Brien S, Freireich EJ, et al. (1995): Cytogenetic and clinical correlates in AML patients with abnormalities of chromosome 16. *Leukemia* 9:965–971.

Marosi C, Köller U, Koller-Weber E, Schwarzinger I, Schneider B, Jäger U, et al. (1992): Prognostic impact of karyotype and immunologic phenotype in 125 adult patients with de novo AML. *Cancer Genet Cytogenet* 61:14–25.

Martelli MP, Sportoletti P, Tiacci E, Martelli MF, Falini B (2013): Mutational landscape of AML with normal cytogenetics: biological and clinical implications. *Blood Rev* 27:13–22.

Martineau M, Berger R, Lillington DM, Moorman AV, Secker-Walker LM (1998): The t(6;11)(q27;q23) translocation in acute leukemia: a laboratory and clinical study of 30 cases. *Leukemia* 12:788–791.

Martinez-Climent JA, Lane NJ, Rubin CM, Morgan E, Johnstone HS, Mick R, et al. (1995): Clinical and prognostic significance of chromosomal abnormalities in childhood acute myeloid leukemia de novo. *Leukemia* 9:95–101.

Marukawa O, Akao Y, Inazawa J, Ariyama T, Abe T, Naoe T, et al. (1996): Molecular cloning of the breakpoint of t(11;22) (q23;q11) chromosome translocation in an adult acute myelomonocytic leukaemia. *Br J Haematol* 92:687–691.

Masetti R, Pigazzi M, Togni M, Astolfi A, Indio V, Manara E, et al. (2013): CBFA2T3-GLIS2 fusion transcript is a novel common feature in pediatric, cytogenetically normal AML, not restricted to FAB M7 subtype. *Blood* 121:3469–3472.

Massaad L, Prieur M, Leonard C, Dutrillaux B (1990): Biclonal chromosome evolution of chronic myelomonocytic leukemia in a child. *Cancer Genet Cytogenet* 44:131–137.

Matsuda A, Jinnai I, Yagasaki F, Ito Y, Ito K, Kusumoto S, et al. (2000): The pathogenetic mechanism of myeloid malignancies associated with deletions of the long arm of chromosome 20 cannot be explained by a "one hit" model. An acute myeloid leukemia patient who developed with 20q- clone during complete remission for 9 years. *Eur J Haematol* 65:210–211.

Mauritzson N, Albin M, Rylander L, Billström R, Ahlgren T, Mikoczy Z, et al. (2002): Pooled analysis of clinical and cytogenetic features in treatment-related and de novo adult acute myeloid leukemia and myelodysplastic syndromes based on a consecutive series of 761 patients analyzed 1976–1993 and on 5098 unselected cases reported in the literature 1974–2001. *Leukemia* 16:2366–2378.

McNerney ME, Brown CD, Wang X, Bartom ET, Karmakar S, Bandlamudi C, et al. (2013): CUX1 is a haploinsufficient tumor suppressor gene on chromosome 7 frequently inactivated in acute myeloid leukemia. *Blood* 121:975–983.

Mecucci C, Vermaelen K, Kulling G, Michaux JL, Noens L, Van Hove W, et al. (1984): Interstitial 9q- deletions in hematologic malignancies. *Cancer Genet Cytogenet* 12:309–319.

Mecucci C, Bosly A, Michaux J-L, Broeckaert-Van Orshoven A, Van Den Berghe H (1985): Acute nonlymphoblastic leukemia with bone marrow eosinophilia and structural anomaly of chromosome 16. *Cancer Genet Cytogenet* 17:359–363.

Mecucci C, Van Orshoven A, Tricot G, Michaux J-L, Delannoy A, Van Den Berghe H (1986): Trisomy 4 identifies a subset of acute nonlymphocytic leukemias. *Blood* 67:1328–1332.

Medeiros BC, Kohrt HE, Arber DA, Bangs CD, Cherry AM, Majeti R, et al. (2010a): Immunophenotypic features of acute myeloid leukemia with inv(3)(q21q26.2)/t(3;3) (q21;q26.2). *Leuk Res* 34:594–597.

Medeiros BC, Othus M, Fang M, Roulston D, Appelbaum FR (2010b): Prognostic impact of monosomal karyotype in young adult and elderly acute myeloid leukemia: the Southwest Oncology Group (SWOG) experience. *Blood* 116:2224–2228.

Megonigal MD, Rappaport EF, Jones DH, Williams TM, Lovett BD, Kelly KM, et al. (1998): t(11;22)(q23;q11.2) in acute myeloid leukemia of infant twins fuses MLL with hCDCrel, a cell division cycle gene in the genomic region of deletion in DiGeorge and velocardiofacial syndromes. *Proc Natl Acad Sci USA* 95:6413–6418.

Mehta AB, Bain BJ, Fitchett M, Shah S, Secker-Walker LM (1998): Trisomy 13 and myeloid malignancy – characteristic blast cell morphology: a United Kingdom Cancer Cytogenetics Group survey. *Br J Haematol* 101:749–752.

Mehta PA, Harris RE, Davies SM, Kim M-O, Mueller R, Lampkin B, et al. (2010): Numerical chromosomal changes and risk of development of myelodysplastic syndrome-acute myeloid leukemia in patients with Fanconi anemia. *Cancer Genet Cytogenet* 203:180–186.

Mercher T, Busson-Le Coniat M, Monni R, Mauchauffe M, Khac FN, Gressin L, et al. (2001): Involvement of a human gene related to the Drosophila spen gene in the recurrent t(1;22) translocation of acute megakaryocytic leukemia. *Proc Natl Acad Sci USA* 98:5776–5779.

Merlat A, Lai JL, Sterkers Y, Demory JL, Bauters F, Preudhomme C, et al. (1999): Therapy-related myelodysplastic syndrome and acute myeloid leukemia with 17p deletion. A report on 25 cases. *Leukemia* 13:250–257.

Mertens F, Johansson B, Mitelman F (1994): Isochromosomes in neoplasia. *Genes Chromosomes Cancer* 10:221–230.

Merzianu M, Medeiros LJ, Cortes J, Yin C, Lin P, Jones D, et al. (2005): inv(16)(p13q22) in chronic myelogenous leukemia in blast phase: a clinicopathologic, cytogenetic, and molecular study of five cases. *Am J Clin Pathol* 124:807–814.

Mesa RA, Hanson CA, Ketterling RP, Schwager S, Knudson RA, Tefferi A (2009): Trisomy 13: prevalence and clinicopathologic correlates of another potentially lenalidomide-sensitive cytogenetic abnormality. *Blood* 113:1200–1201.

Metzeler KH, Becker H, Maharry K, Radmacher MD, Kohischmidt J, Mrozek K, et al. (2011) ASXL1 mutations identify a high-risk subgroup of older patients with primary cytogenetically normal AML within the ELN Favorable genetic category. Blood 118:6920–6929.

Meyer C, Schneider B, Reichel M, Angermueller S, Strehl S, Schnittger S, et al. (2005): Diagnostic tool for the identification of MLL rearrangements including unknown partner genes. *Proc Natl Acad Sci USA* 102:449–454.

Meyer C, Hofmann J, Burmeister T, Gröger D, Park TS, Emerenciano M, et al. (2013): The MLL recombinome of acute leukemias in 2013. *Leukemia* 27:2165–2176.

Micci F, Thorsen J, Panagopoulos I, Nyquist KB, Zeller B, Tierens A, et al. (2013): High-throughput sequencing identifies an NFIA/CBFA2T3 fusion gene in acute erythroid leukemia with t(1;16)(p31;q24). *Leukemia* 27:980–982.

Michaux L, Wlodarska I, Stul M, Dierlamm J, Mugneret F, Herens C, et al. (2000): MLL amplification in myeloid leukemias: a study of 14 cases with multiple copies of 11q23. *Genes Chromosomes Cancer* 29:40–47.

Middeke JM, Beelen D, Stadler M, Göhring G, Schlegelberger B, Baurmann H, et al. (2012): Outcome of high-risk acute myeloid leukemia after allogeneic hematopoietic cell transplantation: negative impact of abnl(17p) and -5/5q-. *Blood* 120:2521–2528.

Middeke JM, Fang M, Cornelissen JJ, Mohr B, Appelbaum FR, Stadler M, et al. (2014): Outcome of patients with abnl(17p) acute myeloid leukemia after allogeneic hematopoietic stem cell transplantation. *Blood* 123:2960–2967.

Mielcarek M, Bryant E, Loken M, Zaucha JM, Torok-Storb B, Storb R (2006): Long-term engraftment and clonal dominance of donor-derived del(20q) hematopoietic cells after allogeneic stem cell transplantation. *Blood* 107:1732–1733.

Minamihisamatsu M, Ishihara T (1988): Translocation (8;21) and its variants in acute nonlymphocytic leukemia. The relative importance of chromosomes 8 and 21 to the genesis of the disease. *Cancer Genet Cytogenet* 33:161–173.

Minelli A, Maserati E, Rossi G, Bernardo ME, De Stefano P, Cecchini MP, et al. (2004): Familial platelet disorder with propensity to acute myelogenous leukemia: genetic heterogeneity and progression to leukemia via acquisition of clonal chromosome anomalies. *Genes Chromosomes Cancer* 40:165–171.

Mitelman F, Levan G (1978): Clustering of aberrations to specific chromosomes in human neoplasms. III. Incidence and geographic distribution of chromosome aberrations in 856 cases. *Hereditas* 89:207–232.

Mitelman F, Brandt L, Levan G (1973): Identification of isochromosome 17 in acute myeloid leukaemia. *Lancet* 2:972.

Mitelman F, Nilsson PG, Brandt L, Alimena G, Gastaldi R, Dallapiccola B (1981): Chromosome pattern, occupation, and clinical features in patients with acute non-lymphocytic leukemia. *Cancer Genet Cytogenet* 4:197–214.

Mitelman F, Johansson B, Mertens F (2014): Mitelman Database of Chromosome Aberrations and Gene Fusions in Cancer. Available at http://cgap.nci.nih.gov/Chromosomes/Mitelman.

Mitterbauer M, Laczika K, Novak M, Mitterbauer G, Hilgarth B, Pirc-Danoewinata H, et al. (2000): High concordance of karyotype analysis and RT-PCR for CBF beta/MYH11 in unselected patients with acute myeloid leukemia. A single center study. *Am J Clin Pathol* 113:406–410.

Miyoshi H, Shimizu K, Kozu T, Maseki N, Kaneko Y, Ohki M (1991): t(8;21) breakpoints on chromosome 21 in acute myeloid leukemia are clustered within a limited region of a single gene, AML1. *Proc Natl Acad Sci USA* 88:10431–10434.

Mochizuki N, Shimizu S, Nagasawa T, Tanaka H, Taniwaki M, Yokota J, et al. (2000): A novel gene, MEL1, mapped to 1p36.3 is highly homologous to the MDS1/EVI1 gene and is transcriptionally activated in t(1;3)(p36;q21)-positive leukemia cells. *Blood* 96:3209–3214.

Mohr B, Schetelig J, Schäfer-Eckart K, Schmitz N, Hänel M, Rösler W, et al. (2013): Impact of allogeneic haematopoietic stem cell transplantation in patients with abnl(17p) acute myeloid leukaemia. *Br J Haematol* 161:237–244.

Moir DJ, Jones PAE, Pearson JJ, Duncan JR, Cook P, Buckle VJ (1984): A new translocation, t(1;3)(p36;q21), in myelodysplastic disorders. *Blood* 64:553–555.

Möllgård L, Saft L, Treppendahl MB, Dybedal I, Nørgaard JM, Astermark J, et al. (2011): Clinical effect of increasing doses of lenalidomide in high-risk myelodysplastic syndrome and acute myeloid leukemia with chromosome 5 abnormalities. *Haematologica* 96:963–971.

Moorman AV, Hagemeijer A, Charrin C, Rieder H, Secker-Walker LM (1998): The translocations, t(11;19)(q23;p13.1) and t(11;19)(q23;p13.3): a cytogenetic and clinical profile of 53 patients. *Leukemia* 12:805–810.

Moorman AV, Roman E, Cartwright RA, Morgan GJ (2002): Smoking and the risk of acute myeloid leukaemia in cytogenetic subgroups. *Br J Cancer* 86:60–62.

Morgan R, Chen Z, Stone JF, Cohen J, Gustafson E, Jolly PC, et al. (1996): Trisomy 10: age and leukemic lineage associations. *Cancer Genet Cytogenet* 89:173–174.

Morishita K, Parganas E, William CL, Whittaker MH, Drabkin H, Oval J, et al. (1992): Activation of EVI1 gene expression in human acute myelogenous leukemias by translocations spanning 300–400 kilobases on chromosome band 3q26. *Proc Natl Acad Sci USA* 89:3937–3941.

Mrózek K, Heinonen K, Lawrence D, Carroll AJ, Koduru PRK, Rao KW, et al. (1997): Adult patients with de novo acute myeloid leukemia and t(9;11)(p22;q23) have a superior outcome to patients with other translocations involving band 11q23: a Cancer and Leukemia Group B Study. *Blood* 90:4532–4538.

Mrózek K, Heinonen K, Theil KS, Bloomfield CD (2002): Spectral karyotyping in patients with acute myeloid leukemia and a complex karyotype shows hidden aberrations, including recurrent overrepresentation of 21q, 11q, and 22q. *Genes Chromosomes Cancer* 34:137–153.

Murati A, Adélaide J, Mozziconacci M-J, Popovici C, Carbuccia N, Letessier A, et al. (2004): Variant MYST4-CBP gene fusion in a t(10;16) acute myeloid leukaemia. *Br J Haematol* 125:601–604.

Murati A, Gervais C, Carbuccia N, Finetti P, Cervera N, Adélaïde J, et al. (2009): Genome profiling of acute myelomonocytic leukemia: alteration of the MYB locus in MYST3-linked cases. *Leukemia* 23:85–94.

Nacheva EP, Grace CD, Brazma D, Gancheva K, Howard-Reeves J, Rai L, et al. (2013): Does BCR/ABL1 positive acute myeloid leukaemia exist? *Br J Haematol* 161:541–550.

Nagamachi A, Matsui H, Asou H, Ozaki Y, Aki D, Kanai A, et al. (2013): Haploinsufficiency of SAMD9L, an endosome fusion facilitator, causes myeloid malignancies in mice mimicking human diseases with monosomy 7. *Cancer Cell* 24:305–317.

Najfeld V, Seremetis S, Troy K, Uehlinger J, Schwartz P, Cuttner J (1986): Trisomy 22 – a new abnormality found in acute leukemia characterized by eosinophilia and monocytoid blasts expressing immature differentiation antigens. *Cancer Genet Cytogenet* 23:105–114.

Nakamura T, Alder H, Gu Y, Prasad R, Canaani O, Kamada N, et al. (1993): Genes on chromosomes 4, 9 and 19 involved in 11q23 abnormalities in acute leukemia share sequence homology and/or common motifs. *Proc Natl Acad Sci USA* 90:4631–4635.

Nakamura T, Largaespada DA, Lee MP, Johnson LA, Ohyashiki K, Toyama K, et al. (1996): Fusion of the nucleoporin gene NUP98 to HOXA9 by the chromosome translocation t(7;11)(p15;p15) in human myeloid leukaemia. *Nat Genet* 12:154–158.

Nakamura H, Kuriyama K, Sadamori N, Mine M, Itoyama T, Sasagawa I, et al. (1997): Morphological subtyping of acute myeloid leukemia with maturation (AML-M2): homogeneous pink-colored cytoplasm of mature neutrophils is most characteristic of AML-M2 with t(8;21). *Leukemia* 11:651–655.

Nakazato H, Shiozaki H, Zhou M, Nakatsu M, Motoji T, Mizoguchi H, et al. (2001): TEL/MN1 fusion in a de novo acute myeloid leukaemia-M2 patient who showed strong resistance to treatment. *Br J Haematol* 113:1079–1081.

Nebral K, König M, Schmidt HH, Lutz D, Sperr WR, Kalwak K, et al. (2005): Screening for NUP98 rearrangements in hematopoietic malignancies by fluorescence in situ hybridization. *Haematologica* 90:746–752.

von Neuhoff C, Reinhardt D, Sander A, Zimmermann M, Bradtke J, Betts DR, et al. (2010): Prognostic impact of specific chromosomal aberrations in a large group of pediatric patients with acute myeloid leukemia treated uniformly according to trial AML-BFM 98. *J Clin Oncol* 28:2682–2689.

Niemeyer MMG, Haak HL, Augustinus E, den Nijs-van Weert JI, Leeksma CHW (1986): Trisomy of chromosome 22 in acute myelomonocytic leukemia. *Cancer Genet Cytogenet* 20:371–374.

Nofrini V, Berchicci L, La Starza R, Gorello P, Di Giacomo D, Arcioni F, et al. (2011): MN1-ETV6 fusion gene arising from MDS with 5q-. *Leuk Res* 35:e123–e126.

Nucifora G, Rowley JD (1995): AML1 and the 8;21 and 3;21 translocations in acute and chronic myeloid leukemia. *Blood* 86:1–14.

O'Riordan ML, Berry EW, Tough IM (1970): Chromosome studies on bone marrow from a male control population. *Br J Haematol* 19:83–90.

Ohyashiki K (1984): Nonrandom cytogenetic changes in human acute leukemia and their clinical implications. *Cancer Genet Cytogenet* 11:453–471.

Ohyashiki K, Ohyashiki JH, Iwabuchi A, Ito H, Toyama K (1988): Central nervous system involvement in acute non-lymphocytic leukemia with inv(16)(p13q22). *Leukemia* 2:398–399

Ohyashiki K, Kodama A, Nakamura H, Wakasugi K, Uchida H, Shirota T, et al. (1996): Trisomy 10 in acute myeloid leukemia. *Cancer Genet Cytogenet* 89:114–117.

Okada M, Miyazaki T, Kumota K (1977): 15/17 translocation in acute promyelocytic leukaemia. *Lancet* 1:961.

Okada M, Suto Y, Hirai M, Shiseki M, Usami A, Okajima K, et al. (2012): Microarray CGH analyses of chromosomal 20q deletions in patients with hematopoietic malignancies. *Cancer Genet* 205:18–24.

Olopade OI, Thangavelu M, Larson RA, Mick R, Kowal-Vern A, Schumacher HR, et al. (1992): Clinical, morphologic, and cytogenetic characteristics of 26 patients with acute erythroblastic leukemia. *Blood* 80:2873–2882.

Ono R, Taki T, Taketani T, Kawaguchi H, Taniwaki M, Okamura T, et al. (2002a): SEPTIN6, a human homologue to mouse Septin6, is fused to MLL in infant acute myeloid leukemia with complex chromosomal abnormalities involving 11q23 and Xq24. *Cancer Res* 62:333–337.

Ono R, Taki T, Taketani T, Taniwaki M, Kobayashi H, Hayashi Y (2002b): LCX, leukemia-associated protein with a CXXC domain, is fused to MLL in acute myeloid leukemia with trilineage dysplasia having t(10;11)(q22;q23). *Cancer Res* 62:4075–4080.

Osaka M, Rowley JD, Zeleznik-Le NJ (1999): MSF (MLL septin-like fusion), a fusion partner gene of MLL, in a therapy-related acute myeloid leukemia with a t(11;17) (q23;q25). *Proc Natl Acad Sci USA* 96:6428–6433.

Oshimura M, Hayata I, Kakati S, Sandberg AA (1976): Chromosomes and causation of human cancer and leukemia. XVII. Banding studies in acute myeloblastic leukemia (AML). *Cancer* 38:748–761.

Otsubo K, Horie S, Nomura K, Miyawaki T, Abe A, Kanegane H (2012): Acute promyelocytic leukemia following aleukemic leukemia cutis harboring NPM/RARA fusion gene. *Pediatr Blood Cancer* 59:959–960.

Oyarzo MP, Lin P, Glassman A, Bueso-Ramos CE, Luthra R, Medeiros LJ (2004): Acute myeloid leukemia with t(6;9) (p23;q34) is associated with dysplasia and a high frequency of flt3 gene mutations. *Am J Clin Pathol* 122:348–358.

Panagopoulos I, Åman P, Fioretos T, Höglund M, Johansson B, Mandahl N, et al. (1994): Fusion of the FUS gene with ERG in acute myeloid leukemia with t(16;21)(p11;q22). *Genes Chromosomes Cancer* 11:256–262.

Panagopoulos I, Teixeira MR, Micci F, Hammerstrom J, Isaksson M, Johansson B, et al. (2000): Acute myeloid leukemia with inv(8)(p11q13). *Leuk Lymphoma* 39:651–656.

Panagopoulos I, Fioretos T, Isaksson M, Samuelsson U, Billström R, Strömbeck B, et al. (2001): Fusion of the MORF and CBP genes in acute myeloid leukemia with the t(10;16)(q22;p13). *Hum Mol Genet* 10:395–404.

Panagopoulos I, Isaksson M, Billström R, Strömbeck B, Mitelman F, Johansson B (2003): Fusion of the NUP98 gene and the homeobox gene HOXC13 in acute myeloid leukemia with t(11;12)(p15;q13). *Genes Chromosomes Cancer* 36:107–112.

Panagopoulos I, Kitagawa A, Isaksson M, Morse H, Mitelman F, Johansson B (2004): MLL/GRAF fusion in an infant acute monocytic leukemia (AML M5b) with a cytogenetically cryptic ins(5;11)(q31;q23q23). *Genes Chromosomes Cancer* 41:400–404.

Park KU, Lee DS, Lee HS, Kim CJ, Cho HI (2001): Granulocytic sarcoma in MLL-positive infant acute myelogenous leukemia. Fluorescence in situ hybridization study of childhood acute myelogenous leukemia for detecting MLL rearrangement. *Am J Pathol* 159:2011–2016.

Park J, Kim M, Lim J, Kim Y, Han K, Lee J, et al. (2009): Three-way complex translocations in infant acute myeloid leukemia with t(7;12)(q36;p13): the incidence and correlation of a HLXB9 overexpression. *Cancer Genet Cytogenet* 191:102–105.

Parkin JL, Arthur DC, Abramson CS, McKenna RW, Kersey JH, Heideman RL, et al. (1982): Acute leukemia associated with the t(4;11) chromosome rearrangement: ultrastructural and immunologic characteristics. *Blood* 60:1321–1331.

Parkin B, Erba H, Ouillette P, Roulston D, Purkayastha A, Karp J, et al. (2010): Acquired genomic copy number aberrations and survival in adult acute myelogenous leukemia. *Blood* 116:4958–4967.

Paschka P, Marcucci G, Ruppert AS, Mrózek K, Chen H, Kittles RA, et al. (2006): Adverse prognostic significance of KIT mutations in adult acute myeloid leukemia with inv(16) and t(8;21): a Cancer and Leukemia Group B study. *J Clin Oncol* 24:3904–3911.

Paschka P, Du J, Schlenk RF, Gaidzik VI, Bullinger L, Corbacioglu A, et al. (2013): Secondary genetic lesions in acute myeloid leukemia with inv(16) or t(16;16): a study of the German-Austrian AML Study Group (AMLSG). *Blood* 121:170–177.

Patel KP, Khokhar FA, Muzzafar T, You MJ, Bueso-Ramos CE, Ravandi F, et al. (2013): TdT expression in acute myeloid leukemia with minimal differentiation is associated with distinctive clinicopathological features and better overall survival following stem cell transplantation. *Mod Pathol* 26:195–203.

Paulsson K, Johansson B (2007): Trisomy 8 as the sole chromosomal aberration in acute myeloid leukemia and myelodysplastic syndromes. *Pathol Biol* 55:37–48.

Paulsson K, Békássy AN, Olofsson T, Mitelman F, Johansson B, Panagopoulos I (2006a): A novel and cytogenetically cryptic t(7;21)(p22;q22) in acute myeloid leukemia results in fusion of RUNX1 with the ubiquitin-specific protease gene USP42. *Leukemia* 20:224–229.

Paulsson K, Heidenblad M, Strömbeck B, Staaf J, Jönsson G, Borg Å, et al. (2006b): High-resolution genome-wide array-based comparative genome hybridization reveals cryptic chromosome changes in AML and MDS cases with trisomy 8 as the sole cytogenetic aberration. *Leukemia* 20:840–846.

Pedersen-Bjergaard J, Philip P, Olesen Larsen S, Jensen G, Byrsting K (1990): Chromosome aberrations and prognostic factors in therapy-related myelodysplasia and acute nonlymphocytic leukemia. *Blood* 76:1083–1091.

Pedersen-Bjergaard J, Johansson B, Philip P (1994): Translocation (3;21)(q26;q22) in therapy-related myelodysplasia following drugs targeting DNA-topoisomerase II combined with alkylating agents, and in myeloproliferative disorders undergoing spontaneous leukemic transformation. *Cancer Genet Cytogenet* 76:50–55.

Pedersen-Bjergaard J, Christiansen DH, Desta F, Andersen MK (2006): Alternative genetic pathways and cooperating genetic abnormalities in the pathogenesis of therapy-related myelodysplasia and acute myeloid leukemia. *Leukemia* 20:1943–1949.

Pedersen-Bjergaard J, Andersen MK, Andersen MT, Christiansen DH (2008): Genetics of therapy-related myelodysplasia and acute myeloid leukemia. *Leukemia* 22:240–248.

Peeters P, Wlodarska I, Baens M, Criel A, Selleslag D, Hagemeijer A, et al. (1997): Fusion of ETV6 to MDS1/

EVI1 as a result of t(3;12)(q26;p13) in myeloproliferative disorders. *Cancer Res* 57:564–569.

Peniket A, Wainscoat J, Side L, Daly S, Kusec R, Buck G, et al. (2005): Del (9q) AML: clinical and cytological characteristics and prognostic implications. *Br J Haematol* 129:210–220.

Perea G, Domingo A, Villamor N, Palacios C, Junca J, Torres P, et al. (2005): Adverse prognostic impact of CD36 and CD2 expression in adult de novo acute myeloid leukemia patients. *Leuk Res* 29:1109–1116.

Perrot A, Luquet I, Pigneux A, Mugneret F, Delaunay J, Harousseau JL, et al. (2011): Dismal prognostic value of monosomal karyotype in elderly patients with acute myeloid leukemia: a GOELAMS study of 186 patients with unfavorable cytogenetic abnormalities. *Blood* 118:679–685.

Petit P, Alexander M, Fondu P (1973): Monosomy 7 in erythroleukaemia. *Lancet* 2:1326–1327.

Pierre RV, Hoagland HC (1972): Age-associated aneuploidy: loss of Y chromosome from human bone marrow cells with aging. *Cancer* 30:889–894.

Pollard JA, Alonzo TA, Gerbing RB, Ho PA, Zeng R, Ravindranath Y, et al. (2010): Prevalence and prognostic significance of KIT mutations in pediatric patients with core binding factor AML enrolled on serial pediatric cooperative trials for de novo AML. *Blood* 115:2372–2379.

Poppe B, Vandesompele J, Schoch C, Lindvall C, Mrózek K, Bloomfield CD, et al. (2004): Expression analyses identify MLL as a prominent target of 11q23 amplification and support an etiologic role for MLL gain of function in myeloid malignancies. *Blood* 103:229–235.

Poppe B, Dastugue N, Vandesompele J, Cauwelier B, De Smet B, Yigit N, et al. (2006): EVI1 is consistently expressed as principal transcript in common and rare recurrent 3q26 rearrangements. *Genes Chromosomes Cancer* 45:349–356.

Powell H, Curtis A, Bown N, Taylor P (2005): No correlation between trisomy 13 and FLT3 duplication in acute myeloid leukemia. *Cancer Genet Cytogenet* 156:92–93.

Prasad R, Gu Y, Alder H, Nakamura T, Canaani O, Saito H, et al. (1993): Cloning of the ALL-1 fusion partner, the AF-6 gene, involved in acute myeloid leukemias with the t(6;11) chromosome translocation. *Cancer Res* 53:5624–5628.

Prasad R, Leshkowitz D, Gu Y, Alder H, Nakamura T, Saito H, et al. (1994a): Leucine-zipper dimerization motif encoded by the AF17 gene fused to ALL-1 (MLL) in acute leukemia. *Proc Natl Acad Sci USA* 91:8107–8111.

Prasad DDK, Ouchida M, Lee L, Rao VN, Reddy ESP (1994b): TLS/FUS fusion domain of TLS/FUS-erg chimeric protein resulting from the t(16;21) chromosomal translocation in human myeloid leukemia functions as a transcriptional activation domain. *Oncogene* 9: 3717–3729.

Prébet T, Boissel N, Reutenauer S, Thomas X, Delaunay J, Cahn J-Y, et al. (2009): Acute myeloid leukemia with translocation (8;21) or inversion (16) in elderly patients treated with conventional chemotherapy: a collaborative study of the French CBF-AML intergroup. *J Clin Oncol* 27:4747–4753.

Preudhomme C, Warot-Loze D, Roumier C, Grardel-Duflos N, Garand R, Lai JL, et al. (2000): High incidence of biallelic point mutations in the Runt domain of the AML1/PEBP2αB gene in Mo acute myeloid leukemia and in myeloid malignancies with acquired trisomy 21. *Blood* 96:2862–2869.

Preudhomme C, Sagot C, Boissel N, Cayuela J-M, Tigaud I, de Botton S, et al. (2002): Favorable prognostic significance of CEBPA mutations in patients with de novo acute myeloid leukemia: a study from the Acute Leukemia French Association (ALFA). *Blood* 100:2717–2723.

Pui C-H, Behm FG, Raimondi SC, Dodge RK, George SL, Rivera GK, et al. (1989): Secondary acute myeloid leukemia in children treated for acute lymphoid leukemia. *N Engl J Med* 321:136–142.

Pullarkat ST, Pullarkat V, Lagoo A, Brynes R, Weiss LM, Bedell V, et al. (2013): Characterization of bone marrow mast cells in acute myeloid leukemia with t(8;21) (q22;q22); RUNX1-RUNX1T1. *Leuk Res* 37:1572–1575.

Quelen C, Lippert E, Struski S, Demur C, Soler G, Prade N, et al. (2011): Identification of a transforming MYB-GATA1 fusion gene in acute basophilic leukemia: a new entity in male infants. *Blood* 117:5719–5722.

Quentin S, Cuccuini W, Ceccaldi R, Nibourel O, Pondarre C, Pagès M-P, et al. (2011): Myelodysplasia and leukemia of Fanconi anemia are associated with a specific pattern of genomic abnormalities that includes cryptic RUNX1/AML1 lesions. *Blood* 117:e161–e170.

Quesnel B, Kantarjian H, Pedersen Bjergaard J, Brault P, Estey E, Lai JL, et al. (1993): Therapy-related acute myeloid leukemia with t(8;21), inv(16), and t(8;16): a report on 25 cases and review of the literature. *J Clin Oncol* 11:2370–2379.

Radtke I, Mullighan CG, Ishii M, Su X, Cheng J, Ma J, et al. (2009): Genomic analysis reveals few genetic alterations in pediatric acute myeloid leukemia. *Proc Natl Acad Sci USA* 106:12944–12949.

Raghavan M, Lillington DM, Skoulakis S, Debernardi S, Chaplin T, Foot NJ, et al. (2005): Genome-wide single nucleotide polymorphism analysis reveals frequent partial uniparental disomy due to somatic recombination in acute myeloid leukemias. *Cancer Res* 65:375–378.

Raimondi SC, Dubé ID, Valentine MB, Mirro J Jr, Watt HJ, Larson RA, et al. (1989a): Clinicopathologic manifestations and breakpoints of the t(3;5) in patients with acute nonlymphocytic leukemia. *Leukemia* 3:42–47.

Raimondi SC, Kalwinsky DK, Hayashi Y, Behm FG, Mirro J Jr, Williams DL (1989b): Cytogenetics of childhood acute nonlymphocytic leukemia. *Cancer Genet Cytogenet* 40: 13–27.

Raimondi SC, Chang MN, Ravindranath Y, Behm FG, Gresik MV, Steuber CP, et al. (1999): Chromosomal abnormalities in 478 children with acute myeloid leukemia: clinical characteristics and treatment outcome in a cooperative Pediatric Oncology Group study-POG 8821. *Blood* 94:3707–3716.

Ratain MJ, Kaminer LS, Bitran JD, Larson RA, Le Beau MM, Skosey C, et al. (1987): Acute nonlymphocytic leukemia following etoposide and cisplatin combination chemotherapy for advanced non-small-cell carcinoma of the lung. *Blood* 70:1412–1417.

Raynaud SD, Baens M, Grosgeorge J, Rodgers K, Reid CDL, Dainton M, et al. (1996): Fluorescence in situ hybridization analysis of t(3;12)(q26;p13): a recurring chromosomal abnormality involving the TEL gene (ETV6) in myelodysplastic syndromes. *Blood* 88:682–689.

Raza-Egilmez SZ, Jani-Sait SN, Grossi M, Higgins MJ, Shows TB, Aplan PD (1998): NUP98-HOXD13 gene fusion in therapy-related acute myelogenous leukemia. *Cancer Res* 58:4269–4273.

Redei I, Mangan KF, Ming PL, Mullaney MT, Rao PN, Goldberg SL, et al. (1997): Detection of a dormant 20q-leukemia clone in bone marrow cultures with hematopoietic growth factors: implications for secondary leukemia post-transplant. *Bone Marrow Transplant* 19:521–523.

Redner RL, Rush EA, Faas S, Rudert WA, Corey SJ (1996): The t(5;17) variant of acute promyelocytic leukemia expresses a nucleophosmin-retinoic acid receptor fusion. *Blood* 87:882–886.

Rege-Cambrin G, Giugliano E, Michaux L, Stul M, Scaravaglio P, Serra A, et al. (2005): Trisomy 11 in myeloid malignancies is associated with internal tandem duplication of both MLL and FLT3 genes. *Haematologica* 90:262–264.

Riske CB, Morgan R, Ondreyco S, Sandberg AA (1994): X and Y chromosome loss as sole abnormality in acute nonlymphocytic leukemia (ANLL). *Cancer Genet Cytogenet* 72:44–47.

Rochowski A, Olson SB, Alonzo TA, Gerbing RB, Lange BJ, Alter BP (2012): Patients with Fanconi anemia and AML have different cytogenetic clones than de novo cases of AML. *Pediatr Blood Cancer* 59:922–924.

Rogers HJ, Vardiman JW, Anastasi J, Raca G, Savage NM, Cherry AM, et al. (2014): Complex or monosomal karyotype and not blast percentage are associated with poor survival in acute myeloid leukemia and myelodysplastic syndrome patients with inv(3)(q21q26.2)/t(3;3)(q21;q26.2): a Bone Marrow Pathology Group study. *Haematologica* 99:821–829.

Röllig C, Bornhäuser M, Thiede C, Taube F, Kramer M, Mohr B, et al. (2011): Long-term prognosis of acute myeloid leukemia according to the new genetic risk classification of the European LeukemiaNet recommendations: evaluation of the proposed reporting system. *J Clin Oncol* 29:2758–2765.

Romana SP, Radford-Weiss I, Ben Abdelali R, Schluth C, Petit A, Dastugue N, et al. (2006): NUP98 rearrangements in hematopoietic malignancies: a study of the Groupe Francophone de Cytogénétique Hématologique. *Leukemia* 20:696–706.

de Rooij JD, Hollink IHIM, Arentsen-Peters STCJM, van Galen JF, Beverloo HB, Baruchel A, et al. (2013): NUP98/JARID1A is a novel recurrent abnormality in pediatric acute megakaryoblastic leukemia with a distinct HOX gene expression pattern. *Leukemia* 27:2280–2288.

Roulston D, Espinosa III R, Stoffel M, Bell GI, Le Beau MM (1993): Molecular genetics of myeloid leukemia: identification of the commonly deleted segment of chromosome 20. *Blood* 82:3424–3429.

Roulston D, Anastasi J, Rudinsky R, Nucifora G, Zeleznik-Le N, Rowley JD, et al. (1995): Therapy-related acute leukemia associated with t(11q23) after primary acute myeloid leukemia with t(8;21): a report of two cases. *Blood* 86:3613–3614.

Roulston D, Espinosa III R, Nucifora G, Larson RA, Le Beau MM, Rowley JD (1998): CBFA2(AML1) translocations with novel partner chromosomes in myeloid leukemias: association with prior therapy. *Blood* 92:2879–2885.

Rowley JD (1973a): Deletions of chromosome 7 in haematological disorders. *Lancet* 2:1385–1386.

Rowley JD (1973b): Identification of a translocation with quinacrine fluorescence in a patient with acute leukemia. *Ann Genet* 16:109–112.

Rowley JD (1976): 5q- acute myelogenous leukemia: reply. *Blood* 48:626.

Rowley JD, Potter D (1976): Chromosomal banding patterns in acute nonlymphocytic leukemia. *Blood* 47:705–721.

Rowley JD, Golomb HM, Dougherty C (1977a): 15/17 translocation, a consistent chromosomal change in acute promyelocytic leukaemia. *Lancet* 1:549–550.

Rowley JD, Golomb HM, Vardiman J (1977b): Nonrandom chromosomal abnormalities in acute non-lymphocytic leukemia in patients treated for Hodgkin disease and non-Hodgkin lymphomas. *Blood* 50:759–770.

Rowley JD, Reshmi S, Sobulo O, Musvee T, Anastasi J, Raimondi S, et al. (1997): All patients with the t(11;16)(q23;p13.3) that involves MLL and CBP have treatment-related hematologic disorders. *Blood* 90:535–541.

Rubin CM, Larson RA, Bitter MA, Carrino JJ, Le Beau MM, Diaz MO, et al. (1987): Association of a chromosomal 3;21 translocation with the blast phase of chronic myelogenous leukemia. *Blood* 70:1338–1342.

Rubin CM, Larson RA, Anastasi J, Winter JN, Thangavelu M, Vardiman JW, et al. (1990): t(3;21)(q26;q22): a recurring chromosomal abnormality in therapy-related myelodysplastic syndrome and acute myeloid leukemia. *Blood* 76:2594–2598.

Rubnitz JE, Raimondi SC, Tong X, Srivastava DK, Razzouk BI, Shurtleff SA, et al. (2002): Favorable impact of the t(9;11) in childhood acute myeloid leukemia. *J Clin Oncol* 20:2302–2309.

Rubnitz JE, Inaba H, Dahl G, Ribeiro RC, Bowman WP, Taub J, et al. (2010): Minimal residual disease-directed therapy for childhood acute myeloid leukaemia: results of the AML02 multicentre trial. *Lancet Oncol* 11:543–552.

Rücker FG, Schlenk RF, Bullinger L, Kayser S, Teleanu V, Kett H, et al. (2012): TP53 alterations in acute myeloid leukemia with complex karyotype correlate with specific copy number alterations, monosomal karyotype, and dismal outcome. *Blood* 119:2114–2121.

Sadamori N, Yao E, Tagawa M, Nakamura H, Sasagawa I, Itoyama T, et al. (1990): 16;21 translocation in acute non-lymphocytic leukemia with abnormal eosinophils: a unique subtype. *Acta Haematol* 84:212–216.

Sainty D, Liso V, Cantu-Rajnoldi A, Head D, Mozziconacci M-J, Arnoulet C, et al. (2000): A new morphologic classification system for acute promyelocytic leukemia distinguishes cases with underlying PLZF/RARA gene rearrangements. *Blood* 96:1287–1296.

Sakai I, Tamura T, Narumi H, Uchida N, Yakushijin Y, Hato T, et al. (2005): Novel RUNX1-PRDM16 fusion transcripts in a patient with acute myeloid leukemia showing t(1;21) (p36;q22). *Genes Chromosomes Cancer* 44:265–270.

Sakurai M, Sandberg AA (1973): Prognosis of acute myeloblastic leukemia: chromosomal correlation. *Blood* 41:93–104.

Sakurai M, Sandberg AA (1976): Chromosomes and causation of human cancer and leukemia. XI. Correlation of karyotypes with clinical features of acute myeloblastic leukemia. *Cancer* 37:285–299.

Sanada M, Uike N, Ohyashiki K, Ozawa K, Lili W, Hangaishi A, et al. (2007): Unbalanced translocation der(1;7) (q10;p10) defines a unique clinicopathological subgroup of myeloid neoplasms. *Leukemia* 21:992–997.

Sandahl JD, Coenen EA, Forestier E, Harbott J, Johansson B, Kerndrup G, et al. (2014a): t(6;9)(p22;q34)/DEK-NUP214 rearranged pediatric myeloid leukemia: an international study on 62 patients. *Haematologica* 99:865–872.

Sandahl JD, Kjeldsen E, Abrahamsson J, Ha S-Y, Heldrup J, Jahnukainen K, et al. (2014b): Ploidy and clinical characteristics of childhood acute myeloid leukemia: a NOPHO-AML study. *Genes Chromosomes Cancer.* 53:667–675

Sandberg AA, Sakurai M (1973): The missing Y chromosome and human leukaemia. *Lancet* 1:375.

Sandberg AA, Abe S, Kowalczyk JR, Zedgenidze A, Takeuchi J, Kakati S (1982): Chromosomes and causation of human cancer and leukemia. L. Cytogenetics of leukemias complicating other diseases. *Cancer Genet Cytogenet* 7:95–136.

Sanderson RN, Johnson PRE, Moorman AV, Roman E, Willett E, Taylor PR, et al. (2006): Population-based demographic study of karyotypes in 1709 patients with adult acute myeloid leukemia. *Leukemia* 20:444–450.

Sandler DP, Shore DL, Anderson JR, Davey FR, Arthur A, Mayer RJ, et al. (1993): Cigarette smoking and risk of acute leukemia: associations with morphology and cytogenetic abnormalities in bone marrow. *J Natl Cancer Inst* 85: 1994–2003.

Santos J, Cerveira N, Correia C, Lisboa S, Pinheiro M, Torres L, et al. (2010): Coexistence of alternative MLL-SEPT9 fusion transcripts in an acute myeloid leukemia with t(11;17)(q23;q25). *Cancer Genet Cytogenet* 197:60–64.

Sasaki M, Muramoto J, Makino S, Hara Y, Okada M, Tanaka E (1975): Two cases of acute myeloblastic leukemia associated with a 9/22 translocation. *Proc Jpn Acad* 51:193–197.

Sasaki M, Okada M, Kondo I, Muramoto J (1976): Chromosome banding patterns in 27 cases of acute myeloblastic leukemia. *Proc Jpn Acad* 52:505–508.

Sasaki M, Kondo K, Tomiyasu T (1983): Cytogenetic characterization of ten cases of Ph1-positive acute myelogenous leukemia. *Cancer Genet Cytogenet* 9:119–128.

Sato Y, Abe S, Mise K, Sasaki M, Kamada N, Kouda K, et al. (1987): Reciprocal translocation involving the short arms of chromosomes 7 and 11, t(7p-;11p+), associated with myeloid leukemia with maturation. *Blood* 70:1654–1658.

Sato Y, Suto Y, Pietenpol J, Golub TR, Gilliland DG, Davis EM, et al. (1995): TEL and KIP1 define the smallest region of deletions on 12p13 in hematopoietic malignancies. *Blood* 86:1525–1533.

Schaich M, Harbich-Brutscher E, Pascheberg U, Mohr B, Soucek S, Ehninger G, et al. (2002): Association of specific cytogenetic aberrations with mdr1 gene expression in adult myeloid leukemia and its implication in treatment outcome. *Haematologica* 87:455–464.

Schaich M, Schlenk RF, Al-Ali HK, Döhner H, Ganser A, Heil G, et al. (2007): Prognosis of acute myeloid leukemia patients up to 60 years of age exhibiting trisomy 8 within a non-complex karyotype: individual patient data-based meta-analysis of the German Acute Myeloid Leukemia Intergroup. *Haematologica* 92:763–770.

Scheres JMJC, Hustinx TWJ, Geraedts JPM, Leeksma CHW, Meltzer PS (1985): Translocation 1;7 in hematologic disorders: a brief review of 22 cases. *Cancer Genet Cytogenet* 18:207–213.

Schlenk RF, Benner A, Krauter J, Büchner T, Sauerland C, Ehninger G, et al. (2004): Individual patient data-based meta-analysis of patients aged 16 to 60 years with core binding factor acute myeloid leukemia: a survey of the German Acute Myeloid Leukemia Intergroup. *J Clin Oncol* 22:3741–3750.

Schnittger S, Kinkelin U, Schoch C, Heinecke A, Haase D, Haferlach T, et al. (2000): Screening for MLL tandem duplication in 387 unselected patients with AML identify a prognostically unfavorable subset of AML. *Leukemia* 14:796–804.

Schnittger S, Kohl TM, Haferlach T, Kern W, Hiddemann W, Spiekermann K, et al. (2006): KIT-D816 mutations in

AML1-ETO-positive AML are associated with impaired event-free and overall survival. *Blood* 107:1791–1799.

Schnittger S, Bacher U, Kern W, Haferlach T, Haferlach C (2007): JAK2V617F as progression marker in CMPD and as cooperative mutation in AML with trisomy 8 and t(8;21): a comparative study on 1103 CMPD and 269 AML cases. *Leukemia* 21:1843–1845.

Schnittger S, Eder C, Jeromin S, Alpermann T, Fasan A, Grossmann V, et al. (2013): ASXL1 exon 12 mutations are frequent in AML with intermediate risk karyotype and are independently associated with an adverse outcome. *Leukemia* 27:82–91.

Schoch C, Haase D, Fonatsch C, Haferlach T, Löffler H, Schlegelberger B, et al. (1997): The significance of trisomy 8 in de novo acute myeloid leukaemia: the accompanying chromosome aberrations determine the prognosis. *Br J Haematol* 99:605–611.

Schoch C, Haferlach T, Haase D, Fonatsch C, Löffler H, Schlegelberger B, et al. (2001): Patients with de novo acute myeloid leukaemia and complex karyotype aberrations show a poor prognosis despite intensive treatment: a study of 90 patients. *Br J Haematol* 112:118–126.

Schoch C, Haferlach T, Bursch S, Gerstner D, Schnittger S, Dugas M, et al. (2002): Loss of genetic material is more common than gain in acute myeloid leukemia with complex aberrant karyotype: a detailed analysis of 125 cases using conventional chromosome analysis and fluorescence in situ hybridization including 24-color FISH. *Genes Chromosomes Cancer* 35:20–29.

Schoch C, Kern W, Kohlmann A, Hiddemann W, Schnittger S, Haferlach T (2005a): Acute myeloid leukemia with a complex aberrant karyotype is a distinct biological entity characterized by genomic imbalances and a specific gene expression profile. *Genes Chromosomes Cancer* 43:227–238.

Schoch C, Kohlmann A, Dugas M, Kern W, Hiddemann W, Schnittger S, et al. (2005b): Genomic gains and losses influence expression levels of genes located within the affected regions: a study on acute myeloid leukemias with trisomy 8, 11, or 13, monosomy 7, or deletion 5q. *Leukemia* 19:1224–1228.

Schouten HC, vanPutten WLJ, Hegemeijer A, Blijham GH, Sonneveld P, Willemze R, et al. (1991): The prognostic significance of chromosomal findings in patients with acute myeloid leukemia in a study comparing the efficacy of autologous and allogeneic bone marrow transplantation. *Bone Marrow Transplant* 8:377–381.

Schütte J, Opalka B, Becher R, Bardenheuer W, Szymanski S, Lux A, et al. (1993): Analysis of the p53 gene in patients with isochromosome 17q and Ph1-positive or -negative myeloid leukemia. *Leuk Res* 17:533–539.

Scott AA, Head DR, Kopecky KJ, Appelbaum FR, Theil KS, Grever MR, et al. (1994): HLA-DR-, CD33+, CD56+, CD16- myeloid/natural killer cell acute leukemia: a previously unrecognized form of acute leukemia potentially misdiagnosed as French-American-British acute myeloid leukemia-M3. *Blood* 84:244–255.

Secker-Walker LM (1971): The chromosomes of bone-marrow cells of haematologically normal men and women. *Br J Haematol* 21:455–461.

Secker-Walker LM, Mehta A, Bain B (1995): Abnormalities of 3q21 and 3q26 in myeloid malignancy: a United Kingdom Cancer Cytogenetic Group study. *Br J Haematol* 91:490–501.

Secker-Walker LM, Moorman AV, Bain BJ, Mehta AB (1998): Secondary acute leukemia and myelodysplastic syndrome with 11q23 abnormalities. *Leukemia* 12:840–844.

Seifert H, Mohr B, Thiede C, Oelschlägel U, Schäkel U, Illmer T, et al. (2009): The prognostic impact of 17p (p53) deletion in 2272 adults with acute myeloid leukemia. *Leukemia* 23:656–663.

Sekeres MA, Gundacker H, Lancet J, Advani A, Petersdorf S, Liesveld J, et al. (2011): A phase 2 study of lenalidomide monotherapy in patients with deletion 5q acute myeloid leukemia: Southwest Oncology Group Study S0605. *Blood* 118:523–528.

Shago M, Bouman D, Kamel-Reid S, Minden M, Chun K (2004): Cryptic insertion of MLL gene into 9p22 leads to MLL-MLLT3 (AF9) fusion in a case of acute myelogenous leukemia. *Genes Chromosomes Cancer* 40:349–354.

Shali W, Helias C, Fohrer C, Struski S, Gervais C, Falkenrodt A, et al. (2006): Cytogenetic studies of a series of 43 consecutive secondary myelodysplastic syndromes/acute myeloid leukemias: conventional cytogenetics, FISH, and multiplex FISH. *Cancer Genet Cytogenet* 168:133–145.

Shannon KM, Watterson J, Johnson P, O'Connell P, Lange B, Shah N, et al. (1992): Monosomy 7 myeloproliferative disease in children with neurofibromatosis, type 1: epidemiology and molecular analysis. *Blood* 79:1311–1318.

Shiba N, Ichikawa H, Taki T, Park M-J, Jo A, Mitani S, et al. (2013): NUP98-NSD1 gene fusion and its related gene expression signature are strongly associated with a poor prognosis in pediatric acute myeloid leukemia. *Genes Chromosomes Cancer* 52:683–693.

Shihadeh F, Reed V, Faderl S, Medeiros LJ, Mazloom A, Hadziahmetovic M, et al. (2012): Cytogenetic profile of patients with acute myeloid leukemia and central nervous system disease. *Cancer* 118:112–117.

Shikami M, Miwa H, Nishii K, Takahashi T, Shiku H, Tsutani H, et al. (1999): Myeloid differentiation antigen and cytokine receptor expression on acute myelocytic leukaemia cells with t(16;21)(p11;q22): frequent expression of CD56 and interleukin-2 receptor α chain. *Br J Haematol* 105:711–719.

Shimada A, Taki T, Tabuchi K, Tawa A, Horibe K, Tsuchida M, et al. (2006): KIT mutations, and not FLT3 internal tandem duplication, are strongly associated with a poor prognosis in pediatric acute myeloid leukemia with t(8;21): a study of the Japanese Childhood AML Cooperative Study Group. *Blood* 107:1806–1809.

Shimizu H, Yokohama A, Hatsumi N, Takada S, Handa H, Sakura T, et al. (2014): Philadelphia chromosome-positive mixed phenotype acute leukemia in the imatinib era. *Eur J Haematol* 934:297–301.

Shing DC, McMullan DJ, Roberts P, Smith K, Chin S-F, Nicholson J, et al. (2003): FUS/ERG gene fusions in Ewing's tumors. *Cancer Res* 63:4568–4576.

Silva FPG, Lind A, Brouwer-Mandema G, Valk PJM, Giphart-Gassler M (2007): Trisomy 13 correlates with RUNX1 mutation and increased FLT3 expression in AML-M0 patients. *Haematologica* 92:1123–1126.

Simmons HM, Oseth L, Nguyen P, O'Leary M, Conklin KF, Hirsch B (2002): Cytogenetic and molecular heterogeneity of 7q36/12p13 rearrangements in childhood AML. *Leukemia* 16:2408–2416.

Slack JL, Arthur DC, Lawrence D, Mrózek K, Mayer RJ, Davey FR, et al. (1997): Secondary cytogenetic changes in acute promyelocytic leukemia—prognostic importance in patients treated with chemotherapy alone and association with the intron 3 breakpoint of the PML gene: a Cancer and Leukemia Group B study. *J Clin Oncol* 15:1786–1795.

Slater RM, von Drunen E, Kroes WG, Weghuis DO, van den Berg E, Smit EM, et al. (2001): t(7;12)(q36;p13) and t(7;12) (q32;p13) – translocations involving ETV6 in children 18 months of age or younger with myeloid disorders. *Leukemia* 15:915–920.

Slovak ML, Traweek ST, Willman CL, Head DR, Kopecky KJ, Magenis RE, et al. (1995): Trisomy 11: an association with stem/progenitor cell immunophenotype. *Br J Haematol* 90:266–273.

Slovak ML, Kopecky KJ, Cassileth PA, Harrington DH, Theil KS, Mohamed A, et al. (2000): Karyotypic analysis predicts outcome of preremission and postremission therapy in adult acute myeloid leukemia: a Southwest Oncology Group/Eastern Cooperative Oncology Group study. *Blood* 96:4075–4083.

Slovak ML, Bedell V, Popplewell L, Arber DA, Schoch C, Slater R (2002): 21q22 balanced chromosome aberrations in therapy-related hematopoietic disorders: report from an international workshop. *Genes Chromosomes Cancer* 33:379–394.

Slovak ML, Gundacker H, Bloomfield CD, Dewald G, Appelbaum FR, Larson RA, et al. (2006): A retrospective study of 69 patients with t(6;9)(p23;q34) AML emphasizes the need for a prospective, multicenter initiative for rare 'poor prognosis' myeloid malignancies. *Leukemia* 20:1295–1297.

Slovak ML, O'Donnell M, Smith DD, Gaal K (2009): Does MDS with der(1;7)(q10;p10) constitute a distinct risk group? A retrospective single institutional analysis of

clinical/pathologic features compared to -7/del(7q) MDS. *Cancer Genet Cytogenet* 193:78–85.

Smith SM, Le Beau MM, Huo D, Karrison T, Sobecks RM, Anastasi J, et al. (2003): Clinical-cytogenetic associations in 306 patients with therapy-related myelodysplasia and myeloid leukemia: the University of Chicago series. *Blood* 102:43–52.

Snaddon J, Neat M, Fitzgibbon J, Smith ML, Rohatiner AZ, Lister TA, et al. (2002): Mutations in the runt homology domain of CBFα2 in myeloid malignancies with acquired trisomy 21. *Cancer Genet Cytogenet* 136:151–152.

Sobulo OM, Borrow J, Tomek R, Reshmi S, Harden A, Schlegelberger B, et al. (1997): MLL is fused to CBP, a histone acetyltransferase, in therapy-related acute myeloid leukemia with a t(11;16)(q23;p13.3). *Proc Natl Acad Sci USA* 94:8732–8737.

Soenen V, Preudhomme C, Roumier C, Daudignon A, Lai J-L, Fenaux P (1998): 17p deletion in acute myeloid leukemia and myelodysplastic syndrome. Analysis of breakpoints and deleted segments by fluorescence in situ. *Blood* 91:1008–1015.

Soni M, Brody J, Allen SL, Schulman P, Kolitz J, Rai K, et al. (1996): Clinical and morphological features of cases of trisomy 13 in acute non-lymphocytic leukemia. *Leukemia* 10:619–623.

Soupir CP, Vergilio J-A, Dal Cin P, Muzikansky A, Kantarjian H, Jones D, et al. (2007): Philadelphia chromosome-positive acute myeloid leukemia: a rare aggressive leukemia with clinicopathologic features distinct from chronic myeloid leukemia in myeloid blast crisis. *Am J Clin Pathol* 127:642–650.

Sreekantaiah C, Baer MR, Preisler HD, Sandberg AA (1989): Involvement of bands 9q21-q22 in five cases of acute non-lymphocytic leukemia. *Cancer Genet Cytogenet* 39:55–64.

Steensma DP, Dewald GW, Hodnefield JM, Tefferi A, Hanson CA (2003): Clonal cytogenetic abnormalities in bone marrow specimens without clear morphologic evidence of dysplasia: a form fruste of myelodysplasia? *Leuk Res* 27:235–242.

Sterkers Y, Preudhomme C, Lai J-L, Demory J-L, Caulier M-T, Wattel E, et al. (1998): Acute myeloid leukemia and myelodysplastic syndromes following essential thrombocythemia treated with hydroxyurea: high proportion of cases with 17p deletion. *Blood* 91:616–622.

Steudel C, Wermke M, Schaich M, Schäkel U, Illmer T, Ehninger G, et al. (2003): Comparative analysis of MLL partial tandem duplication and FLT3 internal tandem duplication mutations in 956 adult patients with acute myeloid leukemia. *Genes Chromosomes Cancer* 37: 237–251.

Stevens-Kroef M, Poppe B, van Zelderen-Bhola S, van den Berg E, van der Blij-Philipsen M, Geurts van Kessel A, et al. (2004): Translocation t(2;3)(p15-23;q26-27) in myeloid malignancies: report of 21 new cases, clinical, cytogenetic and molecular genetic features. *Leukemia* 18:1108–1114.

Stevens-Kroef MJPL, Schoenmakers EFPM, van Kraaij M, Huys E, Vermeulen S, van der Reijden B, et al. (2006): Identification of truncated RUNX1 and RUNX1-PRDM16 fusion transcripts in a case of t(1;21)(p36;q22)-positive therapy-related AML. *Leukemia* 20:1187–1189.

Stoddart A, Fernald AA, Wang J, Davis EM, Karrison T, Anastasi J, et al. (2014): Haploinsufficiency of del(5q) genes, Egr1 and Apc, cooperate with Tp53 loss to induce acute myeloid leukemia in mice. *Blood* 123:1069–1078.

Storlazzi CT, Fioretos T, Surace C, Lonoce A, Mastrorilli A, Strömbeck B, et al. (2006): MYC-containing double minutes in hematologic malignancies: evidence in favor of the episome model and exclusion of MYC as the target gene. *Hum Mol Genet* 15:933–942.

van der Straaten HM, van Biezen A, Brand R, Schattenberg AVMB, Egeler RM, Barge RM, et al. (2005): Allogeneic stem cell transplantation for patients with acute myeloid leukemia or myelodysplastic syndrome who have chromosome 5 and/or 7 abnormalities. *Haematologica* 90:1339–1345.

Strehl S, Borkhardt A, Slany R, Fuchs UE, König M, Haas OA (2003): The human LASP1 gene is fused to MLL in an acute myeloid leukemia with t(11;17)(q23;q21). *Oncogene* 22:157–160.

Strehl S, König M, Meyer C, Schneider B, Harbott J, Jäger U, et al. (2006): Molecular dissection of t(11;17) in acute myeloid leukemia reveals a variety of gene fusions with heterogeneous fusion transcripts and multiple splice variants. *Genes Chromosomes Cancer* 45:1041–1049.

Streubel B, Valent P, Jäger U, Edelhäuser M, Wandt H, Wagner T, et al. (2000): Amplification of the MLL gene on double minutes, a homogeneously staining region, and ring chromosomes in five patients with acute myeloid leukemia or myelodysplastic syndrome. *Genes Chromosomes Cancer* 27:380–386.

Suenaga M, Sanada I, Tsukamoto A, Sato M, Kawano F, Shido T, et al. (1993): Trisomy 4 in a case of acute myelogenous leukemia accompanied by subcutaneous soft tissue tumors. Report of a case and review of the literature. *Cancer Genet Cytogenet* 71:71–75.

Sun J, Konoplev SN, Wang X, Cui W, Chen SS, Medeiros LJ, et al. (2011): De novo acute myeloid leukemia with inv(3)(q21q26.2) or t(3;3)(q21;q26.2): a clinicopathologic and cytogenetic study of an entity recently added to the WHO classification. *Mod Pathol* 24:384–389.

Suzukawa K, Parganas E, Gajjar A, Abe T, Takahashi S, Tani K, et al. (1994): Identification of a breakpoint cluster region 3′ of the ribophorin I gene at 3q21 associated with the transcriptional activation of the EVI1 gene in acute myelogenous leukemias with inv(3)(q21q26). *Blood* 84:2681–2688.

Suzuki A, Kimura Y, Ohyashiki K, Kitano K, Kageyama S, Kasai M, et al. (2000): Trisomy 10 in acute myeloid leukemia: three additional cases from the database of the Japan Adult Leukemia Study Group (JALSG) AML-92 and AML-95. *Cancer Genet Cytogenet* 120:141–143.

Swansbury GJ, Slater R, Bain BJ, Moorman AV, Secker-Walker LM (1998): Hematological malignancies with t(9;11)(p21-22;q23) – a laboratory and clinical study of 125 cases. *Leukemia* 12:792–800.

Sweet DL, Golomb HM, Rowley JD, Vardiman JM (1979): Acute myelogenous leukemia and thrombocythemia associated with an abnormality of chromosome no. 3. *Cancer Genet Cytogenet* 1:33–37.

Sweetser DA, Peniket AJ, Haaland C, Blomberg AA, Zhang Y, Zaidi ST, et al. (2005): Delineation of the minimal commonly deleted segment and identification of candidate tumor-suppressor genes in del(9q) acute myeloid leukemia. *Genes Chromosomes Cancer* 44:279–291.

Swerdlow SH, Campo E, Harris NL, Jaffe ES, Pileri SA, Stein H, et al., editors (2008): *WHO classification of Tumours of the Haematopoietic and Lymphoid Tissues.* Lyon: IARC.

Swirsky DM, Li YS, Matthews JG, Flemans RJ, Rees JKH, Hayhoe FGJ (1984): 8;21 translocation in acute granulocytic leukaemia: cytological, cytochemical and clinical features. *Br J Haematol* 56:199–213.

Taketani T, Taki T, Ono R, Kobayashi Y, Ida K, Hayashi Y (2002a): The chromosome translocation t(7;11)(p15;p15) in acute myeloid leukemia results in fusion of the NUP98 gene with a HOXA cluster gene, HOXA13, but not HOXA9. *Genes Chromosomes Cancer* 34:437–443.

Taketani T, Taki T, Shibuya N, Ito E, Kitazawa J, Terui K, et al. (2002b): The HOXD11 gene is fused to the NUP98 gene in acute myeloid leukemia with t(2;11)(q31;p15). *Cancer Res* 62:33–37.

Taketani T, Taki T, Shibuya N, Kikuchi A, Hanada R, Hayashi Y (2002c): Novel NUP98-HOXC11 fusion gene resulted from a chromosomal break within exon 1 of HOXC11 in acute myeloid leukemia with t(11;12)(p15;q13). *Cancer Res* 62:4571–4574.

Taketani T, Taki T, Takita J, Tsuchida M, Hanada R, Hongo T, et al. (2003): AML1/RUNX1 mutations are infrequent, but related to AML-M0, acquired trisomy 21, and leukemic transformation in pediatric hematologic malignancies. *Genes Chromosomes Cancer* 38:1–7.

Taki T, Sako M, Tsuchida M, Hayashi Y (1997): The t(11;16)(q23;p13) translocation in myelodysplastic syndrome fuses the MLL gene to the CBP gene. *Blood* 89:3945–3950.

Taki T, Ohnishi H, Shinohara K, Sako M, Bessho F, Yanagisawa M, et al. (1999): AF17q25, a putative septin family gene, fuses the MLL gene in acute myeloid leukemia with t(11;17)(q23;q25). *Cancer Res* 59:4261–4265.

Tallman MS, Hakimian D, Shaw JM, Lissner GS, Russell EJ, Variakojis D (1993): Granulocytic sarcoma is associated with the 8;21 translocation in acute myeloid leukemia. *J Clin Oncol* 11:690–697.

Tallman MS, Dewald GW, Gandham S, Logan BR, Keating A, Lazarus HM, et al. (2007): Impact of cytogenetics on outcome of matched unrelated donor hematopoietic stem cell transplantation for acute myeloid leukemia in first or second complete remission. *Blood* 110:409–417.

Tanaka K, Arif M, Eguchi M, Kyo T, Dohy H, Kamada N (1997): Frequent jumping translocations of chromosomal segments involving the ABL oncogene alone or in combination with CD3-MLL genes in secondary leukemias. *Blood* 89:596–600.

Tatsumi K, Taki T, Taniwaki M, Nakamura H, Taguchi J, Chen YZ, et al. (2001): The CDCREL1 gene fused to MLL in de novo acute myeloid leukemia with t(11;22)(q23;q11.2) and its frequent expression in myeloid leukemia cell lines. *Genes Chromosomes Cancer* 30:230–235.

The Cancer Genome Atlas Research (2013): Genomic and epigenomic landscapes of adult de novo acute myeloid leukemia. *N Engl J Med* 368:2059–2074.

de Thé H, Chomienne C, Lanotte M, Degos L, Dejean A (1990): The t(15;17) translocation of acute promyelocytic leukaemia fuses the retinoic acid receptor α gene to a novel transcribed locus. *Nature* 347:558–561.

Thiollier C, Lopez CK, Gerby B, Ignacimouttou C, Poglio S, Duffourd Y, et al. (2012): Characterization of novel genomic alterations and therapeutic approaches using acute megakaryoblastic leukemia xenograft models. *J Exp Med* 209:2017–2031.

Thirman MJ, Gill HJ, Burnett RC, Mbangkollo D, McCabe NR, Kobayashi H, et al. (1993): Rearrangement of the MLL gene in acute lymphoblastic and acute myeloid leukemias with 11q23 chromosomal translocations. *N Engl J Med* 329:909–914.

Thirman MJ, Levitan DA, Kobayashi H, Simon MC, Rowley JD (1994): Cloning of ELL, a gene that fuses to MLL in a t(11;19)(q23;p13.1) in acute myeloid leukemia. *Proc Natl Acad Sci USA* 91:12110–12114.

Thol F, Kölking B, Hollink IHI, Damm F, van den Heuvel-Eibrink MM, Zwaan CM, et al. (2013): Analysis of NUP98/NSD1 translocations in adult AML and MDS patients. *Leukemia* 27:750–754.

Tien H-F, Wang C-H, Chuang S-M, Lee F-Y, Liu M-C, Chen YC, et al. (1992): Characterization of Philadelphia-chromosome-positive acute leukemia by clinical, immunocytochemical, and gene analysis. *Leukemia* 6:907–914.

Tien H-F, Wang C-H, Lin M-T, Lee F-Y, Liu M-C, Chuang S-M, et al. (1995): Correlation of cytogenetic results with immunophenotype, genotype, clinical features, and ras mutation in acute myeloid leukemia. A study of 235 Chinese patients in Taiwan. *Cancer Genet Cytogenet* 84:60–68.

Tiu RV, Gondek LP, O'Keefe CL, Huh J, Sekeres MA, Elson P, et al. (2009): New lesions detected by single nucleotide polymorphism array-based chromosomal analysis have important clinical impact in acute myeloid leukemia. *J Clin Oncol* 27:5219–5226.

Tkachuk DC, Kohler S, Cleary ML (1992): Involvement of a homolog of Drosophila trithorax by 11q23 chromosomal translocations in acute leukemias. *Cell* 71:691–700.

Tosi S, Giudici G, Mosna G, Harbott J, Specchia G, Grosveld G, et al. (1998): Identification of new partner chromosomes involved in fusions with the ETV6 (TEL) gene in hematologic malignancies. *Genes Chromosomes Cancer* 21:223–229.

Tosi S, Harbott J, Teigler-Schlegel A, Haas OA, Pirc-Danoewinata H, Harrison CJ, et al. (2000): t(7;12)(q36;p13), a new recurrent translocation involving ETV6 in infant leukemia. *Genes Chromosomes Cancer* 29:325–332.

Tosi S, Hughes J, Scherer SW, Nakabayashi K, Harbott J, Haas OA, et al. (2003): Heterogeneity of the 7q36 breakpoints in the t(7;12) involving ETV6 in infant leukemia. *Genes Chromosomes Cancer* 38:191–200.

Tošić N, Stojiljković M, Colović N, Ćolović M, Pavlović S (2009): Acute myeloid leukemia with NUP98-HOXC13 fusion and FLT3 internal tandem duplication mutation: case report and literature review. *Cancer Genet Cytogenet* 193:98–103.

Traweek ST, Slovak ML, Nademanee AP, Brynes RK, Niland JC, Forman SJ (1994): Clonal karyotypic hematopoietic cell abnormalities occurring after autologous bone marrow transplantation for Hodgkin's disease and non-Hodgkin's lymphoma. *Blood* 84:957–963.

Trubia M, Albano F, Cavazzini F, Cambrin GR, Quarta G, Fabbiano F, et al. (2006): Characterization of a recurrent translocation t(2;3)(p15-22;q26) occurring in acute myeloid leukaemia. *Leukemia* 20:48–54.

Trujillo JM, Cork A, Hart JS, George SL, Freireich EJ (1974): Clinical implications of aneuploid cytogenetic profiles in adult acute leukemia. *Cancer* 33:824–834.

Tse W, Zhu W, Chen HS, Cohen A (1995): A novel gene, AF1q, fused to MLL in t(1;11)(q21;q23), is specifically expressed in leukemic and immature hematopoietic cells. *Blood* 85:650–656.

Tsukimoto I, Tawa A, Horibe K, Tabuchi K, Kigasawa H, Tsuchida M, et al. (2009): Risk-stratified therapy and the intensive use of cytarabine improves the outcome in childhood acute myeloid leukemia: the AML99 trial from the Japanese Childhood AML Cooperative Study Group. *J Clin Oncol* 27:4007–4013.

UKCCG (United Kingdom Cancer Cytogenetics Group) (1992a): Primary, single, autosomal trisomies associated with haematological disorders. *Leuk Res* 16:841–851.

UKCCG (United Kingdom Cancer Cytogenetics Group) (1992b): Loss of the Y chromosome from normal and neoplastic bone marrows. *Genes Chromosomes Cancer* 5:83–88.

Van Den Berghe H, David G, Michaux J-L, Sokal G, Verwilghen R (1976): 5q- acute myelogenous leukemia. *Blood* 48:624–625.

Van Limbergen H, Poppe B, Michaux L, Herens C, Brown J, Noens L, et al. (2002): Identification of cytogenetic subclasses and recurring chromosomal aberrations in AML and MDS with complex karyotypes using M-FISH. *Genes Chromosomes Cancer* 33:60–72.

Vardiman JW, Arber DA, Brunning RD, Larson RA, Matutes E, Baumann I, et al. (2008): Therapy-related myeloid neoplasms. In: Swerdlow SH, Campo E, Harris NL, Jaffe ES, Pileri SA, Stein H, et al., editors (2008): *WHO classification of Tumours of the Haematopoietic and Lymphoid Tissues.* Lyon: IARC.

Vardiman JW, Thiele J, Arber DA, Brunning RD, Borowitz MJ, Porwit A, et al. (2009): The 2008 revision of the World Health Organization (WHO) classification of myeloid neoplasms and acute leukemia: rationale and important changes. *Blood* 114:937–951.

Vizmanos JL, Larráyoz MJ, Lahortiga I, Floristán F, Álvarez C, Odero MD, et al. (2003): t(10;16)(q22;p13) and MORF-CREBBP fusion is a recurrent event in acute myeloid leukemia. *Genes Chromosomes Cancer* 36:402–405.

Volkert S, Kohlmann A, Schnittger S, Kern W, Haferlach T, Haferlach C (2014): Association of the type of 5q loss with complex karyotype, clonal evolution, TP53 mutation status, and prognosis in acute myeloid leukemia and myelodysplastic syndrome. *Genes Chromosomes Cancer* 53:402–410.

Voutsadakis IA, Maillard N (2003): Acute myelogenous leukemia with the t(3;12)(q26;p13) translocation: case report and review of the literature. *Am J Hematol* 72:135–137.

Walker A, Marcucci G (2012): Molecular prognostic factors in cytogenetically normal acute myeloid leukemia. *Expert Rev Hematol* 5:547–558.

Walter MJ, Payton JE, Ries RE, Shannon WD, Deshmukh H, Zhao Y, et al. (2009): Acquired copy number alterations in adult acute myeloid leukemia genomes. *Proc Natl Acad Sci USA* 106:12950–12955.

Wang P, Spielberger RT, Thangavelu M, Zhao N, Davis EM, Iannantuoni K, et al. (1997): dic(5;17): a recurring abnormality in malignant myeloid disorders associated with mutations of TP53. *Genes Chromosomes Cancer* 20:282–291.

Wang L, Ogawa S, Hangaishi A, Qiao Y, Hosoya N, Nanya Y, et al. (2003): Molecular characterization of the recurrent unbalanced translocation der(1;7)(q10;p10). *Blood* 102:2597–2604.

Weber E, Nowotny H, Haas OA, Kasparu H, Grois N, Lutz D (1990): Trisomy 4: a specific karyotype anomaly in primary and secondary acute myeloid leukemia. *Leukemia* 4:219–221.

Weh HJ, Kuse R, Hoffmann R, Seeger D, Suciu S, Kabisch H, et al. (1988): Prognostic significance of chromosome analysis in de novo acute myeloid leukemia (AML). *Blut* 56:19–26.

Weh HJ, Kuse R, Hossfeld DK (1990): Acute nonlymphocytic leukemia (ANLL) with isochromosome i(17q) as the sole chromosomal anomaly: a distinct entity? *Eur J Haematol* 44:312–314.

Wei S, Wang S, Qiu S, Qi J, Mi Y, Lin D, et al. (2013): Clinical and laboratory studies of 17 patients with acute myeloid leukemia harboring t(7;11)(p15;p15) translocation. *Leuk Res* 37:1010–1015.

Weinfeld A, Westin J, Ridell B, Swolin B (1977): Polycythemia vera terminating in acute leukaemia. A clinical, cytogenetic and morphologic study in 8 patients treated with alkylating agents. *Scand J Haematol* 19:255–272.

Weisser M, Haferlach C, Haferlach T, Schnittger S (2007): Advanced age and high initial WBC influence the outcome of inv(3)(q21q26)/t(3;3)(q21;q26) positive AML. *Leuk Lymphoma* 48:2145–2151.

Welborn J (2004): Constitutional chromosome aberrations as pathogenetic events in hematologic malignancies. *Cancer Genet Cytogenet* 149:137–153.

Welborn JL, Lewis JP, Jenks H, Walling P (1987): Diagnostic and prognostic significance of t(1;3)(p36;q21) in the disorders of hematopoiesis. *Cancer Genet Cytogenet* 28:277–285.

Wells RA, Catzavelos C, Kamel-Reid S (1997): Fusion of retinoic acid receptor α to NuMA, the nuclear mitotic apparatus protein, by a variant translocation in acute promyelocytic leukaemia. *Nat Genet* 17:109–113.

Westman MK, Pedersen-Bjergaard J, Andersen MT, Andersen MK (2013): IDH1 and IDH2 mutations in therapy-related myelodysplastic syndrome and acute myeloid leukemia are associated with a normal karyotype and with der(1;7)(q10;p10). *Leukemia* 27:957–959.

Wiernik PH, Dutcher JP, Paietta E, Hittelman WN, Vyas R, Strack M, et al. (1991): Treatment of promyelocytic blast crisis of chronic myelogenous leukemia with all trans-retinoic acid. *Leukemia* 5:504–509.

Wiktor A, Rybicki BA, Piao ZS, Shurafa M, Barthel B, Maeda K, et al. (2000): Clinical significance of Y chromosome loss in hematologic disease. *Genes Chromosomes Cancer* 27:11–16.

Wiktor AE, Van Dyke DL, Hodnefield JM, Eckel-Passow J, Hanson CA (2011): The significance of isolated Y chromosome loss in bone marrow metaphase cells from males over age 50 years. *Leuk Res* 35:1297–1300.

Wilda M, Perez AV, Bruch J, Woessmann W, Metzler M, Fuchs U, et al. (2005): Use of MLL/GRAF fusion mRNA for measurement of minimal residual disease during chemotherapy in an infant with acute monoblastic leukemia (AML-M5). *Genes Chromosomes Cancer* 43:424–426.

Wildenhain S, Ruckert C, Röttgers S, Harbott J, Ludwig W-D, Schuster FR, et al. (2010): Expression of cell-cell interacting genes distinguishes HLXB9/TEL from MLL-positive childhood acute myeloid leukemia. *Leukemia* 24:1657–1660.

Wilmoth D, Feder M, Finan J, Nowell P (1985): Preleukemia and leukemia with 12p- and 19q+chromosome alterations following alkeran therapy. *Cancer Genet Cytogenet* 15:95–98.

Winick NJ, McKenna RW, Shuster JJ, Schneider NR, Borowitz MJ, Bowman WP, et al. (1993): Secondary acute myeloid leukemia in children with acute lymphoblastic leukemia treated with etoposide. *J Clin Oncol* 11:209–217.

Wlodarska I, Marynen P, La Starza R, Mecucci C, Van den Berghe H (1996): The ETV6, CDKN1B and D12S178 loci are involved in a segment commonly deleted in various 12p aberrations in different hematological malignancies. *Cytogenet Cell Genet* 72:229–235.

Wlodarska I, La Starza R, Baens M, Dierlamm J, Uyttebroeck A, Selleslag D, et al. (1998): Fluorescence in situ hybridization characterization of new translocations involving TEL (ETV6) in a wide spectrum of hematologic malignancies. *Blood* 91:1399–1406.

Wolman SR, Gundacker H, Appelbaum FR, Slovak ML (2002): Impact of trisomy 8 (+8) on clinical presentation, treatment response, and survival in acute myeloid leukemia: a Southwest Oncology Group study. *Blood* 100:29–35.

Won D, Shin SY, Park C-J, Jang S, Chi H-S, Lee K-H, et al. (2013): OBFC2A/RARA: a novel fusion gene in variant acute promyelocytic leukemia. *Blood* 121:1432–1435.

Wong KF, Kwong YL (1999): Trisomy 22 in acute myeloid leukemia: a marker for myeloid leukemia with monocytic features and cytogenetically cryptic inversion 16. *Cancer Genet Cytogenet* 109:131–133.

Wong KF, Kwong YL, So CC (1998): De novo AML with tri-lineage myelodysplasia and a novel t(11;12)(p15;q13). *Cancer Genet Cytogenet* 100:49–51.

Wong AK, Fang B, Zhang L, Guo X, Lee S, Schreck R (2008): Loss of the Y chromosome: an age-related or clonal phenomenon in acute myelogenous leukemia/myelodysplastic syndrome? *Arch Pathol Lab Med* 132:1329–1332.

Wu Y, Slovak ML, Snyder DS, Arber DA (2006): Coexistence of inversion 16 and the Philadelphia chromosome in acute and chronic myeloid leukemias: report of six cases and review of literature. *Am J Clin Pathol* 125:260–266.

Xu W, Zhou H-F, Fan L, Qian S-X, Chen L-J, Qiu H-R, et al. (2008): Trisomy 22 as the sole abnormality is an important marker for the diagnosis of acute myeloid leukemia with inversion 16. *Onkologie* 31:440–444.

Yamada Y, Furusawa S (1976): Preferential involvement of chromosomes No. 8 and No. 21 in acute leukemia and pre-leukemia. *Blood* 47:679–686.

Yamamoto K, Nagata K, Hamaguchi H (2002): A new case of CD7-positive acute myeloblastic leukemia with trisomy 21 as a sole acquired abnormality. *Cancer Genet Cytogenet* 133:183–184.

Yamamoto Y, Tsuzuki S, Tsuzuki M, Handa K, Inaguma Y, Emi N (2010): BCOR as a novel fusion partner of retinoic acid receptor alpha in a t(X;17)(p11;q12) variant of acute promyelocytic leukemia. *Blood* 116:4274–4283.

Yanada M, Kurosawa S, Yamaguchi T, Yamashita T, Moriuchi Y, Ago H, et al. (2012): Prognosis of acute myeloid leukemia harboring monosomal karyotype in patients treated with or without allogeneic hematopoietic cell transplantation after achieving complete remission. *Haematologica* 97:915–918.

Yang XF, Sun A-N, Yin J, Cai C-S, Tian X-P, Qian J, et al. (2012): Monosomal karyotypes among 1147 Chinese patients with acute myeloid leukemia: prevalence, features and prognostic impact. *Asian Pac J Cancer Prev* 13:5421–5426.

Yao E-I, Sadamori N, Nakamura H, Sasagawa I, Itoyama T, Ichimaru M, et al. (1988): Translocation t(16;21) in acute nonlymphocytic leukemia with abnormal eosinophils. *Cancer Genet Cytogenet* 36:221–223.

Yi JH, Huh J, Kim H-J, Kim S-H, Kim H-J, Kim Y-K, et al. (2011): Adverse prognostic impact of abnormal lesions detected by genome-wide single nucleotide polymorphism array-based karyotyping analysis in acute myeloid leukemia with normal karyotype. *J Clin Oncol* 29:4702–4708.

Yoneda-Kato N, Look AT, Kirstein MN, Valentine MB, Raimondi SC, Cohen KJ, et al. (1996): The t(3;5)(q25.1;q34) of myelodysplastic syndrome and acute myeloid leukemia produces a novel fusion gene, NPM-MLF1. *Oncogene* 12:265–275.

Yuan J, McDonough C, Kulharya A, Ramalingam P, Manaloor E (2010): Isolated trisomy 10 in an infant with acute myeloid leukemia: a case report and review of literature. *Int J Clin Exp Pathol* 3:718–722.

Yunis JJ (1984): Recurrent chromosomal defects are found in most patients with acute nonlymphocytic leukemia. *Cancer Genet Cytogenet* 11:125–137.

Yunis JJ, Bloomfield CD, Ensrud K (1981): All patients with acute nonlymphocytic leukemia may have a chromosomal defect. *N Engl J Med* 305:135–139.

Yunis JJ, Brunning RD, Howe RB, Lobell M (1984): High-resolution chromosomes as an independent prognostic indicator in adult acute nonlymphocytic leukemia. *N Engl J Med* 311:812–818.

Zaccaria A, Rosti G, Testoni N (1982): Reciprocal translocation (11q+;17q-) in a patient with acute monoblastic leukemia. *Nouv Rev Fr Hematol* 24:389–390.

Zatkova A, Merk S, Wendehack M, Bilban M, Muzik EM, Muradyan A, et al. (2009): AML/MDS with 11q/MLL amplification show characteristic gene expression signature and interplay of DNA copy number changes. *Genes Chromosomes Cancer* 48:510–520.

Zhou J, Zhang Y, Li J, Li X, Hou J, Zhao Y, et al. (2010): Single-agent arsenic trioxide in the treatment of children with newly diagnosed acute promyelocytic leukemia. *Blood* 115:1697–1702.

van Zutven LJCM, Önen E, Velthuizen SCJM, van Drunen E, von Bergh ARM, van den Heuvel-Eibrink MM, et al. (2006): Identification of NUP98 abnormalities in acute leukemia: JARID1A (12p13) as a new partner gene. *Genes Chromosomes Cancer* 45:437–446.

CHAPTER 7

Myelodysplastic syndromes

Harold J. Olney[1] and Michelle M. Le Beau[2]

[1] Centre Hospitalier de l'Universitié de Montréal (CHUM), Universite de Montreal, Montréal, Quebec, Canada

[2] Section of Hematology/Oncology, University of Chicago, Chicago, IL, USA

Myelodysplastic syndromes (MDS) are a heterogeneous group of clonal bone marrow (BM) disorders characterized by the presence of dysplastic maturation of hematopoietic cells coupled with one or more peripheral cytopenias and a propensity to progress to acute myeloid leukemia (AML) (Vardiman, 2003; Cazzola and Malcovati, 2005). The incidence of MDS increases with age (over 85% of patients are more than 60 years of age), and the disease affects more men than women (4.5 vs. 2.3 per 100 000) (Strom et al., 2008). The exact number of incident and prevalent cases is probably underestimated given difficulties with diagnostic ascertainment and reporting (Goldberg et al., 2010; McQuilten et al., 2014). Although exposure to tobacco, solvents, and farming chemicals is associated with MDS, most cases occur without explanation (Strom et al., 2008). Approximately 10–15% of MDS follow treatment (therapy-related MDS (t-MDS)) with chemotherapy and/or radiation for both neoplastic as well as benign disorders (Vallespi et al., 1998; Godley and Larson, 2002). Although dysplasia is the cardinal feature of MDS, there are a number of other conditions that present a similar histopathologic picture. Nutritional deficiencies (e.g., vitamin B12 and folate), toxins, infections, and congenital conditions must be excluded. In contrast, documenting the clonality of the abnormal cells supports the diagnosis (Vardiman et al., 2009).

The current diagnostic entities are established following the World Health Organization (WHO) criteria, based on BM histological findings, blast count, and cytogenetic findings (Table 7.1). Chronic myelomonocytic leukemia (CMML) was previously considered an MDS but is now considered an overlap disorder with a dysplastic subtype possessing many of the clinical characteristics of the other dysplasias (Bennett et al., 1982). The natural history of the disease, including the risk of leukemic transformation, is significantly worsened with an increasing marrow blast count. In patients with low blast counts, the presence of dysplasia in a single cell line, most commonly erythroid, is distinguished from cases with multilineage dysplasia, which have a worse prognosis. The presence of ring sideroblasts is recognized when ≥15% of erythroid precursors are ring sideroblasts.

The cytogenetic evaluation of a BM sample from patients with MDS has become an integral part of clinical care. Not only does this analysis confirm the diagnosis, it is invaluable in defining the prognosis and median survival, as well as the risk for progression to AML. On a more fundamental level, cytogenetic analysis has been instrumental in establishing the clonality of these syndromes as well as providing insights into their pathobiology. This chapter will

Cancer Cytogenetics: Chromosomal and Molecular Genetic Aberrations of Tumor Cells, Fourth Edition.
Edited by Sverre Heim and Felix Mitelman.
© 2015 John Wiley & Sons, Ltd. Published 2015 by John Wiley & Sons, Ltd.

Table 7.1 World Health Organization MDS classification system

Disease	Marrow blasts (%)	Clinical presentation	Cytogenetic abnormalities (%)
Refractory anemia (RA)	<5	Anemia	25
RA with ring sideroblasts (RARS)	<5	Anemia, ≥15% ring sideroblasts in erythroid precursors	10
5q- syndrome	<5	Anemia, normal platelets	100
Refractory cytopenia with multilineage dysplasia (RCMD)	<5	Bicytopenia or pancytopenia	50
RCMD with ring sideroblasts	<5	Bicytopenia or pancytopenia, ≥15% ring sideroblasts	50
Refractory anemia with excess blasts 1	5–9	Cytopenias +/− blasts (<5%)	50–70
Refractory anemia with excess blasts 2	10–20	Cytopenias, blasts present	50–70
Myelodysplastic syndrome—unclassified	<5	Neutropenia or thrombocytopenia	50
Chronic myelomonocytic leukemia (CMML)—nonproliferative type	<20	Monocytosis (>1000/μl), total leukocytes ≤13 000/μl	25–50

review the most frequently encountered abnormalities exploring their clinical and genetic features.

Diagnosis

The diagnosis of all hematological malignancies, including MDS, begins with the appropriate clinical evaluation combined with expert pathological and genetic analysis. An accurate diagnosis can be crucial in management decisions. In cases of MDS with multilineage dysplasia and an elevated blast count characterized by typical laboratory findings, the diagnosis of MDS is relatively straightforward. Given the varied pathological and clinical picture of MDS, however, more sophisticated testing may be necessary in establishing the diagnosis.

The most widely available and standardized technique for identifying clonality in MDS is chromosome banding analysis. The WHO has included recurring cytogenetic abnormalities in the classification of several subtypes of MDS with distinct clinical presentations and natural histories as discussed later (Vardiman et al., 2009). The analysis of mutated genes has been used to confirm the clonal nature of MDS and in some cases to add prognostic information (Bejar et al., 2011; Walter et al., 2012). Aberrant *in vitro* growth patterns of stem cells can be characteristic of MDS (Spitzer et al., 1979), yet this evaluation is restricted to laboratories with

expertise with this technique and is not routinely available. Immunophenotyping protocols (Wells et al., 2003; Kussick et al., 2005; van de Loosdrecht et al., 2013) and microarray techniques including array comparative genomic hybridization (CGH) and single-nucleotide polymorphism (SNP) arrays (Shaffer et al., 2013) to detect copy-neutral loss of heterozygosity (LOH) may become diagnostically and prognostically useful in the future.

Clinical correlations

For the clinical management of MDS patients, cytogenetic analysis continues to play a vital role. At the time of diagnosis, recurring chromosomal abnormalities are found in 40–70% of patients with primary MDS and in 95% of patients with t-MDS (Vallespi et al., 1998), confirming the presence of a neoplastic process.

The value of cytogenetic analysis in predicting survival and risk of leukemic transformation during a patient's clinical course has been well established (Toyama et al., 1993; Sole et al., 2005; Haase et al., 2007; Malcovati et al., 2007). Among the few independent variables identified that predict clinical outcome in MDS, cytogenetic findings form the cornerstone of successful prognostic scoring systems. The most validated systems, the International Prognostic Scoring System (IPSS) for

Table 7.2 MDS cytogenetic scoring system—Revised International Prognostic Scoring System

Prognostic subgroups (% patients)	Cytogenetic abnormalities	Survival years, median	AML evolution, 25% years, median	Hazard ratio OS/AML
Very good (4%)	–Y, del(11q)	5.4	NR	0.7/0.4
Good (72%)	Normal, del(5q), del(12p), del(20q), 2 abnormalities incl del(5q)	4.8	9.5	1/1
Intermediate (13%)	del(7q), +8, i(17q), +19, any other one or two abnormalities, independent clones	2.7	2.6	1.5/1.8
Poor (4%)	inv(3)/t(3q)/del(3q), –7, two abnormalities incl –7/del(7q), complex: 3 abn	1.5	1.7	2.3/2.3
Very poor (7%)	Complex: >3 abn	0.9	0.7	3.8/3.6

MDS and the Revised International Prognostic Scoring System (IPSS-R), identify marrow blast count, the number of peripheral cytopenias, as well as cytogenetic findings as the variables most useful in prognostication (Table 7.2) (Greenberg et al., 2012). Their application is limited to the time of diagnosis. The WHO diagnostic classification integrates the characteristics of the first two elements into the diagnosis. In the WHO prognostic scoring system (WPSS), the grouping of these entities can be used with the IPSS cytogenetic risk groups as well as the clinical need for blood transfusion to determine a dynamic prognostic score having the advantage of applicability throughout the course of the disease (Malcovati et al., 2007). In lower-risk patients, additional laboratory findings (such as ferritin and β2-microglobulin levels) may help identify those patients with a worse prognosis who may benefit from early therapeutic intervention (Garcia-Manero et al., 2008; Kikuchi et al., 2012). With larger datasets, more rare recurring cytogenetic abnormalities may be examined allowing a refining of the cytogenetic risk groups and providing the clinician with more information to predict the expected outcome for their patients (Haase et al., 2007).

The frequency of cytogenetic abnormalities increases with the severity of disease, as does the risk of leukemic transformation. Clonal chromosome abnormalities can be detected in marrow cells of 25% of patients with refractory anemia (RA), 10% of patients with refractory anemia with ring sideroblasts (RARS), 50% of patients with refractory cytopenias with multilineage dysplasia (RCMD), 50–70% of patients with refractory anemia with excess blasts 1,2 (RAEB-1,2), and (not surprisingly) 100% of patients with MDS with isolated del(5q).

Therapeutic options are increasing in MDS patients as several agents are now approved for their care by various regulatory agencies. Although cytogenetic analysis has always been used to establish prognosis, which dictated therapeutic decisions in a general sense (supportive care vs. remission-inducing cytotoxic chemotherapy regimens), a new era of targeted therapy was launched with the recognition of the sensitivity of MDS with platelet-derived growth factor receptor beta (*PDGFRB*) translocations to the tyrosine kinase inhibitor imatinib mesylate (Apperley et al., 2002) and of del(5q)-positive cases to the immunomodulating drug lenalidomide (List et al., 2006). With further molecular understanding of the underlying abnormalities, treatment of patients will ideally be individualized to the specific chromosomal abnormalities underlying the disease process in each patient, and novel treatments are currently being developed toward this end.

Cytogenetic analysis

A number of recurring cytogenetic abnormalities are seen in MDS (Table 7.3). These findings are not exclusive to MDS as they may also be seen in AML. Most recurring cytogenetic abnormalities found in MDS are unbalanced, most commonly the result of the loss of a whole chromosome or a deletion of

Table 7.3 Recurring chromosomal abnormalities in the myelodysplastic syndromes

Disease	Chromosome abnormality	Frequency	Involved genes*		Consequence
MDS	**Unbalanced**				
	+8	10%			
	−7/del(7q)†	10%			
	del(5q)/t(5q)†	10%			
	del(20q)	5–8%			
	−Y	5%			
	i(17q)/t(17p)†	3–5%	TP53		Loss of function, DNA damage response
	−13/del(13q)†	3%			
	del(11q)†	3%			
	del(12p)/t(12p)†	3%			
	del(9q)†	1–2%			
	idic(X)(q13)†	1–2%			
	Balanced				
	t(1;3)(p36.3;q21.3)†	1%	MMEL1	RPN1	Deregulation of MMEL1—transcriptional activation?
	t(2;11)(p21;q23.3) /t(11q23.3)†	1%		KMT2A/MLL	KMT2A fusion protein—altered transcriptional regulation
	inv(3)(q21.3q26.2) /t(3;3)(q21.3;q26.2)†	1%	RPN1	MECOM/EVI1	Increased expression and altered transcriptional regulation by MECOM
	t(6;9)(p22.3;q34.1)†	1%	DEK	NUP214	Fusion protein—nuclear pore protein
Therapy-related MDS	−7/del(7q)†	50%			
	del(5q)/t(5q)†	40–45%			
	dic(5;17)(q11.1–13.3; p11.1–13)†	5%		TP53	Loss of function, DNA damage response
	der(1;7)(q10;p10)†	3%			
	t(3;21)(q26.2;q22.1)†	3%	MECOM	RUNX1	MECOM–RUNX1 fusion gene leading to loss of RUNX1 and overexpression of MECOM—altered transcriptional regulation
	t(11;16)(q23.3;p13.3) /t(11q23.3)†	2%	KMT2A/MLL	CREBBP	KMT2A fusion protein—altered transcriptional regulation
CMML	t(5;12)(q32;p13.2)	~2%	PDGFRB	ETV6/TEL	Fusion protein—altered signaling pathway

CMML, chronic myelomonocytic leukemia; MDS, myelodysplastic syndrome.

*Genes are listed in order of citation in the karyotype, for example, for the t(11;16), KMT2A is at 11q23.3 and CREBBP at 16p13.3.

†Cytogenetic abnormalities considered in the WHO 2008 classification as presumptive evidence of MDS in patients with persistent cytopenias(s), but with no dysplasia or increased blasts.

part of a chromosome, but unbalanced translocations and more complex derivative (rearranged) chromosomes can also be found (Figures 7.1 and 7.2). The most common cytogenetic abnormalities encountered in MDS are del(5q), −7, and +8, which have been incorporated into the more robust prognostic scoring systems of MDS. Clones with unrelated abnormalities, one of which typically

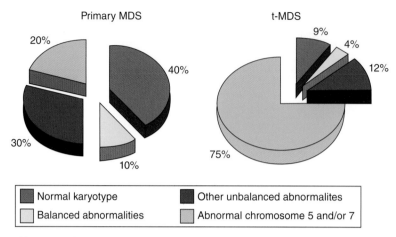

Figure 7.1 Type of karyotypic abnormalities in MDS.

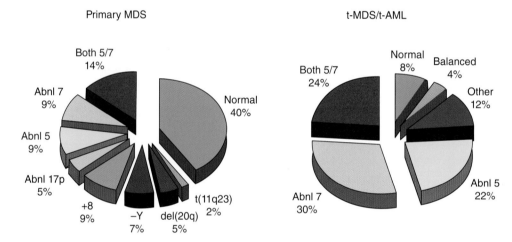

Figure 7.2 Recurring chromosomal abnormalities in MDS.

has a gain of chromosome 8, are seen at a greater frequency (~5% vs. ~1%) in patients with MDS than in AML.

A handful of specific cytogenetic abnormalities, including 5q- (Giagounidis et al., 2004), 17p-, and idic(X) chromosome (associated with RARS), are typically associated with morphologically and clinically distinct subsets of MDS. In rare cases, recurring balanced translocations have been reported. Abnormalities characteristic of acute leukemia without a prior myelodysplastic phase, such as t(15;17), inv(16), and t(8;21), are rare in MDS (Vardiman et al., 2009). The t(9;22), diagnostic of chronic myelogenous leukemia (CML) and a subtype of acute lymphoblastic leukemia (ALL), is exceedingly rare in MDS.

In contrast to classical chromosome banding analysis, fluorescence *in situ* hybridization (FISH) can evaluate interphase as well as metaphase cells in a rapid and efficient manner (Gozzetti and Le Beau, 2000). The primary advantage of FISH is the simplified analysis permitting evaluation of a higher number of cells, thereby greatly increasing sensitivity. It can also be applied to histologically stained cells, allowing a direct correlation of the status of the genetic target within morphologically characterized cells. However, the technique evaluates specific alterations based on probe selection, rather than the entire chromosomal complement. Probes suitable for clinical use are not available for all recurring abnormalities of interest, and variation in the cytogenetic abnormality (with either complex rearrangements or differences in break-points) may not be detected with conventional probes. Commercially available probes have been developed for the detection of MDS-relevant changes such as 11q23.3 translocations involving *KMT2A/MLL*, −Y, del(5q), −7/del(7q), +8, del(11q), del(13q), −17/del(17p), and del(20q).

Cytogenetic findings in MDS

Normal karyotype

In MDS, 50–60% of patients have a normal karyotype. This subset is almost certainly genetically heterogeneous including many cases where technical factors precluded the detection of chromosomally abnormal cells or where leukemogenic alterations occurred at the molecular level and so were undetectable with standard cytogenetic methods. For example, *TET2* mutations are more frequent in MDS patients with a normal karyotype. Despite this heterogeneity, normal cases are a standard reference for comparison of outcomes and fall within the IPSS-R good-risk group. The median survival for these patients is 4.8 years, and the time to progression to AML of 25% of this cohort was 9.4 years (Greenberg et al., 2012; Schanz et al., 2012).

−Y

The clinical and biological significance of loss of the Y chromosome, −Y, is unknown. Loss of the Y has been observed in a number of malignant diseases but has also been reported to be associated with aging. The UK Cancer Cytogenetics Group (UKCCG, 1992) undertook a comprehensive analysis of this abnormality, reporting that a −Y could be identified in 7.7% of patients without a hematologic malignant disease and in 10.7% of patients with MDS and, thus, was not reliable in documenting a malignant process (UKCCG, 1992). In a large series of 215 male patients, Wiktor et al. (2000) found that patients with a hematological disease had a significantly higher percentage of cells with a −Y than did normal controls (52% vs. 37%, $p = 0.036$). The presence of −Y in >75% of metaphase cells accurately predicted a malignant hematological disease. Although loss of a Y chromosome may not be diagnostic of MDS, once the disease is identified by clinical and pathologic means, the IPSS-R found that −Y as the sole abnormality conferred a very good prognosis with a median survival of 5.4 years (Greenberg et al., 2012).

+8

The incidence of trisomy 8 in MDS is ~10%, with half of the patients having +8 as the sole abnormality (Schanz et al., 2012). This abnormality is observed in all MDS subgroups varying with age, gender, and prior treatment with cytotoxic agents or radiation (Vallespi et al., 1998; Paulsson et al., 2001; Schanz et al., 2012). The assessment of the significance of trisomy 8 has been complicated by the finding that +8 is often associated with other recurring abnormalities known to have prognostic significance, for example, del(5q) or −7/del(7q), or may be seen in isolation as a separate clone unrelated to the primary clone in up to 5% of cases. The presence of cryptic abnormalities at other sites within the genome has also been described in some cases examined by molecular techniques (Paulsson et al., 2006). The IPSS-R as well as the WPSS ranked this abnormality in the intermediate-risk group with a median survival of 2.7 years (Greenberg et al., 2012). Nonetheless, several groups have found that patients with +8 as a sole abnormality had a worse disease outcome than that corresponding to an intermediate IPSS risk (Sole et al., 2005; Haase et al., 2007). On the other hand, gain of chromosome 8 as the sole abnormality is in a subset of patients associated with a better response to immunosuppressive therapy, particularly if the patient is younger, diagnosed with RA, and DR15 positive on HLA typing and has a short duration of disease (Sloand and Rezvani, 2008). The gain of chromosome 8 is one of the few examples of gene amplification in MDS and leads to higher levels of expression for many genes on chromosome 8, including *MYC* and several antiapoptotic genes.

Rearrangements of chromosome 5 or del(5q)

In MDS or AML arising de novo, rearrangements leading to loss of the long arm of chromosome 5 are observed in 10–20% of patients, whereas in t-MDS, it is identified in 40% of patients (Figure 7.3) (Vallespi et al., 1998; Godley and Larson, 2002; Smith et al., 2003). Although an interstitial deletion, del(5q), is most common, other rearrangements, such as

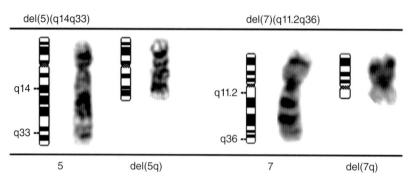

Figure 7.3 Deletions of 5q and 7q in myeloid neoplasms. In this del(5q), breakpoints occur in q14 and q33, resulting in interstitial loss of the intervening chromosomal material. In this del(7q), breakpoints occur in q11.2 and q36. In both cases, the critical commonly deleted segments are lost. Normal chromosome 5 and 7 homologs are shown for comparison.

unbalanced translocations, also occur. Recent studies using FISH and array-based approaches have revealed that −5 does not actually occur, inasmuch as they have identified the presence of chromosome 5 sequences in marker chromosomes or on other rearranged chromosomes. A significant occupational exposure to potential carcinogens can be found in the history of many patients with either a del(5q) or a −7/del(7q) (discussed later), suggesting that abnormalities of chromosome 5 or 7 may be a marker of mutagen-induced malignant hematological disease (West et al., 2000). Abnormalities of 5q are associated with previous exposure to standard- and high-dose treatment with alkylating agents, including use in immunosuppressive regimens (Pedersen-Bjergaard et al., 2000; Godley and Larson, 2002), therapeutic ionizing radiation, and benzene exposure (Irons and Kerzic, 2014).

In primary MDS, abnormalities of chromosome 5, mostly as an isolated del(5q), are the cytogenetic hallmark of the 5q- syndrome, but they may also occur in RAEB 1, 2 of the WHO classification as part of a complex karyotype. Clinically, the patients with an isolated del(5q), or del(5q) plus one additional abnormality, have a good prognosis (IPSS-R median survival of 4.8 years), whereas patients with del(5q) in the setting of a complex karyotype have a poor prognosis with early progression to leukemia, resistance to treatment, and short survival with IPSS-R median survival of 1.5 years for the poor-risk group and 0.7 years for the very poor group with >3 abnormalities (Greenberg et al., 2012). A karyotype review in 866 patients with loss of 5q and a myeloid neoplasia at the University of Chicago

revealed that abnormalities of chromosome 5 were associated with several specific recurring abnormalities: −17/loss of 17p (39%), −3/loss of 3p or 3q (30%), −18/loss of 18q (24%), −12/loss of 12p (24%), +8 (23%), −13/del(13q) (18%), and −20/del(20q) (13%) (Tennant and Le Beau, unpublished data).

MDS with an isolated del(5q) (the 5q- syndrome)

Though the del(5q) in this context is mostly the sole abnormality, it may on occasion be accompanied by a second cytogenetic abnormality (Giagounidis et al., 2004; Mallo et al., 2011; Schanz et al., 2012; Komrokji et al., 2013). Unlike the male predominance in MDS in general, MDS with an isolated del(5q) has an overrepresentation of females (2:1). The initial laboratory findings are usually a macrocytic anemia, often severe and requiring transfusional support, with a normal or elevated platelet count. The diagnosis is usually RA (in two-thirds) or RAEB-1 (in one-third). On BM examination, abnormalities in the megakaryocytic lineage (particularly micromegakaryocytes) are prominent. These patients fall into the IPSS-R good-risk group (median survival of 4.8 years) with low rates of leukemic transformation (Mallo et al., 2011; Greenberg et al., 2012). An immunomodulatory agent, lenalidomide, has transformed the clinical approach to 5q- patients in need of transfusion; treatment with this drug results in dramatic hematological improvement and reduction or elimination of the malignant clone (List et al., 2006). As described later, mutations of *TP53* have emerged as an independent prognostic factor in MDS and are associated with a del(5q)

(Christiansen et al., 2001; Sebaa et al., 2012; Kulasekararaj et al., 2013). Several recent studies employing high-throughput DNA sequencing at a deep coverage have identified *TP53* mutations in 18% of patients with lower-risk MDS with a del(5q), which conferred a higher risk of progression to AML (Jadersten et al., 2011). In addition, these patients have a lower frequency of cytogenetic response to lenalidomide without complete responses documented (Jadersten et al., 2011, Mallo et al., 2011).

Molecular analysis of the del(5q)

Several groups of investigators have defined a minimal commonly deleted segment (CDS) on the long arm of chromosome 5, band 5q31.2, predicted to contain a myeloid tumor suppressor gene (TSG) that is involved in the pathogenesis of the more aggressive forms of MDS and AML (Figure 7.4) (Lai et al., 2001). A second, distal CDS of 1.5 Mb within 5q33.1 has been identified in MDS with an isolated del(5q) (Boultwood et al., 2002). Despite intense efforts, the identification of TSGs on chromosome 5 has been challenging because the deletions of 5q are typically large and encompass both of these regions. Molecular analysis of the 19 candidate genes within the CDS at 5q31.2 and 44 genes in the 5q33.1 CDS did not reveal inactivating

mutations in the remaining alleles, nor was there evidence of transcriptional silencing (Lai et al., 2001; Boultwood et al., 2002; Graubert et al., 2009). Jerez et al. (2012a) used high-density SNP arrays to map the del(5q) in 146 patients with MDS and AML confirming that the deletions were interstitial and hemizygous. Moreover, copy-neutral LOH (also known as acquired uniparental disomy) was rare (4 of 146 patients) (Jerez et al., 2012a). Of interest was that patients who had low-risk MDS typically had smaller deletions, retaining 5q11.1–14.2 and 5q34–35, whereas patients with high-risk MDS, AML, and t-MDS/t-AML typically had larger deletions with loss of these segments. These observations are compatible with a haploinsufficiency model in which loss of one allele of the relevant gene(s) on 5q perturbs cell fate, rather than the biallelic inactivation of a TSG (Shannon and Le Beau, 2008). A number of genes or microRNAs (miRNAs) located on 5q, including *RPS14* (Ebert et al., 2008), miRNA-145 (Kumar et al., 2009; Starczynowski et al., 2010), *EGR1* (Joslin et al., 2007), APC (Wang et al., 2010a), *CTNNA1*, *DIAPH1*, *CSNK1A1*, *SPRY4*, and *TIFAB*, have been implicated in the development of myeloid disorders due to a gene dosage effect, and several of these are reviewed in the following text.

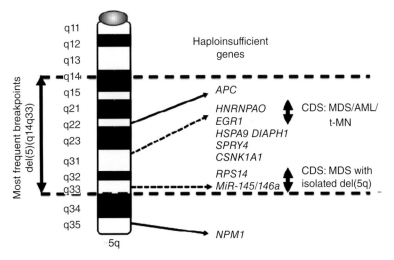

Commonly deleted segments of 5q

Figure 7.4 Idiogram of the long arm of chromosome 5 showing candidate genes within the commonly deleted segments (CDSs) as reported by various investigators. The proximal CDS in 5q31.2 was identified in MDS, AML, and t-MDS/t-AML, whereas the distal CDS in 5q33.1 was identified in MDS with an isolated del(5q).

RPS14

The gene encoding RPS14, which is required for the processing of 18S pre-rRNA, is located at 5q33.1 and is involved in MDS with an isolated del(5q) (Ebert et al., 2008). Downregulation of *RPS14* in CD34+ BM cells blocks differentiation and increases apoptosis of erythroid cells via a TP53-dependent mechanism (Barlow et al., 2010). Of interest, the ribosomal processing defect caused by haploinsufficiency of RPS14 in MDS is highly analogous to the functional ribosomal defect seen in Diamond–Blackfan anemia. Other studies have shown that haploinsufficiency of two miRNAs, miR-145 and miR-146a, encoded by sequences near the *RPS14* gene, cooperates with loss of RPS14 (Kumar et al., 2009; Starczynowski et al., 2010). The Toll–interleukin-1 receptor domain-containing adaptor protein (TIRAP) and *FLI1* are targets of these miRNAs. Haploinsufficiency of miR-145 may account for several features of MDS with an isolated del(5q), including megakaryocytic dysplasia; however, neither *RPS14* nor miR-145 haploinsufficiency is predicted to confer clonal dominance.

APC

APC is a multifunctional tumor suppressor involved in the pathogenesis of colorectal cancer via regulation of the WNT signaling cascade. The *APC* gene is located at 5q22.2 and is deleted in >95% of patients with a del(5q) (Lai et al., 2001). APC is essential for the maintenance and survival of hematopoietic stem and progenitor cells (HSPCs), and conditional inactivation of a single allele of *Apc* in mice leads to the development of severe macrocytic anemia, a block in erythropoiesis at the early stages of differentiation, an expansion of the short-term and long-term HSCs, and increased apoptosis of HSPCs, thus recapitulating several characteristic features of myeloid neoplasms with a del(5q) (Wang et al., 2010a).

EGR1

The early growth response 1 (*EGR1*) gene encodes a member of the WT1 family of Zn finger transcription factors and mediates the cellular response to growth factors and stress stimuli. Egr1 is a direct transcriptional regulator of many known TSGs, for example, *Tp53*, *Cdkn1a/p21*, *Tgfb*, and *Pten*, and acts as a TSG in several human tumors, including breast and non-small cell lung cancer. *Egr1*-null mice show spontaneous mobilization of HSPCs into the periphery, identifying Egr1 as a transcriptional regulator of stem cell migration (Min et al., 2008). Moreover, loss of a single allele of *Egr1* cooperates with mutations induced by an alkylating agent in the development of malignant myeloid diseases (MPD with ineffective erythropoiesis) in mice, indicating that Egr1 is a haploinsufficient TSG (Joslin et al., 2007). Recently, Stoddart et al. (2014) demonstrated that knockdown of *Tp53*, which is mutated in up to 80% of patients with del(5q) MDS or AML, together with haploinsufficiency for both *Egr1* and *Apc* led to an aggressive AML in mice, representing the first mouse model for del(5q) AML and confirming the hypothesis that high-risk MDS/AML associated with a del(5q) results from the cooperative, simultaneous loss of multiple haploinsufficient genes on 5q.

In summary, the data reveal two nonoverlapping CDSs in 5q31.2 and 5q33.1. The proximal segment in 5q31.2 contains a TSG(s) involved in the pathogenesis of high-risk MDS, AML, or t-MDS/t-AML. Band 5q33.1 contains several cooperating TSGs involved in the etiology of MDS with an isolated del(5q). Together, the data support a haploinsufficiency model in which loss of a single allele of more than one gene on 5q (a contiguous deletion syndrome) acts to alter hematopoiesis, promotes self-renewal of HSPCs, induces apoptosis of hematopoietic cells, and disrupts differentiation.

Loss of chromosome 7 or del(7q)

A −7/del(7q) (Figure 7.3) is observed as the sole abnormality in ~5% of adult patients with de novo MDS (Haase et al., 2007; Schanz et al., 2012) but in ~50% of children with MDS (Kardos et al., 2003) and in ~55% of patients with t-MDS (Godley and Larson, 2002; Smith et al., 2003). In constitutional disorders associated with a predisposition to myeloid neoplasms, including Fanconi anemia, neurofibromatosis type 1, and severe congenital neutropenia, a −7/del(7q) is the most frequent BM cytogenetic abnormality detected. As with del(5q), exposure to mutagens, whether occupational (benzene), environmental (smoking), or therapeutic (cytotoxic therapy), has been associated with −7/del(7q) (Smith et al., 2003; Strom et al., 2008; Irons and Kerzic, 2014). The similar clinical and biological features of the myeloid disorders associated with −7/del(7q) suggest that the same gene(s) is altered in each of these contexts. The IPSS-R considers del(7q) as a sole abnormality to have an intermediate prognosis (median overall survival (OS) of 2.7 years), whereas −7 alone or −7/del(7q) with one additional abnormality or as part of a complex karyotype with three abnormalities has a poor prognosis (median OS of 1.5 years), and −7/del(7q) as a component of a complex karyotype with >3 abnormalities has a very poor prognosis (median OS of 0.7 years) (Greenberg et al., 2012).

"Monosomy 7 syndrome" in young children is characterized by a preponderance of males (~4:1), hepatosplenomegaly, leukocytosis, thrombocytopenia, and a poor prognosis (Hasle and Niemeyer, 2011). Juvenile myelomonocytic leukemia (JMML, previously known as juvenile chronic myelogenous leukemia), classified by the WHO as a MDS/MPD disease, shares many features with this entity, with −7 observed either at diagnosis or as a new cytogenetic finding associated with disease acceleration on marrow examination (Loh and Mullighan, 2012). A −7/del(7q) cooperates with activation of the RAS signaling pathway in the pathogenesis of JMML. Activation of the RAS pathway occurs as a result of mutations in the *NRAS* or *KRAS* genes, inactivating mutations in the gene encoding NF1, a negative regulator of RAS proteins, activating mutations in the gene encoding the PTPN11/SHP2 phosphatase, a positive regulator of RAS proteins, or mutations in *CBL*. Collectively, RAS pathway mutations have been identified in ~85% of JMML patients (Christiansen et al., 2003; Side et al., 2004; Loh et al., 2004, 2009). Other mutations in JMML include *RUNX1* mutations and methylation silencing of the *CDKN2B*(*p15^{INK4B}*) gene (Christiansen et al., 2003; Loh et al., 2004; Side et al., 2004).

The molecular mutations underlying the development of MDS and AML with del(7q) are only beginning to be elucidated, with multiple studies having identified a CDS within 7q22. We previously identified a 2.52 CDS within 7q22 spanning the interval containing *LRCC17* and *SRPK2* (Le Beau et al., 1996). Each of the candidate genes within the CDS at 7q22 has been evaluated for mutations; however, no inactivating mutations have been identified in the remaining allele (Wong et al., 2010; Jerez et al., 2012b). Mice with a conditional heterozygous deletion of this region in murine HSPCs

had no apparent alterations of hematopoiesis; however, the HSCs had a functional defect in self-renewal, suggesting that mutations in cooperating genes are required (Wong et al., 2010; Wong and Shannon, unpublished results). Dohner et al. (2006) identified an ~2 Mb deleted segment in proximal q22 that overlaps with the proximal portion of the CDS defined by Le Beau et al. (1996) but extends more proximally, which includes the *CUX1*, *RASA4*, *EPO*, and *FBXL13* genes in 7q22.1. Similarly, Jerez et al. (2012b) used SNP arrays to identify several CDSs on 7q, including one at 7q22, encompassing *CUX1*. Using transcriptome sequencing and SNP array analysis of t-MDS/t-AML and AML de novo, McNerney et al. (2013) identified a 2.17 Mb CDS at 7q22.1 that contained the gene encoding CUX1, a homeodomain transcription factor. Moreover, *CUX1* was disrupted by a translocation in one case, resulting in a loss-of-function fusion mRNA, and *CUX1* transcripts and protein were expressed at haploinsufficient levels in −7/del(7q) myeloid diseases. Knockdown of the conserved homolog in developing *Drosophila*, *Cut*, resulted in melanotic tumors (the equivalent of AML). Similar knockdowns in human HSCs led to an engraftment advantage in NSG mouse xenografts, suggesting that *CUX1* is a haploinsufficient TSG. The recognition of mutations in *EZH2* (7q36.1) is intriguing; however, myeloid neoplasms with *EZH2* mutations typically do not have −7/del(7q), and the del(7q) does not always result in loss of one *EZH2* allele (Ernst et al., 2010; Nikoloski et al., 2010).

Loss of 17p

Loss of the short arm of chromosome 17—del(17p)/t(17p)/i(17q)/−17—has been reported in ~5% of patients with MDS. The loss can result from various abnormalities, including simple deletions, unbalanced translocations, dicentric rearrangements (particularly with chromosome 5) or, less often, −17 or isochromosome formation. The dic(5;17)(q11.1–13.3;p11.1–13) is a frequently recurring rearrangement of 17p, and ~30% of the patients with this change have t-MDS (Wang et al., 1997; Merlat et al., 1999). Patients with loss of 17p typically have complex karyotypes—the most frequent additional changes are del(5q), del(7q), −7, +8, and −18/del(18q) in decreasing frequency—and fall into the poor or very poor IPSS-R groups (median survival of 1.5 years and 0.7 years, respectively) (Sanchez-Castro et al., 2013). Rare patients with i(17q) as the sole abnormality have an intermediate prognosis (Greenberg et al., 2012; Schanz et al., 2012). The *TP53* gene, an important TSG that functions in the cellular response to DNA damage, is located at 17p13.1. One allele of *TP53* is typically lost as a result of the abnormality of 17p; an inactivating mutation in the second allele on the remaining morphologically normal chromosome 17 occurs in ~70% of cases (Wang et al., 1997; Merlat et al., 1999).

Several groups have proposed that the 17p- syndrome is a distinct entity within MDS associated with a characteristic form of dysgranulopoiesis combining pseudo-Pelger–Huët hypolobulation and the presence of small granules in granulocytes (Merlat et al., 1999). Because these features may be observed in MDS also without loss of 17p, the 17p-syndrome is not recognized as a distinct entity by the WHO classification (Vardiman et al., 2009).

del(20q)

A deletion of the long arm of chromosome 20, del(20q), is a common recurring abnormality in malignant myeloid disorders, noted in ~5% of MDS cases and 7% of t-MDS cases (Vallespi et al., 1998; Schanz et al., 2012). Morphologically, the presence of a del(20q) is associated with prominent dysplasia in the erythroid and megakaryocytic lineages. The IPSS-R noted that patients with a del(20q) observed in association with a complex karyotype identified a poor- or very poor-risk group with a median survival for the entire group of 1.5 years or 0.7 years, respectively, whereas the prognosis for patients with an isolated del(20q) was good (median survival of 4.8 years) (Greenberg et al., 2012). These data suggest that the del(20q) in MDS may be associated with a favorable outcome when noted as the sole abnormality but with a less favorable prognosis in the setting of a complex karyotype, a phenomenon that is analogous to that observed for del(5q) in MDS (discussed previously) (Pan et al., 2014).

The deletions of 20q are interstitial and typically large with loss of most of the long arm; a del(20)(q11.2q13.3) is the most common followed by del(20)(q11.2q13.1). Using FISH and molecular

analysis, investigators have identified an interstitial CDS of 4 Mb within 20q12 that is flanked by D20S206 proximally and D20S424 distally and contains a number of genes; however, the identity of a myeloid TSG(s) on 20q is unknown (Bench et al., 2000; Wang et al., 2000). Recent studies have implicated the genes encoding topoisomerase I and a protein related to the polycomb group family of transcriptional repressors, namely, lethal (3) malignant brain tumor (L3MBTL1). Although *L3MBTL1* is not mutated in MDS or AML with del(20q), reduced or absent L3MBTL1 expression may be relevant in that knockdown of *L3MBTL1* in primary human HSPCs (CD34+) results in enhanced sensitivity to EPO, as well as enhanced commitment to, and acceleration of, erythroid differentiation (Perna et al., 2010).

Complex karyotypes

Complex karyotypes are variably defined but generally have ≥3 chromosomal abnormalities. The majority of cases with complex karyotypes involve unbalanced chromosomal abnormalities leading to loss of genetic material. Complex karyotypes are observed in 10% of patients with primary MDS and in as many as 90% of patients with t-MDS (Smith et al., 2003; Schanz et al., 2012). Abnormalities involving chromosome 5 are identified in most cases with complex karyotypes, often with the co-occurrence of 17p loss, but abnormalities leading to loss of 7q are also relatively common. A complex karyotype carries a poor prognosis (IPSS-R median survival of 1.5 years and 0.7 years for the poor- and very poor-risk groups, respectively) (Malcovati et al., 2007; Greenberg et al., 2012).

A monosomal karyotype (MK) is defined by the presence of two or more autosomal monosomies or a single monosomy with at least one structural abnormality. MK MDS is associated with high-risk features, including higher marrow blasts, poor-risk or very poor-risk IPSS-R scores, and complex karyotypes with high-risk abnormalities (−7, del(5q), and −17/loss of 17p). Whether MK provides additional prognostic information is controversial. Some reports suggest that the level of complexity, or *TP53* mutations, may define subsets with a particularly poor outcome (Patnaik et al., 2011; Schanz et al., 2013). The conflicting findings may be influenced, in part, by the imprecision of a classification based solely on cytogenetic analysis, as the application of molecular cytogenetic methods has revealed that up to 46% of cases classified as MK by chromosome banding analysis alone had no actual monosomies. Pending further studies, MK is not recognized as a cytogenetic entity in the upcoming WHO 2014 update.

Rare recurring translocations

Translocations have been identified in ~4% of MDS patients, substantially lower than the frequency in AML (Costa et al., 2013). Costa et al. (2013) reviewed the karyotypes of 5654 patients with MDS and identified 155 novel translocations, nine of which were recurrent, suggesting that our compendium of recurring translocations in MDS is incomplete. The consequence of the recurring translocations is the deregulation of gene expression with increased production of a normal protein product common in lymphoid neoplasms or the generation of a novel fusion gene and production of a fusion protein common in myeloid neoplasms. To date, all of the recurring translocations cloned in malignant myeloid disorders resulted in fusion proteins (Mitelman et al., 2014). In MDS, several such translocations have been identified and examined by molecular analysis.

Translocations of 11q23.3

The *KMT2A/MLL* gene is involved in rearrangement with over 70 partner genes in leukemia (Marschalek, 2011). Translocations involving 11q23.3 are rarely (0.2%) the sole abnormality in MDS (Schanz et al., 2012). In a European workshop study of 550 patients with 11q23.3 abnormalities, 28 cases (5.1%) presented with an MDS, and five others with such an abnormality had evolved from t-MDS to t-AML prior to cytogenetic analysis, for a total of 6% of all examined cases. Onefourth of these cases were t-MDS (Bain et al., 1998). Other abnormalities, including complex karyotypes and a −7/del(7q), frequently accompany the 11q23.3 abnormalities in both primary MDS and t-MDS. No association with FAB subgroup was identified, although RA was overrepresented and RARS underrepresented as compared to most series of MDS patients. The median survival was short (19 months) with leukemic transformation in ~ 20% of cases.

Just under 12% of the 162 patients with 11q23.3 involvement included in an international workshop on MDS and leukemia following cytotoxic treatment presented with a t-MDS (Bloomfield et al., 2002). One-third (6/19) of these patients had progression to an acute leukemia (5 AML, 1 ALL). No clear association with FAB subtype was found. The most common translocations were t(9;11) (p21.3;q23.3) in 6 cases, t(11;19)(q23.3;p13.1) in 3 cases, and t(11;16)(q23.3;p13.3) in 3 cases.

t(11;16)

The t(11;16)(q23.3;p13.3) occurs primarily in t-MDS, but rare cases have presented as t-AML or AML de novo (Rowley et al., 1997). The t(11;16) is unique among the recurring translocations of *KMT2A/MLL* in myeloid malignancies (with AML predominating) in that most patients have t-MDS. The *KMT2A* gene on chromosome 11 is fused with the *CREBBP* (CREB-binding protein, or *CBP*) gene on chromosome 16. The KMT2A protein is a histone H3 lysine 4 methyltransferase that assembles in protein complexes that regulate gene transcription, for example, *HOX* genes during embryonic development, via chromatin remodeling. Transcriptional targets of the fusion proteins include *HOXA9, MEIS1, MYB, MECOM, MYC,* and *EPHA7*. CREBBP is an adapter protein involved in transcriptional control via histone acetylation that mediates chromosome decondensation, thereby facilitating transcription.

PDGFRB translocations

The t(5;12)(q32;p13.2) is observed in <1% of patients with CMML. The molecular consequence of the t(5;12) is fusion of the gene encoding the beta chain of the platelet-derived growth factor receptor (*PDGFRB*) at 5q32 with a novel erythroblastosis virus-transforming sequence (ETS)-like transcription factor, *ETV6* (also known as *TEL*), on chromosome 12. The encoded fusion protein contains the 5′ portion of *ETV6* and the 3′ portion of *PDGFRB* (Golub et al., 1994). Biochemical studies have revealed that the PDGFRB kinase activity is perturbed contributing to the transformed phenotype. *ETV6* encodes a transcriptional repressor and is promiscuously involved in translocations with some 40 genes in hematologic malignancies (Zhang and Rowley, 2006). Interest has increased in identifying this translocation because it predicts for a response to imatinib mesylate, a selective inhibitor of the PDGFRB tyrosine kinase activity (Apperley et al., 2002). Similarly, *PDGFRB* participates in other rare translocations involving genes encoding the membrane-associated protein huntingtin-interacting protein 1 (HIP1) in the t(5;7)(q32;q11.2); the small GTPase RABEP1 (Rabaptin 5) in the t(5;17) (q32;p13.2); and H4, a ubiquitous protein of unknown function, in the t(5;10)(q32;q21) in CMML; and thyroid receptor-interacting protein 11 (TRIP11) in the t(5;14)(q32;q32.1) in a case of AML. A unifying feature of these various translocations is the presence of eosinophilia.

Abnormalities of 3q

Recurring abnormalities of 3q are rare in MDS (~2%). They include the inv(3)(q21.3q26.2)/t(3;3) (q21.3;q26.2) associated with normal or increased platelet counts and the t(3;21)(q26.2;q22.1). Common features of myeloid diseases with abnormalities of 3q are a previous history of cytotoxic exposure, prominent BM dysplasia, and a poor prognosis. Abnormalities of chromosome 7, −7/ del(7q), are observed in most cases. These abnormalities result in overexpression of the *MECOM/ EVI1* gene at 3q26.2, which was originally predicted (but not experimentally validated) to result from juxtaposition with the cryptic enhancer of the housekeeping gene encoding the ribosome-binding protein RPN1 (Martinelli et al., 2003). *MECOM* encodes a zinc finger transcription factor that interacts with a number of transcriptional and epigenetic regulators (CREBBP, CTBP, HDAC, KAT2B (P/CAF), SMAD3, GATA1, GATA2, DNMT3A, and DNMT3B) and mediates chromatin modifications and DNA hypermethylation. Depending on its binding partners, MECOM can act as a transcriptional activator to promote the proliferation of HSPCs, for example, when bound to GATA2, or as a transcriptional repressor inhibiting erythroid differentiation, for example, when bound to GATA1. In addition, MECOM impairs myelopoiesis by deregulation of multiple transcription factor genes, including *RUNX1* and *SPI1/PU.1* (Laricchia-Robbio et al., 2009). Recently, several groups have elucidated a novel molecular mechanism and described a new paradigm for the pathogenesis of MDS/AML, whereby the inv(3)/t(3;3) repositions a distal *GATA2* enhancer to activate *MECOM* expression and

simultaneously confer *GATA2* haploinsufficiency (also recently identified as the etiology of sporadic familial MDS/AML and MonoMac/Emberger syndromes) (Groschel et al., 2014; Yamazaki et al., 2014). The t(3;21)(q26.2;q22.1) has been linked to acute leukemia arising after cytotoxic therapy. It was first recognized in CML in blast crisis and later in t-MDS/t-AML (Rubin et al., 1990). The translocation leads to an out-of-frame fusion of *MECOM* with *RUNX1* at 21q22, with loss of function of *RUNX1* and *MECOM* overexpression.

Evolution of the karyotype

Although individual cases of MDS or AML may be remarkably complex, the parent clone (initiating clone) or "mainline" and its derivative subclones share a set of chromosomal abnormalities, whereas unique subclones have acquired additional aberrations after disease initiation, aberrations that may contribute to progression. Cytogenetic evolution can take several forms. It may include the appearance of an abnormal clone where only normal cells have been seen previously, the acquisition of additional abnormalities in one or more clones, or the progression from the presence of a single clone (often with a simple karyotype) to multiple related or, occasionally, unrelated abnormal clones. The identification of new abnormalities in the karyotype often coincides with a change in the behavior of the disease, usually to a more aggressive course, and may herald incipient leukemia. Hence, serial evaluations can be informative, particularly when there is a change in the clinical features of a patient.

The natural history of MDS is generally characterized by one of three clinical scenarios: (i) a gradual worsening of pancytopenia where the marrow blast count is found to be increasing, (ii) a relatively stable clinical course followed by an abrupt change with a clear leukemic transformation, and (iii) a stable course over many years without significant change in the marrow blast counts when reevaluated. In the first group, the karyotype typically remains stable, and the progression to leukemia is based on the relatively arbitrary finding of more than 20% blasts in the marrow, making the transition to AML a relatively ill-defined event. In the second group, a change in the karyotype with the appearance of subclones or increased karyotypic complexity is typical. Both the karyotype and the disease tend to remain stable in the third group.

Recent studies of paired samples of MDS and AML evolving from an antecedent MDS (sAML) have led to new insights (Walter et al., 2012). First, nearly all cells in the BM (~85%) in patients with MDS and sAML are clonally derived. Second, most cases have a founder clone and ≥1 derivative subclone, with an average of 2.4 clones in MDS and 3.1 clones in sAML. Genomic evolution in MDS proved to be a dynamic process that is shaped by multiple cycles of mutation acquisition followed by clonal selection (Walter et al., 2012).

Molecular pathogenesis of MDS

The pathogenesis and progression of MDS are driven by multiple, cooperating, somatically acquired genetic abnormalities that include chromosomal abnormalities as well as gene mutations, the diversity of which gives rise to the clinical and morphological heterogeneity characteristic of this disease. Recent technological advances, particularly next-generation sequencing, have enabled the identification of a number of mutated genes and have implicated novel pathways in the pathogenesis of MDS. Molecular mutations can be identified in up to 70% of unselected patients with MDS—the frequency may be higher in those patients with a normal karyotype—and showing increases from low-risk to high-risk MDS or AML evolving from MDS; all this provides new insights into the complexity of this disease.

Bejar et al. (2011) demonstrated that the integration of mutation analysis into prognostic scoring systems in MDS has the potential to stratify a diverse disease into discrete subsets with more consistent clinical phenotypes and prognosis. For example, mutations in RUNX1, TP53, and NRAS were associated with severe thrombocytopenia and an elevated blast percentage. In multivariate analysis, mutations in five genes, occurring in one-third of patients, retained independent prognostic significance: TP53, EZH2, ETV6, RUNX1, and ASXL1 predicted poor OS and stratified low-IPSS-risk and intermediate-1- and intermediate-2-IPSS-risk groups into two risk groups each, identifying patients within these subgroups with a poorer prognosis who may require a more intensive therapeutic approach.

The genes involved in MDS fall into four main classes, namely, genes encoding hematopoietic transcription factors, epigenetic regulators of gene transcription, RNA splicing factors, or proteins that regulate cytokine signaling pathways. A detailed review is beyond the scope of this chapter but has been provided elsewhere (Itzykson et al., 2013; Lindsley and Ebert, 2013). Table 7.4 provides a partial list and overview of some of the salient features of genes implicated in the pathogenesis of MDS. The most commonly mutated genes are TET2, ASXL1, EZH2, RUNX1, NRAS, SF3B1, SRSF2, U2AF1, and TP53, which are described briefly in the following text.

Transcription factors

Hematopoiesis is a tightly regulated, dynamic process driven by the coordinated action of transcription factors that regulate lineage-specific gene expression. Not surprisingly, genes encoding transcription factors are commonly mutated in hematological malignancies. RUNX1 (Runt-related transcription factor 1 gene) is the most commonly mutated gene in this class in MDS, whereas TP53 is the most commonly mutated gene in t-MDS. Point mutations in RUNX1 have been reported in 10–20% of MDS, particularly in t-MDS, and increase with the severity of the disease (Steensma et al., 2005b; Chen et al., 2007). RUNX1, also known as AML1, encodes the DNA-binding subunit of the heterodimeric core-binding factor (CBF) complex, essential for definitive hematopoiesis (Speck and Gilliland, 2002). RUNX1 missense mutations predominate and are commonly located in the DNA-binding (or Runt) domain, thereby impairing DNA binding and creating dominant negative proteins. RUNX1 mutations are associated with severe thrombocytopenia (<50 000), increased BM blasts, activating mutations of the RAS pathway, −7/del(7q), and decreased OS (Chen et al., 2007). Germline mutations of RUNX1 cause a rare disease called familial platelet disorder; affected individuals have an MDS-like phenotype with thrombocytopenia and/or dysfunctional platelets and a predisposition to AML (Song et al., 1999).

TP53 (17p13.1) encodes a transcription factor that mediates the cellular response to diverse stresses, including oncogene activation, and can induce cell cycle arrest, activate DNA repair

Table 7.4 Frequency and significance of mutated genes in MDS

Mutated gene	Frequency*	Biological features and clinical significance
Transcription factors		
CEBPA	2–5%	• TF involved in hematopoiesis; loss of function impairs granulopoiesis • Biallelic (N-terminal and C-terminal mutations) • No apparent effect on time to progression to AML or overall survival (OS)
TP53	5–10% (25% in t-MDS)	• The TP53 transcription factor mediates the cellular response to stress stimuli, including DNA damage, by inducing cell cycle arrest, activating DNA repair pathways to maintain the integrity of the genome, and inducing apoptosis • Associated with chromosomal instability, del(5q), loss of 17p, and complex karyotypes • Independent risk factor, associated with rapid progression and poor outcome • Significantly differentiates worse prognosis within each IPSS subgroup
RUNX1	10–20%	• Encodes the DNA-binding subunit of the heterodimeric core-binding factor transcription factor required for hematopoiesis • Point mutations in the RUNT (DNA-binding) domain result in loss of function and a dominant negative effect • Associated with mutations of the RAS pathway and –7/del(7q) • Independent risk factor, associated with severe thrombocytopenia, increased BM blasts, decreased OS, and increased risk of progression to AML
Others	<2%	• Includes *PHF6, WT1, ETV6*
Epigenetic regulators		
ASXL1	10–15%	• Polycomb group protein involved in transcriptional regulation • Prevalence of frameshift mutations predicted to result in a truncated protein suggests a dominant negative function • More common in MDS with an intermediate-risk cytogenetic pattern • Independent risk factor, associated with decreased OS and shorter time to progression to AML
DNMT3A	5%	• Encodes a de novo DNA methyltransferase • Missense, nonsense, and frameshift mutations have been identified throughout the coding region of the *DNMT3A* gene but most commonly (up to 60%) in R882H within the methyltransferase domain that reduces enzymatic activity • Associated with decreased OS and shorter time to progression to AML • Murine *Dnmt3b*-deficient HSCs show bias to self-renewal over differentiation
EZH2	5%	• Encodes a member of the PRC2 complex, a histone 3 lysine 27 methyltransferase that represses transcription • Missense mutations cluster in the C-terminal SET domain and result in loss of function • Mutations may be associated with copy-neutral loss of heterozygosity (UPD) or del(7q) • Independent risk factor, associated with a poor prognosis, decreased OS
IDH1/2	Rare	• Metabolic enzymes catalyzing oxidative decarboxylation of isocitrate to alpha-ketoglutarate (alpha-KG). Missense mutations alter catalytic function converting alpha-KG to 2 hydroxyglutarate while consuming NADPH • Mutations mainly affect codon R132 of IDH1 and codons R140 and R172 of IDH2 and result in altered catalytic function • Associated with advanced MDS and progression to AML • IDH1 mutations are associated with decreased OS

Table 7.4 (*Continued*)

Mutated gene	Frequency*	Biological features and clinical significance
TET2	20%	• Associated with a normal karyotype and may occur with other mutations • Predicted loss of function with compromised catalytic activity demonstrated by decreased levels of 5hmC in genomic DNA from BM cells • 5hmC may serve as an intermediate epigenetic mark in active, replication-independent demethylation, or it may influence transcription directly via specific interactions with nuclear factors. 5hmC is enriched at sites of bivalent histone marks and influences recruitment of the polycomb repressive complex 2 (PRC2) to target genes • No clear prognostic significance
Others	≤1%	• Includes *ATRX* and *UTX*
Receptor tyrosine kinases		
CSF1R	2–5%	• Constitutive activation of the macrophage colony-stimulating factor receptor tyrosine kinase (RTK) • Karyotype predominantly normal • Associated with advanced MDS and progression to AML
CBL	3% 15% of CMML	• *CBL* encodes a multidomain adaptor protein with E3 ubiquitin ligase activity that negatively regulates RTK signaling by modulating receptor degradation • Mutations reduce the enzymatic activity, are frequently biallelic, and are associated with acquired copy-neutral LOH of 11q, implicating wild-type CBL as a tumor suppressor
FLT3 ITD	3–5%	• RTK involved in cytokine signaling, critical in hematopoiesis • Associated with progression to AML and a poor prognosis (decreased OS) • Associated with a complex karyotype and co-occurring RAS mutations
JAK2	3% of RA 60% of RARS-T	• Encodes a tyrosine kinase component of various cytokine signaling pathways • Mutations result in constitutive activation of the tyrosine kinase • Mutated in 60% (V617F) of RARS with thrombocytosis, an unclassified MDS/MPD, mutations in *SF3B1* occur in 70% of RARS-T, often concurrent with *JAK2* mutations • Clinical significance unknown, does not appear to alter prognosis
MPL	5% of RARS-T <1% other	• Encodes the thrombopoietin receptor • Mutations result in constitutive tyrosine kinase activity and are associated with dysmegakaryocytopoiesis • Higher expression in advanced MDS is associated with a poor prognosis
NRAS KRAS	10% 1–2%	• Encodes a GTPase that is activated by cytokine receptors and regulates signaling cascades that are critical for cell growth and survival • Activating mutations result in constitutive signal transduction • NRAS mutations are strongly associated with severe thrombocytopenia and increased BM blasts, increased risk of progression to AML, and decreased OS
PTPN11	Rare	• Encodes the nonreceptor SHP2 tyrosine phosphatase, a positive regulator of RAS proteins. Mutations result in protein activation • Mutated in 30% of JMML • Mutations in *NRAS/KRAS*, *NF1*, and *PTPN11* are mutually exclusive
Others	≤1%	• Includes *GNAS, KIT, CBLB, CDKN2A, BRAF, PTEN*
RNA splicing		
SF3B1	15–30%	• SF3B1 encodes a subunit of the splicing factor 3b complex, which together with the SF3A complex and the U2 snRNA comprise the U2 snRNP • Heterozygous missense mutations predominantly affect conserved residues within the carboxy-terminal HEAT repeats: K700, K666, H662, E622, and R625 • Strongly associated with the presence of ring sideroblasts • Independently associated with prolonged OS and LFS in some studies • Associated with higher platelet counts, lower BM blasts, and higher WBC

(*Continued*)

Table 7.4 (*Continued*)

Mutated gene	Frequency*	Biological features and clinical significance
SRSF2	15%	• Involved in the early steps of U2 snRNP assembly/function • Heterozygous missense mutations • Associated with CMML • Associated with decreased OS
U2AF1	8%	• Encodes a subunit of the U2 small nuclear ribonucleoprotein auxiliary factor (U2AF) that binds the 3′ splice acceptor site • Heterozygous missense substitutions within the conserved zinc finger domains, predominantly at codon S34 and, less commonly, at Q157 • Associated with increased rate of progression to AML, decreased OS
ZRSR2	6%	• Involved in the early steps of U2 snRNP assembly/function • Diverse mutation types throughout the open-reading frame
Others	≤1%	• Includes U2AF65, SF3A1, PRPF8, LUC7L2, SF1, and PRPF40B
Other		
NPM1	Rare	• Nuclear–cytoplasmic shuttling protein, with pleiotropic functions • Terminal frameshift mutations disrupt the nuclear localization signal leading to redistribution to the cytoplasm • Unknown clinical significance in MDS

*Rare mutations occur at a frequency of less than 2%.

pathways, and trigger apoptosis in response to DNA damage. Mutations of *TP53* (exons 4–8) or loss of an allele, typically as a result of a cytogenetic abnormality of 17p, are observed in 5–10% of MDS and 25–30% of patients with t-MDS, particularly in those who have received alkylating agent therapy (Christiansen et al., 2001; Shih et al., 2013). *TP53* mutations may occur as either an early or late event in the course of the disease and are associated with rapid progression and a poor outcome. In both primary MDS and t-MDS, *TP53* mutations are associated with del(5q)/t(5q) and a complex karyotype, although the mutation frequency varies with the disease and cytogenetic abnormality. Kulasekararaj et al. (2013) identified *TP53* mutations in 9.4% of all MDS patients, with the frequency varying from 19% of MDS with an isolated del(5q) to 72% in MDS with a del(5q)/t(5q) and a complex karyotype and correlating with IPSS INT-2/high risk, a higher blast count, and leukemic progression. Similarly, Volkert et al. (2014) noted that *TP53* mutations were more frequent in patients with an unbalanced translocation leading to loss of 5q (95%) than in patients with a del(5q) (40%) or MDS with an isolated del(5q) (22%). Of note is that *TP53* mutations in

myeloid neoplasms are typically accompanied by relatively few mutations in other genes.

Epigenetic regulators

A new paradigm in MDS is the high frequency of mutations in genes involved in the regulation of transcription via chromatin modifications, specifically DNA methylation (*DNMT3A*) and histone methylation (*IDH1/2*, *TET2*, *EZH2*, *ASXL1*), and the intriguing observation that mutations often occur in more than one gene in this class in the same patient, implying functional cooperation (note that *IDH1/2* and *TET2* mutations are mutually exclusive). As such, mutations in epigenetic regulators have the potential to cause widespread and persistent alterations in transcriptional programs.

The most frequently mutated gene in this class in MDS is *TET2* (20% overall, 40% in CMML); point mutations are observed in all cytogenetic subsets but are particularly common in MDS with a normal karyotype (Langemeijer et al., 2009; Bejar et al., 2011). TET2 oxidizes 5-methylcytosine (5-mC) to 5-hydroxymethylcytosine (5hmC), 5-formylcytosine (5fC), and 5-carboxycytosine (5caC), thereby altering the epigenetic mark created by DNA methyltransferases (DNMTs)

(Ito et al., 2011). *TET2* mutations are predicted to result in loss of function, consistent with the observation of reduced levels of 5hmC in genomic DNA from *TET*-mutated malignancies (Ko et al., 2010). In mouse models, *Tet2* mutations cause expansion of the HSPCs as well as enhanced HSC self-renewal and a bias toward myelomonocytic differentiation. At present, the biological role of 5hmC is not completely understood; however, 5hmC may serve as an intermediate species in active, replication-independent demethylation, or it may be an epigenetic mark that influences gene transcription directly via specific interactions with nuclear factors. Recent studies suggest no impact of *TET2* mutations on OS in MDS (Kosmider et al., 2009; Langemeijer et al., 2009; Lindsley and Ebert, 2013).

The DNMTs establish the initial patterns of methylation of cytosine bases in DNA by converting cytosine to 5-mC, primarily in the context of CpG dinucleotides enriched at the site of gene promoters, ultimately reducing gene transcription. Mutations in *DNMT3A* are found in ~5% of MDS and are associated with decreased OS and shorter time to progression to AML (Bejar et al., 2011; Walter et al., 2011). The most common mutation is a missense R882H change within the methyltransferase domain that reduces enzymatic activity. Although the global gene targets of altered DNMT3A activity are poorly understood, murine HSCs that lack Dnmt3a are functionally abnormal with a bias toward self-renewal. They also show increased expression of multipotency "stemness" genes and a decrease in the expression of genes that regulate differentiation (Challen et al., 2012).

ASXL1 mutations are observed in 10–15% of MDS and 40% of CMML and are more common in intermediate-risk MDS (Gelsi-Boyer et al., 2009; Bejar et al., 2011). ASXL1 is a member of the polycomb family of chromatin-binding proteins and is involved in the repression of gene expression. Mutated proteins are predicted to function as dominant negative proteins inhibiting the function of wild-type proteins as well as other members of the polycomb complex. ASXL1 mutations in MDS are an independent risk factor and are associated with decreased OS and shorter time to progression to AML (Bejar et al., 2011; Thol et al., 2011).

EZH2 (enhancer of zeste homolog 2) mutations occur in 5% of MDS (Ernst et al., 2010; Nikoloski et al., 2010; Bejar et al., 2011). *EZH2* encodes a histone methyltransferase that trimethylates histone 3 lysine 27, which is involved in gene silencing. In MDS, the mutations lead to loss of the catalytic activity and are predicted to increase HSC expansion (Majewski et al., 2010). Although *EZH2* is located at 7q36.1, loss or mutation of *EZH2* does not appear to be the major or sole driver of myeloid neoplasms associated with −7/del(7q). *EZH2* mutations are more prevalent in lower-risk MDS but are an independent risk factor associated with a poor prognosis and a shorter OS.

Although the gene targets of mutated epigenetic regulators are poorly understood, the role of epigenetic changes in the pathogenesis and treatment of MDS is becoming increasingly important (Meldi and Figueroa, 2015). For example, we have known for over a decade that transcriptional silencing via DNA methylation of *CDKN2B* ($p15^{INK4B}$) increases with progression from low-risk to high-risk MDS, is observed in a high percentage of patients with t-MDS, and is associated with −7/del(7q) and a poor prognosis (Christiansen et al., 2003). Recent genome-wide studies have shown that increases in promoter hypermethylation are predictive of survival in MDS, even when age, sex, and IPSS risk groups are considered. Aberrant methylation in MDS and sAML affects particular regions and preferentially occurs in genes involved in the WNT and MAPK signaling pathways (Figueroa et al., 2009). Moreover, increases in promoter methylation are seen during progression to AML (Shen et al., 2010). These observations form the rationale for the use of demethylating agents in MDS, which have prolonged the survival of high-risk patients (Fenaux et al., 2009). Similarly, inhibition of histone-modifying enzymes represents another rational approach to MDS therapy.

Receptor tyrosine kinases

Normal hematopoiesis is regulated, in part, by the action of growth factors and cytokines that bind to their cognate cell surface receptors, thereby activating intracellular kinase cascades. Not surprisingly, mutations in these genes can result in constitutive signaling and increased responsiveness to exogenous stimuli, such as growth factors. Recurrent gain-of-function mutations in receptor tyrosine kinases, nonreceptor (intracellular) tyrosine kinases, and other components of cytokine signaling pathways are common in AML (*FLT3, KIT, NRAS/KRAS*) and MPD (*MPL, JAK2*) but are less common in MDS.

The RAS signaling cascade is downstream of a number of activated cytokine receptors, including the FLT3, IL3, and GM-CSF receptors; thus, this signaling pathway plays a pivotal role in hematopoiesis, regulating cellular proliferation, differentiation, and cell death (Ward et al., 2012). Mutant RAS proteins retain an active GTP-bound form, promoting constitutive activation. *NRAS* mutations are present in 10% of MDS cases; the most frequent mutation is a single base change at codon 12 of the protein, but codons 13 and 61 are also frequently mutated. These mutations are associated with severe thrombocytopenia, increased BM blasts, poor prognosis, higher incidence of transformation to AML, and shorter survival (Bacher et al., 2007; Bejar et al., 2011). Many therapeutic molecules, including the MEK and AKT inhibitors as well as imatinib and second-generation tyrosine kinase inhibitors, interrupt various steps in the RAS signaling pathways (Bejar et al., 2011; Ward et al., 2012).

JAK2^{V617F} is a constitutively active cytoplasmic tyrosine kinase that activates JAK–STAT signaling and mediates transformation to cytokine-independent growth in MPDs and has been identified in rare cases of MDS (2–5%) and CMML (3%) (Steensma et al., 2005a). RARS-T is an exception in that 60% of patients have the *JAK2^{V617F}* mutation and present with higher WBCs and platelet counts (Zipperer et al., 2008; Malcovati et al., 2009). Of interest, 70% of RARS-T patients have *SF3B1* mutations, which can co-occur with *JAK2* mutations, providing a possible explanation for the composite MDS/MPD phenotype of RARS-T (Papaemmanuil et al., 2011).

Mutations in the *CBL* gene, encoding a multi-domain adapter protein with E3 ubiquitin ligase activity that negatively regulates signaling from receptor tyrosine kinases via receptor degradation, occur in 15% of CMML but less frequently in MDS (3%) (Lindsley and Ebert, 2013). Mutations are frequently biallelic and are associated with copy-neutral LOH of 11q, raising the possibility that wild-type CBL functions as a tumor suppressor.

RNA splicing

One of the unexpected findings of genomic analysis of MDS using whole-exome or whole-genome sequencing was the identification of recurrent somatic mutations in genes encoding components of the spliceosome, implicating aberrant mRNA splicing in the pathogenesis of MDS (Yoshida et al., 2011). Collectively, these mutations are the most common changes in MDS, occurring in ~50% of patients, and enriched in all myeloid diseases characterized by dysplasia, that is, MDS, t-MDS/t-AML, and AML with myelodysplasia-related changes (Papaemmanuil et al., 2011; Yoshida et al., 2011; Graubert et al., 2012). The RNA splicing machinery, or spliceosome, mediates the processing of pre-mRNA via the excision of introns and ligation of flanking exons to generate mature mRNAs and alternatively spliced mRNA isoforms. The spliceosome consists of multiple small nuclear riboproteins (snRNPs) that perform essential structural and enzymatic functions, as well as accessory proteins. Recurrent mutations in MDS occur in genes involved in the early steps of U2 snRNP assembly (*SF3A1, SF3B1, ZRSR2, SRSF2*) and 3′ splice site recognition (*SF1, U2AF2,* and *U2AF1*). Whether the mutations cause loss of function or altered protein function is unknown, as is also the identity of the mRNA targets that confer the pathogenic function; both aspects are targets of current research. Aberrant splicing could result in the formation of novel protein isoforms with altered function, inappropriate tissue-specific isoforms, or reduced levels of proteins via the introduction of premature stop codons or activation of nonsense-mediated decay.

SF3B1 mutations, the most frequently encountered spliceosomal mutations (~20%), are strongly associated with the presence of ring sideroblasts, higher platelet counts, lower BM blasts, and higher WBC counts. Heterozygous missense mutations predominantly affect five conserved residues within the carboxy-terminal HEAT repeats: K700, K666, H662, E622, and R625 (Papaemmanuil et al., 2011; Yoshida et al., 2011). Initial studies suggested that *SF3B1* mutations were associated with prolonged overall and leukemia-free survival, but other studies did not find mutations of this gene to be an independent prognostic factor (Malcovati et al., 2011; Patnaik et al., 2012).

The *SRSF2* gene at 17q25 encodes a serine-/arginine-rich splicing factor that is critical for assembly of the spliceosome and selection of the correct splice sites. Heterozygous missense mutations of *SRSF2* are detected in ~15% of MDS patients with a higher frequency in elderly males and are associated with decreased OS (Thol et al., 2012).

Mutations in *U2AF1*, which encodes a component of the U2 snRNP auxiliary factor, have been identified in 8–9% of MDS and are associated with an increased rate of progression to AML (Yoshida et al., 2011; Graubert et al., 2012). Heterozygous missense mutations occur within the conserved zinc fingers, predominantly affecting S34 or Q157. Importantly, functional studies of the mutant U2AF1 S34 protein demonstrated increased production of aberrant splice products, and *in vivo* studies in mice showed reduced repopulating capacity of HSCs expressing the mutant protein (Yoshida et al., 2011).

Other gene mutations

Recently, high-throughput sequencing has led to the identification of mutations in a new class of genes in myeloid neoplasms, namely, the cohesin genes. The cohesin complex is involved in the separation of sister chromatids at anaphase, as well as in other long-range chromatin interactions. In MDS, mutations have been identified in four members of the cohesin complex (*STAG2, RAD21, SMC1A,* and *SMC3*) in 8% of MDS patients; however, the prognostic significance of these mutations is not yet known (Kon et al., 2013).

Cytogenetic abnormalities in MDS/MPD

There are no genetic alterations that are specific for this group of diseases. The absence of t(9;22) resulting in the *BCR/ABL1* fusion necessary for the diagnosis of CML, as well as the absence of *PDGFRA* or *PDGFRB* rearrangements, isolated del(5q), and abnormalities of 3q, are key diagnostic elements of these diseases. The abnormalities commonly seen in MDS are also seen in MDS/MPD. There is, however, a markedly lower incidence of del(5q), as well as abnormalities of 11q as compared to the classical forms of MDS (GFCH, 1991; Adeyinka and Dewald, 2003). The most frequent abnormalities include +8 and −7/del(7q). Loss of the Y chromosome is seen in many cases and may represent an age-associated phenomenon rather than any etiologic association. The involvement of 12p in various rearrangements in CMML is also a frequent finding (>5%) (GFCH, 1991). As discussed earlier, translocations of *PDGFRB* (5q32) are noted in rare cases of CMML and aCML (1–2%), and their unifying feature is eosinophilia. In JMML, the only frequently recurring abnormality is the −7/del(7q), which has been reported in 6% of cases, usually as the sole cytogenetic abnormality (Hasle and Niemeyer, 2011). Finally, the MDS/MPD unclassifiable cases do not have specific recurring abnormalities, but cytogenetic analysis is useful in excluding CML and establishing clonality of the disorder.

Other technologies

Recent advances in microarray technology have enabled high-resolution genome-wide genotyping using SNPs for the identification of disease susceptibility loci as well as the identification of acquired genetic imbalances and LOH that occurs without concurrent changes in the gene copy number, which can be attributed to somatic mitotic recombination (referred to as copy-neutral LOH or acquired uniparental disomy). Abnormalities are detected in a higher proportion of cases as compared to what is seen by conventional cytogenetic analysis and are seen also in cases with a normal karyotype; altogether, copy-neutral LOH is reported in ~20% of MDS cases (Shaffer et al., 2013). Moreover, factoring SNP array lesions into the IPSS classification appears to allow for better prognostic resolution, suggesting that SNP array analysis may have future diagnostic application and may complement banding cytogenetics in risk stratification and the selection of therapy.

Emerging paradigms

Extensive experimental evidence indicates that more than one mutation is required for the pathogenesis of hematological malignant diseases. Thus, an important aspect of MDS and leukemia biology is the elucidation of the spectrum of chromosomal abnormalities and molecular mutations that cooperate in the pathways leading to these diseases.

At present, there are a number of unanswered questions regarding the molecular pathogenesis of MDS. For example, we do not yet know the full spectrum of genetic mutations in MDS within each pathway, nor do we know the order in which these mutations occur and the prognostic significance associated with many cooperating mutations. A variety of experimental evidence suggests that the recurring chromosomal abnormalities in MDS and AML are likely to be an early and, in many cases, the initiating event.

Although incompletely understood, emerging data suggest that alterations of the BM microenvironment, or "niche," play a role in the pathogenesis of MDS, making MDS a unique disease of the "tissue" rather than of hematopoietic cells alone (Raaijmakers, 2012; Medyouf et al., 2014). Early histologic studies of MDS identified disruption of the BM architecture, and several features of the early phases of MDS, for example, increased apoptosis, are believed to result from functional alterations in the BM stroma leading to altered expression of inflammatory cytokines such as TNFA, TGFB, IL1B, IL6, and IL8; chemokines; and adhesion molecules (Raaijmakers, 2012). Functional abnormalities of the microenvironment have been reported in MDS and may, in part, account for the poor outcome of stem cell transplantation in MDS, that is, diseased stromal cells remain. A plausible model is that MDS arises in the setting of an abnormal BM microenvironment, creating a permissive environment that promotes the generation of multiple hematopoietic populations with varying genetic events, some of which persist, whereas others may undergo cell death, and yet others may go on to acquire additional mutations necessary to complete malignant transformation. This model would account for the observation of unrelated cytogenetic clones in the BM of MDS patients, as well as the observation of persistent dysplasia in MDS or AML patients following therapy.

A number of different cell types contribute to the HSC niche, including mesenchymal stem cells (MSCs) and their progeny cells such as osteoprogenitors or osteoblast-lineage cells. In an elegant study, Medyouf et al. (2014) demonstrated that MSCs derived from MDS patients display a disturbed differentiation program and are essential for the propagation of MDS stem cells (Lin⁻, CD34⁺, CD38⁻) in an orthotopic xenograft model, mediated by the production of critical niche factors by MDS MSCs such as CDH2, IGFBP2, VEGF2, and LIF. Of note, healthy MSCs adopt MDS MSC-like molecular features when exposed to MDS HSCs, via niche reprogramming.

These studies demonstrate the intricate interplay (bidirectional cross talk) in human MDS between mutant hematopoietic cells and their MSCs. The WNT pathway has emerged as a critical mediator of these microenvironment–stem cell interactions; it regulates the function of BM osteoblasts as well as the maintenance of HSC quiescence and self-renewal (Wang et al., 2010b). Recently, increased β-catenin signaling and nuclear accumulation in stromal osteoblasts was identified in 38% of MDS/AML patients, most (80%) of whom had abnormalities of chromosomes 5 and/or 7 in the hematopoietic cells (Kode et al., 2014). These observations support a mechanism whereby transformation results from the interactions of cell-autonomous and niche-determined events and point to the niche as the site of the initiating event that leads to secondary changes in other cells, that is, "a niche-based" model of oncogenesis. Emerging technologies, such as the ability to examine stromal cells *in vitro* and *in vivo* and to establish *in vivo* models for MDS in mice, will facilitate the evaluation of the role of the microenvironment in the etiology of MDS.

Summary

The role of cytogenetic analysis in MDS remains a pivotal element for establishing the diagnosis, prognosis, and therapeutic decisions, including the initiation of specific treatments and the follow-up of altered clinical behavior of the disease. The recurring abnormalities, while rarely specific for a disease entity, have not only provided insight into prognosis but also the molecular pathogenesis of these heterogeneous disorders. Coupling careful clinical observation with classical cytogenetic techniques, molecular analysis, and newer genomics methods will refine our understanding of these often unpredictable myeloid diseases and, ultimately, identify therapeutic strategies to exploit in the care of the patients suffering from them.

References

Adeyinka A, Dewald GW (2003): Cytogenetics of chronic myeloproliferative disorders and related myelodysplastic syndromes. *Hematol Oncol Clin North Am* 17: 1129–1149.

Apperley JF, Gardembas M, Melo JV, Russell-Jones R, Bain BJ, Baxter EJ, Chase A, et al. (2002): Response to imatinib mesylate in patients with chronic myeloproliferative diseases with rearrangements of the platelet-derived growth factor receptor beta. *N Engl J Med* 347: 481–487.

Bacher U, Haferlach T, Kern W, Haferlach C, Schnittger S (2007): A comparative study of molecular mutations in 381 patients with myelodysplastic syndrome and in 4130 patients with acute myeloid leukemia. *Haematologica* 92: 744–752.

Bain BJ, Moorman AV, Johansson B, Mehta AB, Secker-Walker LM (1998): Myelodysplastic syndromes associated with 11q23 abnormalities. European 11q23 Workshop participants. *Leukemia* 12: 834–839.

Barlow JL, Drynan LF, Hewett DR, Holmes LR, Lorenzo-Abalde S, Lane AL, Jolin HE, et al. (2010): A p53-dependent mechanism underlies macrocytic anemia in a mouse model of human 5q- syndrome. *Nat Med* 16: 59–66.

Bejar R, Stevenson K, Abdel-Wahab O, Galili N, Nilsson B, Garcia-Manero G, et al. (2011): Clinical effect of point mutations in myelodysplastic syndromes. *N Engl J Med* 364: 2496–2506.

Bench AJ, Nacheva EP, Hood TL, Holden JL, French L, Swanton S, et al. (2000): Chromosome 20 deletions in myeloid malignancies: reduction of the common deleted region, generation of a PAC/BAC contig and identification of candidate genes. UK Cancer Cytogenetics Group (UKCCG). *Oncogene* 19: 3902–3913.

Bennett JM, Catovsky D, Daniel MT, Flandrin G, Galton DA, Gralnick HR, et al. (1982): Proposals for the classification of the myelodysplastic syndromes. *Br J Haematol* 51: 189–199.

Bloomfield CD, Archer KJ, Mrozek K, Lillington DM, Kaneko Y, Head DR, et al. (2002): 11q23 balanced chromosome aberrations in treatment-related myelodysplastic syndromes and acute leukemia: report from an international workshop. *Genes Chromosomes Cancer* 33: 362–378.

Boultwood J, Fidler C, Strickson AJ, Watkins F, Gama S, Kearney L, et al. (2002): Narrowing and genomic annotation of the commonly deleted region of the 5q- syndrome. *Blood* 99: 4638–4641.

Cazzola M, Malcovati L (2005): Myelodysplastic syndromes—coping with ineffective hematopoiesis. *N Engl J Med* 352: 536–538.

Challen GA, Sun D, Jeong M, Luo M, Jelinek J, Berg JS, et al. (2012): Dnmt3a is essential for hematopoietic stem cell differentiation. *Nat Genet* 44: 23–31.

Chen CY, Lin LI, Tang JL, Ko BS, Tsay W, Chou WC, et al. (2007): RUNX1 gene mutation in primary myelodysplastic syndrome—the mutation can be detected early at diagnosis or acquired during disease progression and is associated with poor outcome. *Br J Haematol* 139: 405–414.

Christiansen DH, Andersen MK, Pedersen-Bjergaard J (2001): Mutations with loss of heterozygosity of p53 are common in therapy-related myelodysplasia and acute myeloid leukemia after exposure to alkylating agents and significantly associated with deletion or loss of 5q, a complex karyotype, and a poor prognosis. *J Clin Oncol* 19: 1405–1413.

Christiansen DH, Andersen MK, Pedersen-Bjergaard J (2003): Methylation of p15INK4B is common, is associated with deletion of genes on chromosome arm 7q and predicts a poor prognosis in therapy-related myelodysplasia and acute myeloid leukemia. *Leukemia* 17: 1813–1819.

Costa D, Munoz C, Carrio A, Nomdedeu M, Calvo X, Sole F, et al. (2013): Reciprocal translocations in myelodysplastic syndromes and chronic myelomonocytic leukemias: review of 5,654 patients with an evaluable karyotype. *Genes Chromosomes Cancer* 52: 753–763.

Dohner K, Habdank M, Rucker FG, Miller S, Frohling S, Scherer SW, et al. (2006): Molecular characterization of distinct hot spot regions on chromosome 7q in myeloid leukemias. *Blood* 108: 2349.

Ebert BL, Pretz J, Bosco J, Chang CY, Tamayo P, Galili N, et al. (2008): Identification of RPS14 as a 5q- syndrome gene by RNA interference screen. *Nature* 451: 335–339.

Ernst T, Chase AJ, Score J, Hidalgo-Curtis CE, Bryant C, Jones AV, et al. (2010): Inactivating mutations of the histone methyltransferase gene EZH2 in myeloid disorders. *Nat Genet* 42: 722–726.

Fenaux P, Mufti GJ, Hellstrom-Lindberg E, Santini V, Finelli C, Giagounidis A, et al. (2009): Efficacy of azacitidine compared with that of conventional care regimens in the treatment of higher-risk myelodysplastic syndromes: a randomised, open-label, phase III study. *Lancet Oncol* 10: 223–232.

Figueroa ME, Skrabanek L, Li Y, Jiemjit A, Fandy TE, Paietta E, et al. (2009): MDS and secondary AML display unique patterns and abundance of aberrant DNA methylation. *Blood* 114: 3448–3458.

Garcia-Manero G, Shan J, Faderl S, Cortes J, Ravandi F, Borthakur G, et al. (2008): A prognostic score for patients with lower risk myelodysplastic syndrome. *Leukemia* 22: 538–543.

Gelsi-Boyer V, Trouplin V, Adelaide J, Bonansea J, Cervera N, Carbuccia N, et al. (2009): Mutations of polycomb-associated gene ASXL1 in myelodysplastic syndromes and chronic myelomonocytic leukaemia. *Br J Haematol* 145: 788–800.

Groupe Francais de Cytogenetique Hematologique (GFCH) (1991) Chronic myelomonocytic leukemia: single entity or heterogeneous disorder? A prospective multicenter study of 100 patients. *Cancer Genet Cytogenet* 55: 57–65.

Giagounidis AA, Germing U, Haase S, Hildebrandt B, Schlegelberger B, Schoch C, et al. (2004): Clinical, morphological, cytogenetic, and prognostic features of patients with myelodysplastic syndromes and del(5q) including band q31. *Leukemia* 18: 113–119.

Godley LA, Larson R (2002): The syndrome of therapy-related myelodysplasia and myeloid leukemia. In *The Myelodysplastic Syndromes: Pathobiology and Clinical Management*. (Ed: JM Bennett). New York, Marcel Dekker Inc, 136–176.

Goldberg SL, Chen E, Corral M, Guo A, Mody-Patel N, Pecora AL, et al. (2010): Incidence and clinical complications of myelodysplastic syndromes among United States Medicare beneficiaries. *J Clin Oncol* 28: 2847–2852.

Golub TR, Barker GF, Lovett M, Gilliland DG (1994): Fusion of PDGF receptor beta to a novel ets-like gene, tel, in chronic myelomonocytic leukemia with t(5;12) chromosomal translocation. *Cell* 77: 307–316.

Gozzetti A, Le Beau, MM (2000): Fluorescence in situ hybridization: uses and limitations. *Semin Hematol* 37: 320–333.

Graubert TA, Payton MA, Shao J, Walgren RA, Monahan RS, Frater JL, et al. (2009): Integrated genomic analysis implicates haploinsufficiency of multiple chromosome 5q31.2 genes in de novo myelodysplastic syndromes pathogenesis. *PLoS One* 4: e4583.

Graubert TA, Shen D, Ding L, Okeyo-Owuor T, Lunn CL, Shao J, et al. (2012): Recurrent mutations in the U2AF1 splicing factor in myelodysplastic syndromes. *Nat Genet* 44: 53–57.

Greenberg PL, Tuechler H, Schanz J, Sanz G, Garcia-Manero G, Sole F, et al. (2012): Revised international prognostic scoring system for myelodysplastic syndromes. *Blood* 120: 2454–2465.

Groschel S, Sanders MA, Hoogenboezem R, De Wit E, Bouwman BA, Erpelinck C, et al. (2014): A single oncogenic enhancer rearrangement causes concomitant EVI1 and GATA2 deregulation in leukemia. *Cell* 157: 369–381.

Haase D, Germing U, Schanz J, Pfeilstocker M, Nosslinger T, Hildebrandt B, et al. (2007): New insights into the prognostic impact of the karyotype in MDS and correlation with subtypes: evidence from a core dataset of 2124 patients. *Blood* 110: 4385–4395.

Hasle H, Niemeyer CM (2011): Advances in the prognostication and management of advanced MDS in children. *Br J Haematol* 154:185–195.

Irons RD, Kerzic PJ (2014): Cytogenetics in benzene-associated myelodysplastic syndromes and acute myeloid leukemia: new insights into a disease continuum. *Ann N Y Acad Sci* 1310: 84–88.

Ito S, Shen L, Dai Q, Wu SC, Collins LB, Swenberg JA, et al. (2011): Tet proteins can convert 5-methylcytosine to 5-formylcytosine and 5-carboxylcytosine. *Science* 333: 1300–1303.

Itzykson R, Kosmider O, Fenaux P (2013): Somatic mutations and epigenetic abnormalities in myelodysplastic syndromes. *Best Pract Res Clin Haematol* 26: 355–364.

Jadersten M, Saft L, Smith A, Kulasekararaj A, Pomplun S, Gohring G, et al. (2011): TP53 mutations in low-risk myelodysplastic syndromes with del(5q) predict disease progression. *J Clin Oncol* 29: 1971–1979.

Jerez A, Gondek LP, Jankowska AM, Makishima H, Przychodzen B, Tiu RV, et al. (2012a): Topography, clinical, and genomic correlates of 5q myeloid malignancies revisited. *J Clin Oncol* 30: 1343–1349.

Jerez A, Sugimoto Y, Makishima H, Verma A, Jankowska AM, Przychodzen B, et al. (2012b): Loss of heterozygosity in 7q myeloid disorders: clinical associations and genomic pathogenesis. *Blood* 119: 6109–6117.

Joslin JM, Fernald AA, Tennant TR, Davis EM, Kogan SC, Anastasi J, et al. (2007): Haploinsufficiency of EGR1, a candidate gene in the del(5q), leads to the development of myeloid disorders. *Blood* 110: 719–726.

Kardos G, Baumann I, Passmore SJ, Locatelli F, Hasle H, Schultz KR, et al. (2003): Refractory anemia in childhood: a retrospective analysis of 67 patients with particular reference to monosomy 7. *Blood* 102: 1997–2003.

Kikuchi S, Kobune M, Iyama S, Sato T, Murase K, Kawano Y, et al. (2012): Prognostic significance of serum ferritin level at diagnosis in myelodysplastic syndrome. *Int J Hematol* 95: 527–534.

Ko M, Huang Y, Jankowska AM, Pape UJ, Tahiliani M, Bandukwala HS, et al. (2010): Impaired hydroxylation of 5-methylcytosine in myeloid cancers with mutant TET2. *Nature* 468: 839–843.

Kode A, Manavalan JS, Mosialou I, Bhagat G, Rathinam CV, Luo N, et al. (2014): Leukaemogenesis induced by an activating beta-catenin mutation in osteoblasts. *Nature* 506: 240–244.

Komrokji RS, Padron E, Ebert BL, List AF (2013): Deletion 5q MDS: molecular and therapeutic implications. *Best Pract Res Clin Haematol* 26: 365–375.

Kon A, Shih LY, Minamino M, Sanada M, Shiraishi Y, Nagata Y, et al. (2013): Recurrent mutations in multiple components of the cohesin complex in myeloid neoplasms. *Nat Genet* 45: 1232–1237.

Kosmider O, Gelsi-Boyer V, Cheok M, Grabar S, Della-Valle V, Picard F, et al. (2009): TET2 mutation is an independent favorable prognostic factor in myelodysplastic syndromes (MDSs). *Blood* 114: 3285–3291.

Kulasekararaj AG, Smith AE, Mian SA, Mohamedali AM, Krishnamurthy P, Lea NC, et al. (2013): TP53 mutations in myelodysplastic syndrome are strongly correlated with aberrations of chromosome 5, and correlate with adverse prognosis. *Br J Haematol* 160: 660–672.

Kumar M, Narla A, Nomami A, Ball B, Chin C, Chen C, et al. (2009): Coordinate loss of a microRNA mir145 and a protein-coding gene RPS14 cooperate in the pathogenesis of 5q-Syndrome. *Blood* 114: 947.

Kussick SJ, Fromm JR, Rossini A, Li Y, Chang A, Norwood TH, et al. (2005): Four-color flow cytometry shows strong concordance with bone marrow morphology and cytogenetics in the evaluation for myelodysplasia. *Am J Clin Pathol* 124: 170–181.

Lai F, Godley LA, Joslin J, Fernald AA, Liu J, Espinosa R 3rd, et al. (2001): Transcript map and comparative analysis of the 1.5-Mb commonly deleted segment of human 5q31 in malignant myeloid diseases with a del(5q). *Genomics* 71: 235–245.

Langemeijer SM, Kuiper RP, Berends M, Knops R, Aslanyan MG, Massop M, et al. (2009): Acquired mutations in TET2 are common in myelodysplastic syndromes. *Nat Genet* 41: 838–842.

Laricchia-Robbio L, Premanand K, Rinaldi CR, Nucifora G (2009): EVI1 Impairs myelopoiesis by deregulation of PU.1 function. *Cancer Res* 69: 1633–1642.

Le Beau MM, Espinosa R, 3rd, Davis EM, Eisenbart JD, Larson RA, Green ED (1996): Cytogenetic and molecular delineation of a region of chromosome 7 commonly deleted in malignant myeloid diseases. *Blood* 88: 1930–1935.

Lindsley RC, Ebert BL (2013): Molecular pathophysiology of myelodysplastic syndromes. *Annu Rev Pathol* 8: 21–47.

List A, Dewald G, Bennett J, Giagounidis A, Raza A, Feldman E, et al. (2006): Lenalidomide in the myelodysplastic syndrome with chromosome 5q deletion. *N Engl J Med* 355: 1456–1465.

Loh ML, Mulligan CG (2012): Advances in the genetics of high-risk childhood B-progenitor acute lymphoblastic leukemia and juvenile myelomonocytic leukemia: implications for therapy. *Clin Cancer Res* 18: 2754–2767.

Loh ML, Vattikuti S, Schubert S, Reynolds MG, Carlson E, Lieuw KH, et al. (2004): Mutations in PTPN11 implicate the SHP-2 phosphatase in leukemogenesis. *Blood* 103: 2325–2331.

Loh ML, Sakai DS, Flotho C, Kang M, Fliegauf M, Archambeault S, et al. (2009): Mutations in CBL occur frequently in juvenile myelomonocytic leukemia. *Blood* 114: 1859–1863.

Majewski IJ, Ritchie ME, Phipson B, Corbin J, Pakusch M, Ebert A, et al. (2010): Opposing roles of polycomb repressive complexes in hematopoietic stem and progenitor cells. *Blood* 116: 731–739.

Malcovati L, Germing U, Kuendgen A, Della Porta MG, Pascutto C, Invernizzi R, et al. (2007): Time-dependent prognostic scoring system for predicting survival and leukemic evolution in myelodysplastic syndromes. *J Clin Oncol* 25: 3503–3510.

Malcovati L, Della Porta MG, Pietra D, Boveri E, Pellagatti A, Galli A, et al. (2009): Molecular and clinical features of refractory anemia with ringed sideroblasts associated with marked thrombocytosis. *Blood* 114: 3538–3545.

Malcovati L, Papaemmanuil E, Bowen DT, Boultwood J, Della Porta MG, Pascutto C, et al. (2011): Clinical significance of SF3B1 mutations in myelodysplastic syndromes and myelodysplastic/myeloproliferative neoplasms. *Blood* 118: 6239–6246.

Mallo M, Cervera J, Schanz J, Such E, Garcia-Manero G, Luno E, et al. (2011): Impact of adjunct cytogenetic abnormalities for prognostic stratification in patients with myelodysplastic syndrome and deletion 5q. *Leukemia* 25: 110–120.

Marschalek R (2011): Mechanisms of leukemogenesis by MLL fusion proteins. *Br J Haematol* 152: 141–154.

Martinelli G, Ottaviani E, Buonamici S, Isidori A, Borsaru G, Visani G, et al. (2003): Association of 3q21q26 syndrome with different RPN1/EVI1 fusion transcripts. *Haematologica* 88: 1221–1228.

Mcnerney ME, Brown CD, Wang X, Bartom ET, Karmakar S, Bandlamudi C, et al. (2013): CUX1 is a haploinsufficient tumor suppressor gene on chromosome 7 frequently inactivated in acute myeloid leukemia. *Blood* 121: 975–983.

Mcquilten ZK, Wood EM, Polizzotto MN, Campbell LJ, Wall M, Curtis DJ, et al. (2014): Underestimation of myelodysplastic syndrome incidence by cancer registries: results from a population-based data linkage study. *Cancer* 120: 1686–1694.

Medyouf H, Mossner M, Jann JC, Nolte F, Raffel S, Herrmann C, et al. (2014): Myelodysplastic cells in patients reprogram mesenchymal stromal cells to establish a transplantable stem cell niche disease unit. *Cell Stem Cell* 14: 824–837.

Meldi KM, Figueroa ME (2015): Epigenetic deregulation in myeloid malignancies. *Transl Res*, 165: 102–114.

Merlat A, Lai JL, Sterkers Y, Demory JL, Bauters F, Preudhomme C, et al. (1999): Therapy-related myelodysplastic syndrome and acute myeloid leukemia with 17p deletion. A report on 25 cases. *Leukemia* 13: 250–257.

Min IM, Pietramaggiori G, Kim FF, Passegue E, Stevenson KE, Wagers AJ (2008): The transcription factor EGR1 controls both the proliferation and localization of hematopoietic stem cells *Cell Stem Cell* 10: 380–391.

Mitelman F, Johansson B, Mertens F, eds. (2014) *Mitelman Database of Chromosome Aberrations and Gene Fusions in Cancer*. Available at http://cgap.nci.nih.gov/Chromosomes/Mitelman.

Nikoloski G, Langemeijer SM, Kuiper RP, Knops R, Massop M, Tonnissen ER, et al. (2010): Somatic mutations of the histone methyltransferase gene EZH2 in myelodysplastic syndromes. *Nat Genet* 42: 665–667.

Pan J, Wu C, Xue Y, Qiu H, Chen S, Zhang J, et al. (2014): The characteristics and prognostic analysis in 213 myeloid malignancy patients with del(20q): a report of a single-center case series. *Cancer Genet* 207: 51–56.

Papaemmanuil E, Cazzola M, Boultwood J, Malcovati L, Vyas P, Bowen D, et al. (2011): Somatic SF3B1 mutation in myelodysplasia with ring sideroblasts. *N Engl J Med* 365: 1384–1395.

Patnaik MM, Hanson CA, Hodnefield JM, Knudson R, Van Dyke DL, Tefferi A (2011): Monosomal karyotype in myelodysplastic syndromes, with or without monosomy 7 or 5, is prognostically worse than an otherwise complex karyotype. *Leukemia* 25: 266–270.

Patnaik MM, Lasho TL, Hodnefield JM, Knudson RA, Ketterling RP, Garcia-Manero G, et al. (2012): SF3B1 mutations are prevalent in myelodysplastic syndromes with ring sideroblasts but do not hold independent prognostic value. *Blood* 119: 569–572.

Paulsson K, Sall T, Fioretos T, Mitelman F, Johansson B (2001): The incidence of trisomy 8 as a sole chromosomal aberration in myeloid malignancies varies in relation to gender, age, prior iatrogenic genotoxic exposure, and morphology. *Cancer Genet Cytogenet* 130: 160–165.

Paulsson K, Heidenblad M, Strombeck B, Staaf J, Jonsson G, Borg A, et al. (2006): High-resolution genome-wide array-based comparative genome hybridization reveals cryptic chromosome changes in AML and MDS cases with trisomy 8 as the sole cytogenetic aberration. *Leukemia* 20: 840–846.

Pedersen-Bjergaard J, Andersen MK, Christiansen DH (2000): Therapy-related acute myeloid leukemia and myelodysplasia after high-dose chemotherapy and autologous stem cell transplantation. *Blood* 95: 3273–3279.

Perna F, Gurvich N, Hoya-Arias R, Abdel-Wahab O, Levine RL, Asai T, et al. (2010): Depletion of L3MBTL1 promotes the erythroid differentiation of human hematopoietic progenitor cells: possible role in 20q- polycythemia vera. *Blood* 116: 2812–2821.

Raaijmakers MH (2012): Myelodysplastic syndromes: revisiting the role of the bone marrow microenvironment in disease pathogenesis. *Int J Hematol* 95: 17–25.

Rowley JD, Reshmi S, Sobulo O, Musvee T, Anastasi J, Raimondi S, et al. (1997): All patients with the T(11;16)(q23;p13.3) that involves MLL and CBP have treatment-related hematologic disorders. *Blood* 90: 535–541.

Rubin CM, Larson RA, Anastasi J, Winter JN, Thangavelu M, Vardiman JW, et al. (1990): t(3;21)(q26;q22): a recurring chromosomal abnormality in therapy-related myelodysplastic syndrome and acute myeloid leukemia. *Blood* 76: 2594–2598.

Sanchez-Castro J, Marco-Betes V, Gomez-Arbones X, Arenillas L, Valcarcel D, Vallespi T, et al. (2013): Characterization and prognostic implication of 17 chromosome abnormalities in myelodysplastic syndrome. *Leuk Res* 37: 769–776.

Schanz J, Tuchler H, Sole F, Mallo M, Luno E, Cervera J, et al. (2012): New comprehensive cytogenetic scoring system for primary myelodysplastic syndromes (MDS) and oligoblastic acute myeloid leukemia after MDS derived from an international database merge. *J Clin Oncol* 30: 820–829.

Schanz J, Tuchler H, Sole F, Mallo M, Luno E, Cervera J, et al. (2013): Monosomal karyotype in MDS: explaining the poor prognosis? *Leukemia* 27: 1988–1995.

Sebaa A, Ades L, Baran-Marzack F, Mozziconacci MJ, Penther D, Dobbelstein S, et al. (2012): Incidence of 17p deletions and TP53 mutation in myelodysplastic syndrome and acute myeloid leukemia with 5q deletion. *Genes Chromosomes Cancer* 51: 1086–1092.

Shaffer LG, Ballif BC, Schultz RA (2013): The use of cytogenetic microarrays in myelodysplastic syndrome characterization. *Methods Mol Biol* 973: 69–85.

Shannon KM, Le Beau MM (2008): Cancer: hay in a haystack. *Nature* 451: 252–253.

Shen L, Kantarjian H, Guo Y, Lin E, Shan J, Huang X, et al. (2010): DNA methylation predicts survival and response to therapy in patients with myelodysplastic syndromes. *J Clin Oncol* 28: 3098.

Shih AH, Chung SS, Dolezal EK, Zhang SJ, Abdel-Wahab OI, Park CY, et al. (2013): Mutational analysis of therapy-related myelodysplastic syndromes and acute myelogenous leukemia. *Haematologica* 98: 908–912.

Side LE, Curtiss NP, Teel K, Kratz C, Wang PW, Larson RA, et al. (2004): RAS, FLT3, and TP53 mutations in therapy-related myeloid malignancies with abnormalities of chromosomes 5 and 7. *Genes Chromosomes Cancer* 39: 217–223.

Sloand EM, Rezvani K (2008): The role of the immune system in myelodysplasia: implications for therapy. *Semin Hematol* 45: 39–48.

Smith SM, Le Beau MM, Huo D, Karrison T, Sobecks RM, Anastasi J, et al. (2003): Clinical-cytogenetic associations in 306 patients with therapy-related myelodysplasia and myeloid leukemia: the University of Chicago series. *Blood* 102: 43–52.

Sole F, Luno E, Sanzo C, Espinet B, Sanz GF, Cervera J, et al. (2005): Identification of novel cytogenetic markers with prognostic significance in a series of 968 patients with primary myelodysplastic syndromes. *Haematologica* 90: 1168–1178.

Song WJ, Sullivan MG, Legare RD, Hutchings S, Tan X, Kufrin D, et al. (1999): Haploinsufficiency of CBFA2 causes familial thrombocytopenia with propensity to develop acute myelogenous leukaemia. *Nat Genet* 23: 166–175.

Speck NA, Gilliland DG (2002): Core-binding factors in haematopoiesis and leukaemia. *Nat Rev Cancer* 2: 502–513.

Spitzer G, Verma DS, Dicke KA, Smith T, Mccredie KB (1979): Subgroups of oligoleukemia as identified by in vitro agar culture. *Leuk Res* 3: 29–39.

Starczynowski DT, Kuchenbauer F, Argiropoulos B, Sung S, Morin R, Muranyi A, et al. (2010): Identification of miR-145 and miR-146a as mediators of the 5q- syndrome phenotype. *Nat Med* 16: 49–58.

Steensma DP, Dewald GW, Lasho TL, Powell HL, Mcclure RF, Levine RL, et al. (2005a): The JAK2 V617F activating tyrosine kinase mutation is an infrequent event in both "atypical" myeloproliferative disorders and myelodysplastic syndromes. *Blood* 106: 1207–1209.

Steensma DP, Gibbons RJ, Mesa RA, Tefferi A, Higgs DR (2005b): Somatic point mutations in RUNX1/CBFA2/AML1 are common in high-risk myelodysplastic syndrome, but not in myelofibrosis with myeloid metaplasia. *Eur J Haematol* 74: 47–53.

Stoddart A, Fernald AA, Wang J, Davis EM, Karrison T, Anastasi J, et al. (2014): Haploinsufficiency of del(5q) genes, Egr1 and Apc, cooperate with Tp53 loss to induce acute myeloid leukemia in mice. *Blood* 123: 1069–1078.

Strom SS, Velez-Bravo V, Estey EH (2008): Epidemiology of myelodysplastic syndromes. *Semin Hematol* 45: 8–13.

Thol F, Friesen I, Damm F, Yun H, Weissinger EM, Krauter J, et al. (2011): Prognostic significance of ASXL1 mutations in patients with myelodysplastic syndromes. *J Clin Oncol* 29: 2499–2506.

Thol F, Kade S, Schlarmann C, Loffeld P, Morgan M, Krauter J, et al. (2012): Frequency and prognostic impact of mutations in SRSF2, U2AF1, and ZRSR2 in patients with myelodysplastic syndromes. *Blood* 119: 3578–3584.

Toyama K, Ohyashiki K, Yoshida Y, Abe T, Asano S, Hirai H, et al. (1993): Clinical and cytogenetic findings of myelodysplastic syndromes showing hypocellular bone marrow or minimal dysplasia, in comparison with typical myelodysplastic syndromes. *Int J Hematol* 58: 53–61.

United Kingdom Cancer Cytogenetics Group (UKCCG) (1992) Loss of the Y chromosome from normal and neoplastic bone marrows. *Genes Chromosomes Cancer* 5: 83–88.

Vallespi T, Imbert M, Mecucci C, Preudhomme C, Fenaux P (1998): Diagnosis, classification, and cytogenetics of myelodysplastic syndromes. *Haematologica* 83: 258–275.

Van De Loosdrecht AA, Ireland R, Kern W, Della Porta MG, Alhan C, Balleisen JS, et al (2013): Rationale for the clinical application of flow cytometry in patients with myelodysplastic syndromes: position paper of an International Consortium and the European LeukemiaNet Working Group. *Leuk Lymphoma* 54: 472–475.

Vardiman JW (2003): Myelodysplastic syndromes, chronic myeloproliferative diseases, and myelodysplastic/myeloproliferative diseases. *Semin Diagn Pathol* 20: 154–179.

Vardiman JW, Thiele J, Arber DA, Brunning RD, Borowitz MJ, Porwit A, et al. (2009): The 2008 revision of the World Health Organization (WHO) classification of myeloid neoplasms and acute leukemia: rationale and important changes. *Blood* 114: 937–951.

Volkert S, Kohlmann A, Schnittger S, Kern W, Haferlach T, Haferlach C (2014): Association of the type of 5q loss with complex karyotype, clonal evolution, TP53 mutation status, and prognosis in acute myeloid leukemia and myelodysplastic syndrome. *Genes Chromosomes Cancer* 53: 402–410.

Walter MJ, Ding L, Shen D, Shao J, Grillot M, Mclellan M, et al. (2011): Recurrent DNMT3A mutations in patients with myelodysplastic syndromes. *Leukemia* 25: 1153–1158.

Walter MJ, Shen D, Ding L, Shao J, Koboldt DC, Chen K, et al. (2012): Clonal architecture of secondary acute myeloid leukemia. *N Engl J Med* 366: 1090–1098.

Wang P, Spielberger RT, Thangavelu M, Zhao N, Davis EM, Iannantuoni K, et al. (1997): dic(5;17): a recurring abnormality in malignant myeloid disorders associated with mutations of TP53. *Genes Chromosomes Cancer* 20: 282–291.

Wang PW, Eisenbart JD, Espinosa R 3rd, Davis EM, Larson RA, Le Beau MM (2000): Refinement of the smallest commonly deleted segment of chromosome 20 in malignant myeloid diseases and development of a PAC-based physical and transcription map. *Genomics* 67: 28–39.

Wang J, Fernald AA, Anastasi J, Le Beau MM, Qian Z (2010a): Haploinsufficiency of Apc leads to ineffective hematopoiesis. *Blood* 115: 3481–3488.

Wang Y, Krivtsov AV, Sinha AU, North TE, Goessling W, Feng Z, et al. (2010b): The Wnt/beta-catenin pathway is required for the development of leukemia stem cells in AML. *Science* 327: 1650–1653.

Ward AF, Braun BS, Shannon KM (2012): Targeting oncogenic Ras signaling in hematologic malignancies. *Blood* 120: 3397–3406.

Wells DA, Benesch M, Loken MR, Vallejo C, Myerson D, Leisenring WM, et al. (2003): Myeloid and monocytic dyspoiesis as determined by flow cytometric scoring in myelodysplastic syndrome correlates with the IPSS and with outcome after hematopoietic stem cell transplantation. *Blood* 102: 394–403.

West RR, Stafford DA, White AD, Bowen DT, Padua RA (2000): Cytogenetic abnormalities in the myelodysplastic syndromes and occupational or environmental exposure. *Blood* 95: 2093–2097.

Wiktor A, Rybicki BA, Piao ZS, Shurafa M, Barthel B, Maeda K, et al. (2000): Clinical significance of Y chromosome loss in hematologic disease. *Genes Chromosomes Cancer* 27: 11–16.

Wong JC, Zhang Y, Lieuw KH, Tran MT, Forgo E, Weinfurtner K, et al. (2010): Use of chromosome engineering to model a segmental deletion of chromosome band 7q22 found in myeloid malignancies. *Blood* 115: 4524–4532.

Yamazaki H, Suzuki M, Otsuki A, Shimizu R, Bresnick EH, Engel JD, et al. (2014): A remote GATA2 hematopoietic enhancer drives leukemogenesis in inv(3)(q21;q26) by activating EVI1 expression. *Cancer Cel*, 25: 415–427.

Yoshida K, Sanada M, Shiraishi Y, Nowak D, Nagata Y, Yamamoto R, et al. (2011): Frequent pathway mutations of splicing machinery in myelodysplasia. *Nature* 478: 64–69.

Zhang Y, Rowley JD (2006): Chromatin structural elements and chromosomal translocations in leukemia. *DNA Repair (Amst)* 5: 1282–1297.

Zipperer E, Wulfert M, Germing U, Haas R, Gattermann N (2008): MPL 515 and JAK2 mutation analysis in MDS presenting with a platelet count of more than $500 \times 10(9)/l$. *Ann Hematol* 87: 413–415.

CHAPTER 8

Chronic myeloid leukemia

Thoas Fioretos

Department of Clinical Genetics, University of Lund, Lund, Sweden

Chronic myeloid leukemia (CML) is a clonal bone marrow (BM) disease characterized by neoplastic overproduction of, mainly, granulocytes. In the Western world, CML accounts for approximately 15–20% of all cases of leukemia, with an incidence of 1/100 000 per year. CML occurs in all age groups but is most common in older people with a median age of 65 years at the time of diagnosis. There is a slight male preponderance. Studies of atomic bomb survivors exposed to ionizing radiation have shown an excess risk of CML; otherwise, epidemiological studies have failed to find any strong occupational or lifestyle risk factors for developing CML (Ichimaru et al., 1978; Björk et al., 2001).

At the time of diagnosis, the white blood cell (WBC) count is high, typically near 200×10^9/l. The BM morphology is characterized by granulocytic and megakaryocytic hyperplasia, with the megakaryocytes typically being small and often displaying hypolobated nuclei. Eosinophilia and, especially, basophilia are common, and in one-third of the cases, a certain amount of myelofibrosis is present. In contrast to acute lymphoblastic leukemia (ALL) and acute myeloid leukemia (AML), the hematopoietic maturation in CML proceeds in a seemingly orderly manner in the different lineages without any maturation arrest.

The leukemogenic event in CML is thought to occur at the level of the hematopoietic stem cell (HSC). This explains why most hematopoietic lineages, including neutrophils, eosinophils, basophils, erythroid cells, and megakaryocytes, as well as B-cell precursors and early, but not mature, T cells or natural killer cells are involved in the disease process (Takahashi et al., 1998; Jiang et al., 2007).

As will be discussed later in this chapter, the treatment of CML changed dramatically with the introduction of tyrosine kinase inhibitors (TKIs) targeting the product of the underlying cytogenetic and molecular lesion in CML. This also resulted in an entirely altered disease course of CML, with most patients having started therapy with TKI still remaining in clinical and cytogenetic remission. Without novel treatment modalities but also in a fraction of patients receiving such therapies, the initial, relatively benign chronic phase (CP) of CML, which on average (but with wide case-to-case variation) lasts about 3 years, typically then enters a more malignant accelerated phase (AP) and eventually the terminal blast crisis (BC).

CML BC is characterized by an increase in the number of immature cells in the BM and peripheral blood, by progressive anemia and thrombocytopenia, sometimes by extramedullary accumulations

Cancer Cytogenetics: Chromosomal and Molecular Genetic Aberrations of Tumor Cells, Fourth Edition.
Edited by Sverre Heim and Felix Mitelman.
© 2015 John Wiley & Sons, Ltd. Published 2015 by John Wiley & Sons, Ltd.

of blast cells, and by a reduced response to therapy. The morphologic characteristics of the leukemic blasts vary with either myeloblastic or lymphoblastic features predominating. The blasts are in most instances phenotypically indistinguishable from AML cells, but in one-third of the CML BC, they resemble immature lymphoid cells and also express immunophenotypes typical of lymphoblasts.

CML is one of the best-studied human malignancies and has served as a paradigm for the elucidation of how genetic changes cause cells to become malignant. CML is also one of the first malignancies in which a therapy targeting the underlying molecular lesion has improved the clinical outcome of patients. However, despite this progress, many questions remain unanswered. With a focus on cytogenetic and molecular genetic aspects of CML, this chapter will try to address some important issues. How does the t(9;22) or variants of this translocation arise? What are the mechanisms by which this rearrangement causes leukemia? Which are the novel treatment regimens in CML, and how have they affected the way such patients should be monitored clinically? Which secondary genetic changes are responsible for the progression of CP to BC? Whenever possible, clinically relevant issues will be addressed with an emphasis on the implications of cytogenetic and molecular genetic findings in CML.

The discovery and characterization of the Philadelphia chromosome

The Philadelphia chromosome was the first consistent neoplasia-associated chromosomal abnormality reported; its discovery was a milestone in cancer cytogenetics. By studying the leukemic cells of CML patients, Nowell and Hungerford (1960) identified a small G-group chromosome that later was named the Philadelphia chromosome (Ph[1]) after the city in which it was discovered. The use of the superscript anticipated the discovery of new aberrations that would be designated Ph[2], Ph[3], etc., but this naming principle was never implemented and the small derivative chromosome (see later) is now referred to as Ph. The true nature of the Ph chromosome was at first unknown, but with the advent of various chromosome banding techniques around 1970, it was shown to arise as a result of a translocation

between the long arms of chromosomes 9 and 22, that is, t(9;22)(q34;q11), with the Ph chromosome being the der(22)t(9;22) (Rowley, 1973).

De Klein et al. (1982) were able to show that a small segment of chromosome 9, including parts of the *ABL1* (formerly *ABL*) oncogene, was translocated to chromosome 22, thus proving the reciprocal nature of the t(9;22). A subsequent molecular genetic study showed that a chimeric DNA fragment isolated from one CML case, apart from *ABL1*, also contained sequences originating from chromosome 22 (Heisterkamp et al., 1983). These data suggested a role for the *ABL1* gene in CML, a hypothesis that was later supported by the findings of an abnormally sized *ABL1* transcript and ABL1 protein in the CML cell line K562 (Collins et al., 1984; Gale and Canaani, 1984; Konopka et al., 1984) and in CML patients (Stam et al., 1985). Groffen et al. (1984) isolated the area on chromosome 22 involved in the translocation, showing that the breakpoint in 17 patients occurred within a limited region of 5.8 kb, which was termed the "breakpoint cluster region" or bcr. Soon afterward, it was demonstrated that bcr actually was part of a larger gene (Heisterkamp et al., 1985) referred to as *BCR*; the region in which the breakpoints occur in CML was then denoted bcr or M-bcr for "major breakpoint cluster region." Cloning of partial and full-length chimeric *BCR–ABL1* cDNA clones and sequence analyses finally established that the result of the Ph chromosome was the generation of a *BCR–ABL1* fusion gene (Heisterkamp et al., 1985; Shtivelman et al., 1985; Grosveld et al., 1986; Mes-Masson et al., 1986).

When studying t(9;22)-positive ALL, it was noted that only some cases had a detectable rearrangement within M-bcr. The leukemic cells of the other patients were soon found to contain an ABL1 protein of a different size from the one observed in CML (Chan et al., 1987; Clark et al., 1987; Kurzrock et al., 1987). Subsequently, it was demonstrated that this abnormal ABL1 protein also contained antigenic determinants derived from the BCR protein (Walker et al., 1987). Cloning of a chimeric *BCR–ABL1* cDNA containing a smaller part of *BCR* sequences and the localization of the breakpoints to the first *BCR* intron finally proved that a *BCR–ABL1* fusion gene was also present in this subtype of Ph-positive ALL (Feinstein et al., 1987; Hermans et al., 1987).

As will be discussed in detail in the following text, molecular characterization of the chimeric protein later showed that the tyrosine kinase activity of BCR–ABL1 is indispensable for leukemic transformation of t(9;22)-positive leukemias (Lugo et al., 1990). The leukemogenic effects of BCR–ABL1 have now been studied using numerous model systems, which have revealed that BCR–ABL1 affects several signal transduction pathways that influence self-renewal, proliferation, apoptosis, and adhesion of the leukemic cells (Ren, 2005; Cilloni and Saglio, 2012; Ahmed and Van Etten, 2013). A major therapeutic breakthrough finally came with the development of imatinib, a drug that targets the tyrosine kinase activity of the BCR–ABL1 protein (Druker et al., 1996).

Cytogenetic abnormalities in CML CP

Since the discovery that the Ph originated through a t(9;22)(q34;q11), many thousands of CML have been cytogenetically analyzed, and such analyses have clearly established that roughly 85% of cases display a standard, cytogenetically balanced t(9;22) (Figure 8.1). The remainder either harbor variant translocations (see later) or seemingly normal karyotypes, in which the *BCR* and *ABL1* genes recombine through cytogenetically cryptic insertions or other more complex chromosomal rearrangements that can be visualized using fluorescent *in situ* hybridization (FISH) with probes specific for the two genes or through molecular genetic methods. According to prevailing opinions and recent WHO diagnostic guidelines (Swerdlow et al., 2008), CML as a diagnostic entity should be reserved for cases carrying either a standard or variant t(9;22) or its molecular equivalent, the *BCR–ABL1* fusion gene.

Variant translocations are found in 5–10% of patients with newly diagnosed CML (Mitelman et al., 2014). They can be present either in a simple form (involving 22q11 and one additional breakpoint) or in a complex form, involving 22q11, 9q34, and at least one additional breakpoint. In a review of close to 600 CML cases with variant rearrangements, Johansson et al. (2002) reported that the distribution of the breakpoints exhibited a clearly nonrandom pattern, with marked clustering to chromosome bands 1p36, 3p21, 5q13, 6p21, 9q22, 11q13, 12p13, 17p13, 17q21, 17q25, 19q13, 21q22, 22q12, and 22q13. Moreover, some variants were recurrent, with the translocations t(3;9;22)(p21;q34;q11) and t(17;22)(q25;q11) both having been reported in more than 10 cases. Considering that the variant translocations affect additional chromosomal regions, one would perhaps expect that these extra "hits" result in a different disease phenotype. While several studies performed in the preimatinib era arrived at contradictory results (Johansson et al., 2002), recent studies investigating close to 100 cases of variant translocations found no impact on the cytogenetic and molecular response or on outcome compared to cases with a standard Ph chromosome (Fabarius et al., 2011; Marzocchi et al., 2011). Hence, the prevailing opinion is that the clinical, prognostic, and hematologic features of CML with variant translocation are not distinct from those seen in standard t(9;22).

While the standard t(9;22) at the cytogenetic level is seemingly balanced, several FISH analyses have revealed that deletions at the derivative chromosome 9 are present in 10–15% of cases (Sinclair et al., 2000; Huntly et al., 2001, 2003; Lee et al., 2003; Quintas-Cardama et al., 2005; Kreil et al., 2007). Moreover, such deletions are more commonly observed in cases with a variant t(9;22). The deletions have been shown to be of variable size, often involving several megabases both on chromosome 9- and chromosome 22-derived sequences, which means that the reciprocal *ABL1–BCR* fusion and adjacent sequences on the derivative chromosome 9 are lost. Furthermore, several studies have obtained evidence in favor of the deletions taking place at the time of the formation of the t(9;22), that is, they do not occur

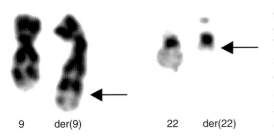

9   der(9)   22   der(22)

Figure 8.1 Partial karyotype showing the t(9;22)(q34;q11). Arrows indicate breakpoints on the derivative chromosomes.

as part of disease evolution (Huntly et al., 2001; Reid and Nacheva, 2005). Numerous investigations have addressed the possible prognostic impact of deletions at the der(9), mainly before the introduction of TKI therapy, with most groups initially reporting adverse prognostic features, including shorter survival times in cases with deletions (Sinclair et al., 2000; Huntly et al., 2001, 2003; Kolomietz et al., 2003; Lee et al., 2003), whereas others failed to detect such differences (Quintas-Cardama et al., 2005; Yoong et al., 2005). To investigate the prognostic value of der(9) deletions in early CP CML, FISH analysis was recently performed on patients included in three prospective Italian imatinib trials (Castagnetti et al., 2010). Deletions at der(9) were identified in 60 (12%) of 521 evaluable patients, but no prognostic impact was identified. According to recent recommendations by the European LeukemiaNet (ELN), deletions at der(9) do not any longer constitute an adverse prognostic factor (Baccarani et al., 2013).

The t(9;22) or its variants are detected as the sole cytogenetic change in 80–90% of CML diagnosed in CP. The remaining cases may display additional karyotypic changes, typically loss of the Y chromosome, +8, +Ph, and i(17q), that is, abnormalities that are similar to the ones detected at quite high frequencies (60–80%; see later) upon disease progression into AP or BC (Johansson et al., 2002). The prognostic impact of additional cytogenetic changes present already at diagnosis of CML CP patients subsequently receiving TKI therapy was initially unclear. Some larger recent studies have shed more light on the matter. Fabarius et al. (2011), investigating 1151 patients from the randomized German CML Study IV, found that 79 patients (7%) displayed additional cytogenetic changes at diagnosis. Of these 79 patients, 38 (48%) displayed loss of the Y chromosome, 16 (20%) showed major route cytogenetic changes (+8, +Ph, i(17q), or +19), whereas 25 (32%) showed minor route changes (all other aberrations). While no prognostic impact was observed when –Y and minor route changes were present, there was a clear negative impact on survival (a 5-year overall survival of only 53%) of major route changes present at diagnosis. Hence, it was concluded that major route changes at diagnosis identify a small group (1.4% in the total material) of patients with

significantly poorer prognosis compared with all other patients (Fabarius et al., 2011). Similarly, Luatti et al. (2012) reported a series of 378 CML patients, 21 (6%) of whom had additional cytogenetic changes. In this subgroup, the overall cytogenetic and molecular response rates were significantly lower and the time to response was significantly longer. Although the long-term outcome of the patients displaying additional cytogenetic changes was inferior, the difference did not reach statistical significance. Based on these two studies, ELN concluded that major route cytogenetic changes present at diagnosis of CML help the identification of patients eligible for investigational approaches, but in daily practice, they do not mandate different initial treatments (Baccarani et al., 2013).

In conclusion, apart from the presence of additional cytogenetic changes at diagnosis of CML, signifying clonal evolution, no other genetic alterations have so far been detected that are clinically relevant. Most likely, in the very near future, next-generation sequencing (NGS) studies in larger cohorts of CML CP patients will become available and may determine whether genetic alterations detected at diagnosis provide important prognostic information in the context of TKI therapy.

Molecular pathology of the t(9;22) (q34;q11) in CML

As a result of the t(9;22) in CML, two main types of fusion genes, designated P210 and P230 BCR–ABL1, are generated that differ depending on the variable numbers of BCR exons included in the fusion genes (Figure 8.2). A shorter variant, P190 BCR–ABL1, which is found in the great majority of patients with Ph-positive ALL, is discussed in Chapter 10. The sizes of the different fusion genes depend on the location of the breakpoints within the BCR gene; the great majority of breaks (>95%) in CML occur in the approximately 4.4 kb M-bcr, which consists of BCR exons 12–15 (also designated b1–b4) and intervening intronic sequences (Deininger et al., 2000; Ross et al., 2013). In a small fraction of the patients, the breakpoints are located further downstream between BCR exons 19 and 21, in the 2.1 kb micro (μ)-bcr. The latter breakpoint, resulting in a P230 BCR–ABL1 fusion transcript

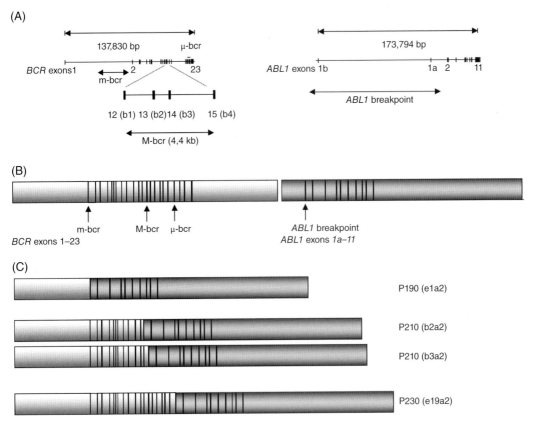

Figure 8.2 Schematic depiction of the main *BCR–ABL1* fusion gene variants. (A) To the left, the genomic structure of the *BCR* gene, spanning approximately 138 kb and containing 23 exons, is displayed. The breakpoints in most Philadelphia-positive ALL fall in the minor breakpoint cluster region (m-bcr), located in the 3′ half of the approximately 72 kb first intron. The great majority of the breaks in CML occur in the approximately 4.4 kb major breakpoint cluster region (M-bcr), which consists of *BCR* exons 12–15 (also designated b1–b4) and intervening intronic sequences. In a small fraction of CML patients, the breakpoints are located further downstream between *BCR* exons 19 and 21 (also designated e19–e21), in the 2.1 kb micro (μ)-bcr. To the right, the genomic structure of the *ABL1* gene, spanning about 174 kb and containing two alternative first exons, 1b and 1a, followed by exons 2 through 11, is shown. The breakpoints in *ABL1* are located in the introns between exons 1b and 1a and 1a and 2 or 5′ of 1b. (B) To the left, approximate sizes of *BCR* exons 1–23, with the different breakpoints at the cDNA level indicated by arrows, are depicted. To the right, the *ABL1* cDNA with exon 1a followed by exons 2–11 is shown. The arrow indicates the breakpoint at the cDNA level upstream of *ABL1* exon 2. (C) Representation of the fusion gene variants P190 *BCR–ABL1* (*BCR* exon 1 fused to *ABL1* exons 2–11; also designated e1a2), P210 *BCR–ABL1* (*BCR* exons 1–13 or 1–14 fused to *ABL1* exons 2–11; also termed b2a2 orb3a2), and P230 *BCR–ABL1* (*BCR* exons 1–19 fused to *ABL1* exons 2–11).

(also termed e19a2), was originally thought to be associated with a better prognosis and chronic neutrophilic leukemia (Pane et al., 1996), but several subsequent reports have identified P230 *BCR–ABL1* also in patients with typical CML. In a review of 23 published cases expressing the P230 *BCR–ABL1* fusion gene, it was concluded that while most such patients display a more indolent disease course, several have shown poor treatment response or have been diagnosed in advanced stages of CML, thus questioning an overall favorable prognosis in this subgroup of patients (Verstovsek et al., 2002). Oshikawa et al. (2010) reviewed 50 published cases of P230 *BCR–ABL1*-positive CML and identified nine patients that had received imatinib treatment. Only three cases were in CML CP and displayed either a complete cytogenetic or hematologic response, while the other cases were diagnosed in advanced phase or harbored additional cytogenetic changes and responded poorly making it difficult to ascertain the prognostic value of P230 *BCR–ABL1*. With the use of RT-PCR, a number of different and unusual in-frame transcripts have also been identified in CML, for example, *BCR* exon 6 fused with *ABL1* exon 2, fusion transcripts in which exon 2 of *ABL1* is missing (e1a3, e13a3, e14a3), or "bizarre" insertions or breakpoints within exons (Barnes and Melo, 2002).

The breakpoints in the *ABL1* gene at 9q34 are distributed over a large area (>300 kb) and, in general, occur 5′ of *ABL* exon 2 in the introns between exons 1b and 1a or exons 1a and 2 (Ross et al., 2013). Regardless of the location of the *ABL1* breakpoints, the first two alternative exons (1a and 1b) are always spliced out during mRNA maturation, with exon 2 of *ABL1* typically becoming juxtaposed to the variable 5′ parts of *BCR*.

Why and how does the t(9;22) or the corresponding *BCR–ABL1* recombination take place? As is the case for most chromosomal translocations, the fundamental mechanisms behind the rearrangement are unknown. The perhaps most widely accepted explanation is that the t(9;22) is a random event that we become aware of when it confers a selective advantage on the cells, namely, their leukemic phenotype. However, many recombinogenic motifs and repetitive elements have been reported to coincide with the breakpoints in *ABL1* and *BCR* and have, hence, been suggested to increase the likelihood of recombination between these two genes, such as *Alu* repeats, heptamer/nonamer sequences, and translin-binding motifs, which could facilitate DNA recombination. A recent study investigating a large number of breakpoints (308 CML cases) failed to demonstrate a critical role of such sequences in the generation of the t(9;22), however (Ross et al., 2013). Because a prerequisite for the joining of *BCR* and *ABL1* is spatial proximity between the broken chromosome ends, the position of 9q34 and 22q11 relative to each other in the nucleus has also been investigated. Evidence in favor of such proximity has indeed been obtained, suggesting that the formation of translocations is at least in part determined by higher-order spatial organization of the genome (Kozubek et al., 1999; Neves et al., 1999; Roix et al., 2003). Yet another feature that may prove important was revealed by the identification of a 76 kb duplicated genomic region (duplicon) present on

9q34 (1.4 Mb 5′ of *ABL1*) and on 22q11 (150 kb 3′ of *BCR*) that could facilitate a mitotic chromosomal exchange by bringing the two genes close to each other (Saglio et al., 2002; Albano et al., 2013). Subsequent random breakage and joining of the two genes, possibly guided by repetitive elements or sequence motifs in the vicinity of the breakpoints, followed by selection for cells producing in-frame *BCR–ABL1* fusion products could be a mechanism by which a combination of different factors would result in a clonal expansion and clinically manifest CML. It is in this context also interesting to note that by using highly optimized and sensitive RT-PCR assays, it has been demonstrated that approximately 25–30% of healthy individuals have detectable P210 *BCR–ABL1* fusion transcripts in their peripheral blood (Biernaux et al., 1995; Bose et al., 1998). This suggests not only that the frequency with which *BCR–ABL1* recombination takes place in the normal hematopoietic system is high, providing circumstantial evidence for the view that the recombination is somehow facilitated by sequence motifs or higher-order spatial organization, but also that a *BCR–ABL1* recombination has to take place in a particularly primed early hematopoietic progenitor cell for clonal expansion to ensue.

Following the formation of the t(9;22) and the fusion of the *BCR* and *ABL1* genes at the DNA level, transcription and splicing will produce an mRNA, approximately 8.5 kb in size, in which *BCR* exons 1–12 or 1–13 become fused to *ABL* exons 2–11 (b2a2 or b3a2 junction) (Figure 8.2). Even in cases where exon 1b or 1a of *ABL1* is included in the chimeric gene and the primary transcript, it is typically spliced out in the mature *BCR–ABL1* mRNA. The 8.5 kb mRNA is translated into a 210 kDa BCR–ABL1 fusion protein (P210) consisting of amino acids 1–902 derived from BCR (or amino acids 1–927 if M-bcr b3 is included), linked to 1096 residues of ABL1. The reciprocal chimeric *ABL1–BCR* gene on the derivative chromosome 9 is also transcribed in approximately 50–70% of CML cases, but its possible pathogenetic role in CML, if any, remains unclear and no distinct correlation to prognostic features has been demonstrated (Melo et al., 1993, 1996; de laFuente et al., 2001).

At the protein level, the P210 and P230 BCR–ABL chimeras include important functional domains derived from the normal BCR and ABL1 proteins. Although the precise normal cellular function of the 160 kDa BCR protein is still largely unknown, it is known that it contains an oligomerization domain and a serine/threonine kinase activity encoded by exon 1, a segment located in the central part that carries a Rho guanine nucleotide exchange factor (RHO-GEF, also designated DBL-like) domain, a pleckstrin homology (PH) domain, and a RAC-GAP domain at the C-terminal end (Ren, 2005; Cilloni and Saglio, 2012; Ahmed and van Etten, 2013). Both P210 and P230 fusion proteins contain the RHO-GEF and PH domains, whereas P230 also harbors a calcium-dependent lipid-binding domain as well as a truncated RAC-GAP domain (Barnes and Melo, 2002). The protein domains of the nonreceptor tyrosine kinase ABL1 included in the P210 and P230 BCR–ABL1 comprise the SRC homology domains SH2 and SH3, a tyrosine kinase domain (SH1), as well as DNA- and actin-binding domains.

In contrast to the normal ABL1 protein, which predominantly is located in the nucleus, the BCR–ABL1 fusion protein is located in the cytoplasm and displays a deregulated and constitutive tyrosine kinase activity, facilitated by the oligomerization domain encoded by the first exon of *BCR* (Lugo et al., 1990; McWhirter and Wang, 1991). During recent years, several studies have identified a number of signaling pathways (e.g., the JAK/STAT, RAS, and PI-3 kinase pathways) and proteins (e.g., CRKL, FAK, and PXN) that become activated or phosphorylated by BCR–ABL1. The molecular signaling pattern that has emerged is highly complex, but it ultimately results in enhanced self-renewal, cellular proliferation, inhibition of apoptosis, and altered adhesion properties that are characteristic features of CML cells (for reviews, see Ren, 2005; Cilloni and Saglio, 2012; Ahmed and van Etten, 2013).

In summary, although we do not know how the t(9;22) or the *BCR–ABL1* fusion arises, detailed molecular genetic and functional studies have resulted in profound insights into how BCR–ABL1 elicits a leukemic response, with mouse experimental models having shown that the fusion gene is capable of initiating a disease closely recapitulating human CML. As will be discussed further in the following text, the introduction of imatinib and other TKIs has not only revolutionized

the treatment of CML but has also opened up new avenues through which an increased understanding of BCR–ABL1-mediated leukemogenesis is emerging.

Treatment of CML

Treatment of CML has changed dramatically over the last decades. Therapy with busulfan was initiated in the 1950s but was then replaced by hydroxyurea, followed by introduction of IFN-α in the early 1980s, the first drug to induce a marked cytogenetic response in CML patients (Goldman, 2007). Treatment with curative intention was subsequently realized through allogeneic stem cell transplantation (SCT) in the 1980s, and this became the treatment of choice for younger patients with HLA-matched donors. The therapy was revolutionized by the arrival of imatinib (imatinib mesylate, formerly STI571) that was first used in clinical trials starting in 1998, in which its limited toxicity and ability to induce hematologic and cytogenetic response were first established (Druker et al., 2001). In a 5-year follow-up of patients receiving imatinib (the IRIS study), the estimated cumulative best rates of a complete hematologic response (CHR) or a complete cytogenetic response (CCR) were 98 and 87%, respectively, and the estimated overall survival of patients who received imatinib as initial therapy was 89% at 60 months (Druker et al., 2006). Further follow-up studies confirmed the excellent results and until recently, imatinib was the standard therapy for newly diagnosed CML CP patients (Baccarani et al., 2013).

The imatinib compound binds to the ATP-binding pocket of the ABL1 domain and stabilizes the inactive, non-ATP-binding conformation of BCR–ABL1. This blocks the tyrosine kinase activity and inhibits both BCR–ABL1-mediated autophosphorylation and substrate phosphorylation, resulting in abrogated downstream cell signaling and reduced proliferation of *BCR–ABL1*-positive cells (O'Hare et al., 2012). Despite the highly promising results of imatinib treatment, problems related to the occurrence of *ABL1* kinase mutations, rendering resistance to imatinib, and its modest activity in more advanced phases of CML prompted the development of second-generation TKIs. In

2010, two new TKIs (nilotinib and dasatinib) received approval as first-line therapies in CML because they resulted in a more rapid and deep molecular response (reviewed by O'Hare et al., 2012; Baccarani et al., 2013). Currently, ELN recommends that outside of clinical trials, the first-line treatment of CML CP can be based on any of the three TKIs approved for this indication (Baccarani et al., 2013). Two additional TKIs (ponatinib and bosutinib) have received approval as a second-line therapy for patients showing resistance or intolerance to the aforementioned therapy. Detailed treatment recommendations for first, second, and subsequent lines of treatment in CML have been published by ELN and are not discussed in this chapter (Baccarani et al., 2013). Because of the success of TKI therapy, the number of patients undergoing allogeneic SCT for CML has dropped significantly.

Following the introduction of imatinib, numerous mutations have been identified in patients displaying resistance. At the protein level, such mutations generally result in an inability of ABL1 to adopt the inactive conformation to which imatinib binds. The most well-known and clinically relevant mutation is T315I, in which threonine is replaced by an isoleucine at amino acid position 315 in the ABL1 part. This mutation is highly resistant to imatinib and also to nilotinib, dasatinib, and bosutinib, while ponatinib remains effective (O'Hare et al., 2012; Baccarani et al., 2013; Soverini et al., 2014). Dasatinib and nilotinib have a smaller spectrum of resistance-conferring mutations than imatinib, but the T315I mutation is also found following treatment with these TKIs (see further in the following text).

Currently available TKIs efficiently eradicate the progenitor cells, while quiescent CML stem cells are insensitive to these drugs (Pellicano et al., 2011). Thus, the persistence of residual CML stem cells offers a source for reestablishment of the disease once treatment is discontinued. Interestingly, however, recent studies have shown that treatment with imatinib can be discontinued in a fraction of CML patients who have been in a sustained and deep molecular remission (MR4.5 or better; for definitions, see in the following text). In the pioneering multicenter Stop Imatinib (STIM) study, it was reported that approximately 40% of the patients at 12 months remained in deep remission and that almost all patients that had a molecular recurrence responded well when treatment was resumed (Mahon et al., 2011). Subsequently, several similar studies have been performed, all reporting that imatinib can be discontinued without a molecular recurrence in a fraction of patients with a sustained and deep molecular response (for review, see Mahon, 2012; Mahon and Etienne, 2014). Within the near future, it will become evident if TKI treatment can be discontinued in a larger proportion of CML patients, following first-line treatment with the more potent inhibitors. However, according to ELN, the data so far are insufficient to make recommendations about treatment discontinuation outside controlled clinical studies (Baccarani et al., 2013).

Because residual leukemic CML stem cells are likely to contribute to relapse following TKI discontinuation, a plethora of novel agents are under development aiming at targeting the leukemic stem cell through various mechanisms (Ahmed and Van Etten, 2013).

Disease monitoring of CML during treatment

Once treatment with TKI has been initiated, regular cytogenetic and molecular monitoring of the *BCR–ABL1* fusion transcript with real-time quantitative (RQ-)PCR should be performed as recommended by ELN (Baccarani et al., 2013). The ELN definitions of cytogenetic and molecular response are outlined in Table 8.1. While chromosome analysis is straightforward, considerable work has been put into efforts to standardize RQ-PCR analysis of BCR–ABL1 fusion transcripts (Cross et al., 2012). Several laboratories have calibrated their RQ-PCR assays to a central reference laboratory and thereby obtained a conversion factor (CF), allowing them to express their results according to the international scale (IS). An important landmark that has been used as a "surrogate end point" in several clinical studies is "major molecular response" (MMR), which corresponds to a threefold log reduction (also designated $MR^{3.0}$) and consequently a BCR–ABL1 expression of less than or equal to 0.1%. Despite ongoing standardization

Table 8.1 Definitions of cytogenetic and molecular response*

Cytogenetic response[†]	Definitions
Complete cytogenetic remission (CCgR or CCyR)	No Ph+ metaphases
Partial cytogenetic remission (PCgR)	1–35% Ph+ metaphases
Minor cytogenetic remission (mCgR)	36–65% Ph+ metaphases
Minimal cytogenetic remission (minCgR)	66–95% Ph+ metaphases
No cytogenetic remission (noCgR)	>95% Ph+ metaphases
Molecular response[††]	**Definitions**
Major molecular response (MMR or MR$^{3.0}$)	BCR–ABL1 expression of $\leq 0.1\%^{IS}$
Molecular response MR$^{4.0}$	BCR–ABL1 expression of $\leq 0.01\%^{IS}$ or undetectable disease in cDNA with >10 000 ABL1 transcripts
Molecular response MR$^{4.5}$	BCR–ABL1 expression of $\leq 0.0032\%^{IS}$ or undetectable disease in cDNA with >32 000 ABL1 transcripts
Molecular response MR$^{5.0}$	BCR–ABL1 expression of $\leq 0.001\%^{IS}$

*Data from Baccarani et al. (2009, 2013) and Cross et al. (2012). For more extensive and detailed definitions, see these references.

[†]At least 20 metaphases should be analyzed. If bone marrow metaphases cannot be obtained or evaluated by chromosome banding analysis, the definition of CCyR may be based on interphase FISH analysis of at least 200 nuclei from peripheral blood cells; CcyR corresponds to <1% BCR–ABL1-positive nuclei.

[††]Molecular response (MR) is assessed with reference to the international scale (IS) and is expressed as a percentage. Hundred percent corresponds to the IRIS standardized baseline and 0.1% corresponds to the upper limit of MMR (MR$^{3.0}$). All log reductions are from the IRIS baseline and not from individual pretreatment levels. The term complete molecular response (CMR) should be avoided and replaced with the term "molecularly undetectable leukemia" with specification of the number of control gene transcript copies.

efforts, there are still some concerns about the reproducibility and interlaboratory variation of the measurements of molecular response, something that will hopefully be improved upon with additional international efforts in standardization and with novel technologies that are under development (Cross et al., 2012; Jennings et al., 2014).

Because the response to TKI therapy has become the most critical prognostic factor in CML, ELN has issued recommendations for assessing the response (Table 8.2). The responses are defined as "optimal" or "failure." An optimal response is associated with a duration of life comparable with that of the general population, indicating that there is no need to change the ongoing treatment. In contrast, "failure" means that the patient should receive a different treatment to limit the risk of progression and death. In between, there is a category called "warning" (previously designated "suboptimal") that implies that the disease characteristics and treatment response require more frequent monitoring to permit timely changes in therapy in case of treatment failure (Baccarani et al., 2013). Importantly, a BCR–ABL1 transcript level close to

a defined cutoff level (i.e., 10%, 1%, 0.1%) is not sufficient to define a failure. Additional tests should therefore be performed before a decision is made to change the therapy.

Issued guidelines by ELN for cytogenetic and molecular monitoring are summarized in Table 8.3 (Baccarani et al., 2013). According to the recommendations, response can be assessed either with RQ-PCR or cytogenetic analysis alone depending on local laboratory facilities, but whenever possible, both cytogenetic and molecular tests are recommended until a CCR and MMR are achieved. Following these landmarks, RQ-PCR alone may be sufficient. However, in case signs of warning, failure, or progression are observed (see Table 8.2), additional workup, including cytogenetic analysis, is mandated.

Despite a high response rate to TKIs, primary and secondary resistance is observed. Primary resistance is defined as a lack of initial response, while secondary resistance is defined as a loss of an established response during treatment (Baccarani et al., 2009, 2013). The frequency with which mutations are detected varies in the literature but

Table 8.2 Definition of response to TKIs as first-line treatment*

	Optimal	Warning	Failure
Baseline/diagnosis	NA	High risk or additional major route cytogenetic changes	NA
3 months	BCR–ABL1 ≤10% and/or Ph+ ≤35%	BCR–ABL1 >10% and/or Ph+ 36–95%	Non-CHR and/or Ph+ >95%
6 months	BCR–ABL1 <1% and/or Ph+ 0%	BCR–ABL1 1–10% and/or Ph+ 1–35%	BCR–ABL1 >10% and/or Ph+ >35%
12 months[†]	BCR–ABL1 ≤0.1% (=MMR)	BCR–ABL1 >0.1–1%	BCR–ABL1 >1% and/or Ph+ >0%
Then and at any time	BCR–ABL1 ≤0.1%	Cytogenetic changes in Ph-negative cells (-7 or 7q-)	Loss of CHR Loss of CCyR Confirmed loss of MMR[††] Mutations CCA/Ph+

*Data from Baccarani et al. (2009, 2013). For more extensive and detailed definitions, see these references. Response can be assessed with either a molecular or cytogenetic technique. Whenever available, both are recommended.
Abbreviations: CCA/Ph+, additional chromosomal abnormalities in Ph-positive cells (clonal cytogenetic evolution); CCyR, complete cytogenetic remission; CHR, complete hematologic remission; MMR, major molecular remission; NA, not applicable.
[†]After 12 months, if MMR is achieved, the response can be assessed by RQ-PCR every 3–6 months. Cytogenetic analysis is required only in case of failure or if RQ-PCR is not available.
[††]Loss of MMR should be confirmed in two consecutive tests, of which one with BCR–ABL1 transcript levels of ≥1%.

Table 8.3 Recommendations for cytogenetic and molecular monitoring of CML*

At diagnosis	Chromosome banding analysis (CBA) of bone marrow metaphases FISH in case of Ph negativity to identify variant translocations or cryptic BCR–ABL1 rearrangements RQ-PCR to identify fusion transcript type
During treatment	RQ-PCR of BCR–ABL1 on the international scale, to be performed every 3 months until an MMR (BCR–ABL1 ≤0.1%, or MR[3.0]) is achieved and then every 3–6 months, and/or CBA of bone marrow metaphases (at least 20 metaphases), to be performed at 3, 6, and 12 months until CCyR has been achieved and then every 12 months. Once CCyR is achieved, FISH on blood cells can be performed. If adequate RQ-PCR can be ensured, cytogenetic analysis can be omitted
Failure, progression	RQ-PCR, mutation analysis, and CBA of bone marrow metaphases. Immunophenotyping in BP
Warning	Molecular and cytogenetic analyses to be performed more frequently. CBA of bone marrow cells recommended in case of myelodysplasia or clonal cytogenetic changes in Ph-negative cells with chromosome 7 abnormalities

*Data from Baccarani et al. (2009, 2013). For more extensive and detailed definitions, see these references. Then RQ-PCR alone may be sufficient: Mutation analysis is recommended in case of progression, failure, and warning (see Soverini et al., 2011). In case of failure, warning, and development of myelodysplastic features, CBA of bone marrow cells is recommended.
Abbreviations: BP, blast phase (crisis); CBA, chromosome banding analysis; FISH, fluorescence in situ hybridization.

has been estimated to be around 50% if treatment failure or progression is observed (Baccarani et al., 2013). In a review of 11 studies in which mutation analysis was performed following imatinib failure, between 21 and 48% of the cases with primary resistance displayed mutations, whereas 10–68% of cases with secondary resistance showed mutations (Soverini et al., 2014). Resistance is typically defined using the ELN criteria for "failure" (see Table 8.2). Mutation analysis, the standard being

Sanger sequencing, is not recommended at diagnosis. However, ELN recommends that during first-line therapy with imatinib, mutation analysis should be performed in case of failure, an increase in BCR–ABL1 transcript levels leading to loss of MMR, in case of suboptimal response, and before changing to other TKIs or other therapies. During second-line therapy with dasatinib or nilotinib, mutation screening should be performed in case of hematologic or cytogenetic failure including no cytogenetic response at 3 months, minimal cytogenetic response (66–95% Ph-positive metaphases) at 6 months, less than partial cytogenetic response (1–35% Ph-positive metaphases) at 12 months, and before changing to other TKIs or other therapies (Soverini et al., 2014). For details on the National Comprehensive Cancer Network (NCCN) guidelines as to when mutation analysis should be performed, which are slightly different from the ELN guidelines, see O'Brien et al. (2013).

So far, more than 80 amino acid substitutions have been reported in association with imatinib resistance (Baccarani et al., 2013). Currently, few mutations are known to confer clinical resistance to nilotinib (Y253H, E255K/V, F359V/C/I) or dasatinib (V299L, T315A, F317L/I/V/C). The T315I mutation, being the most well-known mutation, confers resistance to all currently approved TKIs except ponatinib, which remains clinically active even in the presence of this mutation (O'Hare et al., 2012; Baccarani et al., 2013; Soverini et al., 2014). Depending on the type of mutation identified in a patient developing resistance, ELN and NCCN have recommended appropriate treatment options (for a summary, see O'Hare et al., 2012; Baccarani et al., 2013; Soverini et al., 2014).

Given the increased and sequential use of TKIs and the limited time of follow-up, it is likely that new mutations of clinical relevance will be detected. One concern is the presence of clones with multiple BCR–ABL1 mutations, some with two mutations in the same BCR–ABL1 molecule (compound mutations), including examples of compound mutations that predict resistance to ponatinib at concentrations unlikely to be reached in patients without unacceptable toxicity (Khorashad et al., 2013; Gibbons et al., 2014).

While direct Sanger sequencing currently is the most commonly used method to detect BCR–ABL1 mutations in clinical practice, newer technologies with higher sensitivity are likely to take over. Examples of such methods include mass spectrometry, digital PCR, and NGS-based technologies; especially the latter are likely to be increasingly applied in the near future (Soverini et al., 2014). NGS-based studies will also facilitate the identification of the molecular breakpoints of BCR–ABL1, allowing molecular monitoring of BCR–ABL1-positive cells at the DNA level as described in CML patients discontinuing imatinib treatment (Ross et al., 2010). Finally, since the CML stem cells are likely to contribute to disease relapse following treatment discontinuation, there will be a need to identify markers of these stem cells allowing their detection. In this context, the recent identification of the markers IL1RAP and CD26 on candidate CML stem cells might help identify and quantify such cells at diagnosis, during treatment, and at later follow-up (Järås et al., 2010; Herrmann et al., 2014). Indeed, it was recently demonstrated that a low CML stem cell burden at diagnosis correlates with superior cytogenetic and molecular responses, further suggesting that monitoring leukemic stem cells may become valuable in the future (Mustjoki et al., 2013).

In summary, while therapeutic and diagnostic progress has made treatment of CML more effective, it has become increasingly challenging to keep pace with the optimal clinical management and laboratory practice for monitoring such patients. The reader is hence recommended to regularly consult updated guidelines, for example, issued by the ELN (Baccarani et al., 2009, 2013) or the NCCN (O'Brien et al., 2013).

Cytogenetic evolution in Ph-positive CML

Because of the natural clinical course of CML, with CP eventually progressing into AP and BC, CML has become a well-studied model for the multistep nature of carcinogenesis. Although it is well established that the BCR–ABL1 fusion gene is critical for the initiation of CP and, in most instances, also for the maintenance of BC, less is known about the underlying cellular and genetic events leading to disease progression. However, a growing number of studies have suggested that BCR–ABL1-expressing cells display failures in genomic surveillance and DNA repair, something that could play an important role for the occurrence of secondary genetic changes. In the following text, currently available data regarding cytogenetic and molecular genetic changes observed at disease progression of CML are reviewed.

Even though occasional CML cases harbor other changes early in the disease, as mentioned earlier, the t(9;22) typically remains the sole abnormality throughout most of the CP. When disease progression occurs, however, 60–80% of cases develop additional chromosome aberrations. These secondary changes sometimes precede the hematologic and clinical manifestations of a more malignant disease by several months and thus may serve as valuable prognostic indicators. As will be discussed further in the following text, the treatment given during CP also influences the pattern of secondary genetic changes observed.

Early cytogenetic investigations in the prebanding era indicated that the karyotypic abnormalities occurring in excess of the Ph chromosome were nonrandom, an observation that was corroborated when the various banding techniques became available (Johansson et al., 2002). Based on a series of 10 patients and on a review of 57 published cases with additional cytogenetic aberrations, Mitelman et al. (1976) identified an extra Ph, +8, and i(17q) as the most common secondary changes, present in approximately 90% of cases with additional abnormalities. These changes were referred to as constituting the "major route" of clonal evolution, whereas other less frequently observed changes were designated "minor route" aberrations.

Secondary chromosome aberrations have now been reported in more than 2500 CML cases (Mitelman et al., 2014). The pattern is clearly nonrandom, with the most common chromosomal abnormalities being +8 (34% of cases with additional changes), +Ph (31%), i(17q) (20%), and +19 (13%). All other additional chromosomal changes occur in less than 10%, the most frequent being −Y, +21, −7, +17, and −17; the same aberrations were also the most common in a survey of 180 CML cases with variant translocations (Johansson et al., 2002). Apart from a slightly lower prevalence of +8, +Ph, i(17q), +19, −17, and +14 and a higher frequency of 13q− in CML with variant translocations,

no clear-cut differences between the two groups could be discerned. Combining CML cases with standard and variant translocations, the most common additional chromosomal changes in the study by Johansson et al. (2002) were +8 (30%), +Ph (30%), i(17q) (20%), +19 (12%), −Y (8% of males), +21 (7%), and −7 (5%). Using a cutoff value of 5%, they proposed to expand the major evolutionary route to include all these changes.

As is evident from the compilation earlier, the great majority of the secondary changes observed are genomically unbalanced, that is, trisomies, monosomies, and deletions. There are notable exceptions to this pattern, however; several balanced changes typically found in AML, for example, inv(3)(q21q26)/t(3;3)(q21;q26), t(3;21)(q26;q22), t(7;11)(p15;p15), t(8;21)(q22;q22), t(15;17)(q22;q21), and inv(16)(p13q22), have also been observed at disease progression of CML (Mitelman et al., 2014). As described in Chapter 6, these changes in AML are associated with quite specific phenotypic and clinical features and should, probably, in CML be seen as second primary changes rather than as "ordinary" secondary changes. Notably, as exemplified by t(15;17) and inv(16), the morphologic features of CML BC harboring such changes resemble those found in de novo AML with the same balanced abnormalities (Mitelman et al., 2014). The phenotypic impact of the more common secondary aberrations in CML, in particular whether certain changes are associated with a myeloid or lymphoid BC, is unclear. Reviewing the literature, Johansson et al. (2002) found that the only significant differences in cytogenetic evolution patterns were a higher incidence of i(17q) in myeloid BC and a higher frequency of monosomy 7 and hypodiploidy in lymphoid BC. There were no significant frequency differences of balanced abnormalities in addition to t(9;22) between myeloid and lymphoid BC. Notably, however, whereas most balanced aberrations in myeloid BC are the well-known AML-associated translocations mentioned earlier, balanced changes in lymphoid BC are preferentially nonrecurrent and not characteristic ALL-associated translocations (Johansson et al., 2002).

The type of treatment given during CP seems to influence the patterns of secondary abnormalities observed during AP and BC. For example, +8 is significantly more common after busulfan treatment as compared to CML treated with hydroxyurea (Johansson et al., 2002). Treatment with IFN-α is associated with an aberrant karyotypic evolution pattern displaying increased frequencies of unusual secondary changes, that is, non-major route abnormalities, divergent clones, and cell populations with unrelated aberrations in addition to t(9;22) (Johansson et al., 1996, 2002; Maloisel et al., 1997). The emergence of Ph-negative cells with clonal chromosomal changes, mainly trisomy 8, has been observed after treatment with IFN-α (Johansson et al., 2002), a finding reminiscent of recent reports following treatment with imatinib and other TKIs (see later). In addition, several studies have shown that the cytogenetic evolution pattern is quite distinct after allogeneic SCT (Karrman et al., 2007); major route abnormalities are less frequent, but instead, the changes observed are seemingly random, structurally complex, and sometimes transient, with a high frequency of balanced translocations and divergent clones (Karrman et al., 2007). The occurrence of this "unconventional" cytogenetic evolution pattern following allogeneic SCT has been suggested to be caused by the conditioning regime, that is, a result of the clastogenic effect of total body irradiation and/or alkylating agents (Alimena et al., 1990; Offit et al., 1990; Sessarego et al., 1991; Bilhou-Nabera et al., 1992; Shah et al., 1992; Chase et al., 2000). However, comparing the cytogenetic evolution pattern in CML patients treated with autologous and allogeneic SCT, Karrman et al. (2007) found that balanced changes were more common after allogeneic SCT and that the cytogenetic features after autologous SCT were more similar to the ones observed in nontransplanted CML patients. Because the conditioning regimens are similar in the two settings, it was suggested that the atypical evolution pattern observed after allogeneic SCT rather could be a result of an altered BM microenvironment and/or the immunosuppression given to such patients.

Most patients who have received treatment with TKIs so far remain in complete cytogenetic remission, but when cytogenetic changes appear in Ph-positive cells, they seem to follow the same cytogenetic evolution pattern as before the introduction of TKIs. Haferlach et al. (2010) compared the cytogenetic evolution pattern in 245 CML patients that had received treatment with TKIs and compared this cohort to published cases before the introduction of imatinib (Mitelman et al., 2014). No difference in the cytogenetic evolution pattern was observed between the two groups, regardless whether the additional cytogenetic changes were detected at diagnosis or during follow-up under TKI treatment. Although additional studies clearly are needed, it was concluded that the cytogenetic pathways of clonal evolution in CML are independent of TKI treatment effects and that such drugs do not seem to select specific cytogenetic alterations (Haferlach et al., 2010).

What is the clinical significance of a clonal cytogenetic change detected while a patient is under therapy with imatinib or other TKIs? As discussed earlier, the emergence of additional cytogenetic abnormalities during therapy defines TKI failure according to ELN criteria (see Table 8.2) and should lead to a change of therapy (for details, see Baccarani et al., 2013).

Another cytogenetic phenomenon that has attracted considerable interest in the present era of TKI treatment is the observation of clonal cytogenetic changes in Ph-negative cells in 2–17% of patients in some larger series (Bumm et al., 2003; Medina et al., 2003; O'Dwyer et al., 2003; Terre et al., 2004; Bacher et al., 2005; Abruzzese et al., 2007; Deininger et al., 2007; Jabbour et al., 2007). The most common changes observed in the Ph-negative cells are −7, +8, −5, and −Y. Such changes are also frequent in myelodysplastic syndromes (MDS) and AML, something that has raised concerns about their clinical implications. A growing number of case reports of MDS or AML developing in TKI-treated patients, carrying mainly monosomy 7 or trisomy 8 in their Ph-negative cells, have been published (Mitelman et al., 2014). The frequency with which overt MDS/AML develops in such patients is in the order of 2–10%, emphasizing the importance of continued cytogenetic monitoring of CML patients receiving imatinib (Kovitz et al., 2006; Deininger et al., 2007). Recently, Groves et al. (2011) reviewed 53 patients reported in the literature with monosomy 7 or del(7q) in Ph-negative cells following TKI treatment. Monosomy 7 occurred as the sole abnormality in 29 cases (55%), together with other abnormalities in 14 cases (26%), whereas del(7q) was present in 10 cases (19%). A total of 16 of 51 evaluable patients (31%) developed MDS/AML and the transformation frequency was higher within the first 6 months following detection of monosomy 7. None of the 10 patients with del(7q) developed MDS/AML, suggesting that monosomy 7 is associated with a higher propensity to develop a second myeloid malignancy (Groves et al., 2011). According to ELN guidelines, clonal cytogenetic changes in Ph-negative cells, with the exception of monosomy 7 and del(7q), do not adversely affect the outcome, and BM examination is only recommended in case of cytopenias or dysplastic blood morphology. However, if chromosome 7 abnormalities are observed after TKI treatment, this constitutes a "warning" sign and requires more frequent cytogenetic and molecular genetic monitoring and long-term follow-up with BM biopsies (Baccarani et al., 2013).

The reason(s) for clonal cytogenetic changes in Ph-negative cells is unknown. It could possibly be explained by the (side) effect of imatinib or other TKIs on the normal ABL1 protein, which is involved in DNA damage and repair control. If so, one would expect that similar cytogenetic changes (e.g., +8 or monosomy 7) would be found in other malignant disorders treated with TKIs. One such example is gastrointestinal stromal tumors (also referred to as GIST). In fact, a recent case report described a patient diagnosed with GIST that after imatinib treatment developed MDS with monosomy 7 and a rapid transformation into AML (Pitini et al., 2009). Thus, inhibition of normal ABL1 in CML could favor the selection of cells with random changes, including monosomy 7 or +8, in particular when hematopoiesis is being restored from a limited pool of Ph-negative stem cells.

Molecular genetic evolution in Ph-positive CML

Several molecular genetic changes have been identified during disease progression of CML, but apart from frequent changes that have now been identified in lymphoid BC (see the following text), no single or universal abnormality has been shown to be the critical genetic event for the transition of CP into BC. It is equally unclear if the secondary molecular genetic changes occur at the level of t(9;22)-harboring HSC or in a more mature progenitor, although some support for the latter scenario, at least in myeloid BC, exists (Jamieson et al., 2004). The molecular genetic changes observed can—somewhat simplistically—be divided into those associated with identifiable chromosomal changes, that is, they are the molecular genetic consequences of the major and minor route abnormalities discussed earlier, and those that are cytogenetically cryptic.

Even as regards the most common secondary cytogenetic changes—+8, i(17q), and +Ph—the molecular consequences remain largely unknown. For example, the functional outcome and the pathogenetic effects of trisomy 8, which is found as a sole abnormality in 5–10% of cytogenetically abnormal AML and MDS, are still unclear (Paulsson and Johansson, 2007). Mutations in the well-known tumor suppressor gene (TSG) TP53 in 17p13 have been detected in approximately 10% (0–30%) of CML BC (Hehlmann, 2012). This gene is an attractive candidate for a role in disease progression because of the frequent loss of 17p due to i(17q), −17, or other changes resulting in loss of material from 17p (Johansson et al., 2002; Melo and Barnes, 2007). However, no coding TP53 mutations were detected in a series of CML BC and other hematologic malignancies with i(17q), suggesting that other TSG on 17p or, alternatively, gain of 17q material could be the pathogenetically important event (Fioretos et al., 1999). As to the mechanism by which the i(17q) is formed, some data have been forthcoming suggesting that genomic architectural features may be critical (Barbouti et al., 2004). The i(17q) has been shown to be not a true isochromosome but rather an isodicentric abnormality with the breakpoints occurring in 17p11, either in the very pericentromeric region or in a genetically unstable region denoted the Smith–Magenis syndrome (SMS) common deletion region (Chen et al., 1997; Fioretos et al., 1999; Scheurlen et al., 1999). Thus, the i(17q) should formally be designated idic(17)(p11). The breakpoint region in 17p11 was shown to display a complex genomic architecture characterized by large (38–49 kb), palindromic, low-copy repeats. Palindromic sequences, or inverted repeats, are well-established hot spots of genomic instability, and the identification of such elements at the 17p11 breakpoint, perhaps in combination with a dysfunctional double-strand break repair present in BCR–ABL1-expressing cells (see preceding text), has been suggested to be a critical factor triggering i(17q) formation (Barbouti et al., 2004).

While it seems natural to conclude that the presence of an extra Ph during disease progression results in an increased expression of the *BCR–ABL1* fusion gene, no large studies addressing this issue have been reported. However, it has been shown that the expression level of *BCR–ABL1* increases at AP and BC, suggesting that this may be a critical factor in disease progression (Melo and Barnes, 2007). As to the other major route abnormalities, that is, −7, +19, and +21, no consistent molecular correlates have so far emerged. It was shown that among one CML CP and 13 BC samples with trisomy 21, six (43%) displayed mutations within the DNA-binding domain of *RUNX1* (also known as *AML1*) at 21q22, of which two also harbored a t(1;21)(p36;q22) and a *RUNX1–PRDM16* fusion gene, leading to "biallelic" *RUNX1* mutations (Roche-Lestienne et al., 2008). Thus, *RUNX1* mutations seem to be important alterations associated with CML BC, particularly in cases showing +21, with experimental data also suggesting that this could be a mechanism by which CML BC cells become resistant to imatinib (Miething et al., 2007). More recent studies have confirmed the occurrence of *RUNX1* mutations in CML BC (see following text).

In contrast to our limited understanding of the pathogenetic consequences of major route abnormalities, the molecular consequences of some rarely observed, but nevertheless highly informative, cases of balanced chromosomal changes in BC are better understood. In rare cases of CML BC (see preceding text), balanced changes, such as inv(3)(q21q26), t(3;21)(q26;q22), t(7;11)(p15;p15), t(8;21)(q22;q22), and inv(16) (p13q22), are observed, resulting in the formation of chimeric fusion genes (Mitelman et al., 2014). A notable feature of several of these changes—t(3;21), t(8;21), and inv(16)—is that they rearrange either *RUNX1* or *CBFB*, encoding the heterodimeric core binding factor (CBF) complex, emphasizing the importance of alterations in this regulatory complex in CML disease progression. Another recurring theme is the involvement of homeobox genes, illustrated by the identification of some rarely occurring changes at disease progression: t(7;11)(p15;p15), resulting in *NUP98–HOXA9* and *NUP98–HOXA11* fusions (Borrow et al., 1996; Nakamura et al., 1996; Fujino et al., 2002), the cytogenetically cryptic t(7;17)(p15;q23) that forms a *MSI2–HOXA9* chimera (Barbouti et al., 2003), and the t(1;11)(q23;p15) fusing *NUP98* with the homeobox gene *PMX1* (Nakamura et al., 1999; Roche-Lestienne et al., 2008). The latter changes suggest that deregulation of genes belonging to the *HOX* family could also be a factor in disease progression.

Several molecular genetic changes not correlated to any of the well-known secondary cytogenetic changes, but that were investigated because of their general involvement in tumorigenesis, have also been identified during disease progression. Mutational analyses of 85 unselected CML BC samples, focusing on alterations in key transcription factors involved in regulating normal hematopoiesis (*PU1, CEBPA, GATA1-3, RUNX1, CBFB, MYB, ICSBP, TP53, NRAS,* and *KRAS*), identified novel gain-of-function mutations in *GATA2* in 9 of 85 (10%) cases and confirmed the presence of mutations in *RUNX1* (13%) and *TP53* (4%) (Zhang et al., 2008). Notably, cases with mutations in *GATA2* preferentially displayed a myelomonocytic BC phenotype, with the mutation being associated with an inferior outcome when compared to *RUNX1* mutated cases and those lacking mutations (Zhang et al., 2008). Deletions of *CDKN2A* (also referred to as "*p16*") have been detected in about 30% (14 of 47 cases) of lymphoid BC, whereas such mutations are rare in myeloid BC (Serra et al., 1995; Sill et al., 1995; Hernández-Boluda et al., 2003). Grossmann et al. (2011) used NGS and Sanger sequencing to search for mutations in 11 genes known to be of importance mainly in myeloid malignancies. Investigating 39 CML BC cases, they identified mutations in 30 of 39 (77%) with the most frequent mutations targeting *RUNX1* (33%), *ASXL1* (20%), *WT1* (15%), *NRAS* (5%), *KRAS* (5%), *TET2* (8%), *CBL* (3%), *TP53* (3%), and *IDH1* (8%). In addition, seven cases (18%), mainly of lymphoid BC, displayed intragenic deletions in *IKZF1*, a gene encoding the transcription factor IKAROS that is critical for normal lymphoid differentiation (Grossmann et al., 2011). The importance of *RUNX1* in the disease progression of CML was further confirmed in a series of 85 Chinese CML BC patients, in whom a *RUNX1* mutation frequency of 13% was reported (Zhao et al., 2012).

Genome-wide measurements of DNA copy number changes have contributed to additional insights into mechanisms underlying disease progression in CML. Using (250K) SNP arrays, Mullighan et al. (2008) demonstrated that a significant fraction of Ph-positive ALL (36 of 43 cases, 84%) and 4 of 15 (27%) CML BC samples harbored deletions in the *IKZF1* gene. Overall, 0.5 copy number changes were observed per CML CP sample, whereas about eight alterations were identified on average in each CML BC sample. Frequent codeletions of *PAX5* and *CDKN2A* were also observed in *BCR–ABL1*-positive ALL, indicating that several changes are needed before overt disease develops (Mullighan et al., 2008). Additional studies using SNP arrays have revealed several copy number alterations at disease progression, but no cryptic or recurrent lesions, apart from known submicroscopic deletions at the breakpoints of *BCR* and *ABL1*, were identified in two recent studies (Grossmann et al., 2011; Makishima et al., 2011).

As evident from the aforementioned data, no single cytogenetic or molecular genetic change seems to be responsible for disease transformation in CML. Instead, multiple and different genetic aberrations are likely critical for disease progression. Hopefully, with the introduction of NGS-based technologies, patterns of change also at the molecular level will become established, in analogy with the identification of cytogenetic evolutionary routes. While some "molecular routes" are emerging (e.g., the common deregulation of *RUNX1* in myeloid BC and deletions of *CDKN2A* and *IKZF1* in lymphoid BC), additional studies are clearly needed.

Summary

The t(9;22)(q34;q11) or its variant translocations (seen in 5–10%) are detected in the great majority of BM cells from patients with CML. A minority of CML patients have a seemingly normal karyotype in which the *BCR* and *ABL1* genes fuse through cytogenetically cryptic insertions or other more complex chromosomal rearrangements. Hence, cytogenetically cryptic fusions of *BCR* and *ABL1* should be actively searched for in a diagnostic setting. The introduction of imatinib and other TKIs has dramatically improved the clinical outcome for CML patients, and today, the vast majority of patients receiving TKI treatment in CP remain in complete hematologic and cytogenetic remission with low to undetectable *BCR–ABL1* fusion transcripts. Close monitoring of such patients is mandatory because drug resistance may develop, which can be detected by increased levels of *BCR–ABL1* fusion transcripts in peripheral blood. Mutation analysis of *ABL1* is warranted not only in such instances but also if the initial response to treatment is unsatisfactory, because changes in the dose of imatinib or a shift to second-generation TKI may be advisable. A small percentage (around 8%) of the patients develop additional cytogenetic changes in their Ph-positive cells during the course of treatment, seemingly following the major route of cytogenetic evolution. The emergence of such changes defines TKI failure, mandating change in therapy according to recommendations by ELN. Moreover, 5–10% of patients that receive imatinib develop clonal cytogenetic changes (mainly −7, +8, and −5) in Ph-negative cells that also may pose clinical challenges. Current frequency estimates suggest that only a minority of such patients (2–10%) develop clinically evident MDS/AML. Thus, while clonal cytogenetic evolution in Ph-negative cells may justify regular cytogenetic follow-up, such findings, with the exception of monosomy 7, should not lead to immediate therapeutic intervention in the absence of morphological evidence of MDS/AML. The emergence of monosomy 7 in Ph-negative cells constitutes a "warning" sign, necessitating more frequent cytogenetic and molecular monitoring, and requires long-term follow-up with BM biopsies (Baccarani et al., 2013).

In contrast to the high response rates to imatinib in CP, patients in the more advanced disease stages typically experience only brief remissions. Thus, a major challenge is to keep the disease burden in CML as low as possible to limit the pool of cells from which additional genetic changes can develop and promote disease progression. Given that quiescent CML stem cells are insensitive to currently available TKIs, a permanent cure will require the elimination of such cells. Substantial efforts are now being made to identify new compounds capable of depleting or eradicating CML stem cells. It has become apparent that a relatively large fraction of CML patients that achieve a deep molecular response can discontinue TKI treatment. To identify such patients reliably early in the disease course and to monitor them appropriately are important challenges.

CML continues to serve as a paradigm for how a specific genetic alteration can cause cellular transformation of a normal primitive cell and how multiple different genetic changes eventually result in disease progression. Aided by the detailed molecular and biochemical dissection of CML, several targeted therapies have been designed and clinically approved, and many more drugs are in development aiming at an ultimate cure. CML also serves as model example of how cytogenetic and molecular genetic methods can be used to monitor patients following treatment and how international efforts help daily laboratory and clinical practice by issuing guidelines (Baccarani et al., 2013; O'Brien et al., 2013). CML clearly constitutes a "moving target" and the reader is recommended to regularly consult available guidelines for proper laboratory and clinical management.

Acknowledgments

Financial support from the Swedish Cancer Society, the Swedish Childhood Cancer Foundation, and the Swedish Research Council is gratefully acknowledged.

References

Abruzzese E, Gozzetti A, Galimberti S, Trawinska MM, Caravita T, Siniscalchi A, et al. (2007): Characterization of Ph-negative abnormal clones emerging during imatinib therapy. *Cancer* 109:2466–2472.

Ahmed W, Van Etten RA (2013): Alternative approaches to eradicating the malignant clone in chronic myeloid leukemia: tyrosine-kinase inhibitor combinations and beyond. *Hematology Am Soc Hematol Educ Program* 2013:189–200.

Albano F, Anelli L, Zagaria A, Coccaro N, D'Addabbo P, Liso V, et al. (2013): Genomic segmental duplications on the basis of the t(9;22) rearrangement in chronic myeloid leukemia. *Oncogene* 29:2509–2516.

Alimena G, De Cuia MR, Mecucci C, Arcese W, Mauro F, Screnci M, et al. (1990): Cytogenetic follow-up after allogeneic bone-marrow transplantation for Ph1-positive chronic myelogenous leukemia. *Bone Marrow Transplant* 5:119–127.

Baccarani M, Cortes J, Pane F, Niederwieser D, Saglio G, Apperley J, et al. (2009): European LeukemiaNet. Chronic myeloid leukemia: an update of concepts and management recommendations of European LeukemiaNet. *J Clin Oncol* 27:6041–6051.

Baccarani M, Deininger MW, Rosti G, Hochhaus A, Soverini S, Apperley JF, et al. (2013): European LeukemiaNet recommendations for the management of chronic myeloid leukemia: 2013. *Blood* 122:872–884.

Bacher U, Hochhaus A, Berger U, Hiddemann W, Hehlmann R, Haferlach T, et al. (2005): Clonal aberrations in Philadelphia chromosome negative hematopoiesis in patients with chronic myeloid leukemia treated with imatinib or interferon alpha. *Leukemia* 19:460–463.

Barbouti A, Höglund M, Johansson B, Lassen C, Nilsson PG, Hagemeijer A, et al. (2003): A novel gene, MSI2, encoding a putative RNA-binding protein is recurrently rearranged at disease progression of chronic myeloid leukemia and forms a fusion gene with HOXA9 as a result of the cryptic t(7;17)(p15;q23). *Cancer Res* 63:1202–1206.

Barbouti A, Stankiewicz P, Nusbaum C, Cuomo C, Cook A, Höglund M, et al. (2004): The breakpoint region of the most common isochromosome, i(17q), in human neoplasia is characterized by a complex genomic architecture with large, palindromic, low-copy repeats. *Am J Hum Genet* 74:1–10.

Barnes DJ, Melo JV (2002): Cytogenetic and molecular genetic aspects of chronic myeloid leukemia. *Acta Haematol* 108:180–202.

Biernaux C, Loos M, Sels A, Huez G, Stryckmans P (1995): Detection of major bcr-abl gene expression at a very low level in blood cells of some healthy individuals. *Blood* 86:3118–3122.

Bilhou-Nabera C, Bernard P, Marit G, Viard F, Gharbi MJ, Wen Z, et al. (1992): Serial cytogenetic studies in allografted patients with chronic myeloid leukemia. *Bone Marrow Transplant* 4:263–268.

Björk J, Albin M, Welinder H, Tinnerberg H, Mauritzson N, Kauppinen T, et al. (2001): Are occupational, hobby, or lifestyle exposures associated with Philadelphia chromosome positive chronic myeloid leukaemia? *Occup Environ Med* 58:722–727.

Borrow J, Shearman AM, Stanton VP Jr, Becher R, Collins T, Williams AJ, et al. (1996): The t(7;11)(p15;p15) translocation in acute myeloid leukaemia fuses the genes for nucleoporin NUP98 and class I homeoprotein HOXA9. *Nat Genet* 12:159–167.

Bose S, Deininger M, Gora-Tybor J, Goldman JM, Melo JV (1998): The presence of typical and atypical BCR-ABL fusion genes in leukocytes of normal individuals: biologic significance and implications for the assessment of minimal residual disease. *Blood* 92:3362–3367.

Bumm T, Müller C, Al-Ali HK, Krohn K, Shepherd P, Schmidt E, et al. (2003): Emergence of clonal cytogenetic abnormalities in Ph– cells in some CML patients in cytogenetic remission to imatinib but restoration of polyclonal hematopoiesis in the majority. *Blood* 101:1941–1949.

Castagnetti F, Testoni N, Luatti S, Marzocchi G, Mancini M, Kerim S, et al. (2010): Deletions of the derivative chromosome 9 do not influence the response and the outcome of chronic myeloid leukemia in early chronic phase treated with imatinib mesylate: GIMEMA CML Working Party analysis. *J Clin Oncol* 28:2748–2754.

Chan LC, Karhi KK, Rayter SI, Heisterkamp N, Eridani S, Powles R, et al. (1987): A novel abl protein expressed in Philadelphia positive acute lymphoblastic leukaemia. *Nature* 325:635–637.

Chase A, Pickard J, Szydlo R, Coulthard S, Goldman JM, Cross NCP (2000): Nonrandom involvement of chromosome 13 in patients with persistent or relapsed disease after bonemarrow transplantation for chronic myeloid leukemia. *Genes Chromosomes Cancer* 27:278–284.

Chen KS, Manian P, Koeuth T, Potocki L, Zhao Q, Chinault AC, et al. (1997): Homologous recombination of a flanking repeat gene cluster is a mechanism for a common contiguous gene deletion syndrome. *Nat Genet* 17:154–163.

Cilloni D, Saglio G (2012): Molecular pathways: BCR-ABL. *Clin Cancer Res* 18:930–937.

Clark SS, McLaughlin J, Champlin R, Witte ON (1987): Unique forms of the abl tyrosine kinase distinguish Ph[1]-positive CML from Ph[1]-positive ALL. *Science* 235:85–88.

Collins SJ, Kubonishi I, Miyoshi I, Groudine MT (1984): Altered transcription of the c-abl oncogene in K-562 and other chronic myelogenous leukemia cells. *Science* 225:72–74.

Cross NC, White HE, Müller MC, Saglio G, Hochhaus A (2012): Standardized definitions of molecular response in chronic myeloid leukemia. *Leukemia* 26:2172–2175.

De Klein A, Geurts van Kessel A, Grosveld G, Bartram CR, Hagemeijer A, Bootsma D, et al. (1982): A cellular oncogene is translocated to the Philadelphia chromosome in chronic myelocytic leukemia. *Nature* 300:765–767.

de la Fuente J, Merx K, Steer EJ, Müller M, Szydlo RM, Maywald O, et al. (2001): ABL-BCR expression does not correlate with deletions on the derivative chromosome 9 or survival in chronic myeloid leukemia. *Blood* 98:2879–2880.

Deininger MW, Goldman JM, Melo JV (2000): The molecular biology of chronic myeloid leukemia. *Blood* 96:3343–3356.

Deininger MW, Cortes J, Paquette R, Park B, Hochhaus A, Baccarani M, et al. (2007): The prognosis for patients with chronic myeloid leukemia who have clonal cytogenetic abnormalities in Philadelphia chromosome-negative cells. *Cancer* 110:1509–1519.

Druker BJ, Tamura S, Buchdunger E, Ohno S, Segal GM, Fanning S, et al. (1996): Effects of a selective inhibitor of the Abl tyrosine kinase on the growth of Bcr-Abl positive cells. *Nat Med* 2:561–566.

Druker BJ, Talpaz M, Resta DJ, Peng B, Buchdunger E, Ford JM, et al. (2001): Efficacy and safety of a specific inhibitor of the BCR-ABL tyrosine kinase in chronic myeloid leukemia. *N Engl J Med* 344:1031–1037.

Druker BJ, Guilhot F, O'Brien SG, Gathmann I, Kantarjian H, Gattermann N, et al. (2006): Five-year follow-up of patients receiving imatinib for chronic myeloid leukemia. *N Engl J Med* 355:2408–2417.

Fabarius A, Leitner A, Hochhaus A, Müller MC, Hanfstein B, Haferlach C, et al. (2011): Impact of additional cytogenetic aberrations at diagnosis on prognosis of CML: long-term observation of 1151 patients from the randomized CML Study IV. *Blood* 118:6760–6768.

Feinstein E, Marcelle C, Rosner A, Canaani E, Gale RP, Dreazen O, et al. (1987): A new fused transcript in Philadelphia chromosome positive acute lymphoblastic leukaemia. *Nature* 330:386–388.

Fioretos T, Strömbeck B, Sandberg T, Johansson B, Billström R, Borg Å, et al. (1999): Isochromosome 17q in blast crisis of chronic myeloid leukemia and in other hematologic malignancies is the result of clustered breakpoints in 17p11 and is not associated with coding TP53 mutations. *Blood* 94:225–232.

Fujino T, Suzuki A, Ito Y, Ohyashiki K, Hatano Y, Miura I, et al. (2002): Single-translocation and double-chimeric transcripts: detection of NUP98-HOXA9 in myeloid leukemias with HOXA11 or HOXA13 breaks of the chromosomal translocation t(7;11)(p15;p15). *Blood* 99:1428–1433.

Gale RP, Canaani E (1984): An altered abl RNA transcript in chronic myelogenous leukemia. *Proc Natl Acad Sci U S A* 81:5648–5652.

Gibbons DL, Pricl S, Posocco P, Laurini E, Fermeglia M, Sun H, et al. (2014): Molecular dynamics reveal BCR-ABL1 polymutants as a unique mechanism of resistance to PAN-BCR-ABL1 kinase inhibitor therapy. *Proc Natl Acad Sci U S A* 111:3550–3555.

Goldman JM (2007): How I treat chronic myeloid leukemia in the imatinib era. *Blood* 110:2828–2837.

Groffen J, Stephenson JR, Heisterkamp N, de Klein A, Bartram CR, Grosveld G (1984): Philadelphia chromosomal breakpoints are clustered within a limited region, bcr, on chromosome 22. *Cell* 36:93–99.

Grossmann V, Kohlmann A, Zenger M, Schindela S, Eder C, Weissmann S, et al. (2011): A deep-sequencing study of chronic myeloid leukemia patients in blast crisis (BC-CML) detects mutations in 76.9% of cases. *Leukemia* 25:557–560.

Grosveld G, Verwoerd T, van Agthoven T, de Klein A, Ramachandran KL, Heisterkamp N, et al. (1986): The chronic myelocytic cell line K562 contains a breakpoint in bcr and produces a chimeric bcr/c-abl transcript. *Mol Cell Biol* 6:607–616.

Groves MJ, Sales M, Baker L, Griffiths M, Pratt N, Tauro S (2011): Factors influencing a second myeloid malignancy in patients with Philadelphia-negative -7 or del(7q) clones during tyrosine kinase inhibitor therapy for chronic myeloid leukemia. *Cancer Genet* 204:39–44.

Haferlach C, Bacher U, Schnittger S, Weiss T, Kern W, Haferlach T (2010): Similar patterns of chromosome abnormalities in CML occur in addition to the Philadelphia chromosome with or without tyrosine kinase inhibitor treatment. *Leukemia* 24:638–640.

Hehlmann R (2012): How I treat CML blast crisis. *Blood* 120:737–747.

Heisterkamp N, Stephenson JR, Groffen J, Hansen PF, de Klein A, Bartram CR, et al. (1983): Localization of the c-abl oncogene adjacent to a translocation breakpoint in chronic myelocytic leukemia. *Nature* 306:239–242.

Heisterkamp N, Stam K, Groffen J, de Klein A, Grosveld G (1985): Structural organization of the bcr gene and its role in the Ph' translocation. *Nature* 315:758–761.

Hermans A, Heisterkamp N, von Lindern M, van Baal S, Meijer D, van der Plas D, et al. (1987): Unique fusion of bcr and c-abl genes in Philadelphia chromosome positive acute lymphoblastic leukemia. *Cell* 51:33–40.

Hernández-Boluda JC, Cervantes F, Colomer D, Vela MC, Costa D, Paz MF, et al. (2003): Genomic p16 abnormalities in the progression of chronic myeloid leukemia into blast crisis: a sequential study in 42 patients. *Exp Hematol* 31:204–210.

Herrmann H, Sadovnik I, Cerny-Reiterer S, Rülicke T, Stefanzl G, Willmann M, et al. (2014): Dipeptidyl peptidase IV (CD26) defines leukemic stem cells (LSC) in chronic myeloid leukemia. *Blood* 123(25):3951–3962.

Huntly BJ, Reid AG, Bench AJ, Campbell LJ, Telford N, Shepherd P, et al. (2001): Deletions of the derivative chromosome 9 occur at the time of the Philadelphia translocation and provide a powerful and independent prognostic indicator in chronic myeloid leukemia. *Blood* 98:1732–1738.

Huntly BJ, Guilhot F, Reid AG, Vassiliou G, Hennig E, Franke C, et al. (2003): Imatinib improves but may not fully reverse the poor prognosis of patients with CML with derivative chromosome 9 deletions. *Blood* 102:2205–2212.

Ichimaru M, Ishimaru T, Belsky JL (1978): Incidence of leukemia in atomic bomb survivors belonging to a fixed cohort in Hiroshima and Nagasaki, 1950–71. Radiation dose, years after exposure, age at exposure, and type of leukemia. *J Radiat Res* 19:262–282.

Jabbour E, Kantarjian HM, Abruzzo LV, O'Brien S, Garcia-Manero G, Verstovsek S, et al. (2007): Chromosomal abnormalities in Philadelphia chromosome negative metaphases appearing during imatinib mesylate therapy in patients with newly diagnosed chronic myeloid leukemia in chronic phase. *Blood* 110:2991–2995.

Jamieson CH, Ailles LE, Dylla SJ, Muijtjens M, Jones C, Zehnder JL, et al. (2004): Granulocyte-macrophage progenitors as candidate leukemic stem cells in blast-crisis CML. *N Engl J Med* 351:657–667.

Järås M, Johnels P, Hansen N, Agerstam H, Tsapogas P, Rissler M, et al. (2010): Isolation and killing of candidate chronic myeloid leukemia stem cells by antibody targeting of IL-1 receptor accessory protein. *Proc Natl Acad Sci U S A* 107:16280–16285.

Jennings LJ, George D, Czech J, Yu M, Joseph L (2014): Detection and quantification of BCR-ABL1 fusion transcripts by droplet digital PCR. *J Mol Diagn* 16:174–179.

Jiang X, Smith C, Eaves A, Eaves C (2007): The challenges of targeting chronic myeloid leukemia stem cells. *Clin Lymphoma Myeloma Suppl* 2:S71–S80.

Johansson B, Fioretos T, Billström R, Mitelman F (1996): Aberrant cytogenetic evolution pattern of Philadelphia-positive chronic myeloid leukemia treated with interferon-alpha. *Leukemia* 10:1134–1138.

Johansson B, Fioretos T, Mitelman F (2002): Cytogenetic and molecular genetic evolution of chronic myeloid leukemia. *Acta Haematol* 107:76–94.

Karrman K, Sallerfors B, Lenhoff S, Fioretos T, Johansson B (2007): Cytogenetic evolution patterns in CML post-SCT. *Bone Marrow Transplant* 39:165–171.

Khorashad JS, Kelley TW, Szankasi P, Mason CC, Soverini S, Adrian LT, et al. (2013): BCR-ABL1 compound mutations in tyrosine kinase inhibitor-resistant CML: frequency and clonal relationships. *Blood* 121:489–498.

Kolomietz E, Marrano P, Yee K, Thai B, Braude I, Kolomietz A, et al. (2003): Quantitative PCR identifies a minimal deleted region of 120 kb extending from the Philadelphia chromosome ABL translocation breakpoint in chronic myeloid leukemia with poor outcome. *Leukemia* 17: 1313–1323.

Konopka JB, Watanabe SM, Witte ON (1984): An alteration of the human c-abl protein in K562 leukemia cells unmask associated tyrosine kinase activity. *Cell* 37:1035–1042.

Kovitz C, Kantarjian H, Garcia-Manero G, Abruzzo LV, Cortes J (2006): Myelodysplastic syndromes and acute leukemia developing after imatinib mesylate therapy for chronic myeloid leukemia. *Blood* 108:2811–2813.

Kozubek S, Lukasova E, Mareckova A, Skalnikova M, Kozubek M, Bartova E, et al. (1999): The topological organization of chromosomes 9 and 22 in cell nuclei has a determinative role in the induction of t(9;22) translocations and in the pathogenesis of t(9;22) leukemias. *Chromosoma* 108:426–435.

Kreil S, Pfirrmann M, Haferlach C, Waghorn K, Chase A, Hehlmann R, et al. (2007): Heterogeneous prognostic impact of derivative chromosome 9 deletions in chronic myelogenous leukemia. *Blood* 110:1283–1290.

Kurzrock R, Shtalrid M, Romero P, Kloetzer WS, Talpaz M, Trujillo JM, et al. (1987): A novel c-abl protein product in Philadelphia-positive acute lymphoblastic leukaemia. *Nature* 325:631–635.

Lee DS, Lee YS, Yun YS, Kim YR, Jeong SS, Lee YK, et al. (2003): A study on the incidence of ABL gene deletion on derivative chromosome 9 in chronic myelogenous leukemia by interphase fluorescence in situ hybridization and its association with disease progression. *Genes Chromosomes Cancer* 37:291–299.

Luatti S, Castagnetti F, Marzocchi G, Baldazzi C, Gugliotta G, Iacobucci I, et al. (2012): Additional chromosomal abnormalities in Philadelphia-positive clone: adverse prognostic influence on frontline imatinib therapy: a GIMEMA Working Party on CML analysis. *Blood* 120:761–767.

Lugo TG, Pendergast AM, Muller AJ, Witte ON (1990): Tyrosine kinase activity and transformation potency of bcr-abl oncogene products. *Science* 247:1079–1082.

Mahon FX (2012): Is going for cure in chronic myeloid leukemia possible and justifiable? *Hematology Am Soc Hematol Educ Program* 2012:122–128.

Mahon FX, Etienne G (2014): Deep molecular response in chronic myeloid leukemia: the new goal of therapy? *Clin Cancer Res* 20:310–322.

Mahon FX, Réa D, Guilhot J, Guilhot F, Huguet F, Nicolini F, et al. (2011): Discontinuation of imatinib in patients with chronic myeloid leukaemia who have maintained complete molecular remission for at least 2 years: the prospective, multicentre Stop Imatinib (STIM) trial. *Lancet Oncol* 11:1029–1035.

Makishima H, Jankowska AM, McDevitt MA, O'Keefe C, Dujardin S, Cazzolli H, et al. (2011): CBL, CBLB, TET2, ASXL1, and IDH1/2 mutations and additional chromosomal aberrations constitute molecular events in chronic myelogenous leukemia. *Blood* 117:198–206.

Maloisel F, Laplace A, Uettwiller F, Lioure B, Oberling F (1997): Unusual cytogenetic evolution in CML treated with interferon-alpha. *Leukemia* 11:893–894.

Marzocchi G, Castagnetti F, Luatti S, Baldazzi C, Stacchini M, Gugliotta G, et al. (2011): Variant Philadelphia translocations: molecular-cytogenetic characterization and prognostic influence on frontline imatinib therapy, a GIMEMA Working Party on CML analysis. *Blood* 117: 6793–6800.

McWhirter JR, Wang JY (1991): Activation of tyrosinase kinase and microfilament-binding functions of c-abl by bcr sequences in bcr/abl fusion proteins. *Mol Cell Biol* 11:1553–1565.

Medina J, Kantarjian H, Talpaz M, O'Brien S, Garcia-Manero G, Giles F, et al. (2003): Chromosomal abnormalities in Philadelphia chromosome-negative metaphases appearing during imatinib mesylate therapy in patients with Philadelphia chromosome-positive chronic myelogenous leukemia in chronic phase. *Cancer* 98:1905–1911.

Melo JV, Barnes DJ (2007): Chronic myeloid leukaemia as a model of disease evolution in human cancer. *Nat Rev Cancer* 7:441–453.

Melo JV, Gordon DE, Cross NCP, Goldman JM (1993): The ABL-BCR fusion gene is expressed in chronic myeloid leukemia. *Blood* 81:158–165.

Melo JV, Hochhaus A, Yan XH, Goldman JM (1996): Lack of correlation between ABL-BCR expression and response to interferon-alpha in chronic myeloid leukaemia. *Br J Haematol* 92:684–686.

Mes-Masson AM, McLaughlin J, Daley GQ, Paskind M, Witte ON (1986): Overlapping cDNA clones define the complete coding region for the P210 c-abl gene product associated with chronic myelogenous leukemia cells containing the Philadelphia chromosome. *Proc Natl Acad Sci U S A* 83:9768–9772.

Miething C, Grundler R, Mugler C, Brero S, Hoepfl J, Geigl J, et al. (2007): Retroviral insertional mutagenesis identifies RUNX genes involved in chronic myeloid leukemia disease persistence under imatinib treatment. *Proc Natl Acad Sci U S A* 104:4594–4599.

Mitelman F, Levan G, Nilsson PG, Brandt L (1976): Nonrandom karyotypic evolution in chronic myeloid leukemia. *Int J Cancer* 18:24–30.

Mitelman F, Johansson B, Mertens F, editors (2014): *Mitelman Database of Chromosome Aberrations and Gene Fusions in Cancer*. Available at http://cgap.nci.nih.gov/Chromosomes/Mitelman.

Mullighan CG, Miller CB, Radtke I, Phillips LA, Dalton J, Ma J, et al. (2008): BCR-ABL1 lymphoblastic leukaemia is characterized by the deletion of Ikaros. *Nature* 453: 110–114.

Mustjoki S, Richter J, Barbany G, Ehrencrona H, Fioretos T, Gedde-Dahl T, et al. (2013): Impact of malignant stem cell burden on therapy outcome in newly diagnosed chronic myeloid leukemia patients. *Leukemia* 27:1520–1526.

Nakamura T, Largaespada DA, Lee MP, Johnson LA, Ohyashiki K, Toyama K, et al. (1996): Fusion of the nucleoporin gene NUP98 to HOXA9 by the chromosome translocation t(7;11)(p15;p15) in human myeloid leukaemia. *Nat Genet* 12:154–158.

Nakamura T, Yamazaki Y, Hatano Y, Miura I (1999): NUP98 is fused to PMX1 homeobox gene in human acute myelogenous leukemia with chromosome translocation t(1;11)(q23;p15). *Blood* 94:741–747.

Neves H, Ramos C, daSilva MG, Parreira A, Parreira L (1999): The nuclear topography of ABL, BCR, PML, and RARalpha genes: evidence for gene proximity in specific phases of the cell cycle and stages of hematopoietic differentiation. *Blood* 93:1197–1207.

Nowell P, Hungerford D (1960): A minute chromosome in human granulocytic leukemia. *Science* 132:1497.

O'Brien S, Radich JP, Abboud CN, Akhtari M, Altman JK, Berman E, et al. (2013): Chronic Myelogenous Leukemia, Version 1.2014. *J Natl Compr Canc Netw* 11:1327–1340.

O'Dwyer ME, Gatter KM, Loriaux M, Druker BJ, Olson SB, Magenis RE, et al. (2003): Demonstration of Philadelphia chromosome negative abnormal clones in patients with chronic myelogenous leukemia during major cytogenetic responses induced by imatinib mesylate. *Leukemia* 17:481–487.

Offit K, Burns JP, Cunningham I, Jhanwar SC, Black P, Kernan NA, et al. (1990): Cytogenetic analysis of chimerism and leukemia relapse in chronic myelogenous leukemia patients after T cell-depleted bone marrow transplantation. *Blood* 75:1346–1355.

O'Hare T, Zabriskie MS, Eiring AM, Deininger MW (2012): Pushing the limits of targeted therapy in chronic myeloid leukaemia. *Nat Rev Cancer* 12:513–526.

Oshikawa G, Kurosu T, Arai A, Murakami N, Miura O (2010): Clonal evolution with double Ph followed by tetraploidy in imatinib-treated chronic myeloid leukemia with e19a2 transcript in transformation. *Cancer Genet Cytogenet* 199:56–61.

Pane F, Frigeri F, Sindona M, Luciano L, Ferrara F, Cimino R, et al. (1996): Neutrophilic-chronic myeloid leukemia: a distinct disease with a specific molecular marker (BCR/ABL with C3/A2 junction). *Blood* 88:2410–2414.

Paulsson K, Johansson B (2007): Trisomy 8 as the sole chromosomal aberration in acute myeloid leukemia and myelodysplastic syndromes. *Pathol Biol* 55:37–48.

Pellicano F, Sinclair A, Holyoake T (2011): In search of CML stem cells' deadly weakness. *Curr Hematol Malig Rep* 6:82–87.

Pitini V, Arrigo C, Sauta MG, Altavilla G (2009): Myelodysplastic syndrome appearing during imatinib mesylate therapy in a patient with GIST. *Leuk Res* 33:e143–e144.

Quintas-Cardama A, Kantarjian H, Talpaz M, O'Brien S, Garcia-Manero G, Verstovsek S, et al. (2005): Imatinib mesylate therapy may overcome the poor prognostic significance of deletions of derivative chromosome 9 in patients with chronic myelogenous leukemia. *Blood* 105:2281–2286.

Reid AG, Nacheva EP (2005): Genesis of derivative chromosome 9 deletions in chronic myeloid leukaemia. *Genes Chromosomes Cancer* 43:223–224.

Ren R (2005): Mechanisms of BCR-ABL in the pathogenesis of chronic myelogenous leukaemia. *Nat Rev Cancer* 5:172–183.

Roche-Lestienne C, Deluche L, Corm S, Tigaud I, Joha S, Philippe N, et al. (2008): RUNX1 DNA-binding mutations and RUNX1-PRDM16 cryptic fusions in BCR-ABL+ leukemias are frequently associated with secondary trisomy 21 and may contribute to clonal evolution and imatinib resistance. *Blood* 111:3735–3741.

Roix JJ, McQueen PG, Munson PJ, Parada LA, Misteli T (2003): Spatial proximity of translocation-prone gene loci in human lymphomas. *Nat Genet* 34:287–291.

Ross DM, Branford S, Seymour JF, Schwarer AP, Arthur C, Bartley PA, et al. (2010): Patients with chronic myeloid leukemia who maintain a complete molecular response after stopping imatinib treatment have evidence of persistent leukemia by DNA PCR. *Leukemia* 24:1719–1724.

Ross DM, O'Hely M, Bartley PA, Dang P, Score J, Goyne JM, et al. (2013): Distribution of genomic breakpoints in chronic myeloid leukemia: analysis of 308 patients. *Leukemia* 27:2105–2107.

Rowley JD (1973): A new consistent chromosomal abnormality in chronic myelogenous leukemia identified by quinacrine fluorescence and Giemsa staining. *Nature* 243:290–293.

Saglio G, Storlazzi CT, Giugliano E, Surace C, Anelli L, Rege-Cambrin G, et al. (2002): A 76-kb duplicon maps close to the BCR gene on chromosome 22 and the ABL gene on chromosome 9: possible involvement in the genesis of the Philadelphia chromosome translocation. *Proc Natl Acad Sci U S A* 99:9882–9887.

Scheurlen WG, Schwabe GC, Seranski P, Joos S, Harbott J, Metzke S, et al. (1999): Mapping of the breakpoints on the short arm of chromosome 17 in neoplasms with an i(17q). *Genes Chromosomes Cancer* 25:230–240.

Serra A, Gottardi E, Della Ragione F, Saglio G, Iolascon A (1995): Involvement of the cyclin-dependent kinase-4 inhibitor (CDKN2) gene in the pathogenesis of lymphoid blast crisis of chronic myelogenous leukaemia. *Br J Haematol* 91:625–629.

Sessarego M, Frassoni F, Defferrari R, Bacigalupo A, Fugazza G, Mareni C, et al. (1991): Karyotype evolution of Ph positive chronic myelogenous leukemia patients relapsed in advanced phases of the disease after allogeneic bone marrow transplantation. *Cancer Genet Cytogenet* 57:69–78.

Shah NK, Wagner J, Santos G, Griffin CA (1992): Karyotype at relapse following allogeneic bone marrow transplantation for chronic myelogenous leukemia. *Cancer Genet Cytogenet* 61:183–192.

Shtivelman E, Lifshitz B, Gale RP, Canaani E (1985): Fused transcript of abl and bcr genes in chronic myelogenous leukaemia. *Nature* 315:550–554.

Sill H, Goldman JM, Cross NCP (1995): Homozygous deletions of the p16 tumor-suppressor gene are associated with lymphoid transformation of chronic myeloid leukemia. *Blood* 85:2013–2016.

Sinclair PB, Nacheva EP, Leversha M, Telford N, Chang J, Reid A, et al. (2000): Large deletions at the t(9;22) breakpoint are common and may identify a poor-prognosis subgroup of patients with chronic myeloid leukemia. *Blood* 95:738–743.

Soverini S, Hochhaus A, Nicolini FE, Gruber F, Lange T, Saglio G, et al. (2011): BCR-ABL kinase domain mutation analysis in chronic myeloid leukemia patients treated with tyrosine kinase inhibitors: recommendations from an expert panel on behalf of European LeukemiaNet. *Blood* 118:1208–1215

Soverini S, Branford S, Nicolini FE, Talpaz M, Deininger MW, Martinelli G, et al. (2014): Implications of BCR-ABL1 kinase domain-mediated resistance in chronic myeloid leukemia. *Leuk Res* 38:10–20.

Stam K, Heisterkamp N, Grosveld G, deKlein A, Verma RS, Coleman M, et al. (1985): Evidence of a new bcr/c-abl mRNA in patients with chronic myelocytic leukemia and the Philadelphia chromosome. *N Engl J Med* 313: 1429–1433.

Swerdlow SH, Campo E, Harris NL, Jaffe ES, Pileri SA, Stein H, et al., editors (2008): *WHO Classification of Tumours of Haematopoietic and Lymphoid Tissues.* Lyon, France: IARC.

Takahashi N, Miura I, Saitoh K, Miura AB (1998): Lineage involvement of stem cells bearing the Philadelphia chromosome in chronic myeloid leukemia in the chronic phase as shown by a combination of fluorescence-activated cell sorting and fluorescence in situ hybridization. *Blood* 92:4758–4763.

Terre C, Eclache V, Rousselot P, Imbert M, Charrin C, Gervais C, et al. (2004): Report of 34 patients with clonal chromosomal abnormalities in Philadelphia-negative cells during imatinib treatment of Philadelphia-positive chronic myeloid leukemia. *Leukemia* 18:1340–1346.

Verstovsek S, Lin H, Kantarjian H, Saglio G, DeMicheli D, Pane F, et al. (2002): Neutrophilic-chronic myeloid leukemia: low levels of p230 BCR/ABL mRNA and undetectable BCR/ABL protein may predict an indolent course. *Cancer* 94:2416–2425.

Walker LC, Ganesan TS, Dhut S, Gibbons B, Lister TA, Rothbard J, et al. (1987): Novel chimaeric protein expressed in Philadelphia positive acute lymphoblastic leukaemia. *Nature* 329:851–853.

Yoong Y, Van De Walker TJ, Carlson RO, Dewald GW, Tefferi A (2005): Clinical correlates of submicroscopic deletions involving the ABL-BCR translocation region in chronic myeloid leukemia. *Eur J Haematol* 74:124–127.

Zhang SJ, Ma LY, Huang QH, Li G, Gu BW, Gao XD, et al. (2008): Gain-of-function mutation of GATA-2 in acute myeloid transformation of chronic myeloid leukemia. *Proc Natl Acad Sci U S A* 105:2076–2081.

Zhao LJ, Wang YY, Li G, Ma LY, Xiong SM, Weng XQ, et al. (2012): Functional features of RUNX1 mutants in acute transformation of chronic myeloid leukemia and their contribution to inducing murine full-blown leukemia. *Blood* 119:2873–2882.

CHAPTER 9

Chronic myeloproliferative neoplasms

Peter Vandenberghe and Lucienne Michaux

Centre for Human Genetics, University Hospitals Leuven, University of Leuven, Leuven, Belgium

Myeloproliferative neoplasms (MPN) are clonal hematological malignancies derived from a common stem cell and characterized by proliferation in the bone marrow of one or more myeloid (i.e., granulocytic, erythroid, megakaryocytic, and mast cell) lineages (Fialkow et al., 1981; Raskind et al., 1985). Importantly, the proliferative process occurs with relatively normal and effective maturation, yielding increased numbers of mature erythrocytes, granulocytes, and/or platelets in the peripheral blood. This distinguishes this group of diseases from the myelodysplastic syndromes (MDS), the myelodysplastic/myeloproliferative neoplasms (MDS/MPN), and acute myeloid leukemia (AML).

Polycythemia vera (PV), chronic myeloid leukemia (CML), essential thrombocythemia (ET), and primary myelofibrosis (PMF) (previously called chronic idiopathic myelofibrosis or agnogenic myeloid metaplasia) are the "classic" MPN. Previous classifications of MPN, including the World Health Organization (WHO) classification of 2001 (Jaffe et al., 2001), were mainly based on their clinical and laboratory features: an increased red cell mass as the hallmark of PV, an excessive production of platelets as the distinguishing anomaly of ET, and splenomegaly, narrow fibrosis as well as distinguishing cytological features in PMF. The 2008 WHO classification profoundly revised the diagnostic algorithms for MPN to include also information on molecular abnormalities, such as the *JAK2* V617F and other activating mutations, and relevant histological features as criteria to identify MPN subtypes (Swerdlow et al., 2008; Vardiman et al., 2008).

In the WHO classification of 2008, the term "myeloproliferative neoplasms" superseded the previous "chronic myeloproliferative disorders" so as to emphasize the neoplastic nature of these conditions. In this latest classification, the MPN also encompass mastocytosis, but conversely, neoplasms associated with eosinophilia and abnormalities of the *PDGFRA*, *PDGFRB*, and fibroblast growth factor receptor 1 (*FGFR1*) genes are now classified separately as "myeloid and lymphoid neoplasms with eosinophilia and abnormalities of *PDGFRA*, *PDGFRB*, and *FGFR1*." This again underscores the current trend toward genetic classifications based on disease-specific molecular markers (Table 9.1) (Swerdlow et al., 2008).

The inclusion of molecular and genetic diagnostic criteria in the WHO classification of 2008 reflects the remarkable progress that was made over the past 10 years in the identification of somatic mutations or rearrangements of critical genes in MPN. Several of these involve tyrosine kinases or related molecules and convey a proliferation advantage on

Cancer Cytogenetics: Chromosomal and Molecular Genetic Aberrations of Tumor Cells, Fourth Edition.
Edited by Sverre Heim and Felix Mitelman.
© 2015 John Wiley & Sons, Ltd. Published 2015 by John Wiley & Sons, Ltd.

Table 9.1 2008 World Health Organization (WHO) classification scheme for myeloid neoplasms (data from Vardiman et al., 2008)

(1) *Myeloproliferative neoplasms (MPN)*
Chronic myelogenous leukemia, *BCR–ABL1* positive
Chronic neutrophilic leukemia
Polycythemia vera
Primary myelofibrosis
Essential thrombocythemia
Chronic eosinophilic leukemia, not otherwise categorized
Mastocytosis
MPN, unclassifiable
(2) *Myeloid and lymphoid neoplasms associated with eosinophilia and abnormalities of PDGFRA, PDGFRB, and FGFR1*
Myeloid neoplasms associated with *PDGFRA* rearrangement
Myeloid neoplasms associated with *PDGFRB* rearrangement
Myeloid neoplasms associated with *FGFR1* rearrangement (8p11 myeloproliferative syndrome)
(3) *Myelodysplastic/myeloproliferative neoplasms (MDS/MPN)*
Chronic myelomonocytic leukemia
Juvenile myelomonocytic leukemia
Atypical chronic myeloid leukemia
MDS/MPN, unclassifiable
(4) *Myelodysplastic syndromes (MDS)*
(5) *Acute myeloid leukemia (AML) and related precursor neoplasms*
(6) *Acute leukemias of ambiguous lineage*

the cells harboring them. Such mutations have been termed class I mutations (Tefferi and Gilliland, 2007). At the same time, also additional and unanticipated layers of genetic complexity have been revealed, often involving the epigenetic control of gene expression (Cross, 2011). Most recently, recurrent mutations of calreticulin (*CALR*) were discovered in ET and PMF, and *CALR*-mutated ET appears to be a distinct biological entity with a specific phenotype (Klampfl et al., 2013; Nangalia et al., 2013; Rotunno et al., 2014; Rumi et al., 2014).

As CML is covered separately in Chapter 8, the present review will be dedicated to the cytogenetics of *BCR–ABL1*-negative MPN but will also include coverage of the myeloid and lymphoid neoplasms with abnormalities of *PDGFRA*, *PDGFRB*, and *FGFR1*, as these belonged to the *BCR–ABL1*-negative

MPN in the previous WHO classification. We shall also discuss the place of cytogenetic examinations in the diagnosis and assessment of prognosis of MPN in an era in which the classification of these diseases becomes increasingly driven by analyses of acquired molecular aberrations.

The classic *BCR–ABL1*-negative MPN: PV, ET, and PMF

At diagnosis, cytogenetic abnormalities are reported in only a minority of cases with these disorders. Most of them are recurrent changes in myeloid disorders and not specific for any particular MPN or even MPN in general. The percentage of abnormal karyotypes increases with disease progression and can reach 90% at the time of leukemic transformation. It is not entirely clear to what extent this clonal evolution is inherent in the natural history of these diseases and to what extent it should be attributed to long-term exposure to myelosuppressive agents.

In the past, cytogenetic examinations used to be important in the workup of MPN for several reasons: to exclude the presence of the Philadelphia translocation, to establish clonality when the central blastosis was less than 5%, and to assess prognosis or disease evolution (Vandenberghe et al., 2009). However, the presence of the *BCR–ABL1* fusion gene can also be ruled out by molecular methods. In addition, in the majority of cases, cytogenetic investigations do not yield evidence for clonal hemopoiesis. In 2005, four groups almost simultaneously reported the *JAK2* V617F tyrosine kinase mutation in approximately 95% of PV and in about 50% of ET and PMF cases (Baxter et al., 2005; James et al., 2005; Kralovics et al., 2005; Levine et al., 2005). Given that the *JAK2* V617F mutation is much more prevalent in these MPN than cytogenetic abnormalities, molecular detection of *JAK2* V617F has become the gold standard for demonstrating clonality whenever these diseases are suspected. Nowadays, a diagnosis of PV can often be made without bone marrow examination, diminishing the role of cytogenetic investigations in the diagnostic context of PV. The recent discovery of *CALR* mutations in substantial fractions of *JAK2* wild-type ET and PMF is likely to have an equally strong impact on diagnostic algorithms in the near future. Yet, for the time being, the recommended diagnostic approach for PMF continues to include cytogenetics, because these analyses yield important prognostic information that cannot be obtained otherwise (Barbui et al., 2011a).

Polycythemia vera (PV)

Disease summary

PV is a relatively rare disease (annual incidence 1–2 per 100 000) mainly affecting middle-aged patients (median age of 60 years at diagnosis) and with a slight male predominance (M/F ratio of 1–2:1). The hallmark of PV is excessive and autonomous production of red blood cells resulting in absolute erythrocytosis. In about 25% of patients, the disease presents with circulatory disturbances such as bleeding or venous or arterial thrombotic episodes. Patients may also complain of headache, dizziness, and visual symptoms. Other typical complaints are aquagenic pruritus, erythromelalgia, and gout. However, the course is often insidious with incidental diagnoses in about 50% of cases. Facial plethora and palpable hepato- and/or splenomegaly are the most common physical findings. If correctly treated, PV has an excellent prognosis with a median survival time of 10 years and a normal to near-normal life expectancy. In a recent single-center series, the 5-, 10-, and 15-year survival rates were 93, 79, and 64%, respectively, with a median survival of 24 years (Gangat et al., 2008).

At later stages of the disease, the red cell mass will normalize and decrease with evolution to anemia, and the spleen becomes enlarged. This is usually referred to as the "spent phase" of PV or as postpolycythemic myelofibrosis (PPMF), at which stage the disorder may be difficult to distinguish from PMF. Progression to AML occurs in a minority of patients. It is not entirely clear whether such transition is part of the natural course of PV or caused by the genotoxic treatment received by some patients.

For a long time, PV used to be a diagnosis that strictly required the demonstration of an increased red cell mass and the exclusion of a long list of causes of secondary erythrocytosis. Also required was the presence of one additional major criterion (splenomegaly, clonal cytogenetic abnormalities, or endogenous erythroid colony formation *in vitro*) or two additional minor criteria (thrombocytosis,

neutrophil leukocytosis, typical marrow biopsy, and low serum erythropoietin [EPO]) (Vardiman et al., 2002). In this context, the demonstration of any chromosomal aberration was important as an unequivocal indication of clonality, thus obviating an extensive exclusion of conditions causing secondary erythrocytosis. At the present time, the diagnosis of PV is most often made based on an increased hemoglobin level; the demonstration of the *JAK2* V617F mutation or, if negative, *JAK2* exon12 mutations; and a decreased level of serum EPO. Bone marrow histology and erythroid colony formation studies are done only if a diagnosis cannot be reached using the above criteria. Cytogenetic aberrations no longer constitute either a major or a minor criterion.

Cytogenetics

Bone marrow is the specimen of choice for cytogenetic investigations of PV. The incidence of cytogenetic abnormalities in PV at diagnosis is uncertain, probably reaching 10–25%. The appearance of cytogenetic abnormalities during the course of this disease is difficult to assess, as patients with significant changes in blood counts are more likely to undergo repeat bone marrow examinations. In older series, the frequency of cytogenetic abnormalities increased steeply during later disease phases in treated patients, yielding an overall estimate of 40% (Berger et al., 1984; Rege-Cambrin et al., 1987; Swolin et al., 1988; Diez-Martin et al., 1991; Mertens et al., 1991; Andrieux et al., 2003; Bacher et al., 2005). These high numbers may be partly attributable to the widespread use of P^{32} or alkylators at the time. In fact, Swolin et al. (1988) reported more abnormalities in PV patients treated with chemotherapy than in those treated with phlebotomy. Consistent with this, a more recent series showed a lower transformation rate (Sever et al., 2013). Many cases with terminal evolution toward acute leukemia had an abnormal bone marrow karyotype in older series (Groupe Français de Cytogénétique Hématologique, 1988; Diez-Martin et al., 1991), whereas in a more recent cohort, only two out of four patients evolving to AML displayed an abnormal karyotype (Sever et al., 2013).

The six most common aberrations are 20q–, +8, +9, alterations of 9p, gains of 1q, and 13q– (Figure 9.1). Two-thirds of the cytogenetically

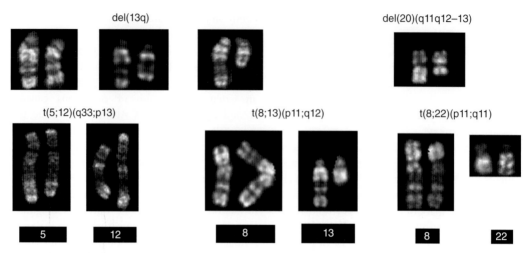

Figure 9.1 Examples of cytogenetic aberrations seen in MPN (R-banding with acridine orange). del(13q) may vary in length: del(13)(q13q21) in a case of ET, del(13)(q13q22) in a case of PMF, and del(13)(q13q33) in a case of ET; del(20)(q11q12-13) in a case of PMF; t(5;12)(q33;p13); t(8;13)(p11;q12); and t(8;22)(p11;q11).

abnormal cases display at least one of these aberrations (Mitelman et al., 2014).

20q−: A deletion of an F-group chromosome in PV was first described in 1966 and subsequently identified as a 20q− (Lawler, 1980). The incidence of the 20q− in PV is between 25 and 30% of the abnormal cases. 20q− is an interstitial deletion of variable extent, usually described as del(20)(q11q12) or del(20)(q11q13) (Roulston et al., 1993; Bench et al., 2000). Cytogenetically cryptic variants have also been reported (Nacheva et al., 1995). The common deleted region still contains six genes, and the putative tumor suppressor gene has not yet been identified (MacGrogan et al., 2001).

Trisomy 8: This is a common and nonspecific aberration in myeloid disorders. It is found in approximately 20% of abnormal karyotypes in PV, mostly as the sole change or associated with trisomy 9.

Trisomy 9 and 9p abnormalities: Trisomy 9 is seen in approximately 20% of abnormal karyotypes. About 5% of PV patients have both trisomy 8 and trisomy 9. FISH studies have shown that gain of 9p is the most frequent change in PV (Chen et al., 1998; Najfeld et al., 2002). Genome-wide screening for loss of heterozygosity (LOH) showed LOH at 9p encompassing *JAK2* at 9p24 in up to 36% of PV and also in some cases of PMF (Kralovics et al., 2002). This observation was one of the leads that converged on the simultaneous discovery by several

groups of the *JAK2* V617F mutation (Baxter et al., 2005; James et al., 2005; Kralovics et al., 2005; Levine et al., 2005).

13q: Deletion of 13q is observed in approximately 10% of abnormal karyotypes in PV. The deletion is interstitial with variable boundaries, most frequently del(13)(q13q21), but del(13)(q13q22) and del(13)(q12q32) are also reported (Pastore et al., 1995; La Starza et al., 1998). The band 13q14 harbors several genes, including the *RB1* gene, which is always deleted. The pathogenetic role of *RB1* in this context is plausible but not yet firmly established (Sinclair et al., 2001).

Gain of 1q: Partial trisomy 1q is found in 10–15% of PV with abnormal karyotypes at diagnosis but becomes the most frequent change (70–90%) in PV evolving to myelofibrotic phase and at the time of acute transformation. Gain of 1q may be the result of a partial interstitial duplication of an additional chromosome 1 with deletion in the short arm or more often of an unbalanced translocation of 1q21-qter material to an acrocentric or other chromosome. A der(1;7)(q10;p10) and a der(1;9)(q10;p10) have been recurrently reported (Swolin et al., 1986; Rege-Cambrin et al., 1991; Chen et al., 1998). The region 1q21–32 is commonly gained. The link between gain of 1q and myelotoxic therapy is debated.

Balanced translocations are rare in PV, seen in only 5–10% of cases.

Evolution of PV to PPMF or AML is usually accompanied by acquisition of (additional) chromosomal aberrations, mainly duplication 1q, deletion 5q, deletion 7q, and deletion 17p. The presence of chromosomal abnormalities may be associated with a higher risk of transformation but does not impact survival (Sever et al., 2013).

Essential thrombocythemia (ET)

Disease summary

ET is characterized by a sustained platelet count of greater than $450 \times 10^9/l$ and megakaryocytic proliferation in the bone marrow with increased numbers of enlarged mature megakaryocytes, without increase of neutrophil granulopoiesis or erythropoiesis. Other MPN, MDS, or myeloid neoplasms must be excluded. Finally, the presence of *JAK2* V617F, *MPL* W515K/L, or another clonal marker should be sought, and if negative, causes of reactive thrombocytosis should be excluded.

The true incidence of ET is unknown but is estimated at $0.6–2.5/10^5$/year, with most cases occurring in the sixth decade and without major sex predilection. The median survival is between 10 and 15 years with a limited risk of developing bone marrow fibrosis or leukemic transformation (<5%). Because ET usually occurs late in middle age, the life expectancy is near normal for many patients.

Early disease is often asymptomatic, with more than half of the cases being discovered incidentally. Arterial and venous thromboembolic events, hemorrhage, and microcirculatory disturbances are frequent complications. The majority of clinical studies on ET were based on previous diagnostic guidelines and also included early prefibrotic stages of PMF with accompanying thrombocytosis. However, when WHO 2008 criteria are strictly applied, extramedullary hematopoiesis and splenomegaly are uncommon (Barbui et al., 2011b; Thiele et al., 2011). It is important to distinguish ET from secondary or reactive thrombocytosis, which is much more common, as well as from early PMF and other MPN and myeloid disorders, and to this end, a bone marrow examination is always required. While the yield of cytogenetic examination is low in ET, it may remain useful in a clinical context of thrombocytosis to exclude the presence of other myeloid disorders (Tefferi, 2012).

Cytogenetics

Chromosome aberrations are found in less than 10% of cases at diagnosis (Third International Workshop on Chromosomes in Leukemia, 1981; Sessarego et al., 1989; Panani, 2006; Gangat et al., 2009), with a spectrum similar to the other BCR–ABL1-negative MPN: del(20q), trisomy 8, trisomy 9, gain of 1q, and del(13q) are the aberrations most commonly seen (Mitelman et al., 2014). del(5q) is more common in ET than in PV. Bone marrow is the specimen of choice for cytogenetic investigations of ET.

As in PV, there are few data on the appearance of cytogenetic abnormalities during the natural history of ET. Development of complex cytogenetic abnormalities, often including chromosomes 7 and 17 (7q–, der(1;7)(q10;p10), 17p–, and i(17q)), is almost invariably seen at the time of leukemic transformation. Conversely, patients with fibrotic transformation most commonly have an unchanged karyotype (Sterkers et al., 1998; Gangat et al., 2009).

Given the low frequency of chromosome aberrations in ET, the role of cytogenetic examination in the diagnosis of this disease lies mainly in the exclusion of other myeloid disorders as the cause of the observed thrombocytosis. For instance, cytogenetic examination may reveal del(5q) or rearrangements involving 3q26, abnormalities associated with thrombocytosis in the setting of MDS or AML. Cytogenetic abnormalities at diagnosis do not predict evolution into more aggressive myeloid disorders or inferior survival (Gangat et al., 2009).

Primary myelofibrosis (PMF)

Disease summary

This condition is also known under the names chronic idiopathic myelofibrosis, myelofibrosis with myeloid metaplasia (MMM), agnogenic myeloid metaplasia, myelosclerosis, and osteosclerosis. It is characterized by bone marrow proliferation of predominantly megakaryocytes and granulocytes and, in fully developed disease, bone marrow fibrosis and extramedullary hematopoiesis (myeloid metaplasia). There is a stepwise evolution from an initial prefibrotic to a fibrotic stage, accompanied by hepatosplenomegaly and a leukoerythroblastic picture with characteristic teardrop forms in the peripheral blood. The incidence of the overt fibrotic phase is estimated at 0.5–1.5/10⁵/year, without clear sex predilection. The majority of patients are between 50 and 70 years of age. PMF carries a 10–20% risk of subsequent development of AML.

Cytogenetics

Sampling of bone marrow is inefficient, especially in the later fibrotic stage ("dry tap"), but cytogenetic data can also be obtained from peripheral blood cultures due to the presence of circulating progenitors. Several series of PMF cases, some of which also include post-PV or post-ET MF, have been reported, totaling more than 600 patients (Demory et al., 1988; Reilly et al., 1994; Dupriez et al., 1996; Reilly et al., 1997; Tefferi et al., 2001; Andrieux et al., 2003; Tefferi et al., 2005; Strasser-Weippl et al., 2006; Djordjevic et al., 2007; Hussein et al., 2009). Chromosomal aberrations are found in 30–55% of PMF. Approximately 30% of cases present with cytogenetic abnormalities, and their frequency increases as the disease progresses. Cytogenetic changes are qualitatively similar to those in PV, albeit with different prevalence. In the larger series, del(20q) and del(13q) are most common and found in 19–33% and 14–23% of the abnormal karyotypes, respectively. Trisomy 8 (8–16%), trisomy 9 (3–14%), and abnormalities of chromosome 1, including gain of 1q (6–28%), are also fairly frequent. Comparative genomic hybridization (CGH) studies have shown gains of cytogenetic material in more than 50% of the PMF patients examined, mostly of 9p, 2q, 3p, chromosome 4, 12q, and 13q, and at higher frequencies than seen by chromosome banding (Al-Assar et al., 2005; Tefferi et al., 2009; Brecqueville et al., 2014).

Disease progression is accompanied by the acquisition of structural changes that may include gain of 1q (3–19%), del(5q) (3–6%), anomalies of chromosome 7 (5–10%), del(17p), and rarely i(17q) (Demory et al., 1988; Reilly et al., 1994, 1997; Dupriez et al., 1996; Tefferi et al., 2001, 2005; Andrieux et al., 2003; Strasser-Weippl et al., 2006; Djordjevic et al., 2007; Hussein et al., 2009). Balanced translocations are rarely seen in PMF; they occur as sole abnormalities rather than in complex karyotypes, and few, if any, seem to be recurrent. A recurrent unbalanced translocation is t(1;6)(q21;p21) leading to partial trisomy

1q and deletion 6p (Dingli et al., 2005; Djordjevic et al., 2007).

In one case each of advanced PMF, secondary MF post-PV, and post-ET, various translocations with a 17q22 breakpoint were detected, involving the *NOG* gene. Deregulated expression of NOG protein may lead to modified expression of bone morphogenetic proteins (BMPs) and hence contribute to myelofibrosis and osteosclerosis (Andrieux et al., 2007).

In contrast to the situation in PV and ET, the prognosis of PMF is, at least in part, determined by cytogenetic aberrations. In one study, patients with an unfavorable karyotype (complex or presence of one or two abnormalities such as +8, −7/7q−, i(17q), inv(3), −5/5q−, 12p−, or 11q23 rearrangements) had a median survival of 2 years compared to 5.2 years for those with a normal karyotype or other cytogenetic aberrations (Caramazza et al., 2011). In the newly devised DIPSS plus score, the presence of an unfavorable karyotype (as defined by Caramazza et al. above), platelet counts, and transfusion need have been incorporated for improved prognostic stratification (Gangat et al., 2011). A monosomal karyotype has also been reported to be associated with a worse prognosis (Vaidya et al., 2011).

Molecular changes in classic MPN

The landmark discovery of the *JAK2* V617F gain-of-function mutation revealed the central role of pathological signaling in the JAK/STAT axis in MPN. *JAK2* V617F is found in about 50–60% of ET, in 95–99% of PV, and in 45–50% of PMF (Baxter et al., 2005; James et al., 2005; Kralovics et al., 2005; Levine et al., 2005). A homozygous, biallelic mutation with LOH at 9p is observed in one-third of PV and 15% of PMF cases but only rarely in ET; it results in duplication of the mutant allele (Kralovics et al., 2005). The variability in the genotype–phenotype relationship has, at least in part, been attributed to the intensity of JAK2 signaling, which is higher in PV than ET, but other factors such as the stage of hematopoietic development at which the mutation is acquired, genetic background, or combination with other unknown somatic mutations could also play a role (Cross, 2011). The mutation has also been found in less than 5% of MDS, AML, and MDS/MPN. However, a substantial fraction of cases with refractory anemia with ring sideroblasts and marked thrombocytosis (MDS-RARS-T) are positive for the *JAK2* V617F mutation (Steensma et al., 2005; Szpurka et al., 2006).

Further underscoring dysregulation of JAK2 signaling as a central theme in the pathogenesis of MPN, mutations of *JAK2* exon 12 are found in about one-third to one-half of *JAK2* V617F-negative PV and are associated with isolated or idiopathic erythrocytosis (Scott et al., 2007). In addition, 5–10% of *JAK2* V617F-negative ET or PMF patients carry an *MPL* W515L/K gain-of-function mutation in exon 10 of *MPL*, the thrombopoietin receptor gene (Pardanani et al., 2006; Pikman et al., 2006). MPL also signals through JAK2 and induces activation of STAT3/STAT5.

In 2013, deletions and insertions in exon 9 of *CALR*, the gene encoding calreticulin, were described in about 70% of ET and 90% of MF without *JAK2* or *MPL* mutations (Klampfl et al., 2013; Nangalia et al., 2013). CALR is a highly conserved protein with multiple functions. Within the endoplasmic reticulum (ER), it ensures proper folding of newly synthesized glycoproteins and modulates calcium homeostasis. Outside the ER, CALR is found in intracellular, cell surface, and extracellular compartments where it has been implicated in diverse processes such as proliferation, apoptosis, immunogenic cell death, and cancer. In spite of all this, somatic *CALR* mutations had not previously been reported in cancer.

CALR mutations in ET and MF are mutually exclusive with *JAK2* and *MPL* mutations. With the exception of MDS/MPN–RARS-T, they are not found in other myeloid malignancies, supporting a causal relationship between *CALR* mutations and excessive platelet production. *CALR* exon 9 deletions/insertions lead to a +1 bp frameshift and to a novel 36-amino-acid carboxy-terminus lacking a KDEL endoplasmic retrieval sequence. Mutant CALR was found to induce growth factor-independent growth *in vitro*. This growth was inhibited by a JAK2 kinase inhibitor, hinting at a link with pathological JAK2 signaling, but the exact mechanisms are unknown at the present time (Klampfl et al., 2013; Nangalia et al., 2013).

Retrospective analyses indicate that *CALR* mutations are associated with a phenotype and clinical course distinct from *JAK2* V617F-positive disease. In particular, ET patients with *CALR* mutations

have lower hemoglobin levels, lower white cell counts, and higher platelet counts. Moreover, MPN with *CALR* mutations had a lower risk of thrombosis and longer overall survival. These findings are consistent with previous studies comparing the course in patients with and without *JAK2* mutations (Rotunno et al., 2014; Rumi et al., 2014).

Somatic mutations in epigenetic regulator genes such as *TET2*, *IDH1*, *IDH2*, *ASXL1*, *DNMT3A*, and *EZH2* occur in a proportion of cases of MPN. They can co-occur with *JAK2*, *MPL*, and *CALR* mutations and are also found in other myeloid malignancies. Hence, they are unlikely to be initial driver mutations in ET (Cross, 2011).

The discovery of *CALR* mutations provides a novel molecular marker for diagnostic and prognostic assessment of MPN. Identification of the remaining drivers in MPN negative for *JAK2*, *CALR*, and *MPL* mutations may further lead to novel diagnostic tools and increased recognition of the clinical heterogeneity within ET (Tefferi and Pardanani, 2014). Eight novel genes, which had been proposed as possible candidate drivers based on the first exome of a *JAK2* V617F-negative ET, were not confirmed to be recurrent in *JAK2* V617F/*MPL* W515K/L-negative ET (Hou et al., 2012; Al Assaf et al., 2014).

The use of JAK inhibitors in *JAK2* V617F mutant as well as nonmutant MF has led to improvements in spleen size, symptom burden, quality of life, and overall survival. However, they seem unable to induce hematologic remissions or to substantially reduce BM fibrosis or the *JAK2* V617F allele burden (Harrison et al., 2012; Verstovsek et al., 2012, 2013). The use of novel inhibitors and combination strategies, their application in additional MPN settings, and the role of signaling in *CALR* mutant MPN merit further study.

"Nonclassic" *BCR–ABL1*-negative MPN

Besides the classic *BCR*–ABL1-negative MPN, there are also other clonal myeloproliferations such as chronic neutrophilic leukemia (CNL), chronic eosinophilic leukemia (CEL), mastocytosis, and the unclassifiable MPN (Vardiman et al., 2008). Mastocytosis is the most common disease in this group. The other "nonclassic" *BCR*–ABL1-negative MPN are rare and only rarely have cytogenetic aberrations. For this reason, they are covered only summarily.

Chronic neutrophilic leukemia (CNL)

CNL is characterized by mature neutrophilic leukocytosis with less than 5% immature cells in the blood. There is granulocytic hyperplasia in the bone marrow but no dysplasia or fibrosis. Splenomegaly is common. CNL is a rare disease, median age is 67 years, and both sexes are equally affected. The prognosis of this clinically indolent disorder is very variable, but acceleration and transformation to AML have been reported. CML and reactive leukocytosis must be excluded to establish the diagnosis.

Cytogenetic studies of bone marrow cells or molecular studies are required to exclude the t(9;22), including rare variants with an e19a2 fusion transcript. The karyotype is abnormal in only a minority of cases with CNL, with +8, +9, +21, del(20q), del(11q), and del(12p) as the most common chromosome aberrations (Bench et al., 1998; Bohm et al., 2003). Interestingly, the *JAK2* V617F mutation was detected in one of the six CNL tested (Steensma et al., 2005). More recently, mutations in *CSF3R* have been identified in about 50% of patients with CNL or atypical CML. They represent a potentially useful criterion for diagnosing these neoplasms, as well as a potential biomarker for responsiveness to JAK or SARK inhibitor therapy (Maxson et al., 2013).

Chronic eosinophilic leukemia/idiopathic hypereosinophilic syndrome (CEL/iHES)

CEL is an MPN characterized by persistent unexplained hypereosinophilia in the blood ($>1500 \times 10^9$/l), bone marrow, and peripheral tissues and signs of peripheral organ damage due to eosinophilic tissue infiltration (mainly of the heart and lungs, splenomegaly, neuropathy, skin rash). A CEL diagnosis also requires the detection of evidence of clonality, for example, the presence of 5–20% blasts in the bone marrow or 2–20% blasts in blood or as per cytogenetic or molecular methods. If clonality cannot be proven, the diagnosis of idiopathic hypereosinophilic syndrome (iHES) is made. The latter diagnosis can be established only after exclusion of an extensive list of benign conditions or syndromes associated with reactive eosinophilia (Valent et al., 2012a). iHES includes eosinophilic leukemias in which clonality cannot (yet) be proven as well as unrecognized cases of immune-driven reactive eosinophilias. Its clinical spectrum may therefore vary from indolent to aggressive. Updated proposals for a global nomenclature and classification of hypereosinophilia-related disorders and conditions have been published, merging previously published proposals and the classification proposal of the WHO (Valent et al., 2012b, c).

CEL is a rare disease. As the category in its current definition dates from 2008 only, its epidemiological features are incompletely known. Causes of death are related to organ damage with congestive heart failure, thromboembolic events, or leukemic progression (Vandenberghe et al., 2004).

Only 15% of iHES/CEL patients show an abnormal karyotype with generally myeloid neoplasia-specific aberrations such as +8 (most frequent), −7, i(17q), del(20q), and −Y (Bain, 2003; Vandenberghe et al., 2004; Gotlib, 2005). Rare cases are *JAK2* V617F positive. The presence of a t(9;22) and rearrangements of *PDGFRA*, *PDGFRB*, and *FGFR1* should be specifically excluded (see section "Myeloid and lymphoid neoplasms with eosinophilia and abnormalities of PDGFRA, PDGFRB, and FGFR1").

Mastocytosis

Mastocytosis is characterized by clonal neoplastic proliferation of abnormal mast cells accumulating in one or more organ systems. Mastocytosis is now considered a true MPN, as mast cells arise from hematopoietic stem cells and share several features with basophils. Subtypes are recognized based on the distribution of the disease and the clinical manifestations. The clinical picture is varied but includes cutaneous mastocytosis, systemic mastocytosis, mast cell leukemia, mast cell sarcoma, and extracutaneous mastocytoma. The symptoms and signs are due to organ invasion on the one hand, inducing osteoporosis, hepatomegaly, ascites, and cytopenia, and release of mast cell mediators on the other, leading to diarrhea, urticaria, pruritus, flushing, and syncope. The clinical course can be indolent or aggressive, associated with another MPN or with mast cell leukemia (Valent et al., 2004).

Cytogenetic data are scarce. + 8, +9, +14, del(7q), del(11q), del(20q), and translocations as well as other structural rearrangements involving chromosome 4 have occasionally been reported (Swolin et al., 2000, 2002).

A large fraction of adult cases with systemic mastocytosis have point mutations of the *KIT* gene in 4q12: the D816V mutation is present in more than 95%. Mutations in exon 10 or 11 are rare but are therapeutically relevant because the latter patients may benefit from imatinib treatment, whereas those with a *KIT* D816V mutant do not (Longley et al., 1996; Macdonald et al., 2002; Garcia-Montero et al., 2006). In addition, Steensma et al. (2005) identified a *JAK2* V617F mutation in two of eight SM cases without *KIT* mutation.

Some cases with manifestations of SM accompanied by eosinophilia have a *FIPIL1–PDGFRA* rearrangement (Pardanani et al., 2003). These cases appear to be very rare but can be classified as "myeloid and lymphoid neoplasms with eosinophilia and abnormalities of *PDGFRA*, *PDGFRB*, and *FGFR1*."

Myeloid and lymphoid neoplasms with eosinophilia and abnormalities of *PDGFRA*, *PDGFRB*, and *FGFR1*

This category includes rare to very rare disease groups associated with rearrangements of *PDGFRA*, *PDGFRB*, and *FGFR1*. Their presentation is often myeloproliferative, but lymphoid components are not uncommon. While they previously belonged to the "chronic myeloproliferative disorders" in the WHO classification of 2001(Vardiman et al., 2001), they are classified separately from the MPN since the WHO classification 2008. Cytogenetic or molecular cytogenetic investigations are key to their diagnosis.

PDGFRA (4q12) rearrangements and mutations

By far, the most frequent aberration in this group is a cytogenetically cryptic deletion of 800 kb at 4q12 (Cools et al., 2003) (Figure 9.2). The deletion fuses

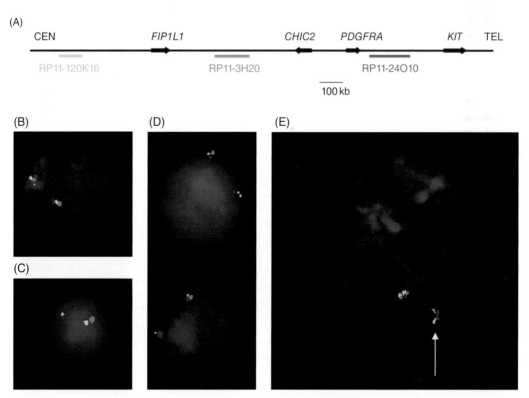

Figure 9.2 FISH detection of the 4q12 deletion associated with the *FIP1L1–PDGFRA* fusion. Genomic map with the FISH probes (A) and examples of three-color FISH analysis performed on a control sample (B) and two patients (C/D–E). A map of the 4q12 region, with relevant genes and selected FISH probes, is drawn to scale. Note loss of the 3H20 (*green*) signal in C–E. (E) *Arrow* indicates a seemingly normal-looking chromosome 4 with the cryptic del(4)(q12) (*Source*: Vandenberghe et al. (2004), reproduced with permission).

the 5′ part of a previously unknown human gene *FIP1L1* and the 3′ part of the *PDGFRA* gene to encode a novel fusion tyrosine kinase, FIP1L1–PDGFRA. The breakpoints are scattered in *FIP1L1* but restricted to exon 12 in *PDGFRA*; the fusion is always in frame and is best detected by RT-PCR or FISH. Due to disruption of an autoinhibitory mechanism mediated by the juxtamembrane domain of PDGFRA, FIP1L1–PDGFRA is a constitutively active tyrosine kinase (Stover et al., 2006).

Reciprocal balanced translocations involving 4q12, the site of *PDGFRA*, have been reported in single cases (see Table 9.2).

Although by far the most frequent clonal aberration in patients with hypereosinophilia, the del(4)(q12q12)/*FIP1L1–PDGFRA* fusion remains extremely rare in unselected patient groups with hypereosinophilia. It is almost exclusively found in males and most often associated with a clinical phenotype of marked hypereosinophilia, splenomegaly, tissue fibrosis, moderately increased serum tryptase and cyanocobalamin level, high risk of cardiac lesions, and thromboembolic events (Klion et al., 2003; Vandenberghe et al., 2004). In addition, this diagnosis has been made in rare patients presenting with AML, T-lymphoblastic lymphoma, and extramedullary localizations or systemic mastocytosis and eosinophilia (Pardanani et al., 2003; Metzgeroth et al., 2007; Lierman et al., 2009; Tang et al., 2012; Chen et al., 2013; Srinivas et al., 2014).

The *FIP1L1–PDGFRA* fusion is present in all myeloid lineages, but eosinophils are particularly sensitive to the proliferative signal. The major interest in identifying *FIP1L1–PDGFRA*-positive CEL lies in the fact that patients with this aberration respond to treatment with imatinib: rapid, complete, and durable hematologic and molecular responses are obtained with doses of 100–400 mg daily (Jovanovic et al., 2007). Retrospective analyses indicate that the disease is refractory to corticosteroids and responds poorly to IFN-α or hydroxyurea, with frequent progression to blast crisis after a few years (Vandenberghe et al., 2004). Nilotinib, too, has been reported to induce hematological, cytogenetic, and molecular responses (Hochhaus et al., 2013).

Secondary resistance of *FIP1L1–PDGFRA*-positive disease to imatinib is rare and associated with progression to acute eosinophilic leukemia, which can be associated with osteolytic lesions, hypercalcemia, skin lesions, and/or leptomeningeal invasion (Ohnishi et al., 2006; Lierman et al., 2009). The mechanism of resistance is based on the selection for or emergence of a T674I kinase domain mutant of *FIPIL1–PDGFRA* (Cools et al., 2003). Other rare resistance variants, such as a *FIP1L1–PDGFRA* D842V or *FIP1L1–PDGFRA* S601P, have been reported (Lierman et al., 2009; Salemi et al., 2009). *In vitro* data suggest that sorafenib, nilotinib, and ponatinib have activity

Table 9.2 Variant translocations leading to *PDGFRA*-related fusion genes

Fusion partner location*	Translocation	Number of cases reported	Presentation	References
STRN (2p22)	t(2;4)(p24;q12)	1	CEL	Curtis et al. (2007)
CDK5RAP2 (9q33)	ins(9;4)(q33;q12q25)	1	CEL (AP)	Walz et al. (2006)
KIF5B (10p11)	der(?)t(?;4)(?;q12) t(4;10)(q28;q11)	1	CEL	Score et al. (2006)
ETV6 (12p13)	t(4;12)(q2?3;p1?2)	1	CEL	Curtis et al. (2007)
BCR (22q11)	t(4;22)(q12;q11)	7	AML, aCML (eo+), aCML → pre-B-ALL, aCML, biphenotypic leukemia	Baxter et al. (2002), Trempat et al. (2003), Safley et al. (2004), Neumann et al. (2007), Wang et al. (2011), and Matikas et al. (2013)

AP, accelerated phase; aCML, atypical CML; eo+, with eosinophilia.

*Cytogenetic location of the gene according to OMIM/HGNC in parentheses.

against T6741 and that disease brought about by the *FIP1L1–PDGFRA* D842V mutant is sensitive to ponatinib (Lierman et al., 2006, 2009, 2012b). Only a few patients with T674I *FIP1L1–PDGFRA* have so far been treated with second-generation tyrosine kinase inhibitors and with varying outcomes (Lierman et al., 2009; Metzgeroth et al., 2012; Al-Riyami et al., 2013).

A fraction of *FIP1L1–PDGFRA*-negative CEL, too, is responsive to imatinib, which strongly suggests that, in these cases, an imatinib-sensitive target is involved. Among them, some alternative fusion genes involving *PDGFRA* or *PDGFRB* have been identified. The most common alternative *PDGFRA* fusion stems from a t(4;22) (q12;q11) encoding a *BCR–PDGFRA* fusion gene, reported in seven patients so far. Most of these cases presented with atypical CML features, splenomegaly, and prominent eosinophilia. One patient presented with atypical CML that evolved into pre-B-ALL. One case presenting with AML and one with mixed-phenotype leukemia have also been reported (Baxter et al., 2002; Trempat et al., 2003; Safley et al., 2004; Neumann et al., 2007; Wang et al., 2011; Matikas et al., 2013). There are several other anecdotical reports of single cases with *PDGFRA* rearrangements involving other partners but presenting with a clinical picture of CEL (Table 9.2). Variant translocations will not be detected by *FIP1L1–PDGFRA* PCR using standard primers, but can be seen in FISH experiments that are designed to detect not only the loss of the *CHIC2* locus but also translocations with breakpoints at 4q12. Alternative PCR approaches measuring the expression of the 3′ region of *PDGFRA* have been proposed to screen for variant translocations involving *PDGFRA* (5q31–33) (Erben et al., 2010). Finally, Elling et al. (2011) reported the occurrence of PDGFRA tyrosine kinase mutations in 7 out of 87 *FIP1L1–PDGFRA*-negative HES patients, providing evidence that imatinib-sensitive *PDGFRA* point mutations may also play a role in the pathogenesis of HES. However, more research should be performed to determine the frequency of *PDGFRA* mutations in *FIP1L1–PDGFRA*-negative HES patients as well as how the response to treatment is in such cases (Elling et al., 2011).

Translocations involving *PDGFRB* (5q33)

The first translocation reported to involve *PDGFRB* was a t(5;12)(q33;p13) encoding the fusion protein ETV6–PDGFRB (Golub et al., 1994) (Figure 9.1). Several *PDGFRB* rearrangements involving other partner chromosomes have been reported since, mostly in only one or at most two patients each (Table 9.3). The chromosomal breakpoint in 5q has not always been interpreted as 5q33 but was more broadly mapped to the 5q31–33 region. All *PDGFRB* rearrangements reported to date were cytogenetically visible, the only exception being a case with uninformative karyotype. A t(5;12)(q33;p13) with an *ERC1–PDGFRB* fusion gene has also been reported, a change that cannot be distinguished from the *ETV6–PDGFRB* rearrangement by banding cytogenetics (Gorello et al., 2008). Dual-color FISH analysis with probes for *PDGFRB* can resolve the breakpoint position even in cases with complex karyotypes. PCR approaches measuring the expression of the 3′ region of *PDGFRB* have been proposed to screen for variant translocations involving *PDGFRB* (Erben et al., 2010).

The disease is exceedingly rare but occurs more often in males (2:1 M/F ratio). Patients most commonly present with CMML-like features, although some were described with features of atypical CML, CEL, MPN with eosinophilia, or AML. While T-lymphoblastic lymphoma has been repeatedly reported among "myeloid and lymphoid neoplasms with eosinophilia and abnormalities of *PDGFRA*, *PDGFRB*, and *FGFR1*," only a single case of a concurrent AML and T-lymphoblastic lymphoma in a patient with rearranged *PDGFRB* was reported so far (Chang et al., 2012). Eosinophilia is usually but not invariably present. Patients have variable splenomegaly, marrow fibrosis, endomyocardial fibrosis, and thrombosis as well as skin infiltration. Before the advent of imatinib, they used to have a poor prognosis under therapy with hydroxyurea and/or IFN-α, with a median survival of 2 years.

As a result of the translocation, the fusion protein exhibits constitutive tyrosine kinase activation due to oligomerization motifs present in the partner gene. The *PDGFRB* fusion induces cytokine-independent growth in cell lines as well as induction of myeloproliferative disease in mice (Magnusson et al., 2001; Schwaller et al., 2001). It is

Table 9.3 Variant translocations leading to *PDGFRB*-related fusion genes

Fusion partner location*	Translocation	Number of cases reported	Presentation	References
TPM3 (1q21)	t(1;5)(q21;q33)	2	CEL	Rosati et al. (2006) and Li et al. (2011)
PDE4DIP (1q21)	t(1;5)(q23;q33)	1	MPN–eo	Wilkinson et al. (2003)
SPTBN1 (2p16)	t(2;5)(p21;q33)	1	MPN-eo	Gallagher et al. (2008)
WDR48 (3p22)	t(1;3;5)(p36;p21;q33)	1	MPN→AML-eo	Hidalgo-Curtis et al. (2010)
GOLGA4 (3p22)	t(3;5)(p21-25;q31-35)	2	CEL	Hidalgo-Curtis et al. (2010)
PRKG2 (4q21)	t(4;5)(q21;q33) or t(4;5;5)(q23;q31;q33)	2	CBL, MPN-eo	Walz et al. (2007) and Gallagher et al. (2008)
CEP85L (6q22)	t(5;6)(q33-34;q23)	2	T-ALL, MPN-eo	Chmielecki et al. (2012) and Winkelmann et al. (2013)
HIP1 (7q11)	t(5;7)(q33;q11.2)	1	aCML with eo	Ross et al. (1998)
KANK1 (9p24)	t(5;9)(31-32;22-24)	1	Thrombocytosis	Medves et al. (2010)
CCDC6 (10q21)	t(5;10)(q33;q21-22)	3	aCML with eo, CMML; CML (AP)	Siena et al. (1999), Kulkarni et al. (2000), Schwaller et al. (2001), and Drechsler et al. (2007)
CAPRIN1 (11p13)	der(11)ins(11;5) (p12;q15q33)	1	CEL	Walz et al. (2007)
ERC1 (12p13)	t(5;12)(q33;p13.3)	1	AML	Gorello et al. (2008)
BIN2 (12q13)	t(5;12)(q33;q13)	1	CEL	Hidalgo-Curtis et al. (2010)
GIT2 (12q24)	t(5;12)(q31–33;q24)	1	CEL	Walz et al. (2007)
SART3 (12q23)	46,XY†	1	MF	Erben et al. (2010)
NIN (14q22)	t(5;14)(q33;q24)	1	MPN-eo	Vizmanos et al. (2004b)
CCDC88C (14q32)	t(5;14)(q33;q32) or t(5;17;14) (q33;q11;q32)	4	CMML-eo, MPN-eo	Levine et al. (2005), Wang et al. (2010), and Gosenca et al. (2014)
TRIP11 (14q32)	t(5;14)(q33;p32)	1	AML relapse	Abe et al. (1997)
TP53BP1 (15q15-21)	t(5;15)(q33;q22)	1	CML-eo	Grand et al. (2004a)
NDE1 (16p13)	t(5;16)(q33;p13)	1	CMML	La Starza et al. (2007)
SPECC1 (17p11)	t(5;17)(q33;p11.2)	1	JMML-eo	Morerio et al. (2004)
RABEP1 (17p13)	t(5;17)(q33;p13)	1	CMML	Magnusson et al. (2001)
MYO18A (17q11)	t(5;17)(q33-34;q11.2)	1	MPN-eo	Walz et al. (2009)
DTD1 (20p11)	t(5;20)(q33;p11)	1	MPN-eo	Gosenca et al. (2014)

aCML, atypical CML; CMML, chronic myelomonocytic leukemia; CBL, chronic basophilic leukemia; JMML, juvenile myelomonocytic leukemia; -eo, associated with eosinophilia.
*Cytogenetic location of the gene according to OMIM/HGNC in parentheses.
†Cytogenetic investigation was uninformative in this case.

inhibited by imatinib in the nanomolar range. Patients with *PDGFRB* fusions have also been shown to enjoy excellent responses to low-dose imatinib. So far, only one case with secondary imatinib resistance was reported (Grand et al., 2004b; Cheah et al., 2014).

Translocations involving *FGFR1* (8p11)

8p11 myeloproliferative syndrome (EMS, also called stem cell leukemic/lymphoma syndrome) is molecularly characterized by a fusion gene that involves the *FGFR1* gene in 8p11. The disease presents a heterogeneous clinical phenotype with features of both MPN with eosinophilia and lymphoma/lymphoblastic leukemia. EMS is extremely rare, with a median patient age of 32 years and only a slight male predominance. Clinical features are eosinophilia, myeloid hyperplasia in the bone marrow, splenomegaly, and a strikingly high incidence of lymphoma either of B- or T-cell phenotype (Macdonald et al., 2002). Eosinophilia is commonly but not invariably present. Lymphadenopathy may be present at diagnosis or develop later. Rare cases present as T-lymphoblastic lymphoma without myeloproliferation, as PV, or with features of systemic mastocytosis. Rapid transformation to acute leukemia, mostly AML, occurs within 1 or 2 years from diagnosis (median 6–9 months). Both myeloid and lymphoid lineage cells exhibit the 8p11 translocation, demonstrating the stem cell origin of the disease.

Balanced translocations between 8p11 and more than 10 partner chromosomes have been reported to date. The most frequent is the t(8;13)(p11;q12) resulting in *ZMYM2–FGFR1* gene fusion (Reiter et al., 1998) (Table 9.3). Other recurrent *FGFR1* fusions are t(6;8)(q27;p11), t(8;9)(p11;q33), and t(8;22)(p11;q11), whereas other fusions yet have been found in single or at most two cases (Table 9.4). In all characterized cases, the tyrosine kinase domain of *FGFR1* is juxtaposed to a dimerization domain of the partner gene, resulting in constitutive activation of *FGFR1*. Some of the fusion mutants have been shown to transform cell lines or induce EMS-like disease in mice (Guasch et al., 2004). Subtly different phenotypes may be associated with different *FGFR1* partner genes; for example, two cases of t(6;8) were initially diagnosed with PV. Thrombocytosis is frequently associated with t(8;9). The incidence of T-cell non-Hodgkin lymphoma has been suggested to be higher in patients with t(8;13) compared to patients with other translocations. The t(8;22) encoding a BCR–FGFR1 fusion protein often leads to a CML-like disease (Cross and Reiter, 2002). Of note, 8p11 breakpoints involving *FGFR1* are distinct from those involving the *MYST3* gene on 8p11, which is associated with AML with monocyte differentiation and erythrophagocytosis (Chapter 6). Three translocations involving the latter gene have been reported, t(8;16)(p11;p13) with a *MYST3–CREBBP* fusion as the most common one and the two rare variants t(8;22)

(p11;q13) and t(8;19)(p11;q13) (Gervais et al., 2008). Another entity not to be confused with EMS is t(8;11)(p11;p15), a rare translocation in AML, which fuses *NUP98* to *NSD3* (Rosati et al., 2002).

Patients with 8p11 syndrome have an extremely poor prognosis and should proceed to allogeneic stem cell transplantation provided they are medically fit and a donor can be found. The FGFR1 fusion kinase is a theoretical target for small molecule inhibitor therapy, and there are data indicating that midostaurin, dovitinib, and ponatinib show activity against *FGFR1* fusion-positive cell lines, FGFR1 fusion-transformed Ba/F3, and/or *FGFR1* fusion-positive leukemia cells. However, published evidence on the activity of these compounds in clinical settings is still lacking (Chase et al., 2007, 2013; Wasag et al., 2011; Lierman et al., 2012b; Ren et al., 2013).

Translocations involving 9p24 (*JAK2*)

Other recurrent genetic abnormalities have been identified in patients with hypereosinophilia, including t(8;9)(p22;p24), leading to a *PCM1–JAK2* fusion gene (Reiter et al., 2005). Almost 25 patients have been reported so far, with a strong male preponderance and a broad age distribution (median age at presentation is 45–50 years). The most common presentation is as a myeloid neoplasm: aCML, AML, CEL, or acute erythroid leukemia, with a strong risk of progression to myeloid or lymphoid blast crisis. Eosinophilia is commonly but not invariably present. At least two cases presented primarily as a lymphoid malignancy, one of T- and one of B-cell origin (Patterer et al., 2013). Cases with a t(9;12)(p24;p13) leading to an *ETV6–JAK2* fusion gene can present in similarly varied ways (Lacronique et al., 1997; Peeters et al., 1997).

Some malignancies with rearrangements of 9p24 (*JAK2*) are not included in the group of "myeloid and lymphoid neoplasms with eosinophilia and abnormalities of *PDGFRA*, *PDGFRB*, and *FGFR1*" in the current WHO 2008 guidelines, but this may be reconsidered in future classification proposals. Indeed, t(8;9)-positive malignancies share several salient features with the disease included in this category including a male preponderance, frequent association with eosinophilia, and variable hematological presentations. Moreover, in two cases,

Table 9.4 *FGFR1* fusions

Fusion partner gene location*	Translocation	Number of cases reported	Presentation	References
TPR (1q25)	t(1;8)(q25;p11)	3	MPN-eo	Li et al. (2012) and Lee et al. (2013)
RANBP2 (2q12)	t(2;8)(q12;p11)	1	MDS/MPN	Gervais et al. (2013)
LRRFIP1 (2q37)	t(2;8)(q37;p11)	1	MPN-eo	Soler et al. (2009)
FGFR1OP (6q27)	t(6;8)(q27;p11)	10	MPN-eo AML PV B-ALL	Chaffanet et al. (1998), Popovici et al. (1999), Sohal et al. (2001), Vizmanos et al. (2004a), Lourenco et al. (2008), and Patnaik et al. (2010)
CUX1 (7q22)	t(7;8)(q22;p11)	1	T-ALL	Wasag et al. (2011)
TIF1 (7q34)	t(7;8)(q34;p11)	1	AML	Belloni et al. (2005)
CEP110 (9q33)	t(8;9)(p11;q33) t(3;8;9)(p25;p21;q34)	23	MPN aCML MPN+T-ALL Mixed-phenotype leukemia (B/My)	Jotterand Bellomo et al. (1992), Chaffanet et al. (1998), Sohal et al. (2001), Mozziconacci et al. (2008), Park et al. (2008), Patnaik et al. (2010), Post et al. (2010), Hu et al. (2011), and Lee et al. (2013)
NUP98 (11p15)	t(8;11)(p11;p15)	1	AML	Sohal et al. (2001)
FGFR1OP2 (12p11)	t(8;12)(p11;q15) or ins(12;8) (p11;p11p21)	6	T-ALL+eo MPN-eo/T-ALL	Sohal et al. (2001), Grand et al. (2004a), Onozawa et al. (2011), and Lee et al. (2013)
CPSF6 (12q15)	t(8;12)(p11;q15)	1	MPN+ T-ALL+ eo	Hidalgo-Curtis et al. (2008)
ZMYM2 (13q12)	t(8;13)(p11;q12)	~35	AML MPN+T-ALL+eo MPN B-ALL+eo MPN+B-ALL +/- eo My/Ly neoplasm with SM	Reiter et al. (1998), Xiao et al. (1998), and Jackson et al. (2010)
MYO18A (17q23)	t(8;17)(p11;q25)	1	MDS/MPN+eo/baso	Walz et al. (2005)
HERVK (19q13)	t(8;19)(p11-12;q13.3)	2	AML SM, KIT D816V positive	Mugneret et al. (2000) and Duckworth et al. (2014)
BCR (22q11)	t(8;22)(p11;q11)	16	MPN+/- eo B-ALL Mixed phenotype, B/myeloid	Fioretos et al. (2001), Pini et al. (2002), Murati et al. (2005), Baldazzi et al. (2010), Kim et al. (2011), Wakim et al. (2011), Dolan et al. (2012), Haslam et al. (2012), Lee et al. (2013), Matikas et al. (2013), Morishige et al. (2013), and Shimanuki et al. (2013)

aCML, atypical CML; CMML, chronic myelomonocytic leukemia; CBL, chronic basophilic leukemia; -eo, associated with eosinophilia.

*Cytogenetic location of the gene according to OMIM/HGNC in parentheses.

hematological and cytogenetic responses to ruxoli-tinib have been reported (Gotlib, 2005; Lierman et al., 2012a; Rumi et al., 2013).

Concluding remarks

The molecular detection of *JAK2*, *MPL*, and *KIT* mutations has superseded cytogenetics as the method of choice to demonstrate clonality in PV, ET, PMF, the so-called classic *BCR–ABL1*-negative MPN, and mastocytosis. The more recent discovery of *CALR* mutations in *JAK2/MPL* wild-type ET and PMF, and of *CSF3R* mutations in CNL, will likely boost this evolution. Yet, cytogenetic investigations remain mandatory for the prognostic stratification of PMF.

In the diagnostic workup of the nonclassic *BCR–ABL1*-negative MPN, the myeloid/lymphoid neoplasms with eosinophilia and abnormalities of *PDGFRA*, *PDGFRB*, and *FGFR1*, and the MDS/MPN, it is essential to recognize those entities in which treatment with small molecule inhibitors can be of value. Cytogenetic investigations are the only practical approach to detect the translocations leading to the numerous fusion genes involving *PDGFRA*, *PDGFRB*, *FGFR1*, and *JAK2*. Karyo-typing remains pivotal in this setting, in combination with FISH/PCR for the cytogenetically cryptic *FIP1L1–PDGFRA* fusion.

Acknowledgments

Peter Vandenberghe is a senior clinical investigator of the Research Foundation—Flanders (FWO-Vlaanderen). This study was supported by grants from FWO (G.0509.10 N), Stichting tegen Kanker (2010-204), and GOA/11/010 from KU Leuven.

References

Abe A, Emi N, Tanimoto M, Terasaki H, Marunouchi T, Saito H (1997): Fusion of the platelet-derived growth factor receptor beta to a novel gene CEV14 in acute myelogenous leukemia after clonal evolution. *Blood* 90:4271–4277.

Al Assaf C, Lierman E, Devos T, Billiet J, Graux C, Papadopoulos P, et al. (2014): Screening of JAK2 V617F and MPL W515 K/L negative essential thrombocythaemia patients for mutations in SESN2, DNAJC17, ST13, TOP1MT, and NTRK1. *Br J Haematol* 165(5):734–737.

Al-Assar O, Ul-Hassan A, Brown R, Wilson GA, Hammond DW, Reilly JT (2005): Gains on 9p are common genomic aberrations in idiopathic myelofibrosis: a comparative genomic hybridization study. *Br J Haematol* 129:66–71.

Al-Riyami AZ, Hudoba M, Young S, Forrest D (2013): Sorafenib is effective for imatinib-resistant FIP1L1/PDGFRA T674I mutation-positive acute myeloid leukemia with eosinophilia. *Leuk Lymphoma* 54:1788–1790.

Andrieux J, Demory JL, Caulier MT, Agape P, Wetterwald M, Bauters F, et al. (2003): Karyotypic abnormalities in mye-lofibrosis following polycythemia vera. *Cancer Genet Cytogenet* 140:118–123.

Andrieux J, Roche-Lestienne C, Geffroy S, Desterke C, Grardel N, Plantier I, et al. (2007): Bone morphogenetic protein antagonist gene NOG is involved in myeloprolifer-ative disease associated with myelofibrosis. *Cancer Genet Cytogenet* 178:11–16.

Bacher U, Haferlach T, Kern W, Hiddemann W, Schnittger S, Schoch C (2005): Conventional cytogenetics of myelopro-liferative diseases other than CML contribute valid information. *Ann Hematol* 84:250–257.

Bain BJ (2003): Cytogenetic and molecular genetic aspects of eosinophilic leukaemias. *Br J Haematol* 122:173–179.

Baldazzi C, Iacobucci I, Luatti S, Ottaviani E, Marzocchi G, Paolini S, et al. (2010): B-cell acute lymphoblastic leu-kemia as evolution of a 8p11 myeloproliferative syndrome with t(8;22)(p11;q11) and BCR-FGFR1 fusion gene. *Leuk Res* 34:e282–e285.

Barbui T, Barosi G, Birgegard G, Cervantes F, Finazzi G, Griesshammer M, et al. (2011a): Philadelphia-negative classical myeloproliferative neoplasms: critical concepts and management recommendations from European LeukemiaNet. *J Clin Oncol* 29:761–770.

Barbui T, Thiele J, Passamonti F, Rumi E, Boveri E, Ruggeri M, et al. (2011b): Survival and disease progression in essential thrombocythemia are significantly influenced by accurate morphologic diagnosis: an international study. *J Clin Oncol* 29:3179–3184.

Baxter EJ, Hochhaus A, Bolufer P, Reiter A, Fernandez JM, Senent L, et al. (2002): The t(4;22):(q12;q11): in atypical chronic myeloid leukaemia fuses BCR to PDGFRA. *Hum Mol Genet* 11:1391–1397.

Baxter EJ, Scott LM, Campbell PJ, East C, Fourouclas N, Swanton S, et al. (2005): Acquired mutation of the tyrosine kinase JAK2 in human myeloproliferative disorders. *Lancet* 365:1054–1061.

Belloni E, Trubia M, Gasparini P, Micucci C, Tapinassi C, Confalonieri S, et al. (2005): 8p11 myeloproliferative syn-drome with a novel t(7;8): translocation leading to fusion of the FGFR1 and TIF1 genes. *Genes Chromosomes Cancer* 42:320–325.

Bench AJ, Nacheva EP, Champion KM, Green AR (1998): Molecular genetics and cytogenetics of myeloproliferative disorders. *Baillieres Clin Haematol* 11:819–848.

Bench AJ, Nacheva EP, Hood TL, Holden JL, French L, Swanton S, et al. (2000): Chromosome 20 deletions in myeloid malignancies: reduction of the common deleted region generation of a PAC/BAC contig and identification of candidate genes. UK Cancer Cytogenetics Group (UKCCG). *Oncogene* 19:3902–3913.

Berger R, Bernheim A, Le Coniat M, Vecchione D, Flandrin G, Dresch C, et al. (1984): Chromosome studies in polycythemia vera patients. *Cancer Genet Cytogenet* 12:217–223.

Bohm J, Kock S, Schaefer HE, Fisch P (2003): Evidence of clonality in chronic neutrophilic leukaemia. *J Clin Pathol* 56:292–295.

Brecqueville M, Rey J, Devillier R, Guille A, Gillet R, Adelaide J, et al. (2014): Array comparative genomic hybridization and sequencing of 23 genes in 80 patients with myelofibrosis at chronic or acute phase. *Haematologica* 99:37–45.

Caramazza D, Begna KH, Gangat N, Vaidya R, Siragusa S, Van Dyke DL, et al. (2011): Refined cytogenetic-risk categorization for overall and leukemia-free survival in primary myelofibrosis: a single center study of 433 patients. *Leukemia* 25:82–88.

Chaffanet M, Popovici C, Leroux D, Jacrot M, Adelaide J, Dastugue N, et al. (1998): t(6;8), t(8;9), and t(8;13) translocations associated with stem cell myeloproliferative disorders have close or identical breakpoints in chromosome region 8p11–12. *Oncogene* 16:945–949.

Chang H, Chuang WY, Sun CF, Barnard MR (2012): Concurrent acute myeloid leukemia and T lymphoblastic lymphoma in a patient with rearranged PDGFRB genes. *Diagn Pathol* 7:19.

Chase A, Grand FH, Cross NC (2007): Activity of TKI258 against primary cells and cell lines with FGFR1 fusion genes associated with the 8p11 myeloproliferative syndrome. *Blood* 110:3729–3734.

Chase A, Bryant C, Score J, Cross NC (2013): Ponatinib as targeted therapy for FGFR1 fusions associated with the 8p11 myeloproliferative syndrome. *Haematologica* 98:103–106.

Cheah CY, Burbury K, Apperley JF, Huguet F, Pitini V, Gardembas M, et al. (2014): Patients with myeloid malignancies bearing PDGFRB fusion genes achieve durable long term remissions with imatinib. *Blood* 123(23):3574–3577.

Chen Z, Notohamiprodjo M, Guan XY, Paietta E, Blackwell S, Stout K, et al. (1998): Gain of 9p in the pathogenesis of polycythemia vera. *Genes Chromosomes Cancer* 22:321–324.

Chen D, Bachanova V, Ketterling RP, Begna KH, Hanson CA, Viswanatha DS (2013): A case of nonleukemic myeloid sarcoma with FIP1L1-PDGFRA rearrangement: an unusual presentation of a rare disease. *Am J Surg Pathol* 37:147–151.

Chmielecki J, Peifer M, Viale A, Hutchinson K, Giltnane J, Socci ND, et al. (2012): Systematic screen for tyrosine kinase rearrangements identifies a novel C6orf204-PDGFRB fusion in a patient with recurrent T-ALL and an associated myeloproliferative neoplasm. *Genes Chromosomes Cancer* 51:54–65.

Cools J, DeAngelo DJ, Gotlib J, Stover EH, Legare RD, Cortes J, et al. (2003): A tyrosine kinase created by fusion of the PDGFRA and FIP1L1 genes as a therapeutic target of imatinib in idiopathic hypereosinophilic syndrome. *N Engl J Med* 348:1201–1214.

Cross NC (2011): Genetic and epigenetic complexity in myeloproliferative neoplasms, *Hematology Am Soc Hematol Educ Program* 2011:208–214.

Cross NC, Reiter A (2002): Tyrosine kinase fusion genes in chronic myeloproliferative diseases. *Leukemia* 16:1207–1212.

Curtis CE, Grand FH, Musto P, Clark A, Murphy J, Perla G, et al. (2007): Two novel imatinib-responsive PDGFRA fusion genes in chronic eosinophilic leukaemia. *Br J Haematol* 138:77–81.

Demory JL, Dupriez B, Fenaux P, Lai JL, Beuscart R, Jouet JP, et al. (1988): Cytogenetic studies and their prognostic significance in agnogenic myeloid metaplasia: a report on 47 cases. *Blood* 72:855–859.

Diez-Martin JL, Graham DL, Petitt RM, Dewald GW (1991): Chromosome studies in 104 patients with polycythemia vera. *Mayo Clin Proc* 66:287–299.

Dingli D, Grand FH, Mahaffey V, Spurbeck J, Ross FM, Watmore AE, et al. (2005): Der(6)t(1;6)(q21-23;p21,3): a specific cytogenetic abnormality in myelofibrosis with myeloid metaplasia. *Br J Haematol* 130:229–232.

Djordjevic V, Dencic-Fekete M, Jovanovic J, Bizic S, Jankovic G, Bogdanovic A, et al. (2007): Cytogenetics of agnogenic myeloid metaplasia: a study of 61 patients. *Cancer Genet Cytogenet* 173:57–62.

Dolan M, Cioc A, Cross NC, Neglia JP, Tolar J (2012): Favorable outcome of allogeneic hematopoietic cell transplantation for 8p11 myeloproliferative syndrome associated with BCR-FGFR1 gene fusion. *Pediatr Blood Cancer* 59:194–196.

Drechsler M, Hildebrandt B, Kundgen A, Germing U, Royer-Pokora B (2007): Fusion of H4/D10S170 to PDGFRbeta in a patient with chronic myelomonocytic leukemia and long-term responsiveness to imatinib. *Ann Hematol* 86:353–354.

Duckworth CB, Zhang L, Li S (2014): Systemic mastocytosis with associated myeloproliferative neoplasm with t(8;19)(p12;q13,1) and abnormality of FGFR1: report of a unique case. *Int J Clin Exp Pathol* 7:801–807.

Dupriez B, Morel P, Demory JL, Lai JL, Simon M, Plantier I, et al. (1996): Prognostic factors in agnogenic myeloid metaplasia: a report on 195 cases with a new scoring system. *Blood* 88:1013–1018.

Elling C, Erben P, Walz C, Frickenhaus M, Schemionek M, Stehling M, et al. (2011): Novel imatinib-sensitive PDGFRA-activating point mutations in hypereosinophilic syndrome induce growth factor independence and leukemia-like disease. *Blood* 117:2935–2943.

Erben P, Gosenca D, Muller MC, Reinhard J, Score J, Del Valle F, et al. (2010): Screening for diverse PDGFRA or PDGFRB fusion genes is facilitated by generic quantitative reverse transcriptase polymerase chain reaction analysis. *Haematologica* 95:738–744.

Fialkow PJ, Faguet GB, Jacobson RJ, Vaidya K, Murphy S (1981): Evidence that essential thrombocythemia is a clonal disorder with origin in a multipotent stem cell. *Blood* 58:916–919.

Fioretos T, Panagopoulos I, Lassen C, Swedin A, Billstrom R, Isaksson M, et al. (2001): Fusion of the BCR and the fibroblast growth factor receptor-1 (FGFR1) genes as a result of t(8;22)(p11;q11) in a myeloproliferative disorder: the first fusion gene involving BCR but not ABL. *Genes Chromosomes Cancer* 32:302–310.

Gallagher G, Horsman DE, Tsang P, Forrest DL (2008): Fusion of PRKG2 and SPTBN1 to the platelet-derived growth factor receptor beta gene (PDGFRB) in imatinib-responsive atypical myeloproliferative disorders. *Cancer Genet Cytogenet* 181:46–51.

Gangat N, Strand J, Lasho TL, Finke CM, Knudson RA, Pardanani A, et al. (2008): Cytogenetic studies at diagnosis in polycythemia vera: clinical and JAK2V617F allele burden correlates. *Eur J Haematol* 80:197–200.

Gangat N, Tefferi A, Thanarajasingam G, Patnaik M, Schwager S, Ketterling R, et al. (2009): Cytogenetic abnormalities in essential thrombocythemia: prevalence and prognostic significance. *Eur J Haematol* 83:17–21.

Gangat N, Caramazza D, Vaidya R, George G, Begna K, Schwager S, et al. (2011): DIPSS plus: a refined Dynamic International Prognostic Scoring System for primary myelofibrosis that incorporates prognostic information from karyotype, platelet count, and transfusion status. *J Clin Oncol* 29:392–397.

Garcia-Montero AC, Jara-Acevedo M, Teodosio C, Sanchez ML, Nunez R, Prados A, et al. (2006): KIT mutation in mast cells and other bone marrow hematopoietic cell lineages in systemic mast cell disorders: a prospective study of the Spanish Network on Mastocytosis (REMA) in a series of 113 patients. *Blood* 108:2366–2372.

Gervais C, Murati A, Helias C, Struski S, Eischen A, Lippert E, et al. (2008): Acute myeloid leukaemia with 8p11 (MYST3) rearrangement: an integrated cytologic cytogenetic and molecular study by the Groupe Francophone de Cytogenetique Hematologique. *Leukemia* 22:1567–1575.

Gervais C, Dano L, Perrusson N, Helias C, Jeandidier E, Galoisy AC, et al. (2013): A translocation t(2;8)(q12;p11) fuses FGFR1 to a novel partner gene RANBP2/NUP358 in a myeloproliferative/myelodysplastic neoplasm. *Leukemia* 27:1186–1188.

Golub TR, Barker GF, Lovett M, Gilliland DG (1994): Fusion of PDGF receptor beta to a novel ets-like gene tel in chronic myelomonocytic leukemia with t(5;12) chromosomal translocation. *Cell* 77:307–316.

Gorello P, La Starza R, Brandimarte L, Trisolini SM, Pierini V, Crescenzi B, et al. (2008): A PDGFRB-positive acute myeloid malignancy with a new t(5;12)(q33;p13,3) involving the ERC1 gene. *Leukemia* 22:216–218.

Gosenca D, Kellert B, Metzgeroth G, Haferlach C, Fabarius A, Schwaab J, et al. (2014): Identification and functional characterization of imatinib-sensitive DTD1-PDGFRB and CCDC88C-PDGFRB fusion genes in eosinophilia-associated myeloid/lymphoid neoplasms. *Genes Chromosomes Cancer* 53:411–421.

Gotlib J (2005): Molecular classification and pathogenesis of eosinophilic disorders: 2005 update. *Acta Haematol* 114:7–25.

Grand EK, Grand FH, Chase AJ, Ross FM, Corcoran MM, Oscier DG, et al. (2004a): Identification of a novel gene FGFR1OP2 fused to FGFR1 in 8p11 myeloproliferative syndrome. *Genes Chromosomes Cancer* 40:78–83.

Grand FH, Burgstaller S, Kuhr T, Baxter EJ, Webersinke G, Thaler J, et al. (2004b): P53-binding protein 1 is fused to the platelet-derived growth factor receptor beta in a patient with a t(5;15)(q33;q22) and an imatinib-responsive eosinophilic myeloproliferative disorder. *Cancer Res* 64:7216–7219.

Groupe Français de Cytogénétique Hématologique (1988): Cytogenetics of acutely transformed chronic myeloproliferative syndromes without a Philadelphia chromosome. A multicenter study of 55 patients. *Cancer Genet Cytogenet* 32:157–168.

Guasch G, Delaval B, Arnoulet C, Xie MJ, Xerri L, Sainty D, et al. (2004): FOP-FGFR1 tyrosine kinase the product of a t(6;8) translocation induces a fatal myeloproliferative disease in mice. *Blood* 103:309–312.

Harrison C, Kiladjian JJ, Al-Ali HK, Gisslinger H, Waltzman R, Stalbovskaya V, et al. (2012): JAK inhibition with ruxolitinib versus best available therapy for myelofibrosis. *N Engl J Med* 366:787–798.

Haslam K, Langabeer SE, Kelly J, Coen N, O'Connell NM, Conneally E (2012): Allogeneic hematopoietic stem cell transplantation for a BCR-FGFR1 myeloproliferative neoplasm presenting as acute lymphoblastic leukemia. *Case Rep Hematol* 2012:620967.

Hidalgo-Curtis C, Chase A, Drachenberg M, Roberts MW, Finkelstein JZ, Mould S, et al. (2008): The t(1;9)(p34;q34) and t(8;12)(p11;q15) fuse pre-mRNA processing proteins SFPQ (PSF) and CPSF6 to ABL and FGFR1. *Genes Chromosomes Cancer* 47:379–385.

Hidalgo-Curtis C, Apperley JF, Stark A, Jeng M, Gotlib J, Chase A, et al. (2010): Fusion of PDGFRB to two distinct loci at 3p21 and a third at 12q13 in imatinib-responsive myeloproliferative neoplasms. *Br J Haematol* 148:268–273.

Hochhaus A, le Coutre PD, Kantarjian HM, Baccarani M, Erben P, Reiter A, et al. (2013): Effect of the tyrosine kinase inhibitor nilotinib in patients with hypereosinophilic syndrome/chronic eosinophilic leukemia: analysis of the phase 2 open-label single-arm A2101 study. *J Cancer Res Clin Oncol* 139:1985–1993.

Hou Y, Song L, Zhu P, Zhang B, Tao Y, Xu X, et al. (2012): Single-cell exome sequencing and monoclonal evolution of a JAK2-negative myeloproliferative neoplasm. *Cell* 148: 873–885.

Hu S, He Y, Zhu X, Li J, He H (2011): Myeloproliferative disorders with t(8;9)(p12;q33): a case report and review of the literature. *Pediatr Hematol Oncol* 28:140–146.

Hussein K, Huang J, Lasho T, Pardanani A, Mesa RA, Williamson CM, et al. (2009): Karyotype complements the International Prognostic Scoring System for primary myelofibrosis. *Eur J Haematol* 82:255–259.

Jackson CC, Medeiros LJ, Miranda RN (2010): 8p11 myeloproliferative syndrome: a review. *Hum Pathol* 41:461–476.

Jaffe ES, Harris NL, Stein H, Vardiman JW, editors (2001): *World Health Organization Classification of Tumours: Pathology and Genetics of Tumours of Haematopoietic and Lymphoid Tissues.* IARC Press; Lyon.

James C, Ugo V, Le Couedic JP, Staerk J, Delhommeau F, Lacout C, et al. (2005): A unique clonal JAK2 mutation leading to constitutive signalling causes polycythaemia vera. *Nature* 434:1144–1148.

Jotterand Bellomo M, Muhlemmatter D, Wicht M, Delacretaz F, Schmidt PM (1992): t(8;9)(p11;q32) in atypical chronic myeloid leukaemia: a new cytogenetic-clinicopathologic association? *Br J Haematol* 81:307–308.

Jovanovic JV, Score J, Waghorn K, Cilloni D, Gottardi E, Metzgeroth G, et al. (2007): Low-dose imatinib mesylate leads to rapid induction of major molecular responses and achievement of complete molecular remission in FIP1L1-PDGFRA-positive chronic eosinophilic leukemia. *Blood* 109:4635–4640.

Kim SY, Oh B, She CJ, Kim HK, Jeon YK, Shin MG, et al. (2011): 8p11 myeloproliferative syndrome with BCR-FGFR1 rearrangement presenting with T-lymphoblastic lymphoma and bone marrow stromal cell proliferation: a case report and review of the literature. *Leuk Res* 35:e30–e34.

Klampfl T, Gisslinger H, Harutyunyan AS, Nivarthi H, Rumi E, Milosevic JD, et al. (2013): Somatic mutations of calreticulin in myeloproliferative neoplasms. *N Engl J Med* 369:2379–2390.

Klion AD, Noel P, Akin C, Law MA, Gilliland DG, Cools J, et al. (2003): Elevated serum tryptase levels identify a subset of patients with a myeloproliferative variant of idiopathic hypereosinophilic syndrome associated with tissue fibrosis poor prognosis and imatinib responsiveness. *Blood* 101:4660–4666.

Kralovics R, Guan Y, Prchal JT (2002): Acquired uniparental disomy of chromosome 9p is a frequent stem cell defect in polycythemia vera. *Exp Hematol* 30:229–236.

Kralovics R, Passamonti F, Buser AS, Teo SS, Tiedt R, Passweg JR, et al. (2005): A gain-of-function mutation of JAK2 in myeloproliferative disorders. *N Engl J Med* 352:1779–1790.

Kulkarni S, Heath C, Parker S, Chase A, Iqbal S, Pocock CF, et al. (2000): Fusion of H4/D10S170 to the platelet-derived growth factor receptor beta in BCR-ABL-negative myeloproliferative disorders with a t(5;10)(q33;q21). *Cancer Res* 60:3592–3598.

La Starza R, Wlodarska I, Aventin A, Falzetti D, Crescenzi B, Martelli MF, et al. (1998): Molecular delineation of 13q deletion boundaries in 20 patients with myeloid malignancies. *Blood* 91:231–237.

La Starza R, Rosati R, Roti G, Gorello P, Bardi A, Crescenzi B, et al. (2007): A new NDE1/PDGFRB fusion transcript underlying chronic myelomonocytic leukaemia in Noonan Syndrome. *Leukemia* 21:830–833.

Lacronique V, Boureux A, Valle VD, Poirel H, Quang CT, Mauchauffe M, et al. (1997): A TEL-JAK2 fusion protein with constitutive kinase activity in human leukemia. *Science* 278:1309–1312.

Lawler SD (1980): Cytogenetic studies in Philadelphia chromosome-negative myeloproliferative disorders particularly, polycythaemia rubra vera. *Clin Haematol* 9:159–174.

Lee H, Kim M, Lim J, Kim Y, Han K, Cho BS, et al. (2013): Acute myeloid leukemia associated with FGFR1 abnormalities. *Int J Hematol* 97:808–812.

Levine RL, Wadleigh M, Sternberg DW, Wlodarska I, Galinsky I, Stone RM, et al. (2005): KIAA1509 is a novel PDGFRB fusion partner in imatinib-responsive myeloproliferative disease associated with a t(5;14)(q33;q32). *Leukemia* 19:27–30.

Li Z, Yang R, Zhao J, Yuan R, Lu Q, Li Q, et al. (2011): Molecular diagnosis and targeted therapy of a pediatric chronic eosinophilic leukemia patient carrying TPM3-PDGFRB fusion. *Pediatr Blood Cancer* 56:463–466.

Li F, Zhai YP, Tang YM, Wang LP, Wan PJ (2012): Identification of a novel partner gene TPR fused to FGFR1 in 8p11 myeloproliferative syndrome. *Genes Chromosomes Cancer* 51:890–897.

Lierman E, Folens C, Stover EH, Mentens N, Van Miegroet H, Scheers W, et al. (2006): Sorafenib is a potent inhibitor of FIP1L1-PDGFRalpha and the imatinib-resistant FIP1L1-PDGFRalpha T674I mutant. *Blood* 108:1374–1376.

Lierman E, Michaux L, Beullens E, Pierre P, Marynen P, Cools J, et al. (2009): FIP1L1-PDGFRalpha D842V, a novel panresistant mutant, emerging after treatment of FIP1L1-PDGFRalpha T674I eosinophilic leukemia with single agent sorafenib. *Leukemia* 23:845–851.

Lierman E, Selleslag D, Smits S, Billiet J, Vandenberghe P (2012a): Ruxolitinib inhibits transforming JAK2 fusion proteins in vitro and induces complete cytogenetic remission in t(8;9)(p22;p24)/PCM1-JAK2-positive chronic eosinophilic leukemia. *Blood* 120:1529–1531.

Lierman E, Smits S, Cools J, Dewaele B, Debiec-Rychter M, Vandenberghe P (2012b): Ponatinib is active against imatinib-resistant mutants of FIP1L1-PDGFRA and KIT and against FGFR1-derived fusion kinases. *Leukemia* 26:1693–1695.

Longley BJ, Tyrrell L, Lu SZ, Ma YS, Langley K, Ding TG, et al. (1996): Somatic c-KIT activating mutation in urticaria pigmentosa and aggressive mastocytosis: establishment of clonality in a human mast cell neoplasm. *Nat Genet* 12:312–314.

Lourenco GJ, Ortega MM, Freitas LL, Bognone RA, Fattori A, Lorand-Metze I, et al. (2008): The rare t(6;8)(q27;p11) translocation in a case of chronic myeloid neoplasm mimicking polycythemia vera. *Leuk Lymphoma* 49:1832–1835.

Macdonald D, Reiter A, Cross NC (2002): The 8p11 myeloproliferative syndrome: a distinct clinical entity caused by constitutive activation of FGFR1. *Acta Haematol* 107:101–107.

MacGrogan D, Alvarez S, DeBlasio T, Jhanwar SC, Nimer SD (2001): Identification of candidate genes on chromosome band 20q12 by physical mapping of translocation breakpoints found in myeloid leukemia cell lines. *Oncogene* 20:4150–4160.

Magnusson MK, Meade KE, Brown KE, Arthur DC, Krueger LA, Barrett AJ, et al. (2001): Rabaptin-5 is a novel fusion partner to platelet-derived growth factor beta receptor in chronic myelomonocytic leukemia. *Blood* 98:2518–2525.

Matikas A, Tzannou I, Oikonomopoulou D, Bakiri M (2013): A case of acute myelogenous leukaemia characterised by the BCR-FGFR1 translocation. BMJ Case Rep pii:bcr2013008834.

Maxson JE, Gotlib J, Pollyea DA, Fleischman AG, Agarwal A, Eide CA, et al. (2013): Oncogenic CSF3R mutations in chronic neutrophilic leukemia and atypical CML. *N Engl J Med* 368:1781–1790.

Medves S, Duhoux FP, Ferrant A, Toffalini F, Ameye G, Libouton JM, et al. (2010): KANK1, a candidate tumor suppressor gene, is fused to PDGFRB in an imatinib-responsive myeloid neoplasm with severe thrombocythemia. *Leukemia* 24:1052–1055.

Mertens F, Johansson B, Heim S, Kristoffersson U, Mitelman F (1991): Karyotypic patterns in chronic myeloproliferative disorders: report on 74 cases and review of the literature. *Leukemia* 5:214–220.

Metzgeroth G, Walz C, Score J, Siebert R, Schnittger S, Haferlach C, et al. (2007): Recurrent finding of the FIP1L1-PDGFRA fusion gene in eosinophilia-associated acute myeloid leukemia and lymphoblastic T-cell lymphoma. *Leukemia* 21:1183–1188.

Metzgeroth G, Erben P, Martin H, Mousset S, Teichmann M, Walz C, et al. (2012): Limited clinical activity of nilotinib and sorafenib in FIP1L1-PDGFRA positive chronic eosinophilic leukemia with imatinib-resistant T674I mutation. *Leukemia* 26:162–164.

Mitelman F, Johansson B, Mertens F (2014): Mitelman Database of Chromosome Aberrations and Gene Fusions in Cancer. Available at http://cgap.nci.nih.gov/Chromosomes/Mitelman.

Morerio C, Acquila M, Rosanda C, Rapella A, Dufour C, Locatelli F, et al. (2004): HCMOGT-1 is a novel fusion partner to PDGFRB in juvenile myelomonocytic leukemia with t(5;17)(q33;p11,2). *Cancer Res* 64:2649–2651.

Morishige S, Oku E, Takata Y, Kimura Y, Arakawa F, Seki R, et al. (2013): A case of 8p11 myeloproliferative syndrome with BCR-FGFR1 gene fusion presenting with trilineage acute leukemia/lymphoma successfully treated by cord blood transplantation. *Acta Haematol* 129:83–89.

Mozziconacci MJ, Carbuccia N, Prebet T, Charbonnier A, Murati A, Vey N, et al. (2008): Common features of myeloproliferative disorders with t(8;9)(p12;q33) and CEP110-FGFR1 fusion: report of a new case and review of the literature. *Leuk Res* 32:1304–1308.

Mugneret F, Chaffanet M, Maynadie M, Guasch G, Favre B, Casasnovas O, et al. (2000): The 8p12 myeloproliferative disorder, t(8;19)(p12;q13,3): a novel translocation involving the FGFR1 gene. *Br J Haematol* 111:647–649.

Murati A, Arnoulet C, Lafage-Pochitaloff M, Adelaide J, Derre M, Slama B, et al. (2005): Dual lympho-myeloproliferative disorder in a patient with t(8;22) with BCR-FGFR1 gene fusion. *Int J Oncol* 26:1485–1492.

Nacheva E, Holloway T, Carter N, Grace C, White N, Green AR (1995): Characterization of 20q deletions in patients with myeloproliferative disorders or myelodysplastic syndromes. *Cancer Genet Cytogenet* 80:87–94.

Najfeld V, Montella L, Scalise A, Fruchtman S (2002): Exploring polycythaemia vera with fluorescence in situ hybridization: additional cryptic 9p is the most frequent abnormality detected. *Br J Haematol* 119:558–566.

Nangalia J, Massie CE, Baxter EJ, Nice FL, Gundem G, Wedge DC, et al. (2013): Somatic CALR mutations in myeloproliferative neoplasms with nonmutated JAK2. *N Engl J Med* 369:2391–2405.

Neumann F, Poelitz A, Hildebrandt B, Fenk R, Haas R, Royer-Pokora B, et al. (2007): The tyrosine-kinase inhibitor imatinib induces long-term remission in a patient with chronic myelogenous leukemia with translocation t(4;22). *Leukemia* 21:836–837.

Ohnishi H, Kandabashi K, Maeda Y, Kawamura M, Watanabe T (2006): Chronic eosinophilic leukaemia with FIP1L1-PDGFRA fusion and T6741 mutation that evolved from Langerhans cell histiocytosis with eosinophilia after chemotherapy *Br J Haematol* 134:547–549.

Onozawa M, Ohmura K, Ibata M, Iwasaki J, Okada K, Kasahara I, et al. (2011): The 8p11 myeloproliferative syndrome owing to rare FGFR1OP2-FGFR1 fusion. *Eur J Haematol* 86:347–349.

Panani AD (2006): Cytogenetic findings in untreated patients with essential thrombocythemia. *In Vivo* 20:381–384.

Pardanani A, Ketterling RP, Brockman SR, Flynn HC, Paternoster SF, Shearer BM, et al. (2003): CHIC2 deletion, a surrogate for FIP1L1-PDGFRA fusion, occurs in systemic mastocytosis associated with eosinophilia and predicts response to imatinib mesylate therapy. *Blood* 102:3093–3096.

Pardanani AD, Levine RL, Lasho T, Pikman Y, Mesa RA, Wadleigh M, et al. (2006): MPL515 mutations in myeloproliferative and other myeloid disorders: a study of 1182 patients. *Blood* 108:3472–3476.

Park TS, Song J, Kim JS, Yang WI, Song S, Kim SJ, et al. (2008): 8p11 myeloproliferative syndrome preceded by t(8;9)(p11;q33), CEP110/FGFR1 fusion transcript: morphologic, molecular, and cytogenetic characterization of myeloid neoplasms associated with eosinophilia and FGFR1 abnormality. *Cancer Genet Cytogenet* 181:93–99.

Pastore C, Nomdedeu J, Volpe G, Guerrasio A, Cambrin GR, Parvis G, et al. (1995): Genetic analysis of chromosome 13 deletions in BCR/ABL negative chronic myeloproliferative disorders. *Genes Chromosomes Cancer* 14:106–111.

Patnaik MM, Gangat N, Knudson RA, Keefe JG, Hanson CA, Pardanani A, et al. (2010): Chromosome 8p11,2 translocations: prevalence, FISH analysis for FGFR1 and MYST3, and clinicopathologic correlates in a consecutive cohort of 13 cases from a single institution. *Am J Hematol* 85:238–242.

Patterer V, Schnittger S, Kern W, Haferlach T, Haferlach C (2013): Hematologic malignancies with PCM1-JAK2 gene fusion share characteristics with myeloid and lymphoid neoplasms with eosinophilia and abnormalities of PDGFRA, PDGFRB, and FGFR1. *Ann Hematol* 92:759–769.

Peeters P, Raynaud SD, Cools J, Wlodarska I, Grosgeorge J, Philip P, et al. (1997): Fusion of TEL, the ETS-variant gene 6 (ETV6), to the receptor-associated kinase JAK2 as a result of t(9;12) in a lymphoid and t(9;15;12) in a myeloid leukemia. *Blood* 90:2535–2540.

Pikman Y, Lee BH, Mercher T, McDowell E, Ebert BL, Gozo M, et al. (2006): MPLW515L is a novel somatic activating mutation in myelofibrosis with myeloid metaplasia. *PLoS Med* 3:e270.

Pini M, Gottardi E, Scaravaglio P, Giugliano E, Libener R, Baraldi A, et al. (2002): A fourth case of BCR-FGFR1 positive CML-like disease with t(8;22) translocation showing an extensive deletion on the derivative chromosome 8p. *Hematol J* 3:315–316.

Popovici C, Zhang B, Gregoire MJ, Jonveaux P, Lafage-Pochitaloff M, Birnbaum D, et al. (1999): The t(6;8)(q27;p11) translocation in a stem cell myeloproliferative disorder fuses a novel gene, FOP, to fibroblast growth factor receptor 1. *Blood* 93:1381–1389.

Post GR, Holloman D, Christiansen L, Smith J, Stuart R, Lazarchick J (2010): Translocation t(3;8;9)(p25;p21;q34) in a patient with features of 8p11 myeloproliferative syndrome: a unique case and review of the literature. *Leuk Res* 34:1543–1544.

Raskind WH, Jacobson R, Murphy S, Adamson JW, Fialkow PJ (1985): Evidence for the involvement of B lymphoid cells in polycythemia vera and essential thrombocythemia. *J Clin Invest* 75:1388–1390.

Rege-Cambrin G, Mecucci C, Tricot G, Michaux JL, Louwagie A, Van Hove W, et al. (1987): A chromosomal profile of polycythemia vera. *Cancer Genet Cytogenet* 25:233–245.

Rege-Cambrin G, Speleman F, Kerim S, Scaravaglio P, Carozzi F, Dal Cin P, et al. (1991): Extra translocation + der(1q9p) is a prognostic indicator in myeloproliferative disorders. *Leukemia* 5:1059–1063.

Reilly JT, Wilson G, Barnett D, Watmore A, Potter A (1994): Karyotypic and ras gene mutational analysis in idiopathic myelofibrosis. *Br J Haematol* 88:575–581.

Reilly JT, Snowden JA, Spearing RL, Fitzgerald PM, Jones N, Watmore A, et al. (1997): Cytogenetic abnormalities and their prognostic significance in idiopathic myelofibrosis: a study of 106 cases. *Br J Haematol* 98:96–102.

Reiter A, Sohal J, Kulkarni S, Chase A, Macdonald DH, Aguiar RC, et al. (1998): Consistent fusion of ZNF198 to the fibroblast growth factor receptor-1 in the t(8;13)(p11;q12) myeloproliferative syndrome. *Blood* 92:1735–1742.

Reiter A, Walz C, Watmore A, Schoch C, Blau I, Schlegelberger B, et al. (2005): The t(8;9)(p22;p24) is a recurrent abnormality in chronic and acute leukemia that fuses PCM1 to JAK2. *Cancer Res* 65:2662–2667.

Ren M, Qin H, Ren R, Cowell JK (2013): Ponatinib suppresses the development of myeloid and lymphoid malignancies associated with FGFR1 abnormalities. *Leukemia* 27:32–40.

Rosati R, La Starza R, Veronese A, Aventin A, Schwienbacher C, Vallespi T, et al. (2002): NUP98 is fused to the NSD3 gene in acute myeloid leukemia associated with t(8;11)(p11,2;p15). *Blood* 99:3857–3860.

Rosati R, La Starza R, Luciano L, Gorello P, Matteucci C, Pierini V, et al. (2006): TPM3/PDGFRB fusion transcript and its reciprocal in chronic eosinophilic leukemia. *Leukemia* 20:1623–1624.

Ross TS, Bernard OA, Berger R, Gilliland DG (1998): Fusion of Huntingtin interacting protein 1 to platelet-derived growth factor beta receptor (PDGFbetaR) in chronic myelomonocytic leukemia with t(5;7)(q33;q11,2). *Blood* 91:4419–4426.

Rotunno G, Mannarelli C, Guglielmelli P, Pacilli A, Pancrazzi A, Pieri L, et al. (2014): Impact of calreticulin mutations on clinical and hematological phenotype and outcome in essential thrombocythemia. *Blood* 123:1552–1555.

Roulston D, Espinosa R, Stoffel M, Bell GI, Le Beau MM (1993): Molecular genetics of myeloid leukemia: identification of the commonly deleted segment of chromosome 20. *Blood* 82:3424–3429.

Rumi E, Milosevic JD, Casetti I, Dambruoso I, Pietra D, Boveri E, et al. (2013): Efficacy of ruxolitinib in chronic eosinophilic leukemia associated with a PCM1-JAK2 fusion gene. *J Clin Oncol* 31:e269–e271.

Rumi E, Pietra D, Ferretti V, Klampfl T, Harutyunyan AS, Milosevic JD, et al. (2014): JAK2 or CALR mutation status defines subtypes of essential thrombocythemia with substantially different clinical course and outcomes. *Blood* 123:1544–1551.

Safley AM, Sebastian S, Collins TS, Tirado CA, Stenzel TT, Gong JZ, et al. (2004): Molecular and cytogenetic characterization of a novel translocation t(4;22) involving the breakpoint cluster region and platelet-derived growth factor receptor-alpha genes in a patient with atypical chronic myeloid leukemia. *Genes Chromosomes Cancer* 40:44–50.

Salemi S, Yousefi S, Simon D, Schmid I, Moretti L, Scapozza L, et al. (2009): A novel FIP1L1-PDGFRA mutant destabilizing the inactive conformation of the kinase domain in chronic eosinophilic leukemia/hypereosinophilic syndrome. *Allergy* 64:913–918.

Schwaller J, Anastasiadou E, Cain D, Kutok J, Wojiski S, Williams IR, et al. (2001): H4(D10S170), a gene frequently rearranged in papillary thyroid carcinoma, is fused to the platelet-derived growth factor receptor beta gene in atypical chronic myeloid leukemia with t(5;10)(q33;q22). *Blood* 97:3910–3918.

Score J, Curtis C, Waghorn K, Stalder M, Jotterand M, Grand FH, et al. (2006): Identification of a novel imatinib responsive KIF5B-PDGFRA fusion gene following screening for PDGFRA overexpression in patients with hypereosinophilia. *Leukemia* 20:827–832.

Scott LM, Tong W, Levine RL, Scott MA, Beer PA, Stratton MR, et al. (2007): JAK2 exon 12 mutations in polycythemia vera and idiopathic erythrocytosis. *N Engl J Med* 356:459–468.

Sessarego M, Defferrari R, Dejana AM, Rebuttato AM, Fugazza G, Salvidio E, et al. (1989): Cytogenetic analysis in essential thrombocythemia at diagnosis and at transformation, A 12-year study. *Cancer Genet Cytogenet* 43:57–65.

Sever M, Quintas-Cardama A, Pierce S, Zhou L, Kantarjian H, Verstovsek S (2013): Significance of cytogenetic abnor-malities in patients with polycythemia vera. *Leuk Lymphoma* 54:2667–2670.

Shimanuki M, Sonoki T, Hosoi H, Watanuki J, Murata S, Mushino T, et al. (2013): Acute leukemia showing t(8;22) (p11;q11) myelodysplasia, CD13/CD33/CD19 expression, and immunoglobulin heavy chain gene rearrangement. *Acta Haematol* 129:238–242.

Siena S, Sammarelli G, Grimoldi MG, Schiavo R, Nozza A, Roncalli M, et al. (1999): New reciprocal translocation t(5;10)(q33;q22) associated with atypical chronic myeloid leukemia. *Haematologica* 84:369–372.

Sinclair EJ, Forrest EC, Reilly JT, Watmore AE, Potter AM (2001): Fluorescence in situ hybridization analysis of 25 cases of idiopathic myelofibrosis and two cases of secondary myelofibrosis: monoallelic loss of RB1 D13S319 and D13S25 loci associated with cytogenetic deletion and trans-location involving 13q14. *Br J Haematol* 113:365–368.

Sohal J, Chase A, Mould S, Corcoran M, Oscier D, Iqbal S, et al. (2001): Identification of four new translocations involving FGFR1 in myeloid disorders. *Genes Chromosomes Cancer* 32:155–163.

Soler G, Nusbaum S, Varet B, Macintyre EA, Vekemans M, Romana SP, et al. (2009): LRRFIP1, a new FGFR1 partner gene associated with 8p11 myeloproliferative syndrome. *Leukemia* 23:1359–1361.

Srinivas U, Barwad A, Pubbaraju SV (2014): Complete response of monoblastic myeloid sarcoma with FIP1L1-PDGFRA rearrangement to imatinib monotherapy. *Br J Haematol* 165(5):583.

Steensma DP, Dewald GW, Lasho TL, Powell HL, McClure RF, Levine RL, et al. (2005): The JAK2 V617F activating tyrosine kinase mutation is an infrequent event in both "atypical" myeloproliferative disorders and myelodysplastic syndromes. *Blood* 106:1207–1209.

Sterkers Y, Preudhomme C, Lai JL, Demory JL, Caulier MT, Wattel E, et al. (1998): Acute myeloid leukemia and myelo-dysplastic syndromes following essential thrombocythemia treated with hydroxyurea: high proportion of cases with 17p deletion. *Blood* 91:616–622.

Stover EH, Chen J, Folens C, Lee BH, Mentens N, Marynen P, et al. (2006): Activation of FIP1L1-PDGFRalpha requires disruption of the juxtamembrane domain of PDGFRalpha and is FIP1L1-independent. *Proc Natl Acad Sci USA* 103:8078–8083.

Strasser-Weippl K, Steurer M, Kees M, Augustin F, Tzankov A, Dirnhofer S, et al. (2006): Prognostic relevance of cyto-genetics determined by fluorescent in situ hybridization in patients having myelofibrosis with myeloid metaplasia. *Cancer* 107:2801–2806.

Swerdlow SH, Campo E, Harris NL, Jaffe ES, Pileri SA, Stein H, et al. (2008): *WHO Classification of Tumours of Haematopoietic and Lymphoid Tissues.* Lyon, IARC Press.

Swolin B, Weinfeld A, Westin J (1986): Trisomy 1q in polycythemia vera and its relation to disease transition. *Am J Hematol* 22:155–167.

Swolin B, Weinfeld A, Westin J (1988): A prospective long-term cytogenetic study in polycythemia vera in relation to treatment and clinical course. *Blood* 72:386–395.

Swolin B, Rodjer S, Roupe G (2000): Cytogenetic studies in patients with mastocytosis. *Cancer Genet Cytogenet* 120:131–135.

Swolin B, Rodjer S, Ogard I, Roupe G (2002): Trisomies 8 and 9 not detected with fish in patients with mastocytosis. *Am J Hematol* 70:324–325.

Szpurka H, Tiu R, Murugesan G, Aboudola S, Hsi ED, Theil KS, et al. (2006): Refractory anemia with ringed sideroblasts associated with marked thrombocytosis (RARS-T): another myeloproliferative condition characterized by JAK2 V617F mutation. *Blood* 108:2173–2181.

Tang TC, Chang H, Chuang WY (2012): Complete response of myeloid sarcoma with FIP1L1-PDGFRA-associated myeloproliferative neoplasms to imatinib mesylate monotherapy. *Acta Haematol* 128:83–87.

Tefferi A (2012): Myeloproliferative neoplasms 2012: the John M Bennett 80th birthday anniversary lecture. *Leuk Res* 36:1481–1489.

Tefferi A, Gilliland DG (2007): Oncogenes in myeloproliferative disorders. *Cell Cycle* 6:550–566.

Tefferi A, Pardanani A (2014): Genetics: CALR mutations and a new diagnostic algorithm for MPN. *Nat Rev Clin Oncol* 11:125–126.

Tefferi A, Mesa RA, Schroeder G, Hanson CA, Li CY, Dewald GW (2001): Cytogenetic findings and their clinical relevance in myelofibrosis with myeloid metaplasia. *Br J Haematol* 113:763–771.

Tefferi A, Dingli D, Li CY, Dewald GW (2005): Prognostic diversity among cytogenetic abnormalities in myelofibrosis with myeloid metaplasia. *Cancer* 104:1656–1660.

Tefferi A, Sirhan S, Sun Y, Lasho T, Finke CM, Weisberger J, et al. (2009): Oligonucleotide array CGH studies in myeloproliferative neoplasms: comparison with JAK2V617F mutational status and conventional chromosome analysis. *Leuk Res* 33:662–664.

Thiele J, Kvasnicka HM, Mullauer L, Buxhofer-Ausch V, Gisslinger B, Gisslinger H (2011): Essential thrombocythemia versus early primary myelofibrosis: a multicenter study to validate the WHO classification. *Blood* 117:5710–5718.

Third International Workshop on Chromosomes in Leukemia (1981): Report on essential thrombocythemia. *Cancer Genet Cytogenet* 4:138–142.

Trempat P, Villalva C, Laurent G, Armstrong F, Delsol G, Dastugue N, et al. (2003): Chronic myeloproliferative disorders with rearrangement of the platelet-derived growth factor alpha receptor: a new clinical target for STI571/Glivec. *Oncogene* 22:5702–5706.

Vaidya R, Caramazza D, Begna KH, Gangat N, Van Dyke DL, Hanson CA, et al. (2011): Monosomal karyotype in primary myelofibrosis is detrimental to both overall and leukemia-free survival. *Blood* 117:5612–5615.

Valent P, Sperr WR, Schwartz LB, Horny HP (2004): Diagnosis and classification of mast cell proliferative disorders: delineation from immunologic diseases and non-mast cell hematopoietic neoplasms. *J Allergy Clin Immunol* 114:3–11.

Valent P, Gleich GJ, Reiter A, Roufosse F, Weller PF, Hellmann A, et al. (2012a): Pathogenesis and classification of eosinophil disorders: a review of recent developments in the field. *Expert Rev Hematol* 5:157–176.

Valent P, Klion AD, Horny HP, Roufosse F, Gotlib J, Weller PF, et al. (2012b): Contemporary consensus proposal on criteria and classification of eosinophilic disorders and related syndromes. *J Allergy Clin Immunol* 130:607–612.

Valent P, Klion AD, Rosenwasser LJ, Arock M, Bochner BS, Butterfield JH, et al. (2012c): ICON: Eosinophil Disorders. *World Allergy Organ J* 5:174–181.

Vandenberghe P, Wlodarska I, Michaux L, Zachee P, Boogaerts M, Vanstraelen D, et al. (2004): Clinical and molecular features of FIP1L1-PDGFRA (+) chronic eosinophilic leukemias. *Leukemia* 18:734–742.

Vandenberghe P, Michaux L, Hagemeijer-Hausman A (2009): Chronic Myeloproliferative Neoplasms. In: Heim S, Mitelman (eds): *Cancer Cytogenetics*. Hoboken, NJ: Wiley & Sons Inc.

Vardiman JW, Brunning RD, Harris NL (2001): WHO histological classification of chronic myeloproliferative diseases. In: Jaffe ES, Harris NL, Stein H, Vardiman JW, eds. WHO Classification of Tumours. Pathology & Genetics of Tumours of Haematopoietic and Lymphoid Tissues. Lyon, IARC Press: 9–15.

Vardiman JW, Harris NL, Brunning RD (2002): The World Health Organization (WHO) classification of the myeloid neoplasms. *Blood* 100:2292–2302.

Vardiman JW, Brunning RD, Arber DA, Le Beau MM, Porwit A, Tefferi A, et al. (2008): In: Swerdlow SH, Campo E, Harris NL, Jaffe ES, Pileri SA, Stein H, Thiele J, Vardiman JW (eds): *WHO Classification of Tumours of Hematopoietic and Lymphoid Tissues*. Lyon: IARC Press.

Verstovsek S, Mesa RA, Gotlib J, Levy RS, Gupta V, DiPersio JF, et al. (2012): A double-blind placebo-controlled trial of ruxolitinib for myelofibrosis. *N Engl J Med* 366:799–807.

Verstovsek S, Mesa RA, Gotlib J, Levy RS, Gupta V, DiPersio JF, et al. (2013): Efficacy safety and survival with ruxolitinib in patients with myelofibrosis: results of a median 2-year follow-up of COMFORT-I. *Haematologica* 98:1865–1871.

Vizmanos JL, Hernandez R, Vidal MJ, Larrayoz MJ, Odero MD, Marin J, et al. (2004a): Clinical variability of patients with the t(6;8)(q27;p12) and FGFR1OP-FGFR1 fusion: two further cases. *Hematol J* 5:534–537.

Vizmanos JL, Novo FJ, Roman JP, Baxter EJ, Lahortiga I, Larrayoz MJ, et al. (2004b): NIN, a gene encoding a CEP110-like centrosomal protein is fused to PDGFRB in a patient with a t(5;14)(q33;q24) and an imatinib-responsive myeloproliferative disorder. *Cancer Res* 64:2673–2676.

Wakim JJ, Tirado CA, Chen W, Collins R (2011): t(8;22)/BCR-FGFR1 myeloproliferative disorder presenting as B-acute lymphoblastic leukemia: report of a case treated with sorafenib and review of the literature. *Leuk Res* 35:e151–e153.

Walz C, Chase A, Schoch C, et al. (2005): The t(8;17)(p11;q23) in the 8p11 myeloproliferative syndrome fuses MYO18A to FGFR1. *Leukemia* 19:1005–1009.

Walz C, Curtis C, Schnittger S, Schultheis B, Metzgeroth G, Schoch C, et al. (2006): Transient response to imatinib in a chronic eosinophilic leukemia associated with ins(9;4)(q33;q12q25) and a CDK5RAP2-PDGFRA fusion gene. *Genes Chromosomes Cancer* 45:950–956.

Walz C, Metzgeroth G, Haferlach C, Schmitt-Graeff A, Fabarius A, Hagen V, et al. (2007): Characterization of three new imatinib-responsive fusion genes in chronic myeloproliferative disorders generated by disruption of the platelet-derived growth factor receptor beta gene. *Haematologica* 92:163–169.

Walz C, Haferlach C, Hanel A, Metzgeroth G, Erben P, Gosenca D, et al. (2009): Identification of a MYO18A-PDGFRB fusion gene in an eosinophilia-associated atypical myeloproliferative neoplasm with a t(5;17)(q33-34;q11,2). *Genes Chromosomes Cancer* 48:179–183.

Wang JR, Yen CC, Gau JP, Hsiao LT, Liu CY, Pai JT, et al. (2010): A case of myeloid neoplasm associated with eosinophilia and KIAA1509-PDGFRbeta responsive to combination treatment with imatinib mesylate and prednisolone. *J Clin Pharm Ther* 35:733–736.

Wang HY, Thorson JA, Broome HE, Rashidi HH, Curtin PT, Dell'Aquila ML (2011): t(4;22)(q12;q11,2) involving presumptive platelet-derived growth factor receptor A and break cluster region in a patient with mixed phenotype acute leukemia. *Hum Pathol* 42:2029–2036.

Wasag B, Lierman E, Meeus P, Cools J, Vandenberghe P (2011): The kinase inhibitor TKI258 is active against the novel CUX1-FGFR1 fusion detected in a patient with T-lymphoblastic leukemia/lymphoma and t(7;8)(q22;p11). *Haematologica* 96:922–926.

Wilkinson K, Velloso ER, Lopes LF, Lee C, Aster JC, Shipp MA, et al. (2003): Cloning of the t(1;5)(q23;q33) in a myeloproliferative disorder associated with eosinophilia: involvement of PDGFRB and response to imatinib. *Blood* 102:4187–4190.

Winkelmann N, Hidalgo-Curtis C, Waghorn K, Score J, Dickinson H, Jack A, et al. (2013): Recurrent CEP85L-PDGFRB fusion in patient with t(5;6) and imatinib-responsive myeloproliferative neoplasm with eosinophilia. *Leuk Lymphoma* 54:1527–1531.

Xiao S, Nalabolu SR, Aster JC, Ma J, Abruzzo L, Jaffe ES, et al. (1998): FGFR1 is fused with a novel zinc-finger gene ZNF198 in the t(8;13) leukaemia/lymphoma syndrome. *Nat Genet* 18:84–87.

CHAPTER 10

Acute lymphoblastic leukemia

Christine J. Harrison[1] and Bertil Johansson[2]

[1]Leukaemia Research Cytogenetics Group, Northern Institute for Cancer Research, Newcastle University, Newcastle upon Tyne, UK
[2]Department of Clinical Genetics, University of Lund, Lund, Sweden

Acute lymphoblastic leukemia (ALL) is characterized by the accumulation of malignant, immature lymphoid cells in the bone marrow and, in most cases, also in peripheral blood. The disease is classified broadly as B-lineage ALL (B-ALL) and T-lineage ALL (T-ALL). It is the most common malignancy in children, representing almost 25% of pediatric cancer. The total incidence of ALL in childhood is 3–4 per 100 000 per year, while for adults, it is less than 1. There is a peak in incidence among children aged 2–5 years, which is approximately four times greater than in infants and almost 10 times greater than in adolescents. The incidence of ALL is almost three times higher in white than black children. Among adults, ALL is more frequent in younger patients, with a median age of less than 30 years. Males are more often affected than females. ALL represents a success story from the point of view of outcome with an overall 5-year survival for children of greater than 90%. Adult survival, although improved, remains at around 50%.

Morphologic, immunophenotypic, and cytogenetic characteristics

B-ALL

B-cell precursor ALL (BCP-ALL) is a malignancy of lymphoblasts committed to the B-cell lineage. The morphology of the cells is largely of the French–American–British (FAB) L1 or L2 type (see following text). A small percentage of patients have a mature B immunophenotype. BCP-ALL is primarily a disease of childhood in that 75% of patients are under the age of 6 years. Bone marrow and peripheral blood are involved in all cases, with frequent extramedullary involvement, primarily of the central nervous system (CNS), lymph nodes, spleen, liver, and testes (Pui et al., 2004). Cytogenetics and molecular testing remain the "gold standard" techniques for the genetic classification of ALL.

T-ALL

T-ALL, which accounts for approximately 15% of childhood and 25% of adult ALL, is a high-risk malignancy of thymocytes (Pui et al., 2004). It is a heterogeneous disease classified according to the expression of specific cytoplasmic or surface markers. The development of normal thymocytes and their regulation mechanisms have been studied extensively, and it has been shown that the significant genes in T-cell development are also rearranged or deregulated in T-ALL (Graux et al., 2006). This is supported by the gene expression signatures of T-ALL, which mirror the specific stages of thymocyte development (Ferrando and Look, 2003). Collectively, these observations indicate a

Cancer Cytogenetics: Chromosomal and Molecular Genetic Aberrations of Tumor Cells, Fourth Edition.
Edited by Sverre Heim and Felix Mitelman.
© 2015 John Wiley & Sons, Ltd. Published 2015 by John Wiley & Sons, Ltd.

multistep process of pathogenesis in T-ALL, further supported by the simultaneous occurrence of multiple genetic changes in the leukemic cells (De Keersmaecker et al., 2005b; Meijerink, 2010).

Morphologic and immunophenotypic features

ALL may be subdivided into subgroups on the basis of cytomorphologic features. The FAB classification (Bennett et al., 1976) constituted the most widely accepted scheme, which provided the basis for the development of current classification systems. The FAB system takes into account both the characteristic morphology of individual cells and the degree of heterogeneity within the leukemic cell population. The salient features of the three ALL subgroups recognized by the FAB classification are as follows:

- L1: Small cells with homogeneous nuclear chromatin, regular nuclear shape, and indistinct nucleoli. This category includes the majority of childhood cases, which may be of B- or T-cell lineage.
- L2: Larger cells of more variable size and distribution of nuclear chromatin than in L1. The nuclear shape is more irregular, and one or more large nucleoli may be present. Approximately 25% of ALL cases are in this category, and they may be of B- as well as T-cell lineage.
- L3: Large, homogeneous cells with finely stippled nuclear chromatin, regular nucleus, prominent nucleoli, and often prominent vacuolation of the basophilic cytoplasm. This category comprises only 1–2% of ALL. There is little association between these cytological features and the immunophenotype, apart from a strong correlation between L3 and a mature B immunophenotype. This is considered as the leukemic equivalent of Burkitt lymphoma and is regarded as a distinct disease entity.

Increased emphasis on the functional aspects of cellular maturation and differentiation led to the proposal of additional classification criteria for ALL. The morphology–immunology–cytogenetics (MIC) classification (First MIC Cooperative Study Group, 1986) was a first attempt to combine information obtained from these three fields of leukemia research into a diagnostic scheme that reflected the intrinsic pathobiology of the various ALL subtypes. Leukemic cells of different types express characteristic nuclear, cytoplasmic, and cell surface antigens, which can be identified with monoclonal antibodies. This is termed the immunophenotype. There are several hundred monoclonal antibodies that allow the detection of more than 260 clusters of differentiation (CD) groupings. The MIC system defines four major immunologic subclasses of B-ALL: (i) In *early B-precursor ALL* (or *early pre-B-ALL*, sometimes known as *pro-B*), the immunophenotype and the beginning of immunoglobulin locus rearrangements strongly indicate that the cells are committed to B-lineage differentiation. They always express CD19, human leukocyte antigen (HLA)-DR, and terminal deoxynucleotidyl transferase (TdT), and the majority express CD22 and CD79a. This leukemia type accounts for approximately 10% of adult and childhood ALL. (ii) When the leukemic cells express the common ALL antigen (CD10) in addition to CD19 and TdT, this is considered to be a sign of further maturation. The leukemia is then classified as *common ALL*, the most frequent ALL subtype accounting for about 60% of childhood and adult ALL. (iii) As the cells start to express immunoglobulin in the cytoplasm as well as CD79b, the leukemia is termed *pre-B-ALL*. The expression of the other markers is identical to common ALL. This subtype accounts for 20–25% of childhood ALL cases. These three subtypes together—early B-precursor ALL, common ALL, and pre-B-ALL—comprise the BCP-ALL category. (iv) The most mature acute leukemia of the B-lineage, *mature B-cell ALL*, is diagnosed when the leukemic cells express immunoglobulins with single light chains on the cell surface. These leukemic cells invariably have L3 morphology and are the leukemic variant of Burkitt lymphoma. They account for approximately 5% of adult and 2% of childhood ALL.

Only two immunological categories of T-ALL are defined by the MIC classification: (i) *early T-precursor ALL* and (ii) the more mature *T-ALL*. All blasts express surface CD7 and cytoplasmic CD3, with variable expression of TdT, CD34, CD2, and CD5. HLA-DR expression in T-ALL is characteristic of an immature clone. T-cell ALL can be subdivided according to the stages of T-cell development into pro-T, pre-T, cortical-T, and mature-T.

The MIC subgroups are associated with non-random karyotypic abnormalities in a manner comparable to the specificity seen between chromosomal rearrangements and morphologic subgroups in acute myeloid leukemia (AML; Chapter 6).

More recently, the World Health Organization (WHO) developed a more advanced classification defining *B-lymphoblastic leukemia/lymphoma and T-lymphoblastic leukemia/lymphoma* (Swerdlow et al., 2008). This system incorporates cytomorphology, immunophenotype, and genetics to define the categories of these two subgroups, with some details of epidemiology, clinical features, and prognosis. The genetic content is restricted to those abnormalities that specifically define a genetic subgroup and thus is rather limited. A new edition is in preparation in which the genetic definitions are being expanded.

Early T-cell precursor ALL

Recently, a subtype of immature T-ALL was described in which the leukemic cells lack expression of mature/cortical thymic markers such as CD1a, CD8, and CD5 and exhibit aberrant expression of myeloid and stem cell markers. These early T-cell precursor (ETP)-ALL comprise an aggressive subtype with a dismal prognosis (Coustan-Smith et al., 2009; Inukai et al., 2012).

Most patients with ALL have characteristic, acquired karyotypic abnormalities in their leukemic cells

An early cytogenetic review undertaken by the Third International Workshop on Chromosomes in Leukemia (1980) found clonal chromosomal aberrations in 66% of the 330 patients (173 adults, 157 children) investigated. Higher aberration frequencies, up to almost 90%, have since been reported by incorporating detection by fluorescence *in situ* hybridization (FISH) and molecular testing of cryptic abnormalities and those hidden within cases with a failed cytogenetic result (Harrison et al., 2005; Moorman et al., 2010b). There are now numerous nonrandom chromosomal rearrangements known with clinical significance in relation to diagnosis and prognosis. Many are also of special interest because they have provided insights into the molecular mechanisms of ALL pathogenesis. The abnormalities may be numerical or structural, with many karyotypes containing both types of change. New abnormalities are added every year, not least because state-of-the-art technologies are increasingly being introduced into leukemia diagnostics. Throughout the 1980s and the 1990s, advancing techniques in FISH, particularly around the Human Genome Mapping Project (McPherson et al., 2001), led to the development of probes for any known human DNA sequence. More recently, studies utilizing array-based comparative genomic hybridization (aCGH) and single-nucleotide polymorphism (SNP) arrays, as well as multiplex ligation-dependent probe amplification (MLPA), have revealed novel chromosomal changes, such as submicroscopic deletions and amplifications, many below the resolution of chromosome banding analysis, which have greatly enhanced the understanding of the genetic mechanisms involved in leukemogenesis (Kuiper et al., 2007; Mullighan et al., 2007; Strefford et al., 2007; Kawamata et al., 2008; Schwab et al., 2013). Classification of childhood BCP-ALL by gene expression profiling has also been used to define significant genetic subgroups, to predict relapse, and to highlight novel molecular targets for therapy (Yeoh et al., 2002; Ross et al., 2003; Harvey et al., 2010b). Currently, novel approaches using next-generation sequencing (NGS) are being introduced into routine practice, for example, to identify important gene mutations within key signaling pathways (Zhang et al., 2011). It is becoming the convention to include these methodologies as complementary cytogenetic techniques, which has brought cytogenetic analysis fashionably back into the 21st century.

Different types of chromosomal rearrangements are predominant in BCP-, mature B-, and T-ALL. Numerical changes affecting ploidy and translocations that produce fusion genes are characteristic of BCP-ALL. These are formed by "in-frame" fusion of parts of the two partner genes located at the chromosomal breakpoints. The fusion gene encodes a new chimeric protein with oncogenic potential (Harrison and Foroni, 2002). These types of translocations are less frequent in T-ALL, which instead often harbor translocations or inversions involving the T-cell receptor (*TCR*) loci: α (*TRA*) and δ (*TRD*) located in chromosomal band 14q11, and β (*TRB*) and γ (*TRG*) located in 7q34 and 7p14, respectively. Such abnormalities are found in approximately 35% of T-ALL by FISH (Cauwelier et al., 2006), with many being cryptic at the banding level. These chromosomal rearrangements result in oncogenes becoming juxtaposed to the promoter and enhancer elements of the *TCR* genes, leading to their aberrant expression (Rabbitts, 1994). Alternatively, aberrant expression of oncogenic transcription factors in T-ALL may result from loss of the upstream transcriptional mechanisms that normally downregulate the expression of these oncogenes during T-cell development (Ferrando et al., 2004a; van Vlierberghe et al., 2006). This mechanism of oncogene upregulation predominates in mature B-ALL, in which the promoters of the immunoglobulin loci upregulate *MYC* as a result of the t(8;14)(q24;q32) and its variant translocations (see following text and Chapter 11).

The cytogenetic, molecular genetic, and clinical features of ALL-associated numerical and structural chromosome abnormalities reported in a sufficient number to allow delineation of clinicogenetic associations are summarized in the following as well as in Table 10.1.

Established ploidy groups in ALL

Ploidy groups representing significant and established cytogenetic entities in ALL comprise high hyperdiploidy (51–65 chromosomes), near haploidy (25–29 chromosomes), low hypodiploidy (30–39 chromosomes), near triploidy (66–79 chromosomes), and near tetraploidy (84–100 chromosomes). Low hyperdiploidy (47–49 chromosomes) or hypodiploidy with 45 chromosomes and single numerical aberrations are increasingly being found as secondary changes associated with specific structural abnormalities, which will be discussed in the following relevant sections.

High hyperdiploidy

High hyperdiploidy is defined as the presence of 51–65 chromosomes with the most frequent modal chromosome number being 55 (Figure 10.1). The gain of chromosomes is nonrandom, and eight chromosomes account for close to 80% of all gains: +4 (78–80% of cases), +6 (85–90%), +10 (63–76%), +14 (84–90%), +17 (68–77%), +18 (76–86%), +21 (99–100%), and +X (89–95%). The gains usually present as trisomies (or two copies of the X chromosome in males). The exceptions are of chromosome 21, which is tetrasomic in approximately 70% of cases, and tetrasomies of chromosomes 14, 10, and 18, which occur in 8–16% of cases (Moorman et al., 2003; Heerema et al., 2007; Paulsson et al., 2010). Structural chromosomal abnormalities are also present in around 50% of cases (Paulsson and Johansson, 2009). Abnormalities of the long arm of chromosome 1 (1q), usually a partial duplication, are the most frequent, being present in approximately 15% of cases. Deletions of 6q are seen in 7% and are usually independent of 1q abnormalities. Isochromosomes occur in about 4%, the most frequent is i(17)(q10) present in 2%. Mutations and deletions of the *PAX5* gene are common in childhood high-hyperdiploid ALL (Mulligan et al., 2007). Mutations of the *FLT3*, *NRAS*, *KRAS*, and *PTPN11* genes have also been found in approximately one-third of cases, where they appear to be mutually exclusive (Case et al., 2008; Paulsson et al., 2008).

There is strong evidence that some childhood leukemias arise *in utero*, including those with high hyperdiploidy (Greaves, 2005). The support comes from the finding of the same leukemia-related abnormalities and clonogenic immunoglobulin gene rearrangements in neonatal blood spots and cord blood prior to the development of overt leukemia. With this in mind, it is also of interest to consider how high hyperdiploidy is acquired. Four possibilities can be envisaged: (1) by initial near haploidy followed by doubling of the chromosomes, (2) the development of tetraploidy followed by losses, (3) sequential gains of chromosomes in consecutive cell divisions, or (4) the simultaneous gain of multiple chromosomes in a single abnormal division. Mechanism 1 occurs, albeit rarely, specifically in association with near haploidy (see following text). Otherwise, there is compelling molecular evidence to indicate that most cases of high hyperdiploidy arise through a simultaneous gain of chromosomes in a single cell division (Paulsson et al., 2005b).

High-hyperdiploid ALL usually has a CD10-positive, early pre-B/common immunophenotype. The incidence differs significantly between children and adults. It has been reported to be as high

Table 10.1 Cytogenetic, molecular genetic, and clinical features of ALL-associated chromosomal aberrations

Aberration	Genes involved	Age group	Characteristic features	Risk
High hyperdiploidy	Whole chromosome gains, *FLT3*, *NRAS*, *KRAS*, *PTPN11*, and *PAX5* mutations	Mostly children, some adults	Common/early pre-B, CD10+	Favorable
Near haploidy	Whole chromosome gains onto the haploid set	Children	Common/pre-B	Poor
Low hypodiploidy	Whole chromosome gains onto the haploid set	Adults	Common/pre-B	Poor
High hypodiploidy	Chromosome loss and structural changes	All	B- and T-lineage	<44, poor
Trisomy 5	Chromosome 5 gain	Older children	Pre-B	Poor
t(1;5)(q21;q33)	*MEF2D*, *CSF1R*	Older children and adults	Pre-B	Unknown
t(1;7)(p34;q34)	*LCK*, *TRB*	Older children and adults	T-ALL	Unknown
t(1;7)(p32;q34)	*TAL1*, *TRB*	Mostly children, some adults	T-ALL	Better than other T-ALL
t(1;11)(p32;q23)	*EPS15*, *MLL*	Mainly infants, some children and adults	Common/pre-B	Variable
t(1;14)(p32;q11)	*TAL1*, *TRA/TRD*	Mostly children, some adults	T-ALL	Better than other T-ALL
TAL1 deletion	*TAL1*, *STIL*	Mostly children, some adults	T-ALL	Better than other T-ALL
dup(1) (q12~21q31~32)	*B4GALT3*, *DAP3*, *RGS16*, *TMEM183A*, and *UCK2*, overexpressed	All	B-lineage	Unknown
t(1;19)(q23;p13.3)	*PBX1*, *TCF3*	All	Pre-B, CD10+, cytoplasmic Ig+	Standard
t(2;8)(p11;q24)	*IGK*, *MYC*	All	Mature B-ALL	Favorable
t(4;11)(q21;q23)	*AFF1*, *MLL*	Mainly infants, some children and adults	Early pre-B, CD10-, CD19+	Poor
del(5)(q32q33.3)	*EBF1*, *PDGFRB*	Older children and adults	Pre-B	Poor
t(5;9)(q22;q34)	*SNX2*, *ABL1*	Older children and adults	Pre-B	Poor
t(5;14)(q31;q32)	*IL3*, *IGH*	Children and adults	Pre-B	Unknown
t(5;14)(q35;q32)	*TLX3*, *BCL11B*	Children and adults	T-ALL	Poor
del(6q)	Unknown	All	Mostly common/pre-B, some T	Variable
t(6;7)(q23;q34)	*MYB*, *TRB*	Young children	T-ALL	Unknown
dup(6)(q23q23)	*MYB*	Young children	T-ALL	Unknown
t(6;11)(q27;q23)	*MLLT4*, *MLL*	All	B- and T-lineage ALL	Poor

Table 10.1 (*Continued*)

Aberration	Genes involved	Age group	Characteristic features	Risk
t(6;14)(p22;q32)	ID4, IGH	Older children and adults	Pre-B	Unknown
inv(7)(p15q34)	HOXA, TRB	All	T-ALL	Unknown
t(7;7)(p15;q34)	HOXA, TRB	All	T-ALL	Unknown
t(7;14)(p15;q11)	HOXA, TRD	All	T-ALL	Unknown
t(7;14)(p15;q32)	HOXA, BCL11B	All	T-ALL	Unknown
dic(7;9)(p11~13; p11~13)	?PAX5	All	B-lineage	Variable
del(7)(p12.2p12.2)	IKZF1	All	Common/pre-B	Poor
i(7)(q10)	Unknown	All	Pre-B	Unknown
t(7;9)(q34;q32)	TRB, TAL2	All	T-ALL	Unknown
t(7;9)(q34;q34.3)	TRB, NOTCH1	All	T-ALL	Unknown
NOTCH1 mutations	NOTCH1	All	T-ALL	Unknown
t(7;10)(q34;q24)	TRB, TLX1	Mainly adults, some children	T-ALL, early cortical	Better than other T-ALL
t(7;11)(q34;p13)	TRB, LMO1	Children and adults	T-ALL	Unknown
t(7;11)(q34;p15)	TRB, LMO2	Children and adults	T-ALL	Unknown
t(7;12)(q34;p13.3)	TRB, CCND2	All	T-ALL	Unknown
t(7;12)(q36;p13)	MNX1, ETV6	Infants	Common/pre-B	Unknown
t(7;19)(q34;p13)	TRB, LYL1	All	T-ALL	Poor
t(8;14)(q11;q32)	CEBPD, IGH	Older children and adults	Pre-B	Unknown
t(8;14)(q24;q11)	MYC, TRA/D	All	T-ALL	Unknown
t(8;14)(q24;q32)	MYC, IGH	All	Mature B-ALL	Favorable
t(8;22)(q24;q11)	MYC, IGL	All	Mature B-ALL	Favorable
del(9p)	CDKN2A	All	B- and T-lineage	Variable
t(9;12)(p24;p13)	JAK2, ETV6	One child	T-ALL	Unknown
dic(9;12) (p11~12;p11~13)	PAX5, ETV6	All	Pre-B	Favorable
dic(9;20)(p13;q11)	PAX5	Young children	Pre-B	Poor
i(9)(q10)	Unknown	Older children and adults	Mostly pre-B	Unknown
t(9;9)(q34;q34)/del(9) (q34q34)	NUP214, ABL1	Adults	T-ALL	Unknown
t(9;10)(q34;q22.3)	ABL1, ZMIZ1	Children	Pre-B	Unknown
t(9;11)(p21;q23)	MLLT3, MLL	All	Pre-B	Unknown
t(9;12)(q34;p13)	PAX5, ETV6	All	Pre-B	Unknown
t(9;14)(q34;q32)	ABL1, EML1	All	T-ALL	Unknown
t(9;22)(q34;q11)	ABL1, BCR	Mainly adults, some children	Pre-B	Extremely poor
t(10;11)(p12;q14)	MLLT10, PICALM	Children and adults	T-ALL	Poor
10p12 and 11q23	MLLT10, MLL	All	Pre-B and T-ALL	Poor
t(10;14)(q24;q11)	TLX1, TRA/TRD	Mainly adults, some children	T-ALL, early cortical	Better than other T-ALL
t(11;14)(p13;q11)	LMO1, TRA/TRD	Children and adults	T-ALL	Unknown

(*Continued*)

Table 10.1 (*Continued*)

Aberration	Genes involved	Age group	Characteristic features	Risk
t(11;14)(p15;q11)	LMO2, TRA/TRD	Children and adults	T-ALL	Unknown
t(11;19)(q23;p13.3)	MLL, MLLT1	Mainly infants, some children and adults	Pre-B	Poor
t(12;14)(p13;q11)	CCND2, TRA	All	T-ALL	Unknown
t(12;17)(p13;q11)	ZNF384, TAF15	Young adults	Early pre-B, CD13+, CD30+	Unknown
t(12;19)(p13;p13)	ZNF384, TCF3; NOL1, TCF3	All	Variant t(1;19)	Unknown
t(12;21)(p13;q22)	ETV6, RUNX1	Young children	Pre-B	Favorable
t(12;22)(p13;q12)	ZNF384, EWSR1	Young adults	As t(12;17)	Unknown
del(13)(q12~14)	Unknown	Children and adults	B-lineage	Unknown
inv(14)(q11q32)	TRA, TCL1	All	T-ALL secondary to AT	Unknown
inv(14)(q11q32)	TRD, BCL11B	All	T-ALL	Unknown
inv(14)(q11q32)	CEBPE, IGH	Older children and adults	Pre-B	Unknown
t(14;14)(q11;q32)	TRA, TCL1	All	T-ALL secondary to AT	Unknown
t(14;14)(q11;q32)	TRD, BCL11B	All	T-ALL	Unknown
t(14;14)(q11;q32)	CEBPE, IGH	Older children and adults	Pre-B	Unknown
t(14;18)(q32;q21)	IGH, BCL2	Adults	Pre-B and mature B	Poor
t(14;19)(q32;q13)	IGH, CEBPA	Older children and adults	Pre-B	Unknown
t(14;20)(q32;q13)	IGH, CEBPB	Older children and adults	Pre-B	Unknown
t(14;21)(q11;q22)	TRA, OLIG2	All	T-ALL	Unknown
15q13~15 rearrangements	Unknown	Mainly infants and some children	B-lineage	Standard
i(17)(q10)	Unknown	All	Secondary change	Unknown
t(17;19)(q22;p13)	HLF, TCF3	All	Pre-B, variant t(1;19)	Extremely poor
del(21)(q22.2q22.2)	ERG	Older children	Pre-B	Good
i(21)(q10)	Unknown	All	Pre-B	Unknown
iAMP21	?RUNX1	Older children	Common/pre-B	Extremely poor
t(X;14)(p22;q32)/ t(Y;14)(p11;q32)	IGH, CRLF2	Older children and adults	Pre-B	Intermediate
del(X)(p22.33p22.33)/ del(Y)(p11.32p11.32)	P2RY8, CRLF2	Older children and adults	Pre-B	Intermediate

as one-third in childhood series (Moorman et al., 2003), whereas among adults, it is found in approximately 10% (Chilton et al., 2014). It was shown by FISH using selected centromeric probes that the incidence of high hyperdiploidy was surprisingly high in cases with a failed or normal cytogenetic result (Harrison et al., 2005). This emphasizes the need to search for hidden high-hyperdiploid clones in such cases.

Children with high-hyperdiploid ALL respond well to standard chemotherapy regimens. They consistently show a superior outcome, along with patients

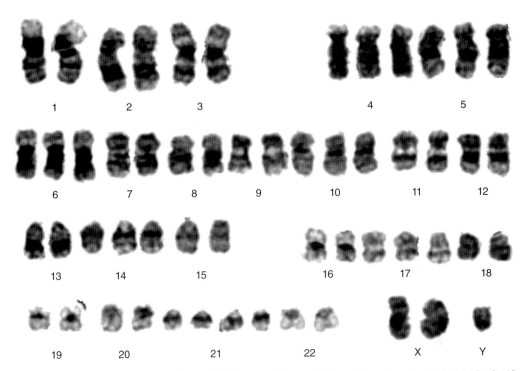

Figure 10.1 Karyogram showing a high-hyperdiploid karyotype from a childhood ALL patient: 55, XY, +X, +4, +5, +6, +10, +14, +17, +21, +21.

with t(12;21)(p13;q22)/*ETV6–RUNX1*, when compared to patients in other cytogenetic subgroups. Recent studies have reported event-free survival rates of greater than 80% at 5 years (Moorman et al., 2010b). The best prognosis is found in younger children (aged 1–9 years) compared to older ones (aged 10–16 years), as well as in those with a higher modal chromosome number (56–67 vs. 51–55 chromosomes) (Raimondi et al., 1996; Dastugue et al., 2013; Paulsson et al., 2013a). The good prognosis associated with the gain of specific chromosomes provides the most likely explanation for the improved outcome among the 56–67 chromosome group. Three early publications and two more recent ones have shown that gains of chromosomes 4, 10 (Harris et al., 1992), and 17 (Heerema et al., 2000b) (referred to as triple trisomies), as well as of chromosome 18 (Moorman et al., 2003), confer improved survival of these patients. Initially, triple (trisomies 4, 10, and 17) and currently double trisomies (chromosomes 4 and 10) are used to classify patients with high-hyperdiploid ALL in the US treatment trials. The presence of structural abnormalities has no effect on the good prognosis of high-hyperdiploid ALL (Raimondi et al., 1996; Moorman et al., 2003; Paulsson et al., 2013a).

Hypodiploid and near-haploid ALL

Hypodiploidy, defined as less than 46 chromosomes, is rare in ALL. It occurs at an overall incidence of approximately 5%, independent of age (Harrison et al., 2004). Based on chromosome number and characteristic cytogenetic features, hypodiploid cases cluster into three distinct subgroups: near haploidy (25–29 chromosomes), low hypodiploidy (30–39 chromosomes), and high hypodiploidy (40–45 chromosomes). The majority (80%) of hypodiploid cases have 45 chromosomes, showing that only a small number exist with less than 45 chromosomes. Among all patients with less than 45 chromosomes, the outcome was extremely poor (Nachman et al., 2007).

Near haploidy (25–29 chromosomes)

Near haploidy has been identified as a rare and unique patient group (Gibbons et al., 1991; Raimondi et al., 2003; Harrison et al., 2004; Nachman et al., 2007; Holmfeldt et al., 2013). Although the range in chromosome number is 25–29, the majority of cases have 26 chromosomes with common chromosomal disomies (Figure 10.2). The most frequent additions to the haploid chromosome set are of chromosome

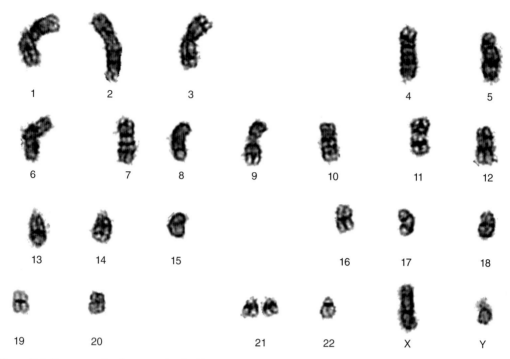

Figure 10.2 Karyogram showing a near-haploid karyotype from a childhood ALL patient: 25<1n>, X, +Y, +21.

21 in all cases, followed by chromosomes X, Y, 14, and 18. This reflects the same pattern of chromosomal gains as seen in high-hyperdiploid ALL (see preceding text). Structural abnormalities are rare within this group (Safavi et al., 2013). A coincident population of hyperdiploid cells with double the chromosome number, representing a duplication of the near-haploid cell line, is frequently present. Cytogenetic evidence has indicated that endoreduplication is the mechanism responsible for this related population (Ma et al., 1998). The distinctive cytogenetic profile of this doubled population, with tetrasomies of most of the gained chromosomes, distinguishes these cases from those with classical high hyperdiploidy. This distinction is extremely important, given the opposing prognostic significance between these two patient groups (see following text) for which treatment decisions are based on the karyotype.

From molecular and genomic profiling studies, including whole-genome and whole-exome sequencing, it was shown that the leukemic cells of patients with near haploidy harbor alterations targeting the lymphoid transcription factor gene *IKZF3* (encoding AIOLOS, 13%), receptor tyrosine kinase signaling, and RAS signaling (71%, affecting

the *NF1* gene in 40% but also *NRAS, KRAS*, and *PTPN11*), leading to activation of the RAS and phosphoinositide 3-kinase (PI3K) signaling pathways (Holmfeldt et al., 2013).

Low hypodiploidy (30–39 chromosomes)

ALL with low hypodiploidy of 30–39 chromosomes is also rare. The original evidence that this group demonstrated consistent with numerical chromosomal changes distinct from near haploidy came from a small study of seven patients described as "severe hypodiploidy" (Callen et al., 1989). They showed a number of chromosomal gains onto the haploid chromosome set in common with near-haploid patients, namely, of chromosomes X, Y, 14, 18, and 21, but with additional gains specific to them: most frequently of chromosomes 1, 11, and 19, followed by chromosomes 5, 6, 8, 10, and 22, and less frequently of chromosomes 2 and 12, while two copies of chromosomes 3, 4, 13, 15, and 16 are rarely seen. Chromosomes 7 and 17 are usually monosomic. Structural chromosomal abnormalities are more frequent than in the near-haploid group (Harrison et al., 2004; Holmfeldt et al., 2013; Mühlbacher et al., 2014). In common with the near-haploid group, the majority of cases show cytogenetic evidence of a population with duplication of the hypodiploid chromosome number, described as near-triploidy (Charrin et al., 2004).

From NGS studies, it has been shown that low-hypodiploid ALL is characterized by inactivating mutations in *IKZF2* (encoding HELIOS, 53%) and aberrations affecting *RB1* (41%), with almost 100% of cases harboring *TP53* mutations (Holmfeldt et al., 2013; Mühlbacher et al., 2014). In approximately 50% of childhood cases with *TP53* mutations, they were also present in matched nontumor DNA, suggesting germline inheritance. These germline mutations were the types indicative of Li–Fraumeni syndrome, a familial condition that greatly increases susceptibility to cancer. These findings implicate for the first time that low-hypodiploid ALL is a manifestation of Li–Fraumeni syndrome (Holmfeldt et al., 2013; Powell et al., 2013), indicating a need to screen for germline *TP53* mutations when low-hypodiploid ALL is diagnosed with a view to genetic counseling of affected families.

As shown for near haploidy, low-hypodiploid leukemic cells show activation of RAS and PI3K signaling pathways. Cells with these abnormalities show sensitivity to PI3K and PI3K/mTOR inhibitors, indicating that these drugs should be explored as a new therapeutic strategy for these aggressive forms of leukemia.

Hidden hypodiploid clones associated with hyperdiploidy or near triploidy

Hyperdiploidy or near triploidy, manifesting with a doubling of gained chromosomes, is likely to be masking a hidden near-haploid or low-hypodiploid clone. FISH with informative centromeric probes, measurement of DNA index, and SNP array analysis revealing multiple uniparental isodisomies have provided useful approaches when the presence of a hidden near-haploid/low-hyperdiploid clone is suspected (Stark et al., 2001; Charrin et al., 2004; Safavi et al., 2013). It is recommended that these tests should be performed in such cases.

High hypodiploidy (40–45 chromosomes)

Some studies have segregated patients with 40–44 chromosomes from those with 45, although their chromosomal changes are similar. Their karyotypes differ significantly from the two groups with less than 40 chromosomes described earlier. They have a high incidence of complex chromosomal abnormalities, with preferential involvement of chromosomes 7, 9, and 12 (Heerema et al., 1999; Harrison et al., 2004; Nachman et al., 2007). The overall reduction in chromosome number may be attributable either to whole chromosome loss or to unbalanced translocations resulting in dicentric chromosomes. The most frequent whole chromosome losses are of chromosomes X, Y, 7, 9, and 13. Chromosome 9 is the one most often involved in the formation of dicentrics, among which the dic(9;20)(p13;q11) is the most common rearrangement (see following text). Chromosomes 7 and 12 are the next most frequently involved. The most commonly observed deletions are of the short arms of chromosomes 7, 9, and 12. Cell populations with duplication of the high-hypodiploid chromosome number are not seen.

Clinical features of the different hypodiploid groups

Patients with near-haploid and low-hypodiploid ALL have common/pre-B immunophenotypes, with the majority having a low white blood cell (WBC) count ($<50 \times 10^9$/l). However, the two groups show different age distributions. Near haploidy is restricted to childhood patients, with a median age of 7 years (range 2–15 years), while patients with low hypodiploidy include adults and children greater than or equal to 9 years old. Although the majority is clustered between 9 and 20 years of age, patients up to the age of 73 years have been described. A particularly poor outcome has been reported for children with near-haploid ALL. Patients with 31–39 chromosomes have a similarly poor outcome, which is unchanged by the presence of a duplicated hyperdiploid population (Gibbons et al., 1991; Harrison et al., 2004; Nachman et al., 2007; Holmfeldt et al., 2013). These observations emphasize the need for accurate diagnosis of near haploidy and low hyperdiploidy to ensure that all cases with less than 40 chromosomes are classified into the appropriate high-risk group for treatment.

Patients with high-hypodiploid ALL are clinically as well as cytogenetically distinct from the near-haploid and low-hypodiploid groups. The age range is 1–52 years with a similar incidence across all ages. The group includes patients with T-ALL in addition to those with BCP-ALL. Patients with ALL with 40–45 chromosomes fare better overall than do the other hypodiploid groups, with no obvious association between the type of chromosomal abnormality and outcome. Although Nachman et al. (2007) indicated a poor outcome for all patients with less than 44 chromosomes, the numbers in their series were small. In terms of understanding the prognosis among high-hypodiploid patients, those known to have established chromosomal abnormalities should be excluded. For example, it is common to find ALL cases with *ETV6–RUNX1* and *BCR–ABL1* fusions having 44 or 45 chromosomes, due to specifically associated chromosomal losses. Once excluded, the variable outcome within the 42–45 chromosome group translates into an overall intermediate risk. Additional contributing factors, maybe at the genetic level, need to be sought to accurately classify this heterogeneous group in terms of outcome.

Near triploidy

Evidence indicates that patients reported to have near triploidy should be included within the low-hyperdiploid group (Charrin et al., 2004; Moorman et al., 2007b). They would be expected to harbor a hidden low-hyperdiploid clone, which would be revealed by FISH with selected centromeric probes, by the measurement of DNA index, or by SNP array analysis (see preceding text).

Near tetraploidy

Near tetraploidy (84–100 chromosomes) has been reported in approximately 1% of childhood BCP-ALL and has been occasionally found in T-ALL (Attarbaschi et al., 2006). It is currently unclear whether this ploidy group constitutes a defined cytogenetic entity. It was shown by Raynaud et al. (1999) that approximately 6% of patients with the cryptic t(12;21)(p13;q22) have a near-tetraploid karyotype, while Attarbaschi et al. (2006) showed that 90% of BCP-ALL patients with near tetraploidy harbored the *ETV6–RUNX1* fusion. Thus, they concluded that near tetraploidy was a specific feature of *ETV6–RUNX1*-positive BCP-ALL, associated with the same excellent outcome afforded to other patients with t(12;21).

Trisomy 5

Although only few cases have been reported with trisomy 5 as a sole cytogenetic abnormality, they are emerging as a specific entity. They have BCP-ALL and show a male predominance. This trisomy occurs mostly in older children, and although the numbers are small, it appears to be associated with a poor outcome (Harris et al., 2004).

Structural rearrangements

The cytogenetic, molecular genetic, and clinical features of ALL-associated structural abnormalities are summarized in the following as well as in Table 10.1 in order of chromosome number. Aberrations involving the same chromosome are listed from pter to qter. For each anomaly, the Mitelman Database of Chromosome Aberrations and Gene Fusions in Cancer (Mitelman et al., 2014) has been searched to identify the number of cases reported, age, and the distribution of the predominant morphologic subtypes. For the sake of brevity, this database is not referred to here nor are the references detailed within as they can be easily resourced from the website. Throughout, we have focused on the cytogenetic features and the clinical implications of the various abnormalities.

t(1;5)(q21;q33)

This translocation was shown by transcriptome sequencing, confirmed by reverse transcription polymerase chain reaction (RT-PCR) and Sanger sequencing, to result in a *MEF2D–CSF1R* fusion between exon 7 of *MEF2D* and exon 12 of *CSF1R* in a single case of BCP-ALL (Lilljebjörn et al., 2014). Alterations of *CSF1R* have been previously reported in myeloid malignancies. The translocation from the index case had originally been described as involving *PDGFRB* based on a positive FISH result using a commercially available probe for *PDGFRB* (see following text). However, *PDGFRB* and *CSF1R* are located in close proximity at only 500 bp apart in 5q33; thus, the probe would not differentiate between them. This observation illustrates the importance of verification of abnormalities involving the 5q33 breakpoints. The *MEF2D–CSF1R* fusion gene was shown to encode a constitutively active tyrosine kinase by demonstrating sensitivity of the patient cells to two tyrosine kinase inhibitors (TKI): imatinib and GW2580, an inhibitor previously shown to have specific activity against CSF1R, implicating a role for TKI in treatment of patients with rearrangements involving this gene, as well as *PDGFRB* (see following text). Although this report presented only a single case, other cases of BCP-ALL with the same breakpoints are emerging, and they are likely to represent additional patients with this fusion. This observation is important as there is increasing interest in rearrangements involving *CSF1R* within the subgroup of patients defined as *BCR–ABL1*-like (see following text).

t(1;7)(p34;q34)

The *LCK* (lymphocyte-specific protein tyrosine kinase) gene in 1p34 is specifically expressed in T cells and is overexpressed in rare cases of T-ALL as a result of t(1;7)(p34;q34), which juxtaposes *LCK* to the *TRB* locus at 7q34 (Burnett et al., 1994). As only few cases of T-ALL with this translocation have been reported to date, no clear clinical associations have emerged.

t(1;7)(p32;q34)

The translocation, t(1;7)(p32;q34), represents a rare variant of the t(1;14)(p32;q11) in which *TRB* rather than *TRA/TRD* upregulates *TAL1* (T-cell lymphocyte leukemia 1, previously known as *TCL5* or *SCL*) in T-ALL (see following text) (Speleman et al., 2005).

t(1;11)(p32;q23)

This reciprocal translocation has been rarely reported in ALL. In the majority of cases, it is the sole karyotypic anomaly. It fuses the *MLL* (myeloid/lymphoid or mixed-lineage leukemia) gene at 11q23 with *EPS15* (epidermal growth factor receptor pathway substrate 15, previously known as *MLLT5* and *AF-1p*). This translocation/gene fusion also occurs, albeit rarely, in AML (Chapter 6). In ALL, the t(1;11) has been reported in patients of all ages and equally often in males and females. The immunophenotypes are common/pre-B-ALL. The specific prognostic association of the t(1;11) is unknown due to its rarity, and reported cases were variable for outcome. For more details of *MLL* translocations in ALL, see the section "t(4;11)(q21;q23)."

t(1;14)(p32;q11)/*TAL1* deletion

In T-ALL, t(1;14)(p32;q11) juxtaposes the *TAL1* gene at 1p32 to *TRA/TRD* at 14q11 (Brown et al., 1990; Carroll et al., 1990; Janssen et al., 1993), leading to deregulated *TAL1* expression, similar to the t(1;7)(p32;q34) (see preceding text). However, the most frequent rearrangement, in 16% of T-ALL, leading to overexpression of *TAL1* is a submicroscopic interstitial deletion of part of 1p32. It involves *STIL* (*SCL/TAL1* interrupting locus, previously known as *SIL* or *SCL*), which lies centromeric of *TAL1*, and the 5′ untranslated region (UTR) of *TAL1* generating a *STIL–TAL1* fusion gene. A second interstitial 1p32 deletion has been observed in about 6% of T-ALL (Bernard et al., 1991). It involves another site within the *TAL1* locus but the same region within *STIL*. *TAL1* and *STIL* are both normally expressed in T-cell development, and high expression levels of *TAL1* in the absence of detectable rearrangements have been described in approximately 40% of T-ALL (Bash et al., 1995; Ferrando et al., 2004a). These abnormalities leading to high *TAL1* expression are common in childhood T-ALL. They are found in 17% of such cases and have been associated with a more favorable outcome (Cavé et al., 2004).

dup(1)(q12 ~ 21 or q31 ~ 32)

Although this duplication has been frequently reported in ALL, it is only rarely found as the sole anomaly. It is therefore mostly regarded as a secondary rather than a primary aberration. The dup(1q) may result from an unbalanced translocation, giving rise to a der(1)t(1;1)(p?;q?). In about one-third of cases with dup(1q), the primary rearrangement is t(8;14)(q24;q32) (see following text). It has been reported in approximately 25% of Burkitt lymphomas. In another third, it is found in high-hyperdiploid karyotypes, often as the only structural abnormality among the many numerical changes. The molecular genetic consequences are unknown, although from a number of cases investigated by aCGH, it was revealed that the proximal breakpoints in all cases were near centromeric, clustering within a 1.4 Mb segment in 1q12 ~ 21.1. The 1q distal breakpoints were heterogeneous. The minimally gained segment in ALL was 57.4 Mb [dup(1)(q22q32.3)] (Davidsson et al., 2007). There is no known association with prognosis, and specifically in high-hyperdiploid ALL, the presence of dup(1q) does not alter the good outcome associated with this cytogenetic subgroup (Moorman et al., 2003; Paulsson et al., 2013a).

t(1;19)(q23;p13.3)

The t(1;19)(q23;p13.3) (Figure 10.3) was first reported to be an ALL-specific abnormality in 1984 by three independent groups (Carroll et al., 1984; Michael et al., 1984; Williams et al., 1984). It may occur in a balanced or an unbalanced form, in which the derivative chromosome 19 only is present (Secker-Walker et al., 1992). The unbalanced form is the most common, accounting for 75% of cases, although some patients display both balanced and unbalanced translocations (Shearer et al., 2005). It has been proposed that the unbalanced form most likely arises from an initial trisomy 1 followed by the translocation event and subsequent loss of the derived chromosome 1 (Paulsson et al., 2005a).

The translocation leads to a fusion of the *TCF3* gene (transcription factor 3, previously known as *E2A* and *ITF1*) at 19p13 with the *PBX1* (pre-B-cell leukemia homeobox 1) gene at 1q23 to form *TCF3–PBX1* (Hunger et al., 1991). In approximately 5–10% of cases with visible translocations, no apparent molecular involvement of *TCF3* and *PBX1* is found (Privitera et al., 1992). This may result from variable breakpoints within the genes, giving rise to an alternative *TCF3–PBX1* fusion transcript (Paulsson et al., 2007). The balanced form of the translocation almost always results in *TCF3–PBX1* fusion, and thus, most *TCF3-PBX1*-negative cases present as der(19)t(1;19). Such *TCF3-PBX1*-negative cases have been shown to coexist with high hyperdiploidy and, more rarely, t(9;22)(q34;q11) (Barber et al., 2007; Paulsson et al., 2013b).

A rare variant, t(17;19)(q22;p13), involving *TCF3* has also been described (see following text). Screening by FISH with break-apart probes specific for *TCF3* has provided an opportunity to accurately detect cases with the *TCF3–PBX1* fusion as well as the rare variants (Barber et al., 2007).

The t(1;19) is one of the most common translocations in ALL, occurring in approximately 6% of cases overall. Interestingly, it is one of the few genetic abnormalities that do not vary in frequency with age. It is generally associated with a pre-B immunophenotype with blasts expressing CD10 and cytoplasmic immunoglobulin. Up to 25% of cases with this immunophenotype are reported to have the translocation (Secker-Walker, 1997). Patients with this abnormality have significantly higher WBC counts than do other ALL patients. The early association of t(1;19) with a poor outcome has been moderated by more aggressive therapy in modern protocols (Hunger, 1996; Kager et al., 2007). It remains unresolved whether the prognosis varies according to the presence of the balanced or unbalanced form of the translocation. Secker-Walker et al. (1992) described an improved outcome for patients with the unbalanced form, but this has not been confirmed in more recent studies (Pui et al., 2009; Andersen et al., 2011).

t(2;8)(p11;q24)

This translocation is a characteristic of Burkitt lymphoma and mature B leukemia. It represents a variant of the t(8;14)(q24;q32) (see following text).

t(4;11)(q21;q23)

The t(4;11) (Figure 10.4) was first detected by Oshimura et al. (1977) and was subsequently described to be consistently associated with ALL

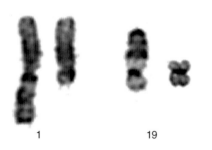

Figure 10.3 Partial karyogram from a BCP-ALL with t(1;19)(q23;p13).

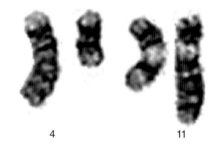

Figure 10.4 Partial karyogram from a BCP-ALL with t(4;11)(q21;q23).

by Van den Berghe et al. (1979). Additional chromosomal changes are often found (~30%) in association with t(4;11). The most common are gain of the X chromosome, i(7)(q10), and trisomy 8 (Johansson et al., 1998).

The t(4;11)(q21;q23) leads to fusion between the *MLL* gene (Rowley et al., 1990) and the AF4/FMR2 family, member 1 gene, *AFF1* (previously known as *AF4*, *MLLT2*, and *PBM1*), generating an *MLL–AFF1* transcript. The breakpoints in *MLL* cluster within an 8.3 kb region between exons 5 and 11. The pathogenetically essential transcript is *MLL–AFF1* on the derivative chromosome 11, in which 5′ *MLL* sequences are fused with 3′ sequences from *AFF1* (Gu et al., 1992; Domer et al., 1993; Downing et al., 1994). However, the reciprocal product may play a more important role than previously thought, especially in relation to treatment response (Marschalek, 2011). Variant and complex translocations as well as submicroscopic insertions have been described.

In addition to t(4;11), there are a number of other well-defined chromosomal abnormalities in ALL involving the *MLL* gene, many of which are also seen in AML (Chapter 6). At least 120 different *MLL* rearrangements have been described, of which about 80 translocation partners are now characterized at the molecular level (Meyer et al., 2013a). The most frequent in ALL are t(6;11) (q27;q23), t(9;11)(p21;q23), rearrangements between 10p12 and 11q23, and t(11;19)(q23;p13.3). The fusion partners are *MLLT4* (*AF6*), *MLLT3* (*AF9*), *MLLT10* (*AF10*), and *MLLT1* (*ENL*), respectively. These will be discussed in the following relevant sections. The different *MLL* fusions encode chimeric proteins in which the N-terminal portion of *MLL* is fused to the C-terminal portion of the new partner. The common translocations involving *MLL* can in most instances be identified by cytogenetics. They may also be detected by RT-PCR using a range of primers (Pallisgaard et al., 1998). However, a dual-color FISH approach has proved to be the most reliable detection method (Harrison et al., 2005). FISH using a break-apart probe flanking *MLL* will detect the multiple partners usually including those of a cryptic nature, for example, those involving insertion events. This method has also been useful for the detection of those translocations, primarily t(4;11) and t(6;11), in which concurrent 3′ *MLL* deletions occur

(Barber et al., 2004a). As the probe is large, covering sequences both 3′ and 5′ of *MLL*, alternative methods may be required (such as high-density SNP arrays) to determine whether the deletion involves only part of or the entire gene.

Chromosomal rearrangements involving *MLL* are strongly associated with infant ALL, accounting for up to 85% of cases in that age group (Biondi et al., 2000; Pieters et al., 2007). Although only 2–3% of pediatric ALL is diagnosed in patients younger than 12 months of age, it has been reported that infants comprise 60% of all t(4;11)-positive childhood cases. In contrast, the incidences in children between the ages of 1 and 15 years and in adults are only around 2 and 5%, respectively (Moorman, 2012). In all age groups, the t(4;11) is the most frequently observed *MLL* rearrangement, whereas it is rare among *MLL*-positive AML (Chapter 6). *MLL* fusions are also rare in T-ALL, accounting for about 5%. The most frequent partners in T-ALL are *MLLT1* in t(11;19)(q23;p13.3) and *MLLT4* in t(6;11)(q27;q23) (Hayette et al., 2002).

ALL with t(4;11) usually have an early B-precursor immunophenotype, being negative for CD10 and positive for CD19. Females are overrepresented, and the patients characteristically have a high WBC count, a high percentage of blasts in the peripheral blood, organomegaly, and CNS involvement. Overall, the outcome is extremely poor, although significantly better in children aged 2–9 years compared to infants, very young children, and patients over the age of 10 years, including adults (Moorman, 2012). The presence of additional chromosomal changes has no impact on outcome in *MLL*-positive childhood ALL (Moorman et al., 2005).

del(5)(q32q33.3)

This deletion of 5q was recently reported to give rise to a fusion of *EBF1* and *PDGFRB* (Figure 10.5). The breakpoints have been defined in *EBF1* exons 14 or 15 and *PDGFRB* exon 11, with overexpression of PDGFRB (Roberts et al., 2012). This deletion is visible by SNP arrays and by loss of the distal *PDGFRB* signal by FISH when using a break-apart probe that flanks the gene. Expression of the fusion transcript has been confirmed by RT-PCR. The fusion is usually mutually exclusive of other established cytogenetic changes. It occurs

(A)

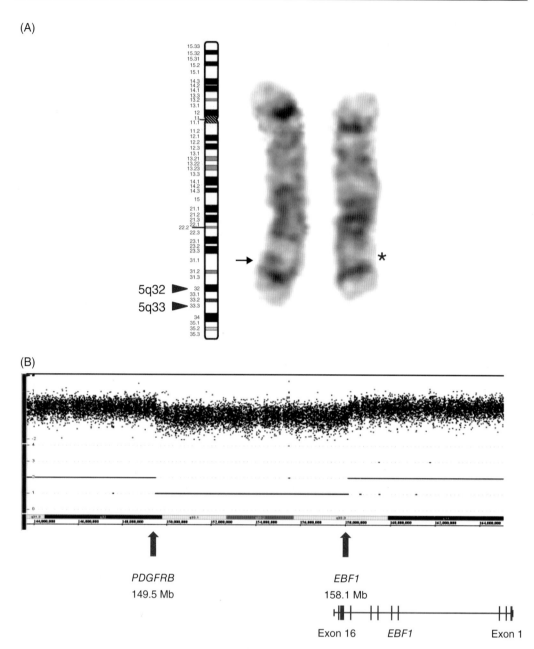

(B)

Figure 10.5 (A) Partial karyogram indicating the del(5)(q32q33) (*red star*) and the related idiogram that gives rise to the *EBF1–PDGFRB* fusion. (B) SNP profile from the 5q3 region of chromosome 5 indicating the relevant breakpoints within *PDGFRB* and *EBF1* and the extent of the deletion. The *red bar* indicates the extent of the *EBF1* gene and shows that the deletion results in loss of exon 16.

in approximately 0.5% of BCP-ALL overall and in 8% of the high-risk BCP-ALL category, which have been classified as *BCR–ABL1*-like (see following text). It defines a high-risk subgroup of patients who are often refractory to conventional therapy. The identification of a *PDGFRB* fusion is of clinical significance, as patients with myeloproliferative neoplasia and activating *PDGFRB* rearrangements show complete hematological and molecular response to imatinib treatment (Apperley et al., 2002). In line with this observation, an increasing number of reports are emerging of responsiveness of refractory *BCR–ABL1*-like ALL, including those with *PDGFRB* rearrangements, to appropriate TKI therapy (see following text), for example, two cases of *EBF1–PDGFRB*-positive ALL showing a response to imatinib have been published (Lengline et al., 2013; Weston et al., 2013).

t(5;9)(q22;q34)

This rare translocation fuses exon 3 of the sorting nexin family gene, *SNX2*, in-frame to *ABL1* exon 4 in the *SNX2–ABL1* fusion. Notably, it highlights another *ABL1* partner gene in BCP-ALL. The one adult and one childhood patients had high WBC counts and a poor outcome, and the child failed treatment with dasatinib with only transient response to imatinib (Ernst et al., 2011; Masuzawa et al., 2014).

t(5;14)(q31;q32)

This translocation leads to the fusion of *IL3* and *IGH*, which, in accordance with other translocations involving *IGH*, leads to overexpression of its partner gene, *IL3* (Grimaldi and Meeker, 1989). Although rarely reported, it defines a specific subtype of B-ALL, comprising less than 1% of such cases, with the striking feature of an increase in circulating eosinophils, representing a reactive population, not part of the leukemic clone. The leukemic blasts are CD19 and CD10 positive. The finding of even a small number of such blasts with this phenotype in a patient with eosinophilia strongly suggests this diagnosis. It is found in both children and adults and is documented as a distinct subtype in the WHO classification (Swerdlow et al., 2008). Its outcome is unknown, but it is likely to reflect the survival pattern described for other patients with translocations involving *IGH* (see following text) (Russell et al., 2014).

t(5;14)(q35;q32)

This cytogenetically cryptic translocation is found only in T-ALL. It comprises approximately 20% of childhood and 13% of adult cases (Berger et al., 2003). The t(5;14) involves the *TLX3* and *BCL11B* genes. *TLX3* (T-cell leukemia homeobox 3, previously known as *HOX11L2* and *RNX*) in 5q35 belongs to the class II homeobox (HOX) gene family. The Krüppel-like zinc finger gene *BCL11B*

(B-cell chronic lymphocytic leukemia (CLL)/lymphoma 11B, zinc finger protein) in 14q32 encodes a transcription factor essential in T-cell development (Wakabayashi et al., 2003). As a result of the translocation, *BCL11B* specifically associates with *TLX3* leading to its upregulation (Bernard et al., 2001; Su et al., 2006b). Rare variants as well as subtle genomic deletions and insertions within 5q have been reported (Berger et al., 2003; Su et al., 2004). *BCL11B* has also been identified as a target of deletion and somatic sequence mutation in T-ALL (De Keersmaecker et al., 2010). Collectively, these observations have highlighted that *TLX3* expression in T-ALL rarely occurs in the absence of 5q abnormalities. Thus, FISH using a break-apart probe targeting *TLX3* provides a reliable detection method (Figure 10.6). The occasional findings of t(5;14)(q35;q11) juxtaposing *TLX3* and *TRA/TRD* (Hansen-Hagge et al., 2002) and t(5;7)(q35;q21) and t(2;5)(p21;q35) involving *TLX3* with *CDK6* (cyclin-dependent kinase 6) and an as yet uncharacterized locus on 2p21, respectively (Berger et al., 2003), indicate that the regulatory elements of *TCR* or other genes may also contribute to the upregulation of *TLX3*. There is an increasing number of reports of the involvement of *BCL11B* in other rearrangements in T-ALL, for example, t(5;14)(q35.1;q32.2), in which *NKX2-5*

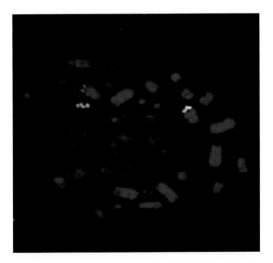

Figure 10.6 A metaphase hybridized with a dual-color break-apart probe specific for *TLX3*. The normal red/green signal is located on the normal chromosome 5. As a result of the t(5;14)(q35;q32), the red signal remains on the derivative chromosome 5, and the green signal is located on the derivative chromosome 14.

(NK2 transcription factor-related locus 5), another HOX gene located to 5q35, is upregulated (Nagel et al., 2003, 2007) with absence of the wild-type *BCL11B* transcript (Przybylski et al., 2005). *TLX3*-expressing T-ALL does not have the favorable outcome generally associated with *TLX1* expression (see following text) (Ballerini et al., 2002; Ferrando et al., 2002; Cavé et al., 2004).

del(6q)

Deletions of the long arm of chromosome 6 occur in 5–13% of ALL in both B-lineage and T-lineage disease, usually in association with other abnormalities, including a strong association with *ETV6–RUNX1*-positive ALL (Lilljebjörn et al., 2010; Borst et al., 2012). They are characteristic of lymphoid malignancies in general, being common also in chronic lymphoproliferative disorders and non-Hodgkin lymphomas (Chapter 11). The breakpoint assignment of del(6q) from a range of studies has varied considerably (Sinclair et al., 2004; Strefford et al., 2007). The bands most frequently reported as the breakpoint sites are 6q15–21. As for all neoplasia-associated terminal deletions examined, the 6q deletions actually are interstitial, even in those cases where the microscopic impression is that it is terminal (Menasce et al., 1994). As the assignment of a commonly deleted region has not been possible, this questions the loss of a single tumor suppressor gene as the pathogenetic consequence of del(6q).

No specific clinical associations have been made with del(6q) in BCP-ALL. Overall, most del(6q)-positive cases occur in the common ALL subgroup. Thus, there is no clear-cut evidence for a prognostic impact of del(6q) in ALL.

t(6;7)(q23;q34) and *MYB* duplication

These abnormalities are found exclusively in T-ALL, occurring in approximately 10% of cases in very young patients (median age of 2.2 years). The *MYB* (v-myb myeloblastosis viral oncogene homolog [avian], previously known as *c-myb*) oncogene in 6q23.3 encodes a nuclear transcription factor that is implicated in proliferation, survival, and differentiation of hematopoietic progenitor cells. In the t(6;7), *MYB* is juxtaposed to *TRB* leading to upregulation of *MYB* expression. A short somatic duplication of 230 kb in 6q23 specifically targeting *MYB* also produces a threefold

overexpression of *MYB* mRNA (Clappier et al., 2007; Lahortiga et al., 2007). These findings identified amplification of *MYB* as an oncogenic event and highlighted *MYB* as a possible therapeutic target in T-ALL. Currently, no clinical associations have been found, likely because of the small number of reported cases.

t(6;11)(q27;q23)

In this translocation, the *MLLT4* gene at 6q27 is the partner of *MLL* at 11q23. It occurs mainly in AML (see Chapter 6) but has also been reported in a handful of ALL of both B- and T-lineages (Martineau et al., 1998; Hayette et al., 2002). The t(6;11) is frequently seen as the sole cytogenetic change. When additional abnormalities are present, they are generally numerical rather than structural. As in t(4;11)-positive cases, the t(6;11) may be accompanied by a concurrent 3′ *MLL* deletion (Barber et al., 2004a). Similar to AML with t(6;11), ALL with this translocation has been associated with a short median overall survival and, hence, a poor prognosis, although the number of patients is usually too small to be analyzed separately from other *MLL* translocations.

t(6;14)(p22;q32)

This translocation may be difficult to visualize by banding analysis; therefore, metaphase FISH with an *IGH* break-apart probe is useful for accurate identification. The karyotypes of t(6;14)-positive ALL are generally complex and often harbor i(9)(q10) (see following text). The t(6;14) brings the *IGH* enhancer at 14q32 into proximity with the *ID4* gene (inhibitor of DNA binding 4, dominant negative helix–loop–helix protein) at 6p22, with breakpoints scattered over a 19 kb region centromeric of this gene. Quantitative PCR shows upregulation of *ID4* mRNA (Russell et al., 2008). The *ID4* gene is one of four members of the basic helix–loop–helix (bHLH) family of transcription factors—ID1, ID2, ID3, and ID4—that act as transcription inhibitory proteins.

Although few cases with the t(6;14) have been described to date (Bellido et al., 2003; Russell et al., 2008; Chapiro et al., 2013), all had BCP-ALL. Their WBC counts were generally low, and the patients were older than expected for ALL (median age of 14 years). This rare subgroup adds to the growing number of *IGH* partners described in BCP-ALL [see "t(14;19)(q32;q13)" for other examples]. As numbers are small, the outcome for these t(6;14) patients was examined together with the other reported *IGH* translocations. Collectively, they define a genetic subgroup that is frequent among adolescents and young adults with ALL. Although associated with an adverse outcome in adults, *IGH* translocations are not an independent prognostic factor in children and adolescents (Russell et al., 2014).

inv(7)(p15q34)/t(7;7)(p15;q34)/t(7;14)(p15;q11)/t(7;14)(p15;q32)

These abnormalities are characteristic of T-ALL. The inv(7), which is often cytogenetically cryptic, and the t(7;7) bring the *TRB* enhancer within the *HOXA* (homeobox A cluster) locus at 7p15 (Soulier et al., 2005; Speleman et al., 2005). There are also rare reports of *HOXA* involved in complex rearrangements with *TCR* genes (Cauwelier et al., 2007). *HOXA* rearrangements have been identified by FISH in up to 3% of T-ALL. They lead to upregulation of genes in the HOXA cluster, especially *HOXA10* and *HOXA11*. *HOXA* has also been seen to be upregulated by *TRD* (Bergeron et al., 2006) and *BCL11B*, specifically *HOXA13* (Su et al., 2006a), in the t(7;14)(p15;q11) and t(7;14)(p15;q32), respectively. Homeobox (*HOX*) genes are divided into two classes. Class 1 *HOX* genes comprise 39 genes distributed in four clusters (A–D) located in 7p15, 17q21, 12q13, and 2q31, respectively. Class II homeobox genes are divergent genes with less homology. Clinical and prognostic associations of *HOX* genes in T-ALL have not been possible to determine due to the rarity of these abnormalities.

dic(7;9)(p11 ~ 13;p11 ~ 13)

Chromosome 9 is frequently involved in the formation of dicentric chromosomes leading to loss of 9p material as well as a deletion of the partner chromosome. The dic(7;9) is a rare abnormality in B-ALL. Although usually seen as the sole abnormality, it has also been reported in association with t(9;22)(q34;q11). The breakpoints are clustered within 9p13.1 and 7p11.2–12.1 (Lundin et al., 2007). It remains unknown whether the pathogenetically important outcome of the dic(7;9) is the formation of a chimeric gene or loss of 7p and/or 9p material. A large comprehensive molecular study of dicentric chromosomes involving 9p identified *PAX5* as the key target gene on chromosome 9 as a consequence of its involvement in multiple fusion genes and by deletion (An et al., 2008). No prognostic associations have been assigned to this abnormality.

del(7)(p12.2p12.2)/*IKZF1* deletion

IKZF1 encodes IKAROS, the founder member of a family of zinc finger transcription factors. It is a master regulator of normal hematopoiesis required for the development of all lymphoid lineages (Georgopoulos et al., 1994). *IKZF1* alterations include focal or large deletions that result in loss of expression of IKZF1. Although a range of *IKZF1* deletion types have been reported, focal deletions of coding exons 4–7 are the most frequent and remove the N-terminal DNA-binding zinc fingers, leading to expression of the dominant negative isoform IK6 (Caye et al., 2013; Schwab et al., 2013). In contrast to changes of *PAX5*, alteration of *IZKF1* is consistently associated with a poor outcome. It is observed in two types of high-risk ALL: Ph/*BCR–ABL1*-positive ALL, where they occur in 70% of cases and are associated with a worse outcome (Mullighan et al., 2008a; Martinelli et al., 2009; Iacobucci et al., 2009), and *BCR–ABL1*-like (Ph-like) ALL, where they are found in about 40% (see following text) (Den Boer et al., 2009; Mullighan et al., 2009b; Roberts et al., 2012). Several groups have also reported that *IKZF1* deletions confer a poor prognostic impact in all risk groups of BCP-ALL (Mullighan et al., 2009b; Waanders et al., 2011; van der Veer et al., 2013; Olsson et al., 2014). In fact, *IKZF1* deletions are the only ones significantly associated with relapse in cases without any known risk-stratifying aberrations.

i(7)(q10)

This isochromosome is relatively common in ALL. It has been reported that i(7)(q10) is not a true isochromosome but an isodicentric abnormality with breakpoints in proximal 7p (Schaad et al., 2006). It is usually associated with other primary cytogenetic changes, most frequently t(1;19), t(4;11) or high hyperdiploidy, indicating that it is a secondary abnormality. The leukemia is mostly BCP-ALL with no other distinguishing laboratory or clinical features.

t(7;9)(q34;q32)

While dysregulation of the *TAL1* gene occurs in almost 25% of patients with T-ALL, upregulation of the *TAL2* gene (T-cell acute lymphocytic leukemia 2) in T-ALL, as a result of the t(7;9)(q34;q32), is rare. This translocation juxtaposes *TAL2* and *TRB* (Xia et al., 1991). The *TAL2* gene product is homologous to those encoded by *TAL1* (see preceding text) and *LYL1* (see following text). Hence, *TAL2*, *TAL1*, and *LYL1* constitute a discrete subgroup of helix–loop–helix protein encoding genes that contribute to the development of T-ALL. *TAL2* transcription is activated ectopically in lymphoid cells, and the upregulated expression of TAL2 in these cells promotes development of T-ALL. Normally, the *TAL* genes are not expressed in the thymus, but become activated and expressed upon chromosomal translocation that ultimately leads to the development of T-ALL. As the properties of *TAL2* broadly resemble those described previously for *TAL1*, this supports the idea that both encoded proteins promote T-ALL by a common mechanism.

t(7;9)(q34;q34.3)

In the rarely occurring t(7;9)(q34;q34.3) of T-ALL, the *NOTCH1* (Notch homolog 1, translocation associated [*Drosophila*], previously known as *TAN1*) gene in 9q34.3 forms a fusion with *TRB*, resulting in aberrant expression of a truncated activated form of *NOTCH1* (Ellisen et al., 1991). This translocation provides a good example that cloning of rare abnormalities is valuable to reveal genes of significance, in this case *NOTCH1*. Activating mutations of the HD (heterodimerization) and PEST domains [polypeptide sequences enriched in proline (P), glutamate (E), serine (S), and threonine (T), proposed to expedite the degradation of proteins] of *NOTCH1* occur frequently in T-ALL, being found in more than 50% of cases. There is evidence that *NOTCH1* mutations are early, prenatal genetic events in T-ALL (Eguchi-Ishimae et al., 2008). *NOTCH1* plays a critical role in T-cell development (Weng et al., 2004). *NOTCH1* acts cooperatively with oncogene transcription factors in T-ALL pathogenesis, providing an example of multistep development of T-ALL (Zhu et al., 2006). The clinical ramification of *NOTCH1* mutations is unclear, with different studies showing either a favorable or nonsignificant prognostic impact.

t(7;10)(q34;q24)

The t(7;10) represents a rare variant of t(10;14) (q24;q11). In t(7;10), *TLX1* (T-cell leukemia homeobox 1, previously known as *HOX11*) is juxtaposed with *TRB* (Cauwelier et al., 2006) (see section "t(10;14)(q24;q11)").

t(7;11)(q34;p13)/t(7;11)(q34;p15)

These translocations occur in T-ALL and recombine *TRB* with the genes *LMO1* (LIM domain only 1[rhombotin 1], previously known as *RBTN1*, *TTG1*, and *RHOM1*) and *LMO2* (LIM domain only 2 [rhombotin-like 1], previously known as *RBTN2*, *TTG2*, and *RHOM2*) in 11p13 and 11p15, respectively (Cauwelier et al., 2006). *LMO1* and *LMO2* are upregulated in T-ALL, and their elevated expression within defined gene expression signatures is indicative of leukemic arrest at specific stages of normal thymocyte development. These are used to define the molecular pathways involved in the pathogenesis of T-ALL (Ferrando et al., 2002) (for more discussion, see section "t(11;14)(p13;q11)/t(11;14)(p15;q11)").

t(7;12)(q34;p13.3)

In T-ALL with t(7;12) or t(12;14)(p13.3;q11) (see following text), massive upregulation of *CCND2* (cyclin D2) is produced by translocation to *TRB* and *TRA*, respectively. These translocations are extremely rare; thus, their clinical associations are unknown. However, their high expression is associated with overexpression of *TAL1*, *TLX1*, *TLX3*, *NOTCH1* mutations, and *CDKN2A* deletions, indicating a role for *CCND2* in the multistep leukemogenesis of T-ALL (Clappier et al., 2006).

t(7;12)(q36;p13)

A small number of infant BCP-ALL cases with a cytogenetically cryptic t(7;12) have been reported (Tosi et al., 2000; Slater et al., 2001; von Bergh et al., 2006). It is often found in association with trisomies of chromosomes 8 and 19, which may provide a marker for the presence of this cryptic abnormality. It is more common in infant AML, in which it is found in approximately 20% of cases. Thus, the cytogenetic associations and clinical implications are described in detail in Chapter 6.

t(7;19)(q34;p13)

The t(7;19) is a rare translocation in T-ALL. It recombines *LYL1* (lymphoblastic leukemia-derived sequence 1) in 19p13 with *TRB* leading to *LYL1* overexpression (Mellentin et al., 1989). *LYL1* is also constitutively overexpressed in a subset of T-ALL without the translocation (Ferrando et al., 2002). T-ALL with *LYL1* overexpression shows an immature phenotype and has been associated with an inferior prognosis.

t(8;14)(q11;q32)

The first t(8;14) found in BCP-ALL was reported by Kardon et al. (1982). The involvement of the *IGH* locus was originally demonstrated by Southern blot (Testoni et al., 1993) and then by FISH analyses (Byatt et al., 2001). The partner gene at 8q11 is *CEBPD*, one of the CCAAT/enhancer-binding protein (*CEBP*) family members, which are a family of six multifunctional basic leucine zipper (bZIP) transcription factors. *CEBPD* is overexpressed as a result of this translocation, revealing an oncogenic role for this gene in BCP-ALL (Akasaka et al., 2007). Four other *CEPB* gene family members have been described as *IGH* partners in ALL, namely, *CEBPA* and *CEBPG* [t(14;19)(q32;q13)], *CEBPE* [inv(14)(q11q32)/t(14;14)(q11;q32)], and *CEBPB* [t(14;20)(q32;q13)], described in the following.

A substantial proportion (25%) of t(8;14)-positive ALL occur in patients with Down syndrome (DS). Furthermore, in a number of non-DS patients, the translocation t(9;22)(q34;q11) has been found (Lundin et al., 2009). In one patient with a relapse, the t(9;22) was present, whereas there was no evidence of t(8;14), providing evidence that the t(8;14) was secondary to the t(9;22) at least in this case (Byatt et al., 2001). All reported cases with t(8;14) were BCP-ALL. The group comprises older children (median age of around 10 years) as well as adults, with variable WBC counts. As for patients with t(6;14)(p22;q32), these t(8;14) patients were examined together with the other *IGH* translocations, which is frequent among adolescents and young adults with ALL. Although associated with an adverse outcome in adults, *IGH* translocations are not an independent prognostic factor in children and adolescents (Russell et al., 2014).

t(8;14)(q24;q11)

The t(8;14)(q24;q11) is a rarely reported translocation in T-ALL. In the majority of cases, the oncogene *MYC* at 8q24 is recombined with *TCRA/TCRD* or, rarely, with *TRB* promoters in t(7;8)(q34;q24). The breakpoint in *MYC* lies 3′ of the third exon as in the variant Burkitt-specific translocations t(2;8) and t(8;22) (see following text and Chapter 11). The molecular characteristics of the translocation are hence similar to those of mature B-cell neoplasms with recombinations between 8q24 and 14q32, 2p11, or 22q11, in which *MYC* is upregulated (see following text).

Patients with t(8;14)-positive T-ALL are more often male than female and tend to have a high WBC count and bulky extramedullary leukemia. The outcome for patients with this translocation is unknown.

t(8;14)(q24;q32)

The t(8;14) and its variants t(2;8)(p11;q24) and t(8;22)(q24;q11) are associated with B-cell neoplasia. The translocations were first described and have been most extensively studied in Burkitt lymphoma, and the reader is referred to Chapter 11 for a detailed description. In summary, the crucial event in all three translocations is the juxtaposing of *MYC* (from 8q24) and either the *IGH* locus (14q32); the *IGK, immunoglobulin kappa light-chain locus (2p12); or the IGL, immunoglobulin lambda light-chain locus* (22q11). Through one of these rearrangements, *MYC* comes under the influence of the transcriptional promoter sequences and enhancer elements in the constitutively active immunoglobulin locus. This in turn leads to deregulation and increased transcription of *MYC*.

ALL with t(8;14) or the variants t(8;22) and t(2;8) is almost always of L3 morphology and mature B-ALL. In fact, no abnormalities other than these three translocations have been associated with L3 leukemia with any consistency. The t(8;14) is most common, found in 85%, whereas t(2;8) and t(8;22) are found in around 5 and 10%, respectively.

t(8;22)(q24;q11)

This translocation is characteristic for Burkitt leukemia/lymphoma. It represents a variant of the t(8;14)(q24;q32) (see preceding text).

del(9p)

Chromosomal abnormalities leading to deletions of 9p in ALL were first described in the 1980s (Kowalczyk and Sandberg, 1983; Chilcote et al., 1985). Sometimes, the loss is homozygous (Heyman et al., 1993). The majority of visible 9p abnormalities result in deletion of 9p21. This chromosome band contains two tandemly linked genes that encode cyclin-dependent kinase inhibitors, namely, *CDKN2A* (previously *p16*) and *CDKN2B* (previously *p15*), while the *CDKN2A* locus also codes for P14ARF (Quelle et al., 1995). It has become clear that *CDKN2A* is the primary target of 9p21 deletions in ALL. Inactivation of *CDKN2A* may occur by hypermethylation or mutation at both the transcriptional and posttranscriptional levels, but deletion is the most frequent event (Chim et al., 2003; Sulong et al., 2009). At the molecular level, the deletions have been shown to vary significantly in size, from single exons to large genomic regions, and to target one or both alleles. Additional genes may be incidentally codeleted. For example, *CDKN2B* is deleted in a significant proportion of ALL but always in association with *CDKN2A* (Bertin et al., 2003). This is also the case for the methylthioadenosine phosphorylase gene, *MTAP*, which is located approximately 100 kb telomeric to *CDKN2A*. FISH provides an excellent method for detecting the majority of both homozygous and hemizygous deletions with the added advantage of providing insight into tumor heterogeneity. However, in some cases, submicroscopic deletions may be too small to be seen by FISH, and SNP arrays are required for their detection. Deletions of 9p usually occur as secondary changes and are associated with all other primary genetic abnormalities in both B-ALL and T-ALL, although in the latter the functional inactivation of *CDKN2A* in the majority of cases implies a direct involvement in T-cell leukemogenesis (De Keersmaecker et al., 2005b).

In childhood ALL, cytogenetically visible 9p abnormalities occur at an incidence of approximately 10%, whereas *CDKN2A* inactivation is found in approximately 25% of B- and up to 88% of T-lineage childhood ALL (De Keersmaecker et al., 2005b; Sulong et al., 2009; Olsson et al., 2014). The frequency of *CDKN2A* inactivation is strongly correlated with cytogenetic subgroups, with lower frequencies being observed among cases with high hyperdiploidy or *ETV6–RUNX1* fusion. Within BCP-ALL, older children (over 10 years) are more likely to have both visible 9p abnormalities and *CDKN2A* inactivation, whereas the reverse is true in T-ALL. Patients with *CDKN2A* deletions have higher WBC counts than other children with ALL.

Survival analysis has shown reduced event-free survival in patients with visible 9p abnormalities (Hann et al., 2001). However, the picture concerning the prognostic significance of *CDKN2A* deletions has been contradictory, likely due to its occurrence within all cytogenetic risk groups regardless of their relative outcome (see following text).

There has been much interest in the *PAX5* gene at 9p13, which is a transcription factor essential for B-lineage development. A SNP array study of a large series of childhood BCP-ALL showed deletion, amplification, point mutation, and structural rearrangement of *PAX5* in 30% of the cases (Mullighan et al., 2007). The majority of *PAX5* deletions involved only a subset of exons, leading to the encoding of an internally deleted PAX5 protein in a dominant leukemic clone, consistent with a role in leukemogenesis. Deletions were also detected in other regulators of B-lymphocyte development and differentiation (see following text).

A number of deletions of 9p include *JAK2* (Janus kinase 2, a protein tyrosine kinase) at 9p24. Although this gene is essential for the transmission of signals from cytokine receptors to downstream signaling and it is known that mutations play a significant role in myeloproliferative neoplasms, it has not been proposed as a target of 9p deletions in ALL. However, a role in DS-associated ALL is emerging with the discovery of *JAK2* mutations in 20% of such cases (see following text).

t(9;12)(p24;p13)

The t(9;12)(p24;p13) has been reported in a small number of B- and T-ALL in both adults and children (Lacronique et al., 1997; Peeters et al., 1997; Zhou et al., 2012) and was shown to fuse the 3′ portion of the tyrosine kinase *JAK2* to the 5′ region of *ETV6* (ETS family member-6, also known as *TEL*), leading to the formation of an *ETV6–JAK2* fusion. Although the precise breakpoints were variable among patients, the fusion protein resulted in the constitutive activation of its tyrosine kinase and conferred cytokine-independent proliferation on the interleukin-3-dependent Ba/F3 hematopoietic cell line.

t(9;11)(p21;q23)

The t(9;11)(p21;q23) is another translocation involving the *MLL* gene at 11q23 with *MLLT3* on the short arm of chromosome 9. Only a small number of cases have been reported in ALL; this abnormality occurs predominantly in AML and is discussed in detail in Chapter 6.

dic(9;12)(p11~12;p11~13)

Since the first report of dic(9;12) (Carroll et al., 1987), many cases have now been described, yielding an incidence of approximately 1% in childhood BCP-ALL. The breakpoint positions in 9p vary considerably at the molecular level, but nevertheless FISH and molecular studies have shown that the abnormality can give rise to a fusion between *ETV6* on 12p13 and the master regulator of B-cell development, *PAX5*, at 9p13 (Cazzaniga et al., 2001; Strehl et al., 2003). These were the first reports of *PAX5* rearrangements in human malignancy resulting in a chimeric transcript. Now, there are many new *PAX5* partners being described. The dic(9;12) contains the NH(2)-terminal region of *PAX5* and most of the *ETV6* gene. The resulting chimeric protein retains the PAX5 paired-box domain and both the helix–loop–helix and DNA-binding domains of ETV6. The PAX5–ETV6 protein acts as an aberrant transcription factor with repressor function, leading to a block in B-cell differentiation (Fazio et al., 2008). As dic(9;12) is an unbalanced translocation, the *ETV6–PAX5* transcript is not present. The dicentric chromosome has been found in association with other chromosomal changes in particular with the *ETV6–RUNX1* fusion (see following text) (Raynaud et al., 1999).

The dic(9;12) occurs in all age groups and has been suggested to have an excellent prognosis (Mahmoud et al., 1992; UKCCG, 1992). The association with the *ETV6–RUNX1* fusion may partly account for the favorable outcome.

Similar to *PAX5*, an increasing range of chromosomal abnormalities are being reported in ALL that involve *ETV6*, many in single reports, for example,

ETV6–ABL2, *ETV6–NCOA2*, and *ETV6–SYK* (Zhou et al., 2012).

dic(9;20)(p13;q11)

The dic(9;20) was first reported in the mid-1990s (Rieder et al., 1995; Slater et al., 1995), and since then, many cases have been described, constituting 2–4% of pediatric BCP-ALL (Forestier et al., 2008a; Zachariadis et al., 2011). FISH with chromosome 9 and 20 centromeric or other selected probes is often required for accurate detection as the dic(9;20) may be difficult to identify at the cytogenetic level. It usually manifests as monosomy 20, sometimes with a 9p deletion (Clark et al., 2000). High-resolution aCGH has shown that although the breakpoints cluster to subbands 9p13.2 and 20q11.2, they are not identical from case to case, suggesting that the functional outcome of the aberration is loss of genetic material rather than a consistent gene rearrangement. Truncation of *PAX5* with a dominant negative effect is the important outcome in at least some cases (An et al., 2008). All cases have modal chromosome numbers between 44 and 50. Additional chromosomal changes are present in 60% of cases, the most frequent of which are homozygous loss of *CDKN2A* (Zachariadis et al., 2012) and gains of chromosomes 21 and X. The dic(9;20) more frequently occurs in pediatric ALL with approximately 90% of the reported cases being children or adolescents. The median age is 3 years, with a female predominance. Although the event-free survival is not particularly favorable, with mostly early relapses, the postrelapse treatment of many patients is successful, yielding a rather favorable overall survival.

i(9)(q10)

The largest series of isochromosomes was reviewed by Pui et al. (1992). Isochromosome for the long arm of chromosome 9 is common, and it is usually associated with other chromosomal aberrations, for example, t(1;19)(q23;p13). As described for i(7)(q10), it is likely that i(9)(q10) is also an isodicentric chromosome. The i(9q) results in hemizygous deletions of *PAX5* (paired box 5) and *CDKN2A* (cyclin-dependent kinase inhibitor 2A). In a number of patients, the deletion of *CDKN2A* is homozygous with the second allele being lost as a result of a cryptic 9p deletion. Children with ALL harboring i(9)(q10) are, on average, older than other children with ALL, and they often have BCP-ALL, although rare cases of T-ALL have been reported. The incidence is equivalent in males and females. The WBC count is highly variable. There are no particular prognostic associations.

t(9;9)(q34;q34)/del(9)(q34q34)

ABL1 is a ubiquitously expressed cytoplasmic tyrosine kinase encoded by the *ABL1* (v-abl, Abelson murine leukemia viral oncogene homolog 1, previously known as *ABL*) gene in 9q34. Although the *BCR–ABL1* fusion of chronic myeloid leukemia (CML) and B-ALL is exceptionally rare in T-ALL, an alternative *ABL1* fusion with *NUP214* (nucleoporin 214 kDa, previously known as *CAN*) has been described as a secondary abnormality in 6% of T-ALL (Burmeister et al., 2006). The primary abnormalities included t(10;14)(q24;q11) (see following text) and t(5;14)(q35;q32) (see preceding text).

This t(9;9)/del(9) was initially discovered by FISH screening for evidence of the *BCR–ABL1* fusion, which revealed multiple extrachromosomal *ABL1* signals on episomes (Figure 10.7) (Barber et al., 2004b; Graux et al., 2004) and, rarely, homogeneously staining regions (hsr) (Ballerini et al., 2005). The episomes are not visible at the cytogenetic level. An in-frame fusion between introns 23–34 of *NUP214* and intron 1 of *ABL1*

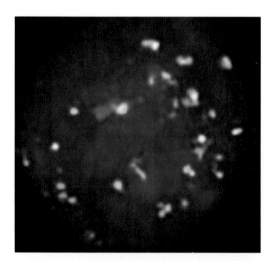

Figure 10.7 Interphase cell hybridized with probes specific for 3′ *ABL1* (*red*) and *NUP214* (*green*) showing episomal amplification of *NUP214–ABL1*.

was identified in cases with this abnormality. This finding was compatible with a model in which the genomic region from *ABL1* to *NUP214* was excised, circularized, and amplified to provide multiple copies of the *NUP214–ABL1* fusion. The episomal copy number is increased due to unequal segregation during cell division and is highly variable between patients (Graux et al., 2008). The *NUP214–ABL1* fusion is associated with increased *HOX* expression (Ferrando et al., 2002) as well as deletion of *CDKN2A* (Hebert et al., 1994), consistent with a multistep pathogenesis of T-ALL. *NUP214–ABL1*-positive and *NUP214–ABL1*-negative T-ALL patients do not differ significantly in their major clinical features, and no significant difference in overall survival has been observed (Burmeister et al., 2006; Graux et al., 2008). Like *BCR–ABL1*, *NUP214–ABL1* acts as a constitutively phosphorylated tyrosine kinase, which is also sensitive to imatinib, a selective inhibitor of *ABL1* kinase activity, as discussed in Chapter 8. However, the response of *NUP214–ABL1*-positive T-ALL patients to imatinib treatment was shown to be highly variable (Stergianou et al., 2005; Clarke et al., 2011).

Five cases of BCP-ALL have now been described with this fusion (Eyre et al., 2012; Roberts et al., 2012). One patient showed episomal amplification similar to that reported in T-ALL (Eyre et al., 2012), whereas the four remaining BCP-ALL cases had gain of only a single copy of this fusion (Roberts et al., 2012). Detection at this level was achieved by transcriptome sequencing or SNP arrays and confirmed by RT-PCR and Sanger sequencing; it would be difficult to identify by FISH. Primary leukemic cells from these latter four patients showed a positive response to dasatinib in experimental *in vitro* and *in vivo* models. In contrast, the cells treated *in vitro* from the patient with the amplified fusion showed no response to a range of TKI. These findings reflect the same variability of response to TKI in BCP-ALL samples as seen in T-ALL patients.

t(9;10)(q34;q22.3)

Six cases of pre-B-ALL with t(9;10)(q34;q22.3) have been reported (Soler et al., 2008; Moorman, 2012). The translocation leads to an in-frame fusion of exon 2 of *ABL1* with exon 14 of *ZMIZ1* (zinc finger, MIZ-type containing 1, previously known as *MIZ*) at 10q22, producing a *ZMIZ1–ABL1* fusion. This translocation adds to the increasing list of *ABL1* fusion partners in acute leukemia. Interestingly, all patients were young females who reached long-term remission on standard therapy, implicating a good outcome.

t(9;12)(q34;p13)

This cryptic translocation fuses *ETV6* intron 5 and *ABL1* intron 2, with transcript variants present in the majority of cases. For an in-frame fusion to occur requires an inverse orientation of both genes with at least three DNA breaks, in part explaining the rarity of the occurrence at approximately 0.5% in ALL. Although it occurs in both childhood and adult ALL, it is more frequent in myeloid malignancies (Zuna et al., 2010; Zhou et al., 2012). Its prenatal origin was demonstrated from the examination of Guthrie cards (Zuna et al., 2010). In BCP-ALL, the prognosis has been shown to be extremely poor. In line with this observation, this translocation has been reported within the newly described BCP-ALL high-risk subgroup, *BCR–ABL1*-like (see following text). In common with other translocations identified within this group and with the *BCR–ABL1* group itself, patients with the *ETV6–ABL1* fusion showed transient or prolonged response to treatment with imatinib and other second-generation TKI (Zuna et al., 2010; Roberts et al., 2012).

t(9;14)(q34;q32)

The cryptic t(9;14)(q34;q32) encoding an EML1–ABL1 fusion protein is another rare *ABL1* fusion with *EML1* (echinoderm microtubule-associated protein-like 1) at 14q32 in T-ALL (De Keersmaecker et al., 2005a). The t(9;14)-positive case also had a deletion of *CDKN2A* and expression of *TLX1* consistent with a multistep pathogenesis of T-ALL.

t(9;22)(q34;q11)

The t(9;22) results in the formation of the Philadelphia (Ph) chromosome seen in CML and, much less frequently, in ALL and AML (see Chapters 6 and 8). Complex and cryptic variant translocations may occur in Ph-positive ALL as they do in CML. As in CML, the translocation joins the 5′ sequences of the *BCR* gene at 22q11 to the 3′ sequences of *ABL1* at 9q34, giving rise to the *BCR–ABL1* fusion.

The breakpoint occurs between exons 1 and 2 (e1a2) of *BCR* in the minor breakpoint cluster region, m-bcr, and between exons 1 and 2 of *ABL1* (e1a2). This generates a 7 kb mRNA and expression of a P190 protein. Alternatively, breakpoints in the *BCR* gene occur within a 5.8 kb region termed the major breakpoint cluster region (M-bcr), between either exons 13 and 14 (b2a2) or exons 14 and 15 (b3a2). This transcribes an aberrant 8.5 kb mRNA encoding a chimeric P210 protein that arises frequently in CML (Chapter 8). Both BCR–ABL1 fusion proteins function as abnormally and constitutively activated tyrosine kinases.

In a small number of ALL patients, the t(9;22) is not visible by conventional cytogenetic analysis, although the *BCR–ABL1* transcript is detectable by RT-PCR (Radich et al., 1994). These are known as Ph-negative/*BCR–ABL1*-positive ALL (Van Rhee et al., 1995). They arise from a submicroscopic rearrangement or are masked within a variant or complex karyotype. As an alternative to RT-PCR, the translocation can be readily identified by dual-color FISH, particularly when it is cryptic. These alternative approaches were reviewed by Kearney (1999). They have been particularly useful in the identification of Ph-negative/*BCR–ABL1*-positive ALL and the presence of *BCR* and/or *ABL1* deletions from the *ABL1–BCR* region of the derived chromosome 9. These deletions have been shown to occur at a similar incidence of 10–15% in Ph-positive ALL as in CML (Robinson et al., 2005). In ALL, the translocation is often accompanied by a second copy of the derived chromosome 22. Other secondary changes differ from those found in CML, including high hyperdiploidy with trisomy for chromosome 2 (Chilton et al., 2014; Paulsson et al., 2013b). It is important that the Ph is identified in these cases, as the prognosis reflects the presence of the t(9;22) rather than the good risk associated with classical high hyperdiploidy (see preceding text). Approximately 70% of Ph-positive ALL have deletions of the B-cell differentiation gene, *IKZF1* (see following text) (Mullighan et al., 2008a).

In ALL, the t(9;22) occurs at a higher incidence in adults (25–30%) than children (~3%), increasing exponentially with age (Secker-Walker, 1997). Patients tend to have a high WBC count and a high incidence of organomegaly and CNS involvement.

The immunophenotype is typically that of pre-B-ALL, although myeloid antigens may be expressed. In all age groups, the outcome is poor despite high-dose intensified chemotherapy regimens. In pediatric Ph-positive ALL, the 3-year event-free survival was about 25% (Arico et al., 2000), and allogeneic stem cell transplantation provided the only curative treatment. However, with the recent introduction of the TKI imatinib, the historically poor outcome of BCR–ABL1-positive ALL has improved. In one study, where a combination of conventional intensive chemotherapy and imatinib was used, a significantly improved event-free survival of 80% was achieved in children (Schultz et al., 2009). In addition, by using second-generation TKI such as dasatinib and nilotinib, the suppression of BCR–ABL1 kinase activity may become even more potent, resulting in further improved outcomes (Kantarjian et al., 2006; Ottmann et al., 2007). Historically, Ph-positive ALL in adults was also associated with a very poor prognosis and a high relapse rate (Secker-Walker et al., 1991). However, the use of imatinib has resulted in improved outcome also for this age group (Liu-Dumlao et al., 2012; Fielding et al., 2014).

t(10;11)(p12;q14)

The t(10;11) fuses the MLLT10 gene at 10p12 with PICALM (phosphatidylinositol-binding clathrin assembly protein, previously known as CALM) at 11q14, giving rise to the PICALM–MLLT10 fusion gene (Dreyling et al., 1998; GFCH, 1991; De Keersmaecker et al., 2005b).

MLLT10 is also the partner of the MLL gene in complex rearrangements between 10p12 and 11q23 (see following text). Distinction between the two translocations can be difficult, and FISH or RT-PCR analysis is often required. The PICALM–MLLT10 fusion may occur in a cryptic rearrangement as expression has been shown in the absence of the translocation (Asnafi et al., 2003). Gene expression arrays showed that T-ALL expressing the PICALM–MLLT10 transcript had a distinctive profile with associated upregulation of HOXA5, HOXA9, and HOXA10 and their coregulator MEIS1 (Meis homeobox 1) (Dik et al., 2005).

The t(10;11) is a rare abnormality, in line with the knowledge that chromosomal rearrangements arising from the in-frame fusion of genes are generally uncommon in T-ALL. It occurs in approximately 10% of childhood and adult T-ALL. There are also reports of this translocation in lymphomas and acute leukemia of several lineages. In T-ALL, it is associated with a poor prognosis, although this has been shown to be dependent on the stage of maturation arrest.

Rearrangements between 10p12 and 11q23

In these rearrangements, the MLLT10 gene recombines with MLL to form the MLLT10–MLL fusion. In contrast to most other genes recombining with MLL, MLLT10 is oriented in the opposite transcriptional direction, making it impossible to generate the 5′ MLL–3′ MLLT10 fusion from a simple reciprocal translocation (Beverloo et al., 1995); an in-frame fusion requires a more complex mechanism of rearrangement. This explains why some cases, which appear to involve a more centromeric breakpoint on chromosome 11 (11q12 ~ 14), rearrange the MLL gene at 11q23. Such cases involve a three-break rearrangement with inversion of 11q and translocation of the inverted segment into 10p. This results in the juxtaposition of 5′ MLL with 3′ MLLT10, which then becomes fused in the correct orientation (Lillington et al., 1998). Alternatively, the fusion may arise from a submicroscopic inversion and insertion. In these complex and insertion cases, FISH or RT-PCR may be required to detect the involvement of MLL.

The MLL–MLLT10 chimera is principally found in acute monoblastic leukemia (Chapter 6), although a small number of ALL cases (comprising ~15% of the total) have been reported in T- and BCP-ALL (Lillington et al., 1998). Due to the small numbers described in ALL, the prognostic association is unknown.

t(10;14)(q24;q11)

The t(10;14) was first associated with T-ALL by Dube et al. (1986). As a result of the translocation, the class II HOX gene TLX1 (T-cell leukemia homeobox 1, formerly known as HOX11) at 10q24 is juxtaposed to the promoter elements of TRA/TRD on chromosome 14 or in rare cases to TRB in the t(7;10)(q34;q24) (see preceding text). It is transcriptionally activated to express the full-length protein at a high level. TLX1 is not normally expressed in developing T cells. *TLX1* is also frequently activated in T-ALL in the absence of visible genetic rearrangement (Ferrando et al., 2002). It is expressed in approximately 30% of T-ALL and more often in adult than in childhood cases. These leukemias show an early cortical phenotype and are reported to have a more favorable outcome than other classes of T-ALL (Ferrando et al., 2004b).

t(11;14)(p13;q11)/t(11;14)(p15;q11)

These translocations are found in T-ALL. The LIM domain-only genes *LMO1* and *LMO2* in 11p15 and 11p13, respectively, are involved in the t(11;14) (p15;q11) and t(11;14)(p13;q11), juxtaposing *LMO1* and *LMO2*, respectively, to the *TRA/TRD* (McGuire et al., 1989). Translocations with *TRB* have also been reported (Cauwelier et al., 2006) (see "t(7;11) (q34;p13)/t(7;11)(q34;p15)"). These rearrangements result in overexpression of *LMO1/LMO2*.

Cryptic deletions of the short arm of chromosome 11, del(11)(p12p13), have been identified in 4% of pediatric T-ALL by aCGH (van Vlierberghe et al., 2006). They lead to activation of the *LMO2* oncogene by deletion of the negative regulatory elements upstream of *LMO2*, which normally downregulate expression of the gene. *LMO2* becomes upregulated by its proximal promoter in the same manner as in the translocations. Together, these rearrangements account for 9% of pediatric T-ALL. Overall, abnormal expression of *LMO1* and *LMO2* occurs in 45% of T-ALL; this includes cases with no evidence of chromosomal changes (Ferrando et al., 2002). Deregulation of *LMO1/LMO2* often occurs in association with deregulation of *LYL1* (*LMO2*) or *TAL1* (*LMO1* and *LMO2*), confirming their involvement within common oncogenic pathways. *LMO1/TAL1* deregulation is more frequent in T-ALL committed to the alpha/beta-lineage. *LMO2*, when coexpressed with *LYL1*, predominantly occurs in immature T-ALL in adults, in which the cells are committed to no particular cell lineage. The prognostic association is unclear.

t(11;19)(q23;p13)

The t(11;19) is one of the more frequently occurring *MLL* translocations. The breakpoint on chromosome 19 may involve 19p13.1 or 19p13.3, more easily detected by G- and R-banding, respectively

(Huret et al., 1993). These alternative breakpoints are the sites of the *ELL* (elongation factor RNA polymerase II, previously known as *ELL1*) and *MLLT1* genes, respectively, which recombine with *MLL*, forming the *MLL–ELL* and *MLL–MLLT10* fusion genes (Yamamoto et al., 1993; Thirman et al., 1994). The t(11;19)(q23;p13.1) has only been found in AML; thus, the reader is referred to Chapter 6 for details.

The t(11;19)(q23;p13.3) occurs in both AML and ALL, although the majority are BCP- and T-ALL. In both diseases, it is frequently accompanied by secondary chromosomal changes, most often gain of an X chromosome and trisomy 8 (Moorman et al., 1998). This translocation predominates in younger patients, particularly infants. As for the other *MLL* rearrangements, the leukemia is associated with a high WBC count, organomegaly, and early leukemic involvement of the CNS. The survival in these ALL patients is poor, remaining unchanged by the presence of additional cytogenetic abnormalities (Moorman et al., 2005).

t(12;14)(p13;q11)

In T-ALL with the rare but recurrent t(12;14) (p13;q11) (see also "t(7;12)(q34;p13.3)"), translocation to *TRA* leads to upregulation of *CCND2*. To investigate the expression of other genes in 12p13, gene expression profiling has been carried out comparing expression data for eight genes surrounding the 12p breakpoint, including *CCND2*, with those in other T-ALL cases. The t(12;14)-positive T-ALL displayed an increased expression of *CCND2* compared to the controls, whereas the expression of the other genes was similar in all T-ALL cases. The t(12;14) was the first neoplasia-associated translocation shown to result in overexpression of cyclin D2. Furthermore, it was the first example of a T-cell neoplasm with targeted deregulation of a member of a cyclin-encoding gene family (Karrman et al., 2006a).

t(12;17)(p13;q12)

The t(12;17)(p13;q12) is rare in ALL. It involves the *ZNF384* gene (zinc finger protein 384, previously known as *CIZ* and *NMP4*) in 12p13, approximately 5 Mb upstream of *ETV6*, and the TATA box binding protein (TBP)-associated factor gene, *TAF15*, in 17q12 (Martini et al., 2002; Nyquist et al., 2011).

The breakpoint in *ZNF384* consistently occurs in intron 2, while the breakpoint in *TAF15* is located either between exons 6 and 7 or exons 9 and 10. These alternative breakpoints correspond to two fusion transcripts of *TAF15*, both coding for the transactivation domain in the N' terminus of the TAF15 protein. Two other translocations that involve *ZNF384* are t(12;22)(p13;q12) (see following text) and the cryptic t(12;19)(p13;p13) (see following text), which rearrange *EWSR1* (Ewing sarcoma breakpoint 1, previously known as *EWS*) and *TCF3* (*E2A*), respectively. Molecular and cytogenetic analyses have provided evidence that the translocations involving *ZNF384* are primary events, playing an early role in the leukemogenic process (La Starza et al., 2005). These rearrangements characterize a specific subset of ALL with an early B-phenotype, myeloid marker expression (CD13 and/or CD33), no bulky disease, and onset in young adults (median age of 22 years). As numbers are small, prognostic associations are difficult to establish, although current data suggest an overall relatively favorable outcome.

t(12;19)(p13;p13)

The t(12;19) is a rare translocation found in B-ALL. It recombines *TCF3* at 19p13 with the *ZNF384* gene at 12p13. The *TCF3* gene is known for its involvement in t(1;19)(q23;p13) (see preceding text) and the variant t(17;19)(q22;p13) (see following text). Thus, t(12;19) likely represents another rare t(1;19) variant in which *ZNF384* emerges as the third transcription factor to be involved in *TCF3* fusions in ALL. *ZNF384* is also the partner in other translocations, namely, t(12;17)(p13;q11) (see preceding text) and t(12;22)(p13;q12) (see following text). The t(12;19) results in two fusion genes, *TCF3–ZNF384* on the der(19)t(12;19) and *NOL1–TCF3* (*NOL1*, nucleolar protein 1) on the der(12)t(12;19), involving duplication of material from 12p (Zhong et al., 2008). The clinical associations and outcome are unknown.

t(12;21)(p13;q22)

The t(12;21) was first discovered by FISH in 1994 (Romana et al., 1994). It is invisible by karyotyping as the banding pattern and the size of the translocated regions between chromosomes 12 and 21 are identical. The translocation involves the ETS-type variant 6 (*ETV6*) gene (previously known as *TEL*, translocated ETS leukemia gene) at 12p13 and the *RUNX1* gene (runt-related transcription factor 1, previously known as *AML1* (acute myeloid leukemia 1), or *CBFA2*) at 21q22, which recombine to form an *ETV6–RUNX1* fusion gene on the derived chromosome 21 (Golub et al., 1995; Romana et al., 1995). It has been convincingly demonstrated that the formation of *ETV6–RUNX1* fusion is a prenatal and initiating event in childhood ALL. Evidence for this came from the finding of the same *ETV6* clonogenic breakpoint in monozygotic twins who both developed *ETV6–RUNX1*-positive ALL and the presence of the fusion in neonatal blood spots of children who later developed *ETV6–RUNX1*-positive ALL (Ford et al., 1998; Greaves, 2005; Hong et al., 2008). Ectopic expression of the erythropoietin receptor, EPOR, contributes critically to the persistence of these covert premalignant *ETV6–RUNX1* clones in children (Inthal et al., 2008; Torrano et al., 2011).

Although rare variant breakpoints have been identified, RT-PCR, using primers for exon 5 of *ETV6* and exon 3 of *RUNX1*, detects the presence of the *ETV6–RUNX1* fusion transcript at the mRNA level in the vast majority of cases. FISH analysis using probes specific for *ETV6* and *RUNX1* enables the *ETV6–RUNX1* fusion to be accurately visualized in interphase and metaphase cells (Harrison et al., 2010). At the same time, the FISH signal pattern indicates the presence of *ETV6* deletions from the chromosome 12 homolog not involved in the translocation and the gain of copies of the normal or derived chromosome 21. All three abnormalities are frequent secondary changes that accompany the t(12;21) (Attarbaschi et al., 2004). Deletion of *ETV6* and a range of other abnormalities have been described as essential second hits to establish leukemia development after the t(12;21) has provided a preleukemic first event (Bateman et al., 2010). The extent of the deletion can be highly variable, ranging from cytogenetically visible deletions to intragenic deletions of *ETV6* (Raynaud et al., 1996). It has been shown that the fusion-positive cell population may be highly heterogeneous in terms of the number and distribution of secondary abnormalities indicating a high level of clonal diversity in these patients (Martineau et al., 2005; Anderson et al., 2011). Near triploidy and near tetraploidy in childhood BCP-ALL are highly characteristic of *ETV6–RUNX1*-positive leukemia, and deletions of 11q23 are also frequent secondary changes (Attarbaschi et al., 2006, 2007; Raimondi et al., 2006), while deletions of the der(12)t(12;21) are rare (Al-Shehhi et al., 2013).

The *ETV6–RUNX1* fusion is the most common translocation in childhood ALL, occurring in 25–30% of BCP-ALL, with a peak incidence at 3–5 years of age (Moorman, 2012). Although not exclusively restricted to children, the incidence in adult ALL is low (1–4%) (Jabber Al-Obaidi et al., 2002). The outlook for children with ALL and this abnormality is generally extremely good, up to 99% on contemporary therapy (Bhojwani et al., 2012). In the rare relapses, it was shown that the diagnostic and relapse clones represented different subclones that evolved from a common *ETV6–RUNX1*-positive progenitor cell, determined from matching genomic *ETV6–RUNX1* breakpoints at both time points. Retrospective analysis revealed that the relapse clone was already present at diagnosis, with a much slower response to therapy compared with the dominant leukemic clone. In all instances, these initially slow-responding clones, after they had developed into the relapse leukemia, were rapidly eradicated by the relapse treatment, underlining their different biology at the two time points of leukemia manifestation. The authors hypothesized that the minor clone was not fully malignant at initial diagnosis but acquired further mutations for the manifestation of relapse (Konrad et al., 2003).

t(12;22)(p13;q12)

The t(12;22) recombines *ZNF384* at 12p13 with *EWSR1* (Ewing sarcoma gene) at 22q12 (Martini et al., 2002). Fusions of the TET proteins (TLS/FUS, EWSR1, and TAF15/RBP56) to different transcription factors are involved in various malignancies including Ewing sarcoma, primitive neuroectodermal tumors, and AML. As a result of a t(12;17)(p13;q12) or its variant t(12;22)(p13;q12), the transcription factor gene *ZNF384* is recurrently involved in acute leukemia through fusion with either *TAF15* or *EWSR1*, respectively. These results extend the involvement of TET-protein fusions to ALL and suggest a role for *ZNF384* in lymphoid and myeloid development (see also sections "t(12;17)(p13;q11)" and "t(12;19)(p13;p13)").

del(13)(q12 ~ 14)

Approximately 3% of childhood and adult B-ALL have abnormalities involving 13q12 ~ 14. Interstitial deletions are the most frequent, although translocations associated with 13q loss have also been described. The centromeric deletion breakpoint is typically in the 13q12 ~ 14 region and the telomeric one between 13q21 and 13qter. Although it occurs as the sole karyotypic abnormality in approximately 10% of cases, it is regarded as a frequent secondary event, occurring across all cytogenetic subtypes (Kovacs et al., 2004; Moorman et al., 2010b). In one report, 13q aberrations were associated with reduced event-free survival (Heerema et al., 2000a). In a more recent study, deletion of 13q within the *ETV6–RUNX1* and high-hyperdiploid groups did not have a significant effect on outcome, while loss of 13q among patients in other cytogenetic groups was associated with an increased risk of relapse. However, this effect was not significant, indicating that del(13q) is not an independent prognostic indicator (Moorman et al., 2010b).

inv(14)(q11q32)/t(14;14)(q11;q32)

The t(14;14) and inv(14) recombine *TRA* at 14q11 with the *TCL1* (T-cell leukemia 1) oncogene at 14q32.1, centromeric of the *IGH* locus (Croce et al., 1985). Rarely, the *TRB* locus is alternatively involved in the t(7;14)(q35;q32). *TCL1* is upregulated by the control elements of the *TCR* gene whether they are positioned 5′ of *TCL1* as for translocations or 3′ as for inversions. A similar situation has been observed in Burkitt lymphoma/leukemia, where the immunoglobulin enhancers can be located either upstream or downstream of the *MYC* oncogene (Chapter 11).

The abnormalities t(14;14) and inv(14) have been detected at high frequency in ataxia telangiectasia (AT), being seen in 7–10% of all AT cases, and in all types of T-lineage lymphoid neoplasias; t(14;14)/inv(14) is considered to be a characteristic chromosomal aberration in T-cell leukemia secondary to AT (Mengle-Gaw et al., 1988), associated with postthymic types of T-ALL such as T-prolymphocytic leukemia (T-PLL) and acute or chronic T-cell leukemia. *TCL1* is overexpressed in the majority of cases of T-PLL. A rarely occurring inv(14)(q11.2q32.31) has also been reported, which results in expression of the *BCL11B–TRD* fusion in association with the absence of the wild-type *BCL11B* transcript (Przybylski et al., 2005) (see previous section on t(5;14)). This inversion is indistinguishable from the inv(14) involving *TCL1*.

A small number of cases have been described with t(14;14) or inv(14) in BCP-ALL (Liu et al., 2004; Akasaka et al., 2007). These abnormalities are significant as they represent another rearrangement involving *IGH* and a member of the *CEBP* gene family, in this case *CEBPE*. Expression of this gene is upregulated as described for the other *IGH* transloca-tions, namely, t(8;14)(q11;q32) (*CEBPD*) (described earlier), t(14;19)(q32;q13) (*CEBPA* and *CEBPG*) (described in the following), and t(14;20)(q32;q13) (*CEBPB*) (described in the following). As for the other ALL subgroups with translocations between *IGH* and a member of the *CEPB* gene family, they have a pre-B immunophenotype, are older children or adults, and have low WBC counts. These patients were examined together with the other *IGH* translocations, which are frequent among adolescents and young adults with ALL. Although associated with an adverse outcome in adults, *IGH* translocations are not an independent prognostic factor in children and adolescents (Russell et al., 2014).

t(14;18)(q32;q21)

The t(14;18) is common in follicle center B-cell lym-phomas, being found in approximately 80% of follic-ular lymphomas and approximately 20% of diffuse large B-cell lymphomas (Chapter 11). The transloca-tion has also been described, albeit rarely, in B-ALL, with the first ones reported 30 years ago (Mufti et al., 1983). The t(14;18) is often associated with other chromosomal abnormalities, particularly with t(8;14)(q24;q32) and its variants t(2;8)(p12;q24) and t(14;22)(q24;q11) (D'Achille et al., 2006).

ALL with t(14;18) is either BCP-ALL or mature B-ALL and usually occurs in older children and adults. These patients have an extremely poor out-come in terms of event-free and overall survival.

t(14;19)(q32;p13)

The rare t(14;19)(q32;p13) is another translocation involving *IGH*, which juxtaposes the erythropoi-etin receptor precursor (*EPOR*) at 19p13 to the *IGH* enhancer, resulting in *IGH–EPOR* and *EPOR* mRNA overexpression. The four cases described by Russell et al. (2009b) and Chapiro et al. (2013)

were one older child (11 years) and three adults with high-risk BCP-ALL. Another case was described as *BCR–ABL1*-like ALL and thus high risk (see following text), in which a cryptic 7.5 kb insertion of *EPOR* into the *IGH* locus, downstream of the IgH enhancer domain, was detected by tran-scriptome sequencing (Roberts et al., 2012).

t(14;19)(q32;q13)

The t(14;19) has been reported in patients with CLL and lymphoma, in which *IGH* is recombined with *BCL3* (Chapter 11). In BCP-ALL, the same translocation breakpoints have been described involving *IGH* and *CEBPA* (Akasaka et al., 2007; Chapiro et al., 2013). The latter gene is one of the CEBP proteins that are a family of six multifunc-tional bZIP transcription factors. *CEBPA* is overex-pressed as a result of the t(14;19), implicating its role as an oncogene in BCP-ALL. *CEBPA* is known to be mutated in AML, in which it operates as a tumor suppressor gene. Thus, *CEBPA* demon-strates opposing functions of CEBP dysregulation in myeloid and lymphoid leukemogenesis.

In one ALL with the same translocation break-points, the *IGH* partner was found to be *CEBPG*, another *CEBP* family member located 71 kb upstream of *CEBPA* in 19q13 (Akasaka et al., 2007). As noted for the t(8;14)(q11;q32), the t(14;19) involving *CEBPG* was shown to be secondary to t(9;22) (q34;q11). Three other *CEBP* gene family members have been described as *IGH* partners in the t(8;14) (q11;q32) (*CEBPD*) (described earlier), inv(14) (q11q32)/t(14;14)(q11;q32) (*CEBPE*) (described earlier), and t(14;20)(q32;q13) (*CEBPB*) (described in the following).

As for t(8;14)(q11;q32) (see preceding text), all t(14;19)-positive ALL have been BCP-ALL. The patients tend to be older children (median age of 15 years) and adults, and the WBC counts are usually low. When grouped together with other patients into the distinctive subtype harboring *IGH* translocations, adults showed an adverse outcome, although these translocations were not an independent prognostic factor in children and adolescents (Russell et al., 2014).

t(14;20)(q32;q13)

Although only few B-ALL cases with the t(14;20) have been reported, it is worthy of note as it repre-sents another translocation formed between *IGH* and a member of the *CEBP* gene family, *CEBPB* (Akasaka et al., 2007; Chapiro et al., 2013). Expression of this gene is upregulated as described earlier for the other *IGH* translocations t(8;14) (q11;q32) (*CEBPD*), inv(14)(q11q32)/t(14;14) (q11;q32) (*CEBPE*), and t(14;19)(q32;q13) (*CEBPA* and *CEBPG*), with the same overall outcome (Russell et al., 2014).

t(14;21)(q11;q22)

OLIG2 (oligodendrocyte lineage transcription factor 2, also known as *bHLHB1*) is upregulated in T-ALL by the rare t(14;21)(q11;q22), which juxtaposes *OLIG2* and *TRA* (Wang et al., 2000). Sequence analysis of the genomic breakpoints indicated that the translocation had been mediated by an illegitimate V(D)J recombination event that disrupted *TRA* and relocated its enhancer elements to the derivative 21 chromosome, close to *OLIG2*. Although *OLIG2* expression is normally restricted to neural tissues, T-cell lymphoblasts with the t(14;21) also express high levels of *OLIG2* mRNA, and it contributes to leukemogenesis in concert with *LMO1* (Lin et al., 2005).

15q13 ~ 15 rearrangements

In childhood ALL, abnormalities with breakpoints in chromosome bands 15q13 ~ 15 have been reported at an incidence of less than 1% (Heerema et al., 2002; Moorman, 2012; De Lorenzo et al., 2014). Of particular note was that the majority were balanced translocations involving a range of chromosomal partners. Patients were BCP-ALL and more frequently infants than older children. Aside from their young age profile, these cases were unremarkable with respect to clinical features and outcome. They were classified as standard-risk ALL, and their outcome was not different from patients without 15q abnormalities; therefore, this abnormality itself does not confer an increased risk of treatment failure.

i(17)(q10)

Although this aberration has been frequently described in ALL, it is rarely seen as the sole anomaly. Together with i(7)(q10) and i(9)(q10), it is the most common isochromosome in ALL (Pui et al., 1992). The overall occurrence of i(17)(q10) as a secondary chromosomal abnormality is particularly common

in leukemia with t(9;22) as the primary aberration (especially in CML; see Chapter 8). However, it is often found in high-hyperdiploid ALL, sometimes as the only structural rearrangement (Herou et al., 2013). In a few cases, it has been seen in association with other primary changes, such as t(4;11)(q21;q23) and t(8;14)(q11;q32). Therefore, it is not surprising that the clinical and hematologic characteristics of ALL with i(17)(q10) do not differ markedly from those of other cytogenetic subtypes.

The molecular consequences of i(17)(q10) remain unknown. One effect is the loss of one allele of each gene on 17p, including the *TP53* (tumor protein p53, previously known as *p53*) tumor suppressor gene, as seen in AML with complex karyotypes (Chapter 6).

t(17;19)(q22;p13)

The t(17;19) is a rare translocation, with an incidence of 0.1% in BCP-ALL (Moorman, 2012). It is a significant variant of t(1;19)(q23;p13) (see preceding text). The leukemic cells with t(17;19) produce a chimeric transcript resulting from the fusion of *TCF3* at 19p13 with the hepatic leukemia factor gene *HLF* at 17q22 (Inaba et al., 1992). *HLF* is a bZIP transcription factor, and two main types of genomic rearrangement enable the fusion of *TCF3* with *HLF*, corresponding to slightly different breakpoint positions (Hunger et al., 1994). Type I rearrangements arise from a breakpoint within intron 13 of *TCF3* and intron 3 of *HLF*, while type II rearrangements involve a breakpoint within intron 12 of *TCF3* and intron 3 of *HLF*. Both types generate novel chimeric proteins with transcription regulating ability.

As for t(1;19), patients with t(17;19) have BCP-ALL. Type I molecular rearrangements have been suggested to be associated with disseminated intravascular coagulation and type II with hypercalcemia. Patients tend to be older with a median age of 13 years and a low WBC count at diagnosis. The prognosis associated with this translocation seems to be extremely poor, with the vast majority of reported patients having died (Hunger 1996; Moorman, 2012).

Another rarely occurring cryptic rearrangement of *TCF3* has also been reported, t(12;19) (p13;p13), that results in the formation of two different fusion genes on the derivative chromosomes (see preceding text).

Submicroscopic del(21)(q22.2q22.2)

Deletions of this region of chromosome 21 specifically target the ETS family transcription factor gene *ERG* (ETS-related gene). *ERG* deletions usually involve an internal subset of exons resulting in loss of the central inhibitory and pointed domains, leading to expression of an aberrant C-terminal ERG fragment that retains the ETS and transactivation domains. It functions as a competitive inhibitor of wild-type ERG. This gene deletion exclusively occurs in cases lacking known chromosomal rearrangements, although it frequently has deletions of exons 4–7 of the *IKZF1* gene (38%) (see preceding text). Thus, this *ERG* deletion defines a distinct subtype of BCP-ALL, occurring in approximately 3%. It is associated with a higher age (median age of 7 years) and aberrant CD2 expression. Notably, despite the presence of *IKZF1* alterations in a proportion of *ERG*-deleted cases, the outcome is favorable, suggesting that *IKZF1* deletions have no impact on prognosis in this genetic subtype (Harvey et al., 2010b; Clappier et al., 2014; Zaliova et al., 2014).

i(21)(q10)

Isochromosome 21q is rare in ALL (Martineau et al., 1996; Cooley et al., 2007). It is often associated with the *ETV6–RUNX1* fusion; thus, the finding of an i(21)(q10) by cytogenetics alone does not indicate whether the abnormal chromosome is i(21)(q10) or ider(21)(q10)t(12;21)(p13;q22). If i(21)(q10) is found as the sole change by banding analysis, it is recommended to search for the presence of the *ETV6–RUNX1* fusion by FISH or RT-PCR, as also suggested when trisomy 21 is found as the sole cytogenetic abnormality (Karrman et al., 2006b). The clinical and prognostic associations of i(21)(q10) in ALL are unclear. Among the 15 cases described by Martineau et al. (1996), the patients characteristically had a low WBC count and BCP-ALL. The large study by Cooley et al. (2007) presented a survival analysis of i(21)(q10) together with other ALL patients harboring abnormalities of 21q. The poor prognosis afforded to the group as a whole may be due to the presence of patients with intrachromosomal amplification of chromosome 21 (iAMP21) among them (see following text), while those with a favorable outcome may harbor the *ETV6–RUNX1* fusion.

Intrachromosomal amplification of chromosome 21 (iAMP21)

This abnormality was first described as multiple copies of the *RUNX1* gene on an abnormal chromosome 21 (Busson-Le Coniat et al., 2001). Two later series described a significant number of patients with this abnormality, defining iAMP21 as a cytogenetic subgroup (Harewood et al., 2003; Soulier et al., 2003). In the majority of cases, amplification of the *RUNX1* gene was detected during routine screening for the presence of the *ETV6–RUNX1* fusion by interphase FISH (Harrison et al., 2005). It manifests as multiple copies of the *RUNX1* gene, which are seen as clusters of signals in interphase cells and in tandem duplication along the long arm of an abnormal chromosome 21 at metaphase. Array CGH and FISH studies defined a minimal region of amplification spanning 5.1 Mb of chromosome 21 from 32.8 to 37.9 Mb. This region always includes *RUNX1*, frequently in association with loss of 21q subtelomeric sequences (Strefford et al., 2006; Robinson et al., 2007; Rand et al., 2011). Gene expression profiling studies showed no significant differentially expressed genes to distinguish iAMP21 patients from other ALL patients with abnormalities of chromosome 21, including those with *ETV6–RUNX1* fusion and high hyperdiploidy with two or more extra copies of chromosome 21 (Strefford et al., 2006). The expression levels of *RUNX1* were highly variable, reflecting the expression of this gene in ALL samples in general. Thus, there is no evidence to indicate that *RUNX1* is the target gene of this abnormality. The abnormal chromosome takes on a surprising variety of morphological forms when examined by karyotyping (Figure 10.8), metaphase FISH, and multicolor banding techniques. These observations, in association with SNP arrays and NGS studies, have shown that the abnormal chromosome 21 arises from highly complex intrachromosomal rearrangements, including inversions, duplications, and deletions, initiated by breakage–fusion–bridge cycles and chromothripsis (Robinson et al., 2007; Li et al., 2014). iAMP21 is defined by the presence of three or more additional copies of *RUNX1* on a single abnormal chromosome 21 (five or more signals in total in interphase) with frequent deletion of subtelomeric 21q sequences, a definition that

(A)

(C)

(B)

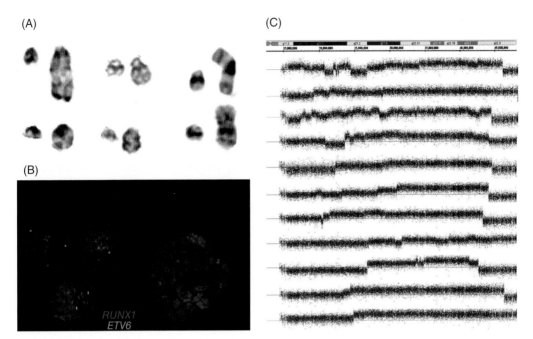

Figure 10.8 (A) Partial karyograms from six patients with iAMP21. The normal chromosome 21 is on the left and the iAMP21 is on the right. The variable morphology and G-banding pattern among individual cells are shown. (B) A metaphase and interphase cells hybridized with probes specific for *ETV6* (*green*) and *RUNX1* (*red*). Multiple copies of *RUNX1* signals are seen clustered in interphase and in tandem duplication on a single abnormal chromosome 21 in metaphase. (C) SNP profiles of chromosome 21 from 11 patients with iAMP21 showing the diversity of copy number abnormalities seen between patients as also reflected in the chromosome morphology.

has now been adopted internationally (Harrison et al., 2010).

From an international study of 530 cases of iAMP21, it was confirmed that the 21q abnormality was a primary genetic change apart from rare associations with *BCR–ABL1* or *ETV6–RUNX1* fusions (Harrison et al., 2014). Karyotypes are pseudodiploid or low hyperdiploid, with gain of chromosome X, loss or deletion of chromosome 7, and *ETV6* and *RB1* deletions as the most frequent recurrent secondary changes. FISH with probes directed to the *RUNX1* gene or SNP arrays provide the only reliable detection method for this abnormality. In cases without metaphases, additional probes should be applied to distinguish iAMP21 from high hyperdiploidy with extra copies of chromosome 21. These might include a subtelomeric probe to chromosome 21 to demonstrate that the number of *RUNX1* signals is greater than the number of chromosomes 21 (Harrison et al., 2010).

In all studies, iAMP21 patients had BCP-ALL; were older, with a median age of 9 years; and generally had low WBC counts. Prospective screening in recent childhood trials has determined the incidence to be 2%. Patients with iAMP21 have a high risk of relapse when treated on standard therapy (Moorman et al., 2007b), although outcome has been dramatically improved with intensive chemotherapy (Heerema et al., 2013; Moorman et al., 2013). The nature of cooperating lesions and the role of iAMP21 in driving an aggressive leukemia are currently poorly understood. However, it has recently been shown that individuals with the rare Robertsonian translocation between chromosomes 15 and 21, rob(15;21)c, have a 2700-fold increased risk of developing iAMP21 BCP-ALL and that the abnormality in these patients always involves both chromosome 15 and 21 of the rob(15;21)c (Li et al., 2014).

t(X;14)(p22;q32) or t(Y;14)(p11;q32)/ del(X)(p22.33p22.33) or del(Y) (p11.32p11.32)

The t(X;14)(p22;q32) and t(Y;14)(p11;q32) juxtapose the cytokine receptor *CRLF2* to the *IGH* enhancer (*IGH–CRLF2*). In the two interstitial deletions del(X)(p22.33p22.33) and del(Y) (p11.32p11.32), *CRLF2* is juxtaposed to the promoter of *P2RY8* (*P2RY8–CRLF2*) (Russell et al., 2009a). *CRLF2*, which is located in the pseudoautosomal region of the sex chromosomes (PAR1) at Xp22.3/Yp11.3, encodes cytokine receptor-like factor 2 (thymic stromal lymphopoietin receptor [TSLPR]). With interleukin-7 receptor alpha, CRLF2 forms a heterodimeric receptor for the ligand TSLP. Both the translocations and the deletions result in aberrant overexpression of CRLF2 on the cell surface of leukemic lymphoblasts that may be detected by flow cytometric immunophenotyping (Mulligan et al., 2009a). Less commonly, a CRLF2 p.Phe232Cys mutation results in receptor dimerization and overexpression (Chapiro et al., 2010). These rearrangements occur in approximately 7% of childhood and adult BCP-ALL and 50% of Down syndrome ALL (DS-ALL) (Kearney et al., 2009; Mulligan et al., 2009a; Russell et al., 2009a; Chapiro et al., 2010).

Approximately half of *CRLF2*-rearranged ALL harbor activating mutations of the Janus kinase genes *JAK1* and *JAK2* (Mulligan et al., 2009a; Russell et al., 2009a; Hertzberg et al., 2010), otherwise uncommon in BCP-ALL. The *JAK* mutations are most often missense mutations at or near R683 in the pseudokinase domain of *JAK2*, distinct from the *JAK2* V617F mutations that are a hallmark of myeloproliferative neoplasms (Chapter 9).

Less common are activating mutations in the kinase domains of *JAK1* and *JAK2*.

In non-DS-ALL, *CRLF2* alterations and *JAK* mutations are associated with *IKZF1* deletions/mutations and poor outcome, particularly in cohorts of high-risk B-ALL (Cario et al., 2010; Harvey et al., 2010a, b; Ensor et al., 2011; Moorman et al., 2012). Notably, elevated *CRLF2* expression in the absence of a rearrangement has also been reported as an adverse prognostic feature (Chen et al., 2012).

Submicroscopic abnormalities

The introduction of high-resolution SNP arrays and NGS technologies has highlighted the significance of DNA copy number alterations (CNA), such as submicroscopic deletions and amplifications, and sequence mutations in ALL. The genes most frequently involved in CNA encode proteins with key roles in lymphoid development (*PAX5*, *IKZF1*, and *EBF1*), cell cycle regulation and tumor suppression (*CDKN2A/B* and *RB1*), putative regulation of apoptosis (*BTG1*), lymphoid signaling, transcriptional regulation and coactivation (*ETV6* and *ERG*), regulation of chromatin structure, and epigenetics (Figure 10.9), while mutations predominantly occur in genes involved in key signaling pathways in BCP-ALL: RAS signaling (*NRAS*, *KRAS*, and *NF1*), cytokine receptor

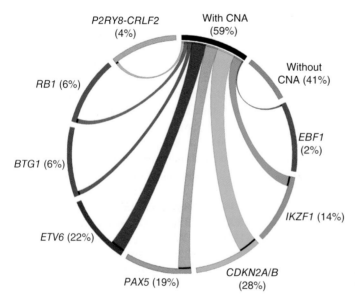

Figure 10.9 This circus plot indicates the distribution of copy number abnormalities in BCP-ALL. The individual colored ribbons represent the proportion of cases showing each abnormality among the total with copy number changes. They are not mutually exclusive.

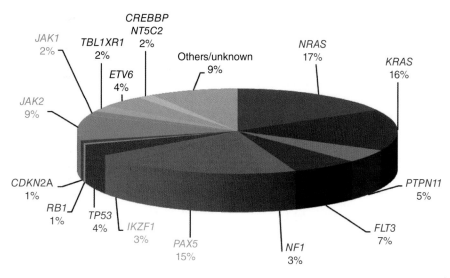

Figure 10.10 Pie chart indicating the distribution of the most common mutations within genes/key signaling pathways in BCP-ALL: RAS signaling (*purple*), B-cell development and differentiation (*blue*), cell cycle control (*red*), JAK (*green*), and others (*black*). These mutations are not mutually exclusive.

signaling (*IL7R* and *JAK2*), and cell cycle control (*TP53* and *RB1*) (Figure 10.10) (Kuiper et al., 2007; Mullighan et al., 2007, 2009b; Zhang et al., 2011). Importantly, several genes are involved in multiple types of genetic aberrations, including CNA, translocations, and sequence mutation, for example, *PAX5*, which also shows intragenic amplification of exons 2 or 5 (Schwab et al., 2013).

Aberrations affecting lymphoid development are the most frequent (e.g., *PAX5* altered in ~35%, *IKZF1* in ~15%, and *EBF1* in ~5%). They are usually loss of function or dominant negative lesions resulting in arrested lymphoid maturation, which is an important characteristic of leukemic cells. Although *PAX5* alterations are the most common genetic alteration in BCP-ALL, they are not associated with outcome (Mullighan et al., 2009b; Iacobucci et al., 2010).

The nature and frequency of genetic lesions are subtype dependent. For example, *MLL*-rearranged leukemia harbors very few additional structural or sequence alterations, while in contrast, the majority of non-*MLL* ALL harbor increased numbers of recurring submicroscopic deletions, at least six to eight per case in *ETV6–RUNX1* and *BCR–ABL1* ALL (Mullighan et al., 2007, 2008a; Dobbins et al., 2013; Schwab et al., 2013).

Relapsed ALL

Although several chromosomal alterations are associated with a higher risk of treatment failure, relapse occurs across the spectrum of ALL subtypes. It has long been recognized that ALL genomes are not static, but exhibit acquisition of chromosomal abnormalities over time (Raimondi et al., 1993); thus, there has been intense interest in genomic profiling of matched diagnosis and relapse samples to dissect the genetic basis of clonal heterogeneity in ALL and the relationship of such heterogeneity to risk of relapse. Although the primary chromosomal abnormality is usually retained between diagnosis and relapse, it has been shown that the majority of ALL show changes in the patterns of their secondary genomic alterations from diagnosis to relapse (Yang et al., 2008; Kawamata et al., 2009) and that many relapse-acquired abnormalities, including deletions of *IKZF1* and *CDKN2A*, are present at low levels at diagnosis (Mullighan et al., 2008b; Yang et al., 2008; Olsson et al., 2014). Recurring mutations have been identified that influence drug sensitivity and risk of relapse. For example, mutations in the transcriptional coactivator and acetyl transferase gene *CREBBP* (CREB-binding protein or CBP) are found in up to 20% of relapsed ALL samples (Mullighan et al., 2011; Inthal et al., 2012). CREBBP acetylates both histone and nonhistone targets and has a role in regulating the transcriptional response to glucocorticoid therapy. Recently, two groups independently identified relapse-associated mutations in the 5′ nucleotidase gene *NT5C2* that conferred increased resistance to purine analogs (Meyer et al., 2013b; Tzoneva et al., 2013). Such mutations associated with resistance to drugs commonly used to treat ALL represent a key mechanism of treatment failure and resistance.

BCR–ABL1-like or Ph-like ALL

Recently, a new subgroup of BCP-ALL has been described, characterized by an expression profile similar to *BCR–ABL1*-positive ALL, deletion of *IKZF1*, and poor outcome, named *BCR–ABL1*-like or Ph-like ALL (Den Boer et al., 2009; Mullighan et al., 2009b; Loh et al., 2013). It is common, comprising up to 10% of childhood and up to one-third of BCP-ALL in adolescents and young adults. Interestingly, the detection of patients in this group based on gene expression profiling showed variation in patient identification; thus, it may be more appropriate to make use of emerging genomic data to identify this poor-risk subgroup. Approximately half of *BCR–ABL1*-like ALL have *CRLF2* rearrangements and concomitant *JAK* mutations (Harvey et al., 2010a). Recent transcriptome and whole-genome sequencing has shown that *BCR–ABL1*-like ALL harbor a diverse range of genomic alterations that activate cytokine receptors and tyrosine kinases including *ABL1*, *ABL2*, *EPOR*, *JAK2*, *PDGFRB*, and *CSF1R* (Roberts et al., 2012). These alterations are enriched in, but not exclusive to, *BCR–ABL1*-like cases. They are most commonly chromosomal rearrangements resulting in chimeric fusion genes deregulating cytokine receptors and tyrosine kinases, a number of which are recurrent: *IGH–EPOR* of the t(14;19) (q32;p13)/ins(14;19)(q32;p13), *EBF1–PDGFRB* of the del(5)(q32q33.3), *NUP214–ABL1* of the t(9;9) (q34;q34)/del(9)(q34q34), and *ETV6–ABL1* of the t(9;12)(q34;p13) (see preceding text), while an increasing number of other partners have been reported in single cases in BCP-ALL, for example, *BCR–JAK2*, *PAX5–JAK2*, *STRN3–JAK2*, *RANBP2–ABL1*, *RCSD1–ABL1*, and *MEF2D–CSF1R* of t(1;5)

(see preceding text), which may become recurrent as further cases are investigated. In up to 20% of *BCR–ABL1*-like cases, alternative alterations activating kinase signaling occur, including activating mutations of *FLT3* and *IL7R*, as well as focal deletions of *SH2B3* (also known as *LNK*), which is a negative regulator of *JAK2*. These diverse genetic alterations activate a limited number of signaling pathways, notably *ABL1*, *PDGFRB*, and JAK–STAT signaling. In addition, primary leukemic cells and xenografts of *BCR–ABL1*-like ALL are highly sensitive to TKI *in vivo* (Maude et al., 2012; Roberts et al., 2012). An increasing number of reports are emerging of responsiveness of refractory *BCR–ABL1*-like ALL to appropriate TKI therapy, for example, two cases of *EBF1–PDGFRB* ALL showing a response to imatinib have been published (Lengline et al., 2013; Weston et al., 2013). Thus, it is predicted that the majority of *BCR–ABL1*-like ALL will be amenable to therapy with a limited number of imatinib-class TKI for *ABL1*, *ABL2*, and *PDGFRB* rearrangements and JAK inhibitors, such as ruxolitinib, for alterations activating JAK–STAT signaling (*EPOR*, *IL7R*, *JAK2*, and *SH2B3*). NGS studies of childhood and adult ALL are ongoing in order to identify comprehensively all kinase-activating alterations in *BCR–ABL1*-like ALL and to implement TKI therapy into clinical trials.

Clinical correlations

Cytogenetic analysis plays an integral part in the diagnosis of ALL. Certain genomic rearrangements are strongly associated with distinctive clinical features, thereby providing a means for improved disease subclassification, as previously discussed in detail. The abnormalities differ between B-ALL and T-ALL with different distributions between age groups. In association with these aspects, the diagnostic karyotype is an important prognostic variable. Modern therapeutic regimens have dramatically improved the survival in ALL. These improvements have increased the need for reliable prognostic indicators to ensure that patients are risk stratified to the most appropriate treatment protocol.

Classification of abnormalities according to lineage

The main patterns of cytogenetic abnormalities, which are characteristic of BCP-ALL, include changes in ploidy: high hyperdiploidy, near haploidy, and low hypodiploidy. The majority of structural rearrangements comprise in-frame translocations leading to the formation of fusion transcripts with oncogenic potential. These include t(1;19)(q23;p13.3) and variants, t(9;22)(q34;q11), *MLL* rearrangements, and t(12;21)(p13;q22), as previously described in detail. An increasing number of patients with 14q32 abnormalities involving *IGH* and overexpression of a range of partner genes have been described (see preceding text), which appear to be linked together as a novel subgroup. In addition, understanding the mechanism behind the intriguing chromosomal abnormality iAMP21 has confirmed that these patients comprise a defined subtype of BCP-ALL. All of these cytogenetic subgroups have distinctive demographic and clinical characteristics as well as prognostic associations. The relative incidence of these changes has now been clarified (Figure 10.11). If patients with a normal karyotype are included along with those having none of the above established cytogenetic changes, approximately

29% of childhood BCP-ALL patients have as yet unclassified chromosomal abnormalities. With further molecular and NGS studies, new genetic subgroups are emerging from within this unclassified group, to which specific clinical features are being assigned, as described earlier for the *BCR–ABL1*-like subgroup.

T-ALL accounts for only 15% of childhood ALL. However, the chromosomal changes are different from BCP-ALL. Cytogenetic abnormalities are seen in approximately 70% of T-ALL, with translocations involving the TCR loci accounting for approximately 35% of them (Cauwelier et al., 2006), a number of which were described previously. Similar to rearrangements of *IGH*, they result in oncogenes becoming juxtaposed to the promoter and enhancer elements of the *TCR* genes, leading to their aberrant expression and the development of T-ALL (Nickoloff et al., 2008). Alternatively, aberrant expression of oncogenic transcription factors in T-ALL may result from loss of the upstream transcriptional elements that normally downregulate the expression of these oncogenes during T-cell development (Ferrando et al., 2004a). The formation of oncogenic fusion transcripts is rare in T-ALL. Translocations of this type include *MLL* fusions and *PICALM–MLLT10* (described earlier) as well as some rare

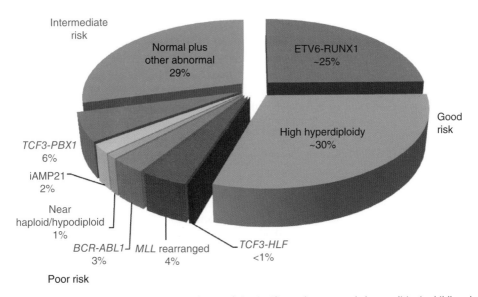

Figure 10.11 Pie chart illustrating the relative incidences of the significant chromosomal abnormalities in childhood BCP-ALL, listed according to their risk group.

rearrangements involving the tyrosine kinase gene *ABL1*. Aberrant expression of one or more transcription factors is a critical component of the molecular pathogenesis of T-ALL, in a mutually exclusive manner (Meijerink, 2010). These have been described as type A mutations and are considered as driver abnormalities that define distinct T-ALL subgroups: (i) *TAL/LMO*, which include the bHLH genes *TAL1*, *TAL2*, *LYL1*, *OLIG2*, and *MYC*, as well as genes involved in transcription regulation, for example, the cysteine-rich LIM-only domain *LMO1* and *LMO2* genes; (ii) abnormalities affecting the homeodomain gene *TLX1*; (iii) *TLX3*; and (iv) members of the *HOXA* cluster, including *MLL* fusions and *PICALM–MLLT10*. T-ALL frequently harbor rearrangements, which occur in more than one of the four subgroups above, referred to as type B abnormalities, including rearrangements of *ABL1*, for example, *NUP214–ABL1* fusion (described earlier), and a spectrum of submicroscopic genetic aberrations commonly involving *CDKN2A/CDKN2B*, *PTEN*, and *MYB* (De Keersmaecker et al., 2005b). Mutations, particularly those involving *NOTCH1*, are highly significant in T-ALL, being found in approximately 60% of cases and across all subgroups. These mutations either occur as activating in *NOTCH1* itself or inactivating in the E3 ubiquitin ligase gene *FBXW7*, and there is evidence of their prenatal origin (Eguchi-Ishimae et al., 2008). Other more recently described novel targets of mutation include the tumor suppressor *CNOT3*, a member of transcriptional regulatory complex, and the ribosomal genes *RPL5* and *RPL10* (De Keersmaecker et al., 2013). Sequence mutations and deletions of *PHF6* result in loss of *PHF6* expression and are associated with *TLX1/3* and *TAL1* rearranged T-ALL (Van Vlierberghe et al., 2010).

Essentially, T-ALL is a highly heterogeneous disease involving the accumulation of multiple oncogenic abnormalities. It has been variously classified according to genetic subtypes. De Keersmaecker et al. (2005b) classified T-ALL-specific abnormalities into subgroups that defined four pathways based on the functions of different classes of mutations: (i) those that provide a proliferative advantage, (ii) those that impair differentiation and survival, (iii) those that affect the cell cycle, and (iv) those that provide self-renewal capacity. Interlaced with

these four major classes of mutations is the molecular classification, which has emerged from gene expression profiling (Ferrando et al., 2002; Ferrando and Look, 2003). It identified several gene expression signatures indicative of arrest at specific stages of thymocyte development; a *LYL1*-positive signature represents immature thymocytes (pro-T), *TLX1*-positivity represents early cortical thymocytes, and *TAL1*-positivity correlates with late cortical thymocytes. More recently, T-ALL has been subdivided into three subtypes based on morphology, immunophenotype, and genetics as (i) pro/pre-T (immature), (ii) cortical, and (iii) mature (Meijerink, 2010).

Studies of immature T-ALL cases delineated a novel genetic entity, named ETP-ALL (Coustan-Smith et al., 2009). Three pathways were shown to be frequently mutated: hematopoietic development, most commonly loss-of-function mutations involving *ETV6*, *GATA3*, *IKZF1*, and *RUNX1*; activating mutations in cytokine receptor and RAS signaling, *NRAS*, *KRAS*, *FLT3*, *JAK1*, *JAK3*, and *IL7R*, with JAK–STAT activation present in the majority of cases (Shochat et al., 2011; Van Vlierberghe et al., 2011; Zenatti et al., 2011; Della Gatta et al., 2012; Neumann et al., 2012; Ntziachristos et al., 2012; Zhang et al., 2012; Neumann et al. 2013a); and a high frequency of mutations of epigenetic regulators. Most common were mutations or deletions of genes encoding components of the polycomb repressor complex 2 (PRC2) (*EZH2*, *SUZ12*, and *EED*) (Neumann et al., 2013b). Interestingly, the mutational spectrum of ETP-ALL is similar to that observed in myeloid leukemias, and the transcriptional profile of ETP-ALL is similar to that of normal and malignant human hematopoietic stem cells and myeloid progenitors. Thus, ETP-ALL may be part of a spectrum of immature leukemias of variable lineage (Zhang et al., 2012).

Age associations

Infants

ALL in infants (i.e., children <1 year of age) is rare. The biological features are different from ALL in older children, with infant ALL having an immature B-lineage phenotype, lacking CD10 expression, and having a high tumor load at presentation (Biondi et al., 2000). At the genetic level, infant

ALL is characterized by a high frequency (~70%) of chromosomal abnormalities involving 11q23 and rearrangements of the *MLL* gene (Heerema et al., 1994; Pieters et al., 2007), indicating a unique cytogenetic profile in this patient group. The t(4;11) (q21;q23) accounts for more than 50% of the *MLL*-positive cases, with the majority of patients being less than 6 months of age. The t(11;19)(q23;p13.3) (20%), t(9;11)(p21;q23) (11%), and rearrangements between 10p12 and 11q23 (4%) are also quite common, while the other *MLL* translocations are much less frequent.

Overall, event-free survival is considerably worse for infants than for older children with ALL. It is heterogeneous and varies according to *MLL* status, CD10 expression, age at diagnosis, presenting WBC count, CNS involvement, coexpression of myeloid markers, and early response to prednisone, with the presence of an *MLL* rearrangement and age less than 6 months being the strongest predictors for poor outcome (Pieters et al., 2007). Infant ALL without *MLL* rearrangements represents a specific subset with an improved prognosis (De Lorenzo et al., 2014). Among these *MLL* germline cases, the common abnormalities seen in older children with ALL are underrepresented. High hyperdiploidy is found in approximately 10% of these patients and is generally associated with the

same improved outcome in this age group as described for older children. The *ETV6–RUNX1* fusion was absent among the relatively small numbers of *MLL*-negative cases screened, indicating that this is not a significant abnormality in infant ALL. The incidence of *BCR–ABL1*-positive cases was also very low, less than 1%. There were a significant number of infant ALL with 15q abnormalities (~10%), while t(7;12)(q36;p13) was found exclusively in infants, although mainly in infant AML. Low *FLT3* expression was also a characteristic feature of infant ALL, which was enriched among *MLL* germline cases (Kang et al., 2012).

Older patients

The relative incidences of the main chromosomal abnormalities according to age are indicated in Figure 10.12. In contrast to the high incidence of *MLL* rearrangements in infants, the proportion seen in older children is low, with a gradual rise occurring with increasing age. Children aged 1–9 years have the highest incidence of high hyperdiploidy and t(12;21)(p13;q22) (Forestier and Schmiegelow, 2006). The incidence of high hyperdiploidy drops to a low level in adolescence, while t(12;21) completely disappears, apart from a few sporadic cases in adulthood. The incidence of the t(1;19)(q23;p13) remains relatively constant

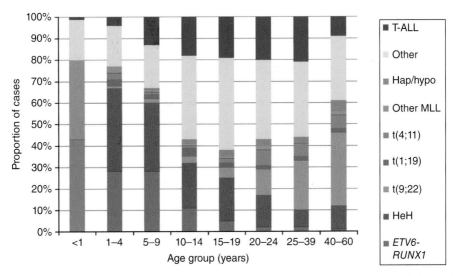

Figure 10.12 Bar chart showing the relative incidences of the significant chromosomal abnormalities (color coded as indicated in the key) according to age. Data taken from UK ALL treatment trials. Provided by Professor Anthony Moorman. Hap/hypo, near haploid, and hypodiploid cases; HeH, high-hyperdiploid cases.

throughout the age groups. Abnormalities involving the *IGH* locus at 14q32 emerge in adolescence with an increasing incidence seen in young adults. iAMP21 is restricted to older children, while the proportion of cases with Ph-positive ALL increases exponentially with age.

Karyotype complexity is a chromosomal subtype shown to have prognostic significance only in adults. It is defined as the presence of five or more chromosomal abnormalities in the absence of an established translocation or ploidy group and occurs in approximately 5% of adult BCP-ALL. There is an indication that the incidence increases with age among adults (Moorman et al., 2007a, 2010a). Most significantly, karyotype complexity in adult ALL is associated with increased risk of relapse and death, with an overall survival of only 20–25% (Granada et al., 2007; Moorman et al., 2007a). In UK adult ALL treatment trials, these patients are now treated as high risk.

Down syndrome (DS)

Children with DS have a greatly increased risk of developing acute leukemia, including ALL. The prevalence is increased almost 20-fold (Hasle et al., 2000), with DS patients comprising up to 3% of childhood ALL. The cytogenetic aberrations characteristic of ALL in DS patients do not differ from those seen in non-DS individuals, although the distribution is different, for example, the incidences of high hyperdiploidy (2–11%) and t(12;21) (10–15%) were lower than those reported for non-DS-ALL (Forestier et al., 2008c, Lundin et al., 2014). Of note was that the DS patients with t(12;21) were older (median age of 6 years) than the non-DS patients (median age of 4.3 years). The DS cases with high hyperdiploidy showed the same chromosomal gains as the non-DS patients, indicating that the same mechanisms are involved in the formation of the karyotype. There was a significant overrepresentation of certain cytogenetic subgroups, for example, the gain of an X chromosome (~40% and as a sole chromosomal abnormality in about 20%), the t(8;14)(q11;q32) leading to upregulation of *CEBPD* (see preceding text) (3%, accounting for 24% of all reported cases with this translocation), and the deletions of 9p (in 20% of cases as the sole visible cytogenetic abnormality).

The t(9;22) was found in approximately 1% of cases. DS patients show a high incidence of rearrangements leading to overexpression of *CRLF2* (50%) compared to non-DS patients (7%), with associated mutations of *JAK2* R683 in half of the *CRLF2*-rearranged cases (see preceding text) (Kearney et al., 2009; Russell et al., 2009a; Hertzberg et al., 2010).

Prognosis

A correlation between prognosis and the karyotype at diagnosis in ALL was first demonstrated by Secker-Walker et al. (1978). The cytogenetic picture is highly informative with regard to disease outcome, and particular significance has been attributed to the presence of specific abnormalities, as detailed in the individual sections earlier. The first large series analyzed for cytogenetic and prognostic correlations was the 330 cases of newly diagnosed ALL, 66% with clonal aberrations, investigated by the Third International Workshop on Chromosomes in Leukemia (1980). The results showed that chromosomal abnormalities identified both high-risk and low-risk ALL patients.

Essentially, there is now international consensus of risk accorded to different cytogenetic subgroups (Harrison et al., 2010). As described in the individual sections earlier, the abnormalities with the most significant impact for treatment and management of BCP-ALL are t(9;22)(q34;q11)/*BCR–ABL1*, t(4;11) (q21;q23)/*MLL–AFF1*, near haploidy/low hypodiploidy (<40 chromosomes), and iAMP21for high risk stratification, as well as those patients with treatment failure and an increased level of minimal residual disease after the first course of induction therapy, usually day 29. To a lesser extent, t(12;21) (p13;q22)/*ETV6–RUNX1* and high hyperdiploidy are stratified as good risk, when there are no associated poor-risk clinical features or detectable minimal residual disease.

Virtually all studies have agreed that in both children and adults, high-hyperdiploid patients have the best prognosis (Moorman, 2012), as described previously. Younger children (aged 1–9 years) fare better compared to older ones (aged 10–16 years) and so do those with a higher modal chromosome number (56–67 vs. 51–55 chromosomes) (Moorman et al., 2003;

Dastugue et al., 2013; Paulsson et al., 2013a). Structural abnormalities impart no change on the good outcome associated with this patient group. Another group associated with a good outcome is children with t(12;21)-positive ALL (Forestier et al., 2008b). Together, high hyperdiploidy and t(12;21) account for more than 50% of childhood ALL, providing a significant input to the overall good prognosis of childhood ALL.

Apart from the numerical abnormalities, these cytogenetic subtypes can be routinely tested for by RT-PCR, providing a basic yet informative screen. However, cytogenetics, particularly FISH, may provide reliable alternative detection methods dependent upon the preferred technical approach within each protocol (Harrison et al., 2010). Currently, FISH with probes specific for *RUNX1* and array-based analyses provide the only reliable detection method for iAMP21, which is vital in view of the requirement of these patients for intensive treatment. The early detection of *BCR–ABL1*-positive patients is also critical for the now routine alternative treatment with TKI, which has dramatically improved outcome and reduced the requirement for allogeneic stem cell transplantation in some adult patients. *MLL* partner identification is also becoming essential as targeted therapies are being developed for their treatment. One example is the methyltransferase DOT1L, which interacts directly or indirectly with several of the *MLL* fusion partners (Daigle et al., 2011).

Although the early association of t(1;19)(q23;p13) with a poor outcome has been moderated by the more aggressive therapy of modern protocols and these patients are now considered as standard risk on current treatment regimens, the prognosis associated with the variant t(17;19)(q22;p13) remains extremely poor. Appropriate detection methods are a prime consideration for their early detection.

In adult ALL, patients with a complex karyotype, comprising five or more unrelated chromosomal abnormalities, have an extremely poor prognosis (Moorman et al., 2007a). This finding is leading to modification of treatment for these patients in new adult ALL treatment trials.

On contemporary protocols, the overall prognosis of T-ALL is now generally similar to B-ALL, particularly when patients are stratified according to their level of minimal residual disease. However,

the prognosis of individual cytogenetic groups in T-ALL remains unclear. It has been reported that patients expressing *TLX3* do not share the favorable outcome associated with *TLX1* expression (see preceding text) (Cavé et al., 2004; Ferrando et al., 2004b) and ETP-ALL comprise an aggressive subtype with a dismal prognosis (Coustan-Smith et al., 2009; Inukai et al., 2012). However, due to the complexity and diversity of T-ALL genetics, it does not currently play a role in treatment stratification.

The genetic diagnosis is of course not the only prognostic factor of importance in ALL, and covariation with already established clinical and hematologic parameters including age, WBC count, percentage of blasts in peripheral blood, immunophenotype, CNS involvement, the presence or absence of mediastinal tumor, and, more recently, the presence of minimal residual disease accounts for some of the observed associations. The most significant fact is that the impact of prognostic factors is heavily dependent on the type of therapy, and so a continuous reassessment of the role of all prognostic factors, including genetics, is needed as the consensus of what constitutes state-of-the-art ALL treatment changes. All of these studies have clearly shown that application of novel agents in the appropriate biological arena to a suitable target can dramatically improve survival. Evolving studies are revealing other potential candidates with promise for future therapies. However, there remain many challenges ahead before these novel drugs become integrated into routine clinical practice.

Summary

Approximately two-thirds of ALL have established acquired chromosomal abnormalities. Although the aberrations are variable, their distribution is distinctly nonrandom, and some rearrangements are associated with hematological, immunophenotypic, and clinical characteristics with remarkable specificity. For an increasing number of translocations, the molecular consequences are now known.

The diagnostic karyotype remains an important independent prognostic factor. With more intensive chemotherapy, however, the adverse prognostic effect of many ALL-associated chromosome abnormalities has been overcome. The prognostically most favorable cytogenetic subgroups in ALL are being considered for therapy reduction, and as more rarely occurring poor-risk abnormalities are identified, there is promise of targeted therapy identified from the molecular consequences of these rearrangements. The discovery of germline mutations, for example, the high incidence of germline *TP53* mutations in patients with hypodiploid ALL (Holmfeldt et al., 2013), has highlighted the role of genetic predisposition to certain subtypes of disease, which are clearly more widespread than previously envisaged. *IKZF1* has also been shown to be linked to disease predisposition. Certain constitutional SNP in *IKZF1* have been associated with childhood BCP-ALL (Papaemmanuil et al., 2009; Prasad et al., 2010; Xu et al., 2013). We should continue to search for novel targets that will surely emerge from the detailed analysis of accumulating data from state-of-the-art NGS technologies in parallel with expression, proteomic, and epigenetic studies to achieve the goal of 100% cure for ALL within the not too distant future.

Acknowledgments

Financial support from the Leukaemia and Lymphoma Research, UK; the Swedish Cancer Society; the Swedish Childhood Cancer Foundation; and the Swedish Research Council is gratefully acknowledged.

References

Akasaka T, Balasas T, Russell LJ, Sugimoto KJ, Majid A, Walewska R, et al. (2007): Five members of the CEBP transcription factor family are targeted by recurrent IGH translocations in B-cell precursor acute lymphoblastic leukemia (BCP-ALL). *Blood* 109:3451–3461.

Al-Shehhi H, Konn ZJ, Schwab CJ, Erhorn A, Barber KE, Wright SL, et al. (2013): Abnormalities of the der(12) t(12;21) in ETV6-RUNX1 acute lymphoblastic leukemia. *Genes Chromosomes Cancer* 52:202–213.

An Q, Wright SL, Konn ZJ, Matheson E, Minto L, Moorman AV, et al. (2008): Variable breakpoints target PAX5 in patients with dicentric chromosomes: a model for the basis of unbalanced translocations in cancer. *Proc Natl Acad Sci USA* 105:17050–17054.

Andersen MK, Autio K, Barbany G, Borgström G, Cavelier L, Golovleva I, et al. (2011): Paediatric B-cell precursor lymphoblastic leukaemia with t(1;19)(q23;p13): clinical and cytogenetic characteristics of 47 cases from the Nordic countries treated according to NOPHO protocols. *Br J Haematol* 155:235–243.

Anderson K, Lutz C, van Delft FW, Bateman CM, Guo Y, Colman SM, et al. (2011): Genetic variegation of clonal architecture and propagating cells in leukaemia. *Nature* 469:356–361.

Apperley JF, Gardembas M, Melo JV, Russell-Jones R, Bain BJ, Baxter EJ, et al. (2002): Response to imatinib mesylate in patients with chronic myeloproliferative diseases with rearrangements of the platelet-derived growth factor receptor beta. *N Engl J Med* 347:481–487.

Arico M, Valsecchi MG, Camitta B, Schrappe M, Chessells J, Baruchel A, et al. (2000): Outcome of treatment in children with philadelphia chromosome-positive acute lymphoblastic leukemia. *N Engl J Med* 342:998–1006.

Asnafi V, Radford-Weiss I, Dastugue N, Bayle C, Leboeuf D, Charrin C, et al. (2003): CALM-AF10 is a common fusion transcript in T-ALL and is specific to the TCRγδ lineage. *Blood* 102:1000–1006.

Attarbaschi A, Mann G, Konig M, Dworzak MN, Trebo MM, Muhlegger N, et al.(2004): Incidence and relevance of secondary chromosome abnormalities in childhood TEL/ AML1+ acute lymphoblastic leukemia: an interphase FISH analysis. *Leukemia* 18:1611–1616.

Attarbaschi A, Mann G, Konig M, Steiner M, Dworzak MN, Gadner H, et al. (2006): Near-tetraploidy in childhood B-cell precursor acute lymphoblastic leukemia is a highly specific feature of ETV6/RUNX1-positive leukemic cases. *Genes Chromosomes Cancer* 45:608–611.

Attarbaschi A, Mann G, Strehl S, Konig M, Steiner M, Jeitler V, et al. (2007): Deletion of 11q23 is a highly specific nonrandom secondary genetic abnormality of ETV6/RUNX1-rearranged childhood acute lymphoblastic leukemia. *Leukemia* 21:584–586.

Ballerini P, Blaise A, Busson-Le Coniat M, Su XY, Zucman-Rossi J, Adam M, et al. (2002): HOX11L2 expression defines a clinical subtype of pediatric T-ALL associated with poor prognosis. *Blood* 100:991–997.

Ballerini P, Busson M, Fasola S, van den Akker J, Lapillonne H, Romana SP, et al. (2005): NUP214-ABL1 amplification in t(5;14)/HOX11L2-positive ALL present with several forms and may have a prognostic significance. *Leukemia* 19:468–470.

Barber KE, Ford AM, Harris RL, Harrison CJ, Moorman AV (2004a): MLL translocations with concurrent 3′ deletions: interpretation of FISH results. *Genes Chromosomes Cancer* 41:266–271.

Barber KE, Martineau M, Harewood L, Stewart M, Cameron E, Strefford JC, et al. (2004b): Amplification of the ABL gene in T-cell acute lymphoblastic leukemia. *Leukemia* 18:1153–1156.

Barber KE, Harrison CJ, Broadfield ZJ, Stewart AR, Wright SL, Martineau M, et al. (2007): Molecular cytogenetic characterization of TCF3 (E2A)/19p13.3 rearrangements in B-cell precursor acute lymphoblastic leukemia. *Genes Chromosomes Cancer* 46:478–486.

Bash RO, Hall S, Timmons CF, Crist WM, Amylon M, Smith RG, et al. (1995): Does activation of the TAL1 gene occur in a majority of patients with T-cell acute lymphoblastic leukemia? A pediatric oncology group study. *Blood* 86:666–676.

Bateman CM, Colman SM, Chaplin T, Young BD, Eden TO, Bhakta M, et al. (2010): Acquisition of genome-wide copy number alterations in monozygotic twins with acute lymphoblastic leukemia. *Blood* 115:3553–3558.

Bellido M, Aventin A, Lasa A, Estivill C, Carnicer MJ, Pons C, et al. (2003): Id4 is deregulated by a t(6;14)(p22;q32) chromosomal translocation in a B-cell lineage acute lymphoblastic leukemia. *Haematologica* 88:994–1001.

Bennett JM, Catovsky D, Daniel MT, Flandrin G, Galton DA, Gralnick HR, et al. (1976): Proposals for the classification of the acute leukaemias. French-American-British (FAB) co-operative group. *Br J Haematol* 33:451–458.

Berger R, Dastugue N, Busson M, van den Akker J, Perot C, Ballerini P, et al. (2003): t(5;14)/HOX11L2-positive T-cell acute lymphoblastic leukemia. A collaborative study of the Groupe Français de Cytogénétique Hématologique (GFCH). *Leukemia* 17:1851–1857.

Bergeron J, Clappier E, Cauwelier B, Dastugue N, Millien C, Delabesse E, et al. (2006): HOXA cluster deregulation in T-ALL associated with both a TCRD-HOXA and a CALM-AF10 chromosomal translocation. *Leukemia* 20:1184–1187.

von Bergh ARM, van Drunen E, van Wering ER, van Zutven LJCM, Hainmann I, Lönnerholm G, et al. (2006): High incidence of t(7;12)(q36;p13) in infant AML but not in infant ALL, with a dismal outcome and ectopic expression of HLXB9. *Genes Chromosomes Cancer* 45:731–739.

Bernard O, Lecointe N, Jonveaux P, Souyri M, Mauchauffe M, Berger R, et al. (1991): Two site-specific deletions and t(1;14) translocation restricted to human T-cell acute leukemias disrupt the 5′ part of the tal-1 gene. *Oncogene* 6:1477–1488.

Bernard OA, Busson-Le Coniat M, Ballerini P, Mauchauffe M, Della Valle V, Monni R, et al. (2001): A new recurrent and specific cryptic translocation, t(5;14)(q35;q32), is associated with expression of the Hox11L2 gene in T acute lymphoblastic leukemia. *Leukemia* 15:1495–1504.

Bertin R, Acquaviva C, Mirebeau D, Guidal-Giroux C, Vilmer E, Cave H (2003): CDKN2A, CDKN2B, and MTAP gene dosage permits precise characterization of mono- and bi-allelic 9p21 deletions in childhood acute lymphoblastic leukemia. *Genes Chromosomes Cancer* 37:44–57.

Beverloo HB, Le Coniat M, Wijsman J, Lillington DM, Bernard O, de Klein A, et al. (1995): Breakpoint heterogeneity in t(10;11) translocations in AML-M4/M5 resulting in fusion of AF10 and MLL is resolved by fluorescent in situ hybridization. *Cancer Res* 55:4220–4224.

Bhojwani D, Pei D, Sandlund JT, Jeha S, Ribeiro RC, Rubnitz JE, et al. (2012): ETV6-RUNX1-positive childhood acute lymphoblastic leukemia: improved outcome with contemporary therapy. *Leukemia* 26:265–270.

Biondi A, Cimino G, Pieters R, Pui CH (2000): Biological and therapeutic aspects of infant leukemia. *Blood* 96:24–33.

Borst L, Wesolowska A, Joshi T, Borup R, Nielsen FC, Andersen MK, et al. (2012): Genome-wide analysis of cytogenetic aberrations in ETV6/RUNX1-positive childhood acute lymphoblastic leukaemia. *Br J Haematol* 157:476–482.

Brown L, Cheng JT, Chen Q, Siciliano MJ, Crist W, Buchanan G, et al. (1990): Site-specific recombination of the tal-1 gene is a common occurrence in human T cell leukemia. *EMBO J* 9:3343–3351.

Burmeister T, Gokbuget N, Reinhardt R, Rieder H, Hoelzer D, Schwartz S (2006): NUP214-ABL1 in adult T-ALL: the GMALL study group experience. *Blood* 108:3556–3559.

Burnett RC, Thirman MJ, Rowley JD, Diaz MO (1994): Molecular analysis of the T-cell acute lymphoblastic leukemia-associated t(1;7)(p34;q34) that fuses LCK and TCRB. *Blood* 84:1232–1236.

Busson-Le Coniat M, Nguyen KF, Daniel MT, Bernard OA, Berger R (2001): Chromosome 21 abnormalities with AML1 amplification in acute lymphoblastic leukemia. *Genes Chromosomes Cancer* 32:244–249.

Byatt SA, Cheung KL, Lillington DM, Mazzullo H, Martineau M, Bennett C, et al. (2001): Three further cases of t(8;14) (q11.2;q32) in acute lymphoblastic leukemia. *Leukemia* 15:1304–1305.

Callen DF, Raphael K, Michael PM, Garson OM (1989): Acute lymphoblastic leukemia with a hypodiploid karyotype with less than 40 chromosomes: the basis for division into two subgroups. *Leukemia* 3:749–752.

Cario G, Zimmermann M, Romey R, Gesk S, Vater I, Harbott J, et al. (2010): Presence of the P2RY8-CRLF2 rearrangement is associated with a poor prognosis in non-high-risk precursor B-cell acute lymphoblastic leukemia in children treated according to the ALL-BFM 2000 protocol. *Blood* 115:5393–5397.

Carroll AJ, Crist WM, Parmley RT, Philips C, Krischer J, Head D, et al. (1984): Pre-B cell leukemia associated with chromosome translocation 1;19. *Blood* 63:721–726.

Carroll AJ, Raimondi SC, Williams DL, Behm FG, Borowitz M, Castleberry RP, et al. (1987): tdic(9;12): a nonrandom chromosome abnormality in childhood B-cell precursor acute lymphoblastic leukemia: a Pediatric Oncology Group Study. *Blood* 70:1962–1965.

Carroll AJ, Crist WM, Link MP, Amylon MD, Pullen DJ, Ragab AH, et al. (1990): The t(1;14)(p34;q11) is nonrandom and restricted to T-cell acute lymphoblastic leukemia: a pediatric oncology group study. *Blood* 76:1220–1224.

Case M, Matheson E, Minto L, Hassan R, Harrison CJ, Bown N, et al. (2008): Mutation of genes affecting the RAS pathway is common in childhood acute lymphoblastic leukemia. *Cancer Res* 68:6803–6809.

Cauwelier B, Dastugue N, Cools J, Poppe B, Herens C, De Paepe A, et al. (2006): Molecular cytogenetic study of 126 unselected T-ALL cases reveals high incidence of TCRβ locus rearrangements and putative new T-cell oncogenes. *Leukemia* 20:1238–1244.

Cauwelier B, Cave H, Gervais C, Lessard M, Barin C, Perot C, et al. (2007): Clinical, cytogenetic and molecular characteristics of 14 T-ALL patients carrying the TCRβ-HOXA rearrangement: a study of the Groupe Francophone de Cytogénétique Hématologique. *Leukemia* 21:121–128.

Cavé H, Suciu S, Preudhomme C, Poppe B, Robert A, Uyttebroeck A, et al. (2004): Clinical significance of HOX11L2 expression linked to t(5;14)(q35;q32), of HOX11 expression, and of SIL-TAL fusion in childhood T-cell malignancies: results of EORTC studies 58881 and 58951. *Blood* 103:442–450.

Caye A, Beldjord K, Mass-Malo K, Drunat S, Soulier J, Gandemer V, et al. (2013): Breakpoint-specific multiplex polymerase chain reaction allows the detection of IKZF1 intragenic deletions and minimal residual disease monitoring in B-cell precursor acute lymphoblastic leukemia. *Haematologica* 98:597–601.

Cazzaniga G, Daniotti M, Tosi S, Giudici G, Aloisi A, Pogliani E, et al. (2001): The paired box domain gene PAX5 is fused to ETV6/TEL in an acute lymphoblastic leukemia case. *Cancer Res* 61:4666–4670.

Chapiro E, Russell L, Lainey E, Kaltenbach S, Ragu C, Della-Valle V, et al. (2010): Activating mutation in the TSLPR gene in B-cell precursor lymphoblastic leukemia. *Leukemia* 24:642–645.

Chapiro E, Radford-Weiss I, Cung HA, Dastugue N, Nadal N, Taviaux S, et al. (2013): Chromosomal translocations involving the IGH@ locus in B-cell precursor acute lymphoblastic leukemia: 29 new cases and a review of the literature. *Cancer Genet* 206:162–173.

Charrin C, Thomas X, Ffrench M, Le QH, Andrieux J, Mozziconacci MJ, et al. (2004): A report from the LALA-94 and LALA-SA groups on hypodiploidy with 30 to 39 chromosomes and near-triploidy: 2 possible expressions of a sole entity conferring poor prognosis in adult acute lymphoblastic leukemia (ALL). *Blood* 104:2444–2451.

Chen IM, Harvey RC, Mullighan CG, Gastier-Foster J, Wharton W, Kang H, et al. (2012): Outcome modeling with CRLF2, IKZF1, JAK, and minimal residual disease in pediatric acute lymphoblastic leukemia: a Children's Oncology Group study. *Blood* 119:3512–3522.

Chilcote RR, Brown E, Rowley JD (1985): Lymphoblastic leukemia with lymphomatous features associated with abnormalities of the short arm of chromosome 9. *N Engl J Med* 313:286–291.

Chilton L, Buck G, Harrison CJ, Ketterling RP, Rowe JM, Tallman MS, et al. (2014): High hyperdiploidy among adolescents and adults with acute lymphoblastic leukaemia (ALL): cytogenetic features, clinical characteristics and outcome. *Leukemia* 28:1511–1518.

Chim CS, Wong AS, Kwong YL (2003): Epigenetic inactivation of INK4/CDK/RB cell cycle pathway in acute leukemias. *Ann Hematol* 82:738–742.

Clappier E, Cuccuini W, Cayuela JM, Vecchione D, Baruchel A, Dombret H, et al. (2006): Cyclin D2 dysregulation by chromosomal translocations to TCR loci in T-cell acute lymphoblastic leukemias. *Leukemia* 20:82–86.

Clappier E, Cuccuini W, Kalota A, Crinquette A, Cayuela JM, Dik WA, et al. (2007): The C-MYB locus is involved in chromosomal translocation and genomic duplications in human T-cell acute leukemia (T-ALL), the translocation defining a new T-ALL subtype in very young children. *Blood* 110:1251–1261.

Clappier E, Auclerc MF, Rapion J, Bakkus M, Caye A, Khemiri A, et al. (2014): An intragenic ERG deletion is a marker of an oncogenic subtype of B-cell precursor acute lymphoblastic leukemia with a favorable outcome despite frequent IKZF1 deletions. *Leukemia* 28:70–77.

Clark R, Byatt SA, Bennett CF, Brama M, Martineau M, Moorman AV, et al. (2000): Monosomy 20 as a pointer to dicentric (9;20) in acute lymphoblastic leukemia. *Leukemia* 14:241–246.

Clarke S, O'Reilly J, Romeo G, Cooney J (2011): NUP214-ABL1 positive T-cell acute lymphoblastic leukemia patient shows an initial favorable response to imatinib therapy post relapse. *Leuk Res* 35:e131–e133.

Cooley LD, Chenevert S, Shuster JJ, Johnston DA, Mahoney DH, Carroll AJ, et al. (2007): Prognostic significance of cytogenetically detected chromosome 21 anomalies in childhood acute lymphoblastic leukemia: a Pediatric Oncology Group study. *Cancer Genet Cytogenet* 175:117–124.

Coustan-Smith E, Mullighan CG, Onciu M, Behm FG, Raimondi SC, Pei D, et al. (2009): Early T-cell precursor leukaemia: a subtype of very high-risk acute lymphoblastic leukaemia. *Lancet Oncol* 10:147–156.

Croce CM, Isobe M, Palumbo A, Puck J, Ming J, Tweardy D, et al. (1985): Gene for alpha-chain of human T-cell receptor: location of chromosome 14 region involved in T-cell neoplasms. *Science* 227:1044–1047.

D'Achille P, Seymour JF, Campbell LJ (2006): Translocation (14;18)(q32;q21) in acute lymphoblastic leukemia: a study of 12 cases and review of the literature. *Cancer Genet Cytogenet* 171:52–56.

Daigle SR, Olhava EJ, Therkelsen CA, Majer CR, Sneeringer CJ, Song J, et al. (2011): Selective killing of mixed lineage leukemia cells by a potent small-molecule DOT1L inhibitor. *Cancer Cell* 20:53–65.

Dastugue N, Suciu S, Plat G, Speleman F, Cavé H, Girard S, et al. (2013): Hyperdiploidy with 58–66 chromosomes in childhood B-acute lymphoblastic leukemia is highly curable: 58951 CLG-EORTC results. *Blood* 121:2415–2423.

Davidsson J, Andersson A, Paulsson K, Heidenblad M, Isaksson M, Borg Å, et al. (2007): Tiling resolution array comparative genomic hybridization, expression and methylation analyses of dup(1q) in Burkitt lymphomas and pediatric high hyperdiploid acute lymphoblastic leukemias reveal clustered near-centromeric breakpoints and overexpression of genes in 1q22-32.3. *Hum Mol Genet* 16:2215–2225.

De Keersmaecker K, Graux C, Odero MD, Mentens N, Somers R, Maertens J, et al. (2005a): Fusion of EML1 to ABL1 in T-cell acute lymphoblastic leukemia with cryptic t(9;14)(q34;q32). *Blood* 105:4849–4852.

De Keersmaecker K, Marynen P, Cools J (2005b): Genetic insights in the pathogenesis of T-cell acute lymphoblastic leukemia. *Haematologica* 90:1116–1127.

De Keersmaecker K, Real PJ, Gatta GD, Palomero T, Sulis ML, Tosello V, et al. (2010): The TLX1 oncogene drives aneuploidy in T cell transformation. *Nat Med* 16:1321–1327.

De Keersmaecker K, Atak ZK, Li N, Vicente C, Patchett S, Girardi T, et al. (2013): Exome sequencing identifies mutation in CNOT3 and ribosomal genes RPL5 and RPL10 in T-cell acute lymphoblastic leukemia. *Nat Genet* 45:186–190.

De Lorenzo P, Moorman AV, Pieters R, Dreyer ZE, Heerema NA, Carroll AJ, et al. (2014): Cytogenetics and outcome of infants with acute lymphoblastic leukemia and absence of MLL rearrangements. *Leukemia* 28:428–430.

Della Gatta G, Palomero T, Perez-Garcia A, Ambesi-Impiombato A, Bansal M, Carpenter ZW, et al. (2012): Reverse engineering of TLX oncogenic transcriptional networks identifies RUNX1 as tumor suppressor in T-ALL. *Nat Med* 18:436–440.

Den Boer ML, van Slegtenhorst M, De Menezes RX, Cheok MH, Buijs-Gladdines JG, Peters ST, et al. (2009): A subtype of childhood acute lymphoblastic leukaemia with poor treatment outcome: a genome-wide classification study. *Lancet Oncol* 10:125–134.

Dik WA, Brahim W, Braun C, Asnafi V, Dastugue N, Bernard OA, et al. (2005): CALM-AF10+ T-ALL expression profiles are characterized by overexpression of HOXA and BMI1 oncogenes. *Leukemia* 19:1948–1957.

Dobbins SE, Sherborne AL, Ma YP, Bardini M, Biondi A, Cazzaniga G, et al. (2013): The silent mutational landscape of infant MLL-AF4 pro-B acute lymphoblastic leukemia. *Genes Chromosomes Cancer* 52:954–960.

Domer PH, Fakharzadeh SS, Chen CS, Jockel J, Johansen L, Silverman GA, et al. (1993): Acute mixed-lineage leukemia t(4;11)(q21;q23) generates an MLL-AF4 fusion product. *Proc Natl Acad Sci USA* 90:7884–7888.

Downing JR, Head DR, Raimondi SC, Carroll AJ, Curcio-Brint AM, Hulshof MG, et al. (1994): The der(11)-encoded MLL/AF-4 fusion transcript is consistently detected in t(4;11)(q21;q23)-containing acute lymphoblastic leukemia. *Blood* 83:330–335.

Dreyling MH, Schrader K, Fonatsch C, Schlegelberger B, Haase D, Schoch C, et al. (1998): MLL and CALM are fused to AF10 in morphologically distinct subsets of acute leukemia with translocation t(10;11): both rearrangements are associated with a poor prognosis. *Blood* 91:4662–4667.

Dube ID, Raimondi SC, Pi D, Kalousek DK (1986): A new translocation, t(10;14)(q24;q11), in T cell neoplasia. *Blood* 67:1181–1184.

Eguchi-Ishimae M, Eguchi M, Kempski H, Greaves M (2008): NOTCH1 mutation can be an early, prenatal genetic event in T-ALL. *Blood* 111:376–378.

Ellisen LW, Bird J, West DC, Soreng AL, Reynolds TC, Smith SD, et al. (1991): TAN-1, the human homolog of the Drosophila Notch gene, is broken by chromosomal translocations in T lymphoblastic neoplasms. *Cell* 66:649–661.

Ensor HM, Schwab C, Russell LJ, Richards SM, Morrison H, Masic D, et al. (2011): Demographic, clinical, and outcome features of children with acute lymphoblastic leukemia and CRLF2 deregulation: results from the MRC ALL97 clinical trial. *Blood* 117: 2129–2136.

Ernst T, Score J, Deininger M, Hidalgo-Curtis C, Lackie P, Ershler WB, et al. (2011): Identification of FOXP1 and SNX2 as novel ABL1 fusion partners in acute lymphoblastic leukaemia. *Br J Haematol* 153:43–46.

Eyre T, Schwab CJ, Kinstrie R, McGuire AK, Strefford J, Peniket A, et al. (2012): Episomal amplification of NUP214-ABL1 fusion gene in B-cell acute lymphoblastic leukemia. *Blood* 120:4441–4443.

Fazio G, Palmi C, Rolink A, Biondi A, Cazzaniga G (2008): PAX5/TEL acts as a transcriptional repressor causing down-modulation of CD19, enhances migration to CXCL12, and confers survival advantage in pre-BI cells. *Cancer Res* 68:181–189.

Ferrando AA, Look AT (2003): Gene expression profiling in T-cell acute lymphoblastic leukemia. *Semin Hematol* 40:274–280.

Ferrando AA, Neuberg DS, Staunton J, Loh ML, Huard C, Raimondi SC, et al. (2002): Gene expression signatures define novel oncogenic pathways in T cell acute lymphoblastic leukemia. *Cancer Cell* 1:75–87.

Ferrando AA, Herblot S, Palomero T, Hansen M, Hoang T, Fox EA, et al. (2004a): Biallelic transcriptional activation of oncogenic transcription factors in T-cell acute lymphoblastic leukemia. *Blood* 103:1909–1911.

Ferrando AA, Neuberg DS, Dodge RK, Paietta E, Larson RA, Wiernik PH, et al. (2004b): Prognostic importance of TLX1 (HOX11) oncogene expression in adults with T-cell acute lymphoblastic leukaemia. *Lancet* 363:535–536.

Fielding AK, Rowe JM, Buck G, Foroni L, Gerrard G, Litzow MR, et al. (2014): UKALLXII/ECOG2993: addition of imatinib to a standard treatment regimen enhances long-term outcomes in Philadelphia positive acute lymphoblastic leukemia. *Blood* 123:843–850.

First MIC Cooperative Study Group (1986): Morphologic, immunologic, and cytogenetic (MIC) working classification of acute lymphoblastic leukemias. *Cancer Genet Cytogenet* 23:189–197.

Ford AM, Bennett CA, Price CM, Bruin MCA, Van Wering ER, Greaves M (1998): Fetal origins of the TEL-AML1 fusion gene in identical twins with leukemia. *Proc Natl Acad Sci USA* 95:4584–4588.

Forestier E, Schmiegelow K (2006): The incidence peaks of the childhood acute leukemias reflect specific cytogenetic aberrations. *J Pediatr Hematol Oncol* 28:486–495.

Forestier E, Gauffin F, Andersen MK, Autio K, Borgström G, Golovleva I, et al. (2008a): Clinical and cytogenetic features of pediatric dic(9;20)(p13.2;q11.2)-positive B-cell precursor acute lymphoblastic leukemias: a Nordic series of 24 cases and review of the literature. *Genes Chromosomes Cancer* 47:149–158.

Forestier E, Heyman M, Andersen MK, Autio K, Blennow E, Borgström G, et al. (2008b): Outcome of ETV6/RUNX1-positive childhood acute lymphoblastic leukaemia in the NOPHO-ALL-1992 protocol: frequent late relapses but good overall survival. *Br J Haematol* 140:665–672.

Forestier E, Izraeli S, Beverloo B, Haas O, Pession A, Michalova K, et al. (2008c): Cytogenetic features of acute lymphoblastic and myeloid leukemias in pediatric patients with Down syndrome: an iBFM-SG study. *Blood* 111:1575–1583.

Georgopoulos K, Bigby M, Wang JH, Molnar A, Wu P, Winandy S, et al. (1994): The Ikaros gene is required for the development of all lymphoid lineages. *Cell* 79:143–156.

Gibbons B, MacCallum P, Watts E, Rohatiner AZS, Webb D, Katz FE, et al. (1991): Near haploid acute lymphoblastic leukemia: seven new cases and a review of the literature. *Leukemia* 5:738–743.

Golub TR, Barker GF, Bohlander SK, Hiebert SW, Ward DC, Bray-Ward P, et al. (1995): Fusion of the TEL gene on 12p13 to the AML1 gene on 21q22 in acute lymphoblastic leukemia. *Proc Natl Acad Sci USA* 92:4917–4921.

Granada I, Sancho J-M, Oriol A, Morgades M, Bethencourt C, Parody R, et al. (2007): The prognostic significance of complex karyotype in Philadelphia chromosome-negative (Ph) acute lymphoblastic leukemia (ALL) in adults is related with risk group. *ASH Annual Meeting Abstracts* 110, 3501.

Graux C, Cools J, Melotte C, Quentmeier H, Ferrando A, Levine R, et al. (2004): Fusion of NUP214 to ABL1 on amplified episomes in T-cell acute lymphoblastic leukemia. *Nat Genet* 36:1084–1089.

Graux C, Cools J, Michaux L, Vandenberghe P, Hagemeijer A (2006): Cytogenetics and molecular genetics of T-cell acute lymphoblastic leukemia: from thymocyte to lymphoblast. *Leukemia* 20:1496–1510.

Graux C, Stevens-Kroef M, Lafage M, Dastugue N, Harrison CJ, Mugneret F, et al. (2008): Heterogeneous patterns of amplification of the NUP214-ABL1 fusion gene in T-cell acute lymphoblastic leukemia. *Leukemia* 23:125–133.

Greaves M (2005): In utero origins of childhood leukaemia. *Early Hum Dev* 81:123–129.

Grimaldi JC, Meeker TC (1989): The t(5;14) chromosomal translocation in a case of acute lymphocytic leukemia joins the interleukin-3 gene to the immunoglobulin heavy chain gene. *Blood* 73:2081–2085.

Groupe Français de Cytogénétique Hématologique (GFCH) (1991): t(10;11)(p13-14;q14-21): a new recurrent translocation in T-cell acute lymphoblastic leukemias. *Genes Chromosomes Cancer* 3:411–415.

Gu Y, Nakamura T, Alder H, Prasad R, Canaani O, Cimino G, et al. (1992): The t(4;11) chromosome translocation of human acute leukemias fuses the ALL-1 gene, related to Drosophila trithorax, to the AF-4 gene. *Cell* 71:701–708.

Hann I, Vora A, Harrison G, Harrison C, Martineau M, Moorman AV, et al. (2001): Determinants of outcome after intensified therapy of childhood lymphoblastic leukaemia: results from Medical Research Council United Kingdom acute lymphoblastic leukaemia XI protocol. *Br J Haematol* 113:103–114.

Hansen-Hagge TE, Schafer M, Kiyoi H, Morris SW, Whitlock JA, Koch P, et al. (2002): Disruption of the RanBP17/Hox11L2 region by recombination with the TCRδ locus in acute lymphoblastic leukemias with t(5;14)(q34;q11). *Leukemia* 16:2205–2212.

Harewood L, Robinson H, Harris R, Al Obaidi MJ, Jalali GR, Martineau M, et al. (2003): Amplification of AML1 on a duplicated chromosome 21 in acute lymphoblastic leukemia: a study of 20 cases. *Leukemia* 17:547–553.

Harris MB, Shuster JJ, Carroll A, Look AT, Borowitz MJ, Crist WM, et al. (1992): Trisomy of leukemic cell chromosomes 4 and 10 identifies children with B-progenitor cell acute lymphoblastic leukemia with a very low risk of treatment failure: a Pediatric Oncology Group study. *Blood* 79:3316–3324.

Harris RL, Harrison CJ, Martineau M, Taylor KE, Moorman AV (2004): Is trisomy 5 a distinct cytogenetic subgroup in acute lymphoblastic leukemia? *Cancer Genet Cytogenet* 148:159–162.

Harrison CJ, Foroni L (2002): Cytogenetics and molecular genetics of acute lymphoblastic leukemia. *Rev Clin Exp Hematol* 6:91–113.

Harrison CJ, Moorman AV, Broadfield ZJ, Cheung KL, Harris RL, Reza Jalali G, et al. (2004): Three distinct subgroups of hypodiploidy in acute lymphoblastic leukaemia. *Br J Haematol* 125:552–559.

Harrison CJ, Moorman AV, Barber KE, Broadfield ZJ, Cheung KL, Harris RL, et al. (2005): Interphase molecular cytogenetic screening for chromosomal abnormalities of prognostic significance in childhood acute lymphoblastic leukaemia: a UK Cancer Cytogenetics Group Study. *Br J Haematol* 129:520–530.

Harrison CJ, Haas O, Harbott J, Biondi A, Stanulla M, Trka J, et al. (2010): Detection of prognostically relevant genetic abnormalities in childhood B-cell precursor acute lymphoblastic leukaemia: recommendations from the Biology and Diagnosis Committee of the International Berlin-Frankfurt-Munster study group. *Br J Haematol* 151:132–142.

Harrison CJ, Moorman AV, Schwab C, Carroll AJ, Raetz EA, Devidas M, et al. (2014): An international study of intra-chromosomal amplification of chromosome 21 (iAMP21): cytogenetic characterization and outcome. *Leukemia* 28:1015–1021.

Harvey RC, Mullighan CG, Chen IM, Wharton W, Mikhail FM, Carroll AJ, et al. (2010a): Rearrangement of CRLF2 is associated with mutation of JAK kinases, alteration of IKZF1, Hispanic/Latino ethnicity, and a poor outcome in pediatric B-progenitor acute lymphoblastic leukemia. *Blood* 115:5312–5321.

Harvey RC, Mullighan CG, Wang X, Dobbin KK, Davidson GS, Bedrick EJ, et al. (2010b): Identification of novel cluster groups in pediatric high-risk B-precursor acute lymphoblastic leukemia with gene expression profiling: correlation with genome-wide DNA copy number alterations, clinical characteristics, and outcome. *Blood* 116:4874–4884.

Hasle H, Clemmensen IH, Mikkelsen M (2000): Risks of leukaemia and solid tumours in individuals with Down's syndrome. *Lancet* 355:165–169.

Hayette S, Tigaud I, Maguer-Satta V, Bartholin L, Thomas X, Charrin C, et al. (2002): Recurrent involvement of the MLL gene in adult T-lineage acute lymphoblastic leukemia. *Blood* 99:4647–4649.

Hebert J, Cayuela JM, Berkeley J, Sigaux F (1994): Candidate tumor-suppressor genes MTS1 (p16INK4A) and MTS2 (p15INK4B) display frequent homozygous deletions in primary cells from T- but not from B-cell lineage acute lymphoblastic leukemias. *Blood* 84:4038–4044.

Heerema NA, Arthur DC, Sather H, Albo V, Feusner J, Lange BJ, et al. (1994): Cytogenetic features of infants less than 12 months of age at diagnosis of acute lymphoblastic leukemia: impact of the 11q23 breakpoint on outcome: a report of the Children's Cancer Group. *Blood* 83:2274–2284.

Heerema NA, Nachman JB, Sather HN, Sensel MG, Lee MK, Hutchinson R, et al. (1999): Hypodiploidy with less than 45 chromosomes confers adverse risk in childhood acute lymphoblastic leukemia: a report from the children's cancer group. *Blood* 94:4036–4045.

Heerema NA, Sather HN, Sensel MG, Lee MK, Hutchinson RJ, Nachman JB, et al. (2000a): Abnormalities of chromosome bands 13q12 to 13q14 in childhood acute lymphoblastic leukemia. *J Clin Oncol* 18:3837–3844.

Heerema NA, Sather HN, Sensel MG, Zhang T, Hutchinson RJ, Nachman JB, et al. (2000b): Prognostic impact of trisomies of chromosomes 10, 17 and 5 among children with acute lymphoblastic leukemia and high hyperdiploidy (>50 chromosomes). *J Clin Oncol* 18:1876–1887.

Heerema NA, Sather HN, Sensel MG, La MK, Hutchinson RJ, Nachman JB, et al. (2002): Abnormalities of chromosome bands 15q13-15 in childhood acute lymphoblastic leukemia. *Cancer* 94:1102–1110.

Heerema NA, Raimondi SC, Anderson JR, Biegel J, Camitta BM, Cooley LD, et al. (2007): Specific extra chromosomes occur in a modal number dependent pattern in pediatric acute lymphoblastic leukemia. *Genes Chromosomes Cancer* 46:684–693.

Heerema NA, Carroll AJ, Devidas M, Loh ML, Borowitz MJ, Gastier-Foster JM, et al. (2013): Intrachromosomal amplification of chromosome 21 is associated with inferior outcomes in children with acute lymphoblastic leukemia treated in contemporary standard-risk children's oncology group studies: a report from the children's oncology group. *J Clin Oncol* 31:3397–3402.

Herou E, Biloglav A, Johansson B, Paulsson K (2013): Partial 17q gain resulting from isochromosomes, unbalanced translocations and complex rearrangements is associated with gene overexpression, older age and shorter overall survival in high hyperdiploid childhood acute lymphoblastic leukemia. *Leukemia* 27:493–496.

Hertzberg L, Vendramini E, Ganmore I, Cazzaniga G, Schmitz M, Chalker J, et al. (2010): Down syndrome acute lymphoblastic leukemia: a highly heterogeneous disease in which aberrant expression of CRLF2 is associated with mutated JAK2: a report from the iBFM Study Group. *Blood* 115:1006–1017.

Heyman M, Grandér D, Bröndum-Nielsen K, Liu Y, Söderhäll S, Einhorn S (1993): Deletions of the short arm of chromosome 9, including the interferon-alpha/-beta genes, in acute lymphocytic leukemia. Studies on loss of heterozygosity, parental origin of deleted genes and prognosis. *Int J Cancer* 54:748–753.

Holmfeldt L, Wei L, Diaz-Flores E, Walsh M, Zhang J, Ding L, et al. (2013): The genomic landscape of hypodiploid acute lymphoblastic leukemia. *Nat Genet* 45:242–252.

Hong D, Gupta R, Ancliff P, Atzberger A, Brown J, Soneji S, et al. (2008): Initiating and cancer-propagating cells in TEL-AML1-associated childhood leukemia. *Science* 319:336–339.

Hunger SP (1996): Chromosomal translocations involving the E2A gene in acute lymphoblastic leukemia: clinical features and molecular pathogenesis. *Blood* 87:1211–1224.

Hunger SP, Galili N, Carroll AJ, Crist WM, Link MP, Cleary ML (1991): The t(1;19)(q23;p13) results in consistent fusion of E2A and PBX1 coding sequences in acute lymphoblastic leukemias. *Blood* 77:687–693.

Hunger SP, Devaraj PE, Foroni L, Secker-Walker LM, Cleary ML (1994): Two types of genomic rearrangements create alternative E2A-HLF fusion proteins in t(17;19)-ALL. *Blood* 83:2970–2977.

Huret JL, Brizard A, Slater R, Charrin C, Bertheas MF, Guilhot F, et al. (1993): Cytogenetic heterogeneity in t(11;19) acute leukemia: clinical, hematological and cytogenetic analyses of 48 patients—updated published cases and 16 new observations. *Leukemia* 7:152–160.

Iacobucci I, Storlazzi CT, Cilloni D, Lonetti A, Ottaviani E, Soverini S, et al.(2009): Identification and molecular characterization of recurrent genomic deletions on 7p12 in the IKZF1 gene in a large cohort of BCR-ABL1-positive acute lymphoblastic leukemia patients: on behalf of Gruppo Italiano Malattie Ematologiche dell'Adulto Acute Leukemia Working Party (GIMEMA AL WP). *Blood* 114:2159–2167.

Iacobucci I, Lonetti A, Paoloni F, Papayannidis C, Ferrari A, Storlazzi CT, et al. (2010): The PAX5 gene is frequently rearranged in BCR-ABL1-positive acute lymphoblastic leukemia but is not associated with outcome. A report on behalf of the GIMEMA Acute Leukemia Working Party. *Haematologica* 95:1683–1690.

Inaba T, Roberts WM, Shapiro LH, Jolly KW, Raimondi SC, Smith SD, et al. (1992): Fusion of the leucine zipper gene HLF to the E2A gene in human acute B-lineage leukemia. *Science* 257:531–534.

Inthal A, Krapf G, Beck D, Joas R, Kauer MO, Orel L, et al. (2008): Role of the erythropoietin receptor in ETV6/RUNX1-positive acute lymphoblastic leukemia. *Clin Cancer Res* 14:7196–7204.

Inthal A, Zeitlhofer P, Zeginigg M, Morak M, Grausenburger R, Fronkova E, et al. (2012): CREBBP HAT domain mutations prevail in relapse cases of high hyperdiploid childhood acute lymphoblastic leukemia. *Leukemia* 26:1797–1803.

Inukai T, Kiyokawa N, Campana D, Coustan-Smith E, Kikuchi A, Kobayashi M, et al. (2012): Clinical significance of early T-cell precursor acute lymphoblastic leukaemia: results of the Tokyo Children's Cancer Study Group Study L99-15. *Br J Haematol* 156:358–365.

Jabber Al-Obaidi MS, Martineau M, Bennett CF, Franklin IM, Goldstone AH, Harewood L, et al. (2002): ETV6/AML1 fusion by FISH in adult acute lymphoblastic leukemia. *Leukemia* 16:669–674.

Janssen JW, Ludwig WD, Sterry W, Bartram CR (1993): SIL-TAL1 deletion in T-cell acute lymphoblastic leukemia. *Leukemia* 7:1204–1210.

Johansson B, Moorman AV, Secker-Walker LM (1998): Derivative chromosomes of 11q23-translocations in hematologic malignancies. *Leukemia* 12:828–833.

Kager L, Lion T, Attarbaschi A, Koenig M, Strehl S, Haas OA, et al. (2007): Incidence and outcome of TCF3-PBX1-positive acute lymphoblastic leukemia in Austrian children. *Haematologica* 92:1561–1564.

Kang H, Wilson CS, Harvey RC, Chen IM, Murphy MH, Atlas SR, et al. (2012): Gene expression profiles predictive of outcome and age in infant acute lymphoblastic leukemia: a Children's Oncology Group study. *Blood* 119:1872–1881.

Kantarjian H, Giles F, Wunderle L, Bhalla K, O'Brien S, Wassmann B, et al. (2006): Nilotinib in imatinib-resistant CML and Philadelphia chromosome-positive ALL. *N Engl J Med* 354:2542–2551.

Kardon NB, Slepowitz G, Kochen JA (1982): Childhood acute lymphoblastic leukemia associated with an unusual 8;14 translocation. *Cancer Genet Cytogenet* 6:339–343.

Karrman K, Andersson A, Björgvinsdottir H, Strömbeck B, Lassen C, Olofsson T, et al (2006a): Deregulation of cyclin D2 by juxtaposition with T-cell receptor alpha/delta locus in t(12;14)(p13;q11)-positive childhood T-cell acute lymphoblastic leukemia. *Eur J Haematol* 77:27–34.

Karrman K, Forestier E, Andersen MK, Autio K, Borgström G, Heim S, et al. (2006b): High incidence of the ETV6/RUNX1 fusion gene in paediatric precursor B-cell acute lymphoblastic leukaemias with trisomy 21 as the sole cytogenetic change: a Nordic series of cases diagnosed 1989–2005. *Br J Haematol* 135:352–354.

Kawamata N, Ogawa S, Zimmermann M, Kato M, Sanada M, Hemminki K, et al. (2008): Molecular allelokaryotyping of pediatric acute lymphoblastic leukemias by high-resolution single nucleotide polymorphism oligonucleotide genomic microarray. *Blood* 111:776–784.

Kawamata N, Ogawa S, Seeger K, Kirschner-Schwabe R, Huynh T, Chen J, et al. (2009): Molecular allelokaryotyping of relapsed pediatric acute lymphoblastic leukemia. *Int J Oncol* 34:1603–1612.

Kearney L (1999): The impact of the new fish technologies on the cytogenetics of haematological malignancies. *Br J Haematol* 104:648–658.

Kearney L, Gonzalez De Castro D, Yeung J, Procter J, Horsley SW, Eguchi-Ishimae M, et al. (2009): Specific JAK2 mutation (JAK2R683) and multiple gene deletions in Down syndrome acute lymphoblastic leukemia. *Blood* 113:646–648.

Konrad M, Metzler M, Panzer S, Ostreicher I, Peham M, Repp R, et al. (2003): Late relapses evolve from slow-responding subclones in t(12;21)-positive acute lymphoblastic leukemia: evidence for the persistence of a preleukemic clone. *Blood* 101:3635–3640.

Kovacs BZ, Niggli FK, Betts DR (2004): Aberrations involving 13q12~q14 are frequent secondary events in childhood acute lymphoblastic leukemia. *Cancer Genet Cytogenet* 151:157–161.

Kowalczyk JP, Sandberg A (1983): A possible subgroup of ALL with 9p abnormalities. *Cancer Genet Cytogenet* 9:383–385.

Kuiper RP, Schoenmakers EF, van Reijmersdal SV, Hehir-Kwa JY, van Kessel AG, van Leeuwen FN, et al. (2007): High-resolution genomic profiling of childhood ALL reveals novel recurrent genetic lesions affecting pathways involved in lymphocyte differentiation and cell cycle progression. *Leukemia* 21:1258–1266.

La Starza R, Aventin A, Crescenzi B, Gorello P, Specchia G, Cuneo A, et al. (2005): CIZ gene rearrangements in acute leukemia: report of a diagnostic FISH assay and clinical features of nine patients. *Leukemia* 19:1696–1699.

Lacronique V, Boureux A, Valle VD, Poirel H, Quang CT, Mauchauffe M, et al. (1997): A TEL-JAK2 fusion protein with constitutive kinase activity in human leukemia. *Science* 278:1309–1312.

Lahortiga I, De Keersmaecker K, Van Vlierberghe P, Graux C, Cauwelier B, Lambert F, et al. (2007): Duplication of the MYB oncogene in T cell acute lymphoblastic leukemia. *Nat Genet* 39:593–595.

Lengline L, Beldjord K, Dombret H, Soulier J, Boissel N, Clappier E (2013): Successful tyrosine kinase inhibitor therapy in a refractory B-cell precursor acute lymphoblastic leukemia with EBF1-PDGFRB fusion. *Haematologica* 98:e146–e148.

Li Y, Schwab C, Ryan SL, Papaemmanuil E, Robinson HM, Jacobs P, et al. (2014): Constitutional and somatic rearrangement of chromosome 21 in acute lymphoblastic leukaemia. *Nature* 508:98–102.

Lillington DM, Young BD, Berger R, Martineau M, Moorman AV, Secker-Walker LM (1998): The t(10;11)(p12;q23) translocation in acute leukaemia: a cytogenetic and clinical study of 20 patients. *Leukemia* 12:801–804.

Lilljebjörn H, Soneson C, Andersson A, Heldrup J, Behrendtz M, Kawamata N, et al. (2010): The correlation pattern of acquired copy number changes in 164 ETV6/RUNX1-positive childhood acute lymphoblastic leukemias. *Hum Mol Genet* 19:3150–3158.

Lilljebjörn H, Ågerstam H, Orsmark-Pietras C, Rissler M, Ehrencrona H, Nilsson L, et al. (2014): RNA-seq identifies clinically relevant fusion genes in leukemia including a novel MEF2D/CSF1R fusion responsive to imatinib. *Leukemia* 28:977–979.

Lin YW, Deveney R, Barbara M, Iscove NN, Nimer SD, Slape C, et al. (2005): OLIG2 (BHLHB1), a bHLH transcription factor, contributes to leukemogenesis in concert with LMO1. *Cancer Res* 65:7151–7158.

Liu S, Bo L, Liu X, Li C, Qin S, Wang J (2004): IGH gene involvement in two cases of acute lymphoblastic leukemia with t(14;14)(q11;q32) identified by sequential R-banding and fluorescence in situ hybridization. *Cancer Genet Cytogenet* 152:141–145.

Liu-Dumlao T, Kantarjian H, Thomas DA, O'Brien S, Ravandi F (2012): Philadelphia-positive acute lymphoblastic leukemia: current treatment options. *Curr Oncol Rep* 14:387–394.

Loh ML, Zhang J, Harvey RC, Roberts K, Payne-Turner D, Kang H, et al. (2013): Tyrosine kinome sequencing of pediatric acute lymphoblastic leukemia: a report from the Children's Oncology Group TARGET Project. *Blood* 121:485–488.

Lundin C, Heidenblad M, Strömbeck B, Borg Å, Hovland R, Heim S, et al. (2007): Tiling resolution array CGH of dic(7;9)(p11~13;p11~13) in B-cell precursor acute lymphoblastic leukemia reveals clustered breakpoints at 7p11.2~12.1 and 9p13.1. *Cytogenet Genome Res* 118:13–18.

Lundin C, Heldrup J, Ahlgren T, Olofsson T, Johansson B (2009): B-cell precursor t(8;14)(q11;q32)-positive acute lymphoblastic leukemia in children is strongly associated with Down syndrome or with a concomitant Philadelphia chromosome. *Eur J Haematol* 82:46–53.

Lundin C, Forestier E, Klarskov Andersen M, Autio K, Barbany G, Cavelier L, et al. (2014): Clinical and genetic features of pediatric acute lymphoblastic leukemia in Down syndrome in the Nordic countries. *J Hematol Oncol* 7:32.

Ma SK, Chan GC, Wan TS, Lam CK, Ha SY, Lau YL, et al. (1998): Near-haploid common acute lymphoblastic leukaemia of childhood with a second hyperdiploid line: a DNA ploidy and fluorescence in-situ hybridization study. *Br J Haematol* 103:750–755.

Mahmoud H, Carroll AJ, Behm F, Raimondi SC, Schuster J, Borowitz M, et al. (1992): The non-random dic(9;12) translocation in acute lymphoblastic leukemia is associated with B-progenitor phenotype and an excellent prognosis. *Leukemia* 6:703–707.

Marschalek R (2011): Mechanisms of leukemogenesis by MLL fusion proteins. *Br J Haematol* 152:141–154.

Martineau M, Clark R, Farrell DM, Hawkins JM, Moorman AV, Secker-Walker LM (1996): Isochromosomes in acute lymphoblastic leukaemia: i(21q) is a significant finding. *Genes Chromosomes Cancer* 17:21–30.

Martineau M, Berger R, Lillington DM, Moorman AV, Secker-Walker LM (1998): The t(6;11)(q27;q23) translocation in acute leukaemia: a laboratory and clinical study of 30 cases. *Leukemia* 12:788–791.

Martineau M, Jalali GR, Barber KE, Broadfield ZJ, Cheung KL, Lilleyman J, et al. (2005): ETV6/RUNX1 fusion at diagnosis and relapse: some prognostic indications. *Genes Chromosomes Cancer* 43:54–71.

Martinelli G, Iacobucci I, Storlazzi CT, Vignetti M, Paoloni F, Cilloni D, et al. (2009): IKZF1 (Ikaros) deletions in BCR-ABL1-positive acute lymphoblastic leukemia are associated with short disease-free survival and high rate of cumulative incidence of relapse: a GIMEMA AL WP report. *J Clin Oncol* 27:5202–5207.

Martini A, La Starza R, Janssen H, Bilhou-Nabera C, Corveleyn A, Somers R, et al. (2002): Recurrent rearrangement of the Ewing's sarcoma gene, EWSR1, or its homologue, TAF15, with the transcription factor CIZ/NMP4 in acute leukemia. *Cancer Res* 62:5408–5412.

Masuzawa A, Kiyotani C, Osumi T, Shioda Y, Iijima K, Tomita O, et al. (2014): Poor responses to tyrosine kinase inhibitors in a child with precursor B-cell acute lymphoblastic leukemia with SNX2-ABL1 chimeric transcript. *Eur J Haematol* 92:263–267.

Maude SL, Tasian SK, Vincent T, Hall JW, Sheen C, Roberts KG, et al. (2012): Targeting JAK1/2 and mTOR in murine xenograft models of Ph-like acute lymphoblastic leukemia. *Blood* 120:3510–3518.

McGuire EA, Hockett RD, Pollock KM, Bartholdi MF, O'Brien SJ, Korsmeyer SJ (1989): The t(11;14)(p15;q11) in a T-cell acute lymphoblastic leukemia cell line activates multiple transcripts, including Ttg-1, a gene encoding a potential zinc finger protein. *Mol Cell Biol* 9:2124–2132.

McPherson JD, Marra M, Hillier L, Waterston RH, Chinwalla A, Wallis J, et al. (2001): A physical map of the human genome. *Nature* 409:934–941.

Meijerink JP (2010): Genetic rearrangements in relation to immunophenotype and outcome in T-cell acute lymphoblastic leukaemia. *Best Pract Res Clin Haematol* 23:307–318.

Mellentin JD, Smith SD, Cleary ML (1989): lyl-1, a novel gene altered by chromosomal translocation in T cell leukemia, codes for a protein with a helix-loop-helix DNA binding motif. *Cell* 58:77–83.

Menasce LP, Orphanos V, Santibanez-Koref M, Boyle JM, Harrison CJ (1994): Deletion of a common region on the long arm of chromosome 6 in acute lymphoblastic leukaemia. *Genes Chromosomes Cancer* 10:26–29.

Mengle-Gaw L, Albertson DG, Sherrington PD, Rabbitts TH (1988): Analysis of a T-cell tumor-specific breakpoint cluster at human chromosome 14q32. *Proc Natl Acad Sci USA* 85:9171–9175.

Meyer C, Hofmann J, Burmeister T, Gröger D, Park TS, Emerenciano M, et al. (2013a): The MLL recombinome of acute leukemias in 2013. *Leukemia* 27:2165–2176.

Meyer JA, Wang J, Hogan LE, Yang JJ, Dandekar S, Patel JP, et al. (2013b): Relapse-specific mutations in NT5C2 in childhood acute lymphoblastic leukemia. *Nat Genet* 45:290–294.

Michael PM, Levin MD, Garson OM (1984): Translocation 1;19—a new cytogenetic abnormality in acute lymphocytic leukemia. *Cancer Genet Cytogenet* 12:333–341.

Mitelman F, Johansson B, Mertens F (2014): Mitelman Database of Chromosome Aberrations and Gene Fusions in Cancer. Available at http://cgap.nci.nih.gov/Chromosomes/Mitelman.

Moorman AV (2012): The clinical relevance of chromosomal and genomic abnormalities in B-cell precursor acute lymphoblastic leukaemia. *Blood Rev* 26:123–135.

Moorman AV, Hagemeijer A, Charrin C, Rieder H, Secker-Walker LM (1998): The translocations, t(11;19)(q23;p13.1) and t(11;19)(q23;p13.3): a cytogenetic and clinical profile of 53 patients. *Leukemia* 12:805–810.

Moorman AV, Richards SM, Martineau M, Cheung KL, Robinson HM, Jalali GR, et al. (2003): Outcome heterogeneity in childhood high-hyperdiploid acute lymphoblastic leukemia. *Blood* 102:2756–2762.

Moorman AV, Raimondi SC, Pui CH, Baruchel A, Biondi A, Carroll AJ, et al. (2005): No prognostic effect of additional chromosomal abnormalities in children with acute lymphoblastic leukemia and 11q23 abnormalities. *Leukemia* 19:557–563.

Moorman AV, Harrison CJ, Buck GA, Richards SM, Secker-Walker LM, Martineau M, et al. (2007a): Karyotype is an independent prognostic factor in adult acute lymphoblastic leukemia (ALL): analysis of cytogenetic data from patients treated on the Medical Research Council (MRC) UKALLXII/Eastern Cooperative Oncology Group (ECOG) 2993 trial. *Blood* 109:3189–3197.

Moorman AV, Richards SM, Robinson HM, Strefford JC, Gibson BE, Kinsey SE, et al. (2007b): Prognosis of children with acute lymphoblastic leukaemia (ALL) and intrachromosomal amplification of chromosome 21 (iAMP21). *Blood* 109:2327–2330.

Moorman AV, Chilton L, Wilkinson J, Ensor HM, Bown N, Proctor SJ (2010a): A population-based cytogenetic study of adults with acute lymphoblastic leukaemia. *Blood* 115:206–214.

Moorman AV, Ensor HM, Richards SM, Chilton L, Schwab C, Kinsey SE, et al. (2010b): Prognostic effect of chromosomal abnormalities in childhood B-cell precursor acute lymphoblastic leukaemia: results from the UK Medical Research Council ALL97/99 randomised trial. *Lancet Oncol* 11:429–438.

Moorman AV, Schwab C, Ensor HM, Russell LJ, Morrison H, Jones L, et al. (2012): IGH@ translocations, CRLF2 deregulation and micro-deletions in adolescents and adults with acute lymphoblastic leukaemia (ALL). *J Clin Oncol* 30:3100–3108.

Moorman AV, Robinson H, Schwab C, Richards SM, Hancock J, Mitchell CD, et al. (2013): Risk-directed treatment intensification significantly reduces the risk of relapse among children and adolescents with acute lymphoblastic leukemia and intrachromosomal amplification of chromosome 21: a comparison of the MRC ALL97/99 and UKALL2003 Trials. *J Clin Oncol* 31: 3389–3396.

Mufti GJ, Hamblin TJ, Oscier DG, Johnson S (1983): Common ALL with pre-B-cell features showing (8;14) and (14;18) chromosome translocations. *Blood* 62:1142–1146.

Mühlbacher V, Zenger M, Schnittger S, Weissmann S, Kunze F, Kohlmann A, et al. (2014): Acute lymphoblastic leukemia with low hypodiploid/near triploid karyotype is a specific clinical entity and exhibits a very high TP53 mutation frequency of 93%. *Genes Chromosomes Cancer* 53:524–536.

Mulligan CG, Goorha S, Radtke I, Miller CB, Coustan-Smith E, Dalton JD, et al. (2007): Genome-wide analysis of genetic alterations in acute lymphoblastic leukaemia. *Nature* 446:758–764.

Mullighan CG, Miller CB, Radtke I, Phillips LA, Dalton J, Ma J, et al. (2008a): BCR-ABL1 lymphoblastic leukaemia is characterized by the deletion of Ikaros. *Nature* 453:110–114.

Mullighan CG, Phillips LA, Su X, Ma J, Miller CB, Shurtleff SA, et al. (2008b): Genomic analysis of the clonal origins of relapsed acute lymphoblastic leukemia. *Science* 322:1377–1380.

Mullighan CG, Collins-Underwood JR, Phillips LAA, Loudin MG, Liu W, Zhang J, et al. (2009a): Rearrangement of CRLF2 in B-progenitor- and Down syndrome-associated acute lymphoblastic leukaemia. *Nat Genet* 41:1243–1246.

Mullighan CG, Su X, Zhang J, Radtke I, Phillips LA, Miller CB, et al. (2009b): Deletion of IKZF1 and prognosis in acute lymphoblastic leukaemia. *N Engl J Med* 360:470–480.

Mullighan CG, Zhang J, Kasper LH, Lerach S, Payne-Turner D, Phillips LA, et al. (2011): CREBBP mutations in relapsed acute lymphoblastic leukaemia. *Nature* 471:235–239.

Nachman JB, Heerema NA, Sather H, Camitta B, Forestier E, Harrison CJ, et al. (2007): Outcome of treatment in children with hypodiploid acute lymphoblastic leukemia. *Blood* 110:1112–1115.

Nagel S, Kaufmann M, Drexler HG, MacLeod RA (2003): The cardiac homeobox gene NKX2-5 is deregulated by juxtaposition with BCL11B in pediatric T-ALL cell lines via a novel t(5;14)(q35.1;q32.2). *Cancer Res* 63:5329–5334.

Nagel S, Scherr M, Kel A, Hornischer K, Crawford GE, Kaufmann M, et al. (2007): Activation of TLX3 and NKX2-5 in t(5;14)(q35;q32) T-cell acute lymphoblastic leukemia by remote 3′-BCL11B enhancers and coregulation by PU.1 and HMGA1. *Cancer Res* 67:1461–1471.

Neumann M, Heesch S, Gokbuget N, Schwartz S, Schlee C, Benlasfer O, et al. (2012): Clinical and molecular characterization of early T-cell precursor leukemia: a high-risk subgroup in adult T-ALL with a high frequency of FLT3 mutations. *Blood Cancer J* 2:e55.

Neumann M, Coskun E, Fransecky L, Mochmann LH, Bartram I, Sartangi NF, et al. (2013a): FLT3 mutations in early T-cell precursor ALL characterize a stem cell like leukemia and imply the clinical use of tyrosine kinase inhibitors. *PLoS One* 8:e53190.

Neumann M, Heesch S, Schlee C, Schwartz S, Gokbuget N, Hoelzer D, et al. (2013b): Whole-exome sequencing in adult ETP-ALL reveals a high rate of DNMT3A mutations. *Blood* 121:4749–4752.

Nickoloff JA, De Haro LP, Wray J, Hromas R (2008): Mechanisms of leukemia translocations. *Curr Opin Hematol* 15:338–345.

Ntziachristos P, Tsirigos A, Van Vlierberghe P, Nedjic J, Trimarchi T, Flaherty MS, et al. (2012): Genetic inactiva-

tion of the polycomb repressive complex 2 in T cell acute lymphoblastic leukemia. *Nat Med* 18:298–303.

Nyquist KB, Thorsen J, Zeller B, Haaland A, Troen G, Heim S, et al. (2011): Identification of the TAF15-ZNF384 fusion gene in two new cases of acute lymphoblastic leukemia with a t(12;17)(p13;q12). *Cancer Genet* 204:147–152.

Olsson L, Castor A, Behrendtz M, Biloglav A, Forestier E, Paulsson K, et al. (2014): Deletions of IKZF1 and SPRED1 are associated with poor prognosis in a population-based series of pediatric B-cell precursor acute lymphoblastic leukemia diagnosed between 1992 and 2011. *Leukemia* 28:302–310.

Oshimura M, Freeman AI, Sandberg AA (1977): Chromosomes and causation of human cancer and leukemia. XXVI. Banding studies in acute lymphoblastic leukemia (ALL). *Cancer* 40:1161–1172.

Ottmann O, Dombret H, Martinelli G, Simonsson B, Guilhot F, Larson RA, et al. (2007): Dasatinib induces rapid hematologic and cytogenetic responses in adult patients with Philadelphia chromosome-positive acute lymphoblastic leukemia with resistance or intolerance to imatinib: interim results of a phase 2 study. *Blood* 110:2309–2315.

Pallisgaard N, Hokland P, Riishoj DC, Pederson B, Jorgensen P (1998): Multiplex reverse transcription-polymerase chain reaction for simultaneous screening of 29 translocations and chromosomal aberrations in acute leukemia. *Blood* 92:574–588.

Papaemmanuil E, Hosking FJ, Vijayakrishnan J, Price A, Olver B, Sheridan E, et al. (2009): Loci on 7p12.2, 10q21.2 and 14q11.2 are associated with risk of childhood acute lymphoblastic leukemia. *Nat Genet* 41:1006–1010.

Paulsson K, Johansson B (2009): High hyperdiploid childhood acute lymphoblastic leukemia. *Genes Chromosomes Cancer* 48:637–660.

Paulsson K, Horvat A, Fioretos T, Mitelman F, Johansson B (2005a): Formation of der(19)t(1;19)(q23;p13) in acute lymphoblastic leukemia. *Genes Chromosomes Cancer* 42:144–148.

Paulsson K, Mörse H, Fioretos T, Behrendtz M, Strömbeck B, Johansson B (2005b): Evidence for a single-step mechanism in the origin of hyperdiploid childhood acute lymphoblastic leukemia. *Genes Chromosomes Cancer* 44:113–122.

Paulsson K, Jonson T, Øra I, Olofsson T, Panagopoulos I, Johansson B (2007): Characterisation of genomic translocation breakpoints and identification of an alternative TCF3/PBX1 fusion transcript in t(1;19)(q23;p13)-positive acute lymphoblastic leukaemias. *Br J Haematol* 138:196–201.

Paulsson K, Horvat A, Strömbeck B, Nilsson F, Heldrup J, Behrendtz M, et al. (2008): Mutations of FLT3, NRAS, KRAS, and PTPN11 are frequent and possibly mutually exclusive in high hyperdiploid childhood acute lymphoblastic leukemia. *Genes Chromosomes Cancer* 47:26–33.

Paulsson K, Forestier E, Lilljebjörn H, Heldrup J, Behrendtz M, Young BD, et al. (2010): Genetic landscape of high hyperdiploid childhood acute lymphoblastic leukemia. *Proc Natl Acad Sci USA* 107:21719–21724.

Paulsson K, Forestier E, Andersen MK, Autio K, Barbany G, Borgström G, et al. (2013a): High modal number and triple trisomies are highly correlated favorable factors in childhood B-cell precursor high hyperdiploid acute lymphoblastic leukemia treated according to the NOPHO ALL 1992/2000 protocols. *Haematologica* 98:1424–1432.

Paulsson K, Harrison CJ, Andersen MK, Chilton L, Nordgren A, Moorman AV, et al. (2013b): Distinct patterns of gained chromosomes in high hyperdiploid acute lymphoblastic leukemia with t(1;19)(q23;p13), t(9;22) (q34;q22) or MLL rearrangements. *Leukemia* 27:974–977.

Peeters P, Raynaud SD, Cools J, Wlodarska I, Grosgeorge J, Philip P, et al. (1997): Fusion of TEL, the ETS-variant gene 6 (ETV6), to the receptor-associated kinase JAK2 as a result of t(9;12) in a lymphoid and t(9;15;12) in a myeloid leukemia. *Blood* 90:2535–2540.

Pieters R, Schrappe M, De Lorenzo P, Hann I, De Rossi G, Felice M, et al. (2007): A treatment protocol for infants younger than 1 year with acute lymphoblastic leukaemia (Interfant-99): an observational study and a multicentre randomised trial. *Lancet* 370:240–250.

Powell BC, Jiang L, Muzny DM, Trevino LR, Dreyer ZE, Strong LC, et al. (2013): Identification of TP53 as an acute lymphocytic leukemia susceptibility gene through exome sequencing. *Pediatr Blood Cancer* 60:E1–E3.

Prasad RB, Hosking FJ, Vijayakrishnan J, Papaemmanuil E, Eoehler R, Greaves M, et al. (2010): Verification of the susceptibility loci on 7p12.2, 10q21.2, and 14p11.2 in precursor B-cell acute lymphoblastic leukemia of childhood. *Blood* 115:1765–1767.

Privitera E, Kamps MP, Hayashi Y, Inaba T, Shapiro LH, Raimondi SC, et al. (1992): Different molecular consequences of the 1;19 chromosomal translocation in childhood B-cell precursor acute lymphoblastic leukemia. *Blood* 79:1781–1788.

Przybylski GK, Dik WA, Wanzeck J, Grabarczyk P, Majunke S, Martin-Subero JI, et al. (2005): Disruption of the BCL11B gene through inv(14)(q11.2q32.31) results in the expression of BCL11B-TRDC fusion transcripts and is associated with the absence of wild-type BCL11B transcripts in T-ALL. *Leukemia* 19:201–208.

Pui C-H, Carroll AJ, Raimondi SC, Schell MJ, Head DR, Shuster JJ, et al. (1992): Isochromosomes in childhood acute lymphoblastic leukemia: a collaborative study of 83 cases. *Blood* 79:2384–2391.

Pui CH, Relling MV, Downing JR (2004): Acute lymphoblastic leukemia. *N Engl J Med* 350:1535–1548.

Pui CH, Campana D, Pei D, Bowman WP, Sandlund JT, Kaste SC, et al. (2009): Treating childhood acute lymphoblastic leukemia without cranial irradiation. *N Engl J Med* 360:2730–2741.

Quelle DE, Zindy F, Ashmun RA, Sherr CJ (1995): Alternative reading frames of the INK4a tumor suppressor gene encode two unrelated proteins capable of inducing cell cycle arrest. *Cell* 83:993–1000.

Rabbitts TH (1994): Chromosomal translocations in human cancer. *Nature* 372:143–149.

Radich JP, Kopecky KJ, Boldt DH, Head D, Slovak ML, Babu R, et al. (1994): Detection of BCR-ABL fusion genes in adult acute lymphoblastic leukemia by the polymerase chain reaction. *Leukemia* 8:1688–1695.

Raimondi SC, Pui C-H, Head DR, Rivera GK, Behm FG (1993): Cytogenetically different leukemic clones at relapse of childhood acute lymphoblastic leukemia. *Blood* 82:576–580.

Raimondi SC, Pui C-H, Hancock ML, Behm FG, Filatov L, Rivera GK (1996): Heterogeneity of hyperdiploid (51-67) childhood acute lymphoblastic leukemia. *Leukemia* 10:213–224.

Raimondi SC, Zhou Y, Mathew S, Shurtleff SA, Sandlund JT, Rivera GK, et al. (2003): Reassessment of the prognostic significance of hypodiploidy in pediatric patients with acute lymphoblastic leukemia. *Cancer* 98:2715–2722.

Raimondi SC, Zhou Y, Shurtleff SA, Rubnitz JE, Pui C-H, Behm FG (2006): Near-triploidy and near-tetraploidy in childhood acute lymphoblastic leukemia: association with B-lineage blast cells carrying the ETV6-RUNX1 fusion, T-lineage immunophenotype, and favorable outcome. *Cancer Genet Cytogenet* 169:50–57.

Rand V, Parker H, Russell LJ, Schwab C, Ensor H, Irving J, et al. (2011): Genomic characterization implicates iAMP21 as a likely primary genetic event in childhood B-cell precursor acute lymphoblastic leukemia. *Blood* 117:6848–6855.

Raynaud S, Cave H, Baens M, Bastard C, Cacheux V, Grosgeorge J, et al. (1996): The 12;21 translocation involving TEL and deletion of the other TEL allele: Two frequently associated alterations found in childhood acute lymphoblastic leukemia. *Blood* 87:2891–2899.

Raynaud SD, Dastugue N, Zoccola D, Shurtleff SA, Mathew S, Raimondi SC (1999): Cytogenetic abnormalities associated with the t(12;21): a collaborative study of 169 children with t(12;21)-positive acute lymphoblastic leukemia. *Leukemia* 13:1325–1330.

van Rhee F, Kasprzyk A, Jamil A, Dickinson H, Lin F, Cross NC, et al. (1995): Detection of the BCR-ABL gene by reverse transcription/polymerase chain reaction and fluorescence in situ hybridization in a patient with Philadelphia chromosome negative acute lymphoblastic leukaemia. *Br J Haematol* 90:225–228.

Rieder H, Schnittger S, Bodenstein H, Schwonzen M, Wörmann B, Berkovic D, et al. (1995): dic(9;20): a new recurrent chromosome abnormality in adult acute lymphoblastic leukemia. *Genes Chromosomes Cancer* 13:54–61.

Roberts KG, Morin RD, Zhang J, Hirst M, Zhao Y, Su X, et al. (2012): Genetic alterations activating kinase and cytokine receptor signaling in high-risk acute lymphoblastic leukemia. *Cancer Cell* 22:153–166.

Robinson HM, Martineau M, Harris RL, Barber KE, Jalali GR, Moorman AV, et al. (2005): Derivative chromosome 9 deletions are a significant feature of childhood Philadelphia chromosome positive acute lymphoblastic leukaemia. *Leukemia* 19:564–571.

Robinson HM, Harrison CJ, Moorman AV, Chudoba I, Strefford JC (2007): Intrachromosomal amplification of chromosome 21 (iAMP21) may arise from a breakage-fusion-bridge cycle. *Genes Chromosomes Cancer* 46:318–326.

Romana SP, Le Coniat M, Berger R (1994): t(12;21): a new recurrent translocation in acute lymphoblastic leukemia. *Genes Chromosomes Cancer* 9:186–191.

Romana SP, Poirel H, Leconiat M, Flexor M-A, Mauchauffé M, Jonveaux P, et al. (1995): High frequency of t(12;21) in childhood B-lineage acute lymphoblastic leukemia. *Blood* 86:4263–4269.

Ross ME, Zhou X, Song G, Shurtleff SA, Girtman K, Williams WK, et al. (2003): Classification of pediatric acute lymphoblastic leukemia by gene expression profiling. *Blood* 102:2951–2959.

Rowley JD, Diaz MO, Espinosa RIII, Patel YD, Van Melle E, Ziemin S, et al. (1990): Mapping chromosome band 11q23 in human acute leukemia with biotinylated probes: identification of 11q23 translocation breakpoints with a yeast artificial chromosome. *Proc Natl Acad Sci USA* 87:9358–9362.

Russell LJ, Akasaka T, Majid A, Sugimoto K-J, Karran EL, Nagel I, et al. (2008): t(6;14)(p22;q32): a new recurrent IGH@ translocation involving ID4 in B-cell precursor acute lymphoblastic leukemia (BCP-ALL). *Blood* 111:387–391.

Russell LJ, Capasso M, Vater I, Akasaka T, Bernard OA, Calasanz MJ, et al. (2009a): Deregulated expression of cytokine receptor gene, CRLF2, is involved in lymphoid transformation in B-cell precursor acute lymphoblastic leukemia. *Blood* 114:2688–2698.

Russell LJ, De Castro DG, Griffiths M, Telford N, Bernard O, Panzer-Grümayer R, et al. (2009b): A novel translocation, t(14;19)(q32;p13), involving IGH@ and the cytokine receptor for erythropoietin. *Leukemia* 23:614–617.

Russell LJ, Enshaei A, Jones L, Erhorn A, Masic D, Bentley H, et al. (2014): IGH@ translocations are prevalent in teenagers and young adults with acute lymphoblastic leukemia and are associated with a poor outcome. *J Clin Oncol* 32:1453–1462.

Safavi S, Forestier E, Golovleva I, Barbany G, Nord KH, Moorman AV, et al. (2013): Loss of chromosomes is the primary event in near-haploid and low-hypodiploid acute lymphoblastic leukemia. *Leukemia* 27:248–250.

Schaad K, Strömbeck B, Mandahl N, Andersen MK, Heim S, Mertens F, et al. (2006): FISH mapping of i(7q) in acute leukemias and myxoid liposarcoma reveals clustered breakpoints in 7p11.2: implications for formation and pathogenetic outcome of the idic(7)(p11.2). *Cytogenet Genome Res* 114:126–130.

Schultz KR, Bowman WP, Aledo A, Slayton WB, Sather H, Devidas M, et al. (2009): Improved early event-free survival with imatinib in Philadelphia chromosome-positive acute lymphoblastic leukemia: a children's oncology group study. *J Clin Oncol* 27:5175–5181.

Schwab CJ, Chilton L, Morrison H, Jones L, Al-Shehhi H, Erhorn A, et al. (2013): Genes commonly deleted in childhood B-cell precursor acute lymphoblastic leukemia: association with cytogenetics and clinical features. *Haematologica* 98:1081–1088.

Secker-Walker LM (1997): *Chromosomes and Genes in Acute Lymphoblastic Leukaemia*. New York: Chapman and Hall.

Secker-Walker LM, Lawler SD, Hardisty RM (1978): Prognostic implications of chromosomal findings in acute lymphoblastic leukaemia at diagnosis. *Br Med J* 2:1529–1530.

Secker-Walker LM, Craig JM, Hawkins JM, Hoffbrand AV (1991): Philadelphia positive acute lymphoblastic leukemia in adults: age distribution, BCR breakpoint and prognostic significance. *Leukemia* 5:196–199.

Secker-Walker LM, Berger R, Fenaux P, Lai JL, Nelken B, Garson M, et al. (1992): Prognostic significance of the balanced t(1;19) and unbalanced der(19)t(1;19) translocations in acute lymphoblastic leukemia. *Leukemia* 6:363–369.

Shearer BM, Flynn HC, Knudson RA, Ketterling RP (2005): Interphase FISH to detect PBX1/E2A fusion resulting from the der(19)t(1;19)(q23;p13.3) or t(1;19)(q23;p13.3) in paediatric patients with acute lymphoblastic leukaemia. *Br J Haematol* 129:45–52.

Shochat C, Tal N, Bandapalli OR, Palmi C, Ganmore I, te Kronnie G, et al. (2011): Gain-of-function mutations in interleukin-7 receptor-alpha (IL7R) in childhood acute lymphoblastic leukemias. *J Exp Med* 208:901–908.

Sinclair PB, Sorour A, Martineau M, Harrison CJ, Mitchell WA, O'Neill E, et al. (2004): A fluorescence in situ hybridization map of 6q deletions in acute lymphocytic leukemia: identification and analysis of a candidate tumor suppressor gene. *Cancer Res* 64:4089–4098.

Slater R, Smit E, Kroes W, Jotterand Bellomo M, Mühlematter D, Harbott J, et al. (1995): A non-random chromosome abnormality found in precursor-B lineage acute lymphoblastic leukaemia: dic(9;20)(p1?3;q11). *Leukemia* 9:1613–1619.

Slater RM, von Drunen E, Kroes WG, Weghuis DO, van den Berg E, Smit EM, et al. (2001): t(7;12)(q36;p13) and t(7;12)(q32;p13) – translocations involving ETV6 in children 18 months of age or younger with myeloid disorders. *Leukemia* 15:915–920.

Soler G, Radford-Weiss I, Ben-Abdelali R, Mahlaoui N, Ponceau JF, Macintyre EA, et al. (2008): Fusion of ZMIZ1 to ABL1 in a B-cell acute lymphoblastic leukaemia with a t(9;10)(q34;q22.3) translocation. *Leukemia* 22:1278–1280.

Soulier J, Trakhtenbrot L, Najfeld V, Lipton JM, Mathew S, Avet-Loiseau H, et al. (2003): Amplification of band q22 of chromosome 21, including AML1, in older children with acute lymphoblastic leukemia: an emerging molecular cytogenetic subgroup. *Leukemia* 17:1679–1682.

Soulier J, Clappier E, Cayuela J-M, Regnault A, Garcia-Peydro M, Dombret H, et al. (2005): HOXA genes are included in genetic and biologic networks defining human acute T-cell leukemia (T-ALL). *Blood* 106:274–286.

Speleman F, Cauwelier B, Dastugue N, Cools J, Verhasselt B, Poppe B, et al. (2005): A new recurrent inversion, inv(7) (p15q34), leads to transcriptional activation of HOXA10 and HOXA11 in a subset of T-cell acute lymphoblastic leukemias. *Leukemia* 19:358–366.

Stark B, Jeison M, Gobuzov R, Krug H, Glaser-Gabay L, Luria D, et al. (2001): Near haploid childhood acute lymphoblastic leukemia masked by hyperdiploid line: detection by fluorescence in situ hybridization. *Cancer Genet Cytogenet* 128:108–113.

Stergianou K, Fox C, Russell NH (2005): Fusion of NUP214 to ABL1 on amplified episomes in T-ALL—implications for treatment. *Leukemia* 19:1680–1681.

Strefford JC, van Delft FW, Robinson HM, Worley H, Yiannikouris O, Selzer R, et al. (2006): Complex genomic alterations and gene expression in acute lymphoblastic leukemia with intrachromosomal amplification of chromosome 21. *Proc Natl Acad Sci USA* 103:8167–8172.

Strefford JC, Worley H, Barber K, Wright S, Stewart ARM, Robinson HM, et al. (2007): Genome complexity in acute lymphoblastic leukemia is revealed by array-based comparative genomic hybridization. *Oncogene* 26:4306–4318.

Strehl S, König M, Dworzak MN, Kalwak K, Haas OA (2003): PAX5/ETV6 fusion defines cytogenetic entity dic(9;12) (p13;p13). *Leukemia* 17:1121–1123.

Su XY, Busson M, Della Valle V, Ballerini P, Dastugue N, Talmant P, et al. (2004): Various types of rearrangements target TLX3 locus in T-cell acute lymphoblastic leukemia. *Genes Chromosomes Cancer* 41:243–249.

Su XY, Drabkin H, Clappier E, Morgado E, Busson M, Romana S, et al. (2006a): Transforming potential of the T-cell acute lymphoblastic leukemia-associated homeobox genes HOXA13, TLX1, and TLX3. *Genes Chromosomes Cancer* 45:846–855.

Su XY, Della-Valle V, Andre-Schmutz I, Lemercier C, Radford-Weiss I, Ballerini P, et al. (2006b): HOX11L2/ TLX3 is transcriptionally activated through T-cell regulatory elements downstream of BCL11B as a result of the t(5;14)(q35;q32). *Blood* 108:4198–4201.

Sulong S, Moorman AV, Irving JA, Strefford JC, Konn ZJ, Case MC, et al. (2009): A comprehensive analysis of the CDKN2A gene in childhood acute lymphoblastic leukemia reveals genomic deletion, copy number neutral loss of heterozygosity, and association with specific cytogenetic subgroups. *Blood* 113:100–107.

Swerdlow SH, Campo E, Harris NL, Jaffe ES, Pileri SA, Stein H, et al., editors (2008): *WHO Classification of Tumours of the Haematopoietic and Lymphoid Tissues*. Lyon: IARC.

Testoni N, Zaccaria A, Martinelli G, Pelliconi S, Buzzi M, Farabegoli P, et al. (1993): t(8;14)(q11;q32) in acute lymphoid leukemia: description of two cases. *Cancer Genet Cytogenet* 67:55–58.

Third International Workshop on Chromosomes in Leukemia (1980): Chromosomal abnormalities in acute lymphoblastic leukemia: structural and numerical changes in 234 cases. *Cancer Genet Cytogenet* 4:101–110.

Thirman MJ, Levitan DA, Kobayashi H, Simon MC, Rowley JD (1994): Cloning of ELL, a gene that fuses to MLL in a t(11;19)(q23;p13.1) in acute myeloid leukemia. *Proc Natl Acad Sci USA* 91:12110–12114.

Torrano V, Procter J, Cardus P, Greaves M, Ford AM (2011): ETV6-RUNX1 promotes survival of early B lineage progenitor cells via a dysregulated erythropoietin receptor. *Blood* 118:4910–4918.

Tosi S, Harbott J, Teigler-Schlegel A, Haas OA, Pirc-Danoewinata H, Harrison CJ, et al. (2000): t(7;12)(q36;p13), a new recurrent translocation involving ETV6 in infant leukemia. *Genes Chromosomes Cancer* 29:325–332.

Tzoneva G, Perez-Garcia A, Carpenter Z, Khiabanian H, Tosello V, Allegretta M, et al. (2013): Activating mutations in the NT5C2 nucleotidase gene drive chemotherapy resistance in relapsed ALL. *Nat Med* 19:368–371.

United Kingdom Cancer Cytogenetics Group (UKCCG) (1992): Translocations involving 9p and/or 12p in acute lymphoblastic leukemia. *Genes Chromosomes Cancer* 5:255–259.

Van Den Berghe H, David G, Broeckaert-Van Orshoven A, Louwagie A, Verwilghen R, Casteels-Van Daele M, et al. (1979): A new chromosome anomaly in acute lymphoblastic leukemia (ALL). *Hum Genet* 46:173–180.

Van Vlierberghe P, van Grotel M, Beverloo HB, Lee C, Helgason T, Buijs-Gladdines J, et al. (2006): The cryptic chromosomal deletion del(11)(p12p13) as a new activation mechanism of LMO2 in pediatric T-cell acute lymphoblastic leukemia. *Blood* 108:3520–3529.

Van Vlierberghe P, Palomero T, Khiabanian H, Van der Meulen J, Castillo M, Van Roy N, et al. (2010): PHF6 mutations in T-cell acute lymphoblastic leukemia. *Nat Genet* 42:338–342.

Van Vlierberghe P, Ambesi-Impiombato A, Perez-Garcia A, Haydu JE, Rigo I, Hadler M, et al. (2011): ETV6 mutations in early immature human T cell leukemias. *J Exp Med* 208:2571–2579.

van der Veer A, Waanders E, Pieters R, Willemse ME, Van Reijmersdal SV, Russell LJ, et al. (2013): Independent prognostic value of BCR-ABL1-like signature and IKZF1 deletion, but not high CRLF2 expression, in children with B-cell precursor ALL. *Blood* 122:2622–2629.

Waanders E, van der Velden VH, van der Schoot CE, van Leeuwen FN, van Reijmersdal SV, de Haas V, et al. (2011): Integrated use of minimal residual disease classification and IKZF1 alteration status accurately predicts 79% of relapses in pediatric acute lymphoblastic leukemia. *Leukemia* 25:254–258.

Wakabayashi Y, Watanabe H, Inoue J, Takeda N, Sakata J, Mishima Y, et al. (2003): Bcl11b is required for differentiation and survival of αβ T lymphocytes. *Nat Immunol* 4:533–539.

Wang J, Jani-Sait SN, Escalon EA, Carroll AJ, de Jong PJ, Kirsch IR, et al. (2000): The t(14;21)(q11.2;q22) chromosomal translocation associated with T-cell acute lymphoblastic leukemia activates the BHLHB1 gene. *Proc Natl Acad Sci USA* 97:3497–3502.

Weng AP, Ferrando AA, Lee W, Morris JP, Silverman LB, Sanchez-Irizarry C, et al. (2004): Activating mutations of NOTCH1 in human T cell acute lymphoblastic leukemia. *Science* 306:269–271.

Weston BW, Hayden MA, Roberts KG, Bowyer S, Hsu J, Fedoriw G, et al. (2013): Tyrosine kinase inhibitor therapy induces remission in a patient with refractory EBF1-PDGFRB-positive acute lymphoblastic leukemia. *J Clin Oncol* 31:e413–e416.

Williams DL, Look AT, Melvin SL, Roberson PK, Dahl G, Flake T, et al. (1984): New chromosomal translocations correlate with specific immunophenotypes of childhood acute lymphoblastic leukemia. *Cell* 36:101–109.

Xia Y, Brown L, Yang CY-C, Tsan JT, Siciliano MJ, Espinosa R III, et al. (1991): TAL2, a helix-loop-helix gene activated by the (7;9)(q34;q32) translocation in human T-cell leukemia. *Proc Natl Acad Sci USA* 88:11416–11420.

Xu H, Yang W, Perez-Andreu V, Devidas M, Fan Y, Cheng C, et al. (2013): Novel susceptibility variants at 10p12.31-12.2 for childhood acute lymphoblastic leukemia in ethnically diverse populations. *J Natl Cancer Inst* 105:733–742.

Yamamoto K, Seto M, Komatsu H, Iida S, Akao Y, Kojima S, et al. (1993): Two distinct portions of LTG19/ENL at 19p13 are involved in t(11;19) leukemia. *Oncogene* 8:2617–2625.

Yang JJ, Bhojwani D, Yang W, Cai X, Stocco G, Crews K, et al. (2008): Genome-wide copy number profiling reveals molecular evolution from diagnosis to relapse in childhood acute lymphoblastic leukemia. *Blood* 112:4178–4183.

Yeoh EJ, Ross ME, Shurtleff SA, Williams WK, Patel D, Mahfouz R, et al. (2002): Classification, subtype discovery, and prediction of outcome in pediatric acute lymphoblastic leukemia by gene expression profiling. *Cancer Cell* 1:133–143.

Zachariadis V, Gauffin F, Kuchinskaya E, Heyman M, Schoumans J, Blennow E, et al. (2011): The frequency and prognostic impact of dic(9;20)(p13.2;q11.2) in childhood B-cell precursor acute lymphoblastic leukemia: results from the NOPHO ALL-2000 trial. *Leukemia* 25:622–628.

Zachariadis V, Schoumans J, Barbany G, Heyman M, Forestier E, Johansson B, et al. (2012): Homozygous deletions of CDKN2A are present in all dic(9;20)(p13.2;q11.2)-positive B-cell precursor acute lymphoblastic leukaemias and may be important for leukaemic transformation. *Br J Haematol* 159: 488–491.

Zaliova M, Zimmermannova O, Dörge P, Eckert C, Möricke A, Zimmermann M, et al. (2014): ERG deletion is associated with CD2 and attenuates the negative impact of IKZF1 deletion in childhood acute lymphoblastic leukemia. *Leukemia* 28:182–185.

Zenatti PP, Ribeiro D, Li W, Zuurbier L, Silva MC, Paganin M, et al. (2011): Oncogenic IL7R gain-of-function mutations in childhood T-cell acute lymphoblastic leukemia. *Nat Genet* 43:932–939.

Zhang J, Mullighan CG, Harvey RC, Wu G, Chen X, Edmonson M, et al. (2011): Key pathways are frequently mutated in high-risk childhood acute lymphoblastic leukemia: a report from the Children's Oncology Group. *Blood* 118:3080–3087.

Zhang J, Ding L, Holmfeldt L, Wu G, Heatley SL, Payne-Turner D, et al. (2012): The genetic basis of early T-cell precursor acute lymphoblastic leukaemia. *Nature* 481:157–163.

Zhong C-H, Prima V, Liang X, Frye C, McGavran L, Meltesen L, et al. (2008): E2A-ZNF384 and NOL1-E2A fusion created by a cryptic t(12;19)(p13.3;p13.3) in acute leukemia. *Leukemia* 22:723–729.

Zhou M-H, Gao L, Jing Y, Xu Y-Y, Ding Y, Wang N, et al. (2012): Detection of ETV6 gene rearrangements in adult acute lymphoblastic leukemia. *Ann Hematol* 91:1235–1243.

Zhu YM, Zhao WL, Fu JF, Shi JY, Pan Q, Hu J, et al. (2006): NOTCH1 mutations in T-cell acute lymphoblastic leukemia: prognostic significance and implication in multifactorial leukemogenesis. *Clin Cancer Res* 12:3043–3049.

Zuna J, Zaliova M, Muzikova K, Meyer C, Lizcova L, Zemanova Z, et al. (2010): Acute leukemias with ETV6/ABL1 (TEL/ABL) fusion: Poor prognosis and prenatal origin. *Genes Chromosomes Cancer* 49:873–884.

CHAPTER 11

Mature B- and T-cell neoplasms and Hodgkin lymphoma

Reiner Siebert and Sietse M. Aukema

Institute of Human Genetics, University Hospital Schleswig-Holstein Campus Kiel, Christian-Albrechts University Kiel, Germany

Mature lymphoid neoplasms are an extremely heterogeneous group of malignancies with regard to biological, clinical, and morphological features (Jaffe et al., 2001; Swerdlow et al., 2008). The clinical presentation mainly includes leukemic forms and tumors affecting predominantly lymphatic organs, such as the lymph nodes or spleen, or nonlymphatic organs, such as the skin or central nervous system (CNS). Both solid and circulating phases are not infrequently present together in lymphoid neoplasms rendering distinction between "leukemia" and "lymphoma" artificial in many cases. The natural course run by the different diseases ranges from the rather indolent, like in some types of chronic lymphocytic leukemia (CLL) or follicular lymphoma (FL), to the highly aggressive, as exemplified by Burkitt lymphoma (BL).

Historically, the main division of mature lymphoid neoplasms has been between Hodgkin disease, nowadays called Hodgkin lymphoma (HL), and non-Hodgkin lymphoma (NHL). More than 99% of HL and approximately 85% of mature lymphoid neoplasms generally derive from lymphoid cells of the B-lineage, the remainder being derived from the T/natural killer (NK)-cell lineage.

Considering this biological and clinical heterogeneity as well as the relatively easy access to samples from lymphatic malignancies, it is not surprising that a huge number of chromosomal aberrations have been described in mature lymphoid neoplasms and also that many of them are nonrandom or even specific (Mitelman et al., 2014). Since Manolov and Manolova (1972) first described a 14q+ marker chromosome in BL and Zech et al. (1976) identified the marker as stemming from a t(8;14)(q24;q32), the first characteristic translocation to be identified in a malignant lymphoma, the karyotypes of several thousand mature lymphoid neoplasms have been made publicly available, and many of the recurrent aberrations have been molecularly characterized. Novel cryptic chromosomal rearrangements are continuously being identified using molecular cytogenetic approaches such as fluorescence *in situ* hybridization (FISH); microarray-based technologies, including array comparative genomic hybridization (aCGH); and lately also high-throughput sequencing (for reviews, see Martín-Subero et al., 2003a, 2003b; Schwaenen et al., 2003; Dewald et al., 2004; Kearney and Horsley, 2005; Ventura et al., 2006; Nieländer et al., 2007; Wolff

Cancer Cytogenetics: Chromosomal and Molecular Genetic Aberrations of Tumor Cells, Fourth Edition.
Edited by Sverre Heim and Felix Mitelman.
© 2015 John Wiley & Sons, Ltd. Published 2015 by John Wiley & Sons, Ltd.

et al., 2007; Kluin and Schuuring, 2011; Campo, 2013). The new information obtained via a variety of recently introduced techniques is constantly refining our picture of the chromosome aberrations of malignant lymphomas and chronic lymphoproliferative disorders, deepening our understanding of how molecular and chromosomal rearrangements are crucial events in tumorigenesis. Nevertheless, the new technologies in no way render superfluous the cytogenetic analysis of banded chromosomes in metaphase plates: also, high-throughput sequencing suffers from limitations in, among other things, the ability to detect chromosomal fusions with the breakpoints in repetitive-rich sequences (e.g., Robertsonian translocations or rearrangements involving immunoglobulin loci). The new technological approaches refine our diagnostic abilities rather than supplant the time-honored, older techniques.

Classification of mature lymphoid neoplasms

The identification and characterization of recurrent chromosomal changes in the tumor cells has influenced and continues to have a major impact on the classification of mature lymphoid neoplasms (Harris et al., 1994; Jaffe et al., 2001, Swerdlow et al, 2008; Kluin and Schuuring, 2011). For example, mantle cell lymphoma (MCL) was only accepted as a separate entity once the translocation t(11;14)(q13;q32) leading to cyclin D1 activation through the juxtaposition of *CCND1* to *IGH* was identified as a genetic hallmark of this disease (Banks et al., 1992).

A problem when assessing the many cytogenetic studies providing the data on which this chapter is based is that most of them were performed before the publication and widespread acceptance of the "WHO classification of tumors of hematopoietic and lymphoid tissues" (Jaffe et al., 2001; Swerdlow et al., 2008). Thus, in many instances, the diagnosis then given is no longer considered valid, or it may not even exist anymore; in fact, it is for this very reason that the title of the present chapter has been changed from that of the earliest editions of *Cancer Cytogenetics*. Usually, the new classification reflects an increased understanding of disease biology; for example, what was formerly called t(11;14)-positive

CLL or B-cell prolymphocytic leukemia (B-PLL) is today, based on modern immunophenotyping analyses, mostly diagnosed as (leukemic) MCL or "MCL-like" disease (van der Velden et al., 2014), and cases of true t(11;14)-positive CLL or B-PLL are hardly recognized any longer. In addition, the detection of novel cytogenetic correlations and the increased use of new gene expression and sequencing technologies make regular revisions of the WHO classification necessary. The present chapter widely relies on the 2001 and 2008 WHO classifications (Swerdlow et al., 2008). However, as we write, a new update of the WHO classification is already being prepared. We therefore try to comment also on such genetic findings that are likely to be featured there.

The WHO classification groups lymphoid neoplasms according to four main criteria, namely, their clinical, morphologic, immunophenotypic, and genetic features. The relative diagnostic importance of these parameters differs among diseases; there is no one "gold standard" (Jaffe et al., 2001; Swerdlow et al., 2008). For each neoplasm, a cell of origin (COO) is postulated. Often, this putative COO represents the stage of differentiation rather than the cell in which the actual initial transforming event occurred, since the latter is not known with certainty. Therefore, the classification is widely based on how we perceive normal B- and T-cell developments to proceed.

The cytogenetic findings will be presented under the main headings "Mature B-cell neoplasms," "Mature T-cell and NK-cell neoplasms," and "HL." For the convenience of the reader, at the beginning of each section, a tabular comparison of the most important relevant classification systems is provided.

B- and T-cell development and physiological B- and T-cell receptor rearrangements

The development and maturation of B and T lymphocytes are tightly regulated processes that take place in the bone marrow, peripheral blood, and lymphoid organs. Every maturation stage is characterized by physiological genetic rearrangements and expression of certain surface molecules and cytokines (for reviews, see Küppers et al., 1999;

Küppers and Dalla-Favera, 2001; Küppers, 2005; Seifert et al., 2013).

The cells of the immune system are able to recognize multiple antigens through a multitude of different antigen-specific receptors. This diversity is generated through programmed intrachromosomal rearrangements of the genes encoding immunoglobulins (*IG*) in B lymphocytes and T-cell receptors (*TCR*) in T lymphocytes. These genes contain all or part of gene segments for variability (*V*), diversity (*D*), joining (*J*), and constant (*C*) sequences. Rearrangements of the V, D, and J genes are responsible for the great variability and specificity of the immune system.

Immunoglobulin molecules, also called antigen receptors or antibodies, are composed of Ig heavy chains (IgH) and light chains, either kappa (Igκ) or lambda (Igλ). These proteins are encoded by the *IGH* locus at chromosome band 14q32, *IGK* at 2p12, and *IGL* at 22q11. The *IGH* gene is composed of *V*, *D*, *J*, and *C* gene segments (Figure 11.1), whereas *IG* light-chain genes lack *D* segments. In the bone marrow, B-cell development is initiated by rearrangements of *IGH* and *IGK/L* loci in B-cell progenitors. The so-called *V(D)J* in *IGH* (Figure 11.1) and *VJ* in *IGK/L* recombinations create a functional Ig. This Ig, of IgM isotype but also IgD in mature B cells, is expressed on the surface of B cells and is essential for cell development and survival. Those cells that produce nonfunctional rearrangements die by apoptosis. B cells leave the bone marrow to become mature, naive (not exposed to antigen) cells that travel through the bloodstream to secondary lymphoid organs such as the lymph nodes, spleen, and mucosa-associated lymphoid tissue (MALT). There, the B cells that interact with antigens through membrane-bound Ig are clonally selected and undergo a process of proliferation and differentiation to create a germinal center. The genomic DNA is then modified by receptor editing, class switching, and somatic hypermutation.

Receptor editing is a process by which an originally expressed antibody polypeptide chain, usually a light chain, is replaced by another one. The process is mediated by secondary rearrangements

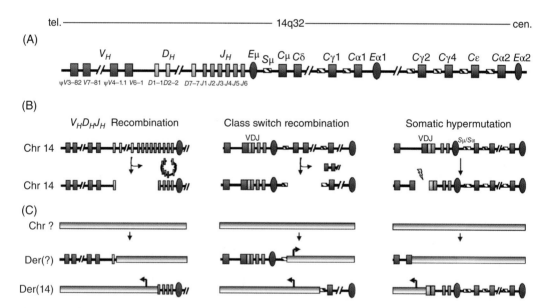

Figure 11.1 Schematic representation of the mechanisms leading to *IGH* translocations in B-cell malignancies (based on Willis and Dyer, 2000; Küppers and Dalla-Favera, 2001). (A) *IGH* locus germline configuration displaying variable (V_H), joining (J_H), diversity (D_H), and constant (*C*) regions. Switch regions (black and white rectangles) lie upstream of each constant region with the exception of Cδ. Eμ and Eα enhancers are shown in red. (B) Schematic representation of the *VDJ* recombination, class switch recombination, and somatic hypermutation mechanisms. (C) Formation of *IGH* translocations. Depending on the breakpoint location at 14q32, the *IGH* locus may deregulate proto-oncogenes in both partner chromosomes through the translocation (elbowed arrows).

of the variable region segments. Some B cells change their Ig isotype from IgM and IgD to IgG, IgA, or IgE, a process called class switching (Figure 11.1). This event is mediated through further recombinations of the *IGH* locus, by which DNA between switch regions immediately upstream of the constant regions is deleted. Somatic hypermutation is the process by which mutations are introduced into the variable sequences of *IG* genes to increase the affinity for the antigen. Eventually, some of these cells with mutant antibodies expressing increased affinity are released to the peripheral blood as antibody-secreting cells, plasma cells, or long-lived memory cells.

The T-cell receptor is a heterodimer composed of either α and β or γ and δ chains. The genes encoding these proteins are *TCRA/D* located at 14q11, *TCRB* at 7q34, and *TCRG* at 7p14. The process by which these genes are assembled to make a functional T-cell receptor is similar to that occurring at *IG* loci in B cells. However, in contrast to B lymphocytes, T lymphocytes proliferate and differentiate along several different developmental pathways generating distinct subpopulations of mature T cells.

Chromosomal translocations involving IG and TCR loci

The IG loci, including both the *IGH* locus in 14q32 and the *IGK* and *IGL* light-chain loci in 2p12 and 22q11, respectively, are recurrently involved in many chromosomal translocations in mature B-cell malignancies (Table 11.1). In contrast, the TCR loci are rather seldom involved in structural aberrations in mature T-cell neoplasms with the notable exception of T-cell prolymphocytic leukemia (T-PLL), in which *inv(14)(q11q32)* and its variant *t(14;14)(q11;q32)* are present in approximately 80%, with some of the remaining cases showing the rare but recurrent t(X;14)(q28;q11) (discussed in the following).

The frequency of IG translocations in different subtypes of mature B-cell malignancies is quite variable. For some diseases, like BL with its *t(8;14) (q24;q32)* and light-chain variants or MCL with its *t(11;14)(q13;q32)*, one or a group of distinct IG translocations are pathognomonic for the disease and, hence, detectable in more than 95% of all cases

(Fu et al., 2005; Hummel et al., 2006; Jares et al., 2007; Salaverria and Siebert, 2011). In other instances, like diffuse large B-cell lymphoma (DLBCL) or multiple myeloma (MM), IG translocations are detectable in roughly half of the cases but recombining with a large number of partners (Siebert et al., 2001; Kuehl and Bergsagel, 2002; Lenz et al., 2007; Martin et al., 2010; Walker et al., 2013a). At the other end of the spectrum, CLL is notable for its lack of IG translocations, and when breaks do occur at 14q32 in this disease, they do not always involve the *IGH* locus (Nowakowski et al., 2005; Wlodarska et al., 2007). IG translocations in malignant B cells may be multiple and may involve both *IGH* and a light-chain locus. A common combination is that of a *t(14;18)(q32;q21)* in FL being followed by a t(8;14) or a corresponding t(2;8) or t(8;22) variant at transformation to DLBCL (Knezevich et al., 2005; Martín-Subero et al., 2005). Such cases, known as "double-hit" lymphomas if they involve IG translocations to *MYC* and either *BCL2* or *BCL6*, are usually clinically aggressive and respond poorly to chemotherapy (Aukema et al., 2011). The latter example also shows that hardly any of the IG translocations in mature B-cell neoplasms is completely specific for a certain lymphoma subtype. For example, t(11;14) (q13;q32) is recurrent in both MCL and MM and t(14;18)(q32;q21) is recurrent in both FL and DLBCL but also recurrently occurs, in addition to trisomy 12, in CLL. The t(8;14)(q24;q32) and its variants can occur, besides in BL, in almost any kind of mature B-cell neoplasm, including CLL, MCL, FL, and DLBCL (Karsan et al., 1993; Au et al., 1999, 2000, 2002, 2004; Sen et al., 2002; Majid et al., 2007; Aukema et al., 2011, 2014; Horn et al., 2011; Put et al., 2012; de Oliveira et al., 2014).

Chromosomal translocations affecting IG loci that look identical at the cytogenetic level are also often identical in terms of which genes they target. In contrast, sometimes different partner genes are involved in seemingly identical translocations, like *BCL2* and *MALT1*, which recombine with *IGH* in t(14;18)(q32;q21) in FL and MALT lymphoma, respectively (Tsujimoto et al., 1985; Sanchez-Izquierdo et al., 2003; Streubel et al., 2003).

As outlined earlier, all IG loci are subject to multiple physiological breaks as part of recombination events during B-cell development. Chromosomal

Table 11.1 Chromosomal translocations and other structural aberrations affecting the *IGH* locus in 14q32, the *IGK* locus in 2p12, or the *IGL* locus in 22q11 in mature B-cell malignancies other than multiple myeloma

Translocation	Lymphoma/leukemia subtype	Translocation partner	References
t(1;14)(p22;q32)*	Mucosa-associated lymphoid tissue (MALT) lymphoma	BCL10	Willis et al. (1999) and Zhang et al. (1999)
t(1;14)(q21;32)	Diffuse large B-cell lymphoma	MUC1	Dyomin et al. (2000) and Gilles et al. (2000)
t(1;14)(q21;32)	Diffuse large B-cell lymphoma	IRTA1	Sonoki et al. (2004)
t(1;14)(q21;32)	Follicular lymphoma	FCGR2B	Chen et al. (2001a)
t(1;22)(q21;q11)	Follicular lymphoma	FCGR2B	Callanan et al. (2000)
t(2;7)(p11;q21)	Indolent B-cell lymphoproliferative disorders, splenic marginal zone lymphoma	CDK6	Corcoran et al. (1999) and Parker et al. (2011, 2013)
t(2;14)(p13;q32)	B-CLL, immunocytoma	BCL11A	Satterwhite et al. (2001)
t(3;14)(p14;q32)	MALT lymphoma, diffuse large B-cell lymphoma	FOXP1	Streubel et al. (2005)
t(3;14)(q27;q32)*	Diffuse large B-cell lymphoma, follicular lymphoma	BCL6	Kerckaert et al. (1993) and Ye et al. (1993a)
t(4;14)(q24;q32)	Posttransplant lympho-proliferative disorder	BANK1	Yan et al. (2014)
t(6;14)(p21;q32)*	Diffuse large B-cell lymphoma, other B-cell lymphomas	CCND3	Sonoki et al. (2001)
t(6;14)(p25;q32)	(Pediatric) diffuse large B-cell lymphoma/FL3B	IRF4	Salaverria et al. (2011)
t(6;14)(q15;q32)	Aggressive B-cell lymphoma, NOS	BACH2	Kobayashi et al. (2011)
t(7;14)(q21;q32)*	Splenic lymphoma with villous lymphocytes	CDK6	Corcoran et al. (1999)
t(8;14)(q24;q32)*	Burkitt lymphoma/leukemia, diffuse large B-cell lymphoma, B-cell prolymphocytic leukemia, multiple myeloma	MYC	Taub et al. (1982)
t(9;14)(p13;q32)	Lymphoplasmacytoid immunocytoma, other B-NHL	PAX5	Busslinger et al. (1996) and Iida et al. (1996)
t(9;14)(q33;q32)	Pediatric chronic myeloid leukemia (blast crisis)	LHX2	Nadal et al. (2012)
t(10;14)(q24;q32)	Diffuse large B-cell lymphoma	NFKB2 (LYT10)	Neri et al. (1991)
t(11;14)(p13;q32)	Diffuse large B-cell lymphoma, follicular lymphoma	CD44	Hu et al. (2012)
t(11;14)(q13;q32)*	Mantle cell lymphoma, B-cell chronic lymphocytic leukemia, B-cell prolymphocytic leukemia, splenic lymphoma with villous lymphocytes	CCND1 (BCL1)	Motokura et al. (1991) and Rosenberg et al. (1991)
t(11;14)(q23;q32)	Primary mediastinal B-cell lymphoma	PAFAH1A2	Lecointe et al. (1999)
t(11;14)(q23;q32)	Diffuse large B-cell lymphoma	RCK	Akao et al. (1992)
t(12;14)(p13;q32)*	Mantle cell lymphoma	CCND2	Gesk et al. (2006) and Herens et al. (2008)
t(12;14)(q24;q32)	Burkitt lymphoma/leukemia, multiple myeloma	BCL7A	Zani et al. (1996)

(Continued)

Table 11.1 (*Continued*)

Translocation	Lymphoma/leukemia subtype	Translocation partner	References
del(14)(q24q32)	Chronic lymphocytic leukemia, low-grade B-NHL	ZFP36L1	Pospisilova et al. (2007) and Nagel et al. (2009a)
t(14;15)(q32;q11–13)	Diffuse large B-cell lymphoma	BCL8	Dyomin et al. (1997)
t(14;16)(q32;q24)	B-ALL (L3), aggressive B-cell lymphoma, NOS	CBFA2T3/ACSF3	Salaverria et al. (2012)
t(14;16)(q32.33;q24.1)	Diffuse large B-cell lymphoma	IRF8	Bouamar et al. (2013) and Tinguely et al. (2014)
t(14;18)(q32;q21)*	Follicular lymphoma, diffuse large B-cell lymphoma	BCL2	Tsujimoto et al. (1985)
t(14;18)(q32;q21)	Marginal zone lymphoma	MALT1	Sanchez-Izquierdo et al. (2003) and Streubel et al. (2003)
t(14;19)(q32;q12)	Diffuse large B-cell lymphoma	CCNE1	Nagel et al. (2009b)
t(14;19)(q32;q13)	Diffuse large B-cell lymphoma	SPIB	Lenz et al. (2007)
t(14;19)(q32;q13)*	B-cell chronic lymphocytic leukemia, other B-NHL	BCL3	Ohno et al. (1990)
t(14;22)(q32;q11)	Low-grade B-NHL	IGL?	Aamot et al. (2005a)
t(X;14)(p11;q32)	MALT lymphoma	GPR34	Ansell et al. (2012)

Modified from Willis and Dyer (2000), Siebert et al. (2001), and Dyer (2013). Only those translocations are shown in which the partner genes have been identified by molecular cloning or equivalent technique(s). Several other IG translocations have been identified and in part FISH mapped, like t(14;19)(q32;p13) (Micci et al., 2007), but await unambiguous identification of the partners.
*Variants with IG light-chain loci in 2p12 and 22q11 have been described.

translocations are supposed to derive from mistakes in these recombination processes. Depending on whether mistakes occur in the V(D)J joining process, during class switching, or as by-products of somatic hypermutation, the chromosomal breakpoints are found in different regions of the IG loci (Figure 11.1). With regard to the heavy-chain locus, class switch-associated translocations affect the centromeric part of *IGH* in 14q32 containing the segments for the constant Ig regions, VDJ-associated translocations mostly affect the middle part of *IGH* that contains the J-segments, and somatic hypermutation-associated translocations predominantly affect the telomeric part of the *IGH* locus containing the V-segments (Willis and Dyer, 2000; Küppers and Dalla-Favera, 2001; Kuehl and Bergsagel, 2002; Dyer, 2003; Küppers, 2005).

The location of the IG breakpoint is supposed to reflect the developmental stage at which the translocation occurs in a B cell. In line with this hypothesis, the t(11;14)(q13;q32) of MCL, which is supposed to occur in a pregerminal center cell in

the bone marrow through an unsuccessful *VDJ* rearrangement, mostly involves a J-segment. In contrast, the cytogenetically identical translocation in a subset of MM stems from a failed class switch recombination event supposed to take place in or after the germinal center and affects the region containing the constant genes (Walker et al., 2013a). Similarly, IG translocations in FL are, with very rare exceptions (Fenton et al., 2002), supposed to derive from mistakes in the *VDJ*-recombination process, whereas those occurring in DLBCL, MM, or CLL mostly involve class switch regions (Willis and Dyer, 2000; Küppers and Dalla-Favera, 2001; Kuehl and Bergsagel, 2002; Dyer, 2003; Küppers, 2005). Remarkably, the t(8;14)(q24;q32) in endemic BL mostly involves the J, whereas the same translocation in sporadic BL mostly affects a constant region, indicating that different pathogenetic mechanisms are at work in the two situations (reviewed in Boxer and Dang, 2001; Küppers and Dalla-Favera, 2001).

The consequences of the IG translocations are activation of intact oncogenes through deregulation mediated by enhancer segments within the IG loci. Only on rare occasions are fusion transcripts of the IG and oncogenes generated (Willis and Dyer, 2000). Although *VDJ*-associated translocations of the *IGH* locus lead to activation of the oncogene on the der(14) through juxtaposition of the translocated oncogene with the *IGH* enhancer, class switch translocations in principle can activate oncogenes on both derivative chromosomes because the centromeric *IGH* enhancer(s) remains on der(14), whereas the telomeric IGH enhancer(s) translocates to the derivative partner chromosome (Figure 11.1). This explains why recurrent loss of the der(11) t(11;14) in MCL or der(14)t(4;14) in MM does not affect deregulation of the *CCND1* and *MMSET* genes in 11q13 and 4p16, respectively (Santra et al., 2003). In translocations affecting the *IGK* and *IGL* light-chain loci, the oncogenic activation usually takes place on the derivative partner chromosomes to which the enhancer elements were translocated (Willis and Dyer, 2000; Küppers and Dalla-Favera, 2001; Kuehl and Bergsagel, 2002; Dyer, 2003; Küppers, 2005; Kroenlein et al., 2012; Shimanuki et al., 2013).

The breakpoint on the derivative partner chromosome can be located 3′ or 5′ of the target oncogene because the transforming mechanism is deregulated expression through aberrant juxtaposition with the IG enhancer rather than creation of a gene fusion or promoter substitution. Enhancers can exert their activity over distances of several hundred kilobases. In BL, for example, the breakpoints affecting the *MYC* gene can be located up to almost 1 Mb centromeric of *MYC* in t(8;14) and telomeric of *MYC* in t(8;22) and t(2;8) (Joos et al., 1992a, 1992b; Einerson et al., 2006; Kroenlein et al., 2012). Remarkably, the breakpoints of the t(8;14) in 8q24 vary between endemic and sporadic BL with the former more frequently affecting the far 5′ (centromeric) part of the *MYC* locus (reviewed in Boxer and Dang, 2001; Küppers and Dalla-Favera, 2001). This variability of the breakpoints, which can also be observed in *MYC* translocations affecting non-IG loci, can pose considerable diagnostic problems if FISH is applied for their detection (Bertrand et al., 2007; May et al., 2010).

Gene deregulation may occasionally be a consequence of an insertion rather than a translocation. Thus, both *BCL2* and *CCND1* have been observed to be inserted into the *IGH* locus in cases of FL and MCL in rearrangements that functionally mimic the t(14;18) and t(11;14), respectively (Vaandrager et al., 2000; Fenton et al., 2004). Although the biological consequences of such insertions appear to be identical to those of regular translocations, their pathogenetic origins would appear to involve different DNA breaks.

Exceptions to the general rule that the recurrent translocations of mature lymphoid neoplasms rarely give rise to fusion genes occur predominantly in MALT lymphoma and T-cell lymphomas. In the former, the specific *t(11;18)(q21;q21)* leads to *API2–MALT1* fusion (Akagi et al., 1999; Dierlamm et al., 1999). In the latter, *t(2;5)(p23;q35)* as well as its rare variants lead to fusion of the anaplastic lymphoma kinase (*ALK*) gene in 2p23 with the nucleophosmin (*NPM*) gene or, in the case of variants, other partners (Morris et al., 1994). Finally, rare cases of peripheral T-cell lymphoma with an *ITK–SYK* fusion due to a *t(5;9)(q33;q22)* have been reported (Streubel et al., 2006b). Recent data from high-throughput sequencing studies suggest that a number of rare fusion genes remain to be discovered in lymphatic neoplasms.

The most common rearrangement of a non-IG locus in mature lymphoid neoplasms is the targeting of the *BCL6* gene in 3q27 that takes place in a variety of translocations with a multitude of chromosomal partners (Ueda et al., 2002a; Ohno, 2006) (Table 11.2). Common to all these translocations is that they lead to promoter substitution and, consequently, deregulation of the *BCL6* gene (Ohno, 2004, 2006; Jardin et al., 2007). Other oncogenes known to be targets of IG translocations are sometimes juxtaposed directly next to each other through translocations, such as *PAX5* and *MYC* through a t(8;9)(q24;p13) and *BCL6* and *MYC* through t(3;8)(q27;q24) in t(14;18)-positive FL (Bertrand et al., 2007; Sonoki et al., 2007; Johnson et al., 2009; Aukema et al., 2011). How the supposed *MYC* deregulation in these translocations occurs is so far unknown though an enhancer mechanism seems likely. There is no evidence for interposition of IG sequences like in t(8;14;18) (q24;q32;q21), a recurrent aberration in FL progression, in which both *MYC* and *BCL2* are deregulated from a common IG fragment between them (Dyer et al., 1996; Knezevich et al., 2005).

Table 11.2 Chromosomal translocations affecting the *BCL6* locus in 3q27 in mature B-cell neoplasms

Translocation	Band of partner locus	BCL6 partner gene	References
t(1;3)(q25;q27)	1q25	GAS5	Nakamura et al. (2008)
t(2;3)(p12;q27)	2p12	IGK	Bastard et al. (1992), Deweindt et al. (1993), and Akasaka et al. (2000a, 2000b)
t(3;3)(q25;q27)	3q25	MBNL1	Akasaka et al. (2003)
	3q26	SIATI	Akasaka et al. (2003)
t(3;3)(q27;q27)	3q27	ST6GAL1	Akasaka et al. (2003)
t(3;3)(q27;q27)	3q27	EIF4A2	Yoshida et al. (1999a) and Akasaka et al. (2003)
t(3;3)(q27;q29)	3q29	TFRC	Yoshida et al. (1999a), Akasaka et al. (2000a, 2000b), and Chen et al. (2006)
t(3;4)(q27;p11–13)	4p11–13	RhoH/TTF	Dallery et al. (1995) and Akasaka et al (2000a, 2000b), (2003)
t(3;6)(q27;p22)	6p21–22	HIST1H4I	Akasaka et al. (1997), (2000a, 2000b), Kurata et al. (2002), and Schwindt et al. (2006)
t(3;6)(q27;p21)	6p21	PIM1	Yoshida et al. (1999a), Akasaka et al. (2000a, 2000b), and Kaneita et al. (2001)
t(3;6)(q27;p21)	6p21	SFRS3/SRP20	Chen et al. (2001b) and Ohno (2006)
t(3;6)(q27;q15)	6q15	U50HG/SNHG5	Tanaka et al. (2000) and Akasaka et al. (2003)
t(3;7)(q27;p12)	7p12	IKZF1	Hosokawa et al. (2000) and Kaneita et al. (2001)
t(3;7)(q27;q32)	7q32	MIR29/FRA7H	Schneider et al. (2008)
t(3;8)(q27;q24.1)	8q24	MYC	Bertrand et al. (2007) and Sonoki et al. (2007)
t(3;9)(q27;p24)	9p24	DMRT1	Chen et al. (2006)
t(3;9)(q27;p11)	9p11	GRHPR	Akasaka et al. (2003)
t(3;11)(q27;q23)	11q23	BOB1/OBF1/POU2AF1	Galiègue-Zouitina et al. (1996) and Ohno (2006)
t(3;12)(q27;p13)	12p13	GAPDH	Montesinos-Rongen et al. (2003) and Chen et al. (2006)
t(3;12)(q27;q12)	12q12	LRMP	Akasaka et al. (2003)
t(3;12)(q27;q23–24)	12q23	NACA	Akasaka et al. (2000a, 2000b)
t(3;13)(q27;q14)	13q14	LCP1	Galiègue-Zouitina et al. (1999)
t(3;14)(q27;q32)	14q32	IGH	Bastard et al. (1992), Deweindt et al. (1993), Kerckaert et al. (1993), Ye et al. (1993b), and Akasaka et al. (2003)
t(3;14)(q27;q32)	14q32	HSP89A	Akasaka et al. (2000a, 2000b), Xu et al. (2000), Montesinos-Rongen et al. (2003), and Chen et al. (2006)
t(3;16)(q27;p13)	16p13	CIITA	Yoshida et al. (1999a, Kaneita et al. (2001), and Akasaka et al. (2003)
t(3;16)(q27;p11)	16p11	IL21R	Ueda et al. (2002b)
t(3;19)(q27;q13)	19q13	NAPA	Akasaka et al. (2003)
t(3;22)(q27;q11)	22q11	IGL	Bastard et al. (1992), Deweindt et al. (1993), Miki et al. (1994b), and Schimanuki et al. (2013)

Data from http://atlasgeneticsoncology.org/Genes/BCL6ID20.html, Ueda et al. (2002a), and Ohno (2006). Chromosomal bands of *BCL6* partner genes and gene annotations may in individual cases be mapped to different chromosomal bands in various publications.

Cytogenetic evolution in lymphoid neoplasms

Several cytogenetic and subsequent molecular genetic studies have led to the concept that the neoplastic process in many mature lymphoid malignancies follows a multistep model similar to that proposed for colorectal cancer and other malignancies. It is widely assumed that a primary genetic alteration of a tumor clone initiates lymphomagenesis. Primary alterations are usually present in the stemline of a tumor. Chromosomal translocations, like several of the *IG* and *TCR* translocations, are most common as primary genetic alterations and can serve as valuable diagnostic markers. However, it should be noted that what in one disease setting may constitute a primary change in another may occur as a secondary abnormality.

As shown in mouse transgenic models, the primary genetic alteration is often not sufficient to drive lymphomagenesis (reviewed in Willis and Dyer, 2000). Moreover, by sensitive molecular techniques, several primary genetic alterations like t(14;18), t(11;14), or t(2;5) can also be detected in healthy individuals, sometimes at surprisingly high levels (Limpens et al., 1995; Maes et al., 2001; Bäsecke et al., 2002; Biagi and Seymour, 2002; Roulland et al., 2004, 2014). Although our understanding is limited as to what extent the cells carrying the translocations are susceptible to neoplastic transformation, it has been shown that the presence of t(14;18)-positive precursors is predictive for the later development of FL and the precursors can actually progress into FL (Roulland et al., 2014). These findings have contributed to the view that additional genetic changes are required for the full neoplastic phenotype of a mature lymphoid malignancy to emerge. The aberrations that bring about this phenotypic transformation are usually called secondary genetic changes. Consequently, the vast majority of lymphomas with a defined primary change, like t(14;18)-positive FL or t(11;14)-positive MCL, carry also secondary alterations (Johansson et al., 1995). The so-called tertiary genetic events may occur in some lymphomas and are associated with the transformation of an indolent malignancy to more aggressive

forms. As will be described subsequently, secondary and tertiary chromosomal alterations in lymphoid malignancies predominantly lead to gain or loss of genetic material, whereas recurrent, balanced translocations—with the exception of translocations affecting the *MYC* locus in chromosome band 8q24—seem to be uncommon as secondary events. The number of secondary genetic aberrations, be they driver or passenger mutations, usually increases during disease progression (Knight et al., 2012; Beà et al., 2013; Landau et al., 2013; Bauer et al., 2014). As a rule of thumb, within a given lymphoma subtype, the prognosis is inversely related to the complexity of the karyotype or the extent of the secondary changes.

Secondary genetic aberrations may be present in only a subset of cells of a given tumor, and different secondary aberrations may be present in different subclones that may become the dominant clone during disease progression or at relapse (Knight et al., 2012; Landau et al., 2013; de Rossi et al., 2014). Tumors of the same type (and harboring the same primary event) might thus show variation in terms of secondary aberrations. Nevertheless, the pattern of secondary changes in mature lymphoid neoplasms is not random but rather seems to depend on the nature of the primary event. Some primary genetic alterations like t(11;18)(q21;q21) are hardly ever associated with cytogenetically detectable secondary aberrations (Horsman et al., 1992; Ott et al., 1997b; Barth et al., 2001). Other translocations such as t(1;14)(p22;q32) are associated with a highly conserved set of secondary events, including trisomy of chromosomes 3, 12, and 18. FL with t(14;18)(q32;q21) show different, distinctive patterns of secondary changes suggesting different pathways of germinal center B-cell transformation (Höglund et al., 2004). T-PLL is characterized by an extraordinary conservation of both primary and secondary genetic changes (reviewed by Dürig et al., 2007).

The mutational pattern in a given lymphoma might not only depend on the primary aberration but also on the mutational mechanisms active in this particular case (Alexandrov et al., 2013). Several mutational mechanisms have been shown to be operative in lymphomas contributing to the mutational landscape of the tumors. Indeed, the genome of a lymphatic neoplasm usually contains between 1000 and several thousand mutations (Puente et al., 2011; Richter et al., 2012; Alexandrov et al., 2013). Based on the mutational patterns detected, it has been shown for FL that disease progression can occur from the initial tumor or from a clonal progenitor not found at initial diagnosis (Okosun et al., 2014; Pasqualucci et al., 2014). Remarkably, at least in FL, chromosomal, molecular, and epigenetic changes seem to evolve, concordantly suggesting that a chromatin-acting factor like *CREBBP* or *MLL2* may be one of the regulators of clonal evolution (Loeffler et al., 2015). Tumor heterogeneity and its impact on progression and clinical outcome will become a major topic for future studies in lymphoma genetics (Knight et al., 2012; Schuh et al., 2012; Landau et al., 2013; Rossi et al, 2014; Suguro et al., 2014).

Chromosomal aberrations common to multiple subtypes of mature lymphoid neoplasms

In the following sections, the most common cytogenetic changes in mature lymphoid neoplasms will be discussed in the context of the disease subtypes in which they are most prominent. It should nevertheless be emphasized that many aberrations are recurrent in several or even all kinds of mature lymphoid neoplasms. These might constitute primary aberrations in some of them but are more likely to be secondary or even tertiary aberrations in the majority. Probably, the best example of such a low-specific change is deletion of 6q.

Deletions of the long arm of chromosome 6 are frequent in all types of mature lymphoid neoplasms including HL. The incidence in different studies varies from roughly 5% in CLL to 30% in DLBCL up to even higher frequencies in T/NK-cell disorders. The deletions have mostly been interpreted as terminal. Band 6q21 seems to be the one most often affected. Offit et al. (1993) reviewed the chromosome 6 abnormalities in 459 consecutively ascertained karyotypically abnormal cases of NHL and suggested that three minimally common deleted regions could be discerned: a distal one encompassing 6q25–27, a second one involving the

more proximal band 6q21, and the third one located between the two others involving band 6q23. Several loss of heterozygosity (LOH), molecular cytogenetic, and aCGH studies have meanwhile narrowed down critical regions in 6q to 6q21, 6q23.3, and 6q27. These studies have identified recurrent inactivation of the *PRDM1/BLIMP1* gene in 6q21 in activated B-cell-type (ABC-DLBCL) and T-cell lymphomas (Pasqualucci et al., 2006; Tam et al., 2006; Iqbal et al., 2009). Moreover, a minimally common deleted region in 6q23.3 containing the *TNFAIP3 (A20)* and *PERP* genes has been identified in FL and ocular adnexal marginal zone B-cell lymphoma (MZL), and mutations inactivating *TNFAIP3* have been detected in classical Hodgkin lymphoma (cHL) and primary mediastinal B-cell lymphomas (PMBCL) (Ross et al., 2007; Giefing et al., 2008; Honma et al., 2008; Schmitz et al., 2009).

The descriptions in this chapter will focus on chromosomal changes as they are detected by chromosome banding techniques. It needs to be stressed that the "real" frequencies of chromosomal aberrations may be underestimated if this approach is the only one taken, without help from molecular cytogenetic techniques like FISH and CGH, which can also be used to examine paraffin-embedded samples. Therefore, though the contribution of these techniques is not the prime concern of this book, data thus obtained will often be referred to as they have contributed mightily to the current picture of the cytogenetic changes of mature lymphoid neoplasms. For reviews focusing on the application of FISH and CGH in lymphoid neoplasms, the reader may be well advised to consult Martín-Subero et al. (2003a), Dewald et al. (2004), Kearney and Horsley (2005), Ventura et al. (2006), Wolff et al. (2007), and Kluin and Schuuring (2011). Finally, the exponentially fast-growing number of studies using aCGH and single-nucleotide polymorphism (SNP) chip-based technologies as well as next-generation sequencing will not be discussed in detail here. A review of the findings obtained by array-based technologies was published by Nieländer et al. (2007), and databasing of the findings has been initiated (http://www.progenetix. net/). For mutational patterns derived from high-throughput sequencing, the reader is referred to constantly updated databases such as COSMIC http://cancer.sanger.ac.uk/cancergenome/projects/cosmic/) and the reports from the ICGC project (http://www.icgc.org/).

Mature B-cell neoplasms

A comparative overview of the different subtypes of mature B-cell neoplasms recognized by the Kiel, REAL, and WHO classifications is provided in Table 11.3. The clinically most relevant chromosomal aberrations are summarized in Table 11.4.

Chronic lymphocytic leukemia/small lymphocytic lymphoma, B-PLL

Chronic lymphocytic leukemia and its nodal variant, small lymphocytic lymphoma (CLL/SLL, here covered together under the acronym CLL), account for 7% of all B- and T/NK-cell lymphomas. A variant of CLL is Mu heavy-chain disease (Jaffe et al., 2001; Swerdlow et al., 2008). B-PLL is an extremely rare disease (1% of lymphocytic leukemias) in which prolymphocytes exceed 55% of lymphoid cells in the blood. CLL/SLL (including variant CLL) and B-PLL are distinct entities within the WHO classification (Jaffe et al., 2001). Nevertheless, from the cytogenetic point of view, since these two diseases show considerable overlap, they are discussed together here.

Chromosome aberrations can be detected in more than 80% of CLL/B-PLL cases studied after appropriate stimulation (Dicker et al., 2006; Mayr et al., 2006; Haferlach et al., 2007). The different frequencies of abnormal clones that have been reported in CLL/B-PLL are attributable to differences in disease stage, treatment, and culture conditions, as well as to which mitogens were used by the various investigators.

The neoplastic cells of CLL (and, to a somewhat less extent, of B-PLL) have very low spontaneous mitotic activity, and their response to conventional mitogens is poor. In earlier studies, 40–50% of CLL showed clonal chromosome aberrations, and common recurrent abnormalities such as *trisomy 12*, *del(13q)*, *del(11q)*, and *del(17p)* could be identified (reviewed by Döhner et al., 1997a, 1997b, 1999; Stilgenbauer et al., 2000). Interphase cytogenetic studies using CGH and locus-specific FISH probes showed that the true incidences of

chromosomal aberrations in CLL differed from what was seen by chromosome banding analysis (Döhner et al., 1993, 1997a, 1997b; Stilgenbauer et al., 1993; Bentz et al., 1995). On the one hand, the percentage of cases showing aberrations at all was significantly higher using interphase cytogenetics (>80%), mostly due to the lack of aberrant metaphases identified by banding analysis and the presence of cytogenetically cryptic deletions. On the other hand, the relative proportion of CLL with trisomy 12 was higher and of deletions was lower by banding cytogenetics than by interphase FISH. Again, this might reflect proliferation advantages or disadvantages of the aberrant clone as well as the fact that some of the deletions are cryptic (Stockero et al., 2006). Particularly pronounced was this difference for del(13q), which can be detected in approximately half of all CLL by FISH but only in some 10% by banding studies (Stilgenbauer et al., 2000).

The introduction of new mitogenic agents, CD40L, and, probably most importantly, immunostimulatory CpG-oligonucleotide DSP30 and IL-2 has dramatically improved the figures (Buhmann et al., 2002; Dicker et al., 2006; Mayr et al., 2006; Haferlach et al., 2007). In a study of 506 CLL samples comparing FISH and banding analysis, 500 cases (99%) were successfully stimulated for metaphase generation (Haferlach et al., 2007). Aberrations were detected in 415 of 500 (83%) cases by banding cytogenetics and in 392 of 500 (78%) cases by FISH. Whereas chromosome banding analysis detected 832 abnormalities, FISH detected only 502, demonstrating that the latter approach underestimates the cytogenetic complexity of CLL (Haferlach et al., 2007). This study confirmed that CLL is characterized mainly by genomic imbalances and that reciprocal translocations are rare. A subgroup of CLL with complex aberrant karyotype (16%) was identified. Mayr et al. (2006), using last-generation mitogen stimulation, found translocations in 33 of 96 (34%) CLL. The majority of the chromosomal translocations occurred within complex karyotypes and were unbalanced. A similar conclusion was drawn also by Van Den Neste et al. (2007) who detected translocations in 42% of CLL with 73% of them being unbalanced. Patients with translocations presented with more complex

Table 11.3 Comparison of the Kiel, REAL, and WHO classifications of B-cell malignancies*

Kiel classification	REAL classification	WHO classification (2001)	WHO classification (2008)
Peripheral B-cell neoplasms	Mature (peripheral) B cell neoplasms		
B-lymphocytic, B-CLL, B-PLL	B-CLL/B-PLL/small lymphocytic lymphoma	**B-CLL**/small lymphocytic lymphoma	**B-CLL**/small lymphocytic lymphoma
Lymphoplasmacytoid immunocytoma	Variant B-CLL: with plasmacytoid differentiation	Variant B-CLL: with monoclonal gammopathy/ plasmacytoid differentiation B-PLL	Variant B-CLL: with monoclonal gammopathy/ plasmacytoid differentiation B-PLL
Lymphoplasmacytic immunocytoma	Lymphoplasmacytoid lymphoma	Lymphoplasmacytoid lymphoma	Lymphoplasmacytic lymphoma
Centrocytic	Mantle cell lymphoma	Mantle cell lymphoma Variant: blastoid	Mantle cell lymphoma
Centroblastic, centrocytoid subtype			Morphologic variants: blastoid, pleomorphic, small cell, marginal zone-like
Centroblastic–centrocytic, follicular	Follicular center lymphoma, follicular grades I and II	**Follicular lymphoma, grades I and II**	**Follicular lymphoma, grades I and II**
Centroblastic–centrocytic, diffuse	Follicular center lymphoma, diffuse, small cell*		
Centroblastic, follicular	Follicular center lymphoma, follicular grade III	Follicular lymphoma, grade III	Follicular lymphoma, grade III
		Cutaneous follicle center lymphoma	Cutaneous follicle center lymphoma
	Extranodal marginal zone B-cell lymphoma (low-grade B-cell lymphoma or MALT)	**Extranodal marginal zone B-cell lymphoma of MALT type**	**Extranodal marginal zone B-cell lymphoma of MALT type**
Monocytoid lymphoma, including marginal zone lymphoma	Nodal marginal zone B-cell lymphoma*	Nodal marginal zone B-cell lymphoma*	Nodal marginal zone B-cell lymphoma*
	Splenic marginal zone B-cell lymphoma*	Splenic marginal zone B-cell lymphoma*	Splenic marginal zone B-cell lymphoma*
Hairy cell leukemia	Hairy cell leukemia	Hairy cell leukemia	Hairy cell leukemia
Plasmacytic	Plasmacytoma/myeloma	**Plasma cell myeloma/ plasmacytoma**	**Plasma cell myeloma/ plasmacytoma**
Centroblastic (monomorphic, polymorphic, and multilobated subtypes)	Diffuse large B-cell lymphoma	**Diffuse large B-cell lymphoma**, variants: centroblastic, immunoblastic, T cell/ histiocyte rich, lymphomatoid granulomatosis type, anaplastic large B cell, plasmablastic	**Diffuse large B-cell lymphoma, NOS**
			Morphologic variants: centroblastic, immunoblastic, anaplastic **Subtypes:** T cell/ histiocyte rich

(Continued)

Table 11.3 (*Continued*)

Kiel classification	REAL classification	WHO classification (2001)	WHO classification (2008)
			Primary CNS Primary cutaneous, leg type EBV-positive DLBCL of the elderly **Other**: DLBCL associated with chronic inflammation Lymphomatoid granulomatosis type ALK+ DLBCL HHV8-associated multicentric Castleman disease
B-immunoblastic B-large cell anaplastic lymphoma			
	Primary mediastinal large B-cell lymphoma	Subtypes: mediastinal (thymic) large B-cell, primary effusion lymphoma, intravascular large B-cell lymphoma	Primary mediastinal (thymic) large B-cell lymphoma
			Primary effusion lymphoma Intravascular large B-cell lymphoma
Burkitt lymphoma	Burkitt lymphoma High-grade B-cell lymphoma, Burkitt-like*	Burkitt lymphoma Burkitt cell leukemia	Burkitt lymphoma Burkitt cell leukemia/B-ALL L3
		Atypical Burkitt lymphoma	**B-cell lymphoma, unclassifiable, with features intermediate between DLBCL and BL**

Data from Lennert et al. (1975), Harris et al. (1994), Jaffe et al. (2001), and Swerdlow et al. (2008).
Bold letters represent the most common subtypes.
*Provisional entity.

karyotypes ($P < 0.001$). It has to be stressed that the chromosomal translocations in CLL seem to be quite heterogeneous. A common theme is nevertheless that many breakpoints are located in regions showing recurrent loss in CLL, like 13q14, and are associated with microdeletions (Herholz et al., 2007). Particularly in CLL with complex karyotypes, translocations often lead to loss of the *TP53* locus in 17p13; vice versa, complex karyotypes are associated with 17p abnormalities and *TP53* mutations (Fink et al., 2006).

Although trisomy 12, del(13q), del(11q), and del(17p), the major aberrations in CLL (Figure 11.2), mostly are seen independently of one another, any combination of the four may be detected. Moreover, del(11q) and del(17p) are recurrently observed as secondary changes that occur during disease progression.

Trisomy 12 is the most frequently reported chromosome abnormality in CLL based on chromosome banding analysis, where it has been detected in nearly one-third of all cytogenetically abnormal cases. By FISH, around 15% of all CLL show trisomy 12. Partial trisomy 12 can be detected in 10–20% of cases (Döhner et al., 1993), and a minimal common gained region has been confined

Table 11.4 Overview of frequent and diagnostically relevant chromosomal aberrations in the most common mature B-lymphoid neoplasms

Neoplasm	Cytogenetic aberration	Frequency (%)
B-cell chronic lymphocytic leukemia/small lymphocytic lymphoma	del(13q)	~50
	+12	~15
	del(11q)	15–20
	del(6q), del(17p)	~5
	t/der(14)(q32)	4–20
Mantle cell lymphoma	t(11;14)(q13;q32)	>95
	del(11q), del(13q), der(3q)	10–50
	+12, del(1p), del(6q), del(9p), del(17p)	5–15
Extranodal marginal zone B-cell lymphoma of MALT type	t(11;18)(q21;q21)	15
	t(14;18)(q32;q21) involving *MALT1*	11
	t(3;14)(p14;q32)	<10
	t(1;14)(p22;q32)	<2
	+3/3q, +18/18q	30
Follicular lymphoma	t(14;18)(q32;q21) and variants involving *BCL2*	80–90
	t(3q27)	<10 (FL1/2)–55 (FL3b)
	+X, +7, +12/12q, +18/18q, +der(18)t(14;18), del(6q), del(10q), del(17p), dup(1q), der(1p)	>10
Diffuse large B-cell lymphoma	t(3q27)	20–40
	t(14;18)(q32;q21)	20–30 (GCB)
	t(8;14)(q24;32)/t(8q24)	5–15 (GCB > ABC)
	+3/3q, +18/18q, +19q, del(6q), del(9p)	10–40 (ABC)
	+1q, +2p13–16, +7, +11q, +12/12q	10–40 (GCB)
	+9/9p23–24, +2p13–16	50–90 (PMBCL)
B-cell lymphoma, unclassifiable, with features intermediate between DLBCL and BL	t(8q24)/*MYC*	40–60 (FISH)
	t(14;18)/*IGH–BCL2*	35–50 (FISH)
	t(3q27)/*BCL6*	10–30 (FISH)
Burkitt lymphoma	t(8;14)(q24;q32) and variants	100
	dup(1q)	~30–50
	+7, +12	~10–30
Plasma cell myeloma/ plasmacytoma	t(4;14)(p16;q32), t(11;14)(q13;q32), t(14;16)(q32;q23)	~20
	t(6;14)(p25;q32), t(8;14)(q24;q32)	5
	Other t(14q32)	
	Total t(14q32)	~40–60
	−13, del(13q)	15–50
	dup(1q), del(6q), del(11q)	5–20

to 12q13 (Dierlamm et al., 1997; Schwaenen et al., 2004). Some cases with trisomy 12 also have other chromosomal aberrations. Among the recurrent additional changes are *t(14;19)(q32;q13)* leading to *IGH–BCL3* fusion (Martín-Subero et al., 2007), *t(14;18)(q32;q21)* leading to *IGH–BCL2* fusion (Karsan et al., 1993; Sen et al., 2002), and a *del(14) (q24q32)* with one breakpoint in the *IGH* locus (Tilly et al., 1988; Pospisilova et al., 2007) (Figures 11.3 and 11.4). Moreover, *trisomy 19* and/ or *trisomy 18* can be seen in a subset of cases

(Schwaenen et al., 2004; Sellmann et al., 2007). It is unknown whether trisomy 12 in those cases that have additional changes is the primary or secondary abnormality; there are data supporting both views. Trisomy 12 has sometimes been associated with atypical morphology that may resemble MCL (Döhner et al., 1999; Matutes et al., 1999; Athanasiadou et al., 2006; Fink et al., 2006).

Structural abnormalities of 13q, t/del(13q), are found in approximately 20% of all cytogenetically abnormal cases (Stilgenbauer et al., 2000; Stockero

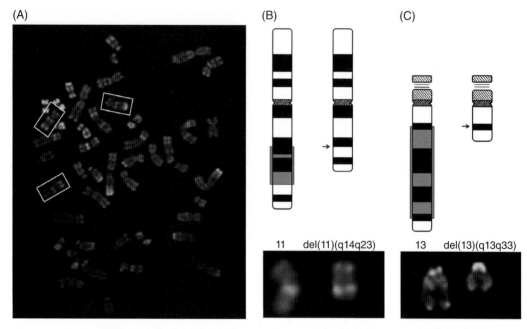

Figure 11.2 Recurrent chromosomal aberrations in CLL and related lymphoid neoplasms. Fluorescence R-banding. (A) Metaphase with trisomy 12. (B) Ideogram and partial karyotype showing del(11)(q14q23). (C) Ideogram and partial karyotype showing del(13)(q13q33).

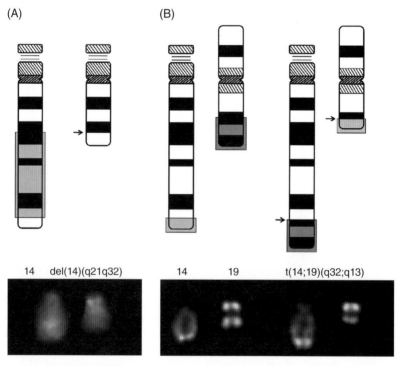

Figure 11.3 Recurrent chromosomal aberrations in CLL and related lymphoid neoplasms. Fluorescence R-banding. (A) Ideogram and partial karyotype with interstitial deletion in 14q cytogenetically assigned to 14q21q32. (B) Ideogram and partial karyotype showing t(14;19)(q32;q13) involving *IGH* and *BCL3*.

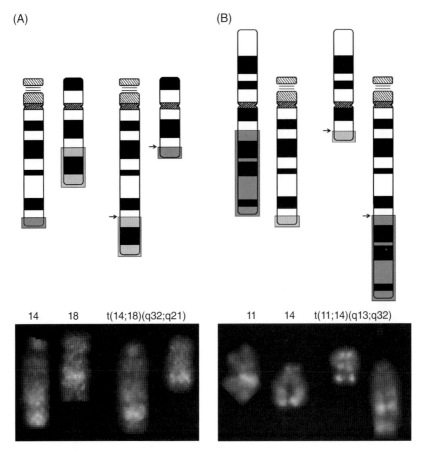

(A)   (B)

14   18   t(14;18)(q32;q21)   11   14   t(11;14)(q13;q32)

Figure 11.4 Translocations t(14;18)(q32;q21) and t(11;14) (q13;q32). Fluorescence R-banding. (A) Ideogram and partial karyotype with t(14;18)(q32;q21) involving *IGH* and *BCL2*. (B) Ideogram and partial karyotype with t(11;14) (q13;q32) involving *IGH* and *CCND1*.

et al., 2006; Herholz et al., 2007). By FISH, the deletion is detectable in 50% of CLL (Döhner et al., 2000). The deletions target the band 13q14, and several nonoverlapping minimal regions of loss have been described. FISH analyses usually apply probes spanning the markers *D13S25*, *D13S319*, or *D13S272* and have detected biallelic losses in 13q14 in a considerable number of cases. Molecular targets of the deletions might be the noncoding genes *miR-15*, *miR-16*, *DLEU1/BCMS*, or *DLEU2* (Wolf et al., 2001; Calin et al., 2002). Elegant mouse model studies suggest the named microRNAs to be major players in CLL initiation (Klein et al., 2010), but there is also good evidence that other genes in 13q14 play a role in CLL progression. Larger (type II) deletions in 13q14 encompassing the *RB1* gene have been associated with an unfavorable

prognosis in CLL as compared to smaller (type I) deletions not affecting *RB1* (Ouillette et al., 2011). Although the *RB1* gene does not seem to be a major pathogenetic target of 13q14 deletions in this disease, it still may play a progressional role (Stilgenbauer et al., 1995; Migliazza et al., 2001; Wolf et al., 2001; Ouillette et al., 2008).

Deletions of 11q, with a minimal region of loss in 11q22, have in earlier studies been detected in only 5% of cases. The deletions are usually small and interstitial, del(11)(q21–22q22–23). By FISH, these deletions can be detected in 15–20%. Most deletions lead to loss of the *ATM* gene, which shows mutation of the second allele in a sizable subset (Döhner et al., 1997b, 2000; Schaffner et al., 1999; Austen et al., 2007). Notably, a few deletions do not encompass the *ATM* gene but instead affect the closely telomeric *FDX* locus (Stilgenbauer et al., 1996).

Structural abnormalities of 17p, t/del(17p), are found in approximately 5% of all cytogenetically abnormal CLL, especially in complex karyotypes (Fink et al., 2006; Mayr et al., 2006). By FISH using a probe for the *TP53* gene, the deletion is found in 5–10%, and mutations of the second allele can be detected in a subset of these cases (Döhner et al., 2000). In B-PLL, the frequency of *TP53* alterations appears to be much higher, perhaps 50%.

Depending on the strictness of the diagnostic criteria, including whether chromosome alterations are used to make a diagnosis, the percentage of *translocations targeting the IG loci* in CLL/B-PLL, that is, t(14q32) and the two variants t(2p12) and t(22q11), has varied between a few percent and up to 20% (Döhner et al., 2000; Nowakowski et al., 2005; Nelson et al., 2007). The translocation *t(11;14)(q13;q32)* leading to *IGH–CCND1* recombination has been reported to be present in 20% of B-PLL and somewhat less commonly in CLL (Figure 11.4). Today, however, most of these cases would be diagnosed as MCL though rare cases of true t(11;14)-positive CLL/B-PLL might exist (van der Velden et al., 2014). *t(14;19)(q32;q13)*, often associated with trisomy 12, is a recurrent translocation in CLL but also occurs in many other B-cell malignancies, where the spectrum of additional chromosomal alterations is mostly more complex (Martín-Subero et al., 2007). *t(2;14)(p13;q32)* leading to *IGH–BCL11A* fusion is another rare but recurrent translocation in CLL (Satterwhite et al., 2001; Küppers et al., 2002). *t(14;18)(q32;q21)* leading to *IGH–BCL2* recombination and the variants *t(18;22)(q21;q11)* and *t(2;18)(p12;q21)* are secondary alterations in a subset of CLL with trisomy 12 but can also be observed in cases of benign lymphocytosis. *t(8;14)(q24;q32)* leading to *IGH–MYC* as well as the corresponding light-chain variants targeting *MYC* can also be observed in CLL, albeit rarely; all these changes seem to be somewhat more common in B-PLL (Merchant et al., 2003; Reddy et al., 2006). Other t(14q32) with rare or private partners are continuously being identified in CLL. A recurrent t(1;6)(p35.3;p25.2) involving the *IRF4* gene has been reported in a series of CLL with unmutated *IGHV* genes and might constitute a primary change in this context

(Michaux et al., 2005). Finally, trisomies for chromosomes 3, 8, and 18 as well as del(6q) and changes leading to gains of 3q26–27, 2p24–25, and 8q24 are among the broad spectrum of changes that have been observed rarely, but recurrently, in CLL (Döhner et al., 1999; Stilgenbauer et al., 1999).

Since the first fully sequenced CLL genomes were published in 2011, a wealth of novel molecular data on this disease has emerged (Puente et al., 2011; Quesada et al., 2011). Nevertheless and perhaps remarkably, these whole-genome sequencing studies have not added major findings to the cytogenetic landscape. The various chromosomal imbalances described earlier seem to be considerably more prevalent than any recurrent gene mutation. The sequencing studies confirmed that *TP53* and *ATM* are recurrently mutated in CLL, but with the notable exception of *SF3B1* and probably *NOTCH1*, no gene seems to be mutated in more than 10% of cases. One of the conclusions of sequencing studies has been that CLL is genetically heterogeneous, with a relatively large number of genes being recurrently mutated at low frequencies and only a few genes being mutated in up to 10–15 % of all patients (Puente et al., 2011; Martínez-Trillos et al., 2013; Quesada et al., 2013). Novel candidate genes implicated in the pathogenesis of CLL emerging from these studies also include *POT1*, *MYD88*, and *DDX3X* (Puente et al., 2011; Quesada et al., 2011, 2013; Martínez-Trillos et al., 2013).

Clinical correlations in CLL/SLL and B-PLL

The prognostic impact of chromosomal aberrations in CLL/B-PLL is well established through several extensive studies within or outside clinical trials (Juliusson et al., 1990; Döhner et al., 1995, 1997a, 1997b, 2000; Chevallier et al., 2002; Caballero et al., 2005; Kröber et al., 2006; Ripollés et al., 2006; Grever et al., 2007; Nelson et al., 2007; Stilgenbauer et al., 2007). Consistently, del(17p)/loss of the *TP53* locus has been described as an unfavorable prognostic marker indicating bad response or even resistance to various kinds of therapy. del(11q) has been shown to be associated with nodal disease and also constitutes an unfavorable marker. The study by Döhner et al. (2000) showed 17p deletion, 11q deletion, trisomy 12, normal karyotype, and 13q deletion as the sole abnormality to be associated with a median survival of 32, 79, 114, 111, and 133 months, respectively. Patients in the 17p– and 11q–groups had more advanced disease than did those in the three other groups. Patients with 17p deletions had the shortest median treatment-free interval, and those with 13q deletions had the longest. In multivariate analysis, the presence or absence of a 17p deletion, the presence or absence of an 11q deletion, age, Binet stage, the serum lactate dehydrogenase level, and the white cell count gave significant prognostic information. These findings have been confirmed in various independent studies, and clinical trials have been initiated treating patients with del(17p) and del(11q) according to high-risk protocols. Moreover, the unfavorable cytogenetic changes have been shown to be associated also with other poor prognostic features such as lack of somatic hypermutation of the *VH* region and CD38 and ZAP70 expression (Kröber et al., 2002; Hallek et al., 2008). Whether the size of 13q deletions influences prognosis in patients participating in clinical trials warrants further investigation.

In the more recent cytogenetic studies using new stimulants, chromosomal translocations were found to be associated with 17p abnormalities and *TP53* mutations, that is, unfavorable prognostic features. Correspondingly, patients with translocations had a significantly higher therapy failure rate and displayed significantly shorter treatment-free and overall survival as compared to patients without translocations (Mayr et al., 2006; Haferlach et al., 2007). Multivariate analyses showed the prognostic impact of translocations to be independent of established clinical and laboratory risk factors. Haferlach et al. (2007) showed the subgroup with complex aberrant karyotypes to be significantly associated with an unmutated VH status and CD38 expression. Thus, all these studies indicate (unbalanced) chromosomal translocations and/or chromosomal complexity to be novel and independent prognostic markers in CLL. Nevertheless, the results of clinical trials comparing the prognostic relevance of conventional and interphase cytogenetic findings are pending.

Sequencing studies point to some degree of association between cytogenetic and molecular genetic disease features although the overall interaction picture seems to be rather complex.

NOTCH1 mutations have been associated with trisomy 12, whereas *SF3B1* mutations were associated with 11q deletions (Villamor et al., 2013; Wang et al., 2011). Alterations of *TP53*, *NOTCH1*, and *SF3B1* have been recurrently associated with inferior outcome and may constitute independent prognostic factors depending on the clinical features and treatment of the patient cohort (Baliakas et al., 2015). In contrast, *MYD88* mutations might characterize a subset of predominately young CLL patients with favorable outcome (Martínez-Trillos et al., 2014). Presumably, future genomic risk profiling in CLL will combine the detection of recurrent imbalances with mutational analysis of a set of recurrently altered genes.

NOTCH1 mutation has been associated with the most common type of acute transformation of CLL, that is, the development of a diffuse large cell malignant lymphoma known as *Richter's syndrome* (Fabbri et al., 2011). Remarkably, the (epi)genetic makeup of Richter's transformed DLBCL is heterogeneous and differs from de novo DLBCL (Scandurra et al., 2010; Chigrinova et al., 2013; Fabbri et al., 2013; Rinaldi et al., 2013a). No specific chromosome aberrations have yet been described in this entity though trisomy 12 and del(11q) seem to be recurrent. In line with other B-cell lymphomas showing progression, high-risk aberrations including del(17p), t(8q24)/+8q24, inactivation of the *CDKN2A* gene in 9p21, and chromosomal complexity seem to be common findings during transformation of CLL (Beà et al., 2002; Chigrinova et al., 2013; Fabbri et al., 2013). Frequently mutated genes in Richter's syndrome include those involved in CLL progression and resistance to chemotherapy (*TP53* disruption and *NOTCH1* activation) as well as some not previously implicated in CLL or Richter's syndrome pathogenesis such as genes involved in chromatin remodeling (*ARID1A/B*, *MLL2*, *IRX5*) (Fabbri et al., 2013).

Mantle cell lymphoma (MCL)

MCL comprises 3–10% of all NHL. The incidence increases with age and there is a strong male predominance (Jaffe et al., 2001; Swerdlow et al., 2008). Though its composition of monomorphous small- to medium-sized lymphoid cells resembling centrocytes led to the historical assignment of MCL to "low-grade" lymphomas, this disease is characterized by a progressive clinical course. MCL has been largely incurable with conventional chemotherapy though modern strategies using immunotherapy and transplantation seem to be promising (Kluin-Nelemans et al., 2012). Remarkably, nearly all MCL show some level of leukemic disease, and there is ample evidence that many MCL in the past have been incorrectly classified as CLL or other low-grade lymphomas. The morphology is variable and a blastic variant of MCL exists, which morphologically mimics acute lymphoblastic leukemia. Indeed, MCL was not recognized as a distinct lymphoma entity until the cytogenetic hallmark of the disease, t(11;14) (q13;q32), was identified (Banks et al., 1992).

The *t(11;14)(q13;q32)* is present in virtually all cases of MCL independent of their morphologic or clinical presentation (Fu et al., 2005). In approximately 20% of the cases, the translocation is part of a more complex rearrangement, and loss of the der(11) is a recurrent phenomenon (Gazzo et al., 2005; Siebert et al., unpublished results). Chromosome numbers are mostly in the diploid or hyperdiploid range except in blastic variants, which have been associated with polyploidy (Ott et al., 1997a). By interphase FISH, the t(11;14) can be detected in the peripheral blood or bone marrow at a level of at least 1% of the cells in around 60% of cases (Böttcher et al., 2008).

The translocation t(11;14)(q13;q32) juxtaposes the *CCND1* (formerly *BCL1*, *PRAD1*) gene next to the *IGH* locus leading to overexpression of cyclin D1, something that is also detectable by immunohistochemistry. The breakpoints in the *IGH* locus mostly affect the region containing the *J*-segments and, thus, differ from the breakpoints of the cytogenetically identical translocation t(11;14) in plasma cell disorders (MM, monoclonal gammopathy of undetermined significance (MGUS)), which cluster to the region containing the *IGH* constant segments. The breakpoints in 11q13 in MCL spread out over more than 150 kb, though some clustering to, for example, the major translocation cluster (MTC) is seen (Willis and Dyer, 2000; Küppers and Dalla-Favera, 2001; Kuehl and Bergsagel, 2002; Dyer, 2003; Küppers, 2005; Jares et al., 2007). Nevertheless, the heterogeneity of the 11q13 breakpoints prevents reliable detection of the t(11;14) by conventional PCR methods, and FISH is recommended if the translocation cannot be

identified by chromosome banding analysis (Martín-Subero et al., 2003a; van Dongen et al., 2003).

Extremely rare variants of the t(11;14) are sometimes seen, namely, t(2;11)(p12;q13) involving *IGK* and *CCND1* and t(11;22)(q13;q11) involving *IGL* and *CCND1* (Brito-Babapulle et al., 1987; Komatsu et al., 1993; Wlodarska et al., 2004; Rocha et al., 2011).

Gene expression profiling studies have recently identified very occasional cases of true t(11;14)-negative MCL, which instead of activation of *CCND1* show expression of the other D-type cyclins (Fu et al., 2005). These cases of t(11;14)-negative MCL show frequent *IG–CCND2* rearrangements, most commonly with an *IGK* or *IGL* partner, and overall show a profile of genomic imbalances and clinical behavior that is similar to that of t(11;14)-positive MCL (Salaverria et al., 2013a).

In addition to the t(11;14)-negative MCL with *IG–CCND2* rearrangements (Gesk et al., 2006; Herens et al., 2008; Wlodarska et al., 2008; Quintanilla-Martinez et al., 2009; Salaverria et al., 2013a), some cases with *t(6;14)(p21;q32)* and the corresponding light-chain variants (breakpoints in 6p21 and 2p12 or 22q11) targeting *CCND3* in 6p21 have also been identified (Wlodarska et al., 2008); however, these translocations do not seem to be specific for MCL but rather occur in plasma cell disorders and DLBCL (Shaughnessy et al., 2001; Sonoki et al., 2001). Finally, a t(14;19)(q32;q13) involving *CCNE1* was identified in a DLBCL (Nagel et al., 2009b).

Au et al. (2002) reviewed data on 78 MCL from British Columbia as well as 167 cases of t(11;14)-associated lymphoproliferative disease retrieved from the literature. Common aneuploidies included −Y, −13, −9, −18, +3, and +12. Frequent structural rearrangements included +3q, +12q, del(6q), del(1p), del(13q), del(10q), del(11q), del(9p), and del(17p). The most common breakpoint clusters were 1p21–22, 1p31–32, 1q21, 6q11–15, 6q23–25, 8q24, 9p21–24, 11q13–23, 13q12–14, and 17p12–13. These findings are not only generally representative of the pattern of secondary chromosome aberrations in t(11;14)(q13;q32)-positive MCL but also show marked resemblance to the pattern of secondary changes in CLL, not least with regard to the structural chromosome aberrations leading to deletions of 13q14, 11q22, and 17p. In contrast to what is seen in CLL, the deletions of 13q14 in some cases affect the *RB1* gene in MCL (Pinyol et al., 2007). The deletions of 11q22 and 17p target the *ATM* and *TP53* genes, respectively, in subsets of cases (Greiner et al., 2006). Complete or partial trisomy 3 leading to gain of 3q27 as well as trisomy 12 is common. Other recurrent structural aberrations lead to deletions of 1p22, 8p21, 9p21, 9q22, and 10p12–13 and high-level amplifications of, for example, the *BMI1* gene in 10p12. t(8q24) with various partners and gain of 8q24 have been described, particularly during disease progression (Hao et al., 2002; Michaux et al., 2004).

From a series of chromosomal CGH (cCGH) and, more recently, aCGH studies, a consistent pattern of chromosomal imbalances in MCL has emerged largely confirming the gain–loss pattern seen by banding cytogenetics and underscoring the nonrandom nature of the genomic imbalances that characterize this disease (de Leeuw et al., 2004; Kohlhammer et al., 2004; Rubio-Moscardo et al., 2005; Tagawa et al., 2005a; Salaverria et al., 2007). Moreover, partial uniparental disomy is common and recurrently targets regions of common chromosomal deletions in MCL (Nieländer et al., 2006; Bea et al., 2009; Vater et al., 2009). These array-based data and the molecular consequences of the detected imbalances have been comprehensively reviewed by Nieländer et al. (2007). As compared to classical MCL, the nonnodal indolent form shows significantly less chromosomal imbalances as seen by array-based profiling (Royo et al., 2012; Navarro et al, 2012). Whole-genome and whole-exome sequencing has revealed many recurrently mutated genes including *NOTCH1/NOTCH2*, *ATM*, *CCND1*, *TP53*, and *BIRC3* and the chromatin modifier genes *WHSC1*, *MLL2*, and *MEF2B* (Kridel et al., 2012; Beà et al., 2013; Rahal et al., 2014).

Clinical correlations in MCL

From the clinical point of view, detection of t(11;14) (q13;q32) is important to differentiate MCL from other low-grade B-cell lymphomas, in particular if immunophenotyping is inconclusive. One should keep in mind, however, that also some few cases of true CLL and splenic lymphoma with villous lymphocytes (SLVL) seem to exist with this translocation, cases that run a more indolent course.

The prognostic impact of secondary chromosomal aberrations in t(11;14)(q13;q32)-positive MCL has not yet been rigorously tested. In general, the nonnodal variant associated with leukemic and splenic presentation and favorable outcome shows a significantly lower number of genomic imbalances than classical MCL, but 17p deletions indicate a poor prognosis in both (Royo et al., 2012; Navarro et al., 2012). This is in line with other studies showing gains of 3q as well as losses in 9q22 and 17p to be prognostically unfavorable karyotype abnormalities (Rubio-Moscardo et al., 2005; Salaverria et al., 2007; Espinet et al., 2010; Sarkozy et al., 2014). One FISH study has suggested that loss of 13q14 was associated with an inferior outcome (Sander et al., 2008). The analyses comparing prognosis and karyotypic complexity in classical MCL are still inconclusive (Katzenberger et al., 2008; Espinet et al., 2010; Sarkozy et al., 2014). The data were largely retrieved from retrospective series of patients who had not been treated according to modern strategies, and so all apparent correlations shall have to await confirmation in new prospective trials.

Lymphoplasmacytic lymphoma (Waldenström macroglobulinemia)

Lymphoplasmacytic lymphoma (LPL) (Waldenström macroglobulinemia (WM)) is characterized by excessive proliferation of an IgM-producing clone of malignant plasmacytoid cells. The cells typically have both surface and cytoplasmic IgM. They also secrete substantial amounts of IgM resulting in a monoclonal spike on serum protein electrophoresis. A variant is gamma heavy-chain disease (Jaffe et al., 2001).

The translocation *t(9;14)(p13;q32)* juxtaposing the *PAX5* gene from 9p13 next to the *IGH* locus has been claimed to be specific for LPL and to be present in up to 50% of cases (Iida et al., 1996). Recent studies have shown that this frequency was dramatically overestimated and that t(9;14) can also occur in other types of mature B-lymphoid neoplasms (Ohno et al., 2000; Cook et al., 2004; Poppe et al., 2005; Baró et al., 2006). Other translocations described in mature B-cell neoplasms seem to be rare in LPL/WM though cases with t(11;18) (q21;q21) have been described; however, these cases might constitute variants of marginal zone lymphoma (see following text).

LPL/WM shows the whole spectrum of aberrations already described in CLL, though generally at lower frequencies. The most frequently detected change in LPL/WM is del(6q), and a deletion of 6q21 has been identified by FISH in 42% of cases (Schop et al., 2002). As outlined earlier, this 6q−aberration is rather unspecific. Losses in *PLEKHG1*, *HIVEP2*, *ARID1B*, and *BCLAF1* constitute the most common deletions within chromosome 6 in WM (Hunter et al., 2014). Recent high-resolution studies have shown also losses of *PRDM2* (93%), *BTG1* (87%), *MKLN1* (77%), *LYN* (60%), and *FOXP1* (37%) (Hunter et al., 2014).

Significant advances in our understanding of WM have come from genome sequencing studies that showed the L265P mutation in *MYD88* in more than 90% of patients with WM and also in half of all patients with IgM MGUS, which may be a precursor of WM (Treon et al., 2012; Xu et al., 2013). *MYD88* mutations have been suggested to be associated with 6q deletions (Kim et al., 2014). Other recurrently altered genes in WM include *CXCR4* and *ARID1A* in 27 and 17% of patients, respectively (Hunter et al., 2014).

Hairy cell leukemia

Hairy cell leukemia (HCL) comprises only 2% of all lymphoid leukemias. It is a neoplasm of small B-lymphoid cells with oval nuclei and abundant cytoplasm with "hairy" projections strongly expressing CD103, CD22, and CD11c. It is mainly a disease of middle-aged men; only 20% of the patients are female (Jaffe et al., 2001).

Not only because of the rarity of the disease but also because the hairy cells exhibit low spontaneous mitotic activity and are difficult to stimulate into mitosis, cytogenetic studies in HCL have been few. A normal karyotype, sometimes with nonclonal aberrations, was found in most cases. Structural rearrangements of the long arm of chromosome 14, *t/del(14q)*, are the changes most frequently reported (Sambani et al., 2001). t(14q32) with various partners but also recurrent interstitial deletions leading to loss of 14q22−24 have been recurrently described (Forconi et al., 2008; Nordgren et al., 2010). Structural aberrations of chromosome 5 also seem to be recurrent, and three CGH studies identified gains of or in 5q13−31 in 10−20% of HCL (Nessling et al., 1999; Ostergaard et al., 2001; Nordgren et al.,

2010). Nevertheless, in line with what was found in the cytogenetic studies, most cases show a balanced or near-balanced genome as documented by SNP array analysis (Rinaldi et al., 2013b).

In contrast to the rarity of copy number abnormalities, all or nearly all HCL patients carry the *BRAF* V600E (or other) mutation (Tiacci et al., 2011; Arcaini et al., 2012; Tschernitz et al., 2014).

Splenic marginal zone lymphoma

Splenic marginal zone lymphoma (SMZL) is a B-cell neoplasm of small lymphocytes that surround and replace the splenic white pulp germinal centers, efface the follicle mantle, and merge with a peripheral (marginal) zone of large cells. Lymphoma cells may be found in the peripheral blood as villous lymphocytes (SLVL) (Jaffe et al., 2001). Without analysis of the spleen, differential diagnosis from other low-grade leukemic B-cell neoplasms may be difficult.

Up to 40% of SMZL carry a *del(7q)* (Oscier et al., 1994; Troussard et al., 1998; Ott et al., 2000; Hernández et al., 2001; Solé et al., 2001; Gazzo et al., 2003). The breakpoints of the deletion vary, but most losses include the bands 7q31−32 (Gruszka-Westwood et al., 2003). A *miRNA-29* locus in 7q32 has been proposed as a target of the deletion and so has *IRF5* (Mateo et al., 1999; Ruiz-Ballesteros et al., 2007; Fresquet et al., 2012). Another region of recurrent loss has been defined in 7q22 (Robledo et al., 2011). More recently, whole-exome sequencing has identified three mutated candidate genes targeted by 7q deletions (*CUL1*, *EZH2*, and *FLNC*), with *FLNC* positioned within the 7q minimally deleted region (Parry et al., 2013). A second group of SZML seems to be characterized by *gain of 3q* (Solé et al., 2001). In addition, a recurrent *t(2;7) (p12;q21)* has been identified in a minority of SMZL cases activating the *CDK6* gene through juxtaposition next to the *IGK* locus (Corcoran et al., 1999; Brito-Babapulle et al., 2002) (Figure 11.5).

The *t(11;14)(q13;q32)* so typical of MCL has been identified also in SMZL. Though it cannot be ruled out that some of these cases may have been MCL, there seems to exist a true t(11;14)-positive SMZL in which this translocation is the sole change or at least part of a simple karyotype, contrasting what is seen in MCL (Brito-Babapulle et al., 1992; Troussard et al., 1998). Other recurrent

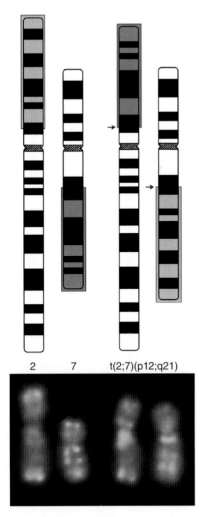

2   7   t(2;7)(p12;q21)

Figure 11.5 Translocation t(2;7)(p12;q21) in splenic marginal zone lymphoma. Fluorescence R-banding.

IGH translocations listed in Table 11.1 have also been observed in rare instances of SMZL. The wide range of additional chromosome aberrations that can be observed in SMZL seems to be rather unspecific.

The spectrum of imbalances in SMZL includes, besides 7q deletions, rearrangements of chromosomes 3 (20%), 6 (20%), 12 (20%), and 14 (10%) though also regions of minimal alteration in 4q22.1, 1q21.3–q22, 20q13.33, 2q23.3–q24.1, and 17p13 have been reported (Andersen et al., 2005; Robledo et al., 2011). Deletions in 7q and 6q have been proposed to be significantly associated (Traverse-Glehen et al., 2013).

Whole-exome sequencing studies identified mutations in *NOTCH2* as the most frequent (20–25%) lesion in SMZL (Parry et al., 2013). In addition to *NOTCH2*, other modulators or members of the NOTCH pathway are also recurrently targeted, including *NOTCH1*, *SPEN*, and *DTX1*. Additional recurrently mutated genes in SMZL are *CREBBP*, *CBFA2T3*, *AMOTL1*, *FAT4*, *FBXO11*, *PLA2G4D*, *TRRAP*, and *USH2A* (Rossi et al., 2012; Kiel et al., 2012; Parry et al., 2013; Martínez et al., 2014). *NOTCH2* mutations have been proposed to be associated with adverse clinical outcomes: relapse, histological transformation, and/or death in SMZL (Kiel et al., 2012).

Extranodal marginal zone B-cell lymphoma of MALT type

Extranodal marginal zone B-cell lymphoma of MALT comprises 7–8% of all B-cell lymphomas and up to 50% of primary gastric lymphomas (Jaffe et al., 2001). A role of antigenic stimulation by *Helicobacter pylori* in gastric MALT lymphoma, particularly in the initial phase of the disease, is nowadays taken for granted (Isaacson and Du, 2004, 2005; Du, 2007). *H. pylori* eradication by antibiotic treatment can cure at least 70% of patients with gastric MALT lymphomas of limited stages. A role of infectious agents has also been claimed for MZL at other sites like *Borrelia burgdorferi* in cutaneous MZL and *Chlamydia psittaci* in ocular adnexal MALT lymphomas. A special subtype previously known as alpha-chain disease but now called immunoproliferative small intestinal disease (IPSID) occurring in the Middle East and the Cape region of South Africa is associated with *Campylobacter jejuni* infection (Jaffe et al., 2001).

Chromosome banding analyses of extranodal MALT lymphomas, in particular gastrointestinal and pulmonal cases, are today limited by the fact that these lymphomas are now diagnosed from endoscopically obtained small biopsies. Resection of the stomach is no longer the preferred treatment in most cases since the introduction of antibiotic therapy, whereas most of the banding data derive from the time when gastrectomy was still performed (Horsman et al., 1992; Ott et al., 1997a). In addition to the banding studies, MALT lymphomas have been extensively characterized by interphase cytogenetic analyses.

There are three recurrent translocations associated with MALT lymphomas that are mutually exclusive but all of which target the same cellular complex that links B-cell receptor signaling to activation of *NFKB*. These translocations are t(11;18)(q21;q21), t(14;18)(q32;q21), and t(1;14)(p22;q32) (Figure 11.6). The *t(11;18)(q21;q21)* results in an *API2–MALT1* fusion gene (Akagi et al., 1999; Dierlamm et al., 1999). This translocation is almost always the only chromosomal abnormality (Horsman et al., 1992; Ott et al., 1997b; Barth et al., 2001). When molecular or molecular cytogenetic techniques are used, the t(11;18) can be detected in around 15% of all MALT lymphomas. It is seen in MALT lymphomas of all sites but particularly frequently in pulmonal (38–53%) and gastric (22–24%) cases (Streubel et al., 2004b; Ye et al., 2005).

t(14;18)(q32;q21) in MALT lymphomas deregulates the *MALT1* gene through juxtaposing it next to the *IGH* locus (Sanchez-Izquierdo et al., 2003; Streubel et al., 2003). This translocation is cytogenetically identical to the t(14;18)(q32;q21) involving *IGH* and *BCL2* and can only be discerned by molecular (cytogenetic) means. The t(14;18) is present in 11% of MALT lymphomas but probably more often in ocular adnexal (7–24%) and liver (17%) lymphomas than in the others (Streubel et al., 2004b; Ye et al., 2005).

The *t(1;14)(p22;q32)* is detectable in less than 2% of MALT lymphomas but might be more common in pulmonal cases (7–9%) (Streubel et al., 2004b; Ye et al., 2005). It juxtaposes the *BCL10* gene next to the *IGH* locus (Willis et al., 1999; Zhang et al., 1999). A variant t(1;2)(p22;p12)

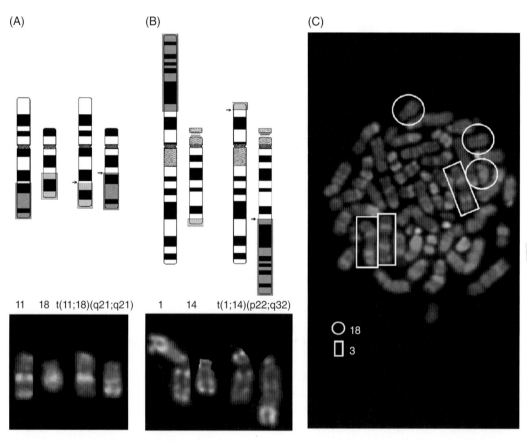

Figure 11.6 Recurrent chromosomal aberrations in marginal zone lymphomas of MALT type and related lymphoid neoplasms. Fluorescence R-banding. (A) Ideogram and partial karyotype with t(11;18)(q21;q21) involving *API2* and *MALT1*. (B) Ideogram and partial karyotype with t(1;14)(p22;q32) involving *BCL10* and *IGH*. (C) Metaphase with trisomy 3 and trisomy 18.

involving the *IGK* locus has been described (Chuang et al., 2007). Lymphomas with t(1;14) show a remarkably conserved pattern of additional changes comprising trisomies for chromosomes 3, 12, and 18 (Willis et al., 1999; Zhang et al., 1999; Siebert et al., unpublished results).

Trisomy 3 and *trisomy 18* can also be observed in translocation-negative MALT lymphomas (Figure 11.6). These changes are detected in 30% of all MALT lymphomas, particularly in intestinal (75%), salivary gland (57%), and orbital adnexal (35%) lymphomas (Ott et al., 1997a; Streubel et al., 2004b). In addition, chromosomal changes leading to partial gains of 3q (3q27), 9q (9q34), and 18q are common in MALT lymphomas (Zhou et al., 2006, 2007; Braggio et al., 2012). Array-based studies have shown MALT lymphoma to present significantly more often gains at 3p, 6p, and 18p as well as deletions at 6q23 than do other marginal zone lymphomas (Rinaldi et al., 2011). Indeed, the interstitial del(6q) is highly recurrent in MALT lymphomas and targets the *TNFAIP3* (*A20*) gene, in particular in ocular adnexal MALT lymphoma (Honma et al., 2008; Chanudet et al., 2010, 2011; Bi et al., 2012).

Streubel et al. (2005) identified a *t(3;14) (p14.1;q32)* in 10% of MALT lymphomas of the thyroid, ocular adnexa, and skin. Subsequent studies showed that this translocation, which juxtaposes the *FOXP1* gene from 3p14 next to the *IGH* locus, and other chromosomal changes targeting *FOXP1* also occasionally occur in other B-cell neoplasms, including DLBCL (Wlodarska et al., 2005; Fenton et al., 2006). Overall, *FOXP1* seems to be a promiscuous translocation partner, and a series of non-*IG* translocations involving *FOXP1* have been described leading to aberrant expression of N-truncated isoforms of the FOXP1 protein (Rouhigharabaei et al., 2014).

There is growing evidence that additional, hitherto unknown t(14q32) involving the *IGH* locus exist in lymphomas occurring at MALT sites. These include a t(X;14)(p11;q32) involving the *GPR34* gene and translocations involving genes in 1p (*CNN3*), 5q (*ODZ2*), and 9p (*JMJD2C*) (Vinatzer et al., 2008; Ansell et al., 2012).

A subset of MALT lymphomas acquire a wide variety of changes typically associated with disease progression such as high-level amplifications, t(8q24) affecting the *MYC* locus, del(17p) leading to loss of *TP53*, or del(9p) leading to loss of the *CDKN2A* locus and can then transform into DLBCL (Barth et al., 2001). Although the t(14;18) and t(1;14) also occur in transformed or high-grade lymphomas involving the MALT, the presence of t(11;18) is restricted to low-grade variants (Barth et al., 2001; Streubel et al., 2004b; Ye et al., 2005).

Clinical correlations in MALT lymphoma

It has been proven for t(11;18) and suggested for t(1;14) that the presence of these translocations indicates a lower probability of cure by antibiotic therapy. Once a translocation occurs, the malignant clone seems to gain a degree of independence from the antigenic stimulus provided by, for example, *H. pylori* (Isaacson and Du, 2003). Liu et al. (2001, 2002) showed that 60% of stage IE and 80% of higher-stage gastric MALT lymphomas that did not respond to *H. pylori* eradication carried a t(11;18), whereas only a single responder displayed this change. The findings were corroborated by other studies (Nakamura et al., 2012; Choi et al., 2013). Lymphomas with t(1;14) mostly present at advanced clinical stages, and immunohistochemistry for BCL10 suggests that cases carrying this abnormality do not respond to eradication (Ye et al., 2006). Partial or complete trisomy 18 also appears to predict adverse clinical behavior (Krugmann et al., 2004; Nakamura et al., 2007).

Nodal marginal zone B-cell lymphoma (including pediatric marginal zone lymphoma)

Nodal marginal zone lymphoma is rare and comprises only 1.8% of lymphoid neoplasms. Cytogenetically, nodal marginal zone lymphoma has not yet been well studied. Karyotypes of less than 100 cases are publicly available, but the consistency of diagnoses has to be questioned (Dierlamm et al., 1996; Ott et al., 2000; Aamot et al., 2005b; Callet-Bauchu et al., 2005). *t(14;19)(q32;q13)* leading to *IGH–BCL3* recombination has been reported as a recurrent change (Martín-Subero et al., 2007). Stary et al. (2013) reported a case of nodal MZL with t(11;14)(q23;q32) involving the *IGH* and *DDX6* genes. Structural changes affecting various regions of *chromosome 3* also seem to be common as does complete or partial *trisomy 18*. The karyotypes are frequently complex and contain various structural rearrangements but as yet no or few specific changes. The aberrations typical of extranodal marginal zone lymphomas, like t(11;18), do not seem to be frequent in nodal marginal zone lymphoma. Array-based studies suggest recurrent gains of chromosomes 3, 12, and 18 but loss of 6q23–24 (*TNFAIP3*) like in other MZL, as well as specific loss of 11q21–22 (*ATM*) (Braggio et al., 2012).

FL (including pediatric FL and primary cutaneous follicle center lymphoma)

FL comprises 22% of all lymphomas worldwide but shows significant geographic variation. FL is rare in children, and the median age of incidence is 59 years. It is a neoplasm resembling follicle center B cells, that is, centrocytes and centroblasts. There is heterogeneity with regard to growth pattern (follicular, follicular and diffuse, and minimally follicular) and the proportion of centroblasts, the latter being reflected in three different grades (FL grades 1–3) with grade 1 showing the lowest numbers of centroblasts. Grade 3 shows the highest number of centroblasts and is subdivided into grade 3a in which centrocytes are present and grade 3b with solid sheets of centroblasts (Jaffe et al., 2001; Swerdlow et al., 2008). Variants include diffuse follicle center lymphoma and cutaneous follicle center lymphoma. Particularly, if considering the prominence of centroblasts in grade 3b and variants with diffuse growth patterns, it is not surprising that at this end of the morphologic spectrum, FL shows considerable overlap with DLBCL (Jaffe et al., 2001; Swerdlow et al., 2008). Moreover, there is a steady rate (3% per year) of transformation of FL mostly to DLBCL (Montoto et al., 2007; Montoto and Fitzgibbon, 2011). Finally, FL and DLBCL might coexist in a patient even in the same lymph node, rendering a clear distinction between the karyotypic features of the two diseases difficult.

Approximately 80–90% of FL carry a *t(14;18) (q32;q21)* or very seldom one of its variants, *t(2;18) (p12;q21)* or *t(18;22)(q21;q11)* (Johansson et al., 1995; Hillion et al., 1991; Bentley et al., 2005; Lin et al., 2008). It is noteworthy that the t(14;18) is extremely rare in FL patients below 18 years of age and virtually absent in children below the age of 14 years (Oschlies et al., 2010; Louissaint et al., 2012; Liu et al., 2013).

Pediatric-type FL is recognized as a distinct but provisional entity in the 2008 WHO classification (Harris et al., 2008; Swerdlow et al., 2008) and is characterized by the absence of *t(14;18)(q32;q21)* and *BCL6* rearrangements and an overall indolent clinical behavior (Oschlies et al., 2010; Louissaint et al., 2012; Attarbaschi et al, 2013; Martin-Guerrero et al., 2013). A subset of cases (mainly FL3 with or without DLBCL component) shows *IG–IRF4* translocations with frequent chromosomal imbalances (Salaverria et al., 2011, 2013b). In FL lacking *IG–IRF4* translocations, two subgroups may be distinguished: one "genetically normal" group with no DLBCL component and no copy number abnormalities and a "genetically aberrant group" (often with a DLBCL component) with more frequent copy number abnormalities, LOH at 1p36, and recurrent *TNFRSF14* and *EZH2* mutations (Salaverria et al., 2011; Martin-Guerrero et al., 2013). Pediatric-type PL is also encountered in young adults; then too it is characterized by a high proliferation rate but indolent clinical behavior (Louissaint et al., 2012; Liu et al., 2013).

In primary cutaneous follicle center lymphoma, conflicting data on the frequency of t(14;18) have been published. Variations among studies may be related to differences among patient cohorts and technique used (PCR vs. FISH) to detect the translocation; however, if any real frequency differences exist at all, the translocation seems to be less common in cutaneous than in nodal FL (Mirza et al., 2002; Vergier et al., 2004; Kim et al., 2005; Streubel et al., 2006a; Belaud-Rotureau et al., 2008; Gulia et al., 2011; Abdul-Wahab et al., 2014).

In nodal FL, there is evidence that the t(14;18) is more frequent in FL grades 1 and 2 (88% according to Katzenberger et al., 2004) than in FL 3, particularly FL 3b. Horn et al. (2011) identified using FISH *BCL2* breaks in 22/25 (88%), 7/12 (58%), and 2/23 (9%) of FL1/2, FL3A, and FL3B, respectively. Ott et al. (2002) found t(14;18) in 8 of 11 (73%) FL3a but only in 2 of 16 (13%) FL3b with or without a DLBCL component. Similarly, Katzenberger et al. (2004) found t(14;18) in only 1 of 27 FL3b (4%). Bosga-Bouwer et al. (2003) claimed the existence of three distinctive subgroups of FL3b based on the presence of breakpoints in 3q27, a translocation t(14;18), or the absence of both. None of their FL grade 3B cases harbored both a t(14;18) and a 3q27 aberration. Indeed, *trisomy 3 and breakpoints in*

3q27 affecting the *BCL6* locus are the most prominent findings in t(14;18)-negative FL. As there is convincing evidence for a biological difference between t(14;18)-positive and t(14;18)-negative FL, these two groups will in the following be treated separately (Leich et al., 2009).

The nonrandom occurrence of *t(14;18)(q32;q21)* in NHL was first pointed out by Fukuhara et al. (1979). Yunis et al. (1984) mapped the breakpoints to subbands 14q32.3 and 18q21.1. The t(14;18) has since turned out to be the most common translocation in NHL (15% of the total) but with considerable geographic differences (Biagi and Seymour, 2002). When tested for molecularly, the translocation can also be detected in tissues from healthy donors to some extent depending on their age and external factors such as smoking habits and exposure to pesticides (Limpens et al., 1995; Biagi and Seymour, 2002; Roulland et al., 2004; Agopian et al., 2009; Tellier et al., 2014). t(14;18) is not restricted to FL but may also be detected in 30% of DLBCL. In that lymphoma, the translocation seems to be largely restricted to the germinal center B-cell-like type (GCB) as defined by gene expression profiling (Rosenwald et al., 2002; Visco et al., 2013). The frequent transformation of FL to DLBCL has led to the suggestion that perhaps those diffuse lymphomas that carry a t(14;18) are the ones that have evolved from follicular NHL (Kneba et al., 1991).

The t(14;18)(q32;q21) in FL juxtaposes the *BCL2* oncogene next to the *IGH* locus (Tsujimoto et al., 1984). In molecular terms, the translocation is therefore different from the cytogenetically identical aberration involving *MALT1* in MALT lymphomas. In FL, the 18q21 breaks in 60–70% of the cases cluster within a 2.8 kb major breakpoint region (MBR) located in an untranslated part of the third and last (3′) exon of *BCL2*; most of these breaks occur within much smaller subregions of the MBR (reviewed by Willis and Dyer, 2000; van Dongen et al., 2003). Some 10% of the breakpoints are found in the more distal minor cluster region (MCR). Variant breakpoints have also been described, including 3′ *BCL2* (12%) and 5′ MCR (6%) (Buchonnet et al., 2000, 2002). The breakpoints in the *IGH* locus fall within the region containing the *J*-segments. Indeed, the translocation is supposed to originate from a failed *VDJ* rearrangement, which in turn argues that this lym-phoma derives from a precursor cell in the bone marrow rather than from a germinal center cell. Remarkably, the t(14;18)-positive clone seems to be characterized by considerable plasticity allowing the tumor cells to become microvascular endothelial cells (Streubel et al., 2004a). The *BCL2* gene deregulated by the translocation encodes an inhibitor of apoptosis (for reviews, see Thomadaki and Scorilas, 2006; Zinkel et al., 2006; Letai, 2008). A subset of t(14;18)-positive lymphomas do not express intact BCL2 due to somatic mutations of the gene (Schraders et al., 2005; Johnson et al., 2009; Adam et al., 2013). Vice versa, BCL2 expression is not restricted to tumor cells of FL but can be observed in a wide range of B-cell lymphoid neoplasms including CLL and DLBCL.

Less common variants of t(14;18) are the *t(2;18) (p12;q21)* and *t(18;22)(q21;q11)* that juxtapose the *BCL2* gene next to the *IGK* and *IGL* loci, respectively (Lin et al., 2008). The breakpoints in these variants are located in the 5′ end of the *BCL2* locus and not in the 3′ end that typically is involved in t(14;18) (Adachi et al., 1990; Hillion et al., 1991). Like t(14;18), both these translocations also occasionally occur in CLL, mostly secondarily to trisomy 12 (Leroux et al., 1991; Bentley et al., 2005). Indeed, they might even be more common in that disease (Adachi et al, 1990; Lin et al., 2008). Due to their rarity, it is not yet proven whether FL with these variants show the same clinical course as do t(14;18)-positive FL.

Only in 10% of t(14;18)-positive cases is this the sole cytogenetic change (Johansson et al., 1995). Recurrent secondary alterations seen in 10% or more are +X, +1q21–44, +7, +12q, +18q, del(1)(p36), del(6q), del(10)(q22–24), and the development of polyploidy. The most frequent secondary event arising after the t(14;18) seems to be the duplication of the der(18)t(14;18) (Johansson et al., 1995; Horsman et al., 2001; Höglund et al., 2004; Aamot et al., 2007). The secondary chromosomal changes in t(14;18)-positive FL arise nonrandomly and in an apparently distinct temporal order. Four possible cytogenetic pathways have been shown to characterize the early stages of clonal evolution, which converge on a common route during later stages. Based on these pathways, FL with t(14;18) may be classified into cytogenetic subgroups defined by the presence or absence of 6q−, +7, or + der(18)t(14;18). These subgroups do not seem to be associated with distinctive prognostic features, however (Höglund et al., 2004).

The most prominent changes in t(14;18)-negative FL are numerical and structural *changes of chromosome 3*. Horsman et al. (2003) showed the average number of chromosomal aberrations to be similar in t(14;18)-positive and t(14;18)-negative FL, namely, 7.9 and 8.2, respectively. *t(14q32)* other than t(14;18) is present in 28% of t(14;18)-negative FL. *Rearrangements of 1p36* are significantly less frequent than in t(14;18)-positive FL (8% versus 18%), whereas *trisomy 3* is significantly more frequent (17% vs. 2%). Trisomy 3 may be part of a distinct cytogenetic pattern in t(14;18)-negative FL, which also includes *trisomy 18*. As described earlier, trisomies for chromosomes 3 and 18 are quite common in marginal zone lymphomas, and it must be questioned whether some of the +3 and +18 single- or double-positive lymphomas are not indeed marginal zone lymphomas with a follicular growth pattern rather than true FL.

In line with the higher frequency of FL grade 3 in t(14;18)-negative FL, several studies have documented *t(3q27)* to be highly recurrent in this disease. Horsman et al. (2003) found that *t(3;14)(q27;q32)* was significantly more frequent in lymphomas without than with t(14;18). The overall frequency of t(3q27) has been reported to be below 10% in t(14;18)-positive FL and FL of grades 1 and 2 but to reach 55% in FL3b with a DLBCL (Horsman et al., 2003; Katzenberger et al., 2004; Horn et al., 2011). In contrast to t(14;18)-positive FL, t(3q27)-positive FL less frequently express CD10 and BCL2 (Jardin et al., 2002).

The target of t(3q27) is *BCL6*, which encodes a transcriptional regulator involved in germinal center formation (Jardin et al., 2007). The *BCL6* (formerly also called *BCL5* or *LAZ3*) gene was identified through cloning of the recurrent t(3;14)(q27;q32) involving *IGH* and was shown to be involved also in its light-chain variants *t(2;3)(p12;q27)* and *t(3;22)(q27;q11)* (Kerckaert et al., 1993; Ye et al., 1993a, 1993b; Miki et al., 1994a, 1994b). A steadily growing number of other t(3q27) translocations and intrachromosomal changes in chromosome 3 are also being cytogenetically identified and molecularly characterized, all of which juxtapose *BCL6* next to various partners

(Table 11.2); for referencing and steady updates, the reader is referred to http://atlasgeneticson cology.org/Genes/BCL6ID20.html. Indeed, *BCL6* seems to be one of the most promiscuous loci in B-cell lymphomas, and translocations affecting 3q27 are highly recurrent in various subtypes of B-cell disorders including particularly DLBCL or nodular lymphocyte predominance HL (discussed subsequently). The common theme of all these translocations is that the *BCL6* promoter is substituted by the promoter of the partner that interrupts its negative autoregulation, a similar effect to that reported for somatic *BCL6* mutations (Chen et al., 1998; Pasqualucci et al., 2003). Despite this supposed common mechanism of action, considerable molecular heterogeneity of the breakpoints has been observed. First, an MBR in the 5′ region of the gene is distinguished from the alternative breakpoint region (ABR) that is located more than 200 kb telomeric (Butler et al., 2002). With regard to the latter, it has not yet been ruled out that also other genes or regulatory elements than *BCL6* may be involved. Remarkably, *BCL6* breakpoints in t(14;18)-negative FL seem to predominantly affect the ABR, whereas those in DLBCL mostly affect the MBR (Bosga-Bouwer et al., 2005; Gu et al, 2009). Though the vast majority of t(3;14)(q27;q32) affects the constant regions of the *IGH* locus, switch gamma translocations seem to be more prominent in FL (70%), whereas switch μ translocations are more frequent in DLBCL (89%) (Ruminy et al., 2006).

A distinctive subtype of t(14;18)-negative FL is characterized by a predominantly diffuse growth pattern and deletions in 1p36 (Katzenberger et al., 2008, 2009).

Clinical correlations and disease progression in FL

The early steps of clonal evolution and disease progression during lymphomagenesis have to be distinguished from the secondary changes that take place when already manifest FL transform to either higher-grade FL or high-grade NHL (e.g., DLBCL or DLBCL–BL intermediate). Several features are notable regarding the initial steps of FL lymphomagenesis:

1 The t(14;18)(q32;q21) can, in up to two-thirds of healthy individuals, be detected in nonmalignant B cells in the peripheral blood. Multiple clones may

be present and can persist and expand over time (Limpens et al., 1995; Roulland et al., 2006a, 2014). The t(14;18) can also be found in reactive lymphoid tissue of healthy individuals (Limpens et al., 1991). At present, these cells may best be described as "follicular lymphoma-like cells" (FLLCs) (Roulland et al., 2006b).

2 The t(14;18)-positive FLLCs (and possibly also follicular lymphoma *in situ* (FLIS) cells; see following text) probably are able to reenter the germinal center and undergo additional rounds of somatic hypermutation there, after which they may circulate between the germinal center and bone marrow (Roulland et al., 2006b; Kluin, 2013). The recently identified t(14;18)-positive germinal center B cells represent an important missing link between the FLLCs and FLIS (see following text) (Kluin, 2014; Tellier et al., 2014).

3 So-called FLIS has been observed in lymph nodes from healthy individuals (Cong et al., 2002). These FLIS show strong BCL2 expression but preservation of the nodal architecture. During the progression from FLIS to manifest FL, an increase in (epi)genomic complexity has been observed (Mamessier et al., 2014; Schmidt et al., 2014).

A model of nonpediatric FL has emerged, suggesting at least two cytogenetic pathways during the progression of manifest lymphomas:

FL grades 1 and 2 with t(14;18) can progress to FL3a when secondary changes occur or transform to secondary DLBCL through the acquisition of tertiary aberrations of, for example, 17p (*TP53*), 9p21 (*CDKN2A*), or 8q24 (*MYC*) (Christie et al., 2008). Transformation is mostly associated with an unfavorable prognosis (Johnson et al., 2008).

FL, mostly of grade 3b and lacking t(14;18) but frequently showing t(3q27), can also progress to DLBCL through pathways similar to those of the first group (Bosga-Bouwer et al., 2005, 2006).

As for the (cytogenetic) pattern of clonal evolution, two main pathways can be distinguished: One includes linear clonal evolution in which the relapse arises from the previous FL clone (with the acquisition of additional genetic aberrations). The other involves divergent clonal evolution where the relapse originates from an FL precursor common to the tumor present at relapse and the preceding FL (Höglund et al., 2004; Berglund et al.,

2007; Johnson et al, 2008; Green et al., 2013; Okosun et al., 2014; Pasqualucci et al., 2014; Loeffler et al., 2015). In addition to t(14;18), mutations of *CREBBP* and *MLL2* seem to be early events in FL lymphomagenesis.

A variety of cytogenetic and molecular cytogenetic studies have correlated chromosomal changes in FL with outcome. Tilly et al. (1994) showed that structural alterations of 1p21–22, 6q23–26, 4q, and 17p were significantly associated with reduced 5-year survival in FL. In t(14;18)-positive FL, del(1)(p36), del(6q), del(10)(q22–24), +7, the total number of abnormalities, the number of markers and additions, and the presence of polyploidy have been correlated with morphologic progression. In t(14;18)-positive FL, Höglund et al. (2004) reported +X, 1p−, +1q, +12, 17p−, and 17q− to be correlated with an unfavorable outcome in univariate analysis and +12 and del(17p) also correlated with poor survival in a multivariate analysis that included clinical risk factors. In male patients, gain of the X chromosome (as assessed by karyotyping and/or array CGH) correlated with poor outcome (Johnson et al., 2008; Eide et al., 2010; Bouska et al., 2014). A cCGH study identified loss of 6q25–27 as being associated with unfavorable prognosis (Viardot et al., 2002), and recent aCGH-based reanalyses confirmed these findings and also suggested that deletions of 9p21 and gain of 11q are unfavorable prognostic markers (Schwaenen et al., 2009). In addition, high-resolution analysis has identified common sites of copy number-neutral LOH including 1p36 (with concomitant somatic mutations in *TNFRSF14*), 6p, 12q, and 16p (Cheung et al., 2010a, 2010b, 2012). *TNFRSF14* and *TP53* mutations have been associated with a worse prognosis (O'Shea et al., 2008; Cheung et al., 2010b). Gain/amplification of 2p15–16.1 (including the *REL* oncogene) may play a role in the transformation of FL to DLBCL (Kwiecinska et al., 2014). Several recent whole-genome and whole-exome sequencing studies have indicated an important role for chromatin modifiers, including *MLL2*, *CREBBP*, and *EZH2*, as driver and accelerator mutations in FL transformation (Green et al., 2013; Okosun et al., 2014; Pasqualucci et al., 2014). tDLBCL are more related to GCB-DLBCL than to ABC-DLBCL (Kwiecinska et al., 2014; Pasqualucci et al., 2014). All these studies should be regarded with some caution, however, since they were all retrospective and heterogeneous with regard to both treatment and t(14;18) positivity. Studies of large series of randomized FL patients in prospective trials are still lacking as are studies taking into account the gene expression risk profiles characteristic of this disease (Dave et al., 2004).

Diffuse large B-cell lymphoma (DLBCL)

DLBCL are a morphologically, biologically, and clinically heterogeneous group that constitutes 30–40% of all B-cell lymphomas. Based on the site of involvement, some entities such as primary DLBCL of the CNS and leg-type primary cutaneous DLBCL are distinguished from systemic DLBCL (Jaffe et al., 2001; Swerdlow et al., 2008). Hardly any chromosomal data exist on these site-specific diseases, but interphase cytogenetic studies have indicated a similar spectrum of changes to that of systemic DLBCL (Hallermann et al., 2004a, 2004b).

Some quantitative differences may nevertheless exist, as more than 30% of leg-type DLBCL have been shown by FISH to have t(8;14)(q24;q32) or variants and also in the plasmablastic and immunoblastic variant was t(8q24) often seen by interphase cytogenetics (Hallermann et al., 2004a; Kanungo et al., 2006; Belaud-Rotureau et al., 2008; Aukema et al., 2014; Siebert et al., unpublished results). In addition, deletions of 6p21 involving the MHC region are reported in over 50% of lymphomas of immune-privileged sites (primary CNS and testicular lymphomas) and are more common compared to nodal DLBCL (Riemersma et al., 2000; Booman et al., 2006, 2008; Schwindt et al., 2009). In primary lymphoma of the bone, gains of 1q and amplification of 2p16.1, both associated with a germinal center-like genetic profile, have been identified (Heyning et al., 2010).

Another subtype, ALK-positive DLBCL, in which the tumor cells show a typical immunoblastic morphology with expression of VS38 and IgA, was recognized based on the expression of anaplastic lymphoma kinase. These lymphomas are cytogenetically characterized by a simple or complex t(2;17)(p23;q23) involving the clathrin (CLTC) gene in 17q23 and the ALK gene in 2p23 (Chikatsu et al., 2003; Gascoyne et al., 2003; Gesk et al., 2005). They typically lack MYC rearrangements but instead show MYC gain and amplification (Valera et al., 2013).

Cytogenetic data on T-cell/histiocyte-rich large B-cell lymphoma (THRLBCL), an additional morphologic subtype of DLBCL, are scarce. CGH analysis of 17 THRLBCL showed genomic imbalances in all cases. The most common imbalances were gain of Xq, 4q13–28, Xp11–21, and 18q21 and loss of 17p (Franke et al., 2002).

The nodal and extranodal types of DLBCL mostly show centroblastic or immunoblastic morphology (Jaffe et al., 2001). These common DLBCL must be distinguished from primary mediastinal (thymic) large B-cell lymphoma (PMBCL) (Jaffe et al., 2001). Gene expression studies have shown the latter to be associated with a distinct expression signature related to that of cHL (Rosenwald et al., 2003; Savage et al., 2003). Various expression subgroups of DLBCL were also identified by these studies. Clinically, most relevant were two subgroups of DLBCL identified by gene expression profiling named according to the COO signature, that is, ABC-DLBCL associated with an unfavorable and GCB-DLBCL associated with a more favorable outcome (Alizadeh et al., 2000; Rosenwald et al., 2002; Gutiérrez-García et al., 2011).

No chromosomal aberration is completely specific for DLBCL, but many of the generally lymphoma-associated rearrangements are prominent also in this disease subtype. t(3q27), involving the BCL6 locus and various partners in a manner similar to that in FL, is seen in 20–40% of DLBCL (Table 11.2). Iqbal et al. (2007) detected BCL6 translocations at the MBR by FISH in 25 (19%) of 133 DLBCL cases, with a higher frequency in PMBCL (33%) and ABC-DLBCL (24%) than in GCB-DLBCL (10%).

Translocations of 14q32 involving the IGH locus can be detected in up to half of all DLBCL (Lenz et al., 2007; Bouamar et al., 2013). Approximately 20–30% of DLBCL show a t(14;18)(q32;q21) (Rosenwald et al., 2002; Hummel et al., 2006; Barrans et al., 2010; Visco et al., 2013). These cases are predominantly centroblastic and belong almost exclusively to the GCB-DLBCL subtype (Schlegelberger et al., 1999; Rosenwald et al., 2002; Iqbal et al., 2004; Visco et al., 2013). A t(8;14)(q24;q32) or variant t(8q24) can be detected in around 10% of DLBCL, some of which, especially (pediatric) cases with an *IG–MYC* translocation and lacking *BCL2* and *BCL6* rearrangements, might represent true BL based on their gene expression profile (Dave et al., 2006; Hummel et al., 2006; Klapper et al., 2008a; Aukema et al., 2014). In others, these translocations are supposed to be secondary changes mostly associated with a very aggressive clinical behavior and in part related to transformation into lymphomas intermediate between DLBCL and BL (see following text). In addition to *t(3;14)(q27;q32)* and the light-chain variants *t(2;3)(p12;q27)* and *t(3;22)(q27;q11)* involving *BCL6* and the *MYC*-targeting translocations more typical of BL, a steadily increasing number of other t(14q32) with various partners also exist (Lenz et al., 2007; Bouamar et al., 2013), particularly in the ABC-DLBCL tumor subset (Lenz et al., 2007).

Frequently recurring numerical chromosome aberrations in DLBCL include gains of chromosomes X, 3, 7, 12, and 18 and losses of the Y chromosome and chromosomes 6, 13, 15, and 17. Based on cytogenetic data, commonly gained chromosomal regions are 1q23–31, 3q21–22, 6p, 7p, 7q31–32, 8q22–24, 11q12–13, 12q14–24, and 18q11–21 in centroblastic lymphomas and 1q21–25, 3p24–21, 6p21, 7p12–21, 18q, and 22q12-qter in immunoblastic lymphomas. Commonly deleted chromosomal regions are 1p35-pter, 2p23-pter, 6q21–22, 6q25-qter, 8p12-pter, 9p21-pter, 11q23-qter, 12p12–13, and 17p12–13 in centroblastic lymphomas and 1p35–36, 2q22–24, 4q32-qter, 6q21–25, 7q33, 8q21, 9p24, 9q21–32, 11q21-qter, 14q23-qter, 16p13, and 18q21-qter in immunoblastic lymphomas. These imbalances mostly occur as part of complex karyotypes with many unbalanced translocations. Losses of the whole chromosome 10, deletions in 8q and 14q, as well as structural abnormalities of 4q have been reported to be significantly more frequent in immunoblastic than in centroblastic lymphomas (Johansson et al., 1995; Schlegelberger et al., 1999).

CGH studies suggest that the main effect of the vast majority of cytogenetic changes in DLBCL is to create a set of common imbalances that may, at least in part, form the basis for the subgroups of DLBCL defined by gene expression. ABC-DLBCL frequently show trisomy 3, gains of 3q (including *BCL6*), 18q21–22 (including *MALT1* and mostly *BCL2*), and 19q13 (including *SPIB*), but losses of 9p21 (including *CDKN2A*) and 6q21–22. GCB-DLBCL show frequent gains of 1q, 2p13–16 (including *REL/BCL11A*), chromosome 7, 11q, and 12q12, whereas PMBCL show gains of 9p21-pter (including *JAK2/PDL2*) and 2p14–16 (including *REL/BCL11A*) (Bea et al., 2005; Tagawa et al., 2005b; Kimm et al., 2007; Wessendorf et al., 2007; Lenz et al., 2008; Green et al., 2014). It should be stressed that complete or partial trisomy 9 with a minimal region of gain in 9p23–24 seems to be specific for PMBCL (Bentz et al., 2001). In general, specific chromosomal alterations might be associated with significant changes in gene expression signatures that reflect various aspects of lymphoma cell biology as well as the host response to the lymphoma (Bea et al., 2005).

Next-generation sequencing analyses have revealed a large number of potentially targetable, recurrently mutated genes including *MLL2*, *TP53*, *TNFRSF14*, *CARD11*, *GNA13*, *CD79B*, *EZH2*, *MYD88*, and *CREBPP* (Ngo et al., 2011; Pasqualucci et al., 2011a, 2011b; Lohr et al., 2012; Morin et al., 2013; Zhang et al., 2013; Bohers et al., 2014; Vaqué et al., 2014). Some of these are associated with one of the COO types, for example, *EZH2* (15–30%) and *GNA13* (15–30%) mutations in GCB-DLBCL and *MYD88* (20–35%) and *CD79B* (15–20%) mutations in ABC-DLBCL (Morin et al., 2011; Ngo et al., 2011; Pasqualucci et al., 2011a; Zhang et al., 2013; Bohers et al., 2014).

Clinical correlations in DLBCL

All clinical correlations in DLBCL have to be treated with extreme caution since the data derive from before the introduction of anti-CD20 antibody therapy (Rituxan). Moreover, established clinical risk factors including International Prognostic Index (IPI) (The International Non-Hodgkin's Lymphoma Prognostic Factors Project, 1993), subtyping by gene expression profiling, and evaluation in the context of other chromosomal aberrations were mostly not taken into account. The data on the prognostic importance of t(14;18) (Barrans et al., 2003; Akyurek et al., 2012; Visco et al., 2013; Bellas et al., 2014) and t(3q27) (Akasaka et al., 2000b; Barrans et al., 2002; Ueda et al., 2002a; Niitsu et al., 2007; Shustik et al., 2010; Akyurek et al., 2012; Akay et al., 2014) are conflicting; at present, no convincing evidence exists that one or the other is reliably linked to prognosis. Like in many other lymphomas, there is good evidence that del(17p) and del(9)(p21) in DLBCL are associated with progression and unfavorable prognosis (Tagawa et al., 2005b). In centroblastic DLBCL, deletions and duplications of 1q have been reported to be adverse risk factors independent of IPI, whereas trisomy 5 and changes of 15q seem to be independent indicators of a reduced risk. In immunoblastic lymphomas, changes of 7q and 8q had a stronger impact on survival than did the IPI (Schlegelberger et al., 1999). Gains of *MAPKAPK3* located at 3p21.31 and loss of 9p21.3 (*CDKN2A/B*) have been associated with chemoresistance in DLBCL patients treated with immunochemotherapy (Kreisel et al., 2011). Interestingly, another study using array CGH found that clonal heterogeneity and 9p21.3 loss were associated with poor prognosis (Suguro et al., 2014). In addition to genomic imbalances, also aberrant DNA methylation has been shown to have prognostic impact with heavily methylated DLBCL cases showing a worse clinical outcome (Chambwe et al., 2014).

Recent advances in gene expression profiling and assessment of cytogenetic imbalance patterns offer new ways to classify lymphomas into prognostically meaningful subgroups based on their COO (Masqué-Soler et al., 2013). Gains of 3p11–12 provide prognostic information independently of the gene expression data (Bea et al., 2005). It is not likely, however, that this way of subgrouping patients exhausts the possibilities for clinically meaningful classification. DLBCL can show considerable molecular genetic heterogeneity, including aberrant somatic hypermutation of *IGH*, *BCL6*, *MYC*, and other genes (Pasqualucci et al., 2001). This and frequent uniparental disomy and epigenetic changes are biological parameters also likely to influence outcome. The adverse prognostic impact of *MYC* (in combination with additional *BCL2* and/or *BCL6*) rearrangements in DLBCL has been demonstrated in multiple FISH studies (Klapper et al., 2008b; Savage et al., 2009; Barrans et al., 2010; Aukema et al., 2014; Tzankov et al., 2014). It is therefore advisable to screen all DLBCL in routine diagnostic situations for *MYC* and related breakpoints with both break-apart and dual-color dual fusion probes, in addition to

performing chromosome banding analysis with karyotyping (Klapper et al., 2008b; Savage et al, 2009; Barrans et al., 2010; May et al., 2010; Kluin and Schuuring, 2011; Aukema et al., 2011, 2014; Tzankov et al., 2014). In the near future, these molecular cytogenetic analyses will likely be combined with targeted panel sequencing for diagnostic and prognostic relevant genes and COO classification using dedicated gene expression profiling.

Other large B-cell lymphomas

Other very rare entities of large B-cell lymphoma include intravascular large B-cell lymphoma (ILBL) and primary effusion lymphoma (PEL) (Jaffe et al., 2001; Swerdlow et al., 2008). In the former disease, hardly any cytogenetic studies have been reported though the presence of t(11;14)(q13;q32), t(14;18) (q32;q21), and *BCL6* rearrangements has been described in single cases (Vieites et al., 2005; Rashid et al., 2006; Cui et al., 2014). A recent review by Mandal et al. (2007) suggested that structural aberrations of chromosomes 1, 6, and 10 and, less frequently, chromosomes 4, 5, and 8 might be nonrandom changes with a recurrent site of deletion in 6q21–24. PEL is universally associated with human herpes virus 8 (HHV-8)/Kaposi sarcoma herpesvirus (KSHV) infection. Also, EBV is found in most cases. Cytogenetic analyses mostly show a complex karyotype with structural rearrangements frequently involved in lymphomas in general but without subgroup-specific abnormalities (Boulanger et al., 2001). Trisomy 7, trisomy 12, and aberrations proximally in the long arm of chromosome 1 seem to be recurrent (Wilson et al., 2002). A CGH study identified recurrent gains of the X chromosome and 12q (Mullaney et al., 2000). In another array CGH study, copy number abnormalities involving, among others, 1q, 7q, 8q, 14q32, and chromosome 12 were identified with *SELPLG/ CORO1C* at 12q24.1 showing amplification/low-level gain in 23% of the cases (Luan et al., 2010).

The majority of PEL occur in the setting of HIV infection, which is associated with an increased risk of lymphoma. AIDS-related lymphomas include systemic lymphomas, mostly DLBCL and BL, primary central nervous system lymphomas (PCNSL), PEL, and plasmablastic lymphoma of the oral cavity (Jaffe et al., 2001; Swerdlow et al., 2008). AIDS-related and other lymphomas in immunodeficient patients show a spectrum of chromosomal aberrations similar to that of their counterparts in immunocompetent patients (Vaghefi et al., 2006). Activation of *MYC* and inactivation of *TP53* in conjunction with EBV and other viral infections seem to play a major pathogenetic role (Carbone, 2003). In line with these molecular changes, there seems to be a trend toward more complex karyotypes and a higher frequency of t(8;14)(q24;q32) and the variant translocations t(2;8) and t(8;22). In lymphomatoid granulomatosis, which is also an Epstein–Barr virus (EBV)-driven lymphoproliferative disorder for which immunodeficient patients carry an increased risk, no cytogenetic aberrations have yet been identified in line with the oligo- or polyclonal origin documented particularly in low-grade cases (Jaffe et al., 2001; Swerdlow et al., 2008).

Burkitt lymphoma (BL)

BL is a highly aggressive disease often presenting at extranodal sites or as an acute leukemia. It is the most common B-cell lymphoma in the pediatric age group but is also observed in the adult population (Boerma et al., 2004; Leoncini et al., 2008). Endemic and sporadic BL are recognized as variants manifesting differences in clinical presentation and biology. Immunodeficiency-associated BL is seen primarily in association with HIV infection.

The cytogenetic hallmark of BL is the *t(8;14) (q24;q32)* and its variants, *t(2;8)(p12;q24)* and *t(8;22)(q24;q11)*. These translocations are present both in the endemic, African tumor type and in the sporadic BL occurring in Europe, America, and Japan, both in EBV-infected patients and in EBV-negative BL. The t(8;14) is present in 75–85% of all BL (Johansson et al., 1995). In 15–25%, one of the variant translocations is found with the t(8;22) occurring twice as frequently as t(2;8) (Figure 11.7).

BL was the first lymphoid neoplasm in which the underlying chromosomal rearrangement was characterized. The first cytogenetic study of BL was reported in 1963 by Jacobs and coworkers. After the introduction of banding techniques, Manolov and Manolova (1972) described an additional band at the end of 14q in five of six fresh BL and in seven of nine cell lines from such tumors. The nature of the BL-specific abnormality was clarified by Zech

et al. (1976), who established that the 14q+ arose through the translocation t(8;14)(q24;q32). Based on a high-resolution study, Manolova et al. (1979) reported that the translocation was reciprocal. Further scrutiny of prophase–prometaphase cells from the BL-derived cell line Daudi allowed Zhang et al. (1982) to map the translocation breakpoints to subbands 8q24.13 and 14q32.33. Berger et al. (1979) described the first variant translocation, t(8;22)(q24;q11), and Miyoshi et al. (1979) and van den Berghe et al. (1979) simultaneously reported the second variant, t(2;8)(p12;q24).

The molecular consequence of the t(8;14) and its variants is deregulation of the *MYC* oncogene in 8q24 through juxtaposition next to one of the IG enhancer elements in the *IGH* (14q32), *IGK* (2p12), or *IGL* (22q11) locus. Activation of *MYC* takes place on the der(14) in t(8;14) and on the der(8) in t(2;8) and t(8;22). Correspondingly, the breakpoints on the der(8) differ between the t(8;14) and its variants being telomeric of the *MYC* gene in the latter and centromeric of *MYC* in the former. Breakpoints can scatter over several hundred kilobases on both sides of the *MYC* locus (Joos et al., 1992a, 1992b; Einerson et al., 2006; Kroenlein et al., 2012). Sporadic, endemic, and immunodeficiency-associated BL show different clustering of the breakpoints on der(14) and der(8), indicating that different pathogenetic mechanisms may be behind the generation of the t(8;14) in these different disease settings. Briefly, the breakpoints of t(8;14) in endemic BL frequently fall far centromeric of the *MYC* gene and regularly affect the J-segments of the *IGH* locus. In contrast, t(8;14) in sporadic BL more frequently involves the switch regions of the constant segments of *IGH*, or the breakpoint occurs between exons 1 and 2 or immediately 5′ of the *MYC* gene. This molecular heterogeneity has to be taken into account when diagnosing one of the translocations by molecular or molecular cytogenetic techniques, and therefore, it is advisable always to use both a *MYC* break-apart and *MYC–IGH* fusion FISH assay as far centromeric breakpoints may be missed using a break-apart assay alone (Hummel et al. 2006). In addition, somatic mutation of the *MYC* locus occurs frequently in BL, which might in part be driven by the VH mutation machinery after the juxtaposition of *MYC* next to *IGH*. Some of the mutations in *MYC*, which may also occur

(A)   (B)   (C)

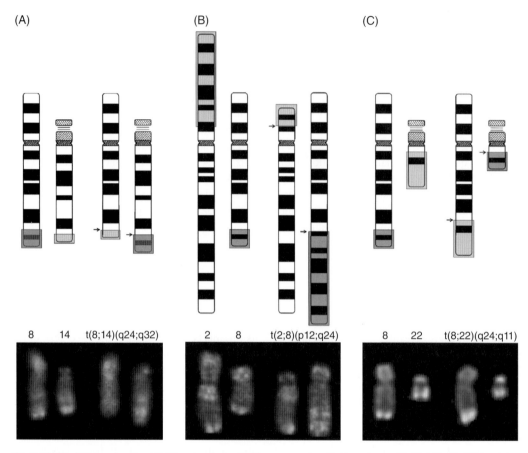

| 8 | 14 | t(8;14)(q24;q32) | | 2 | 8 | t(2;8)(p12;q24) | | 8 | 22 | t(8;22)(q24;q11) |

Figure 11.7 Burkitt translocation t(8;14) and variants. (A) Ideogram and partial karyotype with t(8;14)(q24;q32) involving *MYC* and *IGH*. (B) Ideogram and partial karyotype with t(2;8)(p12;q24) involving *IGK* and *MYC*. (C) Ideogram and partial karyotype with t(8;22)(q24;q11) involving *MYC* and *IGL*. Fluorescence R-banding.

independently of *IGH*-driven hypermutation, might be of pathogenetic relevance. For more details on the molecular characteristics of the Burkitt translocations as well as the pathogenic consequences of *MYC* activation in general, the reader is referred to excellent reviews by, for example, Willis and Dyer (2000), Boxer and Dang (2001), Küppers and Dalla-Favera (2001), Küppers (2005), Klapproth and Wirth (2010), and Ott et al. (2013).

Typically in BL, the t(8;14) or variant translocation is part of a rather simple karyotype; complex karyotypes indicate disease progression and are an adverse prognostic factor (Johansson et al., 1995; Hummel et al., 2006; Salaverria et al., 2008b; Boerma et al., 2009; Poirel et al., 2009). Secondary chromosomal changes are present in around 60% of BL (Berger et al., 1989; Johansson et al., 1995;

Boerma et al., 2009). In a comparison of paired karyotypes from BL patients, complex karyotypes were seen at a higher frequency in relapsed or progressive BL compared to initial diagnostic samples (Aukema and Siebert, in prep.); this may contribute to the very dismal prognosis of patients with progressing and relapsing disease (Woessmann, 2013). The clearly most frequent secondary aberration (>30% of all patients) is *structural rearrangement of chromosome 1*, in particular of the long arm and often leading to partial trisomy for 1q. *Trisomy 7* and *trisomy 12* are other common secondary changes. These three aberrations tend to be mutually exclusive in BL progression (Boerma et al., 2009). Another hot spot for secondary involvement in BL is chromosomal region 13q3, found rearranged in 15% (Johansson et al., 1995). The target is most likely the *miR-17-92* miRNA locus that, like other recurrent molecular changes, seems to interact with *MYC* in transformation (He et al., 2005; O'Donnell et al., 2005). Losses of 13q may be associated with a more unfavorable outcome (Nelson et al., 2010). In addition to secondary chromosomal changes, whole-genome and whole-exome sequencing studies have identified recurrent mutations in *MYC, TP53, ID3, TCF3, CCND3,* and *DDX3X* as common, with mutations targeting *ID3* or *TCF3* occurring in about 70% of sporadic BL cases (Campo, 2012; Love et al., 2012; Richter et al., 2012; Schmitz et al., 2012).

Although the putative existence of BLs lacking a *MYC* translocation has been subject of much discussion (Leucci et al., 2008), it is unlikely that "true" *MYC* translocation-negative BL exist. Recently, in a subset of lymphomas resembling BL by gene expression profile and pathological characteristics but importantly lacking *MYC* translocation, 11q aberrations with proximal gains and telomeric losses were identified (Salaverria et al., 2014).

The view that BL is a homogeneous disease characterized by the presence of one of the three specific translocations is also supported by gene expression profiling studies (Dave et al., 2006; Hummel et al., 2006). Nevertheless, none of the three translocations is completely specific for BL as all of them have been described also in several other B-cell lymphomas. "B-cell lymphoma with features intermediate between DLBCL and BL" is a disease subset strongly enriched for the presence of these translocations and might even present with a typical Burkitt leukemia morphology in the bone marrow (Kluin et al., 2008). In contrast to BL, these intermediate lymphomas, which occur at a significantly older age, mostly show complex karyotypes (Hummel et al., 2006; Boerma et al., 2009; Salaverria and Siebert, 2011; Aukema et al., 2014). Many of them harbor other recurrent *IG* translocations such as t(14;18)(q21;q32) or t(3q27) targeting the *BCL6* locus. These so-called "double-hit" lymphomas are associated with a much more unfavorable outcome, highlighting the clinical relevance of distinguishing both subtypes (Dave et al., 2006; Hummel et al., 2006; Aukema et al., 2011). Moreover, a wide range of t(8q24) that do not involve *IG* loci as partners, such as t(8;9)(q24;p13) juxtaposing *MYC* to *PAX5* and t(3;8)(q27;q24)

juxtaposing *MYC* to *BCL6* (Hummel et al., 2006; Bertrand et al., 2007; Sonoki et al., 2007), may also occur. The detection of a double hit, the presence of a non-*IG–MYC* translocation, and the occurrence of a t(8;14) or variant as part of a complex karyotype should, particularly in nonpediatric patients, lead to a reassessment of the histopathologic diagnosis, especially since each of these three features is associated with an unfavorable outcome (Hummel et al., 2006, Boerma et al., 2009; Aukema et al., 2011, 2014; Salaverria and Siebert, 2011). In cases where a diagnosis of BL is in doubt, profiling for BL-specific genes (the analysis can also be performed on formalin-fixed and paraffin-embedded tissues) as well as mutational analysis (e.g., for *ID3* and *TCF3* mutations that are absent in other *MYC* translocation-positive lymphomas) may be helpful in establishing the correct diagnosis (Love et al., 2012; Richter et al., 2012; Schmitz et al., 2012; Masqué-Soler et al., 2013).

Plasma cell neoplasms

The group of plasma cell neoplasms (PCN) includes solitary plasmacytoma of bone, extraosseous plasmacytoma, and plasma cell myeloma (or MM), the latter including the clinical variants nonsecretory myeloma, smoldering myeloma, indolent myeloma, and plasma cell leukemia (PCL). MGUS is regarded as a precursor state, and approximately 25% of patients with MGUS develop an overt lymphatic, mostly plasma cell, neoplasm after a follow-up of more than 20 years. Also, various kinds of monoclonal immunoglobulin (heavy- and light-chain) deposition diseases related to amyloidosis are included among the PCN (Jaffe et al., 2001; Swerdlow et al., 2008). From the cytogenetic point of view, these plasma cell disorders, as far as they have been characterized, are closely related showing a similar spectrum of changes (Fonseca et al., 2002; Harrison et al., 2002; Chng et al., 2005; Brousseau et al., 2007).

Since the introduction of cytogenetic analyses into the study of plasma cell neoplasias, it has been repeatedly shown that MM is a heterogeneous disease with regard to the underlying chromosomal abnormalities (Dewald et al., 1985; Calasanz et al., 1997a; Nilsson et al., 2003). Karyotyping of MM has been hampered not only by a low level of bone marrow infiltration and a low mitotic index of plasma cells *in vitro* but also by the fact that many of the translocations affecting the *IGH* locus in 14q32 are cytogenetically cryptic in this disease. The 30% of cases showing aberrations therefore grossly underestimates the actual level of karyotypic changes in MM (Dewald et al., 1985; Calasanz et al., 1997b; Nilsson et al., 2003). In addition, poor metaphase quality in many MM cases has prevented the identification of recurrent aberrations, including translocations, by chromosome banding. In those cases that have shown abnormal karyotypes, numerous structural and numerical abnormalities have often been found, and some patients have had multiple abnormal clones. Nevertheless, around 25% of the karyotypes have shown only one or two abnormalities (Calasanz et al., 1997b; Nilsson et al., 2003). The frequency and extent of karyotypic abnormalities seem to correlate with the disease stage. Therefore, most chromosomal changes described by conventional cytogenetics are more likely to be encountered in a highly proliferative clone and are not clearly associated with early disease stages (Hallek et al., 1998).

Two large and independent bioinformatic analyses of the clustering of chromosomal changes have shown that at least three cytogenetic subgroups of plasma cell neoplasias exist (Debes-Marun et al., 2003; Sáez et al., 2004): (i) A hyperdiploid group accounts for 30–50% of the cases and is characterized by gains (mostly trisomy or tetrasomy) of chromosomes and chromosome arms 9/9q, 19, 5, and 15/15q, as well as 3, 11/11q, 7, and 21. These neoplasms show only a low frequency of t(14q32) (9%), −14 (8%), and t/del(22q) (7%). Monosomy 13 is seen in 20% of these cases. (ii) A hypodiploid group accounts for 20–35% of the cases and shows monosomy 13 in around two-thirds. t(14q32) (25%), −14 (42%), and t/del(22q) (34%) are significantly more frequent here than in the hyperdiploid group. (iii) A pseudodiploid group accounting for 20–35% of the cases contains t(14q32) in up to 75%. Monosomy 13 is seen in one-fourth of these cases. There seems to be some overlap between the last two groups, which also show other recurrent aberrations like gains of 9q, 12q, 17q, 18, and 22q; losses of X, 6q, 8, 16, and Y; and structural aberrations involving 16p or 16q, 1p or 1q (partial deletion, trisomy 1q), 11q13, 19q13 or 19p13, 6q,

17q, and 7q (Dewald et al., 1985; Calasanz et al., 1997b; Nilsson et al., 2003).

By means of CGH, Avet-Loiseau et al. (1997) found that losses from 13q and 14q and gains from 1q and 7 occurred in 50–60% of MM patients, with hot spots at 13q12.1–21, 13q32–34, 14q11.2–13, and 14q23–31. Cigudosa et al. (1998) suggested that the most frequent events were gains of chromosome 19 or 19p and complete or partial deletions of chromosome 13. Also, gains of 9q, 11q, 12q, 15q, 17q, and 22q and losses of 6q and 16q have been described in MM based on CGH studies (Gutiérrez et al., 2004).

Using multicolor spectral karyotyping (SKY), several recurring sites of breakage were mapped to chromosomal bands 3q27, 17q24–25, and 20q11 by Rao et al. (1998). Also, new translocations involving 14q32 were identified using this approach, namely, t(12;14)(q24;q32), t(14;20)(q32;q11), t(14;16)(q32;q23), and t(9;14)(p13;q32) (Rao et al., 1998; Sawyer et al., 1998, 2001).

Interphase FISH studies have demonstrated that numerical chromosome abnormalities are present in up to 90% of MM (Drach et al., 1995; Flactif et al., 1995; Zandecki et al., 1996). Among them, partial or complete loss of chromosome 13 is the most common (Shaughnessy et al., 2000; Fonseca et al., 2004). It is worthy of note that in contrast to CLL, the deletions mostly affect the whole 13q arm. Although the monoallelic deletion of *RB1* through monosomy 13 or 13q deletions is a frequent event in MM (Shaughnessy et al., 2000), mutations or rearrangements of *RB1* have not been described, and biallelic loss of the *RB1* gene is infrequent (Juge-Morineau et al., 1995; Zandecki et al., 1995). Deletions of 17p13 occur in up to 10% of MM as detected by interphase FISH (Drach et al., 1998; Fonseca et al., 2003; Chang et al., 2005a, 2005b). Mutations of *TP53* are infrequently found in newly diagnosed MM but occur more often in relapse or in patients with PCL (Neri et al., 1993).

Translocations of 14q32 involving *IGH* are seen in 40–60% of patients with plasma cell neoplasia (Bergsagel and Kuehl, 2001; Avet-Loiseau et al., 2002; Higgins and Fonseca, 2005; Tian et al., 2014). For a long time, the *IGH* translocations have been thought to derive mainly from errors in immunoglobulin class switch recombination (Bergsagel and Kuehl, 2001). However, a recent study found that whereas 100% of t(4;14) were CSR mediated, a considerable subset of t(11;14) and t(14;20) were generated through DH–JH recombination activation gene-mediated mechanisms or receptor revision (Walker et al., 2013a). Thus, some plasma cell disorders may arise at the pro-B-cell hematological progenitor cell level, much earlier in B-cell development than was previously thought. This also supports the view that the said changes are early, if not initiating, pathogenic events (Bergsagel et al., 2005). In addition to t(14q32) involving the IGH locus, variant translocations of 2p12 and 22q11 have also been described in MM involving either the IGK or the IGL light-chain locus. The limited studies available indicate that the prevalence of IGL translocations ranges from around 10% in MM/MGUS to 20% in advanced intramedullary MM tumors, whereas IGK translocations are quite rare, occurring in only a small percentage of intramedullary MM (Bergsagel and Kuehl, 2001; Türkmen et al., 2014). Two separate and independent translocations involving IGH and/or IG light-chain loci seem to occur infrequently and then only in MM tumors but may be present in 5–10% of advanced tumors and primary PCL (Bergsagel and Kuehl, 2001).

Unlike other B-cell malignancies, MM exhibits a wide variety of different IG translocations involving numerous partner chromosomes. Some of these IG translocations are recurrent, whereas others are rare or unique (Table 11.5). The clinical relevance of many of them remains to be determined (Bergsagel and Kuehl, 2001). More than 40% of MM have IG translocations involving seven recurrent chromosomal partners and oncogenes (Table 11.4): 11q13 (CCND1), 4p16 (FGFR3 and MMSET), 6p21 (CCND3), 16q23 (MAF), 20q11 (MAFB), 6p25 (IRF4), and 1q21 (IRTA1/IRTA2). Rare variants include, among others, 2p23 (MYCN), 9p13 (supposedly PAX5), 11q23 (supposedly MLL), 12p13 (supposedly CCND2), and 17q21 (NIK). Recently, also the EGFR gene has been identified as a partner in recombination with the IGH locus (Walker et al., 2013b).

t(11;14)(q13;q32) is the most common (15–20%) translocation found in MM (Laï et al., 1995; Avet-Loiseau et al., 1998; Gertz et al., 2005). The breakpoints in 11q13 are scattered throughout the 360 kb region between the CCND1 gene and the MYEOV gene (myeloma-overexpressed gene) (Ronchetti et al., 1999; Janssen et al., 2000). In 14q32, the breakpoints fall either within the JH or, in contrast to MCL, in the switch region (Bergsagel et al., 1996; Walker et al., 2013a). Similar to MCL, the translocation leads to deregulated expression of CCND1; however, due to the presence of IGH enhancer(s) on der(11) in MM, MYEOV gene expression may also be deregulated. Besides the classical balanced translocation t(11;14)(q13;q32), more complex rearrangements, too, including insertions, have been reported affecting 14q32 (IGH) and 11q13 (CCND1) (Gabrea et al., 1999; Fenton et al., 2004).

The cytogenetically cryptic t(4;14)(p16.3;q32.3) is found in 10–20% of MM when appropriate FISH techniques are used (Avet-Loiseau et al., 1998; Fonseca et al., 2003; Gertz et al., 2005). In the IGH locus, all the breakpoints occur in switch regions (Bergsagel and Kuehl, 2001; Walker et al., 2013a). In 4p16, the breakpoints occur 50–100 kb centromeric of the FGFR3 gene, clustering within a region of about 60 kb within the 5′ exons of the MMSET gene (Chesi et al., 1998a). The MMSET gene on the der(4) becomes deregulated because of the presence of the IGH intronic enhancer. In addition, hybrid mRNA transcripts are formed between IGH (JH and Iμ exons) and the MMSET gene (Chesi et al., 1998a; Keats et al., 2005). On der(14), FGFR3 is juxtaposed to the strong IGH 3′ enhancers, and its expression is consequently deregulated (Chesi

Table 11.5 Recurrent IG translocations in multiple myeloma

Chromosomal band	Oncogene product	Incidence (%)
11q13	CCND1	15–20
6p21	CCND3	5
4p16	FGFR3 and MMSET	10–20
16q23	MAF	5–10
6p25	IRF4	5
20q11	MAFB	2–5
8q24	MYC	1–50
1q21	IRTA1/IRTA2	1–2

Source: Updated from Kuehl and Bergsagel (2002). Reprinted with permission from Macmillan Publishers Ltd.

et al., 1998a). The *FGFR3* gene has been reported to be expressed in only 70–75% of t(4;14)-positive cases, and the lack of *FGFR3* expression normally correlates with loss of the der(14)t(4;14) chromosome (Keats et al., 2003; Santra et al., 2003). *MMSET*, on the other hand, is deregulated by the Eμ enhancer on the der(4) in all t(4;14)-positive MM (Chesi et al., 1998a; Santra et al., 2003).

A *t(14;16)(q32;q23)* has been identified in 5–10% of patients and in about 25% of MM cell lines (Chesi et al., 1998b; Avet-Loiseau et al., 2002; Fonseca et al., 2003). This translocation is difficult to detect by conventional karyotyping but has been reported in 7% of MM patients with abnormal metaphases studied by SKY (Sawyer et al., 1998). The breakpoints in the *IGH* locus mostly occur in switch regions or occasionally in the *JH* region (Chesi et al., 1998b; Bergsagel and Kuehl, 2001). The breakpoints in 16q23 occur in a region 550–1350 kb centromeric to *MAF*, within the 800 kb intron of the oxidoreductase gene *WWOX/FOR* (Bednarek et al., 2000; Ried et al., 2000). As a result of the translocation, *MAF*, the cellular homolog of v-maf that is the transforming gene of the avian maf retrovirus, is juxtaposed to the *IGH* enhancers and highly upregulated (Chesi et al., 1998b). On der(16), the translocation inactivates one allele of the *WWOX/FOR* gene (Bednarek et al., 2000). However, the identification of a cell line carrying a *t(16;22)(q23;q11)* variant translocation affecting *IGL* (22q11) (Chesi et al., 1998b) and with breakpoints telomeric of *MAF* (not involving *WWOX/FOR*) suggests that inactivation of one allele of *WWOX/FOR* by the t(14;16) translocation is not required for MM cell transformation.

The *t(14;20)(q32;q12)* was first identified by spectral karyotyping (Rao et al., 1998) and is present in 2–5% of MM (Hanamura et al., 2001; Kuehl and Bergsagel, 2002; Barillé-Nion et al., 2003). The breakpoints on der(20) occur 0.5–1 Mb centromeric of the *MAFB* gene, scattered within an 800 kb region (Hanamura et al., 2001; Boersma-Vreugdenhil et al., 2004). 25% of t(14;20) are generated through DH–JH recombination activation gene-mediated mechanisms, indicating they occur earlier in B-cell development at the pro-B-cell stage in the bone marrow (Walker et al., 2014).

Deregulation of *CCND3* as a result of *t(6;14) (p21;q32)* is detectable in 5% of MM (Shaughnessy

et al., 2001; Sonoki et al., 2001). All cloned breakpoints in 14q32 have occurred in the *IG* switch regions, whereas the breakpoints in 6p21 cluster to a region no more than 150 kb 5′ (centromeric) to the *CCND3* gene. A variant translocation, *t(6;22) (p21;q11)*, involving *IGL* and *CCND3* has also been described in MM with the breakpoints telomeric to the *CCND3* gene (Shaughnessy et al., 2001).

A steadily growing number of other and less common *IGH* translocations have also been described in MM (Table 11.4), including *t(6;14) (p25;q32)* involving the *IRF4* gene (Yoshida et al., 1999b; Kuehl and Bergsagel, 2002) and *t(1;14) (q21;q32)* involving the *IRTA1/IRTA2* locus (Hatzivassiliou et al., 2001). Among the *IG* translocations in MM are also the *t(8;14)(q24;q32)* and its variants targeting the *MYC* gene (Bergsagel et al., 1997; Avet-Loiseau et al., 2001). They give rise to 10–15% of the *MYC* aberrations in MM (Shou et al., 2000; Avet-Loiseau et al., 2001; Gabrea et al., 2008). In total, the frequency of abnormalities affecting the *MYC* locus in primary tumors ranges from approximately 15% (Avet-Loiseau et al., 2001; Fabris et al., 2003) to 50% (Shou et al., 2000; Affer et al., 2014). The promiscuous *MYC* locus rearrangements hijack enhancers but mostly superenhancers to dysregulate MYC expression (Affer et al., 2014; Walker et al., 2014). These abnormalities involving *MYC* appear late in the course of MM and are considered to be associated with tumor progression (Shou et al., 2000; Bergsagel and Kuehl, 2001). It is worthy of note that the 8q24 aberrations are highly heterogeneous in terms of breakpoint positions (Fabris et al., 2003).

The expression level of *CCND1*, *CCND2*, or *CCND3* mRNA in MGUS and MM is consistently higher than in normal plasma cells (Tarte et al., 2002; Zhan et al., 2002), and almost all MGUS and MM tumors deregulate at least one of the cyclin D genes (Bergsagel et al., 2005). Therefore, the ubiquitous deregulation of cyclin D genes in MGUS and MM, sometimes as a consequence of *IG* translocations but otherwise by presently unknown mechanisms, appears to be a unifying and early, if not initiating, pathogenic event (Bergsagel and Kuehl, 2005; Bergsagel et al., 2005). It has been proposed that the type of cyclin D expressed, together with the pattern of chromosomal changes observed, might be used to classify MM into biologically and clinically relevant subgroups.

Recent whole-genome sequencing studies in MM have revealed mutations in genes involved in protein translation (seen in nearly half of the patients), histone methylation, NF-κB signaling, and blood coagulation (Chapman et al., 2011). Activating mutations of the kinase *BRAF* were observed in 4% of patients. Significantly mutated genes include *NRAS*, *KRAS*, *TP53*, and *CCND1*. Overall and similar to CLL, there seems to be heterogeneity of mutational spectrum across samples, with few recurrent genes (Bolli et al., 2014). Moreover, there is evidence of clonal heterogeneity in MM so that genomic sequence variants can wax and wane with time in progressive tumors (Egan et al., 2012). Overall, chromosomal translocations and imbalances seem to dominate in the pathogenesis of MM as compared to targeted mutations.

Clinical relevance of chromosomal aberrations in plasma cell neoplasias

Dewald et al. (1985) provided evidence that patients with newly diagnosed MM and abnormal metaphases by chromosome banding had active disease and reduced survival compared to patients who had only normal metaphases. This conclusion was later corroborated in several studies. Tricot et al. (1995) found that patients with MM who had metaphase cells with monosomy 13 and/or structural anomalies of chromosome 13 had even shorter survival. Calasanz et al. (1997b) reported that among other chromosomal abnormalities, hypodiploidy and rearrangements of chromosome band 22q11 signified a higher progression rate and shorter survival in MM patients. Independent studies confirmed the importance of these chromosomal aberrations and also pointed toward other aberrations as powerful prognostic markers in MM (Pérez-Simón et al., 1998; Rajkumar et al., 1999; Smadja et al., 2001; Fassas et al., 2002). Among them, translocations affecting *IGH* such as the t(4;14) and t(14;16) and deletions of *TP53* in 17p13 were repeatedly reported to confer a negative outcome in MM (Fonseca et al., 2003; Keats et al., 2003; Chang et al., 2005a, 2005b; Gertz et al., 2005). t(4;14) and t(14;16) were shown to correlate with a poor prognosis not only in untreated patients (Dewald et al., 2005) but also in patients treated with high-dose or conventional chemotherapy (Fonseca et al., 2003; Gertz et al., 2005; Avet-Loiseau et al., 2007; Gutiérrez et al., 2007). The t(11;14) translocation, present in up to 15% of MM, was first associated with an aggressive clinical course (Fonseca et al., 1999), but later studies suggested that these patients do not fare as badly as initially thought (Fonseca et al., 2003; Dewald et al., 2005; Gertz et al., 2005). Several reports have described the importance of deletions of the *TP53* locus for estimating overall survival and time to progression (Chang et al., 2005a, 2005b), but other studies have failed to demonstrate an independent prognostic value of *TP53* deletions in multivariate analyses (Gertz et al., 2005).

The results of studies of the clinical impact of chromosome 13 changes are not clear-cut. Some have claimed that patients with chromosome 13 anomalies in their metaphase or interphase cells have a poor prognosis (Tricot et al., 1995; Avet-Louseau et al., 2000; Kaufmann et al., 2003; Kröger et al., 2004), but others have indicated that chromosome 13 anomalies may not be as important for survival as t(4;14), t(14;16), or del(17)(p13) (Fonseca et al., 2003; Chang et al., 2005a, 2005b; Gertz et al., 2005; Chng et al., 2006). Other reports again indicate a strong association between the presence of chromosome 13 anomalies and t(4;14), t(14;16), or del(17)(p13) (Fonseca et al., 2001; Magrangeas et al., 2005), and one can only conclude that at present the relationship between chromosome 13 anomalies and prognosis is unclear. Some results suggest that the prognostic significance of chromosome 13 anomalies depends on whether they were detected in metaphase or interphase cells (Dewald et al., 2005). In that study, detection of chromosome 13 anomalies in metaphase cells was associated with poor prognosis, whereas patients with chromosome 13 anomalies detected in their interphase nuclei had intermediate survival.

There seems to be a hierarchy of chromosome anomalies in MM that correlate with patient prognosis (Fonseca et al., 2003; Chang et al., 2005a, 2005b; Dewald et al, 2005; Avet-Loiseau et al., 2007). Fonseca et al. (2003), using interphase FISH for the detection of specific anomalies, found that patients with t(4;14), t(14;16), and/or del(17)(p13.1) had a poor prognosis, those with chromosome 13 anomalies without t(4;14), t(14;16), and/or del(17)(p13.1) had intermediate prognosis, and those with other chromosome anomalies, including most patients with t(11;14), had a favorable prognosis. Similar conclusions were drawn by Chang et al. (2005a, 2005b). Dewald et al. (2005) also reached similar results but with a different hierarchy for metaphase and interphase data. For metaphase data, patients with t(4;14), t(14;16), del(17)(p13.1), and/or chromosome 13 anomalies had poorer survival than did patients with t(11;14) and other anomalies. For interphase data, patients with t(4;14) or t(14;16) had poorer survival than did patients with chromosome 13 anomalies, del(17)(p13.1), t(11;14), and other anomalies or who had no anomalies.

Limited data are available on the impact of other recurrent genetic aberrations on prognosis in MM. The prognostic significance of chromosome 11 aberrations is controversial. They have been associated with a poor prognosis in several studies (Tricot et al., 1995; Gutiérrez et al., 2004). On the other hand, Cremer et al. (2005) showed that the response status after autologous stem cell transplantation in patients with 11q aberrations versus those without did not indicate an adverse prognostic significance. Finally, structural aberrations of chromosome 1 have also been associated with an adverse prognostic impact and a poor clinical outcome in MM (Debes-Marun et al., 2003; Segeren et al., 2003; Hanamura et al., 2006; Wu et al., 2007; Hillengass et al., 2008).

Current risk stratification models distinguish between high-, intermediate-, and standard-risk MM. The presence of MAF transcription factor translocations, t(14;16) and t(14;20), as well as 17p deletion indicates high risk, whereas t(4;14), cytogenetic deletion of chromosome 13, and hypodiploidy have been associated with intermediate risk. Hyperdiploidy and the presence of *CCND* translocations, that is, t(11;14) and t(6;14), are indicative of standard risk (Rajkumar, 2012; Bergsagel and Chesi, 2013).

From all these studies have emerged various related recommendations for diagnostic molecular cytogenetic testing of patients with MM. To detect prognostically relevant chromosomal alterations, FISH on immunologically selected plasma cells (e.g., FISH of plasma cells enriched by MACS, ImmunoFISH, FICTION) is nowadays obligatory.

According to the recommendations, as a bare minimum, a FISH panel for MM should enable testing for t(4;14)(p16;q32), t(14;16)(q32;q23), and deletion of *TP53* in 17p13 (Fonseca et al., 2009; Chng et al., 2014). In addition, probes for the detection of t(11;14), possibly together with a probe that detects splitting of *IGH* in general, should also be applied. One may also want to test for losses of 13q as well as gains of 1q. The hyperdiploid variant of MM associated with a favorable outcome can be identified by the use of probes targeting trisomies for chromosomes 5, 9, 15, and/or 19. Conflicting data exist regarding the prognostic value of 1q21 amplification and deletion of 1p21 and/or 1p32; this issue warrants further investigation (Chng et al., 2014). Despite all recent progresses in prognostication relying on interphase FISH and other techniques, chromosome banding analysis can still add independent prognostic information in plasma cell disorders, as demonstrated by Dewald et al. (1985, 2005), and is highly recommended (Rajkumar, 2012; Bergsagel and Chesi, 2013).

Mature T-cell and NK-cell neoplasms

A comparative overview of the different subtypes of mature T-cell neoplasms taking into account the Kiel, REAL, and 2001 WHO classifications is provided in Table 11.6. Data from recent molecular studies including gene expression profiling nevertheless indicate that the current morphology-based classification systems do not adequately reflect the overall heterogeneity of mature T- and NK-cell disorders (de Leval and Gaulard, 2011; Iqbal et al., 2014). Future changes in the classification of these diseases are therefore likely. The clinically most relevant chromosomal aberrations are summarized in Table 11.7.

T-PLL

T-PLL is a rare lymphoproliferative disease with distinctive morphologic appearance, a mostly mature postthymic immunophenotype, and an aggressive clinical course. It comprises cases previously classified as T-cell chronic lymphocytic leukemia (T-CLL) (Jaffe et al., 2001).

The genetic hallmark of T-PLL is *inv(14)(q11q32)*, first associated with T-CLL by Zech et al. (1983),

Table 11.6 Comparison of the Kiel, REAL, and WHO classifications of T- and NK-cell malignant neoplasms*

Kiel classification	REAL classification	WHO classification 2001	WHO classification 2008
	Peripheral T-cell and NK-cell neoplasms	Mature (peripheral) T-cell and NK-cell neoplasms	
T-lymphocytic, CLL type	T-CLL/T-PLL	T-PLL	T-PLL
T-lymphocytic, PLL			
T-lymphocytic, CLL type	Large granular lymphocytic leukemia: T-cell type and NK-cell type	T-cell granular lymphocytic leukemia	T-cell granular lymphocytic leukemia
		Aggressive NK-cell leukemia	Aggressive NK-cell leukemia
			Chronic lymphoproliferative disorders of NK cells*
			EBV+ T-cell lymphoproliferative disorders of childhood
Small cell cerebriform (mycosis fungoides, Sezary syndrome) T-zone	Mycosis fungoides, Sezary syndrome	**Mycosis fungoides,** Sezary syndrome	**Mycosis fungoides,** Sezary syndrome
Lymphoepithelioid, pleomorphic small T-cell, Pleomorphic medium-sized and large T-cell, T-immunoblastic	Peripheral T-cell lymphomas, unspecified (including provisional subtype: subcutaneous panniculitic T-cell lymphoma)	**Peripheral T-cell lymphomas, not otherwise characterized**	**Peripheral T-cell lymphomas, not otherwise characterized**
		Subcutaneous panniculitis-like T-cell lymphoma	Subcutaneous panniculitis-like T-cell lymphoma
	Hepatosplenic γ–δ T-cell lymphoma*	Hepatosplenic γ–δ T-cell lymphoma	Hepatosplenic γ–δ T-cell lymphoma
Angioimmunoblastic (AIDL, LgX)	Angioimmunoblastic T-cell lymphoma	**Angioimmunoblastic T-cell lymphoma**	**Angioimmunoblastic T-cell lymphoma**
	Angiocentric lymphoma	Nasal T-cell and NK-cell lymphoma	Nasal T-cell and NK-cell lymphoma
	Intestinal T-cell lymphoma (with or without enteropathy)	Enteropathy-type T-cell lymphoma	Enteropathy-type T-cell lymphoma
Pleomorphic small T-cellHTLV1+ Pleomorphic medium-sized and large T-cell HTLV1+	Adult T-cell leukemia/ lymphoma (HTLV1+)	Adult T-cell leukemia/ lymphoma (HTLV1+)	Adult T-cell leukemia/ lymphoma (HTLV1+)
T-large cell anaplastic (Ki-1+)	Anaplastic large cell lymphoma, T/null-cell types	**Anaplastic large cell lymphoma, T/null-cell, primary systemic type**	**Anaplastic large cell lymphoma, ALK+**
			Anaplastic large cell lymphoma, ALK-*
		Anaplastic large cell lymphoma, T/null-cell, primary cutaneous type	Anaplastic large cell lymphoma, T/null-cell, primary cutaneous type

Data from Lennert et al. (1975), Harris et al. (1994), Jaffe et al. (2001), and Swerdlow et al. (2008).

Bold letters represent the most common subtypes.

*Provisional entity.

Table 11.7 Overview of frequent and diagnostically relevant chromosomal aberrations in mature T/NK-cell neoplasms*

Neoplasm	Cytogenetic aberration	Frequency (%)
T-cell prolymphocytic leukemia	i(8q) or t(8;8)(p23;q11) or +8	60–90
	inv(14)(q11q32) or t(14;14)(q32;q11)	40–75
	t(X;14)(q28;q11)	<2
	del(6q), del(11q)	10–20
Enteropathy-type T-cell lymphoma	+9q31-qter	70
	del(16)(3q12)	23
Hepatosplenic T-cell lymphoma	i(7q)	>70
	+8	>50
Anaplastic large cell lymphoma	t(2;5)(p23;q35) and variants	40–90
	+X, +7, +9, −Y, del(6q), del(17p)	10–30
Adult T-cell lymphoma/leukemia (HTLV1⁺)	t/der(14q32), t/der(14q11), del(6q)	30–50
Peripheral T-cell lymphomas, NOC	+7/7q, +1q, +3p, +5p, +8q24	20–35
	del(6q), del(10p)	20–30
Angioimmunoblastic T-cell lymphoma	+3	50–80
	+X, +5/5q	20–55
	+21, +3q, del(6q)	20–40

*Only lymphomas with sufficient cytogenetic data are included to estimate frequencies.

which is present in up to 80% of the cases. Its variant, *t(14;14)(q11;q32)*, is detected in 10% of T-PLL. Both chromosomal aberrations juxtapose the *TCL1* locus in 14q32 next to the *TCRAD* locus in 14q11, resulting in upregulation of the *TCL1A* gene (Virgilio et al., 1994). The translocation *t(X;14)(q28;q11)* is the characteristic change in T-PLL lacking inv(14) or t(14;14). It juxtaposes the *MTCP1* (for mature T-cell proliferation-1) gene from Xq28 next to the *TCRAD* locus in 14q11 (Stern et al., 1993). The central importance of T-cell receptor rearrangements in the pathogenesis of T-PLL is further underscored by the fact that deletions and translocations of 7q34–36, the site of the *TCRB* gene locus, are also found repeatedly (15%).

Besides the described TCR-associated translocations that are regarded as the primary oncogenic events in T-PLL, the tumor cells usually harbor also a high load of additional changes. The pattern of these secondary aberrations is highly characteristic for T-PLL and seems to be associated with changes in the gene expression pattern of the tumor cells (Soulier et al., 2001; Dürig et al., 2007; Nowak et al., 2009). In up to 80% of cases, overrepresentations of 8q and deletions of 8p, frequently due to the formation of an isochromosome, *i(8q)*, are present. The breakpoint of the i(8q) is in 8p spread over a large genomic region arguing against a breakpoint-

associated oncogenic mechanism but for a gene dosage effect caused by the resulting imbalances, which is in line with the findings of recent gene expression studies. *Alterations of chromosome 6* leading to gain of or from 6p but losses from 6q as well as *structural changes of 22q* have also been observed in a significant proportion of patients. Other recurrent changes are deletions in 10p and 18p. Finally, del(11q) leads to loss of one copy of the *ATM* gene, while mutations are common in the second allele (Stilgenbauer et al., 1997).

Recent exome sequencing studies have identified a high frequency of mutations in genes encoding members of the JAK–STAT pathway in T-PLL, in particular affecting *JAK1*, *JAK3*, *STAT5B*, and *IL2RG* (Bellanger et al., 2014; Kiel et al., 2014). A mutation in one of these genes has been observed in 76% of all T-PLL. Other recurrently altered genes include *EZH2* and *FBXW10* (Kiel et al., 2014).

T-cell large granular lymphocyte leukemia

T-cell large granular lymphocyte leukemia (T-LGL) is a heterogeneous disorder mostly following an indolent clinical course. Clonal karyotypic abnormalities have been reported in only few cases, some of which might not constitute T-LGL but rather T-PLL, T-ALL, or hepatosplenic T-cell lymphoma. No consistent chromosomal changes have been identified though there is some evidence for breakpoints in regions containing *TCR* loci, that is, 7p, 7q, and 14q11. Deletion 6q has been reported as the only recurrent change (Man et al., 2002). Recent sequencing analyses showed around one-third of all T-LGL to carry somatic mutations of the *STAT3* gene particularly at positions Y640, D661, and N647 in exon 21 encoding the SH2 domain (Koskela et al., 2012). Less common but nevertheless recurrent are mutations affecting the *STAT5B* gene. In *STAT3* mutation-negative cases, changes in other genes encoding members of the JAK–STAT or T-cell activation pathways occur (Andersson et al., 2013).

NK-cell leukemias and lymphomas

Several lymphoma and leukemia types are supposed to derive from a proliferation of NK cells. These include aggressive NK-cell leukemia, extranodal NK/T-cell lymphoma of the nasal type, and blastic NK-cell lymphoma. All of them are rare but with some geographic variation. Extranodal NK/T-cell lymphoma of the nasal type is almost always associated with EBV infection. No specific chromosomal alteration has yet been identified in these diseases. A variety of clonal cytogenetic aberrations have nevertheless been reported, of which del(6q) may be the most common.

CGH studies have shown frequent deletions at 6q16–27, 13q14–34, 11q22–25, and 17p13, loss of the whole X chromosome, as well as DNA amplifications in NK-cell leukemia/lymphoma. Recurrent gains were seen at 1p32-pter, 6p, 11q, 12q, 17q, 19p, 20q, and Xp (Siu et al., 1999). Mao et al. (2003b) reported similar patterns of chromosome imbalances in both blastic NK and cutaneous NK-like T-cell lymphomas. The most frequent DNA copy number changes were losses of 9/9p (83%) followed by loss of 13q and gain of 7 (67%). CGH studies have identified gain of 1q23.1–24.2 and 1q31.3–44 as well as loss of 7p15.1–22.3 and 17p13.1 as recurrent and characteristic of the aggressive NK-cell leukemia group compared with those of extranodal NK/T lymphoma, nasal type. Recurrent changes characteristic of the extranodal NK/T lymphoma, nasal type compared with those of the other group, were gain of 2q and losses of 6q16.1–27, 11q22.3–23.3, 5p14.1–14.3, 5q34–35.3, 1p36.23–36.33, 2p16.1–16.3, 4q12, and 4q31.3–32.1 (Nakashima et al., 2005; Iqbal et al., 2009). *PRDM1*, *FOXO1*, and *AIM1* were proposed as targets for the 6q deletions (Iqbal et al., 2009). Exome sequencing has identified *JAK3* mutations in a subset of NK/T-cell lymphomas (Koo et al., 2012), but also other mechanisms of activation of the JAK–STAT pathway exist in these malignancies (Bouchekioua et al., 2014).

Enteropathy-type T-cell lymphoma

Enteropathy-type T-cell lymphoma (ETL) is a tumor of intraepithelial T lymphocytes with a clear association with celiac disease (Jaffe et al., 2001). No specific cytogenetic aberrations have been identified in the few cases subjected to chromosome banding analysis.

cCGH studies have revealed chromosomal imbalances in 87% of the cases analyzed with recurrent gains from 9q (58%), 7q (24%), 5q (18%), and 1q (16%) and losses from 8p (24%), 13q (24%), and 9p (18%) but with slight geographic variation (Takeshita et al., 2011; Zettl et al., 2002). aCGH studies have confirmed that ETL is characterized by frequent gains of 9q31.3-qter (70%) and loss of 16q12.1 (23%); the two rarely occurred together. Two distinct groups of ETL were delineated by Zettl et al. (2002), Baumgärtner et al. (2003), and De Leeuw et al. (2007): (1) type 1 ETL was linked pathogenetically to celiac disease and characterized cytogenetically by gains of 1q and 5q, and (2) type 2 ETL frequently showed gains of the *MYC* oncogene locus and, more rarely, from chromosome arms 1q and 5q. Recently, *TET2* mutations were described in 2/10 EATL, but comprehensive mutational analyses are yet to be performed (Lemonnier et al., 2012).

Hepatosplenic T-cell lymphoma

Hepatosplenic T-cell lymphoma is a neoplasm derived from cytotoxic T cells usually of gamma/delta T-cell receptor type. An i(7)(q10) or rare variants were present in the vast majority of cases studied so far and are supposed to be the primary genetic change, frequently accompanied by trisomy 8 (Jonveaux et al., 1996; Wlodarska et al., 2002;

Travert et al., 2012). Recently, frequent mutation of the *STAT5B* gene was described in hepatosplenic T-cell lymphoma (Nicolae et al., 2014).

Anaplastic large cell lymphoma

Anaplastic large cell lymphoma (ALCL) is a T-cell lymphoma consisting of CD30 (Ki-1)-positive tumor cells with variable morphologic features. The majority of cases express the anaplastic lymphoma kinase gene due to fusion of this gene with one of several known partners. Therefore, ALK-positive and ALK-negative ALCL are distinguished with the former being associated with a more favorable prognosis (Jaffe et al., 2001). This difference in outcome might be due to the fact that the median age of patients with ALK-positive ALCL is lower than that of patients with ALK-negative disease. According to the 2001 WHO classification, 92% of ALCL in children are ALK positive compared with only 72% of ALCL in adults (Jaffe et al., 2001). The updated WHO classification 2008 treats ALK-positive ALCL as a separate entity (Savage et al., 2008; Swerdlow et al., 2008).

Morgan et al. (1986) analyzed four cases of what was diagnosed as malignant histiocytosis and found in three of them a *t(2;5)(p23;q35)*. Later studies showed that the t(2;5)-carrying tumors actually are high-grade ALCL that express the CD30 (Ki-1) antigen and that, consequently, are often referred to as Ki-1 lymphomas. Many of the tumors have shown evidence of T-lineage differentiation, whereas some lack obvious T-cell markers but are nevertheless derived from T cells. Morris et al. (1994) as well as other investigators showed the molecular consequences of the translocation to be the fusion of a nucleophosmin gene, *NPM*, in band 5q35 with the anaplastic lymphoma kinase gene, *ALK*, in 2p23 leading to a chimeric protein with constitutive tyrosine kinase activity. With the availability of anti-ALK antibodies, it could be shown that the NPM–ALK fusion protein is expressed in the cytoplasm but also often in the nucleus. Up to 20% of ALK-positive ALCL lacked nuclear reactivity of the ALK antibody but instead showed various patterns of cytoplasmic and membranous staining. In the course of these investigations, variants of the t(2;5) were identified that fused the *ALK* gene to other partners. The most frequent of these variants was *t(1;2)(q21–25;p23)*

fusing *ALK* to *TPM3*. Less frequent are *t(2;3) (p23;q12)* leading to *TFG–ALK* fusion, *inv(2) (p23q35)* leading to *ATIC–ALK* fusion, *t(2;17) (p23;q23)* leading to *CLTC–ALK* fusion, *t(X;2) (q11;p23)* leading to *MSN–ALK* fusion, *t(2;17) (p23;q35)* leading to *ALO17–ALK* fusion, and *t(2;22)(p23;q11)* leading to *MYH9–ALK* fusion (Mitev et al., 1998; Hernández et al., 1999; Lamant et al., 1999; Ma et al., 2000; Touriol et al., 2000; Tort et al., 2001; Cools et al., 2002). One can assume that also additional translocations involving the *ALK* gene in 2p23 exist in ALCL.

Secondary chromosomal changes in ALCL are not well studied, but in smaller series, gains of chromosomes 7, 9, and X and losses of Y, 6q, and 17p have been reported (Johansson et al., 1995; Weisenburger et al., 1996). ALK-positive ALCL with *NPM–ALK* or *ALK* variant translocations showed similar profiles of secondary genetic alterations as assessed by CGH. Additional *MYC* translocations transform ALK-positive ALCL into a more aggressive disease as is the case also with other lymphomas (Liang et al., 2013).

Hardly any reliable cytogenetic data on ALK-negative ALCL are at hand that may help distinguish this from ALK-positive disease. Nelson et al. (2008) described gains of 1q (50%) and 3p (30%) and losses of 16pter (50%), 6q13–21 (30%), 15 (30%), 16qter (30%), and 17p13 (30%) as being frequent in ALK-negative ALCL. CGH showed ALK-positive and ALK-negative ALCL to have different secondary genomic aberrations, suggesting that they correspond to different genetic entities. Gains of 17p and 17q24-qter and losses of 4q13–21 and 11q14 were associated with ALK-positive disease, whereas gains of 1q and 6p21 were more frequent in ALK-negative ALCL. Gains of chromosome 7 and 6q and 13q losses were seen in both types (Salaverria et al., 2008a). Zettl et al. (2004) also reported ALK-negative ALCL to display recurrent chromosomal gains of 1q (1q41-qter, 46%) and losses of 6q (6q21, 31%) and 13q (13q21–22, 23%). However, no specific chromosomal alterations were associated with survival. A recent SNP array study identified recurrent losses at 17p13 and at 6q21, involving the *TP53* and *PRDM1* genes, and documented inactivation of PRDM1 by multiple mechanisms, more often in ALK-negative than in ALK-positive ALCL. Losses of *TP53* and/or

PRDM1 were present in 52% of ALK-negative disease compared with 29% of all ALCL cases (Boi et al., 2013).

Primary cutaneous CD30-positive T-cell lymphoproliferative disorders include primary cutaneous ALCL and lymphomatoid papulosis. The former mostly and the latter always lack t(2p23) or its molecular counterpart *ALK* fusion genes and in general show few recurrent chromosomal imbalances (Jaffe et al., 2001). By CGH, the mean number of changes in nonrelapsing disease has been reported to be only 0.33 (range 0–1), compared with 6.29 (range 1–16) in relapsing disease. Chromosomes often found affected by aberrations in relapsing disease have been 6 (86%), 9 (86%), and 18 (43%). Whereas chromosome 9 was mostly affected by gains, chromosomes 6 and 18 mainly showed regions of loss, especially from 6q and 18p. Common regions of loss were 6q21 and 18p11.3 (Prochazkova et al., 2003). An aCGH study identified gains of 7q31 and loss on 6q16–6q21 and 13q34 in 45% of cutaneous ALCL (Szuhai et al., 2013).

Recent sequencing studies have discovered a recurrent t(6;7)(p25.3;q32.3) in ALK-negative ALCL affecting the *IRF4/DUSP22* locus in 6p25 (Feldman et al., 2011). *IRF4* rearrangements may define a subgroup of CD30-positive cutaneous T-cell lymphoma (CTCL) (Pham-Ledard et al., 2010) and *IRF4* translocations also a novel subtype of lymphomatoid papulosis with a benign course (Karai et al., 2013).

Peripheral T-cell lymphoma, unspecified

Peripheral T-cell lymphoma, unspecified (PTCL-US) collectively refers to a number of distinct entities defined by former classifications, such as T-zone, lymphoepithelioid (Lennert), small- to medium-sized, and large cell pleomorphic T-cell lymphoma and T-immunoblastic lymphoma according to the Kiel classification (Jaffe et al., 2001). These tumors account for approximately half of the peripheral T-cell lymphomas seen in Western countries.

In contrast to what is the situation in precursor T-cell neoplasms, translocations t(14q11), t(7q34), and t(7p14) involving the *TCR* gene loci are generally absent in PTCL (Lepretre et al., 2000; Leich et al., 2007). The notable exception is *t(14;19) (q11;q13)* that recurrently translocates *PVRL2* to

the *TCRA* locus in rare cases of PTCL-US, including Lennert lymphoma (Almire et al., 2007; Leich et al., 2007; Shin et al., 2012). The molecular consequence might be the activation of the *BCL3* gene in proximity to the breakpoint in 19q13. In addition, a t(6;14)(p25;q11.2) involving *IRF4* and *TCRAD* was recently reported in a PTCL presenting with massive splenomegaly (Somja et al., 2014). Another recurrent translocation in PTCL-US is *t(5;9)(q33;q22)* resulting in *ITK–SYK* fusion. Streubel et al. (2006b) detected *ITK–SYK* fusion transcripts in 5 of 30 (17%) unspecified PTCL but not in cases of angioimmunoblastic T-cell lymphoma (AITL) (*n* = 9) and anaplastic lymphoma kinase-negative anaplastic large cell lymphoma (*n* = 7). Remarkably, three of the five t(5;9)(q33;q22)-positive unspecified PTCL shared a very similar histological pattern with predominant involvement of lymphoid follicles and the same CD3 + CD5 + CD4+ bcl-6 + CD10+ immunophenotype.

Like in other AITL and ALK-negative ALCL, cytogenetic correlations have not yet come across as very characteristic. Nelson et al. (2008) reported frequent gains involving 7q22–31 (33%), 1q (24%), 3p (20%), 5p (20%), and 8q24-qter (22%) but losses of 6q22–24 (26%) and 10p13-pter (26%) in PTCL-US. A comparable spectrum of imbalances was reported by Schlegelberger et al. (1994a, 1994b) and Lepretre et al. (2000). In 36 de novo PTCL-US, Zettl et al. (2004) identified by CGH recurrent chromosomal losses from 13q (minimally overlapping region 13q21, 36% of cases), 6q and 9p (6q21 and 9p21-pter, in 31% each), 10q and 12q (10q23–24 and 12q21–22, in 28% each), and 5q (5q21, 25%). Recurrent gains were seen of 7q22-qter (31%). In 11 PTCL-US, high-level amplifications were observed, including three cases with amplification of 12p13. Thorns et al. (2007) used aCGH to examine 20 PTCL-US finding gains of or from 17 (17q11–25), 8 (involving the *MYC* locus at 8q24), 11q13, and 22q and losses of or from 13q, 6q (6q16–22), 11p11, and 9 (9p21–33). Interestingly, gains of 4q (4q28–31 and 4q34-qter), 8q24, and 17 were significantly more frequent in PTCL-US than in AITL. Hartmann et al. (2010) used SNP arrays to identify recurrent gains at 1q32–43, 2p15–16, 7, 8q24, 11q14–25, 17q11–21, and 21q11–21 and losses from 1p35–36, 5q33, 6p22, 6q16, 6q21–22,

8p21–23, 9p21, 10p11–12, 10q11–22, 10q25–26, 13q14, 15q24, 16q22, 16q24, 17p11, 17p13, and Xp22 (4 or more cases each). Genomic imbalances affected several regions containing members important in nuclear factor-kappaB signaling with *REL* in 2p being particularly targeted. Nakagawa et al. (2009) identified by aCGH a complex genomic aberration pattern with 32 regions showing frequent genomic imbalances, including high copy number gains at 14q32.2 and homozygous losses at 9p21.3. Gains of 7p and 7q and loss of 9p21.3 showed a significant association with poor prognosis. The authors opined that PTCL-US cases with genomic imbalances showed distinct histopathologic and prognostic features compared with cases without such alterations and showed genetic, histopathologic, and prognostic resemblance to lymphoma-type ATLL.

No certain correlations have been found between the cytogenetic findings and histologic subgroups or clinical outcome in PTCL-US. Schlegelberger et al. (1994b) observed trisomy 3 only in T-zone lymphoma and lymphoepithelioid lymphoma according to the Kiel classification. Zettl et al. (2004) reported high-level amplifications of 12p13 to be restricted to cytotoxic PTCL-NOS. This lack of definite association between genomic aberrations and histological subgroups could be due to the much higher molecular than morphologic complexity. Indeed, recent gene expression profiling studies reclassified 37% of morphologically diagnosed PTCL-US cases into other subtypes according to their molecular signatures (Iqbal et al., 2014). Recent sequencing analyses suggest that this molecular heterogeneity might be determined by genomic mutations often targeting the DNA methylation machinery (Palomero et al., 2014). Mutations affecting *TET2* have been identified in more than a third (38%) of PTCL-US cases and seem to be particularly prevalent when the PTCL derives from TFH cells. The *TET2* mutations were associated with advanced-stage disease, thrombocytopenia, high IPI scores, and short progression-free survival (Lemonnier et al., 2012). In addition, mutation p.Gly17Val in *RHOA* is detectable in 20% of PTCL-US. Other genes potentially involved in the pathogenesis of PTCL-US include *FYN*, *ATM*, *B2M*, and *CD58* (Palomero et al., 2014).

Angioimmunoblastic T-cell lymphoma (AITL)

AITL accounts for 15–20% of peripheral T-cell lymphomas. It was initially felt to be an atypical reactive process, angioimmunoblastic lymphadenopathy (AILD), with an increased risk of progression to lymphoma. Atypical and oligoclonal proliferations may precede the development of lymphoma. EBV can be detected in more than 75% of AITL (Jaffe et al., 2001).

A cytogenetic feature characteristic of AITL is unrelated clones, which can be found in 15% of cases (Kaneko et al., 1988; Schlegelberger et al., 1994a, 1994b). *Trisomy 3, trisomy 5,* and *+X* predominate (Kaneko et al., 1988; Schlegelberger, 1994a, 1994b, 1994d; Lepretre et al., 2000). Using interphase cytogenetics, Schlegelberger et al. (1994d) found that 78% of AITL showed +3 clones and 34% showed +X clones. These frequencies far exceeded those observed with metaphase cytogenetics (+3, 41%; +X, 20%) and may possibly represent an overestimate based on the applied cutoff levels for diagnosing alterations by FISH. Nelson et al. (2008) reported that the most common abnormalities in AITL were gains of or from 5q (55%), 21 (41%), and 3q (36%), trisomies of chromosomes 5 and 21 (41%), and loss of 6q (23%). Translocations affecting *TCR* loci are generally absent (Gesk et al., 2003; Leich et al., 2007). Using aCGH, Thorns et al. (2007) found that the most common changes in AITL were gains of 22q, 19, and 11p11–q14 (11q13) and losses of 13q. Trisomies 3 and 5 were identified in only a small number of cases.

A major breakthrough in the understanding of the pathogenesis of AITL has come from sequencing studies (Palomero et al., 2014; Sakata-Yanagimoto et al., 2014; Yoo et al., 2014). Mutations were frequently found particularly affecting *RHOA*, *TET2*, *IDH2*, and *DNMT3A*. The *RHOA* mutations were detected in 53–68% and mostly led to the change p.Gly17Val. *TET2* mutations were seen in 47–76% (Odejide et al., 2014). The *IDH2* mutations mostly targeted R172 and were found in 20–45% of AITL (Cairns et al., 2012). In contrast, *IDH1* mutations seem to be uncommon in this disease. *DNMT3A* mutations have been observed in around one-third of AITL and often occur together with *TET2* mutations. Other less frequent loss-of-function mutations may be found in *TP53*, *ETV6*,

CCND3, and *EP300*, whereas uncommon gain-of-function mutations may target *JAK2* and *STAT3* (Odejide et al., 2014).

Clinical correlations in AITL

Schlegelberger et al. (1996) reported presence of abnormal metaphases in unstimulated cultures, clones with +X, structural aberrations of the short arm of chromosome 1 (1p31–32), and complex clones with more than four aberrations to be associated with a significantly lower incidence of therapy-induced remission and a significantly shorter survival. Multivariate analysis showed that these cytogenetic findings had a significant influence on survival, whereas therapy modalities did not. Only the presence of complex aberrant clones was an independent prognostic factor. Trisomy 3 had no effect on survival.

The clinical importance of *RHOA*, *IDH2*, *TET2*, and *DNMT3A* mutations warrants investigation. *TET2* mutations have been suggested to be associated with advanced-stage disease, thrombocytopenia, high IPI scores, and a shorter progression-free survival (Lemonnier et al., 2012).

Mycosis fungoides and Sézary syndrome

Mycosis fungoides (MF) is the most common subtype of the T-cell lymphomas that arise primarily in the skin. It is a mature T-cell lymphoma presenting with patches/plaques and is characterized by a dermal infiltration of small- to medium-sized T cells with cerebriform nuclei. Sézary syndrome (SS) is a generalized mature T-cell lymphoma characterized by the presence of erythroderma, lymphadenopathy, and neoplastic T lymphocytes in the blood. It is regarded as a variant of MF though its behavior is usually more aggressive (Jaffe et al., 2001).

Chromosome banding data on both these CTCL are still limited with karyotypes available on only about 150 cases (Mitelman et al., 2014). Chromosome abnormalities, mostly in complex karyotypes, are seen in 40–70% of patients with MF/SS, but there have only been a few instances of recurrent rearrangements (Schlegelberger et al., 1994a, 1994b, 1994d; Mao et al., 2003a; Espinet et al., 2004; Batista et al., 2006). The karyotypes in almost all cases are highly complex with evidence

of chromosomal instability. *Monosomy 10* has been reported as the most frequent cytogenetic change (73% of abnormal cases). *Monosomy 9* and *trisomy 18* have also been recurrently observed. The chromosomes most frequently involved in structural aberrations have been 1, 6, 8, 9, 10, 11, and 17. Recurrent breakpoints have been seen in 1p32–36, 1q, 2q, 6q22–27, 8q22, 17p11.2–13, 10q23–26, and 19p13.3. The aberrations dic(17;8)(p11.2;p11.2), der(1)t(1;10)(p2;q2), and der(14) t(14q;15q) might be recurrent in MF/SS, whereas translocations affecting *TCR* loci seem to be absent (Salgado et al., 2011).

Karenko et al. (2005) identified common clonal deletions or translocations with a breakpoint in 12q21 or 12q22 in SS. These seem to target the *NAV3 (POMFIL1)* gene for inactivation. With locus-specific FISH, *NAV3* deletions were found in the skin lesions of 4 of 8 (50%) patients with early MF and in the skin or lymph nodes of 11 of 13 (85%) patients with advanced MF or SS. The findings were not corroborated in the study by Marty et al. (2008).

CGH studies have revealed common losses of or from 1p, 6q, 10q, 13q, 17p, and 19 and gains of or from 7, 8q, 17q, and 18 (Mao et al., 2002, 2003a; Fischer et al., 2004). The pattern −6q, +7, +8, and −13 was the most frequent combination of imbalances. Later, aCGH analyses confirmed recurrent losses of 17p13.2–p11.2 and 10p12.1–q26.3 in 71% and 68% of cases, respectively, and gains in 17p11.2–q25.3 (64%) and chromosome 8/8q (50%), but also found recurrent loss of 9q13–21.33 and gain of 10p15.3–12.2 (Caprini et al., 2009). In line with these data, gain of 17q has been proposed as an early event in the pathogenesis of CTCL (Barba et al., 2008).

Chromosomal aberrations are more common in advanced and aggressive disease stages and subtypes. A high number of aberrations, gain of 8q, and loss of 6q and 13q have been associated with shorter survival (Fischer et al., 2004). Van Doorn et al. (2009) suggested that the pattern of chromosomal imbalances in MF differed from that of SS with highly recurrent chromosomal alterations in MF including gains of 7q36 and 7q21–22 and losses of 5q13 and 9p21. They also suggested that alterations on 9p21, 8q24, and 1q21–22 were associated with poor prognosis. Besides 9p21.3 (*CDKN2A*,

CDKN2B, and *MTAP*) and 8q24.21 (*MYC*) alterations, changes in 10q26-qter (*MGMT* and *EBF3*) have also been shown to correlate with overall survival. Moreover, two MF genomic subgroups have been described, a stable group (0–5 DNA aberrations) and an unstable group (>5 DNA aberrations), with patients of the genomically unstable group having shorter overall survival (Espinet and Salgado, 2013).

Exome sequencing in a single case of SS identified somatic missense mutations in *TBL1XR1*, *EPHA7*, and *SLFN12*, but these have not been shown to be recurrent (Andersson et al., 2014). Other candidate genes recurrently found inactive in CTCL include *TP53* and *E2A* (Steininger et al., 2011; Lamprecht et al., 2012). There are still no systematic sequencing studies in this disease.

The spectrum of cytogenetic changes in *subcutaneous panniculitis-like T-cell lymphomas* (SPTL)—a rare, difficult-to-diagnose, and poorly characterized subtype of CTCL—has been shown by CGH to overlap with the gain–loss characteristics of MM and SS. Many DNA copy number changes were identified, the most common of which were losses of 1pter, 2pter, 10qter, 11qter, 12qter, 16, 19, 20, and 22, whereas gains of 2q and 4q as well as *NAV3* aberrations were identified in 44% of the SPTL samples. Gains of or from 5q and 13q may characterize SPTL (Hahtola et al., 2008).

Adult T-cell leukemia/lymphoma

Adult T-cell leukemia/lymphoma (ATLL) is a usually widely disseminated peripheral T-cell neoplasm. ATLL is endemic in several regions of the world, in particular Japan, the Caribbean basin, and parts of Central Africa. The distribution of the disease is closely linked to the prevalence of human T-cell leukemia virus-1 (HTLV-1), which is found in all cases and is supposed to be causative for the disease (Jaffe et al., 2001).

Chromosome abnormalities have been found in more than 90% of the ATLL patients examined (Kamada et al., 1992; Itoyama et al., 2001). Although the changes are often both complex and variable, they are undoubtedly nonrandom. Chromosome 14 is the one most frequently rearranged, often as *t(14;14)(q11;q32)*, *inv(14)(q11q32)*, and *del(14)(q11q13)* or recombining 14q11 with several other chromosome arms, including Xq, 1p,

1q, 3p, 3q, 8q, 10p, 11p, 12q, and 18p. *t(14;14) (q11;q32)* has been shown to involve the *TCRAD* and *BCL11B* genes in at least one case, suggesting general involvement of the *TCR* loci (Przybylski et al., 2005). Furthermore, CGH has identified common 14q32 gain/amplification associated with *BCL11B* overexpression (Oshiro et al., 2006) although other groups have described low expression of BCL11B protein in ATLL (Kurosawa et al., 2013). The *BCL11B* gene may also be involved in ATLL through a translocation t(2;14)(q34;q32) recombining it with *HELIOS*; the latter gene has also been implicated in ATL1 pathogenesis of ATLL through various other aberrations (Fujimoto et al., 2012; Asanuma et al., 2013). Other frequently detected imbalances have been gains of 7q and 3p and losses of 6q and 13q (Tsukasaki et al., 2001; Oshiro et al., 2006).

Comparison of the genome profiles of acute and lymphoma types of ATLL detected by CGH revealed that the lymphoma type more frequently had gains from 1q, 2p, 4q, 7p, and 7q and losses from 10p, 13q, 16q, and 18p, whereas the acute type showed gain of 3/3p. Recurrent high-level amplifications were found at 1p36, 6p25, 7p22, 7q, and 14q32 in the lymphoma type, with *CARD11* being a candidate oncogene in 7p22 (Oshiro et al., 2006). Numerous other chromosomal regions have also occasionally been involved in ATLL, including 1p, 1q, 3q, 5p, 5q, 9q, 10p, 10q, 11q, 12q, 18q, and Y. A del(6q) with breakpoints mostly localized to bands q15 and q21 is seen in 25% of ATLL patients, mostly together with changes of 14q11 and/or 14q32. Altogether, aberrations affecting 14q11, 14q32, and/or 6q are seen in half of all karyotypically abnormal ATL.

Clinical correlations in ATLL

Aberrations of 1p, 1q, 1q10–21, 10p, 10p13, 12q, 14q, and 14q32 have been reported to correlate with clinical features like hepatosplenomegaly, elevated lactate dehydrogenase, hypercalcemia, and an unusual immunophenotype, all indicators of clinical severity in ATLL. Multiple changes; abnormalities of 1p, 1p22, 1q, 1q10–21, 2q, 3q, 3q10–12, 3q21, 14q, 14q32, and 17q; and partial losses from chromosome arms 2q, 9p, 14p, 14q, and 17q have correlated with shorter survival (Itoyama et al., 2001).

Hodgkin lymphoma (HL)

HL represents a peculiar subtype of mostly B-cell lymphoid malignancy that has been classified into two main subtypes, cHL and the more rare nodular lymphocyte-predominant HL (nlpHL). One of the main features of HL is that the tumor parenchyma cells only represent 0.1–10% of the total even in representative samples, the rest being derived from an intense inflammatory reaction. Therefore, the cytogenetic examination of HL is very challenging and frequently renders normal karyotypes that are representative only of the abundant nonmalignant cells. When the chromosome analysis is informative, karyotypes are very different from those of NHL (Drexler, 1992; Atkin, 1998).

cHL, including the subtypes nodular sclerosis, lymphocyte rich, mixed cellularity, and lymphocyte depleted

Chromosome analyses in many cHL reveal only normal karyotypes derived from the nonneoplastic bystander cells. A subset of cases particularly in earlier studies also showed single or few aberrations, which nowadays are supposed not to be derived from the tumor parenchyma. The application of chromosome banding analysis and interphase FISH studies in combination with CD30 immunofluorescence staining has unambiguously shown that, in most instances, the neoplastic Hodgkin/Reed–Sternberg (HRS) cells of cHL are characterized by highly complex karyotypes with evidence of ongoing chromosomal instability (i.e., each metaphase may be cytogenetically different), modal chromosome numbers mostly in the tri- or tetraploid range, multiple aneuploidies, and segmental chromosome aberrations (Drexler, 1992; Schlegelberger et al., 1994c; Weber-Matthiesen et al., 1995; Atkin, 1998; MacLeod et al., 2000; Joos et al., 2003; Martín-Subero et al., 2003a). Usually, the karyotype is not fully resolvable. Falzetti et al. (1999) reviewed the karyotypes of 177 cHL and pointed to some clonal nonrandom changes. Breakpoints in 1p36, 6q15–12, 7q22–32, 8q24, 11q23, 12q24, 14q32, and 19p13 were present in more than 5% of cases. Moreover, the short arms of the acrocentric chromosomes were recurrently

involved in translocations, suggesting a pathogenetic role of instability at *rRNA* loci.

Recurrent *deletions of 6q* are seen and the *TNFAIP3* gene has been suggested to be targeted by these deletions with concomitant mutations of the second allele in roughly half of the cases (Giefing et al., 2008; Hartmann et al., 2008). Other tumor suppressor genes inactivated in cHL are particularly *IKBA* in 14q and *SOCS1* in 16p13 (Cabannes et al., 1999; Emmerich et al., 1999; Jungnickel et al., 2000; Weniger et al., 2006; Mottok et al., 2007).

Molecular cytogenetic studies demonstrated that *t(14q32)* involving the *IGH* locus are present in 15–20% of cHL (Martín-Subero et al., 2006). The partners of these translocations are heterogeneous, including 2p16 *(REL)*, 3q27 *(BCL6)*, 8q24 *(MYC)*, 14q24, 16p13 *(C2TA)*, 17q12, and 19q13 *(BCL3)* (Martín-Subero et al., 2006; Szymanowska et al., 2008). Translocations t(14;18)(q32;q21) and t(3q27) occur extremely rarely in cHL with the exception of composite cHL and NHL, in which the HRS cells regularly carry the typical primary chromosomal alteration of the respective NHL (Schmitz et al., 2005; Szymanowska et al., 2008).

CGH of DNA from microdissected HRS cells has identified gains of chromosomal material (e.g., duplications or amplifications) in 2p13–16 (affecting the *REL* oncogene) in 40–50% of the cases and in 9p24 (possibly targeting *JAK2*, *PDL1*, and *PDL2*) in 30–40% (Joos et al., 2000, 2002; Martín-Subero et al., 2002). With regard to 2p, it has been shown that HRS cells with extra copies of the *REL* gene may have accumulation of the REL protein in the nucleus (Barth et al., 2003), which might account for the characteristic REL/NF-κB activation observed in HRS cells (Bargou et al., 1996). Array CGH studies of microdissected HRS cells have shown recurrent imbalances including gains of 2p, 9p, 16p, 17q, 19q, and 20q and losses of 6q, 11q, and 13q (Hartmann et al., 2008; Steidl et al., 2010).

Sequencing studies, besides identifying recurrent mutation of *PTPN1*, have confirmed the involvement of the *C2TA* (*MHC2TA*) gene in chromosomal translocations in cHL (Steidl et al., 2011; Gunawardana et al., 2014). Indeed, 15% of analyzed cHL showed breakpoints in C2TA, which is a partner in in-frame fusions with several other genes, most prominently *PDL2*.

nlpHL

nlpHL shares many features with DLBCL and may indeed be an NHL rather than an HL. Correspondingly, the scarce cytogenetic data suggest the presence of similar chromosomal aberrations in nlpHL to those of DLBCL. Using cytogenetic and molecular cytogenetic techniques, *t(3q27)* involving the *BCL6* locus has been reported in up to 50% of the cases (Wlodarska et al., 2003; Renné et al., 2005). The 3q27 rearrangements as usual include *t(3;14)(q27;q32)* with its light-chain variants but also involve non-IG loci as translocation partners. Recent cell line studies suggest also involvement of *C2TA* and *PDL2* in the pathogenesis of nlpHL similar to the situation in cHL (Steidl et al., 2011; Twa et al., 2014).

Practically no information is available about the prognostic impact of chromosomal findings in HL, particularly if modern therapies with a high likelihood of cure are being considered. One CGH study has associated del(13q) with unfavorable disease outcome in cHL (Chui et al., 2003). These findings were not corroborated by Steidl et al. (2010) who instead showed gains of 16p11.2–13.3 to be significantly associated with a poor prognosis.

Clinical correlations

The cytogenetic changes in mature lymphoid neoplasms and their clinical impact greatly depend on the disease subtype in which they occur. They have therefore mostly been discussed in the respective disease-specific sections.

The most important clinical reason for identifying chromosomal aberrations in suspected mature lymphoid neoplasms is the fact that they provide essential information on which a correct, precise diagnosis can be based. Different histopathologic subtypes of mature lymphoid neoplasms are associated with very different natural courses and show quite different responses to therapy. Modern therapy for mature lymphoid neoplasms relies on the proper classification of the lymphoma, and the patterns of both primary and secondary chromosomal aberrations constitute part of the foundation for that classification. Indeed, comments on the 2001 WHO classification recommend that cytogenetic analysis be performed in all cases and should form part of the pathology report (Harris et al., 1999, 2000).

It has to be emphasized that the same chromosomal aberrations may have different prognostic impact in the various subtypes of mature lymphoid neoplasms. Among NHL, for example, t(11;14) (q13;q32) mostly signifies a MCL that has a poor prognosis, although a subgroup of MCL with this translocation and favorable prognosis exists (Navarro et al., 2012). In contrast, t(11;14) in MM defines a disease subset with a relatively favorable outcome (though compared to t(11;14)-positive MCL, the overall survival of patients with t(11;14)-positive MM is still worse). Moreover, t(11;14) can be detected in preneoplastic disorders like MGUS and in quite indolent diseases like SLVL. These findings point to the need to integrate cytogenetic analysis into an interdisciplinary diagnostic workup of mature lymphoid neoplasms, which, besides histopathologic features and the immunophenotype, also takes into account both the clinical presentation and the neoplastic cells' genetic characteristics. It can be anticipated that the diagnostic process will soon also see the integration of findings made by array-based technologies like gene expression profiling as well as high-throughput sequencing.

Despite the fact that the clinical relevance of cytogenetic changes in mature lymphoid neoplasms always has to be evaluated in the context of the disease subtype, a few common themes generally associated with unfavorable outcome seem to exist: in most instances of mature lymphoid neoplasms, the rule of thumb is that the more complex the karyotype, the worse is the prognosis. A notable exception here is cHL that is characterized by highly complex karyotypes, and yet long-term cure rates far exceeding 80% are reached with modern therapy. Losses of 17p and 9p are supposed to mostly target the *TP53* and *TP16* gene loci. One or both changes are associated with unfavorable outcome in many mature lymphoid neoplasms, including CLL, FL, MCL, and DLBCL. Finally, translocations affecting the band 8q24 mostly target the *MYC* oncogene. In most types of mature lymphoid neoplasms, including FL, MCL, and DLBCL, these changes are associated with increased clinical aggressiveness and an unfavorable prognosis. The notable exception here is BL in which t(8;14) and variants are the pathognomonic alterations. Despite being a biologically highly aggressive disease, BL can be cured in most instances, particularly in children.

The near future will see the increasing introduction of molecular cytogenetic techniques like FISH and array CGH into the diagnosis of mature lymphoid neoplasms. Indeed, interphase FISH is already widely used for the diagnosis of the most recurrent alterations in CLL and MM and is also becoming a routine tool for the detection of diagnostically relevant chromosomal alterations in formalin-fixed, paraffin-embedded tissues (Ventura et al., 2006). Nevertheless, in contrast to chromosome banding analysis, interphase FISH will never provide a full overview of all chromosomal aberrations of a mature lymphoid neoplasm. This carries the very real risk that clinically relevant alterations, like t(8q24) in t(14;18)-positive FL, might be missed simply because they were not searched for. Moreover, a subclone with prognostically unfavorable chromosomal aberrations may be missed by FISH, whereas it might be detected by conventional cytogenetics due to a proliferative advantage of these cells. Finally, complex and variant FISH patterns might be difficult to interpret without knowledge of the metaphase chromosomal picture, the karyotype.

The advent of array CGH and related techniques enables the production of a wealth of new data at a resolution somewhere between the cytogenetic and molecular levels. One should exercise considerable caution when trying to translate findings and conclusions between the microscopic cytogenetic and the array-based information realms. As can be seen from the previous discussion of 13q deletions in MM, the diagnostic impact of a chromosomal change may seemingly depend on the technique with which it was detected (Dewald et al., 2005). Both small and large genetic changes can be missed if one exclusively relies on only one technique, not least if the change in question is present only in a subclone. The results are invariably best if different techniques and investigative principles are allowed to complement each other.

Recent technological developments have allowed high-throughput sequencing to become a part of both scientific and diagnostic analyses of lymphatic neoplasms. These new techniques provide valuable information helping us to understand the pathogenesis of neoplastic diseases better as well as to make more meaningful diagnoses and choose the optimal treatment. Prominent examples are *ID3* mutations in BL, *MYD88* mutations in Waldenström disease, or *RHOA* mutations in ATLL. In principle, sequencing technologies are able to detect all kinds of genomic alterations, be they balanced translocations, imbalances, or mutations. In practice, this may not be so easy, not least when it comes to translocations with repeat-rich breakpoints. In addition, the subclonal composition of tumors is hard to evaluate if these techniques are used alone. Finally, a wealth of bioinformatic challenges need to be resolved for daily use. It nevertheless seems beyond doubt that the future will see an integration of the different tumor genetic techniques also for diagnostic purposes, in lymphatic neoplasms as elsewhere, with important clinical benefits for the patients (Biesecker et al., 2012; Yates and Campbell, 2012; Mwenifumbo and Marra, 2013).

It should finally be stressed that the treatment of many mature lymphoid neoplasms is now undergoing profound changes. Probably, the most important recent improvement in the treatment of the most common lymphomas, including the mature B-cell lymphomas MCL, FL, and DLCBL, was the introduction of anti-CD20 immunotherapy (Rituxan) (Coiffier et al, 2002; Kluin-Nelemans et al., 2012). Almost all cytogenetic studies referred to earlier were performed before the introduction of this therapy, and we do not know whether the cytogenetic–prognostic correlations detected during the pre-Rituxan era still apply when the new antibody treatment is given. Indeed, with the exception of CLL and MM and in part BL and DLBCL, hardly any systematic cytogenetic studies within clinical trials exist. This needs to be changed in future so that cytogenetic studies as well as molecular studies form an essential and integral part of prospective clinical trials; only then can the clinical impact of the various acquired genomic changes in mature lymphoid neoplasms be reliably assessed.

Acknowledgments

The authors' own studies on chromosomal aberrations in lymphoid neoplasms are supported by Bundesministerium für Bildung und Forschung (BMBF), Deutsche Krebshilfe, Wilhelm Sander-Stiftung, KinderKrebsInitiative (KKI) Buchholz/Holm-Seppensen, European Union, Lymphoma Research Foundation (New York), and Schleswig-Holsteinische Krebsgesellschaft. The authors would like to thank Dr. Jose-Ignacio Martin-Subero, Dr. Borja Saez, and Heike Blohm for editorial support and Dr. Lana Harder, Dr. Simone Heidemann, and Claus-Peter Blohm for providing the figures and the graphical design. Finally, the authors acknowledge all colleagues worldwide who have made publicly available their cytogenetic data on lymphoid neoplasms and at the same time apologize to all whose work could not be cited herein. SMA is a fellow of the JSM-UMCG MD-PhD program, a recipient of the "Nijbakker-Morra" and "Hippocrates" Foundations awards, and is supported by the "Foundation de Drie Lichten," the "René Vogels' Foundation," and the framework of a "JSM-Ubbo Emmius Foundation Talent Grant."

References

Aamot HV, Bjørnslett M, Delabie J, Heim S (2005a): t(14;22) (q32;q11) in non-Hodgkin lymphoma and myeloid leukaemia: molecular cytogenetic investigations. *Br J Haematol* 130:845–851.

Aamot HV, Micci F, Holte H, Delabie J, Heim S (2005b): G-banding and molecular cytogenetic analyses of marginal zone lymphoma. *Br J Haematol* 130:890–901.

Aamot HV, Torlakovic EE, Eide MB, Holte H, Heim S (2007): Non-Hodgkin lymphoma with t(14;18): clonal evolution patterns and cytogenetic–pathologic–clinical correlations. *J Cancer Res Clin Oncol* 133:455–470.

Abdul-Wahab A, Tang SY, Robson A, Morris S, Agar N, Wain EM, et al. (2014): Chromosomal anomalies in primary cutaneous follicle center cell lymphoma do not portend a poor prognosis. *J Am Acad Dermatol* 70:1010–1020.

Adachi M, Tefferi A, Greipp PR, Kipps TJ, Tsujimoto Y (1990): Preferential linkage of bcl-2 to immunoglobulin light chain gene in chronic lymphocytic leukemia. *J Exp Med* 171:559–564.

Adam P, Baumann R, Schmidt J, Bettio S, Weisel K, Bonzheim I, et al. (2013): The BCL2 E17 and SP66 antibodies discriminate 2 immunophenotypically and genetically distinct subgroups of conventionally BCL2-"negative" grade 1/2 follicular lymphomas. *Hum Pathol* 44:1817–1826.

Affer M, Chesi M, Chen WD, Keats JJ, Demchenko YN, Tamizhmani K, et al. (2014): Promiscuous MYC locus rearrangements hijack enhancers but mostly super-enhancers to dysregulate MYC expression in myeloma. *Leukemia* 28:1725–1735.

Agopian J, Navarro JM, Gac AC, Lecluse Y, Briand M, Grenot P, et al. (2009): Agricultural pesticide exposure and the molecular connection to lymphomagenesis. *J Exp Med* 206:1473-1483.

Akagi T, Motegi M, Tamura A, Suzuki R, Hosokawa Y, Suzuki H, et al. (1999): A novel gene, MALT1 at 18q21, is involved in t(11;18) (q21;q21) found in low-grade B-cell lymphoma of mucosa-associated lymphoid tissue. *Oncogene* 18:5785–5794.

Akao Y, Seto M, Yamamoto K, Iida S, Nakazawa S, Inazawa J, et al. (1992): The RCK gene associated with t(11;14) translocation is distinct from the MLL/ALL-1 gene with t(4;11) and t(11;19) translocations. *Cancer Res* 52:6083–6087.

Akasaka T, Miura I, Takahashi N, Akasaka H, Yonetani N, Ohno H, et al. (1997): A recurring translocation, t(3;6) (q27;p21), in non-Hodgkin's lymphoma results in replacement of the 5′ regulatory region of BCL6 with a novel H4 histone gene. *Cancer Res* 57:7–12.

Akasaka H, Akasaka T, Kurata M, Ueda C, Shimizu A, Uchiyama T, et al. (2000a): Molecular anatomy of BCL6 translocations revealed by long-distance polymerase chain reaction-based assays. *Cancer Res* 60:2335–2341.

Akasaka T, Ueda C, Kurata M, Akasaka H, Yamabe H, Uchiyama T, et al. (2000b): Nonimmunoglobulin (non-Ig)/BCL6 gene fusion in diffuse large B-cell lymphoma results in worse prognosis than Ig/BCL6. *Blood* 96:2907–2909.

Akasaka T, Lossos IS, Levy R (2003): BCL6 gene translocation in follicular lymphoma: a harbinger of eventual transformation to diffuse aggressive lymphoma. *Blood* 102:1443–1448.

Akay OM, Aras BD, Isiksoy S, Toprak C, Mutlu FS, Artan S, et al. (2014): BCL2, BCL6, IGH, TP53 and MYC protein expression and gene rearrangements as prognostic markers in diffuse large B-cell lymphoma: a study of 44 Turkish patients. *Cancer Genet* 207:87–93.

Akyurek N, Uner A, Benekli M, Barista I (2012): Prognostic significance of MYC, BCL2, and BCL6 rearrangements in patients with diffuse large B-cell lymphoma treated with cyclophosphamide, doxorubicin, vincristine, and prednisolone plus rituximab. *Cancer* 118:4173–183.

Alexandrov LB, Nik-Zainal S, Wedge DC, Aparicio SA, Behjati S, Biankin AV, et al. (2013): Signatures of mutational processes in human cancer. *Nature* 500:415–421.

Alizadeh AA, Eisen MB, Davis RE, Ma C, Lossos IS, Rosenwald A, et al. (2000): Distinct types of diffuse large B-cell lymphoma identified by gene expression profiling. *Nature* 403:503–511.

Almire C, Bertrand P, Ruminy P, Maingonnat C, Wlodarska I, Martín-Subero JI, et al. (2007): PVRL2 is translocated to the TRA@ locus in t(14;19)(q11;q13)-positive peripheral T-cell lymphomas. *Genes Chromosomes Cancer* 46: 1011–1018.

Andersen CL, Gruszka-Westwood A, Atkinson S, Matutes E, Catovsky D, Pedersen RK, et al. (2005): Recurrent genomic imbalances in B-cell splenic marginal-zone lymphoma revealed by comparative genomic hybridization. *Cancer Genet Cytogenet* 156:122–128.

Andersson EI, Rajala HL, Eldfors S, Ellonen P, Olson T, Jerez A, et al. (2013): Novel somatic mutations in large granular lymphocytic leukemia affecting the STAT-pathway and T-cell activation. *Blood Cancer J* 6:e168.

Andersson E, Eldfors S, Edgren H, Ellonen P, Väkevä L, Ranki A, et al. (2014): Novel TBL1XR1, EPHA7 and SLFN12 mutations in a Sezary syndrome patient discovered by whole exome sequencing. *Exp Dermatol* 23:366–368.

Ansell SM, Akasaka T, McPhail E, Manske M, Braggio E, Price-Troska T, et al. (2012): t(X;14)(p11;q32) in MALT lymphoma involving GPR34 reveals a role for GPR34 in tumor cell growth. *Blood* 120:3949–3957.

Arcaini L, Zibellini S, Boveri E, Riboni R, Rattotti S, Varettoni M, et al. (2012): The BRAF V600E mutation in hairy cell leukemia and other mature B-cell neoplasms. *Blood* 119:188–191.

Asanuma S, Yamagishi M, Kawanami K, Nakano K, Sato-Otsubo A, Muto S, et al. (2013): Adult T-cell leukemia cells are characterized by abnormalities of Helios expression that promote T cell growth. *Cancer Sci* 104:1097–1106.

Athanasiadou A, Stamatopoulos K, Tsompanakou A, Gaitatzi M, Kalogiannidis P, Anagnostopoulos A, Fassas A, Tsezou A (2006): Clinical, immunophenotypic, and molecular profiling of trisomy 12 in chronic lymphocytic leukemia and comparison with other karyotypic subgroups defined by cytogenetic analysis. *Cancer Genet Cytogenet* 168:109–119.

Atkin NB (1998): Cytogenetics of Hodgkin's disease. *Cytogenet Cell Genet* 80: 23–27.

Attarbaschi A, Beishuizen A, Mann G, Rosolen A, Mori T, Uyttebroeck A, et al. (2013): Children and adolescents with follicular lymphoma have an excellent prognosis with either limited chemotherapy or with a "Watch and wait" strategy after complete resection. *Ann Hematol* 92:1537–1541.

Au WY, Gascoyne RD, Viswanatha DS, Skinnider BF, Connors JM, Klasa RJ, et al. (1999): Concurrent chromosomal alterations at 3q27, 8q24 and 18q21 in B-cell lymphomas. *Br J Haematol* 105:437–440.

Au WY, Horsman DE, Viswanatha DS, Connors JM, Klasa RJ, Gascoyne RD (2000): 8q24 translocations in blastic transformation of mantle cell lymphoma. *Haematologica* 85:1225–1227.

Au WY, Gascoyne RD, Viswanatha DS, Connors JM, Klasa RJ, Horsman DE (2002): Cytogenetic analysis in mantle cell lymphoma: a review of 214 cases. *Leuk Lymphoma* 43:783–791.

Au WY, Horsman DE, Gascoyne RD, Viswanatha DS, Klasa RJ, Connors JM (2004): The spectrum of lymphoma with 8q24 aberrations: a clinical, pathological and cytogenetic study of 87 consecutive cases. *Leuk Lymphoma* 45:519–528.

Aukema SM, Siebert R, Schuuring E, van Imhoff GW, Kluin-Nelemans HC, Boerma EJ, Kluin PM (2011): Double-hit B-cell lymphomas. *Blood* 117:2319–2331.

Aukema SM, Kreuz M, Kohler CW, Rosolowski M, Hasenclever D, Hummel M, et al. (2014). Biological characterization of adult MYC-translocation-positive mature B-cell lymphomas other than molecular Burkitt lymphoma. *Haematologica* 99:726–735.

Austen B, Skowronska A, Baker C, Powell JE, Gardiner A, Oscier D, et al. (2007): Mutation status of the residual ATM allele is an important determinant of the cellular response to chemotherapy and survival in patients with chronic lymphocytic leukemia containing an 11q deletion. *J Clin Oncol* 25:5448–5457.

Avet-Loiseau H, Andree-Ashley LE, Moore D 2nd, Mellerin MP, Feusner J, et al. (1997): Molecular cytogenetic abnormalities in multiple myeloma and plasma cell leukemia measured using comparative genomic hybridization. *Genes Chromosomes Cancer* 19:124–133.

Avet-Loiseau H, Li JY, Facon T, Brigaudeau C, Morineau N, Maloisel F, et al. (1998): High incidence of translocations t(11;14)(q13;q32) and t(4;14)(p16;q32) in patients with plasma cell malignancies. *Cancer Res* 58:5640–5645.

Avet-Loiseau H, Gerson F, Magrangeas F, Minvielle S, Harousseau JL, Bataille R, et al. (2001): Rearrangements of the c-myc oncogene are present in 15% of primary human multiple myeloma tumors. *Blood* 98:3082–3086.

Avet-Loiseau H, Facon T, Grosbois B, Magrangeas F, Rapp MJ, Harousseau JL, et al. (2002): Oncogenesis of multiple myeloma: 14q32 and 13q chromosomal abnormalities are not randomly distributed, but correlate with natural history, immunological features, and clinical presentation. *Blood* 99:2185–2191.

Avet-Loiseau H, Attal M, Moreau P, Charbonnel C, Garban F, Hulin C, et al. (2007): Genetic abnormalities and survival in multiple myeloma: the experience of the Intergroupe Francophone du Myélome. *Blood* 109:3489–3495.

Avet-Louseau H, Daviet A, Sauner S, Bataille R, Intergroupe Francophone du Myélome (2000): Chromosome 13 abnormalities in multiple myeloma are mostly monosomy 13. *Br J Haematol* 111:1116–1117.

Baliakas P, Hadzidimitriou A, Sutton LA, Rossi D, Minga E, Villamor N, et al. (2015): Recurrent mutations refine prognosis in chronic lymphocytic leukemia. *Leukemia* 29:329–336.

Banks PM, Chan J, Cleary ML, Delsol G, DeWolf-Peeters C, Gatter K, et al. (1992): Mantle cell lymphoma. A proposal for unification of morphologic, immunologic, and molecular data. *Am J Surg Pathol* 16:637–640.

Barba G, Matteucci C, Girolomoni G, Brandimarte L, Varasano E, Martelli MF, et al. (2008): Comparative genomic hybridization identifies 17q11.2 approximately q12 duplication as an early event in cutaneous T-cell lymphomas. *Cancer Genet Cytogenet* 184:48–51.

Bargou RC, Leng C, Krappmann D, Emmerich F, Mapara MY, Bommert K, et al. (1996): High-level nuclear NF-kappa B and Oct-2 is a common feature of cultured Hodgkin/Reed–Sternberg cells. *Blood* 87:4340–4347.

Barillé-Nion S, Barlogie B, Bataille R, Bergsagel PL, Epstein J, Fenton RG, et al. (2003): Advances in biology and therapy of multiple myeloma. Hematology Am Soc Hematol Educ Program 248–278.

Baró C, Salido M, Domingo A, Granada I, Colomo L, Serrano S, et al. (2006): Translocation t(9;14)(p13;q32) in cases of splenic marginal zone lymphoma. *Haematologica* 91:1289–1291.

Barrans SL, O'Connor SJ, Evans PA, Davies FE, Owen RG, Haynes AP, et al. (2002): Rearrangement of the BCL6 locus at 3q27 is an independent poor prognostic factor in nodal diffuse large B-cell lymphoma. *Br J Haematol* 117:322–332.

Barrans SL, Evans PA, O'Connor SJ, Kendall SJ, Owen RG, Haynes AP, et al. (2003): The t(14;18) is associated with germinal center-derived diffuse large B-cell lymphoma and is a strong predictor of outcome. *Clin Cancer Res* 9:2133–2139.

Barrans S, Crouch S, Smith A, Turner K, Owen R, Patmore R, et al. (2010): Rearrangement of MYC is associated with poor prognosis in patients with diffuse large B-cell lymphoma treated in the era of rituximab. *J Clin Oncol* 28:3360–3365.

Barth TF, Bentz M, Leithäuser F, Stilgenbauer S, Siebert R, Schlotter M, et al. (2001): Molecular-cytogenetic comparison of mucosa-associated marginal zone B-cell lymphoma and large B-cell lymphoma arising in the gastro-intestinal tract. *Genes Chromosomes Cancer* 31:316–325.

Barth TF, Martin-Subero JI, Joos S, Menz CK, Hasel C, Mechtersheimer G, et al. (2003): Gains of 2p involving the REL locus correlate with nuclear c-Rel protein accumulation in neoplastic cells of classical Hodgkin lymphoma. *Blood* 101:3681–3686.

Bäsecke J, Griesinger F, Trümper L, Brittinger G (2002): Leukemia- and lymphoma-associated genetic aberrations in healthy individuals. *Ann Hematol* 81:64–75.

Bastard C, Tilly H, Lenormand B, Bigorgne C, Boulet D, Kunlin A, et al. (1992): Translocations involving band 3q27 and Ig gene regions in non-Hodgkin's lymphoma. *Blood* 79:2527–2531.

Batista DA, Vonderheid EC, Hawkins A, Morsberger L, Long P, Murphy KM, et al. (2006): Multicolor fluorescence in situ hybridization (SKY) in mycosis fungoides and Sézary syndrome: search for recurrent chromosome abnormalities. *Genes Chromosomes Cancer* 45:383–391.

Bauer B, Siebert R, Traulsen A. (2014): Cancer initiation with epistatic interactions between driver and passenger mutations. *J Theor Biol*. 358:52–60.

Baumgärtner AK, Zettl A, Chott A, Ott G, Müller-Hermelink HK, Starostik P (2003): High frequency of genetic aberrations in enteropathy-type T-cell lymphoma. *Lab Invest* 83:1509–1516.

Beà S, López-Guillermo A, Ribas M, Puig X, Pinyol M, Carrió A, et al. (2002): Genetic imbalances in progressed B-cell chronic lymphocytic leukemia and transformed large-cell lymphoma (Richter's syndrome). *Am J Pathol* 161:957–968.

Bea S, Zettl A, Wright G, Salaverria I, Jehn P, Moreno V, et al. (2005): Diffuse large B-cell lymphoma subgroups have distinct genetic profiles that influence tumor biology and improve gene-expression-based survival prediction. *Blood* 106:3183–3190.

Bea S, Salaverria I, Armengol L, Pinyol M, Fernandez V, Hartmann EM, et al. (2009): Uniparental disomies, homozygous deletions, amplifications and target genes in mantle cell lymphoma revealed by integrative high-resolution whole genome profiling. *Blood* 26:3059–3069.

Beà S, Valdés-Mas R, Navarro A, Salaverria I, Martín-Garcia D, Jares P, et al. (2013): Landscape of somatic mutations and clonal evolution in mantle cell lymphoma. *Proc Natl Acad Sci USA* 110:18250–18255.

Bednarek AK, Laflin KJ, Daniel RL, Liao Q, Hawkins KA, Aldaz CM (2000): WWOX, a novel WW domain-containing protein mapping to human chromosome 16q23.3–24.1, a region frequently affected in breast cancer. *Cancer Res* 60:2140–2145.

Belaud-Rotureau MA, Marietta V, Vergier B, Mainhaguiet G, Turmo M, Idrissi Y, et al. (2008): Inactivation of p16[INK4a]/CDKN2A gene may be a diagnostic feature of large B cell lymphoma leg type among cutaneous B cell lymphomas. *Virchows Arch* 452:607–620.

Bellanger D, Jacquemin V, Chopin M, Pierron G, Bernard OA, Ghysdael J, et al. (2014): Recurrent JAK1 and JAK3 somatic mutations in T-cell prolymphocytic leukemia. *Leukemia* 28:417–419.

Bellas C, García D, Vicente Y, Kilany L, Abraira V, Navarro B, et al. (2014): Immunohistochemical and molecular characteristics with prognostic significance in diffuse large B-cell lymphoma. *PLoS One* 9:e98169.

Bentley G, Palutke M, Mohamed AN (2005): Variant t(14;18) in malignant lymphoma: a report of seven cases. *Cancer Genet Cytogenet* 157:12–17.

Bentz M, Huck K, du Manoir S, Joos S, Werner CA, Fischer K, et al. (1995): Comparative genomic hybridization in chronic B-cell leukemias shows a high incidence of chromosomal gains and losses. *Blood* 85:3610–3618.

Bentz M, Barth TF, Brüderlein S, Bock D, Schwerer MJ, Baudis M, et al. (2001): Gain of chromosome arm 9p is characteristic of primary mediastinal B-cell lymphoma

(MBL): comprehensive molecular cytogenetic analysis and presentation of a novel MBL cell line. *Genes Chromosomes Cancer* 30:393–401.

Berger R, Bernheim A, Weh HJ, Flandrin G, Daniel MT, Brouet JC, et al. (1979): A new translocation in Burkitt's tumor cells. *Hum Genet* 53:111–112.

Berger R, Le Coniat M, Derré J, Vecchione D (1989): Secondary nonrandom chromosomal abnormalities of band 13q34 in Burkitt lymphoma-leukemia. *Genes Chromosomes Cancer* 1:115–118.

Berglund M, Enblad G, Thunberg U, Amini RM, Sundström C, Roos G, et al. (2007): Genomic imbalances during transformation from follicular lymphoma to diffuse large B-cell lymphoma. *Mod Pathol.* 20:63–75.

Bergsagel PL, Chesi M (2013): Molecular classification and risk stratification of myeloma. *Hematol Oncol Suppl* 1:38–41.

Bergsagel PL, Kuehl WM (2001): Chromosome translocations in multiple myeloma. *Oncogene* 20:5611–5622.

Bergsagel PL, Kuehl WM (2005): Molecular pathogenesis and a consequent classification of multiple myeloma. *J Clin Oncol* 23:6333–6338.

Bergsagel PL, Chesi M, Nardini E, Brents LA, Kirby SL, Kuehl WM (1996): Promiscuous translocations into immunoglobulin heavy chain switch regions in multiple myeloma. *Proc Natl Acad Sci USA* 93:13931–13936.

Bergsagel PL, Nardini E, Brents L, Chesi M, Kuehl WM (1997): IgH translocations in multiple myeloma: a nearly universal event that rarely involves c-myc. *Curr Top Microbiol Immunol* 224:283–287.

Bergsagel PL, Kuehl WM, Zhan F, Sawyer J, Barlogie B, Shaughnessy J Jr (2005): Cyclin D dysregulation: an early and unifying pathogenic event in multiple myeloma. *Blood* 106:296–303.

Bertrand P, Bastard C, Maingonnat C, Jardin F, Maisonneuve C, Courel MN, et al. (2007): Mapping of MYC breakpoints in 8q24 rearrangements involving non-immunoglobulin partners in B-cell lymphomas. *Leukemia* 21:515–523.

Bi Y, Zeng N, Chanudet E, Huang Y, Hamoudi RA, Liu H, et al. (2012): A20 inactivation in ocular adnexal MALT lymphoma. *Haematologica* 97:926–930.

Biagi JJ, Seymour JF (2002): Insights into the molecular pathogenesis of follicular lymphoma arising from analysis of geographic variation. *Blood* 99:4265–4275.

Biesecker LG, Burke W, Kohane I, Plon SE, Zimmern R (2012): Next-generation sequencing in the clinic: are we ready? *Nat Rev Genet* 13:818–824.

Boerma EG, van Imhoff GW, Appel IM, Veeger NJ, Kluin PM, Kluin-Nelemans JC (2004): Gender and age-related differences in Burkitt lymphoma – epidemiological and clinical data from the Netherlands. *Eur J Cancer* 40:2781–2787.

Boerma EG, Siebert R, Kluin PM, Baudis M (2009): Translocations involving 8q24 in Burkitt lymphoma and

other malignant lymphomas: a historical review of cytogenetics in the light of todays knowledge. *Leukemia* 23:225–234.

Boersma-Vreugdenhil GR, Kuipers J, VanStralen E, Peeters T, Michaux L, Hagemeijer A, et al. (2004): The recurrent translocation t(14;20)(q32;q12) in multiple myeloma results in aberrant expression of MAFB: a molecular and genetic analysis of the chromosomal breakpoint. *Br J Haematol* 126:355–363.

Bohers E, Mareschal S, Bouzelfen A, Marchand V, Ruminy P, Maingonnat C, et al. (2014): Targetable activating mutations are very frequent in GCB and ABC diffuse large B-cell lymphoma. *Genes Chromosomes Cancer* 53:144–153.

Boi M, Rinaldi A, Kwee I, Bonetti P, Todaro M, Tabbò F, et al. (2013): PRDM1/BLIMP1 is commonly inactivated in anaplastic large T-cell lymphoma. *Blood* 122: 2683–2693.

Bolli N, Avet-Loiseau H, Wedge DC, Van Loo P, Alexandrov LB, Martincorena I, et al. (2014): Heterogeneity of genomic evolution and mutational profiles in multiple myeloma. *Nat Commun* 5:2997.

Booman M, Douwes J, Glas AM, Riemersma SA, Jordanova ES, Kok K, et al. (2006): Mechanisms and effects of loss of human leukocyte antigen class II expression in immune-privileged site-associated B-cell lymphoma. *Clin Cancer Res* 12:2698–2705.

Booman M, Szuhai K, Rosenwald A, Hartmann E, Kluin-Nelemans H, de Jong D, et al. (2008): Genomic aberrations and gene expression in primary diffuse large B-cell lymphomas of immune-privileged sites: the importance of apoptosis and immunomodulatory pathways. *J Pathol* 216:209–217.

Bosga-Bouwer AG, van Imhoff GW, Boonstra R, van der Veen A, Haralambieva E, van den Berg A, et al. (2003): Follicular lymphoma grade 3B includes 3 cytogenetically defined subgroups with primary t(14;18), 3q27, or other translocations: t(14;18) and 3q27 are mutually exclusive. *Blood* 101:1149–1154.

Bosga-Bouwer AG, Haralambieva E, Booman M, Boonstra R, van den Berg A, Schuuring E, et al. (2005): BCL6 alternative translocation breakpoint cluster region associated with follicular lymphoma grade 3B. *Genes Chromosomes Cancer* 44:301–304.

Bosga-Bouwer AG, van den Berg A, Haralambieva E, de Jong D, Boonstra R, Kluin P, van den Berg E, Poppema S (2006): Molecular, cytogenetic, and immunophenotypic characterization of follicular lymphoma grade 3B; a separate entity or part of the spectrum of diffuse large B-cell lymphoma or follicular lymphoma? *Hum Pathol* 37:528–533.

Böttcher S, Ritgen M, Buske S, Gesk S, Klapper W, Hoster E, et al. (2008): Minimal residual disease detection in mantle cell lymphoma: methods and significance of four-color flow cytometry compared to consensus IGH-polymerase chain reaction at initial staging and for follow-up examinations. *Haematologica* 93:551–559.

Bouamar H, Abbas S, Lin AP, Wang L, Jiang D, Holder KN, et al. (2013): A capture-sequencing strategy identifies IRF8, EBF1, and APRIL as novel IGH fusion partners in B-cell lymphoma. *Blood* 122:726–733.

Bouchekioua A, Scourzic L, de Wever O, Zhang Y, Cervera P, Aline-Fardin A, et al. (2014): JAK3 deregulation by activating mutations confers invasive growth advantage in extranodal nasal-type natural killer cell lymphoma. *Leukemia* 28:338–348.

Boulanger E, Agbalika F, Maarek O, Daniel MT, Grollet L, Molina JM, et al. (2001): A clinical, molecular and cytogenetic study of 12 cases of human herpesvirus 8 associated primary effusion lymphoma in HIV-infected patients. *Hematol J* 2:172–179.

Bouska A, McKeithan TW, Deffenbacher KE, Lachel C, Wright GW, Iqbal J, et al. (2014): Genome-wide copy-number analyses reveal genomic abnormalities involved in transformation of follicular lymphoma. *Blood* 123:1681–1690.

Boxer LM, Dang CV (2001): Translocations involving c-myc and c-myc function. *Oncogene* 20: 5595–5610.

Braggio E, Dogan A, Keats JJ, Chng WJ, Huang G, Matthews JM, et al. (2012): Genomic analysis of marginal zone and lymphoplasmacytic lymphomas identified common and disease-specific abnormalities. *Mod Pathol* 25:651–660.

Brito-Babapulle V, Pittman S, Melo JV, Pomfret M, Catovsky D (1987): Cytogenetic studies on prolymphocytic leukemia. 1. B-cell prolymphocytic leukemia. *Hematol Pathol* 1:27–33.

Brito-Babapulle V, Ellis J, Matutes E, Oscier D, Khokhar T, MacLennan K, et al. (1992): Translocation t(11;14) (q13;q32) in chronic lymphoid disorders. *Genes Chromosomes Cancer* 5:158–165.

Brito-Babapulle V, Gruszka-Westwood AM, Platt G, Andersen CL, Elnenaei MO, Matutes E, et al. (2002): Translocation t(2;7)(p12;q21–22) with dysregulation of the CDK6 gene mapping to 7q21–22 in a non-Hodgkin's lymphoma with leukemia. *Haematologica* 87: 357–362.

Brousseau M, Leleu X, Gerard J, Gastinne T, Godon A, Genevieve F, et al. (2007): Hyperdiploidy is a common finding in monoclonal gammopathy of undetermined significance and monosomy 13 is restricted to these hyperdiploid patients. *Clin Cancer Res* 13:6026–6031.

Buchonnet G, Lenain P, Ruminy P, Lepretre S, Stamatoullas A, Parmentier F, et al. (2000): Characterisation of BCL2-JH rearrangements in follicular lymphoma: PCR detection of 3′ BCL2 breakpoints and evidence of a new cluster. *Leukemia* 14:1563–1569.

Buchonnet G, Jardin F, Jean N, Bertrand P, Parmentier F, Tison S, et al. (2002): Distribution of BCL2 breakpoints in follicular lymphoma and correlation with clinical features: specific subtypes or same disease? *Leukemia* 16:1852–1856.

Buhmann R, Kurzeder C, Rehklau J, Westhaus D, Bursch S, Hiddemann W, et al. (2002): CD40L stimulation enhances the ability of conventional metaphase cytogenetics to detect chromosome aberrations in B-cell chronic lymphocytic leukaemia cells. *Br J Haematol* 118:968–975.

Busslinger M, Klix N, Pfeffer P, Graninger PG, Kozmik Z (1996): Deregulation of PAX-5 by translocation of the Emu enhancer of the IgH locus adjacent to two alternative PAX-5 promoters in a diffuse large-cell lymphoma. *Proc Natl Acad Sci USA* 93:6129–6134.

Butler MP, Iida S, Capello D, Rossi D, Rao PH, Nallasivam P, et al. (2002): Alternative translocation breakpoint cluster region 5′ to BCL-6 in B-cell non-Hodgkin's lymphoma. *Cancer Res* 62:4089–4094.

Caballero D, García-Marco JA, Martino R, Mateos V, Ribera JM, Sarrá J, et al. (2005): Allogeneic transplant with reduced intensity conditioning regimens may overcome the poor prognosis of B-cell chronic lymphocytic leukemia with unmutated immunoglobulin variable heavy-chain gene and chromosomal abnormalities (11q– and 17p–). *Clin Cancer Res* 11:7757–7763.

Cabannes E, Khan G, Aillet F, Jarrett RF, Hay RT (1999): Mutations in the IkBa gene in Hodgkin's disease suggest a tumour suppressor role for IkappaBalpha. *Oncogene* 18:3063–3070.

Cairns RA, Iqbal J, Lemonnier F, Kucuk C, de Leval L, Jais JP, et al. (2012): IDH2 mutations are frequent in angioimmunoblastic T-cell lymphoma. *Blood* 119:1901–1903.

Calasanz MJ, Cigudosa JC, Odero MD, Ferreira C, Ardanaz MT, Fraile A, et al. (1997a): Cytogenetic analysis of 280 patients with multiple myeloma and related disorders: primary breakpoints and clinical correlations. *Genes Chromosomes Cancer* 18:84–93.

Calasanz MJ, Cigudosa JC, Odero MD, García-Foncillas J, Marín J, Ardanaz MT, Rocha E, Gullón A (1997b): Hypodiploidy and 22q11 rearrangements at diagnosis are associated with poor prognosis in patients with multiple myeloma. *Br J Haematol* 98:418–425.

Calin GA, Dumitru CD, Shimizu M, Bichi R, Zupo S, Noch E, et al. (2002): Frequent deletions and down-regulation of micro-RNA genes miR15 and miR16 at 13q14 in chronic lymphocytic leukemia. *Proc Natl Acad Sci USA* 99:15524–15529.

Callanan MB, LeBaccon P, Mossuz P, Duley S, Bastard C, Hamoudi R, et al. (2000): The IgG Fc receptor, Fc gamma RIIB, is a target for deregulation by chromosomal translocation in malignant lymphoma. *Proc Natl Acad Sci USA* 97:309–314.

Callet-Bauchu E, Baseggio L, Felman P, Traverse-Glehen A, Berger F, Morel D, et al. (2005): Cytogenetic analysis delineates a spectrum of chromosomal changes that can distinguish non-MALT marginal zone B-cell lymphomas among mature B-cell entities: a description of 103 cases. *Leukemia* 19:1818–1823.

Campo E (2012): New pathogenic mechanisms in Burkitt lymphoma. *Nat Genet* 44:1288–1289.

Campo E (2013): Whole genome profiling and other high throughput technologies in lymphoid neoplasms: current contributions and future hopes. *Mod Pathol* 26: S97–S110.

Caprini E, Cristofoletti C, Arcelli D, Fadda P, Citterich MH, Sampogna F, et al. (2009): Identification of key regions and genes important in the pathogenesis of Sézary syndrome by combining genomic and expression microarrays. *Cancer Res* 69:8438–8446.

Carbone A (2003): Emerging pathways in the development of AIDS-related lymphomas. *Lancet Oncol* 4: 22–29.

Chambwe N, Kormaksson M, Geng H, De S, Michor F, Johnson NA, et al. (2014): Variability in DNA methylation defines novel epigenetic subgroups of DLBCL associated with different clinical outcomes. *Blood* 123:1699–1708.

Chang H, Qi C, Yi QL, Reece D, Stewart AK (2005a): p53 Gene deletion detected by fluorescence in situ hybridization is an adverse prognostic factor for patients with multiple myeloma following autologous stem cell transplantation. *Blood* 105: 358–360.

Chang H, Qi XY, Samiee S, Yi QL, Chen C, Trudel S, et al. (2005b): Genetic risk identifies multiple myeloma patients who do not benefit from autologous stem cell transplantation. *Bone Marrow Transplant* 36:793–796.

Chanudet E, Huang Y, Ichimura K, Dong G, Hamoudi RA, Radford J, et al. (2010): A20 is targeted by promoter methylation, deletion and inactivating mutation in MALT lymphoma. *Leukemia* 24:483–487.

Chanudet E, Huang Y, Zeng N, Streubel B, Chott A, Raderer M, et al. (2011): TNFAIP3 abnormalities in MALT lymphoma with autoimmunity. *Br J Haematol* 154:535–539.

Chapman MA, Lawrence MS, Keats JJ, Cibulskis K, Sougnez C, Schinzel AC, et al. (2011): Initial genome sequencing and analysis of multiple myeloma. *Nature* 471:467–472.

Chen W, Iida S, Louie DC, Dalla-Favera R, Chaganti RS (1998): Heterologous promoters fused to BCL6 by chromosomal translocations affecting band 3q27 cause its deregulated expression during B-cell differentiation. *Blood* 91:603–607.

Chen W, Palanisamy N, Schmidt H, Teruya-Feldstein J, Jhanwar SC, Zelenetz AD, et al. (2001a): Deregulation of FCGR2B expression by 1q21 rearrangements in follicular lymphomas. *Oncogene* 20:7686–7693.

Chen W, Itoyama T, Chaganti RS (2001b): Splicing factor SRP20 is a novel partner of BCL6 in a t(3;6)(q27;p21) translocation in transformed follicular lymphoma. *Genes Chromosomes Cancer* 32:281–284.

Chen YW, Hu XT, Liang AC, Au WY, So CC, Wong ML, et al. (2006): High BCL6 expression predicts better prognosis, independent of BCL6 translocation partner, or BCL6-deregulating mutations, in gastric lymphoma. *Blood* 108:2373–2383.

Chesi M, Nardini E, Lim RS, Smith KD, Kuehl WM, Bergsagel PL (1998a): The t(4;14) translocation in myeloma dysregulates both FGFR3 and a novel gene, MMSET, resulting in IgH/MMSET hybrid transcripts. *Blood* 92:3025–3034.

Chesi M, Bergsagel PL, Shonukan OO, Martelli ML, Brents LA, Chen T, et al. (1998b): Frequent dysregulation of the c-maf proto-oncogene at 16q23 by translocation to an Ig locus in multiple myeloma. *Blood* 91:4457–4463.

Cheung KJ, Delaney A, Ben-Neriah S, Schein J, Lee T, Shah SP, et al. (2010a): High resolution analysis of follicular lymphoma genomes reveals somatic recurrent sites of copy-neutral loss of heterozygosity and copy number alterations that target single genes. *Genes Chromosomes Cancer* 49:669–681.

Cheung KJ, Johnson NA, Affleck JG, Severson T, Steidl C, Ben-Neriah S, et al. (2010b): Acquired TNFRSF14 mutations in follicular lymphoma are associated with worse prognosis. *Cancer Res* 70:9166–9174.

Cheung KJ, Rogic S, Ben-Neriah S, Boyle M, Connors JM, Gascoyne RD, et al. (2012): SNP analysis of minimally evolved t(14;18)(q32;q21)-positive follicular lymphomas reveals a common copy-neutral loss of heterozygosity pattern. *Cytogenet Genome Res* 136:38–43.

Chevallier P, Penther D, Avet-Loiseau H, Robillard N, Ifrah N, Mahé B, et al. (2002): CD38 expression and secondary 17p deletion are important prognostic factors in chronic lymphocytic leukaemia. *Br J Haematol* 116:142–150.

Chigrinova E, Rinaldi A, Kwee I, Rossi D, Rancoita PM, Strefford JC, et al. (2013): Two main genetic pathways lead to the transformation of chronic lymphocytic leukemia to Richter syndrome. *Blood* 122:2673–2682.

Chikatsu N, Kojima H, Suzukawa K, Shinagawa A, Nagasawa T, Ozawa H, et al. (2003): ALK⁺, CD30⁻, CD20⁻ large B-cell lymphoma containing anaplastic lymphoma kinase (ALK) fused to clathrin heavy chain gene (CLTC). *Mod Pathol* 16:828–832.

Chng WJ, VanWier SA, Ahmann GJ, Winkler JM, Jalal SM, Bergsagel PL, et al. (2005): A validated FISH trisomy index demonstrates the hyperdiploid and nonhyperdiploid dichotomy in MGUS. *Blood* 106:2156–2161.

Chng WJ, Santana-Dávila R, VanWier SA, Ahmann GJ, Jalal SM, Bergsagel PL, et al. (2006): Prognostic factors for hyperdiploid-myeloma: effects of chromosome 13 deletions and IgH translocations. *Leukemia* 20:807–813.

Chng WJ, Dispenzieri A, Chim CS, Fonseca R, Goldschmidt H, Lentzsch S, et al. (2014): IMWG consensus on risk stratification in multiple myeloma. *Leukemia* 28:269–277.

Choi YJ, Kim N, Paik JH, Kim JM, Lee SH, Park YS, et al. (2013): Characteristics of *Helicobacter pylori*-positive and *Helicobacter pylori*-negative gastric mucosa-associated lymphoid tissue lymphoma and their influence on clinical outcome. *Helicobacter* 18:197–205.

Christie L, Kernohan N, Levison D, Sales M, Cunningham J, Gillespie K, et al. (2008): C-MYC translocation in t(14;18) positive follicular lymphoma at presentation: an adverse prognostic indicator? *Leuk Lymphoma* 49:470–476.

Chuang SS, Liu H, Martín-Subero JI, Siebert R, Huang WT, Ye H (2007): Pulmonary mucosa-associated lymphoid tissue lymphoma with strong nuclear B-cell CLL/lymphoma 10 (BCL10) expression and novel translocation t(1;2)(p22;p12)/immunoglobulin kappa chain-BCL10. *J Clin Pathol* 60:727–728.

Chui DT, Hammond D, Baird M, Shield L, Jackson R, Jarrett RF (2003): Classical Hodgkin lymphoma is associated with frequent gains of 17q. *Genes Chromosomes Cancer* 38:126–136.

Cigudosa JC, Rao PH, Calasanz MJ, Odero MD, Michaeli J, Jhanwar SC, et al. (1998): Characterization of nonrandom chromosomal gains and losses in multiple myeloma by comparative genomic hybridization. *Blood* 91:3007–3010.

Coiffier B, Lepage E, Briere J, Herbrecht R, Tilly H, Bouabdallah R, et al. (2002): CHOP chemotherapy plus rituximab compared with CHOP alone in elderly patients with diffuse large-B-cell lymphoma. *N Engl J Med* 346:235–242.

Cong P, Raffeld M, Teruya-Feldstein J, Sorbara L, Pittaluga S, Jaffe ES (2002): In situ localization of follicular lymphoma: description and analysis by laser capture microdissection. *Blood* 99:3376–3382.

Cook JR, Aguilera NI, Reshmi-Skarja S, Huang X, Yu Z, Gollin SM, et al. (2004): Lack of PAX5 rearrangements in lymphoplasmacytic lymphomas: reassessing the reported association with t(9;14). *Hum Pathol* 35: 447–454.

Cools J, Wlodarska I, Somers R, Mentens N, Pedeutour F, Maes B, et al. (2002): Identification of novel fusion partners of ALK, the anaplastic lymphoma kinase, in anaplastic large-cell lymphoma and inflammatory myofibroblastic tumor. *Genes Chromosomes Cancer* 34:354–362.

Corcoran MM, Mould SJ, Orchard JA, Ibbotson RE, Chapman RM, Boright AP, et al. (1999): Dysregulation of cyclin dependent kinase 6 expression in splenic marginal zone lymphoma through chromosome 7q translocations. *Oncogene* 18:6271–6277.

Cremer FW, Kartal M, Hose D, Bila J, Buck I, Bellos F, et al. (2005): High incidence and intraclonal heterogeneity of chromosome 11 aberrations in patients with newly diagnosed multiple myeloma detected by multiprobe interphase FISH. *Cancer Genet Cytogenet* 161:116–124.

Cui J, Liu Q, Cheng Y, Chen S, Sun Q (2014): An intravascular large B-cell lymphoma with a t(3;14)(q27;q32) translocation. *J Clin Pathol* 67:279–281.

Dallery E, Galiègue-Zouitina S, Collyn-d'Hooghe M, Quief S, Denis C, Hildebrand MP, et al. (1995): TTF, a gene encoding a novel small G protein, fuses to the lymphoma-associated LAZ3 gene by t(3;4) chromosomal translocation. *Oncogene* 10:2171–2178.

Dave SS, Wright G, Tan B, Rosenwald A, Gascoyne RD, Chan WC, et al. (2004): Prediction of survival in follicular lymphoma based on molecular features of tumor-infiltrating immune cells. *N Engl J Med* 351:2159–2169.

Dave SS, Fu K, Wright GW, Lam LT, Kluin P, Boerma EJ, et al. (2006): Molecular diagnosis of Burkitt's lymphoma. *N Engl J Med* 354:2431–2442.

De Leeuw RJ, Davies JJ, Rosenwald A, Bebb G, Gascoyne RD, Dyer MJ, et al. (2004): Comprehensive whole genome array CGH profiling of mantle cell lymphoma model genomes. *Hum Mol Genet* 13: 1827–1837.

De Leeuw RJ, Zettl A, Klinker E, Haralambieva E, Trottier M, Chari R, et al. (2007): Whole-genome analysis and HLA genotyping of enteropathy-type T-cell lymphoma reveals 2 distinct lymphoma subtypes. *Gastroenterology* 132:1902–1911.

De Leval L, Gaulard P (2011): Tricky and terrible T-cell tumors: these are thrilling times for testing: molecular pathology of peripheral T-cell lymphomas. *Hematology Am Soc Hematol Educ Program* 2011:336–343.

De Oliveira FM, Rodrigues-Alves AP, Lucena-Araújo AR, de Paula Silva F, da Silva FB, Falcão RP (2014): Mantle cell lymphoma harboring Burkitt's-like translocations presents differential expression of aurora kinase genes compared with other 8q abnormalities. *Med Oncol* 31:931.

Debes-Marun CS, Dewald GW, Bryant S, Picken E, Santana-Dávila R, González-Paz N, et al. (2003): Chromosome abnormalities clustering and its implications for pathogenesis and prognosis in myeloma. *Leukemia* 17:427–436.

Dewald GW, Kyle RA, Hicks GA, Greipp PR (1985): The clinical significance of cytogenetic studies in 100 patients with multiple myeloma, plasma cell leukemia, or amyloidosis. *Blood* 66:380–390.

Dewald GW, Brockman SR, Paternoster SF (2004): Molecular cytogenetic studies for hematological malignancies. *Cancer Treat Res* 121: 69–112.

Dewald GW, Therneau T, Larson D, Lee YK, Fink S, Smoley S, et al. (2005): Relationship of patient survival and chromosome anomalies detected in metaphase and/or interphase cells at diagnosis of myeloma. *Blood* 106:3553–3558.

Deweindt C, Kerckaert JP, Tilly H, Quief S, Nguyen VC, Bastard C (1993): Cloning of a breakpoint cluster region at band 3q27 involved in human non-Hodgkin's lymphoma. *Genes Chromosomes Cancer* 8:149–154.

Dicker F, Schnittger S, Haferlach T, Kern W, Schoch C (2006): Immunostimulatory oligonucleotide-induced metaphase cytogenetics detect chromosomal aberrations in 80% of CLL patients: a study of 132 CLL cases with correlation to FISH, IgVH status, and CD38 expression. *Blood* 108:3152–3160.

Dierlamm J, Pittaluga S, Wlodarska I, Stul M, Thomas J, Boogaerts M, et al. (1996): Marginal zone B-cell lymphomas of different sites share similar cytogenetic and morphologic features. *Blood* 87:299–307.

Dierlamm J, Wlodarska I, Michaux L, Vermeesch JR, Meeus P, Stul M, et al. (1997): FISH identifies different types of duplications with 12q13–15 as the commonly involved segment in B-cell lymphoproliferative malignancies characterized by partial trisomy 12. *Genes Chromosomes Cancer* 20:155–166.

Dierlamm J, Baens M, Wlodarska I, Stefanova-Ouzounova M, Hernandez JM, Hossfeld DK, et al. (1999): The apoptosis inhibitor gene API2 and a novel 18q gene, MLT, are recurrently rearranged in the t(11;18)(q21;q21) associated with mucosa-associated lymphoid tissue lymphomas. *Blood* 93:3601–3609.

Döhner H, Pohl S, Bulgay-Mörschel M, Stilgenbauer S, Bentz M, Lichter P (1993): Trisomy 12 in chronic lymphoid leukemias: a metaphase and interphase cytogenetic analysis. *Leukemia* 7:516–520.

Döhner H, Fischer K, Bentz M, Hansen K, Benner A, Cabot G, et al. (1995): p53 gene deletion predicts for poor survival and non-response to therapy with purine analogs in chronic B-cell leukemias. *Blood* 85:1580–1589.

Döhner H, Stilgenbauer S, Fischer K, Bentz M, Lichter P (1997a): Cytogenetic and molecular cytogenetic analysis of B cell chronic lymphocytic leukemia: specific chromosome aberrations identify prognostic subgroups of patients and point to loci of candidate genes. *Leukemia* 11 (S2) 19–24.

Döhner H, Stilgenbauer S, James MR, Benner A, Weilguni T, Bentz M, et al. (1997b): 11q deletions identify a new subset of B-cell chronic lymphocytic leukemia characterized by extensive nodal involvement and inferior prognosis. *Blood* 89:2516–2522.

Döhner H, Stilgenbauer S, Döhner K, Bentz M, Lichter P (1999): Chromosome aberrations in B-cell chronic lymphocytic leukemia: reassessment based on molecular cytogenetic analysis. *J Mol Med* 77:266–281.

Döhner H, Stilgenbauer S, Benner A, Leupolt E, Kröber A, Bullinger L, et al. (2000): Genomic aberrations and survival in chronic lymphocytic leukemia. *N Engl J Med* 343:1910–1916.

van Doorn R, van Kester MS, Dijkman R, Vermeer MH, Mulder AA, Szuhai K, et al. (2009): Oncogenomic analysis of mycosis fungoides reveals major differences with Sézary syndrome. *Blood* 113:127–136.

Drach J, Schuster J, Nowotny H, Angerler J, Rosenthal F, Fiegl M, et al. (1995): Multiple myeloma: high incidence of chromosomal aneuploidy as detected by interphase fluorescence in situ hybridization. *Cancer Res* 55:3854–3859.

Drach J, Ackermann J, Fritz E, Krömer E, Schuster R, Gisslinger H, et al. (1998): Presence of a p53 gene deletion in patients with multiple myeloma predicts for short survival after conventional-dose chemotherapy. *Blood* 92:802–809.

Drexler HG (1992): Recent results on the biology of Hodgkin and Reed–Sternberg cells. I. Biopsy material. *Leuk Lymphoma* 8:283–313.

Du MQ (2007): MALT lymphoma: recent advances in aetiology and molecular genetics. *J Clin Exp Hematop* 47:31–42.

Dürig J, Bug S, Klein-Hitpass L, Boes T, Jöns T, Martin-Subero JI, et al. (2007): Combined single nucleotide polymorphism-based genomic mapping and global gene expression profiling identifies novel chromosomal imbalances, mechanisms and candidate genes important in the pathogenesis of T-cell prolymphocytic leukemia with inv(14)(q11q32). *Leukemia* 21:2153–2163.

Dyer MJ (2003): The pathogenetic role of oncogenes deregulated by chromosomal translocation in B-cell malignancies. *Int J Hematol* 77:315–320.

Dyer MJ (2013): The detection of chromosomal translocations involving the immunoglobulin loci in B-cell malignancies. *Methods Mol Biol* 971:123–133.

Dyer MJ, Lillington DM, Bastard C, Tilly H, Lens D, Heward JM, et al. (1996): Concurrent activation of MYC and BCL2 in B cell non-Hodgkin lymphoma cell lines by translocation of both oncogenes to the same immunoglobulin heavy chain locus. *Leukemia* 10:1198–1208.

Dyomin VG, Rao PH, Dalla-Favera R, Chaganti RS (1997): BCL8, a novel gene involved in translocations affecting band 15q11–13 in diffuse large-cell lymphoma. *Proc Natl Acad Sci USA* 94:5728–5732.

Dyomin VG, Palanisamy N, Lloyd KO, Dyomina K, Jhanwar SC, Houldsworth J, et al. (2000): MUC1 is activated in a B-cell lymphoma by the t(1;14)(q21;q32) translocation and is rearranged and amplified in B-cell lymphoma subsets. *Blood* 95:2666–2671.

Egan JB, Shi CX, Tembe W, Christoforides A, Kurdoglu A, Sinari S, et al. (2012): Whole-genome sequencing of multiple myeloma from diagnosis to plasma cell leukemia reveals genomic initiating events, evolution, and clonal tides. *Blood* 120:1060–1066.

Eide MB, Liestøl K, Lingjaerde OC, Hystad ME, Kresse SH, Meza-Zepeda L, et al. (2010): Genomic alterations reveal potential for higher grade transformation in follicular lymphoma and confirm parallel evolution of tumor cell clones. *Blood* 116:1489–1497.

Einerson RR, Law ME, Blair HE, Kurtin PJ, McClure RF, Ketterling RP, et al. (2006): Novel FISH probes designed to detect IGK-MYC and IGL-MYC rearrangements in B-cell lineage malignancy identify a new breakpoint cluster region designated BVR2. *Leukemia* 20:1790–1799.

Emmerich F, Meiser M, Hummel M, Demel G, Foss HD, Jundt F, et al. (1999): Overexpression of I kappa B alpha without inhibition of NF-kappaB activity and mutations in the I kappa B alpha gene in Reed–Sternberg cells. *Blood* 94:3129–3134.

Espinet B, Salgado R (2013): Mycosis fungoides and Sézary syndrome. *Methods Mol Biol* 973:175–188.

Espinet B, Salido M, Pujol RM, Florensa L, Gallardo F, Domingo A, et al. (2004): Genetic characterization of Sézary's syndrome by conventional cytogenetics and cross-species color banding fluorescent in situ hybridization. *Haematologica* 89:165–173.

Espinet B, Salaverria I, Beà S, Ruiz-Xivillé N, Balagué O, Salido M, et al. (2010): Incidence and prognostic impact of secondary cytogenetic aberrations in a series of 145 patients with mantle cell lymphoma. *Genes Chromosomes Cancer* 49:439–451.

Fabbri G, Rasi S, Rossi D, Trifonov V, Khiabanian H, Ma J, et al. (2011): Analysis of the chronic lymphocytic leukemia coding genome: role of NOTCH1 mutational activation. *J Exp Med* 208:1389–1401.

Fabbri G, Khiabanian H, Holmes AB, Wang J, Messina M, Mullighan CG, et al. (2013): Genetic lesions associated with chronic lymphocytic leukemia transformation to Richter syndrome. *J Exp Med* 210:2273–2288.

Fabris S, Storlazzi CT, Baldini L, Nobili L, Lombardi L, Maiolo AT, et al. (2003): Heterogeneous pattern of chromosomal breakpoints involving the MYC locus in multiple myeloma. *Genes Chromosomes Cancer* 37:261–269.

Falzetti D, Crescenzi B, Matteuci C, Falini B, Martelli MF, Van Den Berghe H, et al. (1999): Genomic instability and recurrent breakpoints are main cytogenetic findings in Hodgkin's disease. *Haematologica* 84:298–305.

Fassas AB, Spencer T, Sawyer J, Zangari M, Lee CK, Anaissie E, et al. (2002): Both hypodiploidy and deletion of chromosome 13 independently confer poor prognosis in multiple myeloma. *Br J Haematol* 118: 1041–1047.

Feldman AL, Dogan A, Smith DI, Law ME, Ansell SM, Johnson SH, et al. (2011): Discovery of recurrent t(6;7) (p25.3;q32.3) translocations in ALK-negative anaplastic large cell lymphomas by massive parallel genomic sequencing. *Blood* 117:915–919.

Fenton JA, Vaandrager JW, Aarts WM, Bende RJ, Heering K, van Dijk M, et al. (2002): Follicular lymphoma with a novel t(14;18) breakpoint involving the immunoglobulin heavy chain switch mu region indicates an origin from germinal center B cells. *Blood* 99:716–718.

Fenton JA, Pratt G, Rothwell DG, Rawstron AC, Morgan GJ (2004): Translocation t(11;14) in multiple myeloma: analysis of translocation breakpoints on der(11) and der(14) chromosomes suggests complex molecular mechanisms of recombination. *Genes Chromosomes Cancer* 39:151–155.

Fenton JA, Schuuring E, Barrans SL, Banham AH, Rollinson SJ, Morgan GJ, et al. (2006): t(3;14)(p14;q32) results in aberrant expression of FOXP1 in a case of diffuse large B-cell lymphoma. *Genes Chromosomes Cancer* 45:164–168.

Fink SR, Smoley SA, Stockero KJ, Paternoster SF, Thorland EC, Van Dyke DL, et al. (2006): Loss of TP53 is due to rearrangements involving chromosome region 17p10–p12 in chronic lymphocytic leukemia. *Cancer Genet Cytogenet* 167:177–181.

Fischer TC, Gellrich S, Muche JM, Sherev T, Audring H, Neitzel H, et al. (2004): Genomic aberrations and survival in cutaneous T cell lymphomas. *J Invest Dermatol* 122:579–586.

Flactif M, Zandecki M, Laï JL, Bernardi F, Obein V, Bauters F, et al. (1995): Interphase fluorescence in situ hybridization (FISH) as a powerful tool for the detection of aneuploidy in multiple myeloma. *Leukemia* 9:2109–2114.

Fonseca R, Hoyer JD, Aguayo P, Jalal SM, Ahmann GJ, Rajkumar SV, et al. (1999): Clinical significance of the translocation (11;14)(q13;q32) in multiple myeloma. *Leuk Lymphoma* 35: 599–605.

Fonseca R, Oken MM, Greipp PR, Eastern Cooperative Oncology Group Myeloma Group (2001): The t(4;14) (p16.3;q32) is strongly associated with chromosome 13 abnormalities in both multiple myeloma and monoclonal gammopathy of undetermined significance. *Blood* 98:1271–1272.

Fonseca R, Bailey RJ, Ahmann GJ, Rajkumar SV, Hoyer JD, Lust JA, et al. (2002): Genomic abnormalities in monoclonal gammopathy of undetermined significance. *Blood* 100:1417–1424.

Fonseca R, Blood E, Rue M, Harrington D, Oken MM, Kyle RA, et al. (2003): Clinical and biologic implications of recurrent genomic aberrations in myeloma. *Blood* 101: 4569–4575.

Fonseca R, Barlogie B, Bataille R, Bastard C, Bergsagel PL, Chesi M, et al. (2004): Genetics and cytogenetics of multiple myeloma: a workshop report. *Cancer Res* 64:1546–1558.

Fonseca R, Bergsagel PL, Drach J, Shaughnessy J, Gutierrez N, Stewart AK, et al. (2009): International Myeloma Working Group molecular classification of multiple myeloma: spotlight review. *Leukemia* 23:2210–2221.

Forconi F, Poretti G, Kwee I, Sozzi E, Rossi D, Rancoita PM, et al. (2008): High density genome-wide DNA profiling reveals a remarkably stable profile in hairy cell leukaemia. *Br J Haematol* 141:622–630.

Franke S, Wlodarska I, Maes B, Vandenberghe P, Achten R, Hagemeijer A, et al. (2002): Comparative genomic hybridization pattern distinguishes T-cell/histiocyte-rich B-cell lymphoma from nodular lymphocyte predominance Hodgkin's lymphoma. *Am J Pathol* 161:1861–1867.

Fresquet V, Robles EF, Parker A, Martinez-Useros J, Mena M, Malumbres R, et al. (2012): High-throughput sequencing analysis of the chromosome 7q32 deletion reveals IRF5 as a potential tumour suppressor in splenic marginal-zone lymphoma. *Br J Haematol* 158:712–726.

Fu K, Weisenburger DD, Greiner TC, Dave S, Wright G, Rosenwald A, et al. (2005): Cyclin D1-negative mantle cell lymphoma: a clinicopathologic study based on gene expression profiling. *Blood* 106: 4315–4321.

Fujimoto R, Ozawa T, Itoyama T, Sadamori N, Kurosawa N, Isobe M (2012): HELIOS-BCL11B fusion gene involvement in a t(2;14)(q34;q32) in an adult T-cell leukemia patient. *Cancer Genet* 205:356–364.

Fukuhara S, Rowley JD, Variakojis D, Golomb HM (1979): Chromosome abnormalities in poorly differentiated lymphocytic lymphoma. *Cancer Res* 39:3119–3128.

Gabrea A, Bergsagel PL, Chesi M, Shou Y, Kuehl WM (1999): Insertion of excised IgH switch sequences causes overexpression of cyclin D1 in a myeloma tumor cell. *Mol Cell* 3:119–123.

Gabrea A, Martelli ML, Qi Y, Roschke A, Barlogie B, Shaughnessy JD Jr, et al. (2008): Secondary genomic rearrangements involving immunoglobulin or MYC loci show similar prevalences in hyperdiploid and nonhyperdiploid myeloma tumors. *Genes Chromosomes Cancer* 47:573–590.

Galième-Zouitina S, Quief S, Hildebrand MP, Denis C, Lecocq G, Collyn-d'Hooghe M, et al. (1996): The B cell transcriptional coactivator BOB1/OBF1 gene fuses to the LAZ3/BCL6 gene by t(3;11)(q27;q23.1) chromosomal translocation in a B cell leukemia line (Karpas 231). *Leukemia* 10:579–587.

Galiègue-Zouitina S, Quief S, Hildebrand MP, Denis C, Detourmignies L, Laï JL, et al. (1999): Nonrandom fusion of L-plastin(LCP1) and LAZ3(BCL6) gene by t(3;13)(q27;q14) chromosome translocation in two cases of B-cell non-Hodgkin lymphoma. *Genes Chromosomes Cancer* 26:97–105.

Gascoyne RD, Lamant L, Martin-Subero JI, Lestou VS, Harris NL, Müller-Hermelink HK, et al. (2003): ALK-positive diffuse large B-cell lymphoma is associated with clathrin-ALK rearrangements: report of 6 cases. *Blood* 102:2568–2573.

Gazzo S, Baseggio L, Coignet L, Poncet C, Morel D, Coiffier B, et al. (2003): Cytogenetic and molecular delineation of a region of chromosome 3q commonly gained in marginal zone B-cell lymphoma. *Haematologica* 88:31–38.

Gazzo S, Felman P, Berger F, Salles G, Magaud JP, Callet-Bauchu E (2005): Atypical cytogenetic presentation of t(11;14) in mantle cell lymphoma. *Haematologica* 90:1708–1709.

Gertz MA, Lacy MQ, Dispenzieri A, Greipp PR, Litzow MR, Henderson KJ, et al. (2005): Clinical implications of t(11;14)(q13;q32), t(4;14)(p16.3;q32), and −17p13 in myeloma patients treated with high-dose therapy. *Blood* 106:2837–2840.

Gesk S, Martín-Subero JI, Harder L, Luhmann B, Schlegelberger B, Calasanz MJ, et al. (2003): Molecular cytogenetic detection of chromosomal breakpoints in T-cell receptor gene loci. *Leukemia* 17:738–745.

Gesk S, Gascoyne RD, Schnitzer B, Bakshi N, Janssen D, Klapper W, et al. (2005): ALK-positive diffuse large B-cell lymphoma with ALK-clathrin fusion belongs to the spectrum of pediatric lymphomas. *Leukemia* 19:1839–1840.

Gesk S, Klapper W, Martín-Subero JI, Nagel I, Harder L, Fu K, et al. (2006): A chromosomal translocation in cyclin D1-negative/cyclin D2-positive mantle cell lymphoma fuses the CCND2 gene to the IGK locus. *Blood* 108:1109–1110.

Giefing M, Arnemann J, Martin-Subero JI, Nieländer I, Bug S, Hartmann S, et al. (2008): Identification of candidate tumour suppressor gene loci for Hodgkin and Reed-Sternberg cells by characterisation of homozygous deletions in classical Hodgkin lymphoma cell lines. *Br J Haematol* 142:916–924.

Gilles F, Goy A, Remache Y, Shue P, Zelenetz AD (2000): MUC1 dysregulation as the consequence of a t(1;14)(q21;q32) translocation in an extranodal lymphoma. *Blood* 95:2930–2936.

Green MR, Gentles AJ, Nair RV, Irish JM, Kihira S, Liu CL, et al. (2013): Hierarchy in somatic mutations arising during genomic evolution and progression of follicular lymphoma. *Blood* 121:1604–1611.

Green MR, Vicente-Dueñas C, Romero-Camarero I, Long Lui C, Dai B, González-Herrero I, et al. (2014): Transient expression of BCL6 is sufficient for oncogenic function and induction of mature B-cell lymphoma. *Nat Commun* 5:3904.

Greiner TC, Dasgupta C, Ho VV, Weisenburger DD, Smith LM, Lynch JC, et al. (2006): Mutation and genomic deletion status of ataxia telangiectasia mutated (ATM) and p53 confer specific gene expression profiles in mantle cell lymphoma. *Proc Natl Acad Sci USA* 103:2352–2357.

Grever MR, Lucas DM, Dewald GW, Neuberg DS, Reed JC, Kitada S, et al. (2007): Comprehensive assessment of genetic and molecular features predicting outcome in patients with chronic lymphocytic leukemia: results from the US Intergroup Phase III Trial E2997. *J Clin Oncol* 25:799–804.

Gruszka-Westwood AM, Hamoudi R, Osborne L, Matutes E, Catovsky D (2003): Deletion mapping on the long arm of chromosome 7 in splenic lymphoma with villous lymphocytes. *Genes Chromosomes Cancer* 36: 57–69 (Erratum in Genes Chromosomes Cancer, 2004, 39:170).

Gu K, Fu K, Jain S, Liu Z, Iqbal J, Li M, et al. (2009): t(14;18)-negative follicular lymphomas are associated with a high frequency of BCL6 rearrangement at the alternative breakpoint region. *Mod Pathol* 22:1251–1257.

Gulia A, Saggini A, Wiesner T, Fink-Puches R, Argenyi Z, Ferrara G, et al. (2011): Clinicopathologic features of early lesions of primary cutaneous follicle center lymphoma, diffuse type: implications for early diagnosis and treatment. *J Am Acad Dermatol* 65:991–1000.

Gunawardana J, Chan FC, Telenius A, Woolcock B, Kridel R, Tan KL, et al. (2014): Recurrent somatic mutations of PTPN1 in primary mediastinal B cell lymphoma and Hodgkin lymphoma. *Nat Genet* 46:329–335.

Gutiérrez NC, García JL, Hernández JM, Lumbreras E, Castellanos M, Rasillo A, et al. (2004): Prognostic and biologic significance of chromosomal imbalances assessed by comparative genomic hybridization in multiple myeloma. *Blood* 104:2661–2666.

Gutiérrez NC, Castellanos MV, Martín ML, Mateos MV, Hernández JM, Fernández M, et al. (2007): Prognostic and biological implications of genetic abnormalities in multiple myeloma undergoing autologous stem cell transplantation: t(4;14) is the most relevant adverse prognostic factor, whereas RB deletion as a unique abnormality is not associated with adverse prognosis. *Leukemia* 21:143–150.

Gutiérrez-García G, Cardesa-Salzmann T, Climent F, González-Barca E, Mercadal S, Mate JL, et al. (2011): Gene-expression profiling and not immunophenotypic algorithms predict prognosis in patients with diffuse large B-cell lymphoma treated with immunochemotherapy. *Blood* 117:4836–4843.

Haferlach C, Dicker F, Schnittger S, Kern W, Haferlach T (2007): Comprehensive genetic characterization of CLL: a study on 506 cases analysed with chromosome banding analysis, interphase FISH, IgV(H) status and immunophenotyping. *Leukemia* 21:2442–2451.

Hahtola S, Burghart E, Jeskanen L, Karenko L, Abdel-Rahman WM, Polzer B, et al. (2008): Clinicopathological characterization and genomic aberrations in subcutaneous panniculitis-like T-cell lymphoma. *J Invest Dermatol* 128:2304–2309.

Hallek M, Bergsagel PL, Anderson KC (1998): Multiple myeloma: increasing evidence for a multistep transformation process. *Blood* 91:3–21.

Hallek M, Cheson BD, Catovsky D, Caligaris-Cappio F, Dighiero G, Dohner H, et al. (2008): Guidelines for the diagnosis and treatment of chronic lymphocytic leukemia: a report from the International Workshop on Chronic Lymphocytic Leukemia (IWCLL) updating the National Cancer Institute-Working Group (NCI-WG) 1996 guidelines. *Blood* 111:5446–5456.

Hallermann C, Kaune KM, Gesk S, Martin-Subero JI, Gunawan B, Griesinger F, et al. (2004a): Molecular cytogenetic analysis of chromosomal breakpoints in the IGH, MYC, BCL6, and MALT1 gene loci in primary cutaneous B-cell lymphomas. *J Invest Dermatol* 123:213–219.

Hallermann C, Kaune KM, Siebert R, Vermeer MH, Tensen CP, Willemze R, et al. (2004b): Chromosomal aberration patterns differ in subtypes of primary cutaneous B cell lymphomas. *J Invest Dermatol* 122:1495–1502.

Hanamura I, Iida S, Akano Y, Hayami Y, Kato M, Miura K, et al. (2001): Ectopic expression of MAFB gene in human myeloma cells carrying (14;20)(q32;q11) chromosomal translocations. *Jpn J Cancer Res* 92:638–644.

Hanamura I, Stewart JP, Huang Y, Zhan F, Santra M, Sawyer JR, et al. (2006): Frequent gain of chromosome band 1q21

in plasma-cell dyscrasias detected by fluorescence in situ hybridization: incidence increases from MGUS to relapsed myeloma and is related to prognosis and disease progression following tandem stem-cell transplantation. *Blood* 108: 1724–1732.

Hao S, Sanger W, Onciu M, Lai R, Schlette EJ, Medeiros LJ (2002): Mantle cell lymphoma with 8q24 chromosomal abnormalities: a report of 5 cases with blastoid features. *Mod Pathol* 15:1266–1272.

Harris NL, Jaffe ES, Stein H, Banks PM, Chan JK, Cleary ML, et al. (1994): A revised European–American classification of lymphoid neoplasms: a proposal from the International Lymphoma Study Group. *Blood* 84:1361–1392.

Harris NL, Jaffe ES, Diebold J, Flandrin G, Muller-Hermelink HK, Vardiman J, et al. (1999): World Health Organization classification of neoplastic diseases of the hematopoietic and lymphoid tissues: report of the Clinical Advisory Committee Meeting, Airlie House, Virginia, November 1997. *J Clin Oncol* 17:3835–3849.

Harris NL, Jaffe ES, Diebold J, Flandrin G, Muller-Hermelink HK, Vardiman J, et al. (2000): The World Health Organization classification of hematological malignancies report of the Clinical Advisory Committee Meeting, Airlie House, Virginia, November 1997. *Mod Pathol* 13:193–207.

Harris NL, Swerdlow S, Jaffe ES, Ott G, Nathwani BN, de Jong D, et al. (2008): Follicular lymphoma. In: Swerdlow S, Campo E, Harris N, et al, eds. *WHO Classification of Tumours of Haematopoietic and Lymphoid Tissues* IARC:220–226.

Harrison CJ, Mazzullo H, Ross FM, Cheung KL, Gerrard G, Harewood L, et al. (2002): Translocations of 14q32 and deletions of 13q14 are common chromosomal abnormalities in systemic amyloidosis. *Br J Haematol* 117:427–435.

Hartmann S, Martin-Subero JI, Gesk S, Hüsken J, Giefing M, Nagel I, et al. (2008): Detection of genomic imbalances in microdissected Hodgkin and Reed-Sternberg cells of classical Hodgkin's lymphoma by array-based comparative genomic hybridization. *Haematologica* 93:1318–1326.

Hartmann S, Gesk S, Scholtysik R, Kreuz M, Bug S, Vater I, et al. (2010): High resolution SNP array genomic profiling of peripheral T cell lymphomas, not otherwise specified, identifies a subgroup with chromosomal aberrations affecting the REL locus. *Br J Haematol* 148:402–412.

Hatzivassiliou G, Miller I, Takizawa J, Palanisamy N, Rao PH, Iida S, et al. (2001): IRTA1 and IRTA2, novel immunoglobulin superfamily receptors expressed in B cells and involved in chromosome 1q21 abnormalities in B cell malignancy. *Immunity* 14:277–289.

He L, Thomson JM, Hemann MT, Hernando-Monge E, Mu D, Goodson S, et al. (2005): A microRNA polycistron as a potential human oncogene. *Nature* 435:828–833.

Herens C, Lambert F, Quintanilla-Martinez L, Bisig B, Deusings C, deLeval L (2008): Cyclin D1-negative mantle cell lymphoma with cryptic t(12;14)(p13;q32) and cyclin D2 overexpression. *Blood* 111:1745–1746.

Herholz H, Kern W, Schnittger S, Haferlach T, Dicker F, Haferlach C (2007): Translocations as a mechanism for homozygous deletion of 13q14 and loss of the ATM gene in a patient with B-cell chronic lymphocytic leukemia. *Cancer Genet Cytogenet* 174:57–60.

Hernández L, Pinyol M, Hernández S, Beà S, Pulford K, Rosenwald A, et al. (1999): TRK-fused gene (TFG) is a new partner of ALK in anaplastic large cell lymphoma producing two structurally different TFG–ALK translocations. *Blood* 94:3265–3268.

Hernández JM, Garcia JL, Gutiérrez NC, Mollejo M, Martinez-Climent JA, Flores T, et al. (2001): Novel genomic imbalances in B-cell splenic marginal zone lymphomas revealed by comparative genomic hybridization and cytogenetics. *Am J Pathol* 158:1843–1850.

Heyning FH, Jansen PM, Hogendoorn PC, Szuhai K (2010): Array-based comparative genomic hybridisation analysis reveals recurrent chromosomal alterations in primary diffuse large B cell lymphoma of bone. *J Clin Pathol* 63:1095–1100.

Higgins MJ, Fonseca R (2005): Genetics of multiple myeloma. *Best Pract Res Clin Haematol* 18:525–536.

Hillengass J, Zechmann CM, Nadler A, Hose D, Cremer FW, Jauch A, et al. (2008): Gain of 1q21 and distinct adverse cytogenetic abnormalities correlate with increased microcirculation in multiple myeloma. *Int J Cancer* 122:2871–2875.

Hillion J, Mecucci C, Aventin A, Leroux D, Wlodarska I, Van Den Berghe H, et al. (1991): A variant translocation t(2;18) in follicular lymphoma involves the 5′ end of bcl-2 and Igκ light chain gene. *Oncogene* 6:169–172.

Höglund M, Sehn L, Connors JM, Gascoyne RD, Siebert R, Säll T, et al. (2004): Identification of cytogenetic subgroups and karyotypic pathways of clonal evolution in follicular lymphomas. *Genes Chromosomes Cancer* 39:195–204.

Honma K, Tsuzuki S, Nakagawa M, Karnan S, Aizawa Y, Kim WS, et al. (2008): TNFAIP3 is the target gene of chromosome band 6q23.3–q24.1 loss in ocular adnexal marginal zone B cell lymphoma. *Genes Chromosomes Cancer* 47:1–7.

Horn H, Schmelter C, Leich E, Salaverria I, Katzenberger T, Ott MM, et al. (2011): Follicular lymphoma grade 3B is a distinct neoplasm according to cytogenetic and immunohistochemical profiles. *Haematologica* 96:1327–1334.

Horsman D, Gascoyne R, Klasa R, Coupland R (1992): t(11;18)(q21;q21.1): a recurring translocation in lymphomas of mucosa-associated lymphoid tissue (MALT)? *Genes Chromosomes Cancer* 4:183–187.

Horsman DE, Connors JM, Pantzar T, Gascoyne RD (2001): Analysis of secondary chromosomal alterations in 165 cases of follicular lymphoma with t(14;18). *Genes Chromosomes Cancer* 30:375–382.

Horsman DE, Okamoto I, Ludkovski O, Le N, Harder L, Gesk S, et al. (2003): Follicular lymphoma lacking the t(14;18)(q32;q21): identification of two disease subtypes. *Br J Haematol* 120: 424–433.

Hosokawa Y, Maeda Y, Ichinohasama R, Miura I, Taniwaki M, Seto M (2000): The Ikaros gene, a central regulator of lymphoid differentiation, fuses to the BCL6 gene as result of t(3;7)(q27;p12) translocation in a patient with diffuse large B-cell lymphoma. *Blood* 95:2719–2721.

Hu XT, Chen YW, Liang AC, Au WY, Wong KY, Wan TS, et al. (2012): CD44 activation in mature B-cell malignancies by a novel recurrent IGH translocation. *Blood* 115:2458–2461.

Hummel M, Bentink S, Berger H, Klapper W, Wessendorf S, Barth TF, et al. (2006): A biologic definition of Burkitt's lymphoma from transcriptional and genomic profiling. *N Engl J Med* 354:2419–2430.

Hunter ZR, Xu L, Yang G, Zhou Y, Liu X, Cao Y, et al. (2014): The genomic landscape of Waldenstrom macroglobulinemia is characterized by highly recurring MYD88 and WHIM-like CXCR4 mutations, and small somatic deletions associated with B-cell lymphomagenesis. *Blood* 123:1637–1646.

Iida S, Rao PH, Nallasivam P, Hibshoosh H, Butler M, Louie DC, et al. (1996): The t(9;14)(p13;q32) chromosomal translocation associated with lymphoplasmacytoid lymphoma involves the PAX-5 gene. *Blood* 88:4110–4117.

Iqbal J, Sanger WG, Horsman DE, Rosenwald A, Pickering DL, Dave B, et al. (2004): BCL2 translocation defines a unique tumor subset within the germinal center B-cell-like diffuse large B-cell lymphoma. *Am J Pathol* 165: 159–166.

Iqbal J, Greiner TC, Patel K, Dave BJ, Smith L, Ji J, et al. (2007): Distinctive patterns of BCL6 molecular alterations and their functional consequences in different subgroups of diffuse large B-cell lymphoma. *Leukemia* 21: 2332–2343.

Iqbal J, Kucuk C, Deleeuw RJ, Srivastava G, Tam W, Geng H, et al. (2009): Genomic analyses reveal global functional alterations that promote tumor growth and novel tumor suppressor genes in natural killer-cell malignancies. *Leukemia* 23:1139–1151.

Iqbal J, Wright G, Wang C, Rosenwald A, Gascoyne RD, Weisenburger DD, et al. (2014): Gene expression signatures delineate biological and prognostic subgroups in peripheral T-cell lymphoma. *Blood* 123:2915–2923.

Isaacson PG, Du MQ (2003): Gastric lymphomas: genetics and resistance to *H. pylori* eradication. *Verh Dtsch Ges Pathol* 87:116–122.

Isaacson PG, Du MQ (2004): MALT lymphoma: from morphology to molecules. *Nat Rev Cancer* 4: 644–653.

Isaacson PG, Du MQ (2005): Gastrointestinal lymphoma: where morphology meets molecular biology. *J Pathol* 205:255–274.

Itoyama T, Chaganti RS, Yamada Y, Tsukasaki K, Atogami S, Nakamura H, et al. (2001): Cytogenetic analysis and clinical significance in adult T-cell leukemia/lymphoma: a study of 50 cases from the human T-cell leukemia virus type-1 endemic area, Nagasaki. *Blood* 97:3612–3620.

Jaffe ES, Harris NL, Stein H, Vardiman JW, editors (2001): *The World Health Organization Classification of Tumours: Pathology & Genetics. Tumours of Haematopoietic and Lymphoid Tissues.* Lyon: IACR Press.

Janssen JW, Vaandrager JW, Heuser T, Jauch A, Kluin PM, Geelen E, et al. (2000): Concurrent activation of a novel putative transforming gene, myeov, and cyclin D1 in a subset of multiple myeloma cell lines with t(11;14) (q13;q32). *Blood* 95: 2691–2698.

Jardin F, Gaulard P, Buchonnet G, Contentin N, Leprêtre S, Lenain P, et al. (2002): Follicular lymphoma without t(14;18) and with BCL-6 rearrangement: a lymphoma subtype with distinct pathological, molecular and clinical characteristics. *Leukemia* 16:2309–2317.

Jardin F, Ruminy P, Bastard C, Tilly H (2007): The BCL6 proto-oncogene: a leading role during germinal center development and lymphomagenesis. *Pathol Biol* (Paris)55:73–83.

Jares P, Colomer D, Campo E (2007): Genetic and molecular pathogenesis of mantle cell lymphoma: perspectives for new targeted therapeutics. *Nat Rev Cancer* 7:750–762.

Johansson B, Mertens F, Mitelman F (1995): Cytogenetic evolution patterns in non-Hodgkin's lymphoma. *Blood* 86:3905–3914.

Johnson NA, Al-Tourah A, Brown CJ, Connors JM, Gascoyne RD, Horsman DE (2008): Prognostic significance of secondary cytogenetic alterations in follicular lymphomas. *Genes Chromosomes Cancer* 47:1038–1048.

Johnson NA, Savage KJ, Ludkovski O, Ben-Neriah S, Woods R, Steidl C, et al. (2009): Lymphomas with concurrent BCL2 and MYC translocations: the critical factors associated with survival. *Blood* 114:2273–2279.

Jonveaux P, Daniel MT, Martel V, Maarek O, Berger R (1996): Isochromosome 7q and trisomy 8 are consistent primary, non-random chromosomal abnormalities associated with hepatosplenic T gamma/delta lymphoma. *Leukemia* 10:1453–1455.

Joos S, Falk MH, Lichter P, Haluska FG, Henglein B, Lenoir GM, et al. (1992a): Variable breakpoints in Burkitt lymphoma cells with chromosomal t(8;14) translocation separate c-myc and the IgH locus up to several hundred kb. *Hum Mol Genet* 1:625–632.

Joos S, Haluska FG, Falk MH, Henglein B, Hameister H, Croce CM, et al. (1992b): Mapping chromosomal breakpoints of Burkitt's t(8;14) translocations far upstream of c-myc. *Cancer Res* 52:6547–6552.

Joos S, Küpper M, Ohl S, von Bonin F, Mechtersheimer G, Bentz M, et al. (2000): Genomic imbalances including amplification of the tyrosine kinase gene JAK2 in CD30+ Hodgkin cells. *Cancer Res* 60:549–552.

Joos S, Menz CK, Wrobel G, Siebert R, Gesk S, Ohl S, et al. (2002): Classical Hodgkin lymphoma is characterized by recurrent copy number gains of the short arm of chromosome 2. *Blood* 99:1381–1387.

Joos S, Granzow M, Holtgreve-Grez H, Siebert R, Harder L, Martín-Subero JI, et al. (2003): Hodgkin's lymphoma cell lines are characterized by frequent aberrations on chromosomes 2p and 9p including REL and JAK2. *Int J Cancer* 103:489–495.

Juge-Morineau N, Mellerin MP, Francois S, Rapp MJ, Harousseau JL, Amiot M, et al. (1995): High incidence of deletions but infrequent inactivation of the retinoblastoma gene in human myeloma cells. *Br J Haematol* 91:664–667.

Juliusson G, Oscier DG, Fitchett M, Ross FM, Stockdill G, Mackie MJ, et al. (1990): Prognostic subgroups in B-cell chronic lymphocytic leukemia defined by specific chromosomal abnormalities. *N Engl J Med* 323:720–724.

Jungnickel B, Staratschek-Jox A, Bräuninger A, Spieker T, Wolf J, Diehl V, et al. (2000): Clonal deleterious mutations in the IkappaBalpha gene in the malignant cells in Hodgkin's lymphoma. *J Exp Med* 191:395–402.

Kamada N, Sakurai M, Miyamoto K, Sanada I, Sadamori N, Fukuhara S, et al. (1992): Chromosome abnormalities in adult T-cell leukemia/lymphoma: a karyotype review committee report. *Cancer Res* 52:1481–1493.

Kaneita Y, Yoshida S, Ishiguro N, Sawada U, Horie T, Mori S, et al. (2001): Detection of reciprocal fusion 5′-BCL6/partner-3′ transcripts in lymphomas exhibiting reciprocal BCL6 translocations. *Br J Haematol* 113:803–806.

Kaneko Y, Maseki N, Sakurai M, Takayama S, Nanba K, Kikuchi M, et al. (1988): Characteristic karyotypic pattern in T-cell lymphoproliferative disorders with reactive "angioimmunoblastic lymphadenopathy with dysproteinemia-type" features. *Blood* 72:413–421.

Kanungo A, Medeiros LJ, Abruzzo LV, Lin P (2006): Lymphoid neoplasms associated with concurrent t(14;18) and 8q24/c-MYC translocation generally have a poor prognosis. *Mod Pathol* 19:25–33.

Karai LJ, Kadin ME, Hsi ED, Sluzevich JC, Ketterling RP, Knudson RA, et al. (2013): Chromosomal rearrangements of 6p25.3 define a new subtype of lymphomatoid papulosis. *Am J Surg Pathol* 37:1173–1181.

Karenko L, Hahtola S, Päivinen S, Karhu R, Syrjä S, Kähkönen M, et al. (2005): Primary cutaneous T-cell lymphomas show a deletion or translocation affecting NAV3, the human UNC-53 homologue. *Cancer Res* 65:8101–8110.

Karsan A, Gascoyne RD, Coupland RW, Shepherd JD, Phillips GL, Horsman DE (1993): Combination of t(14;18) and a Burkitt's type translocation in B-cell malignancies. *Leuk Lymphoma* 10:433–441.

Katzenberger T, Ott G, Klein T, Kalla J, Müller-Hermelink HK, Ott MM (2004): Cytogenetic alterations affecting BCL6 are predominantly found in follicular lymphomas grade 3B with a diffuse large B-cell component. *Am J Pathol* 165: 481–490.

Katzenberger T, Kienle D, Stilgenbauer S, Höller S, Schilling C, Mäder U, et al. (2008): Delineation of distinct tumour profiles in mantle cell lymphoma by detailed cytogenetic, interphase genetic and morphological analysis. *Br J Haematol* 142:538–550.

Katzenberger T, Kalla J, Leich E, Stocklein H, Hartmann E, Barnickel S, et al. (2009): A distinctive subtype of t(14;18) negative nodal follicular non-Hodgkin lymphoma characterized by a predominantly diffuse growth pattern and deletions in the chromosomal region 1p36. *Blood* 113:1052–1061.

Kaufmann H, Krömer E, Nösslinger T, Weltermann A, Ackermann J, Reisner R, et al. (2003): Both chromosome 13 abnormalities by metaphase cytogenetics and deletion of 13q by interphase FISH only are prognostically relevant in multiple myeloma. *Eur J Haematol* 71: 179–183.

Kearney L, Horsley SW (2005): Molecular cytogenetics in haematological malignancy: current technology and future prospects. *Chromosoma* 114: 286–294.

Keats JJ, Reiman T, Maxwell CA, Taylor BJ, Larratt LM, Mant MJ, et al. (2003): In multiple myeloma, t(4;14)(p16;q32) is an adverse prognostic factor irrespective of FGFR3 expression. *Blood* 101:1520–1529.

Keats JJ, Maxwell CA, Taylor BJ, Hendzel MJ, Chesi M, Bergsagel PL, et al. (2005): Overexpression of transcripts originating from the MMSET locus characterizes all t(4;14)(p16;q32)-positive multiple myeloma patients. *Blood* 105:4060–4069.

Kerckaert JP, Deweindt C, Tilly H, Quief S, Lecocq G, Bastard C (1993): LAZ3, a novel zinc-finger encoding gene, is disrupted by recurring chromosome 3q27 translocations in human lymphomas. *Nat Genet* 5:66–70.

Kiel MJ, Velusamy T, Betz BL, Zhao L, Weigelin HG, Chiang MY, et al. (2012): Whole-genome sequencing identifies recurrent somatic NOTCH2 mutations in splenic marginal zone lymphoma. *J Exp Med* 209:1553–1565.

Kiel MJ, Velusamy T, Rolland D, Sahasrabuddhe AA, Chung F, Bailey NG, et al. (2014): Integrated genomic sequencing reveal mutational landscape of T-cell prolymphocytic leukemia. *Blood* 124:1460–1472.

Kim BK, Surti U, Pandya A, Cohen J, Rabkin MS, Swerdlow SH (2005): Clinicopathologic, immunophenotypic, and molecular cytogenetic fluorescence in situ hybridization analysis of primary and secondary cutaneous follicular lymphomas. *Am J Surg Pathol* 29:69–82.

Kim JA, Im K, Park SN, Kwon J, Choi Q, Hwang SM, et al. (2014). MYD88 L265P mutations are correlated with 6q deletion in Korean patients with Waldenström macroglobulinemia. Biomed Res Int. 2014:363540.

Kimm LR, deLeeuw RJ, Savage KJ, Rosenwald A, Campo E, Delabie J, et al. (2007): Frequent occurrence of deletions in primary mediastinal B-cell lymphoma. *Genes Chromosomes Cancer* 46:1090–1097.

Klapper W, Szczepanowski M, Burkhardt B, Berger H, Rosolowski M, Bentink S, et al. (2008a): Molecular profiling of pediatric mature B-cell lymphoma treated in population-based prospective clinical trials. *Blood* 112:1374–1381.

Klapper W, Stoecklein H, Zeynalova S, Ott G, Kosari F, Rosenwald A, et al. (2008b): Structural aberrations affecting the MYC locus indicate a poor prognosis independent of clinical risk factors in diffuse large B-cell lymphomas treated within randomized trials of the German High-Grade Non-Hodgkin's Lymphoma Study Group (DSHNHL). *Leukemia* 22:2226–2229.

Klapproth K, Wirth T (2010): Advances in the understanding of MYC-induced lymphomagenesis. *Br J Haematol* 149:484–497.

Klein U, Lia M, Crespo M, Siegel R, Shen Q, Mo T, et al. (2010): The DLEU2/miR-15a/16-1 cluster controls B cell proliferation and its deletion leads to chronic lymphocytic leukemia. *Cancer Cell* 17:28–40.

Kluin PM (2013): Origin and migration of follicular lymphoma cells. *Haematologica* 98:1331–1333.

Kluin PM (2014): The missing link in early follicular lymphoma development. *Blood* 123:3371–3372.

Kluin P, Schuuring E (2011): Molecular cytogenetics of lymphoma: where do we stand in 2010? *Histopathology* 58: 128–144.

Kluin PM, Harris NL, Stein H, Leoncini L, Raphaël M, Campo E, et al. (2008): B-cell lymphoma, unclassifiable, with features intermediate between diffuse large B-cell lymphoma and Burkitt lymphoma. In: Swerdlow S, Campo E, Harris N, Jaffe ES, Pileri S, Stein H, et al., eds. *WHO Classification of Tumours of Haematopoietic and Lymphoid Tissues*. IARC, Lyon:265–266.

Kluin-Nelemans HC, Hoster E, Hermine O, Walewski J, Trneny M, Geisler CH, et al. (2012): Treatment of older patients with mantle-cell lymphoma. *N Engl J Med* 367:520–531.

Kneba M, Eick S, Herbst H, Willigeroth S, Pott C, Bolz I, et al. (1991): Frequency and structure of t(14;18) major breakpoint regions in non-Hodgkin's lymphomas typed according to the Kiel classification: analysis by direct DNA sequencing. *Cancer Res* 51:3243–3250.

Knezevich S, Ludkovski O, Salski C, Lestou V, Chhanabhai M, Lam W, et al. (2005): Concurrent translocation of BCL2 and MYC with a single immunoglobulin locus in high-grade B-cell lymphomas. *Leukemia* 19:659–663.

Knight SJ, Yau C, Clifford R, Timbs AT, Sadighi Akha E, Dréau HM, et al. (2012): Quantification of subclonal distributions of recurrent genomic aberrations in paired pre-treatment and relapse samples from patients with B-cell chronic lymphocytic leukemia. *Leukemia* 26:1564–1575.

Kobayashi S, Taki T, Chinen Y, Tsutsumi Y, Ohshiro M, Kobayashi T, et al. (2011): Identification of IGHCδ-BACH2 fusion transcripts resulting from cryptic chromosomal rearrangements of 14q32 with 6q15 in aggressive

B-cell lymphoma/leukemia. *Genes Chromosomes Cancer* 50:207–216.

Kohlhammer H, Schwaenen C, Wessendorf S, Holzmann K, Kestler HA, Kienle D, et al. (2004): Genomic DNA-chip hybridization in t(11;14)-positive mantle cell lymphomas shows a high frequency of aberrations and allows a refined characterization of consensus regions. *Blood* 104:795–801.

Komatsu H, Yoshida K, Seto M, Iida S, Aikawa T, Ueda R, et al. (1993): Overexpression of PRAD1 in a mantle zone lymphoma patient with a t(11;22)(q13;q11) translocation. *Br J Haematol* 85:427–429.

Koo GC, Tan SY, Tang T, Poon SL, Allen GE, Tan L, et al. (2012): Janus Kinase 3-activating mutations identified in natural killer/T-cell lymphoma . *Cancer Discov* 2:591–597.

Koskela HL, Eldfors S, Ellonen P, van Adrichem AJ, Kuusanmäki H, Andersson EI, et al. (2012): Somatic STAT3 mutations in large granular lymphocytic leukemia. *N Engl J Med* 366:1905–1913.

Kreisel F, Kulkarni S, Kerns RT, Hassan A, Deshmukh H, Nagarajan R, et al. (2011): High resolution array comparative genomic hybridization identifies copy number alterations in diffuse large B-cell lymphoma that predict response to immuno-chemotherapy. *Cancer Genet* 204:129–137.

Kridel R, Meissner B, Rogic S, Boyle M, Telenius A, Woolcock B, et al. (2012): Whole transcriptome sequencing reveals recurrent NOTCH1 mutations in mantle cell lymphoma. *Blood* 119:1963–1971.

Kröber A, Seiler T, Benner A, Bullinger L, Brückle E, Lichter P, et al. (2002): V(H) mutation status, CD38 expression level, genomic aberrations, and survival in chronic lymphocytic leukemia. *Blood* 100:1410–1416.

Kröber A, Bloehdorn J, Hafner S, Bühler A, Seiler T, Kienle D, et al. (2006): Additional genetic high-risk features such as 11q deletion, 17p deletion, and V3-21 usage characterize discordance of ZAP-70 and VH mutation status in chronic lymphocytic leukemia. *J Clin Oncol* 24:969–975.

Kroenlein H, Schwartz S, Reinhardt R, Rieder H, Molkentin M, Gökbuget N, et al. (2012): Molecular analysis of the t(2;8)/MYC-IGK translocation in high-grade lymphoma/leukemia by long-distance inverse PCR. *Genes Chromosomes Cancer* 51:290–299.

Kröger N, Schilling G, Einsele H, Liebisch P, Shimoni A, Nagler A, et al. (2004): Deletion of chromosome band 13q14 as detected by fluorescence in situ hybridization is a prognostic factor in patients with multiple myeloma who are receiving allogeneic dose-reduced stem cell transplantation. *Blood* 103:4056–4061.

Krugmann J, Tzankov A, Dirnhofer S, Fend F, Greil R, Siebert R, et al. (2004): Unfavourable prognosis of patients with trisomy 18q21 detected by fluorescence in situ hybridisation in t(11;18) negative, surgically resected, gastrointestinal B cell lymphomas. *J Clin Pathol* 57:360–364.

Kuehl WM, Bergsagel PL (2002): Multiple myeloma: evolving genetic events and host interactions. *Nat Rev Cancer* 2:175–187.

Küppers R (2005): Mechanisms of B-cell lymphoma pathogenesis. *Nat Rev Cancer* 5: 251–262.

Küppers R, Dalla-Favera R (2001): Mechanisms of chromosomal translocations in B cell lymphomas. *Oncogene* 20:5580–5594.

Küppers R, Klein U, Hansmann ML, Rajewsky K (1999): Cellular origin of human B-cell lymphomas. *N Engl J Med* 341:1520–1529.

Küppers R, Sonoki T, Satterwhite E, Gesk S, Harder L, Oscier DG, et al. (2002): Lack of somatic hypermutation of IG V(H) genes in lymphoid malignancies with t(2;14)(p13;q32) translocation involving the BCL11A gene. *Leukemia* 16:937–939.

Kurata M, Maesako Y, Ueda C, Nishikori M, Akasaka T, Uchiyama T, et al. (2002): Characterization of t(3;6)(q27;p21) breakpoints in B-cell non-Hodgkin's lymphoma and construction of the histone H4/BCL6 fusion gene, leading to altered expression of BCL6. *Cancer Res* 62:6224–6230.

Kurosawa N, Fujimoto R, Ozawa T, Itoyama T, Sadamori N, Isobe M (2013): Reduced level of the BCL11B protein is associated with adult T-cell leukemia/lymphoma. *PLoS One* 8:e55147.

Kwiecinska A, Ichimura K, Berglund M, Dinets A, Sulaiman L, Collins VP, et al. (2014): Amplification of 2p as a genomic marker for transformation in lymphoma. *Genes Chromosomes Cancer* 53:750–768.

Laï JL, Zandecki M, Mary JY, Bernardi F, Izydorczyk V, Flactif M, et al. (1995): Improved cytogenetics in multiple myeloma: a study of 151 patients including 117 patients at diagnosis. *Blood* 85:2490–2497.

Lamant L, Dastugue N, Pulford K, Delsol G, Mariamé B (1999): A new fusion gene TPM3–ALK in anaplastic large cell lymphoma created by a (1;2)(q25;p23) translocation. *Blood* 93:3088–3095.

Lamprecht B, Kreher S, Möbs M, Sterry W, Dörken B, Janz M, et al. (2012): The tumour suppressor p53 is frequently nonfunctional in Sézary syndrome. *Br J Dermatol* 167:240–246.

Landau DA, Carter SL, Stojanov P, McKenna A, Stevenson K, Lawrence MS, et al. (2013): Evolution and impact of subclonal mutations in chronic lymphocytic leukemia. *Cell.* 152:714–726.

Lecointe N, Meerabux J, Ebihara M, Hill A, Young BD (1999): Molecular analysis of an unstable genomic region at chromosome band 11q23 reveals a disruption of the gene encoding the alpha2 subunit of platelet-activating factor acetylhydrolase (Pafah1a2) in human lymphoma. *Oncogene* 18:2852–2859.

Leich E, Haralambieva E, Zettl A, Chott A, Rüdiger T, Höller S, et al. (2007): Tissue microarray-based screening for chromosomal breakpoints affecting the T-cell receptor gene loci in mature T-cell lymphomas. *J Pathol* 213:99–105.

Leich E, Salaverria I, Bea S, Zettl A, Wright G, Moreno V, et al. (2009): Follicular lymphomas with and without translocation t(14;18) differ in gene expression profiles and genetic alterations. *Blood* 114:826–834.

Lemonnier F, Couronné L, Parrens M, Jaïs JP, Travert M, Lamant L, et al. (2012): Recurrent TET2 mutations in peripheral T-cell lymphomas correlate with T_{FH}-like features and adverse clinical parameters. *Blood* 120:1466–1469.

Lennert K, Stein H, Kaiserling E (1975): Cytological and functional criteria for the classification of malignant lymphomata. *Br J Cancer* 2:29–43.

Lenz G, Nagel I, Siebert R, Roschke AV, Sanger W, Wright GW, et al. (2007): Aberrant immunoglobulin class switch recombination and switch translocations in activated B cell-like diffuse large B cell lymphoma. *J Exp Med* 204:633–643.

Lenz G, Wright GW, Emre NC, Kohlhammer H, Dave SS, Davis RE, et al. (2008): Molecular subtypes of diffuse large B-cell lymphoma arise by distinct genetic pathways. *Proc Natl Acad Sci USA* 105:13520–13525.

Leoncini L, Raphael M, Stein H, Harris NL, Jaffe ES, Kluin PM (2008): Burkitt lymphoma. In: Swerdlow S, Campo E, Harris N, Jaffe ES, Pileri S, Stein H, et al., eds. *WHO Classification of Tumours of Haematopoietic and Lymphoid Tissues*. IARC, Lyon:262–264.

Lepretre S, Buchonnet G, Stamatoullas A, Lenain P, Duval C, d'Anjou J, et al. (2000): Chromosome abnormalities in peripheral T-cell lymphoma. *Cancer Genet Cytogenet* 117:71–79.

Leroux D, Hillion J, Monteil M, Le Marc'hadour F, Jacob MC, Sotto JJ, et al. (1991): t(18;22)(q21;q11) with rearrangement of BCL2 as a possible secondary change in a lymphocytic lymphoma. *Genes Chromosomes Cancer* 3:205–209.

Letai AG (2008): Diagnosing and exploiting cancer's addiction to blocks in apoptosis. *Nat Rev Cancer* 8:121–132.

Leucci E, Cocco M, Onnis A, De Falco G, van Cleef P, Bellan C, et al. (2008): MYC translocation-negative Burkitt lymphoma cases: an alternative pathogenic mechanism involving miRNA deregulation. *J Pathol* 216:440–450.

Liang X, Branchford B, Greffe B, McGavran L, Carstens B, Meltesen L, et al. (2013): Dual ALK and MYC rearrangements leading to an aggressive variant of anaplastic large cell lymphoma. *J Pediatr Hematol Oncol* 35:e209–e213.

Limpens J, de Jong D, van Krieken JH, Price CG, Young BD, van Ommen GJ, et al., (1991): Bcl-2/JH rearrangements in benign lymphoid tissues with follicular hyperplasia. *Oncogene* 6:2271–2276.

Limpens J, Stad R, Vos C, de Vlaam C, de Jong D, van Ommen GJ, et al. (1995): Lymphoma-associated translocation t(14;18) in blood B cells of normal individuals. *Blood* 85:2528–2536.

Lin P, Jetly R, Lennon PA, Abruzzo LV, Prajapati S, Medeiros LJ (2008): Translocation (18;22)(q21;q11) in B-cell lymphomas: a report of 4 cases and review of literature. *Hum Pathol* 39:1664–1672.

Liu H, Ruskon-Fourmestraux A, Lavergne-Slove A, Ye H, Molina T, Bouhnik Y, et al. (2001): Resistance of t(11;18) positive gastric mucosa-associated lymphoid tissue lymphoma to *Helicobacter pylori* eradication therapy. *Lancet* 357:39–40.

Liu H, Ye H, Ruskone-Fourmestraux A, DeJong D, Pileri S, Thiede C, et al. (2002): t(11;18) is a marker for all stage gastric MALT lymphomas that will not respond to *H. pylori* eradication. *Gastroenterology* 122:1286–1294.

Liu Q, Salaverria I, Pittaluga S, Jegalian AG, Xi L, Siebert R, et al. (2013): Follicular lymphomas in children and young adults. *Am J Surg Pathol* 37:333–343.

Loeffler M, Kreuz M, Haake A, Hasenclever D, Trautmann H, Arnold C (2015): Genomic and epigenomic co-evolution in follicular lymphomas. *Leukemia* 29:456–463.

Lohr JG, Stojanov P, Lawrence MS, Auclair D, Chapuy B, Sougnez C, et al. (2012): Discovery and prioritization of somatic mutations in diffuse large B-cell lymphoma (DLBCL) by whole-exome sequencing. *Proc Natl Acad Sci USA* 109:3879–3884.

Louissaint A Jr, Ackerman AM, Dias-Santagata D, Ferry JA, Hochberg EP, Huang MS, et al. (2012): Pediatric-type nodal follicular lymphoma: an indolent clonal proliferation in children and adults with high proliferation index and no BCL2 rearrangement. *Blood* 120:2395–2404.

Love C, Sun Z, Jima D, Li G, Zhang J, Miles R, et al. (2012): The genetic landscape of mutations in Burkitt lymphoma. *Nat Genet* 44:1321–1325.

Luan SL, Boulanger E, Ye H, Chanudet E, Johnson N, Hamoudi RA, et al. (2010): Primary effusion lymphoma: genomic profiling revealed amplification of SELPLG and CORO1C encoding for proteins important for cell migration. *J Pathol* 222:166–179.

Ma Z, Cools J, Marynen P, Cui X, Siebert R, Gesk S, et al. (2000): Inv(2)(p23q35) in anaplastic large-cell lymphoma induces constitutive anaplastic lymphoma kinase (ALK) tyrosine kinase activation by fusion to ATIC, an enzyme involved in purine nucleotide biosynthesis. *Blood* 95:2144–2149.

MacLeod RA, Spitzer D, Bar-Am I, Sylvester JE, Kaufmann M, Wernich A, et al. (2000): Karyotypic dissection of Hodgkin's disease cell lines reveals ectopic subtelomeres and ribosomal DNA at sites of multiple jumping translocations and genomic amplification. *Leukemia* 14:1803–1814.

Maes B, Vanhentenrijk V, Wlodarska I, Cools J, Peeters B, Marynen P, et al. (2001): The NPM–ALK and the ATIC–ALK fusion genes can be detected in non-neoplastic cells. *Am J Pathol* 158:2185–2193.

Magrangeas F, Lodé L, Wuilleme S, Minvielle S, Avet-Loiseau H (2005): Genetic heterogeneity in multiple myeloma. *Leukemia* 19:191–194.

Majid A, Tsoulakis O, Walewska R, Gesk S, Siebert R, Kennedy DB, et al. (2007): BCL2 expression in chronic lymphocytic leukemia: lack of association with the BCL2 938A>C promoter single nucleotide polymorphism. *Blood* 111:874–877.

Mamessier E, Song JY, Eberle FC, Pack S, Drevet C, Chetaille B, et al. (2014): Early lesions of follicular lymphoma: a genetic perspective. *Haematologica* 99:481–488.

Man C, Au WY, Pang A, Kwong YL (2002): Deletion 6q as a recurrent chromosomal aberration in T-cell large granular lymphocyte leukemia. *Cancer Genet Cytogenet* 139:71–74.

Mandal AK, Savvidou L, Slater RM, Cockett W, Wiggins J, Missouris CG (2007): Angiotropic lymphoma: associated chromosomal abnormalities. *Eur J Intern Med* 18:432–434.

Manolov G, Manolova Y (1972): Marker band in one chromosome 14 from Burkitt lymphomas. *Nature* 237:33–34.

Manolova Y, Manolov G, Kieler J, Levan A, Klein G (1979): Genesis of the 14q + marker in Burkitt's lymphoma. *Hereditas* 90:5–10.

Mao X, Lillington D, Scarisbrick JJ, Mitchell T, Czepulkowski B, Russell-Jones R, et al. (2002): Molecular cytogenetic analysis of cutaneous T-cell lymphomas: identification of common genetic alterations in Sézary syndrome and mycosis fungoides. *Br J Dermatol* 147:464–475.

Mao X, Lillington DM, Czepulkowski B, Russell-Jones R, Young BD, Whittaker S (2003a): Molecular cytogenetic characterization of Sézary syndrome. *Genes Chromosomes Cancer* 36:250–260.

Mao X, Onadim Z, Price EA, Child F, Lillington DM, Russell-Jones R, et al. (2003b): Genomic alterations in blastic natural killer/extranodal natural killer-like T cell lymphoma with cutaneous involvement. *J Invest Dermatol* 121:618–627.

Martin LD, Belch AR, Pilarski LM (2010): Promiscuity of translocation partners in multiple myeloma. *J Cell Biochem* 109:1085–1094.

Martínez N, Almaraz C, Vaqué JP, Varela I, Derdak S, Beltran S, et al. (2014): Whole-exome sequencing in splenic marginal zone lymphoma reveals mutations in genes involved in marginal zone differentiation. *Leukemia* 28:1334-1340.

Martínez-Trillos A, Quesada V, Villamor N, Puente XS, López-Otín C, Campo E (2013): Recurrent gene mutations in CLL. *Adv Exp Med Biol* 792:87–107.

Martínez-Trillos A, Pinyol M, Navarro A, Aymerich M, Jares P, Juan M, et al. (2014): Mutations in TLR/MYD88 pathway identify a subset of young chronic lymphocytic leukemia patients with favorable outcome. *Blood* 123:3790–3796.

Martin-Guerrero I, Salaverria I, Burkhardt B, Szczepanowski M, Baudis M, Bens S, et al. (2013): Recurrent loss of heterozygosity in 1p36 associated with TNFRSF14 mutations

in IRF4 translocation negative pediatric follicular lymphoma. *Haematologica* 98:1237–1241.

Martín-Subero JI, Gesk S, Harder L, Sonoki T, Tucker PW, Schlegelberger B, et al. (2002): Recurrent involvement of the REL and BCL11A loci in classical Hodgkin lymphoma. *Blood* 99:1474–1477.

Martín-Subero JI, Gesk S, Harder L, Grote W, Siebert R (2003a): Interphase cytogenetics of hematological neoplasms under the perspective of the novel WHO classification. *Anticancer Res* 23:1139–1148.

Martín-Subero JI, Knippschild U, Harder L, Barth TF, Riemke J, Grohmann S, et al. (2003b): Segmental chromosomal aberrations and centrosome amplifications: pathogenetic mechanisms in Hodgkin and Reed–Sternberg cells of classical Hodgkin's lymphoma? *Leukemia* 17:2214–2219.

Martín-Subero JI, Odero MD, Hernandez R, Cigudosa JC, Agirre X, Saez B, et al. (2005): Amplification of IGH/MYC fusion in clinically aggressive IGH/BCL2-positive germinal center B-cell lymphomas. *Genes Chromosomes Cancer* 43:414–423.

Martín-Subero JI, Klapper W, Sotnikova A, Callet-Bauchu E, Harder L, Bastard C, et al. (2006): Chromosomal breakpoints affecting immunoglobulin loci are recurrent in Hodgkin and Reed–Sternberg cells of classical Hodgkin lymphoma. *Cancer Res* 66:10332–10338.

Martín-Subero JI, Ibbotson R, Klapper W, Michaux L, Callet-Bauchu E, Berger F, et al. (2007): A comprehensive genetic and histopathologic analysis identifies two subgroups of B-cell malignancies carrying a t(14;19)(q32;q13) or variant BCL3-translocation. *Leukemia* 21:1532–1544.

Marty M, Prochazkova M, Laharanne E, Chevret E, Longy M, Jouary T, et al. (2008): Primary cutaneous T-cell lymphomas do not show specific NAV3 gene deletion or translocation. *J Invest Dermatol* 128:2458–2466.

Masqué-Soler N, Szczepanowski M, Kohler CW, Spang R, Klapper W (2013): Molecular classification of mature aggressive B-cell lymphoma using digital multiplexed gene expression on formalin-fixed paraffin-embedded biopsy specimens. *Blood* 122:1985–1986.

Mateo M, Mollejo M, Villuendas R, Algara P, Sanchez-Beato M, Martínez P, et al. (1999): 7q31–32 allelic loss is a frequent finding in splenic marginal zone lymphoma. *Am J Pathol* 154:1583–1589.

Matutes E, Carrara P, Coignet L, Brito-Babapulle V, Villamor N, Wotherspoon A, et al. (1999): FISH analysis for BCL-1 rearrangements and trisomy 12 helps the diagnosis of atypical B cell leukaemias. *Leukemia* 13:1721–1726.

May PC, Foot N, Dunn R, Geoghegan H, Neat MJ (2010): Detection of cryptic and variant IGH-MYC rearrangements in high-grade non-Hodgkin's lymphoma by fluorescence in situ hybridization: implications for cytogenetic testing. *Cancer Genet Cytogenet* 198:71–75.

Mayr C, Speicher MR, Kofler DM, Buhmann R, Strehl J, Busch R, et al. (2006): Chromosomal translocations are associated with poor prognosis in chronic lymphocytic leukemia. *Blood* 107:742–751.

Merchant S, Schlette E, Sanger W, Lai R, Medeiros LJ (2003): Mature B-cell leukemias with more than 55% prolymphocytes: report of 2 cases with Burkitt lymphoma-type chromosomal translocations involving c-myc. *Arch Pathol Lab Med* 127: 305–309.

Micci F, Panagopoulos I, Tjønnfjord GE, Kolstad A, Delabie J, Beiske K, et al. (2007): Molecular cytogenetic characterization of t(14;19)(q32;p13), a new recurrent translocation in B cell malignancies. *Virchows Arch* 450:559–565.

Michaux L, Wlodarska I, Theate I, Stul M, Scheiff JM, Deneys V, et al. (2004): Coexistence of BCL1/CCND1 and CMYC aberrations in blastoid mantle cell lymphoma: a rare finding associated with very poor outcome. *Ann Hematol* 83:578–583.

Michaux L, Wlodarska I, Rack K, Stul M, Criel A, Maerevoet M, et al. (2005): Translocation t(1;6)(p35.3;p25.2): a new recurrent aberration in "unmutated" B-CLL. *Leukemia* 19:77–82.

Migliazza A, Bosch F, Komatsu H, Cayanis E, Martinotti S, Toniato E, et al. (2001): Nucleotide sequence, transcription map, and mutation analysis of the 13q14 chromosomal region deleted in B-cell chronic lymphocytic leukemia. *Blood* 97:2098–2104.

Miki T, Kawamata N, Hirosawa S, Aoki N (1994a): Gene involved in the 3q27 translocation associated with B-cell lymphoma, BCL5, encodes a Krüppel-like zinc-finger protein. *Blood* 83:26–32.

Miki T, Kawamata N, Arai A, Ohashi K, Nakamura Y, Kato A, et al. (1994b): Molecular cloning of the breakpoint for 3q27 translocation in B-cell lymphomas and leukemias. *Blood* 83:217–222.

Mirza I, Macpherson N, Paproski S, Gascoyne RD, Yang B, Finn WG, et al. (2002): Primary cutaneous follicular lymphoma: an assessment of clinical, immunophenotypic, and molecular features. *J Clin Oncol* 20:647–655.

Mitelman F, Johansson B, Mertens F (Eds.) (2014): Mitelman Database of Chromosome Aberrations and Gene Fusions in Cancer. Available at http://cgap.nci.nih.gov/Chromosomes/Mitelman.

Mitev L, Christova S, Hadjiev E, Guenova M, Oucheva R, Valkov I, et al. (1998): A new variant chromosomal translocation t(2;2)(p23;q23) in CD30+/Ki-1+ anaplastic large cell lymphoma. *Leuk Lymphoma* 28:613–616.

Miyoshi I, Hiraki S, Kimura I, Miyamoto K, Sato J (1979): 2/8 translocation in a Japanese Burkitt's lymphoma. *Experientia* 35:742–743.

Montesinos-Rongen M, Akasaka T, Zühlke-Jenisch R, Schaller C, Van Roost D, et al. (2003): Molecular characterization of BCL6 breakpoints in primary diffuse large B-cell lymphoma of the central nervous system identifies GAPD as novel translocation partner. *Brain Pathol* 13:534–538.

Montoto S, Fitzgibbon J (2011): Transformation of indolent B-cell lymphomas. *J Clin Oncol* 29:1827–1834.

Montoto S, Davies AJ, Matthews J, Calaminici M, Norton AJ, Amess J, et al. (2007): Risk and clinical implications of transformation of follicular lymphoma to diffuse large B-cell lymphoma. *J Clin Oncol* 25:2426–2433.

Morgan R, Hecht BK, Sandberg AA, Hecht F, Smith SD (1986): Chromosome 5q35 breakpoint in malignant histiocytosis. *N Engl J Med* 314:1322.

Morin RD, Mendez-Lago M, Mungall AJ, Goya R, Mungall KL, Corbett RD, et al. (2011): Frequent mutation of histone-modifying genes in non-Hodgkin lymphoma. *Nature* 476:298–303.

Morin RD, Mungall K, Pleasance E, Mungall AJ, Goya R, Huff RD, et al. (2013): Mutational and structural analysis of diffuse large B-cell lymphoma using whole-genome sequencing. *Blood* 122:1256–1265.

Morris SW, Kirstein MN, Valentine MB, Dittmer KG, Shapiro DN, Saltman DL, et al. (1994): Fusion of a kinase gene, ALK, to a nucleolar protein gene, NPM, in non-Hodgkin's lymphoma. *Science* 263:1281–1284.

Motokura T, Bloom T, Kim HG, Jüppner H, Ruderman JV, Kronenberg HM, et al. (1991): A novel cyclin encoded by a bcl1-linked candidate oncogene. *Nature* 350: 512–515.

Mottok A, Renné C, Willenbrock K, Hansmann ML, Bräuninger A (2007): Somatic hypermutation of SOCS1 in lymphocyte-predominant Hodgkin lymphoma is accompanied by high JAK2 expression and activation of STAT6. *Blood* 110: 3387–3390.

Mullaney BP, Ng VL, Herndier BG, McGrath MS, Pallavicini MG (2000): Comparative genomic analyses of primary effusion lymphoma. *Arch Pathol Lab Med* 124: 824–826.

Mwenifumbo JC, Marra MA (2013): Cancer genome-sequencing study design. *Nat Rev Genet* 14:321–332.

Nadal N, Chapiro E, Flandrin-Gresta P, Thouvenin S, Vasselon C, Beldjord K, et al. (2012): LHX2 deregulation by juxtaposition with the IGH locus in a pediatric case of chronic myeloid leukemia in B-cell lymphoid blast crisis. *Leuk Res* 36:e195–e198.

Nagel I, Bug S, Tönnies H, Ammerpohl O, Richter J, Vater I, et al. (2009a): Biallelic inactivation of TRAF3 in a subset of B-cell lymphomas with interstitial del(14)(q24.1q32.33). *Leukemia* 23:2153–2155.

Nagel I, Akasaka T, Klapper W, Gesk S, Böttcher S, Ritgen M, et al. (2009b): Identification of the gene encoding cyclin E1 (CCNE1) as a novel IGH translocation partner in t(14;19)(q32;q12) in diffuse large B-cell lymphoma. *Haematologica* 94:1020–1023.

Nakagawa M, Nakagawa-Oshiro A, Karnan S, Tagawa H, Utsunomiya A, Nakamura S, et al. (2009): Array comparative genomic hybridization analysis of PTCL-U reveals a distinct subgroup with genetic alterations similar to lymphoma-type adult T-cell leukemia/lymphoma. *Clin Cancer Res* 15:30–38.

Nakamura S, Ye H, Bacon CM, Goatly A, Liu H, Banham AH, et al. (2007): Clinical impact of genetic aberrations in gastric MALT lymphoma: a comprehensive analysis using interphase fluorescence in situ hybridisation. *Gut* 56:1358–1363.

Nakamura Y, Takahashi N, Kakegawa E, Yoshida K, Ito Y, Kayano H, et al. (2008): The GAS5 (growth arrest-specific transcript 5) gene fuses to BCL6 as a result of t(1;3)(q25;q27) in a patient with B-cell lymphoma. *Cancer Genet Cytogenet* 182:144–149.

Nakamura S, Sugiyama T, Matsumoto T, Iijima K, Ono S, Tajika M, et al. (2012): Long-term clinical outcome of gastric MALT lymphoma after eradication of *Helicobacter pylori*: a multicentre cohort follow-up study of 420 patients in Japan. *Gut* 61:507–513.

Nakashima Y, Tagawa H, Suzuki R, Karnan S, Karube K, Ohshima K, et al. (2005): Genome-wide array-based comparative genomic hybridization of natural killer cell lymphoma/leukemia: different genomic alteration patterns of aggressive NK-cell leukemia and extranodal Nk/T-cell lymphoma, nasal type. *Genes Chromosomes Cancer* 44: 247–255.

Navarro A, Clot G, Royo C, Jares P, Hadzidimitriou A, Agathangelidis A, et al. (2012): Molecular subsets of mantle cell lymphoma defined by the IGHV mutational status and SOX11 expression have distinct biologic and clinical features. *Cancer Res* 72:5307–5316.

Nelson BP, Gupta R, Dewald GW, Paternoster SF, Rosen ST, Peterson LC (2007): Chronic lymphocytic leukemia FISH panel: impact on diagnosis. *Am J Clin Pathol* 128:323–332.

Nelson M, Horsman DE, Weisenburger DD, Gascoyne RD, Dave BJ, Loberiza FR, et al. (2008): Cytogenetic abnormalities and clinical correlations in peripheral T-cell lymphoma. *Br J Haematol* 141:461–469.

Nelson M, Perkins SL, Dave BJ, Coccia PF, Bridge JA, Lyden ER, et al. (2010): An increased frequency of 13q deletions detected by fluorescence in situ hybridization and its impact on survival in children and adolescents with Burkitt lymphoma: results from the Children's Oncology Group study CCG-5961. *Br J Haematol* 148:600–610.

Neri A, Chang CC, Lombardi L, Salina M, Corradini P, Maiolo AT, et al. (1991): B cell lymphoma-associated chromosomal translocation involves candidate oncogene lyt-10, homologous to NF-kappa B p50. *Cell* 67: 1075–1087.

Neri A, Baldini L, Trecca D, Cro L, Polli E, Maiolo AT (1993): p53 gene mutations in multiple myeloma are associated with advanced forms of malignancy. *Blood* 81: 128–135.

Nessling M, Solinas-Toldo S, Lichter P, Reifenberger G, Wolter M, Möller P, et al. (1999): Genomic imbalances are rare in hairy cell leukemia. *Genes Chromosomes Cancer* 26:182–183.

Ngo VN, Young RM, Schmitz R, Jhavar S, Xiao W, Lim KH, et al. (2011): Oncogenetically active MYD88 mutations in human lymphoma. *Nature* 470:115–119.

Nicolae A, Xi L, Pittaluga S, Abdullaev Z, Pack SD, Chen J, et al. (2014): Frequent STAT5B mutations in γδ hepatosplenic T-cell lymphomas. *Leukemia* 28:2244–2248.

Nieläender I, Martín-Subero JI, Wagner F, Martínez-Climent JA, Siebert R (2006): Partial uniparental disomy: a recurrent genetic mechanism alternative to chromosomal deletion in malignant lymphoma. *Leukemia* 20:904–905.

Nieländer I, Bug S, Richter J, Giefing M, Martín-Subero JI, Siebert R (2007): Combining array-based approaches for the identification of candidate tumor suppressor loci in mature lymphoid neoplasms. *APMIS* 115:1107–1134.

Niitsu N, Okamoto M, Nakamura N, Nakamine H, Aoki S, Hirano M, et al. (2007): Prognostic impact of chromosomal alteration of 3q27 on nodal B-cell lymphoma: correlation with histology, immunophenotype, karyotype, and clinical outcome in 329 consecutive patients. *Leuk Res* 31:1191–1197.

Nilsson T, Höglund M, Lenhoff S, Rylander L, Turesson I, Westin J, et al. (2003): A pooled analysis of karyotypic patterns, breakpoints and imbalances in 783 cytogenetically abnormal multiple myelomas reveals frequently involved chromosome segments as well as significant age- and sex-related differences. *Br J Haematol* 120:960–969.

Nordgren A, Corcoran M, Sääf A, Bremer A, Kluin-Nelemans HC, Schoumans J, et al. (2010): Characterisation of hairy cell leukaemia by tiling resolution array-based comparative genome hybridisation: a series of 13 cases and review of the literature. *Eur J Haematol* 84:17–25.

Nowak D, Le Toriellec E, Stern MH, Kawamata N, Akagi T, Dyer MJ, et al. (2009): Molecular allelokaryotyping of T-cell prolymphocytic leukemic cells with high density single nucleotide polymorphism arrays identifies novel common genomic lesions and acquired uniparental disomy. *Haematologica* 94:518–527.

Nowakowski GS, Dewald GW, Hoyer JD, Paternoster SF, Stockero KJ, Fink SR, et al. (2005): Interphase fluorescence in situ hybridization with an IGH probe is important in the evaluation of patients with a clinical diagnosis of chronic lymphocytic leukaemia. *Br J Haematol* 130:36–42.

O'Donnell KA, Wentzel EA, Zeller KI, Dang CV, Mendell JT (2005): c-Myc-regulated microRNAs modulate E2F1 expression. *Nature* 435:839–843.

O'Shea D, O'Riain C, Taylor C, Waters R, Carlotti E, Macdougall F, et al. (2008): The presence of TP53 mutation at diagnosis of follicular lymphoma identifies a high-risk group of patients with shortened time to disease progression and poorer overall survival. *Blood* 112:3126–3129.

Odejide O, Weigert O, Lane AA, Toscano D, Lunning MA, Kopp N, et al. (2014): A targeted mutational landscape of angioimmunoblastic T-cell lymphoma. *Blood* 123:1293–1296.

Offit K, Parsa NZ, Gaidano G, Filippa DA, Louie D, Pan D, et al. (1993): 6q deletions define distinct clinico-pathologic subsets of non-Hodgkin's lymphoma. *Blood* 82:2157–2162.

Ohno H (2004): Pathogenetic role of BCL6 translocation in B-cell non-Hodgkin's lymphoma. *Histol Histopathol* 19:637–650.

Ohno H (2006): Pathogenetic and clinical implications of non-immunoglobulin; BCL6 translocations in B-cell non-Hodgkin's lymphoma. *J Clin Exp Hematop* 46:43–53.

Ohno H, Takimoto G, McKeithan TW (1990): The candidate proto-oncogene bcl-3 is related to genes implicated in cell lineage determination and cell cycle control. *Cell* 60:991–997.

Ohno H, Ueda C, Akasaka T (2000): The t(9;14)(p13;q32) translocation in B-cell non-Hodgkin's lymphoma. *Leuk Lymphoma* 36:435–445.

Okosun J, Bödör C, Wang J, Araf S, Yang CY, Pan C, et al. (2014): Integrated genomic analysis identifies recurrent mutations and evolution patterns driving the initiation and progression of follicular lymphoma. *Nat Genet* 46:176–181.

Oschlies I, Salaverria I, Mahn F, Meinhardt A, Zimmermann M, Woessmann W, et al. (2010): Pediatric follicular lymphoma – a clinico-pathological study of a population-based series of patients treated within the Non-Hodgkin's Lymphoma – Berlin-Frankfurt-Münster (NHL-BFM) multicenter trials. *Haematologica* 95:253–259.

Oscier DG, Matutes E, Gardiner A, Glide S, Mould S, Brito-Babapulle V, et al. (1994): Cytogenetic studies in splenic lymphoma with villous lymphocytes. *Br J Haematol* 85:487–491.

Oshiro A, Tagawa H, Ohshima K, Karube K, Uike N, Tashiro Y, et al. (2006): Identification of subtype-specific genomic alterations in aggressive adult T-cell leukemia/lymphoma. *Blood* 107:4500–4507.

Ostergaard M, Lindbjerg Andersen C, Pedersen B, Koch J, Nielsen B (2001): Recurrent imbalances involving chromosome 5 and 7q22–q35 in hairy cell leukemia: a comparative genomic hybridization study. *Genes Chromosomes Cancer* 30: 218–219.

Ott G, Kalla J, Ott MM, Schryen B, Katzenberger T, Müller JG, et al. (1997a): Blastoid variants of mantle cell lymphoma: frequent bcl-1 rearrangements at the major translocation cluster region and tetraploid chromosome clones. *Blood* 89:1421–1429.

Ott G, Katzenberger T, Greiner A, Kalla J, Rosenwald A, Heinrich U, et al. (1997b): The t(11;18)(q21;q21) chromosome translocation is a frequent and specific aberration in low-grade but not high-grade malignant non-Hodgkin's lymphomas of the mucosa-associated lymphoid tissue (MALT-) type. *Cancer Res* 57:3944–3948.

Ott MM, Rosenwald A, Katzenberger T, Dreyling M, Krumdiek AK, Kalla J, et al. (2000): Marginal zone B-cell lymphomas (MZBL) arising at different sites represent different biological entities. *Genes Chromosomes Cancer* 28:380–386.

Ott G, Katzenberger T, Lohr A, Kindelberger S, Rüdiger T, Wilhelm M, et al. (2002): Cytomorphologic, immunohistochemical, and cytogenetic profiles of follicular lymphoma: 2 types of follicular lymphoma grade 3. *Blood* 99:3806–3812.

Ott G, Rosenwald A, Campo E (2013): Understanding MYC-driven aggressive B-cell lymphomas: pathogenesis and classification. *Blood* 122:3884–3891.

Ouillette P, Erba H, Kujawski L, Kaminski M, Shedden K, Malek SN (2008): Integrated genomic profiling of chronic lymphocytic leukemia identifies subtypes of deletion 13q14. *Cancer Res* 68:1012–1021.

Ouillette P, Collins R, Shakhan S, Li J, Li C, Shedden K, et al. (2011): The prognostic significance of various 13q14 deletions in chronic lymphocytic leukemia. *Clin Cancer Res* 17:6778–6790.

Palomero T, Couronné L, Khiabanian H, Kim MY, Ambesi-Impiombato A, Perez-Garcia A, et al. (2014): Recurrent mutations in epigenetic regulators, RHOA and FYN kinase in peripheral T cell lymphomas. *Nat Genet* 46:166–170.

Parker E, Macdonald JR, Wang C (2011): Molecular characterization of a t(2;7) translocation linking CDK6 to the IGK locus in CD5(–) monoclonal B-cell lymphocytosis. *Cancer Genet* 204:260–264.

Parker EP, Siebert R, Oo TH, Schneider D, Hayette S, Wang C (2013): Sequencing of t(2;7) translocations reveals a consistent breakpoint linking CDK6 to the IGK locus in indolent B-cell neoplasia. *J Mol Diagn* 15:101–109.

Parry M, Rose-Zerilli MJ, Gibson J, Ennis S, Walewska R, Forster J, et al. (2013): Whole exome sequencing identifies novel recurrently mutated genes in patients with splenic marginal zone lymphoma. *PLoS One* 8:e83244.

Pasqualucci L, Neumeister P, Goossens T, Nanjangud G, Chaganti RS, Küppers R, et al. (2001): Hypermutation of multiple proto-oncogenes in B-cell diffuse large-cell lymphomas. *Nature* 412:341–346.

Pasqualucci L, Migliazza A, Basso K, Houldsworth J, Chaganti RS, Dalla-Favera R (2003): Mutations of the BCL6 proto-oncogene disrupt its negative autoregulation in diffuse large B-cell lymphoma. *Blood* 101:2914–2923.

Pasqualucci L, Compagno M, Houldsworth J, Monti S, Grunn A, Nandula SV, et al. (2006): Inactivation of the PRDM1/BLIMP1 gene in diffuse large B cell lymphoma. *J Exp Med* 203: 311–317.

Pasqualucci L, Trifonov V, Fabbri G, Ma J, Rossi D, Chiarenza A, et al. (2011a): Analysis of the coding genome of diffuse large B-cell lymphoma. *Nat Genet* 43:830–837.

Pasqualucci L, Dominguez-Sola D, Chiarenza A, Fabbri G, Grunn A, Trifonov V, et al. (2011b): Inactivating mutations of acetyltransferase genes in B-cell lymphoma. *Nature* 471:189–195.

Pasqualucci L, Khiabanian H, Fangazio M, Vasishtha M, Messina M, Holmes AB, et al. (2014): Genetics of follicular lymphoma transformation. *Cell Rep* 6:130–140.

Pérez-Simón JA, García-Sanz R, Tabernero MD, Almeida J, González M, Fernández-Calvo J, et al. (1998): Prognostic value of numerical chromosome aberrations in multiple myeloma: a FISH analysis of 15 different chromosomes. *Blood* 91:3366–3371.

Pham-Ledard A, Prochazkova-Carlotti M, Laharanne E, Vergier B, Jouary T, Beylot-Barry M, et al. (2010): IRF4 gene rearrangements define a subgroup of CD30-positive cutaneous T-cell lymphoma: a study of 54 cases. *J Invest Dermatol* 130:816–825.

Pinyol M, Bea S, Plà L, Ribrag V, Bosq J, Rosenwald A, et al. (2007): Inactivation of RB1 in mantle-cell lymphoma detected by nonsense-mediated mRNA decay pathway inhibition and microarray analysis. *Blood* 109:5422–5429.

Poirel HA, Cairo MS, Heerema NA, Swansbury J, Aupérin A, Launay E, et al. (2009): Specific cytogenetic abnormalities are associated with a significantly inferior outcome in children and adolescents with mature B-cell non-Hodgkin's lymphoma: results of the FAB/LMB 96 international study. *Leukemia* 23:323–331.

Poppe B, DePaepe P, Michaux L, Dastugue N, Bastard C, Herens C, et al. (2005): PAX5/IGH rearrangement is a recurrent finding in a subset of aggressive B-NHL with complex chromosomal rearrangements. *Genes Chromosomes Cancer* 44:218–223.

Pospisilova H, Baens M, Michaux L, Stul M, Van Hummelen P, Van Loo P, et al. (2007): Interstitial del(14)(q) involving IGH: a novel recurrent aberration in B-NHL. *Leukemia* 21:2079–2083.

Prochazkova M, Chevret E, Beylot-Barry M, Sobotka J, Vergier B, Delaunay M, et al. (2003): Chromosomal imbalances: a hallmark of tumour relapse in primary cutaneous CD30+ T-cell lymphoma. *J Pathol* 201:421–429.

Przybylski GK, Dik WA, Wanzeck J, Grabarczyk P, Majunke S, Martin-Subero JI, et al. (2005): Disruption of the BCL11B gene through inv(14)(q11.2q32.31) results in the expression of BCL11B–TRDC fusion transcripts and is associated with the absence of wild-type BCL11B transcripts in T-ALL. *Leukemia* 19:201–208.

Puente XS, Pinyol M, Quesada V, Conde L, Ordóñez GR, Villamor N, et al. (2011): Whole-genome sequencing identifies recurrent mutations in chronic lymphocytic leukaemia. *Nature* 475:101–105.

Put N, Van Roosbroeck K, Konings P, Meeus P, Brusselmans C, Rack K, et al. (2012): Chronic lymphocytic leukemia and prolymphocytic leukemia with MYC translocations: a subgroup with an aggressive disease course. *Ann Hematol* 91:863–873.

Quesada V, Conde L, Villamor N, Ordóñez GR, Jares P, Bassaganyas L, et al. (2011): Exome sequencing identifies recurrent mutations of the splicing factor SF3B1 gene in chronic lymphocytic leukemia. *Nat Genet* 44:47–52.

Quesada V, Ramsay AJ, Rodríguez D, Puente XS, Campo E, López-Otín C (2013): The genomic landscape of chronic lymphocytic leukemia: clinical implications. *BMC Med* 11:124.

Quintanilla-Martinez L, Slotta-Huspenina J, Koch I, Klier M, Hsi ED, de Leval L, et al. (2009): Differential diagnosis of cyclin D2+ mantle cell lymphoma based on fluorescence in situ hybridization and quantitative real-time-PCR. *Haematologica* 94:1595–1598.

Rahal R, Frick M, Romero R, Korn JM, Kridel R, Chan FC, et al. (2014): Pharmacological and genomic profiling identifies NF-κB-targeted treatment strategies for mantle cell lymphoma. *Nat Med* 20:87–92.

Rajkumar SV (2012): Multiple myeloma: 2012 update on diagnosis, risk-stratification, and management. *Am J Hematol* 87:78–88.

Rajkumar S, Fonseca R, Lacy M, Witzig T, Lust J, Greipp P, et al. (1999): Abnormal cytogenetics predict poor survival after high-dose therapy and autologous blood cell transplantation in multiple myeloma. *Bone Marrow Transplant* 24:497–503.

Rao PH, Cigudosa JC, Ning Y, Calasanz MJ, Iida S, Tagawa S, et al. (1998): Multicolor spectral karyotyping identifies new recurring breakpoints and translocations in multiple myeloma. *Blood* 92:1743–1748.

Rashid R, Johnson RJ, Morris S, Dickinson H, Czyz J, O'Connor SJ, et al. (2006): Intravascular large B-cell lymphoma associated with a near-tetraploid karyotype, rearrangement of BCL6, and a t(11;14)(q13;q32). *Cancer Genet Cytogenet* 171:101–104.

Reddy K, Satyadev R, Bouman D, Hibbard MK, Lu G, Paolo R (2006): Burkitt t(8;14)(q24;q32) and cryptic deletion in a CLL patient: report of a case and review of literature. *Cancer Genet Cytogenet* 166:12–21.

Renné C, Martín-Subero JI, Hansmann ML, Siebert R (2005): Molecular cytogenetic analyses of immunoglobulin loci in nodular lymphocyte predominant Hodgkin's lymphoma reveal a recurrent IGH-BCL6 juxtaposition. *J Mol Diagn* 7:352–356.

Richter J, Schlesner M, Hoffmann S, Kreuz M, Leich E, Burkhardt B, et al. (2012): Recurrent mutations of the ID3 gene in Burkitt lymphoma identified by integrated genome, exome and transcriptome sequencing. *Nat Genet* 44:1316–1320.

Ried K, Finnis M, Hobson L, Mangelsdorf M, Dayan S, Nancarrow JK, et al. (2000): Common chromosomal fragile site FRA16D sequence: identification of the FOR gene spanning FRA16D and homozygous deletions and translocation breakpoints in cancer cells. *Hum Mol Genet* 9:1651–1663.

Riemersma SA, Jordanova ES, Schop RF, Philippo K, Looijenga LH, Schuuring E, et al. (2000): Extensive genetic alterations of the HLA region, including homozygous deletions of HLA class II genes in B-cell lymphomas arising in immune-privileged sites. *Blood* 96:3569–3577.

Rinaldi A, Mian M, Chigrinova E, Arcaini L, Bhagat G, Novak U, et al. (2011): Genome-wide DNA profiling of marginal zone lymphomas identifies subtype-specific lesions with an impact on the clinical outcome. *Blood* 117:1595–1604.

Rinaldi A, Mensah AA, Kwee I, Forconi F, Orlandi EM, Lucioni M, et al. (2013a): Promoter methylation patterns in Richter syndrome affect stem-cell maintenance and cell cycle regulation and differ from de novo diffuse large B-cell lymphoma. *Br J Haematol* 163:194–204.

Rinaldi A, Kwee I, Young KH, Zucca E, Gaidano G, Forconi F, et al. (2013b): Genome-wide high resolution DNA profiling of hairy cell leukaemia. *Br J Haematol* 162:566–569.

Ripollés L, Ortega M, Ortuño F, González A, Losada J, Ojanguren J, et al. (2006): Genetic abnormalities and clinical outcome in chronic lymphocytic leukemia. *Cancer Genet Cytogenet* 171:57–64.

Robledo C, García JL, Benito R, Flores T, Mollejo M, Martínez-Climent JÁ, et al. (2011): Molecular characterization of the region 7q22.1 in splenic marginal zone lymphomas. *PLoS One* 6:e24939.

Rocha CK, Praulich I, Gehrke I, Hallek M, Kreuzer KA (2011): A rare case of t(11;22) in a mantle cell lymphoma like B-cell neoplasia resulting in a fusion of IGL and CCND1: case report. *Mol Cytogenet* 4:8.

Ronchetti D, Finelli P, Richelda R, Baldini L, Rocchi M, Viggiano L, et al. (1999): Molecular analysis of 11q13 breakpoints in multiple myeloma. *Blood* 93:1330–1337.

Rosenberg CL, Wong E, Petty EM, Bale AE, Tsujimoto Y, Harris NL, et al. (1991): PRAD1, a candidate BCL1 oncogene: mapping and expression in centrocytic lymphoma. *Proc Natl Acad Sci USA* 88:9638–9642.

Rosenwald A, Wright G, Chan WC, Connors JM, Campo E, Fisher RI, et al. (2002): The use of molecular profiling to predict survival after chemotherapy for diffuse large-B-cell lymphoma. *N Engl J Med* 346:1937–1947.

Rosenwald A, Wright G, Leroy K, Yu X, Gaulard P, Gascoyne RD, et al. (2003): Molecular diagnosis of primary mediastinal B cell lymphoma identifies a clinically favorable subgroup of diffuse large B cell lymphoma related to Hodgkin lymphoma. *J Exp Med* 198:851–862.

Ross CW, Ouillette PD, Saddler CM, Shedden KA, Malek SN (2007): Comprehensive analysis of copy number and allele status identifies multiple chromosome defects underlying follicular lymphoma pathogenesis. *Clin Cancer Res* 13:4777–4785.

Rossi D, Trifonov V, Fangazio M, Bruscaggin A, Rasi S, Spina V, et al. (2012): The coding genome of splenic marginal zone lymphoma: activation of NOTCH2 and other pathways regulating marginal zone development. *J Exp Med* 209:1537–1551.

Rossi D, Khiabanian H, Spina V, Ciardullo C, Bruscaggin A, Famà R, et al. (2014): Clinical impact of small TP53 mutated subclones in chronic lymphocytic leukemia. *Blood* 123:2139–2147.

Rouhigharabaei L, Finalet Ferreiro J, Tousseyn T, van der Krogt JA, Put N, Haralambieva E, et al. (2014): Non-IG aberrations of FOXP1 in B-cell malignancies lead to an aberrant expression of N-truncated isoforms of FOXP1. *PLoS One* 9:e85851.

Roulland S, Lebailly P, Lecluse Y, Briand M, Pottier D, Gauduchon P (2004): Characterization of the t(14;18) BCL2-IGH translocation in farmers occupationally exposed to pesticides. *Cancer Res* 64:2264–2269.

Roulland S, Lebailly P, Lecluse Y, Heutte N, Nadel B, Gauduchon P (2006a).Long-term clonal persistence and evolution of t(14;18)-bearing B cells in healthy individuals. *Leukemia* 20:158–162.

Roulland S, Navarro JM, Grenot P, Milili M, Agopian J, Montpellier B, et al. (2006b): Follicular lymphoma-like B cells in healthy individuals: a novel intermediate step in early lymphomagenesis. *J Exp Med* 203:2425–2431.

Roulland S, Kelly RS, Morgado E, Sungalee S, Solal-Celigny P, Colombat P, Jouve N, et al. (2014): t(14;18) translocation: a predictive blood biomarker for follicular lymphoma development. *J Clin Oncol* 32:1347–1355.

Royo C, Navarro A, Clot G, Salaverria I, Giné E, Jares P, et al. (2012): Non-nodal type of mantle cell lymphoma is a specific biological and clinical subgroup of the disease. *Leukemia* 26:1895–1898.

Rubio-Moscardo F, Climent J, Siebert R, Piris MA, Martín-Subero JI, Nieländer I, et al. (2005): Mantle-cell lymphoma genotypes identified with CGH to BAC microarrays define a leukemic subgroup of disease and predict patient outcome. *Blood* 105: 4445–4454.

Ruiz-Ballesteros E, Mollejo M, Mateo M, Algara P, Martínez P, Piris MA (2007): MicroRNA losses in the frequently deleted region of 7q in SMZL. *Leukemia* 21: 2547–2549.

Ruminy P, Jardin F, Picquenot JM, Gaulard P, Parmentier F, Buchonnet G, et al. (2006): Two patterns of chromosomal breakpoint locations on the immunoglobulin heavy-chain locus in B-cell lymphomas with t(3;14)(q27;q32): relevance to histology. *Oncogene* 25:4947–4954.

Sáez B, Martín-Subero JI, Guillén-Grima F, Odero MD, Prosper F, Cigudosa JC, et al. (2004): Chromosomal abnormalities clustering in multiple myeloma reveals cytogenetic subgroups with nonrandom acquisition of chromosomal changes. *Leukemia* 18:654–657.

Sakata-Yanagimoto M, Enami T, Yoshida K, Shiraishi Y, Ishii R, Miyake Y, et al. (2014): Somatic RHOA mutation in angioimmunoblastic T cell lymphoma. *Nat Genet* 46:171–175.

Salaverria I, Siebert R (2011): The gray zone between Burkitt's lymphoma and diffuse large B-cell lymphoma from a genetics perspective. *J Clin Oncol* 29: 1835–1843.

Salaverria I, Zettl A, Beà S, Moreno V, Valls J, Hartmann E, et al. (2007): Specific secondary genetic alterations in mantle cell lymphoma provide prognostic information independent of the gene expression-based proliferation signature. *J Clin Oncol* 25:1216–1222.

Salaverria I, Beà S, Lopez-Guillermo A, Lespinet V, Pinyol M, Burkhardt B, et al. (2008a): Genomic profiling reveals different genetic aberrations in systemic ALK-positive and ALK-negative anaplastic large cell lymphomas. *Br J Haematol* 140:516–526.

Salaverria I, Zettl A, Beà S, Hartmann EM, Dave SS, Wright GW, et al. (2008b): Chromosomal alterations detected by comparative genomic hybridization in subgroups of gene expression-defined Burkitt's lymphoma. *Haematologica* 93:1327–1334.

Salaverria I, Philipp C, Oschlies I, Kohler CW, Kreuz M, Szczepanowski M, et al. (2011): Translocations activating IRF4 identify a subtype of germinal center-derived B-cell lymphoma affecting predominantly children and young adults. *Blood* 118:139–147.

Salaverria I, Akasaka T, Gesk S, Szczepanowski M, Burkhardt B, Harder L, et al. (2012): The CBFA2T3/ACSF3 locus is recurrently involved in IGH chromosomal translocation t(14;16)(q32;q24) in pediatric B-cell lymphoma with germinal center phenotype. *Genes Chromosomes Cancer* 51:338–343.

Salaverria I, Royo C, Carvajal-Cuenca A, Clot G, Navarro A, Valera A, et al. (2013a): CCND2 rearrangements are the most frequent genetic events in cyclin D1(−) mantle cell lymphoma. *Blood* 121:1394–1402.

Salaverria I, Martin-Guerrero I, Burkhardt B, Kreuz M, Zenz T, Oschlies I, et al. (2013b): High resolution copy number analysis of IRF4 translocation-positive diffuse large B-cell and follicular lymphomas. *Genes Chromosomes Cancer* 52:150–155.

Salaverria I, Martin-Guerrero I, Wagener R, Kreuz M, Kohler CW, Richter J, et al. (2014): A recurrent 11q aberration pattern characterizes a subset of MYC-negative high-grade B-cell lymphomas resembling Burkitt lymphoma. *Blood* 123:1187–1198.

Salgado R, Gallardo F, Servitje O, Estrach T, García-Muret MP, Romagosa V, et al. (2011): Absence of TCR loci chromosomal translocations in cutaneous T-cell lymphomas. *Cancer Genet* 204:405–409.

Sambani C, Trafalis DT, Mitsoulis-Mentzikoff C, Poulakidas E, Makropoulos V, Pantelias GE, et al. (2001): Clonal chromosome rearrangements in hairy cell leukemia: personal experience and review of literature. *Cancer Genet Cytogenet* 129:138–144.

Sanchez-Izquierdo D, Buchonnet G, Siebert R, Gascoyne RD, Climent J, Karran L, et al. (2003): MALT1 is deregulated by both chromosomal translocation and amplification in B-cell non-Hodgkin lymphoma. *Blood* 101:4539–4546.

Sander S, Bullinger L, Leupolt E, Benner A, Kienle D, Katzenberger T, et al. (2008): Genomic aberrations in mantle cell lymphoma detected by interphase fluorescence in situ hybridization. Incidence and clinicopathological correlations. *Haematologica* 93:680–687.

Santra M, Zhan F, Tian E, Barlogie B, Shaughnessy J Jr (2003): A subset of multiple myeloma harboring the t(4;14) (p16;q32) translocation lacks FGFR3 expression but maintains an IGH/MMSET fusion transcript. *Blood* 101:2374–2376.

Sarkozy C, Terré C, Jardin F, Radford I, Roche-Lestienne C, Penther D, et al. (2014): Complex karyotype in mantle cell lymphoma is a strong prognostic factor for the time to treatment and overall survival, independent of the MCL international prognostic index. *Genes Chromosomes Cancer* 53:106–116.

Satterwhite E, Sonoki T, Willis TG, Harder L, Nowak R, Arriola EL, et al. (2001): The BCL11 gene family: involvement of BCL11A in lymphoid malignancies. *Blood* 98:3413–3420.

Savage KJ, Monti S, Kutok JL, Cattoretti G, Neuberg D, et al. (2003): The molecular signature of mediastinal large B-cell lymphoma differs from that of other diffuse large B-cell lymphomas and shares features with classical Hodgkin lymphoma. *Blood* 102:3871–3879.

Savage KJ, Harris NL, Vose JM, Ullrich F, Jaffe ES, Connors JM, et al. (2008): ALK-negative anaplastic large-cell lymphoma (ALCL) is clinically and immunophenotypically different from both ALK-positive ALCL and peripheral T-cell lymphoma, not otherwise specified: report from the International Peripheral T-Cell Lymphoma Project. *Blood* 111:5496–5504.

Savage KJ, Johnson NA, Ben-Neriah S, Connors JM, Sehn LH, Farinha P, et al. (2009): MYC gene rearrangements are associated with a poor prognosis in diffuse large B-cell lymphoma patients treated with R-CHOP chemotherapy. *Blood* 114:3533–3537.

Sawyer JR, Lukacs JL, Munshi N, Desikan KR, Singhal S, Mehta J, et al. (1998): Identification of new nonrandom translocations in multiple myeloma with multicolor spectral karyotyping. *Blood* 92:4269–4278.

Sawyer JR, Lukacs JL, Thomas EL, Swanson CM, Goosen LS, Sammartino G, et al. (2001): Multicolour spectral karyotyping identifies new translocations and a recurring pathway for chromosome loss in multiple myeloma. *Br J Haematol* 112:167–174.

Scandurra M, Rossi D, Deambrogi C, Rancoita PM, Chigrinova E, Mian M, et al. (2010): Genomic profiling of Richter's syndrome: recurrent lesions and differences with de novo diffuse large B-cell lymphomas. *Hematol Oncol* 28:62–67.

Schaffner C, Stilgenbauer S, Rappold GA, Döhner H, Lichter P (1999): Somatic ATM mutations indicate a pathogenic role of ATM in B-cell chronic lymphocytic leukemia. *Blood* 94:748–753.

Schlegelberger B, Himmler A, Bartles H, Kuse R, Sterry W, Grote W (1994a): Recurrent chromosome abnormalities in peripheral T-cell lymphomas. *Cancer Genet Cytogenet* 78:15–22.

Schlegelberger B, Himmler A, Gödde E, Grote W, Feller AC, Lennert K (1994b): Cytogenetic findings in peripheral T-cell lymphomas as a basis for distinguishing low-grade and high-grade lymphomas. *Blood* 83:505–511.

Schlegelberger B, Weber-Matthiesen K, Himmler A, Bartels H, Sonnen R, Kuse R, et al. (1994c): Cytogenetic findings and results of combined immunophenotyping and karyotyping in Hodgkin's disease. *Leukemia* 8:72–80.

Schlegelberger B, Zhang Y, Weber-Matthiesen K, Grote W (1994d): Detection of aberrant clones in nearly all cases of angioimmunoblastic lymphadenopathy with dysproteinemia-type T-cell lymphoma by combined interphase and metaphase cytogenetics. *Blood* 84:2640–2648.

Schlegelberger B, Zwingers T, Hohenadel K, Henne-Bruns D, Schmitz N, Haferlach T, et al. (1996): Significance of cytogenetic findings for the clinical outcome in patients with T-cell lymphoma of angioimmunoblastic lymphadenopathy type. *J Clin Oncol* 14:593–599.

Schlegelberger B, Zwingers T, Harder L, Nowotny H, Siebert R, Vesely M, et al. (1999): Clinicopathogenetic significance of chromosomal abnormalities in patients with blastic peripheral B-cell lymphoma. *Blood* 94:3114–3120.

Schmidt J, Salaverria I, Haake A, Bonzheim I, Adam P, Montes-Moreno S, et al. (2014): Increasing genomic and epigenomic complexity in the clonal evolution from in situ to manifest t(14;18)-positive follicular lymphoma *Leukemia* 28:1103–1112.

Schmitz R, Renné C, Rosenquist R, Tinguely M, Distler V, Menestrina F, et al. (2005): Insights into the multistep transformation process of lymphomas: IgH-associated translocations and tumor suppressor gene mutations in clonally related composite Hodgkin's and non-Hodgkin's lymphomas. *Leukemia* 19:1452–1458.

Schmitz R, Hansmann ML, Bohle V, Martin-Subero JI, Hartmann S, Mechtersheimer G, et al. (2009): TNFAIP3 (A20) is a tumor suppressor gene in Hodgkin lymphoma and primary mediastinal B cell lymphoma. *J Exp Med* 206:981–989.

Schmitz R, Young RM, Ceribelli M, Jhavar S, Xiao W, Zhang M, et al. (2012): Burkitt lymphoma pathogenesis and therapeutic targets from structural and functional genomics. *Nature* 490:116–120.

Schneider B, Nagel S, Kaufmann M, Winkelmann S, Bode J, Drexler HG, et al. (2008): t(3;7)(q27;q32) fuses BCL6 to a non-coding region at FRA7H near miR-29. *Leukemia* 22:1262–1266.

Schop RF, Kuehl WM, VanWier SA, Ahmann GJ, Price-Troska T, Bailey RJ, et al. (2002): Waldenström macroglobulinemia neoplastic cells lack immunoglobulin heavy chain locus translocations but have frequent 6q deletions. *Blood* 100:2996–3001.

Schraders M, de Jong D, Kluin P, Groenen P, van Krieken H (2005): Lack of Bcl-2 expression in follicular lymphoma may be caused by mutations in the BCL2 gene or by absence of the t(14;18) translocation. *J Pathol* 205:329–335.

Schuh A, Becq J, Humphray S, Alexa A, Burns A, Clifford R, et al. (2012): Monitoring chronic lymphocytic leukemia progression by whole genome sequencing reveals heterogeneous clonal evolution patterns. *Blood* 120:4191–4196.

Schwaenen C, Wessendorf S, Kestler HA, Döhner H, Lichter P, Bentz M (2003): DNA microarray analysis in malignant lymphomas. *Ann Hematol* 82:323–332.

Schwaenen C, Nessling M, Wessendorf S, Salvi T, Wrobel G, Radlwimmer B, et al. (2004): Automated array-based genomic profiling in chronic lymphocytic leukemia: development of a clinical tool and discovery of recurrent genomic alterations. *Proc Natl Acad Sci USA* 101:1039–1044.

Schwaenen C, Viardot A, Berger H, Barth TF, Bentink S, Döhner H, et al. (2009): Microarray-based genomic profiling reveals novel genomic aberrations in follicular lymphoma which associate with patient survival and gene expression status. *Genes Chromosomes Cancer* 48:39–54.

Schwindt H, Akasaka T, Zühlke-Jenisch R, Hans V, Schaller C, Klapper W, et al. (2006): Chromosomal translocations fusing the BCL6 gene to different partner loci are recurrent in primary central nervous system lymphoma and may be associated with aberrant somatic hypermutation or defective class switch recombination. *J Neuropathol Exp Neurol* 5:776–782.

Schwindt H, Vater I, Kreuz M, Montesinos-Rongen M, Brunn A, Richter J, et al. (2009): Chromosomal imbalances and partial uniparental disomies in primary central nervous system lymphoma. *Leukemia* 23:1875–1884.

Segeren CM, Sonneveld P, van derHolt B, Vellenga E, Croockewit AJ, Verhoef GE, et al. (2003): Overall and event-free survival are not improved by the use of myeloablative therapy following intensified chemotherapy in previously untreated patients with multiple myeloma: a prospective randomized phase 3 study. *Blood* 101:2144–2151.

Seifert M, Scholtysik R, Küppers R (2013): Origin and pathogenesis of B cell lymphomas. *Methods Mol Biol* 971:1–25.

Sellmann L, Gesk S, Walter C, Ritgen M, Harder L, Martín-Subero JI, et al. (2007): Trisomy 19 is associated with trisomy 12 and mutated IGHV genes in B-chronic lymphocytic leukaemia. *Br J Haematol* 138:217–220.

Sen F, Lai R, Albitar M (2002): Chronic lymphocytic leukemia with t(14;18) and trisomy 12. *Arch Pathol Lab Med* 126:1543–1546.

Shaughnessy J, Tian E, Sawyer J, Bumm K, Landes R, Badros A, et al. (2000): High incidence of chromosome 13 deletion in multiple myeloma detected by multiprobe interphase FISH. *Blood* 96: 1505–1511.

Shaughnessy J Jr, Gabrea A, Qi Y, Brents L, Zhan F, Tian E, et al. (2001): Cyclin D3 at 6p21 is dysregulated by recurrent chromosomal translocations to immunoglobulin loci in multiple myeloma. *Blood* 98:217–223.

Shimanuki M, Sonoki T, Hosoi H, Watanuki J, Murata S, Kawakami K, et al. (2013): Molecular cloning of IGλ rearrangements using long-distance inverse PCR (LDI-PCR). *Eur J Haematol* 90:59–67.

Shin SY, Jang S, Park CJ, Chi HS, Lee KH, Huh J, et al. (2012): A rare case of Lennert's type peripheral T-cell lymphoma with t(14;19)(q11.2;q13.3). *Int J Lab Hematol* 34:328–332.

Shou Y, Martelli ML, Gabrea A, Qi Y, Brents LA, Roschke A, et al. (2000): Diverse karyotypic abnormalities of the c-myc locus associated with c-myc dysregulation and tumor progression in multiple myeloma. *Proc Natl Acad Sci USA* 97:228–233.

Shustik J, Han G, Farinha P, Johnson NA, Ben Neriah S, Connors JM, et al. (2010): Correlations between BCL6 rearrangements and outcome in patients with diffuse large B-cell lymphoma treated with CHOP or R-CHOP. *Haematologica* 95:96–101.

Siebert R, Rosenwald A, Staudt LM, Morris SW (2001): Molecular features of B-cell lymphoma. *Curr Opin Oncol* 13:316–324.

Siu LL, Wong KF, Chan JK, Kwong YL (1999): Comparative genomic hybridization analysis of natural killer cell lymphoma/leukemia. Recognition of consistent patterns of genetic alterations. *Am J Pathol* 155:1419–1425.

Smadja NV, Bastard C, Brigaudeau C, Leroux D, Fruchart C, Groupe Français de Cytogénétique Hématologique (2001): Hypodiploidy is a major prognostic factor in multiple myeloma. *Blood* 98:2229–2238.

Solé F, Salido M, Espinet B, Garcia JL, Martinez Climent JA, Granada I, et al. (2001): Splenic marginal zone B-cell lymphomas: two cytogenetic subtypes, one with gain of 3q and the other with loss of 7q. *Haematologica* 86:71–77.

Somja J, Bisig B, Bonnet C, Herens C, Siebert R, de Leval L (2014): Peripheral T-cell lymphoma with t(6;14)(p25;q11.2) translocation presenting with massive splenomegaly. *Virchows Arch* 464:735–741.

Sonoki T, Harder L, Horsman DE, Karran L, Taniguchi I, Willis TG, et al. (2001): Cyclin D3 is a target gene of t(6;14)(p21.1;q32.3) of mature B-cell malignancies. *Blood* 98:2837–2844.

Sonoki T, Willis TG, Oscier DG, Karran EL, Siebert R, Dyer MJ (2004): Rapid amplification of immunoglobulin heavy chain switch (IGHS) translocation breakpoints using long-distance inverse PCR. *Leukemia* 18:2026–2031.

Sonoki T, Tatetsu H, Nagasaki A, Hata H (2007): Molecular cloning of translocation breakpoint from der(8)t(3;8)(q27;q24) defines juxtaposition of downstream of C-MYC and upstream of BCL6. *Int J Hematol* 86:196–198.

Soulier J, Pierron G, Vecchione D, Garand R, Brizard F, Sigaux F, et al. (2001): A complex pattern of recurrent chromosomal losses and gains in T-cell prolymphocytic leukemia. *Genes Chromosomes Cancer* 31:248–254.

Stary S, Vinatzer U, Müllauer L, Raderer M, Birner P, Streubel B (2013): t(11;14)(q23;q32) involving IGH and DDX6 in nodal marginal zone lymphoma. *Genes Chromosomes Cancer* 52:33–43.

Steidl C, Telenius A, Shah SP, Farinha P, Barclay L, Boyle M, et al. (2010): Genome-wide copy number analysis of Hodgkin Reed-Sternberg cells identifies recurrent imbalances with correlations to treatment outcome. *Blood* 116:418–427.

Steidl C, Shah SP, Woolcock BW, Rui L, Kawahara M, Farinha P, et al. (2011): MHC class II transactivator CIITA is a recurrent gene fusion partner in lymphoid cancers. *Nature* 471:377–3781.

Steininger A, Möbs M, Ullmann R, Köchert K, Kreher S, Lamprecht B, et al. (2011): Genomic loss of the putative tumor suppressor gene E2A in human lymphoma. *J Exp Med* 208:1585–1593.

Stern MH, Soulier J, Rosenzwajg M, Nakahara K, Canki-Klain N, Aurias A, et al. (1993): MTCP-1: a novel gene on the human chromosome Xq28 translocated to the T cell receptor alpha/delta locus in mature T cell proliferations. *Oncogene* 8:2475–2483.

Stilgenbauer S, Döhner H, Bulgay-Mörschel M, Weitz S, Bentz M, Lichter P (1993): High frequency of monoallelic retinoblastoma gene deletion in B-cell chronic lymphoid leukemia shown by interphase cytogenetics. *Blood* 81: 2118–2124.

Stilgenbauer S, Leupolt E, Ohl S, Weiss G, Schröder M, Fischer K, et al. (1995): Heterogeneity of deletions involving RB-1 and the D13S25 locus in B-cell chronic lymphocytic leukemia revealed by fluorescence in situ hybridization. *Cancer Res* 55:3475–3477.

Stilgenbauer S, Liebisch P, James MR, Schröder M, Schlegelberger B, Fischer K, et al. (1996): Molecular cytogenetic delineation of a novel critical genomic region in chromosome bands 11q22.3–923.1 in lymphoproliferative disorders. *Proc Natl Acad Sci USA* 93:11837–11841 (Erratum in Proc Natl Acad Sci USA, 1996, 93:14992).

Stilgenbauer S, Schaffner C, Litterst A, Liebisch P, Gilad S, Bar-Shira A, et al. (1997): Biallelic mutations in the ATM gene in T-prolymphocytic leukemia. *Nat Med* 3:1155–1159.

Stilgenbauer S, Bullinger L, Benner A, Wildenberger K, Bentz M, Döhner K, et al. (1999): Incidence and clinical significance of 6q deletions in B cell chronic lymphocytic leukemia. *Leukemia* 13:1331–1334.

Stilgenbauer S, Lichter P, Döhner H (2000): Genetic features of B-cell chronic lymphocytic leukemia. *Rev Clin Exp Hematol* 4:48–72.

Stilgenbauer S, Sander S, Bullinger L, Benner A, Leupolt E, Winkler D, et al. (2007): Clonal evolution in chronic lymphocytic leukemia: acquisition of high-risk genomic aberrations associated with unmutated VH, resistance to therapy, and short survival. *Haematologica* 92:1242–1245.

Stockero KJ, Fink SR, Smoley SA, Paternoster SF, Shanafelt TD, Call TG, et al. (2006): Metaphase cells with normal G-bands have cryptic interstitial deletions in 13q14 detectable by fluorescence in situ hybridization in B-cell chronic lymphocytic leukemia. *Cancer Genet Cytogenet* 166:152–156.

Streubel B, Lamprecht A, Dierlamm J, Cerroni L, Stolte M, Ott G, et al. (2003): t(14;18)(q32;q21) involving IGH and MALT1 is a frequent chromosomal aberration in MALT lymphoma. *Blood* 101:2335–2339.

Streubel B, Chott A, Huber D, Exner M, Jäger U, Wagner O, et al. (2004a): Lymphoma-specific genetic aberrations in microvascular endothelial cells in B-cell lymphomas. *N Engl J Med* 351:250–259.

Streubel B, Simonitsch-Klupp I, Müllauer L, Lamprecht A, Huber D, Siebert R, et al. (2004b): Variable frequencies of MALT lymphoma-associated genetic aberrations in MALT lymphomas of different sites. *Leukemia* 18:1722–1726.

Streubel B, Vinatzer U, Lamprecht A, Raderer M, Chott A (2005): t(3;14)(p14.1;q32) involving IGH and FOXP1 is a novel recurrent chromosomal aberration in MALT lymphoma. *Leukemia* 19:652–658.

Streubel B, Scheucher B, Valencak J, Huber D, Petzelbauer P, Trautinger F, et al. (2006a): Molecular cytogenetic evidence of t(14;18)(IGH;BCL2) in a substantial proportion of primary cutaneous follicle center lymphomas. *Am J Surg Pathol* 30:529–536.

Streubel B, Vinatzer U, Willheim M, Raderer M, Chott A (2006b): Novel t(5;9)(q33;q22) fuses ITK to SYK in unspecified peripheral T-cell lymphoma. *Leukemia* 20:313–318.

Suguro M, Yoshida N, Umino A, Kato H, Tagawa H, Nakagawa M, et al. (2014): Clonal heterogeneity of lymphoid malignancies correlates with poor prognosis. *Cancer Sci* 105:897–904.

Swerdlow SH, Campo E, Harris NL, Jaffe ES, Pileri SA, Stein H, et al. (Eds.) (2008): *WHO Classification of Tumors of Haematopoietic and Lymphoid Tissues*. Lyon: IARC.

Szuhai K, van Doorn R, Tensen CP, Van Kester (2013): Array-CGH analysis of cutaneous anaplastic large cell lymphoma. Methods Mol Biol 197–212.

Szymanowska N, Klapper W, Gesk S, Küppers R, Martin-Subero JI, Siebert R (2008): BCL2 and BCL3 are recurrent translocation partners of the IGH locus. *Cancer Genet Cytogenet* 186:110–114.

Tagawa H, Karnan S, Suzuki R, Matsuo K, Zhang X, Ota A, et al. (2005a): Genome-wide array-based CGH for mantle cell lymphoma: identification of homozygous deletions of the proapoptotic gene BIM. *Oncogene* 24:1348–1358.

Tagawa H, Suguro M, Tsuzuki S, Matsuo K, Karnan S, Ohshima K, et al. (2005b): Comparison of genome profiles for identification of distinct subgroups of diffuse large B-cell lymphoma. *Blood* 106: 1770–1777 (Erratum in Blood, 2006, 107:3052).

Takeshita M, Nakamura S, Kikuma K, Nakayama Y, Nimura S, Yao T, et al. (2011): Pathological and immunohisto-chemical findings and genetic aberrations of intestinal enteropathy-associated T cell lymphoma in Japan. *Histopathology* 58:395–407.

Tam W, Gomez M, Chadburn A, Lee JW, Chan WC, Knowles DM (2006): Mutational analysis of PRDM1 indicates a tumor-suppressor role in diffuse large B-cell lymphomas. *Blood* 107:4090–4100.

Tanaka R, Satoh H, Moriyama M, Satoh K, Morishita Y, Yoshida S, et al. (2000): Intronic U50 small-nucleolar-RNA (snoRNA) host gene of no protein-coding potential is mapped at the chromosome breakpoint t(3;6) (q27;q15) of human B-cell lymphoma. *Genes Cells* 5:277–287.

Tarte K, DeVos J, Thykjaer T, Zhan F, Fiol G, Costes V, et al. (2002): Generation of polyclonal plasmablasts from peripheral blood B cells: a normal counterpart of malignant plasmablasts. *Blood* 100:1113–1122.

Taub R, Kirsch I, Morton C, Lenoir G, Swan D, Tronick S, et al. (1982): Translocation of the c-myc gene into the immunoglobulin heavy chain locus in human Burkitt lymphoma and murine plasmacytoma cells. *Proc Natl Acad Sci USA* 79:7837–7841.

Tellier J, Menard C, Roulland S, Martin N, Monvoisin C, Chasson L, et al. (2014): Human t(14;18)positive germinal center B cells: a new step in follicular lymphoma pathogenesis? *Blood* 123:3462–3465.

The International Non-Hodgkin's Lymphoma Prognostic Factors Project (1993): A predictive model for aggressive non-Hodgkin's lymphoma. *N Engl J Med* 329:987–994.

Thomadaki H, Scorilas A (2006): BCL2 family of apoptosis-related genes: functions and clinical implications in cancer. *Crit Rev Clin Lab Sci* 43:1–67.

Thorns C, Bastian B, Pinkel D, Roydasgupta R, Fridlyand J, Merz H, et al. (2007): Chromosomal aberrations in angio-immunoblastic T-cell lymphoma and peripheral T-cell lymphoma unspecified: a matrix-based CGH approach. *Genes Chromosomes Cancer* 46:37–44.

Tiacci E, Trifonov V, Schiavoni G, Holmes A, Kern W, Martelli MP, et al. (2011): BRAF mutations in hairy-cell leukemia. *N Engl J Med* 364:2305–2315.

Tian E, Sawyer JR, Heuck CJ, Zhang Q, van Rhee F, Barlogie B, et al. (2014): In multiple myeloma, 14q32 translocations are nonrandom chromosomal fusions driving high expression levels of the respective partner genes. *Genes Chromosomes Cancer* 53:549–557.

Tilly H, Bastard C, Halkin E, Lenormand B, Bizet M, Dauce JP, et al. (1988): Del(14)(q22) in diffuse B-cell lymphocytic lymphoma. *Am J Clin Pathol* 89:109–113.

Tilly H, Rossi A, Stamatoullas A, Lenormand B, Bigorgne C, Kunlin A, et al. (1994): Prognostic value of chromosomal abnormalities in follicular lymphoma. *Blood* 84:1043–1049.

Tinguely M, Thies S, Frigerio S, Reineke T, Korol D, Zimmermann DR (2014): IRF8 is associated with germinal center B-cell-like type of diffuse large B-cell lymphoma and exceptionally translocation t(14;16)(q32.33;q24.1). *Leuk Lymphoma* 55:136–142.

Tort F, Pinyol M, Pulford K, Roncador G, Hernandez L, Nayach I, et al. (2001): Molecular characterization of a new ALK translocation involving moesin (MSN-ALK) in anaplastic large cell lymphoma. *Lab Invest* 81:419–426.

Touriol C, Greenland C, Lamant L, Pulford K, Bernard F, Rousset T, et al. (2000): Further demonstration of the diversity of chromosomal changes involving 2p23 in ALK-positive lymphoma: 2 cases expressing ALK kinase fused to CLTCL (clathrin chain polypeptide-like). *Blood* 95:3204–3207.

Traverse-Glehen A, Bachy E, Baseggio L, Callet-Bauchu E, Gazzo S, Verney A, et al. (2013): Immunoarchitectural patterns in splenic marginal zone lymphoma: correlations with chromosomal aberrations, IGHV mutations, and survival. A study of 76 cases. *Histopathology* 62:876–893.

Travert M, Huang Y, de Leval L, Martin-Garcia N, Delfau-Larue MH, Berger F, et al. (2012): Molecular features of hepatosplenic T-cell lymphoma unravels potential novel therapeutic targets. *Blood* 119:5795–5806.

Treon SP, Xu L, Yang G, Zhou Y, Liu X, Cao Y, et al. (2012): MYD88 L265P somatic mutation in Waldenström's macroglobulinemia. *N Engl J Med* 367:826–833.

Tricot G, Barlogie B, Jagannath S, Bracy D, Mattox S, Vesole DH, et al. (1995): Poor prognosis in multiple myeloma is associated only with partial or complete deletions of chromosome 13 or abnormalities involving 11q and not with other karyotype abnormalities. *Blood* 86:4250–4256.

Troussard X, Mauvieux L, Radford-Weiss I, Rack K, Valensi F, et al. (1998): Genetic analysis of splenic lymphoma with villous lymphocytes: a Groupe Français d'Hématologie Cellulaire (GFHC) study. *Br J Haematol* 101:712–721.

Tschernitz S, Flossbach L, Bonengel M, Roth S, Rosenwald A, Geissinger E (2014): Alternative BRAF mutations in BRAF V600E-negative hairy cell leukemias. *Br J Haematol* 165:529–533.

Tsujimoto Y, Finger LR, Yunis J, Nowell PC, Croce CM (1984): Cloning of the chromosome breakpoint of neoplastic B cells with the t(14;18) chromosome translocation. *Science* 226:1097–1099.

Tsujimoto Y, Gorham J, Cossman J, Jaffe E, Croce CM (1985): The t(14;18) chromosome translocations involved in B-cell neoplasms result from mistakes in VDJ joining. *Science* 229:1390–1393.

Tsukasaki K, Krebs J, Nagai K, Tomonaga M, Koeffler HP, Bartram CR, et al. (2001): Comparative genomic hybridization analysis in adult T-cell leukemia/lymphoma: correlation with clinical course. *Blood* 97: 3875–3881.

Türkmen S, Binder A, Gerlach A, Niehage S, Theodora Melissari M, Inandiklioglu N, et al. (2014): High prevalence of immunoglobulin light chain gene aberrations as revealed by FISH in multiple myeloma and MGUS. *Genes Chromosomes Cancer* 53:650–656.

Twa DD, Chan FC, Ben-Neriah S, Woolcock BW, Mottok A, Tan KL, et al. (2014): Genomic rearrangements involving programmed death ligands are recurrent in primary mediastinal large B-cell lymphoma. *Blood* 123:2062–2065.

Tzankov A, Xu-Monette ZY, Gerhard M, Visco C, Dirnhofer S, Gisin N, et al. (2014): Rearrangements of MYC gene facilitate risk stratification in diffuse large B-cell lymphoma patients treated with rituximab-CHOP. *Mod Pathol* 27:958–971.

Ueda C, Akasaka T, Ohno H (2002a): Non-immunoglobulin/BCL6 gene fusion in diffuse large B-cell lymphoma: prognostic implications. *Leuk Lymphoma* 43:1375–1381.

Ueda C, Akasaka T, Kurata M, Maesako Y, Nishikori M, Ichinohasama R, et al. (2002b): The gene for interleukin-21 receptor is the partner of BCL6 in t(3;16)(q27;p11), which is recurrently observed in diffuse large B-cell lymphoma. *Oncogene* 21:368–376.

Vaandrager JW, Schuuring E, Philippo K, Kluin PM (2000): V(D)J recombinase-mediated transposition of the BCL2 gene to the IGH locus in follicular lymphoma. *Blood* 96:1947–1952.

Vaghefi P, Martin A, Prévot S, Charlotte F, Camilleri-Broët S, Barli E, et al. (2006): Genomic imbalances in AIDS-related lymphomas: relation with tumoral Epstein–Barr virus status. *AIDS* 20:2285–2291.

Velera A, Coloma L, Martinez A, de Jong D, Balagué O, Matheu G, et al. (2013): ALK-positive large B-cell lymphomas express a terminal B-cell differentiation program and activated STAT3 but lack MYC rearrangements. *Mod Pathol* 26:1329–1337.

Van Den Berghe H, Louwagie A, Broeckaert-Van Orshoven A, David G, Verwilghen R, Michaux JL, et al. (1979): Philadelphia chromosome in human multiple myeloma. *J Natl Cancer Inst* 63:11–16.

Van Den Neste E, Robin V, Francart J, Hagemeijer A, Stul M, Vandenberghe P, et al. (2007): Chromosomal transloca-tions independently predict treatment failure, treatment-free survival and overall survival in B-cell chronic lymphocytic leukemia patients treated with cladribine. *Leukemia* 21:1715–1722.

Van Dongen JJ, Langerak AW, Brüggemann M, Evans PA, Hummel M, Lavender FL, et al. (2003): Design and stan-dardization of PCR primers and protocols for detection of clonal immunoglobulin and T-cell receptor gene recombi-nations in suspect lymphoproliferations: report of the BIOMED-2 Concerted Action BMH4-CT98-3936. *Leukemia* 17:2257–2317.

Vaqué JP, Martínez N, Batlle-López A, Pérez C, Montes-Moreno S, Sánchez-Beato M, et al. (2014). B-cell lym-phoma mutations: improving diagnostics and enabling targeted therapies. *Haematologica* 99:222–231.

Vater I, Wagner F, Kreuz M, Berger H, Martin-Subero JI, Pott C, et al. (2009): GeneChip analyses point to novel patho-genetic mechanisms in mantle cell lymphoma. *Br J Haematol* 144:317–331.

van der Velden VHJ, Hoogeveen PG, de Ridder D, Schnindler-van der Struijk M, van Zelm MC, Sanders M, et al. (2014): B-cell prolymphocytic leukemia: a specific subgroup of mantle cell lymphoma. *Blood* 124:412–419.

Ventura RA, Martin-Subero JI, Jones M, McParland J, Gesk S, Mason DY, et al. (2006): FISH analysis for the detection of lymphoma-associated chromosomal abnormalities in rou-tine paraffin-embedded tissue. *J Mol Diagn* 8:141–151.

Vergier B, Belaud-Rotureau MA, Benassy MN, Beylot-Barry M, Dubus P, Delaunay M, et al (2004): Neoplastic cells do not carry bcl2-JH rearrangements detected in a subset of primary cutaneous follicle center B-cell lymphomas. *Am J Surg Pathol* 28:748–755.

Viardot A, Möller P, Högel J, Werner K, Mechtersheimer G, Ho AD, et al. (2002): Clinicopathologic correlations of genomic gains and losses in follicular lymphoma. *J Clin Oncol* 20:4523–4530.

Vieites B, Fraga M, Lopez-Presas E, Pintos E, Garcia-Rivero A, Forteza J (2005): Detection of t(14;18) translocation in a case of intravascular large B-cell lymphoma: a germinal centre cell origin in a subset of these lymphomas? *Histopathology* 46:466–468.

Villamor N, Conde L, Martínez-Trillos A, Cazorla M, Navarro A, Beà S, et al. (2013): NOTCH1 mutations iden-tify a genetic subgroup of chronic lymphocytic leukemia patients with high risk of transformation and poor out-come. *Leukemia* 27:1100–1106.

Vinatzer U, Gollinger M, Müllauer L, Raderer M, Chott A, Streubel B (2008): Mucosa-associated lymphoid tissue lymphoma: novel translocations including rearrange-ments of ODZ2, JMJD2C, and CNN3. *Clin Cancer Res* 14:6426–6431.

Virgilio L, Narducci MG, Isobe M, Billips LG, Cooper MD, Croce CM, et al. (1994): Identification of the TCL1 gene involved in T-cell malignancies. *Proc Natl Acad Sci USA* 91:12530–12534.

Visco C, Tzankov A, Xu-Monette ZY, Miranda RN, Tai YC, Li Y, et al. (2013): Patients with diffuse large B-cell lym-phoma of germinal center origin with BCL2 transloca-tions have poor outcome, irrespective of MYC status: a report from an International DLBCL rituximab-CHOP Consortium Program Study. *Haematologica* 98:255–263.

Walker BA, Wardell CP, Johnson DC, Kaiser MF, Begum DB, Dahir NB, et al. (2013a): Characterization of IGH locus breakpoints in multiple myeloma indicates a subset of translocations appear to occur in pregerminal center B-cells. *Blood* 121:3413–3419.

Walker BA, Wardell CP, Ross FM, Morgan GJ (2013b): Identification of a novel t(7;14) translocation in multiple myeloma resulting in overexpression of EGFR. *Genes Chromosomes Cancer* 52:817–822.

Walker BA, Wardell CP, Brioli A, Boyle E, Kaiser MF, Begum DB, et al (2014): Translocations at 8q24 juxtapose MYC with genes that harbor superenhancers resulting in over-expression and poor prognosis in myeloma patients. *Blood Cancer J* 4:e191.

Wang L, Lawrence MS, Wan Y, Stojanov P, Sougnez C, Stevenson K, et al. (2011): SF3B1 and other novel cancer genes in chronic lymphocytic leukemia. *N Engl J Med* 365:2497–2506.

Weber-Matthiesen K, Deerberg J, Poetsch M, Grote W, Schlegelberger B (1995): Numerical chromosome aberra-tions are present within the CD30⁺ Hodgkin and Reed–Sternberg cells in 100% of analyzed cases of Hodgkin's disease. *Blood* 86: 1464–1468.

Weisenburger DD, Gordon BG, Vose JM, Bast MA, Chan WC, Greiner TC, et al. (1996): Occurrence of the t(2;5)(p23;q35) in non-Hodgkin's lymphoma. *Blood* 87:3860–3868.

Weniger MA, Melzner I, Menz CK, Wegener S, Bucur AJ, Dorsch K, et al. (2006): Mutations of the tumor suppressor gene SOCS-1 in classical Hodgkin lymphoma are frequent and associated with nuclear phospho-STAT5 accumulation. *Oncogene* 25:2679–2684.

Wessendorf S, Barth TF, Viardot A, Mueller A, Kestler HA, Kohlhammer H, et al. (2007): Further delineation of chromo-somal consensus regions in primary mediastinal B-cell lym-phomas: an analysis of 37 tumor samples using high-resolution genomic profiling (array-CGH). *Leukemia* 21:2463–2469.

Willis TG, Dyer MJ (2000): The role of immunoglobulin translocations in the pathogenesis of B-cell malignancies. *Blood* 96:808–822.

Willis TG, Jadayel DM, Du MQ, Peng H, Perry AR, Abdul-Rauf M, et al. (1999): Bcl10 is involved in t(1;14)(p22;q32) of MALT B cell lymphoma and mutated in multiple tumor types. *Cell* 96:35–45.

Wilson KS, McKenna RW, Kroft SH, Dawson DB, Ansari Q, Schneider NR (2002): Primary effusion lymphomas exhibit complex and recurrent cytogenetic abnormalities. *Br J Haematol* 116:113–121.

Wlodarska I, Martin-Garcia N, Achten R, De Wolf-Peeters C, Pauwels P, Tulliez M, et al. (2002): Fluorescence in situ hybridization study of chromosome 7 aberrations in hepatosplenic T-cell lymphoma: isochromosome 7q as a common abnormality accumulating in forms with features of cytologic progression. *Genes Chromosomes Cancer* 33:243–251.

Wlodarska I, Nooyen P, Maes B, Martin-Subero JI, Siebert R, Pauwels P, et al. (2003): Frequent occurrence of BCL6 rearrangements in nodular lymphocyte predominance Hodgkin lymphoma but not in classical Hodgkin lymphoma. *Blood* 101:706–710.

Wlodarska I, Meeus P, Stul M, Thienpont L, Wouters E, Marcelis L, et al. (2004): Variant t(2;11)(p11;q13) associated with the IgK-CCND1 rearrangement is a recurrent translocation in leukemic small-cell B-non-Hodgkin lymphoma. *Leukemia* 18:1705–1710.

Wlodarska I, Veyt E, De Paepe P, Vandenberghe P, Nooijen P, Theate I, et al. (2005): FOXP1, a gene highly expressed in a subset of diffuse large B-cell lymphoma, is recurrently targeted by genomic aberrations. *Leukemia* 19:1299–1305.

Wlodarska I, Matthews C, Veyt E, Pospisilova H, Catherwood MA, Poulsen TS, et al. (2007): Telomeric IGH losses detectable by fluorescence in situ hybridization in chronic lymphocytic leukemia reflect somatic VH recombination events. *J Mol Diagn* 9:47–54.

Wlodarska I, Dierickx D, Vanhentenrijk V, Van Roosbroeck K, Pospísilová H, Minnei F, et al. (2008): Translocations targeting CCND2, CCND3 and MYCN do occur in t(11;14)-negative mantle cell lymphoma. *Blood* 111:5683–5690.

Woessmann W (2013): How to treat children and adolescents with relapsed non-Hodgkin lymphoma? *Hematol Oncol Suppl* 1:64–68.

Wolf S, Mertens D, Schaffner C, Korz C, Döhner H, Stilgenbauer S, et al. (2001): B-cell neoplasia associated gene with multiple splicing (BCMS): the candidate B-CLL gene on 13q14 comprises more than 560 kb covering all critical regions. *Hum Mol Genet* 10:1275–1285.

Wolff DJ, Bagg A, Cooley LD, Dewald GW, Hirsch BA, Jacky PB, et al. (2007): Guidance for fluorescence in situ hybridization testing in hematologic disorders. *J Mol Diagn* 9:134–143.

Wu KL, Beverloo B, Lokhorst HM, Segeren CM, van der Holt B, Steijaert MM, et al. (2007): Abnormalities of chromosome 1p/q are highly associated with chromosome 13/13q deletions and are an adverse prognostic factor for the outcome of high-dose chemotherapy in patients with multiple myeloma. *Br J Haematol* 136:615–623.

Xu WS, Liang RH, Srivastava G (2000): Identification and characterization of BCL6 translocation partner genes in primary gastric high-grade B-cell lymphoma: heat shock protein 89 alpha is a novel fusion partner gene of BCL6. *Genes Chromosomes Cancer* 27:69–75.

Xu L, Hunter ZR, Yang G, Zhou Y, Cao Y, Liu X, et al. (2013): MYD88 L265P in Waldenström macroglobulinemia, immunoglobulin M monoclonal gammopathy, and other B-cell lymphoproliferative disorders using conventional and quantitative allele-specific polymerase chain reaction. *Blood* 121:2051–2058.

Yan J, Nie K, Mathew S, Tam Y, Cheng S, Knowles DM, et al. (2014): Inactivation of BANK1 in a novel IGH-associated translocation t(4;14)(q24;q32) suggests a tumor suppressor role in B-cell lymphoma. *Blood Cancer J* 4:e215.

Yates LR, Campbell PJ (2012): Evolution of the cancer genome. *Nat Rev Genet* 13:795–806.

Ye BH, Lista F, Lo Coco F, Knowles DM, Offit K, Chaganti RS, et al. (1993a): Alterations of a zinc finger-encoding gene, BCL-6, in diffuse large-cell lymphoma. *Science* 262:747–750.

Ye BH, Rao PH, Chaganti RS, Dalla-Favera R (1993b): Cloning of bcl-6, the locus involved in chromosome translocations affecting band 3q27 in B-cell lymphoma. *Cancer Res* 53:2732–2735.

Ye H, Gong L, Liu H, Hamoudi RA, Shirali S, Ho L, et al. (2005): MALT lymphoma with t(14;18)(q32;q21)/IGH-MALT1 is characterized by strong cytoplasmic MALT1 and BCL10 expression. *J Pathol* 205:293–301.

Ye H, Gong L, Liu H, Ruskone-Fourmestraux A, deJong D, Pileri S, et al. (2006): Strong BCL10 nuclear expression identifies gastric MALT lymphomas that do not respond to *H. pylori* eradication. *Gut* 55:137–138.

Yoo HY, Sung MK, Lee SH, Kim S, Lee H, Park S, et al. (2014): A recurrent mutation in RHOA GTPase in angioimmunoblastic T cell lymphoma. *Nat Genet* 46:371–375.

Yoshida S, Kaneita Y, Aoki Y, Seto M, Mori S, Moriyama M (1999a): Identification of heterologous partner genes fused to the BCL6 gene in diffuse large B-cell lymphomas: 5′-RACE and LA-PCR analyses of biopsy samples. *Oncogene* 18:7994–7999.

Yoshida S, Nakazawa N, Iida S, Hayami Y, Sato S, Wakita A, et al. (1999b): Detection of MUM1/IRF4-IgH fusion in multiple myeloma. *Leukemia* 13:1812–1816.

Yunis JJ, Oken MM, Theologides A, Howe RB, Kaplan ME (1984): Recurrent chromosomal defects are found in most patients with non-Hodgkin's-lymphoma. *Cancer Genet Cytogenet* 13:17–28.

Zandecki M, Facon T, Preudhomme C, Vanrumbeke M, Vachee A, Quesnel B, et al. (1995): The retinoblastoma gene (RB-1) status in multiple myeloma: a report on 35 cases. *Leuk Lymphoma* 18:497–503.

Zandecki M, Laï JL, Facon T (1996): Multiple myeloma: almost all patients are cytogenetically abnormal. *Br J Haematol* 94:217–227.

Zani VJ, Asou N, Jadayel D, Heward JM, Shipley J, Nacheva E, et al. (1996): Molecular cloning of complex chromosomal translocation t(8;14;12)(q24.1;q32.3;q24.1) in a Burkitt lymphoma cell line defines a new gene (BCL7A) with homology to caldesmon. *Blood* 87:3124–3134.

Zech L, Haglund U, Nilsson K, Klein G (1976): Characteristic chromosomal abnormalities in biopsies and lymphoid-cell lines from patients with Burkitt and non-Burkitt lymphomas. *Int J Cancer* 17:47–56.

Zech L, Hammarström L, Smith CI (1983): Chromosomal aberrations in a case of T-cell CLL with concomitant IgA myeloma. *Int J Cancer* 32:431–435.

Zettl A, Ott G, Makulik A, Katzenberger T, Starostik P, Eichler T, et al. (2002): Chromosomal gains at 9q characterize enteropathy-type T-cell lymphoma. *Am J Pathol* 161:1635–1645.

Zettl A, Rüdiger T, Konrad MA, Chott A, Simonitsch-Klupp I, Sonnen R, et al. (2004): Genomic profiling of peripheral T-cell lymphoma, unspecified, and anaplastic large T-cell lymphoma delineates novel recurrent chromosomal alterations. *Am J Pathol* 164:1837–1848.

Zhan F, Hardin J, Kordsmeier B, Bumm K, Zheng M, Tian E, et al. (2002): Global gene expression profiling of multiple myeloma, monoclonal gammopathy of undetermined significance, and normal bone marrow plasma cells. *Blood* 99:1745–1757.

Zhang S, Zech L, Klein G (1982): High-resolution analysis of chromosome markers in Burkitt lymphoma cell lines. *Int J Cancer* 29:153–157.

Zhang Q, Siebert R, Yan M, Hinzmann B, Cui X, Xue L, et al. (1999): Inactivating mutations and overexpression of BCL10, a caspase recruitment domain-containing gene, in MALT lymphoma with t(1;14)(p22;q32). *Nat Genet* 22:63–68.

Zhang J, Grubor V, Love CL, Banerjee A, Richards KL, Mieczkowski PA, et al. (2013): Genetic heterogeneity of diffuse large B-cell lymphoma. *Proc Natl Acad Sci U S A* 110:1398–1403.

Zhou Y, Ye H, Martin-Subero JI, Hamoudi R, Lu YJ, Wang R, et al. (2006): Distinct comparative genomic hybridisation profiles in gastric mucosa-associated lymphoid tissue lymphomas with and without t(11;18)(q21;q21). *Br J Haematol* 133:35–42.

Zhou Y, Ye H, Martin-Subero JI, Gesk S, Hamoudi R, Lu YJ, et al. (2007): The pattern of genomic gains in salivary gland MALT lymphomas. *Haematologica* 92:921–927.

Zinkel S, Gross A, Yang E (2006): BCL2 family in DNA damage and cell cycle control. *Cell Death Differ* 13:1351–1359.

CHAPTER 12

Tumors of the upper aerodigestive tract

Susanne M. Gollin

Department of Human Genetics, University of Pittsburgh Graduate School of Public Health, University of Pittsburgh Cancer Institute, Pittsburgh, PA, USA

Upper aerodigestive tract cancer includes tumors of the head and neck (oral cavity, oropharynx, pharynx, hypopharynx, and larynx), nasal cavity, sinuses, nasopharynx, salivary glands, and esophagus. This chapter presents cytogenetic alterations in the major tumors from this region as well as their molecular correlates and prognostic implications. In light of these genetic alterations, prospects for personalized therapeutics are discussed.

Squamous cell carcinomas of the head and neck

Head and neck squamous cell carcinomas (HNSCC) are the most common tumors of the upper aerodigestive tract and rank as the seventh most common cancer worldwide. They are responsible for 9.2% of all cancer cases and 4.6% of all cancer deaths worldwide (Ferlay et al., 2013) and 3.6% of new cancers and 2% of cancer deaths annually in the USA (Siegel et al., 2014). If identified early, the prognosis of HNSCC is excellent. Although the relative 5-year survival rate from HNSCC has increased over the past 40 years, survival disparities remain between

Caucasians and African Americans (63% vs. 42%, respectively), partly due to late diagnosis in the latter group (Siegel et al., 2014).

HNSCC usually develop as a result of one of two environmental exposures: (i) chewing or smoking tobacco or using betel quid with or without alcohol consumption or (ii) human papilloma virus (HPV) infection (Leemans et al., 2011). From 1983 to 2002, the incidence of oral cancer has declined worldwide, consistent with decreased tobacco use, but oropharyngeal cancer (OPC) has increased dramatically in economically developed countries, primarily in men younger than 60 years of age, and likely as a result of HPV16 infection (Chaturvedi et al., 2013). At least 70% of OPCs in the USA are thought to be caused by HPV infection, compared to 16.3% in 1984–1989 and fewer than 10% today in less economically developed countries (Chaturvedi et al., 2013; Pytynia et al., 2014). Further, likely as a result of decreased smoking, the incidence of HPV-negative HNSCC in the USA declined by 50% from 1988 to 2004, while the incidence of HPV-positive HNSCC increased by 225% (Chung et al., 2014; Pytynia et al., 2014). The racial disparities in head and neck cancer survival may be attributed in part to a lower frequency of HPV-positive OPC in

Cancer Cytogenetics: Chromosomal and Molecular Genetic Aberrations of Tumor Cells, Fourth Edition.
Edited by Sverre Heim and Felix Mitelman.
© 2015 John Wiley & Sons, Ltd. Published 2015 by John Wiley & Sons, Ltd.

African Americans compared to Caucasians (Settle et al., 2009). The frequency of HPV-related tumors is expected to decrease significantly with widespread implementation of prophylactic vaccination of both males and females against the major oncogenic types of the virus.

HPV-infected HNSCC generally have fewer mutations and cytogenetic alterations than other HNSCC because the viral genetic activity is sufficient to block the activity of the critical *RB1* and *TP53* tumor suppressor pathways, resulting in cancer. Probably as a result of less chromosomal instability (CIN) in their tumors due to the presence of fewer mutations, patients with HPV-positive OPC have better disease-free and overall survival than those with HPV-negative tumors (Pytynia et al., 2014). Therefore, it is important to test HNSCC for HPV to fully integrate all prognostic factors. The recommended testing protocol for formalin-fixed, paraffin-embedded (FFPE) tissue specimens is to carry out immunostaining (IHC) for CDKN2A (p16), a surrogate marker for HPV infection, followed by the HPV DNA polymerase chain reaction (PCR) on positive cases (Leemans et al., 2011). The only concern about this protocol is that one of the most frequent findings in HNSCC is heterozygous or homozygous deletion of 9p21 including the *CDKN2A* and *CDKN2B* genes, as discussed in the following. As a consequence, CDKN2A IHC may be negative in spite of the presence of HPV16, giving a false-negative tumor test. The only solution is to carry out CDKN2A IHC plus HPV PCR.

Cytogenetic findings

Numerous cytogenetic analyses of HNSCC have been documented (Mitelman et al., 2014). In general, HNSCC have largely similar chromosomal alterations irrespective of their anatomic location, suggesting that they develop via common pathogenetic pathways (Järvinen et al., 2008).

Like other tumors, HNSCC develop as a result of dysregulation of multiple cancer-related genes, that is, oncogenes, tumor suppressor genes (TSG), and genome integrity or DNA damage response (DDR) genes. A genetic progression model for HNSCC was proposed (Califano et al., 1996; Forastiere et al., 2001) based on the concept that tumors develop and progress as a result of an orderly accumulation of chromosomal deletions (with concomitant TSG losses) and rearrangements and/or amplifications (with associated oncogene activations) that imbue a clonal population of cells with a proliferative advantage. A more recent multistep progression model of oral squamous cell carcinoma (OSCC) was based on analysis of genetic alterations by chromosomal comparative genomic hybridization (cCGH) in primary tumors and adjacent dysplastic lesions from the same biopsy specimen (Noutomi et al., 2006). The studies showed that gains of 3q26-qter, 5p15, 8q11–21, and 8q24.1-qter and loss of 18q22-qter are involved in the transition from mild to moderate dysplasia. Gains of 11q13, 14q, 17q11–22, and 20q and loss of 9p are involved in the transition from moderate to severe dysplasia. Losses of 3p14–21 and 5q12–22 are frequently seen together and were associated with progression from severe dysplasia to invasive cancer. Loss of 4p is linked to lymph node metastasis in patients with OSCC. Wreesmann et al. (2004) showed that several cytogenetic alterations identified by cCGH in nodal metastases are not present in the primary tumors, including gains of 10p11–12 and 11p and losses of 4q22–31, 9p13–24, and 14q. Genes that may be targeted by these imbalances are involved in cell adhesion and/or in the mitogen-activated protein kinase (MAPK) and phosphatidylinositol 3-kinase (PI3K) pathways.

Califano et al. (1996, 2000) and Braakhuis et al. (2004) proposed that these molecular genetic findings support "field cancerization." This concept, first put forward by Slaughter et al. (1953), involves the exposure of epithelial tissue to carcinogenic or cancer-promoting substances, such as cigarette smoke, alcohol, and/or viruses. Neoplasia occurs first where the exposure is maximal, but all exposed tissues have the opportunity to express the neoplastic phenotype. Multiple regions of premalignant change may coalesce to form a large lesion or multicentric foci. The genetic changes in HNSCC may be conceptualized as a series of evolutionary events that may have neutral, deleterious, or advantageous effects on the proliferation of a clone or clones of cells. Neutral or deleterious genetic changes may result in stagnation or cell death, whereas advantageous events may result in a proliferative advantage, an increase in recruitment of blood vessels to the developing tumor, and/or the ability to metastasize. The model of Braakhuis et al.

(2004) advanced this idea by suggesting that the initial genetic alteration occurs in a stem cell, forming first a patch and then an expanding field of cells with the original and subsequent genomic and/or chromosomal alterations. Then, clonal selection of one or more cells within this field of preneoplastic cells leads to the development of a carcinoma(s). Harper et al. (2007) was among the first to show that a small percentage of cultured HNSCC cells meet the criteria for cancer "stem cells," that is, they have the capacity for self-renewal, generate an amplification hierarchy, and produce cells that differentiate appropriately. Metastases may be derived from migrating stem cells from the original field or tumor, and second primaries may develop from newly deranged stem cells (Braakhuis et al., 2004).

Several different molecular subtypes have been proposed for HNSCC. Chung et al. (2004) proposed the first molecular classification scheme for HNSCC, dividing the disease into four categories based upon gene expression patterns. They showed that these subtypes had different recurrence-free and overall survival. Group 1 tumors had high TGFA, an activated EGFR pathway, and poor clinical outcome; group 2 had a strong mesenchymal cell signature, often having undergone epithelial to mesenchymal transition (EMT); group 3 were closest to normal epithelial cells; and group 4 showed an expression pattern similar to cells exposed to cigarette smoke. A more recent subtyping strategy by some of the same authors led to and validated a very similar molecular classification, with types 1 through 4 replaced with the expression subtypes basal, mesenchymal, atypical (often HPV+), and classical, respectively, based on biological characteristics of genes expressed at high levels in each subtype (Walter et al., 2013). Another scheme divided the tumors into three classes based first on HPV infection (positive or negative) status and then divided the HPV-negative tumors based on high or low levels of CIN (Leemans et al., 2011).

Cytogenetic abnormalities have been shown to be useful biomarkers for diagnosis, prognosis, and therapeutic response of malignancies and point to locations of specific genes where molecular disruptions have occurred. Karyotypes are usually prepared from short- or long-term HNSCC cell cultures, since mitoses are usually not observed after direct harvest of dissociated tumor biopsies. Critics may argue that cytogenetic analysis of cell cultures is inherently biased, since specific cell populations are selected for and evolve in culture. Tumors usually are characterized by tremendous CIN, and cultured cell lines are similar in this regard to the tumors from which they originate. Cell lines arise from the same tumor cells as in the tumor, but culturing selects those cells that grow best under our relatively primitive culture conditions. Worsham et al. (1999) and Martin et al. (2008) used fluorescence *in situ* hybridization (FISH) to show that the cytogenetic alterations in metaphases from long-term HNSCC cell cultures reflect aberrations present in interphase nuclei from either direct harvests of biopsies, touch preparations, or paraffin sections of the primary tumors from which they were derived. Reshmi et al. (2004) showed that the karyotypes of HNSCC cell lines are relatively stable over time. Mutations in cell lines reflect most of the mutations in human tumors (Li et al., 2014). These studies all argue in favor of the value of examining short- or long-term cultured HNSCC cells or cell lines, and most concerns over studies of authenticated cell lines should be put to rest. Cell lines represent the tumors from which they were derived and remain critically important preclinical research models for examination of response to therapies, among many other important research applications.

The karyotypes of HNSCC (reviewed by Gollin, 2001; Jin et al., 2006b; Martin et al., 2008) typically are complex, are usually near triploid, and contain multiple clonal numerical and structural chromosome abnormalities (Figure 12.1). There may be considerable cytogenetic variability among cells, reflecting heterogeneity due to clonal evolution within the original tumor, as shown by Worsham et al. (1999) and Martin et al. (2008). The cell-to-cell differences are due in part to cytoskeletal alterations, which result in chromosomal segregational defects and lead to karyotypic differences between daughter cells after mitosis, that is, CIN (Saunders et al., 2000; Gollin, 2005). These spindle defects may be the result of chromosomal aberrations. One example is the amplification and consequent overexpression of the *NUMA1* gene at 11q13, which results in multipolar spindles, leading to daughter cells

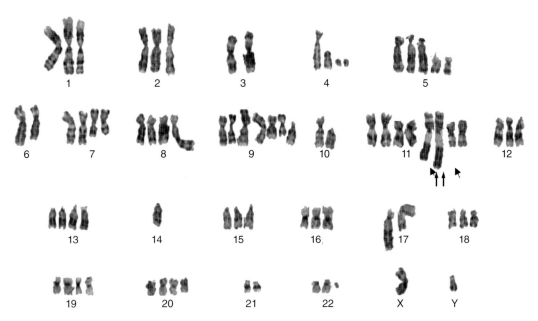

Figure 12.1 Representative trypsin–Giemsa-banded karyotype from a squamous cell carcinoma cell line (UPCI:SCC131, passage 18). In this cell, there are two relatively normal-appearing chromosomes 11 on the left and two very long derivative chromosomes 11, each with a homogeneously staining region (hsr) at 11q13 and nonchromosome 11-derived chromatin distal to the hsr, with a deletion of 11q14 to 11qter.

that differ from each other and their mother cell (Saunders et al., 2000; Huang et al., 2002; Quintyne et al., 2005).

Chromosomal gains and losses in HNSCC have been identified by classical karyotyping after trypsin–Giemsa banding (G-banding) as well as by molecular cytogenetic techniques. The findings by G-banding were refined in some cases using multicolor FISH (M-FISH) or spectral karyotyping (SKY). In addition, cCGH and/or array CGH (aCGH) has been utilized to clarify the copy numbers of chromosomal segments in cell lines and to determine the molecular karyotypes of tumors refractory to karyotyping because they were paraffin embedded or frozen or did not express sufficient metaphase cells. The frequency of chromosomal losses appears to exceed that of gains (Jin et al., 2006b; Martin et al., 2008). Although not discussed frequently in the literature, the most common karyotypic change in HNSCC is tetraploidization (Shackney et al., 1989). Frequently, HNSCC cell cultures express both near-diploid and near-tetraploid subclones (Martin et al., 2008). Tetraploidization in HNSCC occurs after 11q13 amplification as evidenced by the observation that

most cells with 11q13 amplification have four copies of chromosome 11, two of which contain homogeneously staining regions (hsr) and two of which appear to be normal (Martin et al., 2008). Tetraploidization can occur as a result of various cellular defects including dysfunctional TP53 (reviewed by Hayashi and Karlseder, 2013), but in tumor cells with 11q13 amplification, it most likely occurs during cytokinesis as a result of cleavage furrow regression after encountering a dicentric chromosome.

Structural chromosome alterations are common in HNSCC, including deletions, translocations, isochromosomes, and unidentified marker chromosomes. Duplications, insertions, inversions, ring chromosomes, dicentric chromosomes, and endoreduplicated chromosomes have also been reported, but less frequently than those listed previously. Evidence of gene amplification in the form of an hsr is often present (Albertson, 2006), whereas double minute (dmin) chromosomes are much less common. Although many investigators have attempted to identify the one gene "driving" gene amplification, multiple genes within an amplified segment (amplicon) are often overexpressed, suggesting that gain or amplification of chromosomal segments is often "driven" by more than one gene (Huang et al., 2006; Järvinen et al., 2008; Pickering et al., 2013). In spite of the numerous and diverse structural abnormalities, banding analyses of HNSCC have revealed several consistent chromosomal breakpoints, including bands 1p13 and 11q14 (Jin et al., 1990, 1998a, 1998b, 2006b; Åkervall et al., 1997). Structural chromosome rearrangements involving breakage and fusion of pericentromeric chromatin from both participating chromosomes are among the most frequently observed alterations, comprising 58% of breakpoints in OSCC that result in unbalanced whole-arm translocations (41%) and isochromosomes (17%), particularly for 3q, 5p, 7p, 8q, and 9q (Hermsen et al., 2005; Martínez et al., 2012). Formation of these isochromosomes results in loss of the other chromosome arm, contributing to the frequent observation of loss of chromosome arms 3p, 8p, and 9p in HNSCC (Gollin, 2001; Hermsen et al., 2005; Jin et al., 2006b; Martin et al., 2008; Freier et al., 2010a). Numerous other nonrandom chromosome abnormalities have been observed by classical cytogenetics (karyotyping) and molecular cytogenetic analysis by FISH, cCGH, and aCGH of multiple independent tumors from previously untreated patients. In describing primary cytogenetic abnormalities in human tumors or the correlates between chromosome alterations and tumor behavior, it is important to analyze only tumors from patients previously untreated by chemotherapy or radiation, because these modalities may lead to chromosome aberrations that may corrupt the results of the study. On the other hand, one can monitor karyotypic evolution in a tumor over time and identify the cytogenetic alterations that evolve during therapy or as a result of tumor progression and delineate prognostic markers that may change over time in a tumor or its local or distant metastases. These cytogenetic findings (whether identified by classical or molecular cytogenetic methods) may be useful in specifying prognosis, therapeutic response, or pointing to the most efficacious therapy.

The most frequent chromosomal gains in HNSCC are gains of 3q and 8q and the most frequent segmental loss is that of 3p (Tables 12.1 and 12.2). In many cases, these findings result from formation of an isochromosome for 3q and/or 8q,

resulting in duplication of the long arm and loss of the short arm. In contrast, the majority of extra copies of 3q observed in our HNSCC cell lines resulted from unbalanced translocations (Martin et al., 2008). Likewise, some cases of 3p loss appear to be due to breakage at 3p14.2, the site of the most common chromosomal fragile site, FRA3B, and the FHIT gene (reviewed in Karras et al., 2014). By classical cytogenetics, the next most common gains are of chromosome arms 5p, 7p, 9q, and 20q, again frequently as a result of isochromosome formation, along with concomitant losses of the short arms of chromosome 9 and the long arms of chromosomes 5 and 7.

Gene amplification, defined as five or more copies of a gene, genes, or chromosomal segment(s) on a near-diploid background or 10 or more copies on a near-tetraploid background, is common in HNSCC. Copy number gain and amplification are used synonymously and thus confused in the molecular cytogenomics and molecular genomics literature. Amplification is clearly synonymous with high-level gain, as used in this chapter, but certainly signifies more than one or two duplicated copies of a gene, genes, or chromosomal segment(s). Multiple genes in each amplified region have been examined to determine which one is the "driver" of this gain/amplification or the most important gene in the amplicon. It is the strong opinion of this author that there may not be only *one* driver gene per gained or amplified chromosomal segment, but more than one, since, in most cases, multiple genes are amplified and overexpressed. Pickering et al. (2013) appear to concur with this opinion. The multiple amplified genes may have complementary, combined, and/or synergistic oncogenic activity. As mentioned earlier, band 11q13 appears to be amplified (usually in the form of an hsr) in 26% or duplicated in almost half of all HNSCC (Gollin, 2001; Huang et al., 2002, 2006; Jin et al., 2006a). Huang et al. (2002) found 20–80 copies of genes in the 11q13 amplicon core using quantitative PCR. One mechanism for 11q13 amplification, suggested by Gibcus et al. (2007a), involves rearrangement of large, fragile, low-copy repeats (called segmental duplications) flanking the amplified region. We showed that amplification of 11q13 occurs by a slightly different mechanism, breakage–fusion–bridge (BFB) cycles (Reshmi et al., 2007b),

Table 12.1 Meta-analysis of chromosomal gains in HNSCC*

Chromosome segment	CC (%)	CGH<2008 (%)	TCGA gain (%)	TCGA amp. (%)	Genes of interest in or near peak region
1q25–44	21	27	–	–	
2q11.2	–	–	20	–	ANKRD39, SEMA4C, FAM178B
2q31.2	–	–	21	–	NFE2L2
3q11-qter (3q26.33)	25	67	72	21	PIK3CA*, SOX2-OT, SOX2, LINC01206, FLJ46066
5p14–15.3 (5p15.3)	16	48	45	–	TERT, NKD2
6p12.1	–	–	21	–	TINAG
6q22-qter	–	23	–	–	
7p11–22 (7p11.2)	28	29	42	10	EGFR, EGFR-AS1
7q21.2–21.3	18	32	32	–	CALCR
8p11.23	–	–	31	–	WHSC1L1, LETM2, FGFR1
8q11.21	–	–	60	–	CEBPD*, PRKDC*, MCM4*, SNAI2*
8q13–q24.3 (8q24.21)	29	50	74	14	POU5F1B*, MYC*, PVT1*
9p24.1	–	–	24	–	8:JAK2
9p13.3	–	–	26	–	11: RMRP, CA9, TLN1, CREB3
9q (9q34)	19	49	–	–	
11p13	–	–	20	–	EHF, APIP, CD44, SLC1A2
11q13	28	32	44	26	14: CCND1*, ORAOV1*, ANO1*, FADD*, PPFIA1, CTTN*
12p13.33	–	–	31	–	11: KDM5A, WNK1
12q15	–	–	20	–	14: MDM2, YEATS4, FRS2
13q22.1	–	–	20	–	KLF5*, KLF12*
17q11–22 (17q12)	10	25	17	–	ERBB2
18p (18p11.31)	–	24	30	–	LPIN2, MYOM1, MYL112A, MYL12B
18q11.2	–	–	20	–	TMEM241
20q12–13.2	33	48	44	–	ZNF341, CHMP4B

*By classical and molecular cytogenetic analysis, including FISH, oligonucleotide and SNP array CGH, and corresponding genes in the regions. FISH, fluorescence *in situ* hybridization; SNP, single-nucleotide polymorphism. Approximate percent frequency of HNSCC with the particular gain, amplification (amp.), or loss based on classical cytogenetic (CC) analysis or chromosomal or array CGH pre-2008 from Table 11.1 in Avramut and Gollin (2009) and from the 511 HNSCC in The Cancer Genome Atlas (TCGA) SNP array dataset analyzed by Beroukhim et al. (2010) and Mermel et al. (2011) who found 34 peak regions of gain or amplification and 54 peak regions of loss (major peaks listed) (HNSCC, www.broadinstitute/ TCGA; dataset, 2014-04-28 stddata__2014_04_16 [6 July 2014]). Frequencies less than 10% are not listed. Genes noted are those either listed in the website above or not listed but selected by the author (marked*), and if the number of genes in the peak is too high, that number is noted and selected (by author) genes in the region are listed.

the first step of which involves distal 11q loss (11q14-qter), shown by FISH studies in as many as 70% and by aCGH in almost half of HNSCC, thus revealing one of the most common regions of loss in these tumors (Parikh et al., 2007). Other sites of chromosomal amplification include chromosomal bands 3q26.3, 7p11.2, and 8q24.2 according to the author's analysis of The Cancer Genome Atlas (TCGA) HNSCC data (Beroukhim et al., 2010; Mermel et al., 2011).

The most frequent chromosomal losses appear to involve either common chromosomal fragile sites (*FRA3B* at 3p14 and *FRA11F* at 11q14.3) or breakage and rearrangement of centromeres

Table 12.2 Meta-analysis of chromosomal losses in HNSCC*

Chromosome segment	CC (%)	CGH < 2008 (%)	Loss (%)	Genes of interest in or near peak region
1p12–13.2	–	–	25	150:BCL2L15, HIPK1
2q	25	31		
(2q22.1–22.2)			22	LRP1B
(2q35–37.3)			30	206: TWIST2, DOCK10
3p12–25	49	60		
(3p14.3)			71	LINC01212; FHIT*
(3p13)			70	GBE1
(3p12.1)			65	ESRG, LRTM1
4q21–31	29	46		
(4q22.1)			32	CCSER1
4q35.2	–	–	40	FAT1
5q12–23	21	62		
(5q12.1)			41	PDE4B
6q	26	31	–	
7q22-qter	26	22		
(7q36.1)			25	8:KMT2C, XRCC2, ACTR3B
8p23.2	51	47	58	CSMD1
9p21.3–24	30	60		
(9p23–24.1)			46	PTPRD
(9p21.3)			59	MTAP, CDKN2A, CDKN2B
10p11.21–11.22	–	–	30	PARD3, PARD3-AS1
10q22–26	25	30		
(10q23)			26	KLLN, PTEN
11p15.4–15.5	–	–	31	158
11q14-qter	27	30		
(11q14.1)			32	4: TENM4
(11q14.2)			36	4: PICALM, EED
(11q22.3–23.3)			47	64: SDHD, H2AFX*, ATM*
13q12–34	28	53		
(13q12.11)			44	33: SKA3
(13q14.2)			41	RB1
14q	25	14	–	
17p	23	–	–	
18q	41	59		
(18q23)			55	19: ZNF236, GALR1, CTDP1, PARD6G
19p13.3	–	–	32	9: STK11, POLR2E
21q11.2–21	37	69	–	
21q22.3	–	–	38	PCBP3
22	31	20	–	
Xp	59	29	–	
Xq21.33	–	–	15	RPA4

*By classical and molecular cytogenetic analysis, including FISH, oligonucleotide and SNP array CGH, and corresponding genes in the regions. FISH, fluorescence *in situ* hybridization; SNP, single-nucleotide polymorphism. Approximate percent frequency of HNSCC with the particular gain, amplification (amp.), or loss based on classical cytogenetic (CC) analysis or chromosomal or array CGH pre-2008 from Table 11.1 in Avramut and Gollin (2009) and from the 511 HNSCC in The Cancer Genome Atlas (TCGA) SNP array dataset analyzed by Beroukhim et al. (2010) and Mermel et al. (2011) who found 34 peak regions of gain or amplification and 54 peak regions of loss (major peaks listed) (HNSCC, www.broadinstitute/ TCGA; dataset, 2014-04-28 stddata__2014_04_16 [6 July 2014]). Frequencies less than 10% are not listed. Genes noted are those either listed in the website above or not listed but selected by the author (marked*), and if the number of genes in the peak is too high, that number is noted and selected (by author) genes in the region are listed.

resulting in isochromosome formation and loss of 3p, 5q, 8p, and 9p. Additional relatively frequent losses involve the long arms of the acrocentric chromosomes 13 and 21 and the long arms of chromosomes 4 and 18. Van Dyke et al. (1994) observed that the Y chromosome is lost frequently in males as is the inactive X chromosome, particularly Xp, in females, although these were not noted to be frequent findings in the TCGA data. Of interest is the observation that several of the genetic changes (17p13 loss, 14q24 loss, and 6p loss) discovered by molecular genetic methods and noted to be important in the progression of HNSCC were not observed at a high frequency by classical or molecular (CGH) cytogenetic methods. One plausible explanation for this discrepancy is that the molecular deletions may be smaller than the level of resolution of cytogenetic methods or that aCGH probes did not cover the region and, thus, they were not detectable.

In summary, the most frequent cytogenetic alterations in HNSCC are gains of 5p14–15, 8q11–12, and 20q12–13; gains or amplifications of 3q26, 7p11, 8q24, and 11q13; and losses of 3p, 4q35, 5q12, 8p23, 9p21–24, 11q14–23, 13q12–14, 18q23, and 21q22. The chromosomal findings often provide an explanation for the molecular genetic alterations. For example, allelic imbalance at the *CCND1* locus in 11q13 could be mistaken as loss of heterozygosity (LOH) when it is actually FISH analysis-confirmed gene amplification (Califano et al., 1996). Genetic analysis revealed that most instances of 11q13 amplification occur by BFB cycles (Reshmi et al., 2007b) and/or duplicon-mediated rearrangement (Gibcus et al., 2007a). As discussed earlier, cytogenetic observations also suggest that, in many cases, the coordinate gains and losses involving arms of chromosomes 3, 5, 7, and 8 occur as a consequence of isochromosome formation. These results demonstrate that classical and molecular cytogenetic analyses continue to be valuable tools for placing molecular genetic findings in perspective at the cellular level.

Molecular genetic correlates of the key cytogenetic findings in HNSCC and their prognostic significance

Although few classical cytogenetic analyses have been reported on head and neck tumors since the previous edition of this book, several aCGH analyses, some of which are correlated with concurrent gene expression analyses, and multiple next-generation sequencing analyses have been published. It is impossible to discuss all the results of each individual study in this chapter or even cite all that might have merited citation. A number of correlated cytogenetic–molecular genetic studies have been reported that could not be readily placed into the categories of individual chromosome segments discussed in the following. One is that of Snijders et al. (2005) who reported that *TP53* mutation is positively correlated with amplification of *CCND1* and *EGFR*. Indeed, it has become clear that TP53 plays a critical role in the DDR and chromosomal stability. Mutations in *TP53* are common, seen in at least half of HNSCC, and methylation or other mechanisms for downregulating expression of the gene or its protein are present in the vast majority of HNSCC. It follows that CIN, which arises as a result of disruptions in multiple cellular pathways, is one of the most dramatic and prevalent findings in HNSCC (Gollin, 2005; García Martínez et al., 2014).

3q gain

Gain of the long arm of chromosome 3 appears to be one of the most frequent genetic alterations in HNSCC, with the smallest region of gain corresponding to band 3q26 according to the TCGA results and 3q28 according to Pickering et al. (2013) (Table 12.1). 3q gains have been reported in 72% of HNSCC, and amplification is reported in 21% of HNSCC by TCGA SNP arrays (Beroukhim et al., 2010). Gains of 3q25–29 are associated with shortened disease-specific survival (Sticht et al., 2005). Although *TP63*, *CCNL1*, *DCUN1D1*, *SOX2*, and *PIK3CA* are all gained in HNSCC and each could contribute to oncogenesis and/or cancer progression individually, matrix CGH data showed that *PIK3CA* undergoes copy number increase most frequently (Freier et al., 2007). *PIK3CA* is an oncogene that maps to 3q26.3 and codes for the catalytic subunit of PI3K, a protein complex activated by growth factor tyrosine kinases. The gene product stimulates AKT signaling, allowing growth factor-independent growth, cell invasion, and metastasis (Samuels and Ericson, 2006). *PIK3CA* has been considered to be involved in early HNSCC because amplification of this gene was observed in precancerous oral dysplasia (Redon et al., 2002). Kaplan-Meier analysis of results from analysis of 115 HNSCC showed that *PIK3CA* copy number amplification ($n = 37$, 32%) was associated with cancer relapse and a poor prognosis in patients without lymph node metastasis (log-rank test, $p = 0.026$) (Suda et al., 2012). *DCUN1D1* also maps to 3q26.3 and is amplified and overexpressed in HNSCC, and alterations correlate with poor clinical outcome (Sarkaria et al., 2006). Singh and colleagues showed that *DCUN1D1* has oncogenic activity, at least part of which results from activation of the hedgehog-signaling pathway (Sarkaria et al., 2006). Chen et al. (2014) validated *DCUN1D1* as a "driver" gene that codes for an E3 ubiquitin ligase complex subunit required for neddylation. *DCUN1D1* knockdown by RNA interference and antisense (Sarkaria et al., 2006) and shRNA (Chen et al., 2014) resulted in apoptosis. Cyclin L1 (*CCNL1*, 3q25.32) is thought to be involved as an immediate-early gene after growth factor signaling, in pre-mRNA processing, and in G0 to G1 cell cycle signaling and is localized to nuclear speckles (Sticht et al., 2005). *CCNL1* has been shown to be amplified and overexpressed in tumors compared to corresponding normal tissues (Redon et al., 2002; Muller et al., 2006), features that are associated with lymph node metastases independent of anatomic site and T-stage and also with more advanced clinical stage (Sticht et al., 2005; Muller et al., 2006). High-level *CCNL1* amplification is associated with shorter overall survival in HNSCC from all sites except the pharynx (Sticht et al., 2005; Muller et al., 2006). Additional candidate genes at 3q25–27 that are amplified and overexpressed in HNSCC include *TIPARP*, *TERC*, *EIF4G1*, and *DVL3* (reviewed by Wreesmann and Singh, 2005). The *ATR* gene at 3q23 codes for a member of the phosphatidylinositol 3′-kinase-like kinase (PIKK) family and is closely related to ATM, encoded by the gene mutated in ataxia telangiectasia (AT) (see section "11q loss"). ATR and ATM are at the apex of the DDR. ATR activates checkpoint signaling after genotoxic stresses, including ionizing radiation (IR), ultraviolet (UV) light, and DNA replication fork stalling. ATR phosphorylates BRCA1, CHEK1, MCM2, RAD17, RPA2, SMC1, and TP53, which leads to checkpoint activation, arrests DNA replication and mitosis, and promotes DNA repair,

recombination, and apoptosis (Pruitt et al., 2014). Aberrant overexpression of ATR in HNSCC results in CIN through an aberrant DDR, leads to therapeutic resistance, and is likely to result in tumor progression (Smith et al., 1998; Gollin, 2005; Parikh et al., 2007, 2014; Sankunny et al., 2014). An integrated copy number–gene expression microarray analysis of laryngeal SCC by Järvinen et al. (2006) showed overexpression of additional genes associated with 3q gain including *RAB6B* at 3q22, *PDC10* and *GPCR1* at 3q26, *MCCC1* and *LAMP3* at 3q27, and *TRFC* at 3q29. Snijders et al. (2005) reported amplification of *TM4SF1* at 3q24–25 in OSCC. Yet, none of these genes reside in the statistically relevant peak of gain according to TCGA, only *SOX2-OT*, *SOX2* (3q26.33), *LINC01206*, and *FLJ46066*. Freier et al. (2010b) first reported *SOX2* copy number gain by cCGH and mRNA overexpression by qRT-PCR in OSCC and confirmed this gain in 52% (115/223) of OSCC in tissue microarrays by *SOX2* FISH. Of interest, *SOX2*, when combined with three other transcription factors, *POU5F1*, *MYC*, and *KLF4*, is sufficient to reprogram differentiated cells into induced pluripotent stem (iPS) cells (Takahashi and Yamanaka, 2006). Recent examination of 3q gain/amplification in SCC of the lung and esophagus revealed that in these tumors, SOX2 preferentially binds to the transcription factor TP63 (in 3q28), rather than its preferred binding factor in embryonic stem cells, OCT4 (Watanabe et al., 2014). This may maintain a more immature or less differentiated precursor population of tumor cells with gain or amplification of distal 3q. Further, *SOX2* expression is upregulated in a subpopulation of suspected HNSCC stem cells with characteristics of EMT associated with metastasis (Lechner et al., 2013). TP63, coded for by the *TP63* gene, is a *TP53* homolog that plays a role in maintaining epithelial progenitor/stem cell populations as mentioned earlier; it shows copy number gains and is overexpressed in HNSCC (Sticht et al., 2005) correlating with a worse survival rate in OSCC patients (Lo Muzio et al., 2007). The correlation between copy number gains and overexpression of multiple genes on distal 3q, tumor progression, and an aggressive clinical course in HNSCC suggests that multiple genes may be involved and that one or more of these genes/proteins, their interactions, or the biochemical pathways in which they participate may be targets for therapeutic intervention.

7p gain

Copy number gains of 7p12–22 have been observed in nearly 30% of HNSCC cell lines by classical cytogenetics and cCGH (Table 12.1; Gollin, 2001; Martin et al., 2008) and 42% of TCGA HNSCC by SNP aCGH, and *EGFR* at 7p12 is high level amplified in 10% of TCGA HNSCC. The EGFR pathway is one of the most intensively studied biochemical pathways in HNSCC. The epidermal growth factor receptor (EGFR) is a transmembrane glycoprotein that includes an intracellular tyrosine kinase domain. EGFR signaling is initiated by ligand binding to the extracellular ligand-binding domain, leading to receptor homo-/heterodimerization and autophosphorylation by the intracellular kinase domain, resulting in receptor activation. Following activation, EGFR phosphorylates its cytoplasmic substrates, and the resultant signaling cascade drives multiple cellular responses, including altered gene expression, cytoskeletal restructuring, an antiapoptotic response, and cell proliferation (Pruitt et al., 2014). *EGFR* is overexpressed in as many as 90% of HNSCC (Kalyankrishna and Grandis, 2006). Overexpression of *EGFR* in HNSCC contributes to an aggressive and treatment-resistant phenotype with a poor prognosis and arises as a result of several different mechanisms. A frequent cause is increased *EGFR* gene copy number, including some cases of gene amplification and others of polysomy 7. Additional causes include increased mRNA synthesis, decreased downregulation, and expression of EGFRvIII, a constitutively active truncated form of the protein seen in almost half of HNSCC. EGFR plays key roles in HNSCC growth, survival, invasion, metastasis, and angiogenesis (Kalyankrishna and Grandis, 2006). FISH analysis of *EGFR* copy number showed that 58% of HNSCC with high polysomy and/or gene amplification had a statistically significant shorter progression-free and overall survival (Chung et al., 2006). Although EGFR-targeted therapies are useful in some patients with overexpression, response rates are low (Rabinowits and Haddad, 2012; Young et al., 2013).

8p gain

Although 8p11.2 is gained in about 31% of HNSCC and amplified in 8% (Table 12.1), the *WHSC1L1* gene topped the list of cancer-amplified genes with high copy number versus expression correlation or cancer "driver" genes according to Chen et al. (2014). *WHSC1L1* codes for a histone methyltransferase (NSD3) that preferentially methylates "Lys-4," a specific tag for epigenetic transcriptional activation, and "Lys-27" of histone H3, a mark for transcriptional repression (Pruitt et al., 2014). Chen et al. (2014) reported that knockdown by siRNA led to reduced cell proliferation and increased apoptosis in amplified cell lines. They suggested that the structural similarity between NSD1, NSD2, and NSD3 should be used for structure-based drug design to develop a new class of histone methyltransferase inhibitors.

8q gain

Gain of 8q, involving bands 8q23.1–24.22, is among the most frequent (74%) copy number alterations in HNSCC, and 8q24.2 is amplified in about 14% of HNSCC according to TCGA (Table 12.1). Further, 8q gain is an early change seen in high-grade oral dysplasia (Salahshourifar et al., 2014). 8q gain was reported in 47% of HNSCC and cell lines by cCGH (Squire et al., 2002). Agochiya et al. (1999) used FISH to show *MYC* and *PTK2* (8q24) copy number gain or amplification in several primary tumor types, including HNSCC. FISH confirmed the cytogenetic results of a number of groups cited in this chapter by showing that the 8q copy number increase is frequently due to isochromosome formation. Further, Agochiya et al. (1999) observed that increased *PTK2* gene dosage is associated with increased gene expression in most cell lines, although coordinate increase in MYC protein expression was not always present. These investigators therefore suggested that the *PTK2* gene, which plays an important role in adhesion and growth-regulatory signal transduction, might provide selection pressure for maintaining increased gene dosage at distal 8q. Järvinen et al. (2006) identified three additional genes at 8q24 both gained and overexpressed in laryngeal SCC, namely, *SLA*, *WISP1*, and *NDRG1*. Another gene of interest is the *OCT4* pseudogene, *POU5F1B*, which is amplified and overexpressed in gastric cancer and associated with a poor prognosis (Hayashi et al., 2014). Further studies are necessary to clarify the role of 8q gain in HNSCC and to determine whether targeting any of the overexpressed proteins may constitute the backbone of effective therapies.

11q13 amplification

Band 11q13 harbors an amplicon core of 13–14 genes amplified in the form of an hsr in 30–50% of HNSCC by FISH and 26% by TCGA SNP aCGH; it is gained in 42% of TCGA HNSCC and to a lesser degree in a number of other cancers (Table 12.1). This amplification is best visualized with FISH. Izzo et al. (1998) found 11q13 amplification to be an early change in HNSCC, and Noutomi et al. (2006) and Salahshourifar et al. (2014) concluded that it plays a role in the transition from moderate to severe dysplasia. We showed in OSCC cell lines that 11q13 amplification occurs as a result of BFB cycles initiated by a break at the common chromosomal fragile site FRA11F (Shuster et al., 2000; Reshmi et al., 2007a, 2007b), consistent with other studies that demonstrated that gene amplification results from breakage at chromosomal fragile sites (Ciullo et al., 2002; Hellman et al., 2002). Common fragile sites are thought to lead to replication fork stall or collapse, cell cycle checkpoint induction, and DNA repair (Durkin and Glover, 2007). In OSCC, defects in the DDR as a result of genetic loss distal to the 11q13 amplicon and double-strand breakage at FRA11F as a result of replication fork collapse may prompt aberrant DNA repair to occur through sister chromatid fusion, leading to CIN through BFB cycles (Shuster et al., 2000; Reshmi et al., 2007a, 2007b). Alternatively, Gibcus et al. (2007a) proposed that these 11q13 fragile sites are not involved in the breakage necessary for 11q13 amplification, but that the presence of both syntenic transitions and segmental duplications determines the pattern of amplification according to the model proposed by Narayanan et al. (2006).

The core of the 11q13 amplicon contains 13–14 genes (Huang et al., 2002, 2006; Jin et al., 2006a), including CCND1, CTTN, FGF3, FGF4, FADD, ORAOV1, and ANO1. All but three or four of the amplified genes in the amplicon core are overexpressed both in HNSCC tumors and cell lines (Huang et al., 2006; Gibcus et al., 2007b). In

addition, rapid disease recurrence and poor survival in cases with lymph node involvement correlated with cyclin D1 protein overexpression (Jares et al., 1994; Michalides et al., 1995, 1997; Fracchiolla et al., 1997). Freier et al. (2006) noted that several cytoskeleton-associated genes are coamplified at 11q13, a point also discussed by Huang et al. (2006), suggesting that these genes may play a role in motility and invasiveness. CCND1 has been considered to be the most important oncogenic driver in the amplicon given its role in promoting the G1/S transition. At one time, all other genes were ignored. We identified two genes in the amplicon, which we named TAOS1 and TAOS2 (tumor amplified and overexpressed sequence; Huang et al., 2002, 2006); they have since been renamed, ORAOV1 (oral cancer overexpressed) and TMEM16A (transmembrane protein 16a) and now ANO1 (anoctamin 1), respectively. ORAOV1 maps adjacent to CCND1. Silencing of ORAOV1 in HeLa cells inhibits cell growth and colony formation and results in apoptosis. ORAOV1 is conserved evolutionarily across eukaryotes, including baker's yeast, Saccharomyces cerevisiae, where the ortholog of ORAOV1 is an essential yeast gene (Lto1) found recently to be essential for both maturation of the 60S ribosomal subunit and initiation of translation under aerobic conditions, but is not required when cells are maintained anaerobically (Zhai et al., 2014). These authors proposed that Lto1 may be able to mitigate against ROS-induced ribosomal damage, explaining why overexpression of ORAOV1 is selected for in solid tumors (Zhai et al., 2014). This hypothesis becomes somewhat more plausible in light of a recently published study showing that ORAOV1 binds to pyrroline-5-carboxylate reductase (PYCR), an enzyme that catalyzes the last step in proline biosynthesis and plays a role in the cellular response to oxidative stress (Togashi et al., 2014). ANO1 codes for a calcium-dependent chloride channel (CaCC) that plays a role in transepithelial anion and fluid transport. ANO1 protein expression is an independent marker of adverse prognosis in HNSCC patients (Ruiz et al., 2012). The exact role of ANO1 in the "grow" or "go" process of tumor growth or metastasis appears to be controversial. Whether the protein mediates EMT and metastasis when under conditions of decreased expression by stable RNA knockdown or gene promoter methylation and growth when overexpressed as Duvvuri et al. (2012) and Shiwarski et al. (2014) indicate or whether high levels stimulate migration rather than cell proliferation as Ayoub et al. (2010) suggest is still not clear. Cortactin overexpression by immunohistochemistry correlated with lymph node metastasis (Rothschild et al., 2006). These investigators also used RNA interference to show that downregulation of *CTTN* in amplified cells impairs cell motility and invasion. Gibcus et al. (2007b) showed that *FADD* is amplified and overexpressed in laryngeal carcinomas, and they proposed that tumors with high levels of Ser[194]-phosphorylated FADD may respond to Taxol-based combined chemotherapy and radiotherapy. Rothschild et al. (2006) and Timpson et al. (2007) found that HNSCC that overexpress cortactin (*CTTN*) are resistant to the EGFR kinase inhibitor gefitinib and suggested *CTTN* as a possible marker of prognosis, disease progression, and therapeutic responsiveness, especially to EGFR-directed agents. They indicated that this might be related to the modest therapeutic success of this targeted inhibitor in HNSCC.

We proposed that 11q13 amplification is driven by a cassette of genes that provide growth or metastatic advantage to cancer cells. Martin et al. (2008) showed in our series of OSCC cell lines that all of those with 11q13 amplification also showed distal 11q loss. Statistical analyses revealed that amplification of 11q13, identified by the presence of an hsr, and concomitant distal 11q loss were statistically associated with tumor site ($p = 0.0095$). Amplification of 11q13 with distal 11q loss was found to occur more frequently in tumors of the tongue, retromolar trigone, and buccal mucosa. In the 11 OSCC cell lines examined by cCGH, the most significant finding was the correlation of 11q13 amplification/distal 11q loss (11q22-qter) with decreased patient survival ($p = 0.015$). All patients whose tumors lacked 11q13 amplification/distal 11q loss (6/11) survived, compared to only one of five patients whose tumors had 11q13 amplification and distal 11q loss. This observation further validates the use of 11q13 amplification/distal 11q loss as a biomarker for patient prognosis, as has previously been reported by several groups, but does not rule out the possibility that distal 11q loss alone may be associated with a poor prognosis, as these two chromosomal regions could not be ana-

lyzed separately in this set of tumor cell lines. Distal 11q loss is discussed later in this chapter.

20q gain

Amplification of 20q13 in HNSCC is rare, although 20q gain is fairly common. We observed 20q gain in more than half of our OSCC cell lines examined by cCGH (Martin et al., 2008), although our meta-analysis of CGH studies published before 2008 showed 20q gain in 48% of tumors (Avramut and Gollin, 2009). Gain of 20q12–13.2 was reported in 44% of TCGA HNSCC, with *ZNF341* and *CHMP4B* localized to the peak region of gain. Although the function of ZNF341 is not clear, CHMP4B is thought to be a core component of the endosomal sorting required for transport complex III (ESCRT-III), which is involved in formation of multivesicular bodies (MVB) and sorting of endosomal cargo proteins into the MVB. MVB contain intraluminal vesicles (ILV) that are generated by invagination and scission from the limiting membrane of the endosome and generally are delivered to lysosomes, enabling degradation of membrane proteins, such as stimulated growth factor receptors, lysosomal enzymes, and lipids. The MVB pathway appears to require the sequential function of ESCRT-O, ESCRT-I, ESCRT-II, and ESCRT-III complexes. ESCRT-III proteins mostly dissociate from the invaginating membrane before the ILV is released. The ESCRT machinery also functions in topologically equivalent membrane fission events such as the terminal stages of cytokinesis. When overexpressed, membrane-assembled circular arrays of CHMP4B filaments can promote or stabilize negative curvature and outward membrane budding (Pruitt et al., 2014). Further studies are warranted to understand the upregulated genes on 20q, their prognostic significance, and therapeutic potential.

3p loss

Loss of the short arm of chromosome 3 is one of the earliest and most frequent changes in HNSCC, occurring in 56% and 78% of low-grade and high-grade dysplasias, respectively, and in more than 90% of OSCC (Roz et al., 1996; Salahshourifar et al., 2014). As many as 71% of TCGA HNSCC lost one or more segments of 3p (Table 12.2). 3p loss is mediated by either isochromosome formation or chromosome breakage, most frequently at 3p14, the site of the *FHIT* gene and the most common chromosomal fragile site, *FRA3B* (Durkin and Glover, 2007; Ishii et al., 2007). Breakage and loss of function of at least one *FHIT* allele resulting in loss of FHIT protein expression have been reported in precursor lesions and the vast majority of HNSCC compared to matched normal mucosa by our group and others (Virgilio et al., 1996; Gao et al., 2014). FHIT and CHEK1 (often called Chk1 kinase; see also section "11q loss") appear to cooperate to prevent tumor initiation and progression by preventing replication stress-related DNA damage and genome instability, and FHIT may also suppress tumorigenicity through apoptosis of cells that have sustained DNA damage (Saldivar et al., 2013). This is pertinent to HNSCC since we know that *FHIT* spans *FRA3B*, the most common fragile site in the genome that just so happens to be susceptible to breakage by cigarette smoke (Stein et al., 2002) and is also one of the most common chromosomal integration sites of the HPV genome (Ragin et al., 2004). As Ishii et al. (2007) pointed out, the DNA damage-susceptible *FRA3B/FHIT* chromosome fragile region paradoxically encodes a protein, FHIT, that is necessary for protecting cells from accumulation of DNA damage through modulation of checkpoint proteins, HUS1 and phospho-CHEK1. The Fanconi anemia (FA) gene, *FANCD2*, which maps to 3p26.3, may be another hot spot of genetic alterations in HNSCC (Weber et al., 2007). FA patients have a 50-fold higher risk for all solid tumors compared to the general population but a 700-fold higher incidence of head and neck cancers (Rosenberg et al., 2003). Often, patients with FA are first diagnosed after developing HNSCC before the age of 30. FANCD2 is important because it is monoubiquitylated in an FA core complex- and a UBE2T-dependent manner, targeting the protein into nuclear foci where it colocalizes with BRCA1, BRCA2/FANCD1, and other proteins, continuing the FA gene pathway signaling and enabling the cellular response to DNA cross-linking agents (Jacquemont and Taniguchi, 2007). Another potentially important DDR gene on 3p is topoisomerase IIb (*TOP2B*, 3p24) (Hermsen et al., 2005). The topoisomerase II (topo II) protein catalyzes strand passage of double-strand DNA and is essential for chromosomal condensation and sister chromatid exchange. During metaphase, it associates with the centromere, and its inhibition, for example, by means of etoposide, results in cleavage within the centromere. One might speculate that loss of this isoform of topo II in the context of 3p loss may result in breakage and rearrangement at centromeres and the many isochromosomes and centromeric rearrangements that are seen in HNSCC. Numerous other TSG, including *RASSF1*, map to 3p, and it is likely that also these and additional genes will be found to play a role in HNSCC.

4q loss

Two segments of the long arm of chromosome 4 are lost in TCGA HNSCC, 4q35.2 in 40% and 4q21–31, with a peak at 4q22, in 32%. The distal peak includes the *FAT1* gene, an ortholog of the *Drosophila* fat gene, which encodes a tumor suppressor essential for controlling cell proliferation during *Drosophila* development. *FAT1* is expressed highly in fetal epithelia. The gene product is an integral membrane protein containing 34 tandem cadherin-type repeats, five epidermal growth factor (EGF)-like repeats, and one laminin A-G domain (Pruitt et al., 2014). *FAT1* was deleted and mutated in 46% of the HNSCC examined by Pickering et al. (2013) and mutated in 28% of 110 gingivobuccal OSCC examined by the India Project Team of the International Cancer Genome Consortium (2013). Inactivated FAT1 cannot sequester β-catenin at the cell membrane, which leads to WNT signaling and tumor growth (Morris et al., 2013). Loss of 4q22.1 occurs in the common fragile site region *FRA4F* (Rozier et al., 2004) and results in deficiency of *CCSER1* in 35% of HNSCC, esophageal cancers, and other tumors. Patel et al. (2013) reported that *CCSER1* lies at a consensus site of genomic deletions in cancers and that 40% of cancers have in-frame deletions of exons that are conserved evolutionarily. CCSER1 protein localizes to the gamma-tubulin ring complex in early mitosis and to the midbody in late cytokinesis. *CCSER1* knockdown results in cytokinesis failure, multipolar spindles, and multinucleated cells (Patel et al., 2013), suggesting that deletion or copy number loss of this gene may result in CIN.

8p loss

The short arm of chromosome 8 is lost in a large variety of tumors, including 58% of HNSCC (Table 12.2). Some of the losses are the result of submicroscopic deletions not detectable by chromosome banding analysis. Nearly half of all HNSCC show allelic loss in 8p23.2 and even homozygous deletions, suggesting the presence of a TSG, identified to be *CSMD1* (Ishwad et al., 1999; Scholnick and Richter, 2003). The *CSMD1* gene is located within *FRA8B* at 8p23.2, and its expression is aberrant in most HNSCC as a result of deletion, epigenetic silencing, and/or aberrant splicing (Richter et al., 2005). CSMD1 is a transmembrane protein whose function is not entirely clear, but appears to be immune system related. One relatively recent study of melanoma cells indicated an interaction of CSMD1 with the SMAD protein family, proposing a signaling role in apoptosis (Tang et al., 2012). Loss of 8p23 in HNSCC is a statistically significant, independent predictor of poor prognosis (shortened disease-free interval and reduced disease-specific survival) (Bockmuhl et al., 2001).

9p loss

Alterations in band 9p21 are among the most frequent genetic changes in HNSCC (Gollin, 2001). The mechanisms for 9p loss include isochromosome formation for 9q as well as 9p deletions of variable size. van der Riet et al. (1994) first reported a high level of loss (72%) of 9p21–22 at an early stage in HNSCC. Genes in this region include *PTPRD* at 9p23–24 and *CDKN2A*, *CDKN2B*, and *MTAP* at 9p21.3 (Table 12.2). *PTPRD* is lost in approximately 50% of TCGA HNSCC and is mutated in about 13% of HNSCC (Giefing et al., 2011). PTPRD, considered a tumor suppressor protein, is a receptor protein phosphatase that plays a critical role in cellular signaling, including dephosphorylation of STAT3 and inhibition of tumor cell growth (Giefing et al., 2011). The PTPRD protein was not visible in Western blots of laryngeal SCC with 9p deletions compared to normal control tissues (Giefing et al., 2011). Thus, *PTPRD* deletions or mutations can directly drive tumor growth by hyperactivation of the PTPRD substrate, STAT3, which is a powerful and active transcription factor in HNSCC and other tumors (Lui et al., 2014). We and others have observed copy number loss of 9p21.3 by FISH in histopathologically normal oral mucosa and in low-grade dysplasia (reviewed by Mountzios et al., 2014). The *CDKN2A* gene is lost in 59% of TCGA HNSCC with 15% of tumors expressing loss of more than one copy of the gene. Deletions and/or

somatic mutations of *CDKN2A* (21%) and promoter hypermethylation result in inactivation of *CDKN2A* (p16) in as many as 80% of HNSCC. Pickering et al. (2013) observed loss of *CDKN2A* and amplification of *CCND1* in 94% of OSCC (33/35), suggesting that cell cycle alterations are common in OSCC. Alterations in any or all of these genes may lead to uncontrolled cell proliferation through loss of cell cycle checkpoint control, resulting in tumorigenesis. These defects may be useful therapeutic targets in HNSCC.

11q loss

Loss of chromosome 11 distal to the 11q13 amplicon was first reported in HNSCC by Jin et al. (1998a). Distal 11q deletion was shown to be the first step in the 11q13 amplification process in many HNSCC (Reshmi et al., 2007b). cCGH analysis of our OSCC cells revealed both loss of chromosomal material from 11q22 and 11q13 amplification in approximately 50% of the tumors examined (Martin et al., 2008). Distal 11q loss is thought to occur after dysplasia, at an intermediate stage of tumor progression, but before carcinoma *in situ* (Califano et al., 1996). Loss of distal 11q was reported in 45% of TCGA HNSCC and in high frequencies of a variety of HNSCC by Bockmuhl et al. (1998) using cCGH, laryngeal SCC by Järvinen et al. (2006), and OSCC by Freier et al. (2007, 2010a) as shown in Table 12.2. Although the TCGA HNSCC results show several peak regions of loss on distal 11q (Beroukhim et al., 2010; Mermel et al., 2011), Pickering et al. (2013) defined the region of distal 11q loss to span 11q22.3-qter (chr11:103 349 953-135 006 516), with a peak at 11q22.3. Distal 11q contains a block of critical DDR genes, including *ATM* (11q22.3), *MRE11A* (11q21), *H2AFX* (11q23.3), and *CHEK1* (11q24.2). As reviewed in Sankunny et al. (2014), the apex of the DDR to IR is the *ATM* gene, which is mutated in the rare, pleiotropic autosomal recessive disorder AT. *ATM* encodes a 370 kDa protein that is a member of the family of lipid/protein kinases related to PI3K, known as the PI3K-related kinases. In IR-induced double-strand breaks (DSB), the MRE11–RAD50–NBN (MRN) complex plays the role of a "sensor." The primary "transducer" of the DSB signal is ATM. In response to DNA DSB induced by IR, ATM is rapidly phosphorylated at the serine 1981 (ser1981) residue, which facilitates the phosphorylation of various other proteins involved in the regulation and repair of DNA damage. These "effectors" of ATM include ABL1, BRCA1, TP53, and CHEK2. An important substrate of ATM is the histone H2AX, a member of the histone H2A subfamily that maps to distal 11q. ATM activates H2AX at the DSB site, converting it into the phosphorylated form, gamma-H2AX, which then anchors DDR proteins to the sites of damage. The signaling cascade activated by ATM culminates in cell cycle arrest, apoptosis, and DNA repair. Ataxia telangiectasia and Rad3 related (ATR) is another PI3K family protein involved primarily in signaling the presence of stalled replication forks and maintenance of genomic integrity during S phase, along with its partners, ATR-interacting protein (ATRIP) and replication protein A (RPA). Although ATR plays a primary role in responding to UV light and chemotherapy-induced genomic insults, it also appears to play a role in responding to IR-induced DNA damage. The presence of ATR in nuclear foci after IR treatment suggests recruitment of this kinase to sites of DNA damage; ATM is known to regulate the loading of ATR to sites of DNA DSB. Unlike the rapid phosphorylation of ATM after treatment, ATR recruitment and activation are comparatively delayed but also require a functional MRN complex. Even though the ATM and ATR pathways are thought to respond primarily to different types of DNA damage, the two pathways appear to be intimately intertwined. We showed in TP53-defective OSCC cell lines that distal 11q loss measured by relative copy number loss of the ATM gene by FISH is associated with a diminished DDR as measured by a decrease in the size and number of gamma-H2AX foci and increased CIN after treatment with IR, a poor prognosis, and reduced sensitivity (resistance) to IR in OSCC cell lines (Parikh et al., 2007, 2014; Sankunny et al., 2014). Further, our gene and protein expression studies showed upregulation of the ATR–CHEK1 pathway after IR treatment of cell lines with defective TP53 signaling and distal 11q loss. Targeted knockdown of the ATR–CHEK1 pathway in these cells using CHEK1 or ATR siRNA or a CHEK1 small molecule inhibitor (SMI, PF-00477736) resulted in increased sensitivity of the tumor cells to IR. Gadhikar et al. (2013) showed that treatment of TP53-deficient HNSCC cells with the CHEK1/2 inhibitor AZD7762 sensitizes them to cisplatin

therapy. Combined, these results suggest that distal 11q loss is a useful biomarker in OSCC for therapeutic resistance that can be reversed by ATR–CHEK1 pathway inhibition. Thus, distal 11q loss could be used as a biomarker predictive of a less favorable prognosis and a decreased response to conventional chemoradiation therapy, but could be developed as a companion diagnostic to determine response to CHEK1 or ATR inhibition in combination with radiation or chemotherapy in the treatment of OSCC and other tumors.

13q loss

Loss of 13q, with peaks at bands 13q12.11 and 13q14.2, occurs in 44% and 41% of TCGA HNSCC, respectively (Beroukhim et al., 2010; Mermel et al., 2011). The more proximal peak of loss at band 13q12.11 includes 22 genes, one of which is SKA3. SKA3 is a component of the spindle and kinetochore-binding complex (SKA1–3) in the outer kinetochore that mediates kinetochore–microtubule attachment and chromosome alignment and is required for chromatid cohesion and timely anaphase onset (Jeyaprakash et al., 2012; Pruitt et al., 2014; Sivakumar et al., 2014). Aurora B negatively regulates localization of the SKA complex to the kinetochores by phosphorylating SKA1 and SKA3 (Jeyaprakash et al., 2012). Thus, one might speculate that copy number loss of SKA3 may result in CIN.

The critical gene in the more distal peak is thought to be the retinoblastoma gene, RB1, a critical TSG that plays three major roles in cells. The classical role of the RB1 protein is that it prevents a cell from replicating damaged DNA by preventing its progression through cell cycle phase G1 (the first growth or gap phase) into S phase (synthesis phase). Hypophosphorylated RB1 binds to and inhibits the E2F transcription factors, which prevents their release and stalls the cell cycle in G1. Upon phosphorylation by CDK6 and CDK4 and subsequently by CDK2 at Ser567 in G1, RB1 releases E2F1 that then promotes transcription of proteins required for the G1/S phase transition. RB1 is dephosphorylated late in the mitotic phase of the cell cycle. This classical role of RB1 has been expanded recently by the discovery of two additional, independent, nontranscriptional/nontranslational roles: (i) RB1 activates BAX, which binds to and antagonizes the apoptosis repressor, BCL2, resulting in translocation to the mitochondria leading to the release of cytochrome c, which triggers apoptosis (Hilgendorf et al., 2013), and (ii) loss of a single allele of the *Rb1* gene in mice causes telomere attrition and spontaneous CIN in osteoblast lineage cells, which is increased after treatment with IR (Gonzalez-Vasconcellos et al., 2013). Further dissection of the association between CIN and *RB1* revealed that loss of one copy of *RB1* reduced recruitment of the condensin II complex to pericentromeric chromatin, preventing proper replication of this chromatin and resulting in increased gamma-H2AX foci, misshapen kinetochores, CIN, and aneuploidy (Coschi et al., 2014; Hinds, 2014) that can be suppressed by augmentation of cohesion function (Manning et al., 2014). Thus, loss of even one copy of *RB1* may result in CIN and carcinogenesis.

18q loss

Loss of 18q occurs frequently in HNSCC, with 18q23 loss reported in 55% of TCGA HNSCC (Beroukhim et al., 2010; Mermel et al., 2011). There are 19 genes in the peak of loss according to these investigators, including *GALR1* and *PARD6G*. 18q loss is associated with advanced tumor stage and a poor prognosis (Pearlstein et al., 1998; Takebayashi et al., 2004; Misawa et al., 2013). The galanin receptor 1 (*GALR1*) gene that maps to 18q23 often undergoes copy number loss in HNSCC, first shown by Kanazawa et al. (2007). Gene expression is lost as a result of promoter methylation, which is also associated with a poor prognosis in HNSCC patients (Misawa et al., 2013). GALR1 is a G-protein-coupled receptor that inhibits proliferation in keratinocytes by inactivating the MAPK pathway. Antibody blockade of GALR1 enhances proliferation of HNSCC cells, and restoration of expression results in cell cycle arrest and inhibition of colony formation (Misawa et al., 2013). Therefore, these results suggest that *GALR1* is a TSG that inhibits cell proliferation. PARD6G localizes to the older, mother centriole. Depletion results in the absence of a number of proteins from the centriole, resulting in defects in ciliogenesis, interphase and spindle microtubule organization, and centrosome organization and function. PARD6G depleted cells have multipolar spindles (Dormoy et al., 2013). Thus, copy number loss of *PARD6G* at 18q23 could lead to CIN.

The classical and molecular cytogenetic alterations discussed previously are the most common genomic alterations in HNSCC resulting from environmental insults, primarily chewing, smoking, and/or drinking of dried or fermented botanicals. The result is DNA damage, chromosomal breakage, and defective cellular pathways that cause an imbalance between cell proliferation and cell death, CIN, and cancer.

Other tumors of the nasal cavity, sinuses, and nasopharynx

Besides the more prevalent HNSCC, many other benign and malignant tumors arise in the head and neck area. An outstanding review including a discussion of molecular cytogenetic and genetic alterations in sinonasal carcinomas was published recently (Llorente et al., 2014). Genetic and biochemical pathway alterations in mucosal melanoma of the head and neck region were also recently reviewed (Lourenço et al., 2014). Gil and Fliss (2012) reported that the cytogenetic alterations in cranial base tumors were useful not only in developing new grading systems but also as diagnostic and prognostic markers. Lin et al. (2014a) examined the genomic landscape of nasopharyngeal carcinoma (NPC), a tumor caused by Epstein–Barr virus (EBV) infection, and identified a distinct mutational signature different from the APOBEC3B signature seen in HPV-induced carcinomas. They noted that there were fewer copy number alterations in NPC than in other solid tumors. Like other upper aerodigestive cancers, NPC is characterized by copy number loss of *CDKN2A*, mutation and/or deletion of *TP53*, and amplification of the *MYC* and *CCND1* genes (Lin et al., 2014a). The fascinating collection of tumors that develop in the nasal cavity, sinuses, and nasopharynx are ripe for examination to identify genetic alterations that shed light on their etiology and pinpoint therapeutic targets.

Salivary glands

The genomic changes underlying benign and malignant tumors of the salivary glands are less well understood due in part to the lower incidence of these tumors (about 5% of head and neck cancers; Stenman et al., 2014) and their wide histological variation. Recent reviews of cytogenetic and molecular genetic alterations in salivary gland tumors have been published by Weinreb (2013), who discussed translocations in pleomorphic adenoma, mucoepidermoid carcinoma (MEC), adenoid cystic carcinoma, mammary analog secretary carcinoma, and hyalinizing clear cell carcinomas, and Stenman et al. (2014), who focused on pathognomonic gene fusions and driver mutations of clinical significance including translational implications of the genetic findings, with an eye to the development of targeted therapeutics.

Here, we focus on the most common histological subtype of salivary gland cancer, *MECs*. These tumors are invariably characterized by the translocation t(11;19)(q21;p13.1), which leads to a fusion involving *MAML2* and *CRTC1* (Figure 12.2) or, less frequently, *CRTC3* (reviewed in Stenman et al., 2014). The rearrangement fuses exon 1 from *CTRC1* (cAMP response element binding [CREB] protein-regulated transcription coactivator 1) at 19p13.1 with exons 2–5 of *MAML2* [mastermind-like 2 (*Drosophila*), a Notch receptor coactivator] at 11q21, which replaces the Notch-binding domain of *MAML2* with the CREB-binding domain of *CTRC1* or *CTRC3*, which is then fused to the transactivation domain of *MAML2*. This appears to result in activation of EGFR signaling in an autocrine fashion that increases growth and survival of the MEC cells, leaving them highly sensitive to targeted therapy with EGFR inhibitors. MECs have recently been classified into three categories by combining results of classical cytogenetics and/or FISH for the translocation, histopathology, and aCGH: (i) translocation-positive, low- or intermediate-grade tumors with very few or no other copy number alterations and a favorable prognosis; (ii) translocation-positive, high-grade MECs with or without *CDKN2A* deletions, multiple copy number alterations, and a poor prognosis; and (iii) translocation-negative, high-grade MEC-like adenocarcinomas with multiple copy number alterations and a poor prognosis (Jee et al., 2013; Stenman et al., 2014).

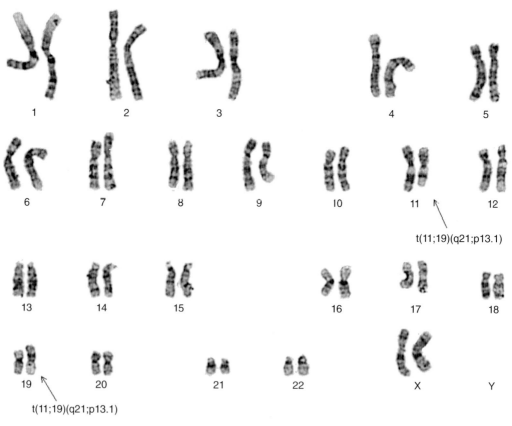

Figure 12.2 A t(11;19)(q21;p13.1) resulting in a *MAML2/CRTC1* gene fusion characterizes mucoepidermoid carcinomas. Arrows indicate derivative chromosomes.

Esophageal cancer

Esophageal cancers make up 3.2% of all cancer cases and account for 4.9% of all cancer deaths according to GLOBOCAN 2012 (Ferlay et al., 2013). In the USA, they comprise 1% of new cancers and account for 2.6% of cancer deaths annually (Siegel et al., 2014). If identified early, the prognosis is excellent. However, esophageal cancer is not often diagnosed early. Although the relative 5-year survival rate from this cancer has increased significantly over the past 40 years, it remains dismal and survival disparities remain between Caucasians and African Americans (18% vs. 11%, respectively), largely thought to be due to late diagnosis (Siegel et al., 2014). Esophageal cancer is three to four times more common in males than females (Jemal et al., 2011). Most esophageal carcinomas are either *esophageal squamous cell carcinomas* (ESCC), which arise in the middle or upper one-third of the esophagus, or *esophageal adenocarcinomas* (EAC). Similar to HNSCC, ESCC is thought to result from alcohol and tobacco consumption, but two recent papers, a review and a meta-analysis of ESCC, suggest that HPV16 may play a role in SCC of the upper esophagus as it does in SCC of the adjacent oropharynx (Syrjänen, 2013; Petrick et al., 2014). However, whether HPV plays a role in the etiology of ESCC remains controversial. EAC develops from intestinal metaplasia of the esophageal epithelium (Barrett's esophagus [BE]) in the lower one-third of the esophagus or the gastroesophageal junction (GEJ). BE usually develops in response to chronic gastroesophageal reflux, which results in inflammation as the contents of the stomach and duodenum bathe the esophagus. The frequency of EAC has risen dramatically (~600%) in developed Western countries over the past 30 years (Dulak et al., 2013).

Molecular genetic correlates of the key cytogenetic findings in esophageal cancer and their prognostic significance

The most frequent cytogenetic findings in ESCC include gains or amplifications of 1q, 3q, 5p, 7p, 7q, 8p, 8q, 11q, 12p, and 17q and losses involving 3p, 4p, 4q, 5q, 8p, 9p, 11p, 11q, 13q, 16q, 18q, 19p, Xp, and Xq (Beroukhim et al., 2010; Mermel et al.,

2011; Shi et al., 2013; Lin et al., 2014b; Song et al., 2014). The major regions of gain or loss in ESCC, the peak bands, and the proposed critical genes are listed in Tables 12.3 and 12.4. High-level amplification of 3q26, 8q24, and 11q13; loss of 3p12–14; and homozygous deletion of 9p21.3 are the most frequent cytogenetic alterations. Comparing dysplasia with ESCC, Shi et al. (2013) found 9p loss to be an early change, seen in both early dysplasia and ESCC, whereas 11q gain or amplification was seen in moderate dysplasia but was also associated with lymph node metastasis and, thus, advanced disease.

11q13 amplification including the *ORAOV1* gene was recently reported in 53% of ESCC and is associated with poorly differentiated histology, tumors in the upper or middle esophagus, and a trend toward shorter disease-free and overall survival after surgery compared to patients without 11q13 amplification (Togashi et al., 2014). The *ANO1* gene also maps to 11q13 and is amplified in ESCC. *ANO1* expression was found elevated relatively early in the development of ESCC, in moderate dysplasia compared to normal esophageal epithelium (Shi et al., 2013). Both *ANO1* mRNA and protein were overexpressed in ESCC (Shi et al., 2013), and as for *ORAOV1*, overexpression correlated with lymph node metastasis and advanced clinical stage. RNAi-mediated knockdown of *ANO1* in two ESCC cell lines with increased *ANO1* expression resulted in inhibition of cell proliferation (Shi et al., 2013). A third 11q13-amplified and overexpressed gene, *CTTN*, was also associated with lymph node metastases in ESCC (Luo et al., 2006). These investigators showed that RNAi treatment decreased *CTTN* expression resulting in impaired cell migration and anoikis resistance.

Examination of EAC reveals gain, amplification, and loss of a variety of chromosomal regions, but a substantially lower percentage of tumors show these chromosomal alterations than ESCC (or HNSCC) as shown in Tables 12.5 and 12.6. This suggests that the etiology is different. The two most frequently mutated genes in EAC are *TP53* and *CDKN2A*, both of which undergo copy number loss in these tumors. Of interest, regulatory control of the cell cycle is frequently defective in EAC, from a relatively high frequency of mutations in and loss of *CDKN2A* to amplification of *CCND1*, *CCNE1*, *CDK6*, and

Table 12.3 Meta-analysis of chromosomal gains in ESCC*

Chromosome segment	CC (%)	aCGH amp. % (Lin et al. [2014b])	TCGA gain (%)	TCGA amp. (%)	Genes of interest in or near peak region
1q21	27	–	52	–	TUFT1
2q14.2	–	–	33	–	13[T]: PTPN4, GLI2, CLASP1
3q11-qter	71	10			PIK3CA[L], SOX2[L]
(3q26.33)			71	27	ACTRT3 [T], MYNN [T]
5p14–15.3 (5p15.3)	52	–	58	18	TERT
6p12	–	–	34	10	4[T]: RSPH9, MRPS18A, VEGFA
7p11–22 (7p11.2)	27	11	65	15	4[T]: EGFR[LT]
7q21.2–21.3	29	–	63	17	10[T]: KRIT1, ANKIB1, GATAD1, PEX1, CDK6
8p11.23	–	11	40	10	21[T]:FGFR1[LT]
8q13–q24.3 (8q24.21)	66	9	79	33	MYC[L], CCAT1[T]
11p13	–	–	29	–	APIP
11q13	70	46	60	40	6: CCND1[L], FGF3/4/19[L], ORAOV1*, ANO1[T], FADD[T], PPFIA1[T], CTTN[TL], CPT1A[L]
12p12.1	23	5	47	13	CASC1, LYRM5, KRAS
17q21.2	–	–	37	12	11[T]: PPP1R1B, STARD3, TCAP, PNMT, PGAP3, ERBB2, MIEN1, GRB7, IKZF3
18q11.2	–	–	26	10	6: LAMA3, CABYR
19q12	–	–	25	–	CCNE1

By classical and molecular cytogenetic analysis, including FISH, oligonucleotide and SNP array CGH, and corresponding genes in the regions. Deletion refers to homozygous or high-level deletion by aCGH or SNP arrays. Approximate percent frequency of ESCC with the particular gain, amplification (amp.), or loss based on classical cytogenetic (CC) analysis pre-2008 from Table 11.1 in Avramut and Gollin (2009), combined data (n = 184) from Supplementary Table 7 from Lin et al. (2014b)[L], and the 126 esophageal carcinomas (NOS) in The Cancer Genome Atlas (TCGA[T]) SNP array dataset analyzed by Beroukhim et al. (2010) and Mermel et al. (2011) who found 33 peak regions of gain or amplification and 57 peak regions of loss (major peaks listed) (www.broadinstitute/TCGA; dataset: 2014-07-08 stddata__2014_06_14 [28 July 2014]). TCGA frequencies less than 10% are not listed. Genes noted are from TCGA[T], Lin et al. (2014b)[L], and those not listed but selected by the author based on the literature (marked), and if the number of genes in the peak is too high, that number is noted and selected genes in the region are listed.

MYC (Dulak et al., 2012, 2013). EAC express frequent loss of chromosomal band 7q21, which appears to be a marker of adenocarcinoma of the GEJ (van Dekken et al., 2008, 2009). These investigators showed a significant correlation between chromosomal gain or amplification and mRNA and protein expression or overexpression for the cell cycle regulatory gene CDK6. Although CDK6 expression was observed by immunohistochemistry in GEJ EAC, they did not detect expression in BE dysplasia or carcinoma in situ, suggesting that CDK6 is associated with frank malignancy (van Dekken et al., 2008). This difference between BE and EAC is interesting and potentially very important, but

Agrawal et al. (2012) nevertheless showed that BE contains most of the genetic alterations present in matched EAC. Additional distinctions between matched BE and EAC are critical to identifying which genetic alterations are responsible for the switch from benign to malignant neoplasia.

The regions of gain, amplification, and loss are remarkably similar between HNSCC, ESCC, and, surprisingly, EAC. A comparison of Tables 12.1 and 12.3 and Tables 12.2 and 12.4 reveals that the majority of regions of gain, amplification, loss, and homozygous loss in HNSCC and ESCC are identical, suggesting similar biochemical pathway disturbances in SCC at these two nearby locations.

Table 12.4 Meta-analysis of chromosomal losses in ESCC*

Chromosome segment	CC	aCGH deletion (Lin et al. [2014b])	TCGA loss	TCGA del.	Genes of interest in or near peak region
1p12–13.2	–	–	35	–	18:PTPN22, HIPK1
2q22.1–2	–	6	36	–	LRP1B
3p12–25	35				
(3p14.2) (3p12.1)		4	70	–	FHIT
			71	–	ESRG, LRTM1
4p15.2	–	–	54	–	KCN1P4
4q22	27	–	53	–	CCSER1
5q12	20	3	57	–	PPDE4D^L
6p25	–	–	35	–	FOXC1, GMDS
7q31.1	–	–	27	–	LRRN3
8p23.2	–	–	45	–	CSMD1
9p21.3–24	17				
(9p23–24.1)		3	–	–	PTPRD
(9p21.3)		33	77	31	CDKN2A/B
10p11.21	–	–	25	–	PARD3
10q23	–	–	37	–	KLLN, PTEN
11p15.4–15.5	–	–	44	–	114 genes
11q22.3–23.3	–	–	43	–	H2AFX*, ATM*
(11q24.3)	–	–	44	–	ZBTB44
13q12–34	20	–			
(13q12.11)	–	–	44	–	81: SKA3
(13q14.2)	–	–	47	–	RB1
16q23.3–q24.1	–	–	42	10	WWOX
18q21.1	–	–	61	–	SMAD4, ELAC1
19p13.3	17	–	45	–	45: POLR2E
21q11.2–q21.3	20	–	–	–	–
Xp11.4–p11.23	–	–	42	–	DUSP21, KDM6A
Xq21.1–2	–	–	41	–	FTHL17

By classical and molecular cytogenetic analysis, including FISH, oligonucleotide and SNP array CGH, and corresponding genes in the regions. Deletion refers to homozygous or high-level deletion by aCGH or SNP arrays. Approximate percent frequency of ESCC with the particular gain, amplification (amp.), or loss based on classical cytogenetic (CC) analysis pre-2008 from Table 11.1 in Avramut and Gollin (2009), combined data (n = 184) from Supplementary Table 7 from Lin et al. (2014b)^L, and the 126 esophageal carcinomas (NOS) in The Cancer Genome Atlas (TCGA^T) SNP array dataset analyzed by Beroukhim et al. (2010) and Mermel et al. (2011) who found 33 peak regions of gain or amplification and 57 peak regions of loss (major peaks listed) (www.broadinstitute/TCGA; dataset: 2014-07-08 stddata__2014_06_14 [28 July 2014]). TCGA frequencies less than 10% are not listed. Genes noted are from TCGA^T, Lin et al. (2014b)^L, and those not listed but selected by the author based on the literature (marked), and if the number of genes in the peak is too high, that number is noted and selected genes in the region are listed.

Moreover, similarities also exist between Tables 12.3 and 12.5 and between Tables 12.4 and 12.6, suggesting that some of the defective pathways in ESCC and EAC are the same, although loss of band 7q21 seems to be unique to EAC, particularly malignancy at the GEJ. Discussion of the genes located in these genomic regions is therefore not repeated, and the reader may wish to refer to the section on HNSCC for more information. Further,

much of the LOH in 17p13.1–13.3 in both HNSCC and ESCC appears to be copy neutral using SNP arrays, meaning that copy number loss is not present yet LOH has occurred as a result of mitotic segregation errors, homologous recombination, or nondisjunction (Marescalco et al., 2014). 8p23 gain or neutral copy number change without LOH of CTSB, GATA4, NEIL2, and FDFT1 is associated with poor survival in EAC compared to loss

Table 12.5 Chromosomal copy number gains in EAC*

Chromosome segment	CC (%)	SNP aCGH gain %	SNP aCGH amp. %	Genes of interest in or near peak region
1q21.1	–	35	–	16: BCL9
3q26.2	–	28	–	6: MDS1, MECOM, MYNN
6p21.1	37	26	–	57: VEGFA, POLH, CCND3, GNMT
7p11.1–22.3	58			
(7p11.2)		22	11	1: EGFR
7q21.3	–	28	–	9: CDK6
8p23.1	50	20	–	5: BLK, CTSB, GATA4, FDFT1
8q11.1–24.3	80			
(8q24.21)		39	13	1: MYC
11q13.3	50	19	–	9: CCND1, ANO1, ORAOV1*, FADD, FGF3/4/19, PPFIA1, CTTN
12p12.1	66	19	15	1: IFLTD1, [KRAS]
13q11–34	–			
(13q22.1)		30	11	KLF5
(13q22.3–31.1)		30	11	MYCBP2, EDRNB
17q12	30	15	15	2: ERBB2, GRB7
18q11.2	–	37	–	1: GATA6
19q12	–	24	11	3: CCNE1, PLEKHF1, URI1
20q13.2	60	46	–	7: ZNF217

*By classical and molecular cytogenetic analysis, including FISH, oligonucleotide and SNP array CGH, and corresponding genes in the regions. FISH, fluorescence in situ hybridization; SNP, single-nucleotide polymorphism. Approximate percent frequency of EAC with the particular gain, amplification (amp.), or loss based on classical cytogenetic (CC) analysis pre-2008 from Table 11.1 in Avramut and Gollin (2009). Del., deletion, refers to homozygous or high-level deletion by SNP arrays. Array CGH data are from Frankel et al. (2014) and analysis of 54 EAC by SNP arrays that show concurrence with those of Dulak et al. (2012, 2013); those genes not specifically mentioned by Frankel et al. that are mentioned by Dulak et al. are in brackets [ ]. *, additional gene added by author. Frequencies less than 10% are not listed. TCGA data for esophageal carcinomas, not separated into ESCC and EAC, are shown in Tables 12.3 and 12.4.

or copy-neutral LOH (Frankel et al., 2014). Further application of SNP arrays will undoubtedly reveal additional copy-neutral LOH in regions harboring TSG.

The mechanisms involved in chromosomal gains, losses, amplification, and instability have been investigated for many years (reviewed in Gollin, 2005). They involve chromosomal segregational defects resulting from cytoskeletal alterations, defects in the DDR, telomere dysfunction, cell cycle disturbances, and CIN leading to LOH, which begets more CIN. Some investigators have noted that a few of the consistent deletions in esophageal tumors overlap with or border common chromosomal fragile sites (Gu et al., 2010; Boonstra et al., 2012), many of which were discussed earlier in the context of HNSCC. It is clear that common

fragile sites are heterogeneous but unstable genomic regions that share sensitivity to the replication stress that occurs during the early stages of cancer development (Ozeri-Galai et al., 2012). Examination of the data presented here for HNSCC, ESCC, and EAC shows loss of 3p14 involving FRA3B and the FHIT gene, 4q22 involving FRA4F and the CCSER1 gene (Rozier et al., 2004), FRA11F at 11q14 and distal 11q loss involving critical DDR genes in HNSCC, and FRA16D and WWOX in ESCC and EAC. Boonstra et al. (2012) reported evidence that these deletions occur early in the development of EAC. Understanding the effects of these nonrandom chromosomal gains and losses will not only inform us about cancer, but about how the disrupted cellular processes occur in normal cells.

Table 12.6 Chromosomal copy number losses in EAC*

Chromosome segment	CC (%)	SNP aCGH loss %	SNP aCGH del. %	Genes of interest in or near peak region
1q44	–	22	–	–
3p14.2	–	30	61	FHIT
4q22.1	50	24	13	CCSER1*
5q11.2	43	41	–	PPDE4D
6p25	–	28	11	FOXC1
9p21.3–24	43			
(9p23)		41	19	PTPRD
(9p21.3)		44	17	CDKN2A/B
16q23.1	–	22	32	WWOX
18q21.2	54	41	–	SMAD4
19p13.11	–	30	–	NDUFA13, PBX4, TSSK6, LPAR2
21q22.12	65	33	–	RUNX1

*By classical and molecular cytogenetic analysis, including FISH, oligonucleotide and SNP array CGH, and corresponding genes in the regions. FISH, fluorescence *in situ* hybridization; SNP, single-nucleotide polymorphism. Approximate percent frequency of EAC with the particular gain, amplification (amp.), or loss based on classical cytogenetic (CC) analysis pre-2008 from Table 11.1 in Avramut and Gollin (2009). Del., deletion, refers to homozygous or high-level deletion by SNP arrays. Array CGH data are from Frankel et al. (2014) and analysis of 54 EAC by SNP arrays that show concurrence with those of Dulak et al. (2012, 2013); those genes not specifically mentioned by Frankel et al. that are mentioned by Dulak et al. are in brackets [ ]. *, additional gene added by author. Frequencies less than 10% are not listed. TCGA data for esophageal carcinomas, not separated into ESCC and EAC, are shown in Tables 12.3 and 12.4.

Translational integration of cytogenetic alterations as biomarkers of upper aerodigestive tract cancer

Nonrandom cytogenetic alterations in HNSCC are likely to serve as useful biomarkers. These might include (i) *cancer risk biomarkers*, as in the rare patients with *RB1* deletions and retinoblastoma; (ii) *diagnostic biomarkers*, as in the case of unique translocations; (iii) *predictive biomarkers*, as in (a) *ERBB2* amplification and Herceptin® (trastuzumab) therapy or (b) distal 11q loss marked by *ATM* loss and/or dysfunction and/or ATR–CHEK1 pathway upregulation in the setting of a defective G1 cell cycle checkpoint (as from defective TP53 signaling) and therapy with an ATR or CHEK1 small molecule inhibitor like AZD6738, VE822, or LY2606368 (Parikh et al., 2007, 2014; Sankunny et al., 2014); and (iv) *prognostic biomarkers* for (a) outcome, such as using FISH panels in chronic lymphocytic leukemia, or (b) tumor surveillance by copy number analysis of cell-free DNA in plasma from cancer patients.

One of the most pressing and potentially impactful aims of cancer genetics research at this time is to identify the best therapy for each patient, that is, personalized cancer genomic medicine. An important contribution to this goal was the first integrated genomic analysis of OSCC, a subset of HNSCC (Pickering et al., 2013). Integration of gene expression, copy number, methylation, and point mutations revealed four major driver pathways (mitogenic signaling, NOTCH, cell cycle, and TP53) and two additional, highly mutated genes (*FAT1* and *CASP8*). Mutated caspase 8 defined a new molecular subtype of OSCC with fewer copy number alterations. Lin et al. (2014b) and Song et al. (2014) characterized the genomic landscape of about 300 ESCC using whole-genome/whole-exome sequencing, targeted sequencing, and copy number analysis to identify aberrant genes, pathways, and therapeutic targets (reviewed by Lin et al., 2014c). Already known mutated genes implicated in ESCC include *TP53*, *CDKN2A*, *RB1*, *PTEN*, *NFE2L2*, *PIK3CA*, and *NOTCH1*, and the new genes *FAT1*, *FAT2*, *ZNF750*, *KMT2D*, *ADAM29*, and *FAM135B* also command attention. Copy number gain of *FGFR1* is present in both HNSCC (31%) and ESCC (40%) and it is amplified in 7% and 10% of these tumors, respectively

(Beroukhim et al., 2010; Mermel et al., 2011; Lin et al., 2014c). Clinical trials of several FGF receptor small molecule inhibitors are underway (Lin et al., 2014c). The newfound knowledge from these and similar studies is likely to lead to new, targeted therapies for both HNSCC and ESCC.

A major problem in the treatment of cancer patients is the emergence of tumor cell resistance to the therapeutic drugs. Several references have been made throughout the HNSCC section to biomarkers of therapeutic resistance. One of the most common markers of poor prognosis and resistance to chemotherapy and radiotherapy in HNSCC is distal 11q loss (Parikh et al., 2007, 2014; Gadhikar et al., 2013; Sankunny et al., 2014). Treatment of tumor cells with siRNA or targeted small molecule inhibitors to CHEK1 or ATR reverses this resistance (Gadhikar et al., 2013; Sankunny et al., 2014), and clinical trials based on these findings are underway. Other chromosomal gains and losses inform us as to the efficacy of targeted therapies for HNSCC, ESCC, EAC, and other cancers. For example, copy number gains of the *PIK3CA* gene suggest that tumors may respond to PI3 kinase inhibitors, while loss of *PTPRS* suggests decreased efficacy of EGFR inhibitors (reviewed in Ow et al., 2013). The first targeted therapy used on EAC based on genomic findings was trastuzumab in GEJ adenocarcinomas with *ERBB2* gene amplification. Mutations have since been observed in 3% of specimens and so also serve as possible predictive biomarkers. Cost-effective and therapeutically efficacious utilization of the new, targeted therapies being developed at a rapid rate requires validated predictive biomarkers, which are being identified for each of these cancers and advanced toward the marketplace as a consequence of the decreased cost of aCGH and DNA and RNA sequencing. The future looks brighter for patients diagnosed with upper aerodigestive tract tumors as a result of personalized cancer genomic medicine.

Summary

Tumors of the upper aerodigestive tract are among the most devastating in terms of morbidity and mortality. However, the numbers of HNSCC, ESCC, and EAC being examined at present using molecular cytogenetic and molecular genetic tools enable robust correlations of cytogenetic biomarkers with therapeutic response and outcome. The cytogenetic findings in upper aerodigestive tract tumors are now increasingly being placed into the context of biochemical pathways in order to understand how the genetic alterations in the tumor affect cell biology. The cytogenetic findings thus lead to more accurate diagnosis, prognosis, and patient selection to identify the optimal treatment for each individual patient. This will ultimately result in more efficacious targeted therapies administered to the right patients based on a detailed molecular understanding of carcinogenesis in the upper aerodigestive tract.

References

Agochiya, M., Brunton, V.G., Owens, D.W., Parkinson, E.K., Paraskeva, C., Keith, W.N., et al. (1999): Increased dosage and amplification of the focal adhesion kinase gene in human cancer cells. *Oncogene* 18, 5646–5653.

Agrawal, N., Jiao, Y., Bettegowda, C., Hutfless, S.M., Wang, Y., David, S., et al. (2012): Comparative genomic analysis of esophageal adenocarcinoma and squamous cell carcinoma. *Cancer Discov* 2, 899–905.

Åkervall, J.A., Michalides, R.J., Mineta, H., Balm, A., Borg, A., Dictor, M.R., et al. (1997): Amplification of cyclin D1 in squamous cell carcinoma of the head and neck and the prognostic value of chromosomal abnormalities and cyclin D1 overexpression. *Cancer* 79, 380–389.

Albertson, D.G. (2006): Gene amplification in cancer. *Trends Genet* 22, 447–455.

Avramut, M., Gollin, S.M. (2009): Tumors of the upper aerodigestive tract. In: Heim S., Mitelman F., editors. 3rd edition. *Cancer Cytogenetics*. Hoboken, NJ: John Wiley & Sons, pp 375–412.

Ayoub, C., Wasylyk, C., Li, Y., Thomas, E., Marisa, L., Robé, A., et al. (2010): ANO1 amplification and expression in HNSCC with a high propensity for future distant metastasis and its functions in HNSCC cell lines. *Br J Cancer* 103, 715–726.

Beroukhim, R., Mermel, C.H., Porter, D., Wei, G., Raychaudhuri, S., Donovan, J., et al. (2010): The landscape of somatic copy-number alteration across human cancers. *Nature* 463, 899–905, http://www.broadinstitute/TCGA; HNSCC dataset: 2014-04-28 stddata__2014_04_16 examined on [6 July 2014]; Esophageal Cancer (NOS) dataset: 2014-07-08 stddata__2014_06_14 [28 July 2014] (accessed on February 2, 2015).

Bockmuhl, U., Wolf, G., Schmidt, S., Schwendel, A., Jahnke, V., Dietel, M., et al. (1998): Genomic alterations associated with malignancy in head and neck cancer. *Head Neck* 20, 145–151.

Bockmuhl, U., Ishwad, C.S., Ferrell, R.E., Gollin, S.M. (2001): Association of 8p23 deletions with poor survival in head and neck cancer. *Otolaryngol Head Neck Surg* 124, 451–455.

Boonstra, J.J., van Marion, R., Douben, H.J., Lanchbury, J.S., Timms, K.M., Abkevich, V., et al. (2012): Mapping of homozygous deletions in verified esophageal adenocarcinoma cell lines and xenografts. *Genes Chromosomes Cancer* 51, 272–282.

Braakhuis, B.J., Leemans, C.R., Brakenhoff, R.H. (2004): A genetic progression model of oral cancer: current evidence and clinical implications. *J Oral Pathol Med* 33, 317–322.

Califano, J., van der Riet, P., Westra, W., Nawroz, H., Clayman, G., Piantadosi, S., et al. (1996): Genetic progression model for head and neck cancer: implications for field cancerization. *Cancer Res* 56, 2488–2492.

Califano, J., Westra, W.H., Meininger, G., Corio, R., Koch, W.M., Sidransky, D. (2000): Genetic progression and clonal relationship of recurrent premalignant head and neck lesions. *Clin Cancer Res* 6, 347–352.

Chaturvedi, A.K., Anderson, W.F., Lortet-Tieulent, J., Curado, M.P., Ferlay, J., Franceschi, S., et al. (2013): Worldwide trends in incidence rates for oral cavity and oropharyngeal cancers. *J Clin Oncol* 31, 4550–4559.

Chen, Y., McGee, J., Chen, X., Doman, T.N., Gong, X., Zhang, Y., et al. (2014): Identification of druggable cancer driver genes amplified across TCGA datasets. *PLoS One* 9(5), e98293.

Chung, C.H., Parker, J.S., Karaca, G., Wu, J., Funkhouser, W.K., Moore, D., et al. (2004): Molecular classification of head and neck squamous cell carcinomas using patterns of gene expression. *Cancer Cell* 5, 489–500.

Chung, C.H., Ely, K., McGavran, L., Varella-Garcia, M., Parker, J., Parker, N., et al. (2006): Increased epidermal growth factor receptor gene copy number is associated with poor prognosis in head and neck squamous cell carcinomas. *J Clin Oncol* 24, 4170–4176.

Chung, C.H., Bagheri, A., D'Souza, G. (2014): Mutations in the retinoblastoma-related gene RB2/p130 in primary nasopharyngeal carcinoma. *Oral Oncol* 50, 364–369.

Ciullo, M., Debily, M.A., Rozier, L., Autiero, M., Billault, A., Mayau, V., et al. (2002): Initiation of the breakage-fusion-bridge mechanism through common fragile site activation in human breast cancer cells: the model of PIP gene duplication from a break at FRA7I. *Hum Mol Genet* 11, 2887–2894.

Coschi, C.H., Ishak, C.A., Gallo, D., Marshall, A., Talluri, S., Wang, J., et al. (2014): Haploinsufficiency of an RB-E2F1-condensin II complex leads to aberrant replication and aneuploidy. *Cancer Discov* 4, 840–853.

van Dekken, H., van Marion, R., Vissers, K.J., Hop, W.C., Dinjens, W.N., Tilanus, H.W., et al. (2008): Molecular dissection of the chromosome band 7q21 amplicon in gastroesophageal junction adenocarcinomas identifies cyclin-dependent

kinase 6 at both genomic and protein expression levels. *Genes Chromosomes Cancer* 47, 649–656.

van Dekken, H., Tilanus, H.W., Hop, W.C., Dinjens, W.N., Wink, J.C., Vissers, K.J., et al. (2009): Array comparative genomic hybridization, expression array, and protein analysis of critical regions on chromosome arms 1q, 7q, and 8p in adenocarcinomas of the gastroesophageal junction. *Cancer Genet Cytogenet* 189, 37–42.

Dormoy, V., Tormanen, K., Sütterlin, C. (2013): Par6γ is at the mother centriole and controls centrosomal protein composition through a Par6α-dependent pathway. *J Cell Sci* 126, 860–870.

Dulak, A.M., Schumacher, S.E., van Lieshout, J., Imamura, Y., Fox, C., Shim, B., et al. (2012): Gastrointestinal adenocarcinomas of the esophagus, stomach, and colon exhibit distinct patterns of genome instability and oncogenesis. *Cancer Res* 72, 4383–4393.

Dulak, A.M., Stojanov, P., Peng, S., Lawrence, M.S., Fox, C., Stewart, C., et al. (2013): Exome and whole-genome sequencing of esophageal adenocarcinoma identifies recurrent driver events and mutational complexity. *Nat Genet* 45, 478–486.

Durkin, S.G., Glover, T.W. (2007): Chromosome fragile sites. *Annu Rev Genet* 41, 169–192.

Duvvuri, U., Shiwarski, D.J., Xiao, D., Bertrand, C., Huang, X., Edinger, R.S., et al. (2012): TMEM16A induces MAPK and contributes directly to tumorigenesis and cancer progression. *Cancer Res* 72, 3270–3281.

Ferlay, J., Soerjomataram, I., Ervik, M., Dikshit, R., Eser, S., Mathers, C., et al. (2013): GLOBOCAN 2012 v1.0, Cancer Incidence and Mortality Worldwide: IARC CancerBase No. 11. Lyon: IARC, http://globocan.iarc.fr (accessed on July 2, 2014).

Forastiere, A., Koch, W., Trotti, A., Sidransky, D. (2001): Head and neck cancer. *N Engl J Med* 345, 1890–1900.

Fracchiolla, N.S., Pruneri, G., Pignataro, L., Carboni, N., Capaccio, P., Boletini, A., et al. (1997): Molecular and immunohistochemical analysis of the bcl-1/cyclin D1 gene in laryngeal squamous cell carcinomas: correlation of protein expression with lymph node metastases and advanced clinical stage. *Cancer* 79, 1114–1121.

Frankel, A., Armour, N., Nancarrow, D., Krause, L., Hayward, N., Lampe, G., et al. (2014): Genome-wide analysis of esophageal adenocarcinoma yields specific copy number aberrations that correlate with prognosis. *Genes Chromosomes Cancer* 53, 324–338.

Freier, K., Sticht, C., Hofele, C., Flechtenmacher, C., Stange, D., Puccio, L., et al. (2006): Recurrent coamplification of cytoskeleton-associated genes EMS1 and SHANK2 with CCND1 in oral squamous cell carcinoma. *Genes Chromosomes Cancer* 45, 118–125.

Freier, K., Schwaenen, C., Sticht, C., Flechtenmacher, C., Muhling, J., Hofele, C., et al. (2007): Recurrent FGFR1 amplification and high FGFR1 protein expression in oral squamous cell carcinoma (OSCC). *Oral Oncol* 43, 60–66.

Freier, K., Hofele, C., Knoepfle, K., Gross, M., Devens, F., Dyckhoff, G., et al. (2010a): Cytogenetic characterization of head and neck squamous cell carcinoma cell lines as model systems for the functional analyses of tumor-associated genes. *J Oral Pathol Med* 39, 382–389.

Freier, K., Knoepfle, K., Flechtenmacher, C., Pungs, S., Devens, F., Toedt G., et al. (2010b): Recurrent copy number gain of transcription factor *SOX2* and corresponding high protein expression in oral squamous cell carcinoma. *Genes Chromosomes Cancer* 49, 9–16.

Gadhikar, M.A., Sciuto, M.R., Alves, M.V., Pickering, C.R., Osman, A.A., Neskey, D.M., et al. (2013): Chk1/2 inhibition overcomes the cisplatin resistance of head and neck cancer cells secondary to the loss of functional p53. *Mol Cancer Ther* 12, 1860–1873.

Gao, G., Kasperbauer, J.L., Tombers, N.M., Wang, V., Mayer, K., Smith, D.I. (2014): A selected group of large common fragile site genes have decreased expression in oropharyngeal squamous cell carcinomas. *Genes Chromosomes Cancer* 53, 392–401.

García Martínez, J., García-Inclán, C., Suárez, C., Llorente, J.L., Hermsen, M.A. (2014): DNA aneuploidy-specific therapy for head and neck squamous cell carcinoma. *Head Neck*. doi:10.1002/hed.23687

Gibcus, J.H., Kok, K., Menkema, L., Hermsen, M.A., Mastik, M., Kluin, P.M., et al. (2007a): High-resolution mapping identifies a commonly amplified 11q13.3 region containing multiple genes flanked by segmental duplications. *Hum Genet* 121, 187–201.

Gibcus, J.H., Menkema, L., Mastik, M.F., Hermsen, M.A., deBock, G.H., vanVelthuysen, M.L., et al. (2007b): Amplicon mapping and expression profiling identify the Fas-associated death domain gene as a new driver in the 11q13.3 amplicon in laryngeal/pharyngeal cancer. *Clin Cancer Res* 13, 6257–6266.

Giefing, M., Zemke, N., Brauze, D., Kostrzewska-Poczekaj, M., Luczak, M., Szaumkessel, M., et al. (2011): High resolution arrayCGH and expression profiling identifies PTPRD and PCDH17/PCH68 as tumor suppressor gene candidates in laryngeal squamous cell carcinoma. *Genes Chromosomes Cancer* 50, 154–166.

Gil, Z., Fliss, D.M. (2012): Cytogenetic analysis of skull base tumors: where do we stand? *Curr Opin Otolaryngol Head Neck Surg* 20, 130–136.

Gollin, S.M. (2001): Chromosomal alterations in squamous cell carcinomas of the head and neck: window to the biology of disease. *Head Neck* 23, 238–353.

Gollin, S.M. (2005): Mechanisms leading to chromosomal instability. *Semin Cancer Biol* 15, 33–42.

Gonzalez-Vasconcellos, I., Anastasov, N., Sanli-Bonazzi, B., Klymenko, O., Atkinson, M.J., Rosemann, M. (2013): Rb1 haploinsufficiency promotes telomere attrition and radiation-induced genomic instability. *Cancer Res* 73, 4247–4255.

Gu, J., Ajani, J.A., Hawk, E.T., Ye, Y., Lee, J.H., Bhutani, M.S., et al. (2010): Genome-wide catalogue of chromosomal aberrations in barrett's esophagus and esophageal adeno-carcinoma: a high-density single nucleotide polymorphism array analysis. *Cancer Prev Res (Phila)* 3, 1176–1186.

Harper, L.J., Piper, K., Common, J., Fortune, F., Mackenzie, I.C. (2007): Stem cell patterns in cell lines derived from head and neck squamous cell carcinoma. *J Oral Pathol Med* 36, 594–603.

Hayashi, M.T., Karlseder, J. (2013): DNA damage associated with mitosis and cytokinesis failure. *Oncogene* 32, 4593–4601.

Hayashi, H., Arao, T., Togashi, Y., Kato, H., Fujita, Y., De Velasco, M.A., et al. (2014): The OCT4 pseudogene POU5F1B is amplified and promotes an aggressive phenotype in gastric cancer. *Oncogene* 34(2):199–208.

Hellman, A., Zlotorynski, E., Scherer, S.W., Cheung, J., Vincent, J.B., Smith, D.I., et al. (2002): A role for common fragile site induction in amplification of human oncogenes. *Cancer Cell* 1, 89–97.

Hermsen, M., Snijders, A., Guervos, M.A., Taenzer, S., Koerner, U., Baak, J., et al. (2005): Centromeric chromosomal translocations show tissue-specific differences between squamous cell carcinomas and adenocarcinomas. *Oncogene* 24, 1571–1579.

Hilgendorf, K.I., Leshchiner, E.S., Nedelcu, S., Maynard, M.A., Calo, E., Ianari, A., et al. (2013): The retinoblastoma protein induces apoptosis directly at the mitochondria. *Genes Dev* 27, 1003–1015.

Hinds, P.W. (2014): A little pRB can lead to big problems. *Cancer Discov* 4, 764–765.

Huang, X., Gollin, S.M., Raja, S., Godfrey, T.E. (2002): High-resolution mapping of the 11q13 amplicon and identification of a gene, TAOS1, that is amplified and overexpressed in oral cancer cells. *Proc Natl Acad Sci USA* 99, 11369–11374.

Huang, X., Godfrey, T.E., Gooding, W.E., McCarty, K.S. Jr., Gollin, S.M. (2006): Comprehensive genome and transcriptome analysis of the 11q13 amplicon in human oral cancer and synteny to the 7 F5 amplicon in murine oral carcinoma. *Genes Chromosomes Cancer* 45, 1058–1069.

India Project Team of the International Cancer Genome Consortium (2013): Mutational landscape of gingivo-buccal oral squamous cell carcinoma reveals new recurrently-mutated genes and molecular subgroups. *Nat Commun* 4, 2873.

Ishii, H., Wang, Y., Huebner, K. (2007): A Fhit-ing role in the DNA damage checkpoint response. *Cell Cycle* 6, 1044–1048.

Ishwad, C.S., Shuster, M., Bockmuhl, U., Thakker, N., Shah, P., Toomes, C., et al. (1999): Frequent allelic loss and homozygous deletion in chromosome band 8p23 in oral cancer. *Int J Cancer* 80, 25–31.

Izzo, J.G., Papadimitrakopoulou, V.A., Li, X.Q., Ibarguen, H., Lee, J.S., Ro, J.Y., et al. (1998): Dysregulated cyclin D1 expression early in head and neck tumorigenesis: in vivo evidence for an association with subsequent gene amplification. *Oncogene* 17, 2313–2322.

Jacquemont, C., Taniguchi, T. (2007): The Fanconi anemia pathway and ubiquitin. *BMC Biochem* 8 (Suppl 1), S10.

Jares, P., Fernandez, P.L., Campo, E., Nadal, A., Bosch, F., Aiza, G., et al. (1994): PRAD-1/cyclin D1 gene amplification correlates with messenger RNA overexpression and tumor progression in human laryngeal carcinomas. *Cancer Res* 54, 4813–4817.

Järvinen, A.K., Autio, R., Haapa-Paananen, S., Wolf, M., Saarela, M., Grenman, R., et al. (2006): Identification of target genes in laryngeal squamous cell carcinoma by high-resolution copy number and gene expression microarray analyses. *Oncogene* 25, 6997–7008.

Järvinen, A.-K., Autio, R., Kilpinen, S., Saarela, M., Leivo, I., Grénman, R., et al. (2008): High-resolution copy number and gene expression microarray analyses of head and neck squamous cell carcinoma cell lines of tongue and larynx. *Genes Chromosomes Cancer* 47, 500–509.

Jee, K.J., Persson, M., Heikinheimo, K., Passador-Santos, F., Aro, K., Knuutila, S., et al. (2013): Genomic profiles and CRTC1-MAML2 fusion distinguish different subtypes of mucoepidermoid carcinoma. *Mod Pathol* 26, 213–222.

Jemal, A., Bray, F., Center, M.M., Ferlay, J., Ward, E., Forman, D. (2011): Global cancer statistics. *CA Cancer J Clin* 61, 69–90.

Jeyaprakash, A.A., Santamaria, A., Jayachandran, U., Chan, Y.W., Benda, C., Nigg, E.A., et al. (2012): Structural and functional organization of the Ska complex, a key component of the kinetochore-microtubule interface. *Mol Cell* 46, 274–286.

Jin, Y.S., Higashi, K., Mandahl, N., Heim, S., Wennerberg, J., Biörklund, A., et al. (1990): Frequent rearrangement of chromosomal bands 1p22 and 11q13 in squamous cell carcinomas of the head and neck. *Genes Chromosomes Cancer* 2, 198–204.

Jin, Y., Höglund, M., Jin, C., Martins, C., Wennerberg, J., Åkervall, J., et al. (1998a): FISH characterization of head and neck carcinomas reveals that amplification of band 11q13 is associated with deletion of distal 11q. *Genes Chromosomes Cancer* 22, 312–320.

Jin, Y., Jin, C., Wennerberg, J., Mertens, F., Hoglund, M. (1998b): Cytogenetic and fluorescence in situ hybridization characterization of chromosome 1 rearrangements in head and neck carcinomas delineate a target region for deletions within 1p11–1p13. *Cancer Res* 58, 5859–5865.

Jin, C., Jin, Y., Gisselsson, D., Wennerberg, J., Wah, T.S., Strömback, B., et al. (2006a): Molecular cytogenetic characterization of the 11q13 amplicon in head and neck squamous cell carcinoma. *Cytogenet Genome Res* 115, 99–106.

Jin, C., Jin, Y., Wennerberg, J., Annertz, K., Enoksson, J., Mertens, F. (2006b): Cytogenetic abnormalities in 106 oral squamous cell carcinomas. *Cancer Genet Cytogenet* 164, 44–53.

Kalyankrishna, S., Grandis, J.R. (2006): Epidermal growth factor receptor biology in head and neck cancer. *J Clin Oncol* 24, 2666–2672.

Kanazawa, T., Iwashita, T., Kommareddi, P., Nair, T., Misawa, K., Misawa, Y., et al. (2007): Galanin and galanin receptor type 1 suppress proliferation in squamous carcinoma cells: activation of the extracellular signal regulated kinase pathway and induction of cyclin-dependent kinase inhibitors. *Oncogene* 26, 5762–5771.

Karras, J.R., Paisie, C.A., Huebner, K. (2014): Replicative stress and the FHIT gene: Roles in tumor suppression, genome stability and prevention of carcinogenesis. *Cancers* 6, 1208–1219.

Lechner, M., Frampton, G.M., Fenton, T., Feber, A., Palmer, G., Jay, A., et al. (2013): Targeted next-generation sequencing of head and neck squamous cell carcinoma identifies novel genetic alterations in HPV+ and HPV– tumors. *Genome Med* 5, 49.

Leemans, C.R., Braakjuis, B.J.M., Brakenhoff, R.H. (2011): The molecular biology of head and neck cancer. *Nat Rev Cancer* 11, 9–22.

Li, H., Wawrose, J.S., Gooding, W.E., Garraway, L.A., Lui, V.W., Peyser, N.D., et al. (2014): Genomic analysis of head and neck squamous cell carcinoma cell lines and human tumors: a rational approach to preclinical model selection. *Mol Cancer Res* 12, 571–582.

Lin, D.C., Meng, X., Hazawa, M., Nagata, Y., Varela, A.M., Xu, L., et al. (2014a): The genomic landscape of nasopharyngeal carcinoma. *Nat Genet* 46, 866–871.

Lin, D.C., Hao, J.J., Nagata, Y., Xu, L., Shang, L., Meng, X., et al. (2014b): Genomic and molecular characterization of esophageal squamous cell carcinoma. *Nat Genet* 46, 467–473.

Lin, D.C., Wang, M.R., Koeffler, H.P. (2014c): Targeting genetic lesions in esophageal cancer. *Cell Cycle* 13, 2013–2014c.

Llorente, J.L., López, F., Suárez, C., Hermsen, M.A. (2014): Sinonasal carcinoma: clinical, pathological, genetic and therapeutic advances. *Nat Rev Clin Oncol* 11, 460–472.

Lo Muzio, L., Campisi, G., Farina, A., Rubini, C., Pastore, L., Giannone, N., et al. (2007): Effect of p63 expression on survival in oral squamous cell carcinoma. *Cancer Invest* 25, 464–469.

Lourenço, S.V., Fernandes, J.D., Hsieh, R., Coutinho-Camillo, C.M., Bologna, S., Sangueza, M., et al. (2014): Head and neck mucosal melanoma: a review. *Am J Dermatopathol* 36, 578–587.

Lui, V.W., Peyser, N.D., Ng, P.K., Hritz, J., Zeng, Y., Lu, Y., et al. (2014): Frequent mutation of receptor protein tyrosine phosphatases provides a mechanism for STAT3 hyperactivation in head and neck cancer. *Proc Natl Acad Sci USA* 111, 1114–1119.

Luo, M.L., Shen, X.M., Zhang, Y., Wei, F., Xu, X., Cai, Y., et al. (2006): Amplification and overexpression of CTTN (*EMS1*) contribute to the metastasis of esophageal squamous cell carcinoma by promoting cell migration and anoikis resistance. *Cancer Res* 66, 11690–11699.

Manning, A.L., Yazinski, S.A., Nicolay, B., Bryll, A., Zou, L., Dyson, N.J. (2014): Suppression of genome instability in pRB-deficient cells by enhancement of chromosome cohesion. *Mol Cell* 53, 993–1004.

Marescalco, M.S., Capizzi, C., Condorelli, D.F., Barresi, V. (2014): Genome-wide analysis of recurrent copy-number alterations and copy-neutral loss of heterozygosity in head and neck squamous cell carcinoma. *J Oral Pathol Med* 43, 20–27.

Martin, C.L., Reshmi, S.C., Ried, T., Gottberg, W., Wilson, J.W., Reddy, J.K., et al. (2008): Chromosomal imbalances in oral squamous cell carcinoma: examination of 31 cell lines and review of the literature. *Oral Oncol* 44, 369–382.

Martínez, J.G., Pérez-Escuredo, J., Llorente, J.L., Suárez, C., Hermsen, M.A. (2012): Localization of centromeric breaks in head and neck squamous cell carcinoma. *Cancer Genet* 205, 622–629.

Mermel, C.H., Schumacher, S.E., Hill, B., Meyerson, M.L., Beroukhim, R., Getz, G. (2011): GISTIC2.0 facilitates sensitive and confident localization of the targets of focal somatic copy-number alteration in human cancers. *Genome Biol* 12:R41.

Michalides, R., vanVeelen, N., Hart, A., Loftus, B., Wientjens, E., Balm, A. (1995): Overexpression of cyclin D1 correlates with recurrence in a group of forty-seven operable squamous cell carcinomas of the head and neck. *Cancer Res* 55, 975–978.

Michalides, R.J., vanVeelen, N.M., Kristel, P.M., Hart, A.A., Loftus, B.M., Hilgers, F.J., et al. (1997): Overexpression of cyclin D1 indicates a poor prognosis in squamous cell carcinoma of the head and neck. *Arch Otolaryngol Head Neck Surg* 123, 497–502.

Misawa, K., Kanazawa, T., Misawa, Y., Uehara, T., Imai, A., Takahashi, G., et al. (2013): Galanin has tumor suppressor activity and is frequently inactivated by aberrant promoter methylation in head and neck cancer. *Transl Oncol* 6, 338–346.

Mitelman, F., Johansson, B., Mertens, F., editors (2014): Mitelman Database of Chromosome Aberrations and Gene Fusions in Cancer, http://cgap.nci.nih.gov/Chromosomes/Mitelman.

Morris, L.G., Kaufman, A.M., Gong, Y., Ramaswami, D., Walsh, L.A., Turcan, Ş., et al. (2013): Recurrent somatic mutation of FAT1 in multiple human cancers leads to aberrant Wnt activation. *Nat Genet* 45, 253–261.

Mountzios, G., Rampias, T., Psyrri, A. (2014): The mutational spectrum of squamous-cell carcinoma of the head and neck: targetable genetic events and clinical impact. *Ann Oncol* 25:1889–1900.

Muller, D., Millon, R., Theobald, S., Hussenet, T., Wasylyk, B., du Manoir, S., et al. (2006): Cyclin L1 (CCNL1) gene alterations in human head and neck squamous cell carcinoma. *Br J Cancer* 94, 1041–1044.

Narayanan, V., Mieczkowski, P.A., Kim, H.M., Petes, T.D., Lobachev, K.S. (2006): The pattern of gene amplification is determined by the chromosomal location of hairpin-capped breaks. *Cell* 125, 1283–1296.

Noutomi, Y., Oga, A., Uchida, K., Okafuji, M., Ita, M., Kawauchi, S., et al. (2006): Comparative genomic hybridization reveals genetic progression of oral squamous cell carcinoma from dysplasia via two different tumourigenic pathways. *J Pathol* 210, 67–74.

Ow, T.J., Sandulache, V.C., Skinner, H.D., Myers, J.N. (2013): Integration of cancer genomics with treatment selection: from the genome to predictive biomarkers. *Cancer* 119, 3914–3928.

Ozeri-Galai, E., Bester, A.C., Kerem, B. (2012): The complex basis underlying common fragile site instability in cancer. *Trends Genet* 28, 295-302.

Parikh, R.A., White, J.S., Huang, X., Schoppy, D.W., Baysal, B.E., Baskaran, R., et al. (2007): Loss of distal 11q is associated with DNA repair deficiency and reduced sensitivity to ionizing radiation in head and neck squamous cell carcinoma. *Genes Chromosomes Cancer* 46, 761–775.

Parikh, R.A., Appleman, L.J., Bauman, J.E., Sankunny, M., Lewis, D.W., Vlad, A., et al. (2014): Upregulation of the ATR-CHEK1 pathway in head and neck squamous cell carcinomas. *Genes Chromosomes Cancer* 53, 25–37.

Patel, K., Scrimieri, F., Ghosh, S., Zhong, J., Kim, M.S., Ren, Y.R., et al. (2013): FAM190A deficiency creates a cell division defect. *Am J Pathol* 183, 296–303.

Pearlstein, R.P., Benninger, M.S., Carey, T.E., Zarbo, R.J., Torres, F.X., Rybicki, B.A., et al. (1998): Loss of 18q predicts poor survival of patients with squamous cell carcinoma of the head and neck. *Genes Chromosomes Cancer* 21, 333–339.

Petrick, J.L., Wyss, A.B., Butler, A.M., Cummings, C., Sun, X., Poole, C., et al. (2014): Prevalence of human papillomavirus among oesophageal squamous cell carcinoma cases: systemic review and meta-analysis. *Br J Cancer* 110, 2369–2377.

Pickering, C.R., Zhang, J., Yoo, S.Y., Bengtsson, L., Moorthy, S., Neskey, D.M., et al. (2013): Integrative genomic characterization of oral squamous cell carcinoma identifies frequent somatic drivers. *Cancer Discov* 3, 770–781.

Pruitt, K.D., Brown, G.R., Hiatt, S.M., Thibaud-Nissen, F., Astashyn, A., Ermolaeva, O., et al. (2014): RefSeq: an update on mammalian reference sequences. *Nucleic Acids Res* 42: D756–D763.

Pytynia, K.B., Dahlstrom, K.R., Sturgis, E.M. (2014): Epidemiology of HPV-associated oropharyngeal cancer. *Oral Oncol* 50, 380–386.

Quintyne, N.J., Reing, J.E., Hoffelder, D.R., Gollin, S.M., Saunders, W.S. (2005): Spindle multipolarity is prevented by centrosomal clustering. *Science* 307, 127–129.

Rabinowits, G., Haddad, R.I. (2012): Overcoming resistance to EGFR inhibitor in head and neck cancer: a review of the literature. *Oral Oncol* 48, 1085–1089.

Ragin, C.C., Reshmi, S.C., Gollin, S.M. (2004): Mapping and analysis of HPV16 integration sites in a head and neck cancer cell line. *Int J Cancer* 110, 701–709.

Redon, R., Hussenet, T., Bour, G., Caulee, K., Jost, B., Muller, D., et al. (2002): Amplicon mapping and transcriptional analysis pinpoint cyclin L as a candidate oncogene in head and neck cancer. *Cancer Res* 62, 6211–6217.

Reshmi, S.C., Saunders, W.S., Kudla, D.M., Ragin, C.R., Gollin, S.M. (2004): Chromosomal instability and marker chromosome evolution in oral squamous cell carcinoma. *Genes Chromosomes Cancer* 41, 38–46.

Reshmi, S.C., Huang, X., Schoppy, D.W., Black, R.C., Saunders, W.S., Smith, D.I., et al. (2007a): Relationship between FRA11F and 11q13 gene amplification in oral cancer. *Genes Chromosomes Cancer* 46, 143–154.

Reshmi, S.C., Roychoudhury, S., Yu, Z., Feingold, E., Potter, D., Saunders, W.S., et al. (2007b): Inverted duplication pattern in anaphase bridges confirms the breakage-fusion-bridge (BFB) cycle model for 11q13 amplification. *Cytogenet Genome Res* 116, 46–52.

Richter, T.M., Tong, B.D., Scholnick, S.B. (2005): Epigenetic inactivation and aberrant transcription of *CSMD1* in squamous cell carcinoma cell lines. *Cancer Cell Int* 5, 29.

van der Riet, P., Nawroz, H., Hruban, R.H., Corio, R., Tokino, K., Koch, W., et al. (1994): Frequent loss of chromosome 9p21–22 early in head and neck cancer progression. *Cancer Res* 54, 1156–1158.

Rosenberg, P.S., Greene, M.H., Alter, B.P. (2003): Cancer incidence in persons with Fanconi anemia. *Blood* 101, 822–826.

Rothschild, B.L., Shim, A.H., Ammer, A.G., Kelley, L.C., Irby, K.B., Head, J.A., et al. (2006): Cortactin overexpression regulates actin-related protein 2/3 complex activity, motility, and invasion in carcinomas with chromosome 11q13 amplification. *Cancer Res* 66, 8017–8025.

Roz, L., Wu, C.L., Porter, S., Scully, C., Speight, P., Read, A., et al. (1996): Allelic imbalance on chromosome 3p in oral dysplastic lesions: an early event in oral carcinogenesis. *Cancer Res* 56, 1228–1231.

Rozier, L., El-Achkar, E., Apiou, F., Debatisse, M. (2004): Characterization of a conserved aphidicolin-sensitive common fragile site at human 4q22 and mouse 6C1: possible association with an inherited disease and cancer. *Oncogene* 23, 6872–6880.

Ruiz, C., Martins, J.R., Rudin, F., Schneider, S., Dietsche, T., Fischer, C.A., et al. (2012): Enhanced expression of ANO1 in head and neck squamous cell carcinoma causes cell migration and correlates with poor prognosis. *PLoS One* 7, e43265.

Salahshourifar, I., Vincent-Chong, V.K., Kallarakkal, T.G., Zain, R.B. (2014): Genomic DNA copy number alterations from precursor oral lesions to oral squamous cell carcinoma. *Oral Oncol* 50, 404–412.

Saldivar, J.C., Bene, J., Hosseini, S.A., Miuma, S., Horton, S., Heerema, N.A., et al. (2013): Characterization of the role of Fhit in suppression of DNA damage. *Adv Biol Regul* 53, 77–85.

Samuels, Y., Ericson, K. (2006): Oncogenic PI3K and its role in cancer. *Curr Opin Oncol* 18, 77–82.

Sankunny, M., Parikh, R.A., Lewis, D.W., Gooding, W.E., Saunders, W.S., Gollin, S.M. (2014): Targeted inhibition of ATR or CHEK1 reverses radioresistance in oral squamous cell carcinoma cells with distal chromosome arm 11q loss. *Genes Chromosomes Cancer* 53, 129–143.

Sarkaria, I., Oc, P., Talbot, S.G., Reddy, P.G., Ngai, I., Maghami, E., Patel, K.N., et al. (2006): Squamous cell carcinoma related oncogene/DCUN1D1 is highly conserved and activated by amplification in squamous cell carcinomas. *Cancer Res* 66, 9437–9444.

Saunders, W.S., Shuster, M., Huang, X., Gharaibeh, B., Enyenihi, A.H., Petersen, I., et al. (2000): Chromosomal instability and cytoskeletal defects in oral cancer cells. *Proc Natl Acad Sci USA* 97, 303–308.

Scholnick, S.B., Richter, T.M. (2003): The role of *CSMD1* in head and neck carcinogenesis. *Genes Chromosomes Cancer* 38, 281–283.

Settle, K., Posner, M.R., Shumaker, L.M., Tan, M., Suntharalingam, M., Goloubeva, O., et al. (2009): Racial survival disparity in head and neck cancer results from low prevalence of human papillomavirus infection in black oropharyngeal cancer patients. *Cancer Prev Res* 2, 776–781.

Shackney, S.E., Smith, C.A., Miller, B.W., Burholt, D.R., Murtha, K., Giles, H.R., et al. (1989): Model for the genetic evolution of human solid tumors. *Cancer Res* 49, 3344–3354.

Shi, Z.Z., Shang, L., Jiang, Y.Y., Hao, J.J., Zhang, Y., Zhang, T.T., et al. (2013): Consistent and differential genetic aberrations between esophageal dysplasia and squamous cell carcinoma detected by array comparative genomic hybridization. *Clin Cancer Res* 19, 5867–5878.

Shiwarski, D.J., Shao, C., Bill, A., Kim, J., Xiao, D., Bertrand, C., et al. (2014): To "grow" or "go": TMEM16A expression as a switch between tumor growth and metastasis in SCCHN. *Clin Cancer Res.* 20, 4673–4688.

Shuster, M.I., Han, L., LeBeau, M.M., Davis, E., Sawicki, M., Lese, C.M., et al. (2000): A consistent pattern of RIN1 rearrangements in oral squamous cell carcinoma cell lines supports a breakage-fusion-bridge cycle model for 11q13 amplification. *Genes Chromosomes Cancer* 28, 153–163.

Siegel, R., Ma, J., Zou, Z., Jemal, A. (2014): Cancer statistics, 2014. *CA Cancer J Clin* 64, 9–29.

Sivakumar, S., Daum, J.R., Tipton, A.R., Rankin, S., Gorbsky, G.J. (2014): The spindle and kinetochore-associated (Ska) complex enhances binding of the anaphase-promoting complex/cyclosome (APC/C) to chromosomes and promotes mitotic exit. *Mol Biol Cell* 25, 594–605.

Slaughter, D.P., Southwick, H.W., Smejkal, W. (1953): Field cancerization in oral stratified squamous epithelium; clinical implications of multicentric origin. *Cancer* 6, 963–968.

Smith, L., Liu, S.J., Goodrich, L., Jacobson, D., Degnin, C., Bentley, N., et al. (1998): Duplication of ATR inhibits Myo D, induces aneuploidy and eliminates radiation-induced G1 arrest. *Nat Genet* 19, 39–46.

Snijders, A.M., Schmidt, B.L., Fridlyand, J., Dekker, N., Pinkel, D., Jordan, R.C., et al. (2005): Rare amplicons implicate frequent deregulation of cell fate specification pathways in oral squamous cell carcinoma. *Oncogene* 24, 4232–4242.

Song, Y., Li, L., Ou, Y., Gao, Z., Li, E., Li, X., et al. (2014): Identification of genomic alterations in oesophageal squamous cell cancer. *Nature* 509, 91–95.

Squire, J.A., Bayani, J., Luk, C., Unwin, L., Tokunaga, J., MacMillan, C., et al. (2002): Molecular cytogenetic analysis of head and neck squamous cell carcinoma: By comparative genomic hybridization, spectral karyotyping, and expression array analysis. *Head Neck* 24, 874–887.

Stein, C.K., Glover, T.W., Palmer, J.L., Glisson, B.S. (2002): Direct correlation between FRA3B expression and cigarette smoking. *Genes Chromosomes Cancer* 34, 333–340.

Stenman, G., Persson, F., Andersson, M.K. (2014): Diagnostic and therapeutic implications of new molecular biomarkers in salivary gland cancers. *Oral Oncol* 50, 683–690.

Sticht, C., Hofele, C., Flechtenmacher, C., Bosch, F.X., Freier, K., Lichter, P., et al. (2005): Amplification of cyclin L1 is associated with lymph node metastases in head and neck squamous cell carcinoma (HNSCC). *Br J Cancer* 92, 770–774.

Suda, T., Hama, T., Kondo, S., Yuza, Y., Yoshikawa, M., Urashima, M., et al. (2012): Copy number amplification of the PIK3CA gene is associated with poor prognosis in non-lymph node metastatic head and neck squamous cell carcinoma. *BMC Cancer* 12, 416.

Syrjänen, K. (2013): Geographic origin is a significant determinant of human papillomavirus prevalence in oesophageal squamous cell carcinoma: systematic review and meta-analysis. *Scand J Infect Dis* 45, 1–18.

Takahashi, K., Yamanaka, S. (2006): Induction of pluripotent stem cells from mouse embryonic and adult fibroblast cultures by defined factors. *Cell* 126, 663–676.

Takebayashi, S., Hickson, A., Ogawa, T., Jung, K.Y., Mineta, H., Ueda, Y., et al. (2004): Loss of chromosome arm 18q with tumor progression in head and neck squamous cancer. *Genes Chromosomes Cancer* 41, 145–154.

Tang, M.R., Wang, Y.X., Guo, S., Han, S.Y., Wang, D. (2012): CSMD1 exhibits antitumor activity in A375 melanoma cells through activation of the Smad pathway. *Apoptosis* 17, 927–937.

Timpson, P., Wilson, A.S., Lehrbach, G.M., Sutherland, R.L., Musgrove, E.A., Daly, R.J. (2007): Aberrant expression of cortactin in head and neck squamous cell carcinoma cells is associated with enhanced cell proliferation and resistance to the epidermal growth factor receptor inhibitor gefitinib. *Cancer Res* 67, 9304–9314.

Togashi, Y., Arao, T., Kato, H., Matsumoto, K., Terashima, M., Hayashi, H., et al. (2014): Frequent amplification of ORAOV1 gene in esophageal squamous cell cancer promotes an aggressive phenotype via proline metabolism and ROS production. *Oncotarget* 5, 2962–2973.

Van Dyke, D.L., Worsham, M.J., Benninger, M.S., Krause, C.J., Baker, S.R., Wolf, G.T., et al. (1994): Recurrent cytogenetic abnormalities in squamous cell carcinomas of the head and neck region. *Genes Chromosomes Cancer* 9, 192–206.

Virgilio, L., Shuster, M., Gollin, S.M., Veronese, M.L., Ohta, M., Huebner, K., et al. (1996): FHIT gene alterations in head and neck squamous cell carcinomas. *Proc Natl Acad Sci USA* 93, 9770–9775.

Walter, V., Yin, X., Wilkerson, M.D., Cabanski, C.R., Zhao, N., Du, Y., et al. (2013): Molecular subtypes in head and neck cancer exhibit distinct patterns of chromosomal gain and loss of canonical cancer genes. *PLoS One* 8, e56823.

Watanabe, H., Ma, Q., Peng, S., Adelmant, G., Swain, D., Song, W., et al. (2014): SOX2 and p63 colocalize at genetic loci in squamous cell carcinomas. *J Clin Invest* 124, 1636–1645.

Weber, F., Xu, Y., Zhang, L., Patocs, A., Shen, L., Platzer, P., et al. (2007): Microenvironmental genomic alterations and clinicopathological behavior in head and neck squamous cell carcinoma. *JAMA* 297, 187–195.

Weinreb, I. (2013): Translocation-associated salivary gland tumors: a review and update. *Adv Anat Pathol* 20, 367–377.

Worsham, M.J., Wolman, S.R., Carey, T.E., Zarbo, R.J., Benninger, M.S., Van Dyke, D.L. (1999): Chromosomal aberrations identified in culture of squamous carcinomas are confirmed by fluorescence in situ hybridisation. *Mol Pathol* 52, 42–46.

Wreesmann, V.B., Singh, B. (2005): Chromosomal aberrations in squamous cell carcinomas of the upper aerodigestive tract: biologic insights and clinical opportunities. *J Oral Pathol Med* 34, 449–459.

Wreesmann, V.B., Wang, D., Goberdhan, A., Prasad, M., Ngai, I., Schnaser, E.A., et al. (2004): Genetic abnormalities associated with nodal metastasis in head and neck cancer. *Head Neck* 26, 10–15.

Young, N.R., Liu, J., Pierce, C., Wei, T.F., Grushko, T., Olopade, O.I., et al. (2013): Molecular phenotype predicts sensitivity of squamous cell carcinoma of the head and neck to epidermal growth factor receptor inhibition. *Mol Oncol* 7, 359–368.

Zhai, C., Li, Y., Mascarenhas, C., Lin, Q., Li, K., Vyrides, I., et al. (2014): The function of ORAOV1/LTO1, a gene that is overexpressed frequently in cancer: essential roles in the function and biogenesis of the ribosome. *Oncogene* 33, 484–494.

CHAPTER 13

Tumors of the lung

Penny Nymark[1,4], Eeva Kettunen[2] and Sakari Knuutila[3]

[1]Department of Toxicogenomics, Maastricht University, Maastricht, The Netherlands
[2]Health and Work Ability, Systems Toxicology, Finnish Institute of Occupational Health, Helsinki, Finland
[3]Department of Pathology, Haartman Institute and HUSLAB, University of Helsinki and Helsinki University Central Hospital, Helsinki, Finland
[4]Institute of Environmental Medicine, Karolinska Institute, Stockholm, Sweden

Cytogenetic information is available on three main types of lung tumors: pulmonary hamartomas, bronchial carcinoids, and the genuine lung cancers.

Pulmonary hamartomas are benign tumors that occur in 0.25% of the population. Cytogenetic studies based on some 300 samples indicate that rearrangements of 6p21.3 and 12q14–15 are common in these tumors (Kazmierczak et al., 1999; Kayser et al., 2003). The breakpoints in chromosomes 6 and 12 target the *HMGA1* and *HMGA2* genes, respectively. Two different translocations, t(6;14)(p21.3;q24) and t(3;12)(q27;q14), make up the bulk of the rearrangements involving these genes (Blank et al., 2001) with *HMGA2–LPP* fusion due to t(3;12)(q27;q14) being seen in 60–80% of the tumors.

Bronchial carcinoids are neuroendocrine tumors that are classified as either high-grade neuroendocrine carcinomas (NEC) or carcinoid tumors (CT) (Swarts et al., 2012). The clinically more aggressive NEC generally display more extensive genomic aberrations compared to CT. Some recurrent cytogenetic aberrations such as trisomy 7 (Johansson et al., 1993) and loss of 11q have been identified in roughly half of all cases, somewhat more frequently in NEC than in CT (Walch et al., 1998). A tumor suppressor gene (TSG) at 11q13.1, *MEN1*, has been shown to be involved in the development of lung carcinoids and

has also been found to be affected by mutations, loss of heterozygosity (LOH), and microsatellite instability (MSI) in such tumors (Ullmann et al., 1998; Walch et al., 1998). *MEN1* mutations are restricted to CT, whereas changes in the *RB1* pathway have been shown to be more common in NEC than in CT (Swarts et al., 2012). The gene *RASSF1A* at 3p21.3 has been found to be methylated in 71% of NEC and in 45% of CT, although methylation and silencing of TSG are otherwise relatively rare events in carcinoids compared to other lung cancers (Toyooka et al., 2001). *TP53* mutations are common in NEC but rare in CT, and indeed, the former, but not CT, is associated with smoking, which in its turn is strongly associated with this type of mutations (Swarts et al., 2012).

The most extensively studied tumors of the lung are the genuine *lung cancers*, which account for nearly one-third of all cancer deaths worldwide (Siegel et al., 2012). They are classified into *non-small cell lung cancer* (NSCLC) and *small cell lung cancer* (SCLC). NSCLC is further divided into *adenocarcinoma* (AdC, 50%), *squamous cell carcinoma* (SCC, 35%), and *large cell lung cancer* (LCLC, 15% but decreasing) as well as other less common types such as *adenosquamous carcinoma* (AdC/SCC) and *sarcomatoid carcinoma* (SC) (Cagle et al., 2013).

Cancer Cytogenetics: Chromosomal and Molecular Genetic Aberrations of Tumor Cells, Fourth Edition.
Edited by Sverre Heim and Felix Mitelman.
© 2015 John Wiley & Sons, Ltd. Published 2015 by John Wiley & Sons, Ltd.

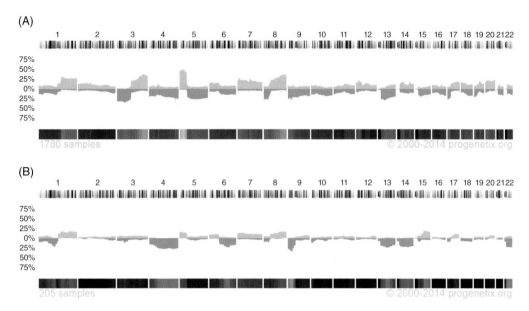

Figure 13.1 Recurrent DNA copy number aberrations in (A) 1780 lung carcinomas and (B) 205 malignant mesotheliomas. Losses are shown in blue and gains in yellow (*Source:* www.progenetix.org; keywords to search under "Search Samples": "lung" and "pleura -> malignant mesothelioma").

Nearly all lung carcinomas exhibit both multiple structural and numerical cytogenetic abnormalities, and comparative genomic hybridization (CGH) (both chromosomal and array) data from 1780 lung carcinomas can be found in the Progenetix database, which also provides data exploration and visualization tools (Cai et al., 2014). In addition, the UCSC Cancer Genome Browser allows for interactive examination of almost 1000 cancer genomes and their associated clinical information (including interactive Kaplan–Meier plots), which is available in The Cancer Genome Atlas (Cline et al., 2013). Finally, the Mitelman Database of Chromosome Aberrations and Gene Fusions in Cancer and the CanGEM database provide data on additional samples (Scheinin et al., 2008; Mitelman et al., 2014). A survey of these databases shows that the most common large aberrations detected by CGH in lung cancer are gains at 1q, 3q, 5p, and 8q and that the most common losses are from 3p, 4, 5q, 13q, and 17p (Figure 13.1A) (Cai et al., 2014). We restrict our summary here to the most recent knowledge on diagnostically relevant aberrations in the respective histological subtypes. In addition, we present some of the strategies for targeted therapy where cytogenetics has proved useful.

Diagnostically relevant genetic biomarkers in lung cancer

Lung carcinomas in patients with no evident exposure to carcinogens have been shown to carry fewer aberrations than those of patients with known exposures to, for example, tobacco smoke (Sanchez-Cespedes et al., 1998; Grepmeier et al., 2005). Mutations of the epidermal growth factor receptor gene (*EGFR*) in 7p12 are specifically associated with cancers in never-smokers, and the frequency of such mutations is higher in AdC, in females, and in Asian patients (Mäki-Nevala et al., 2014). *EGFR* amplification is at least partially independent of mutations and is associated with great sensitivity and prolonged progression-free survival among patients with NSCLC who are treated with EGFR tyrosine kinase inhibitors (TKIs) (Franklin et al., 2002; Zhao et al., 2005; Li et al., 2014). *EGFR* amplification has shown a unique association with in-frame deletions in exon 19 of the gene (Sholl et al., 2009). Also, insertion–deletion variations in *EGFR* have been reported and are thought to lead to sensitivity to TKI treatment (Tuononen et al., 2013). These aberrations are not detectable by RT-PCR kits available for diagnostic purpose, a circumstance that argues for the use of

Table 13.1 Diagnostically and therapeutically important genomic aberrations in lung cancer

Aberration	Target gene	Histological subtype	Molecular/ gene expression subtype*,†	Diagnostic relevance	Therapeutic relevance	References
inv(2)(p21p23)	EML4–ALK	AdC; SCC (rare); LCLC	3.1	Predicts response to therapy	Response to ALK inhibitors (crizotinib)	West et al. (2012), CLCGP and NGM (2013), and Tuononen et al. (2014)
+2p23	ALK	AdC		Associated with acquired resistance to ALK inhibitors		Stella et al. (2013)
+3p21.3	RBM5	AdC; SCLC	—	Predicts response to cisplatin	Possibly resensitizes to cisplatin	Li et al. (2012)
+3q26.3	PIK3CA	AdC; SCC	5.1; mainly classical	Possibly predicts response to therapy	Possible response to, for example, PI3K inhibitors	West et al. (2012)
6q22 rearrangement	ROS1	AdC	7.1	Possibly predicts response to therapy	Possible response to ROS1 inhibitors	West et al. (2012)
+7p12	EGFR	AdC; SCC (rare)	1.1	Predicts response to therapy	Response to TKIs (gefitinib, erlotinib)	West et al. (2012) and CLCGP and NGM (2013)
+7q31	MET	AdC	4.1	Associated with acquired resistance to EGFR inhibitors	Response to MET inhibitors	Stella et al. (2013)
+10q23	PTEN	AdC	5.2	Possibly predicts response to therapy	Possible response to, for example, PI3K inhibitors	West et al. (2012)
+3q26	SOX2	SCC	Mainly classical	Possibly predicts response to therapy	Response to cyclin D1 inhibitors	Drilon et al. (2012)
+8p11	FGFR1	SCC; SCLC	Nonclassical	Possibly predicts response to therapy	FGFR1 inhibitor (AZD4547, BGJ398)	CGARN (2012) and Drilon et al. (2012)

*West et al. (2012).
†Wilkerson et al. (2010).

targeted next-generation sequencing (NGS) for screening purposes (Tuononen et al., 2013). The power of NGS in this context is also illustrated by the recent finding that ephrin gene mutations are recurrent and common in AdC (Mäki-Nevala et al., 2013). In a small proportion of nonsmokers, oncogenic fusion genes such as *EML4–ALK* and other types of rearrangements involving *ALK*, *KIF5B–RET*, and fusions with *ROS1*, *FGFR1*, and *NTRK1* have been reported (Vaishnavi et al., 2013). The *EML4–ALK*

fusion is the result of a paracentric inversion in the short arm of chromosome 2, inv(2)(p21p23), first reported by Soda et al. (2007). It is present in 2–12% of lung carcinomas depending largely on the study population, and it is associated with younger age and AdC histology although a few positive SCC and LCLC cases have also been reported (Table 13.1) (Calio et al., 2014; Tuononen et al., 2014). *ALK* fusions and mutations of *EGFR* and *KRAS* have been shown to be mutually exclusive, while *MET* mutations seem to be recurrent (in 36%) and also *PIK3CA*, *CTNNB1*, and *TP53* mutations have been found in these tumors (Tuononen et al., 2014).

A large study of 371 AdC analyzed by single-nucleotide polymorphism (SNP) arrays identified a total of 31 recurrent focal aberrations, of which amplification of 14q13.3 was the most frequent (12%). Additionally, the study identified a proto-oncogene (*NKX2-1*) in this subband as well as LOH at 17p and 19p (Weir et al., 2007). *NKX2-1* has since been explored for its potential as a therapeutic target (Winslow et al., 2011). Loss and downregulation of genes at 19p13 have been linked to AdC and asbestos exposure in lung cancer (Wikman et al., 2007; Ruosaari et al., 2008). The region contains the *KEAP1* TSG, which may constitute an early biomarker due to its role in the interaction between the aryl hydrocarbon receptor (AhR) and the transcription factor NRF2 (Anttila et al., 2011). Interestingly, gain at 12p13.3 in lung cancer has been related to the overexpression of two microRNAs (miRNAs; miR-141 and miR-200c) that regulate *KEAP1*, demonstrating another mechanisms for downregulation of this gene (Nymark et al., 2011; van Jaarsveld et al., 2013). Decreased expression of *KEAP1*, coupled with increased expression of *NFE2L2*, has been associated with poor prognosis (Drilon et al., 2012). In addition, a t(15;19)(q11;p13) interrupting *NOTCH3* at 19p13 was detected in a lung tumor of a nonsmoking young woman, and overexpression of *NOTCH3* has been significantly associated with abnormalities in chromosome 19 in seven lung cancer cell lines (Dang et al., 2000). Loss of 13q14.1 and gain of 8q24.2 (*MYC*) have been associated with disease-free survival in AdC. Furthermore, gain of *MYC*, co-occurrence of *EGFR* mutations, and amplification as well as simple gains at 16p (*FUS*) have been shown to be frequent in AdC of never-smokers (Job et al., 2010). LOH at 16p (*TSC2*) has been associated with adenomatous hyperplasia preceding AdC (Takamochi et al., 2001). AdC in never-smokers is characterized by frequent loss of *RB1* (13q14.2) and *WRN* (8p12) and has been associated with scar-like fibrosis (Job et al., 2010). Gain of 19q13.1 as well as loss of 22q12.2 has been linked with current or former smoking history in AdC (Shibata et al., 2005).

SCC, which is most strongly associated with smoking, exhibits similarities with AdC as far as acquired genomic aberrations are concerned. Nevertheless, differences in response to treatment between the two tumor types suggest the existence of substantial dissimilarities in biology (Drilon et al., 2012). The classical *EGFR* mutations have been reported to be extremely rare in SCC, but they nevertheless exist, and a distinct *EGFR* deletion mutation has been described in a few SCC (5–8%) supporting the inclusion of all subtypes in genomic diagnosis (Drilon et al., 2012; CLCGP and NGM, 2013; Calio et al., 2014). However, the most striking difference between AdC and SCC is seen for gain of 3q23–29 (Kettunen et al., 2000; Tonon et al., 2005b; Garnis et al., 2006; CGARN, 2012; Drilon et al., 2012; Stella et al., 2013). Amplification (>88%) and overexpression of the gene *TP63* (3q28) as well as amplification (~43%) and mutations in *PIK3CA* (3q26.3) have been found in SCC (Tonon et al., 2005a; Kawano et al., 2006; Drilon et al. 2012; Stella et al., 2013). Copy number aberrations (CNA) of *PIK3CA* predict response to PI3K inhibitors (Table 13.1), and *TP63* (3q27–28) amplification has been associated with improved survival as well as with the so-called classical gene expression subtype in SCC (Wilkerson et al., 2010; Drilon et al., 2012; Stella et al., 2013). Also, amplification (70%) of *SOX2*, at 3q26.3, has been associated with increased overall survival (Drilon et al., 2012). In contrast to AdC, which typically show loss at 8p11-p12, SCC has been shown to harbor gains of this region in 22%, and the gene *FGFR1* is thought to be a target (Drilon et al., 2012; Stella et al., 2013). In addition, *SKP2* (5p13) has been found to be more frequently amplified in SCC than in AdC (Jiang et al., 2004), and overexpression of this gene has been related to metastasis and poor prognosis (Yokoi et al., 2004; Takanami, 2005). Smoking has been shown to cause more gains as well as losses in regions containing genes, whereas tumors in nonsmoking or light-smoking patients more often have losses but typically of regions without genes (Huang et al., 2011). Furthermore, inactivation of *CDKN2A* (9p21.3) by multiple mechanisms, including deletion (30–60%), occurs frequently in NSCLC and apparently exclusively in smokers (Merlo et al., 1995; Brambilla et al., 1999; Panani and Roussos, 2006; Wikman and Kettunen, 2006). Deletion of *CDKN2A* together with lack of *p16INK4* and *ARF* expression has been described in 29% of SCC (CGARN, 2012).

Finally, gains at 1q21–25 and 8q11–25 as well as losses at 3p12–14, 4p15–16, 8p22–23, 10q, and 21q have been associated with a metastatic SCC phenotype (Petersen et al., 2000).

The karyotypes of *nonneuroendocrine types of LCLC* exhibit several similarities with AdC and SCC and were recently reassigned almost completely to either of these subtypes based on immunohistochemical and genomic analyses (CLCGP and NGM, 2013). *ALK* fusions have also been identified in LCLC (Tuononen et al., 2014). Large cell neuroendocrine carcinoma (LCNEC) exhibits similarities with SCLC (discussed in the following text) (Ullmann et al., 1998, 2001; CLCGP and NGM, 2013). In AdC/SCC, aberrations in each histologic component are characteristic for AdC and SCC, respectively, whereas SCs are generally characterized by gains rather than losses of genomic material (Torenbeek et al., 1999; Blaukovitsch et al., 2006).

SCLC account for one-fifth of all lung cancers and are, together with LCNEC and carcinoids, considered to be neuroendocrine tumors. *EGFR* and *KRAS* are rarely altered in SCLC, but *FGFR1* (8p11) has been found to be affected by focal amplification (Peifer et al., 2012). The first recurrent aberration to be identified in almost 100% of SCLC was loss of 3p (Whang-Peng et al., 1982), with subband 3p21.3 currently commanding the greatest interest as the site of a pathogenetically important suppressor gene. These losses are not specific for SCLC as they also occur in the majority (>70%) of NSCLC and even in premalignant SCLC (Sutherland et al., 2010). Several potential TSG have been identified in the region, such as *RASSF1A*, *FUS*, *CACNA2D2*, and *RBM5* (Liu et al., 2007; Sutherland et al., 2010). *RBM5* has been shown to resensitize cisplatin-resistant lung cancer cells to cisplatin, and loss of the gene may serve as a biomarker for prediction of response to this drug (Li et al., 2012). LOH at 3p21 has been associated with an early age of smoking onset (Hirao et al., 2001), and loss of 3p21.3, as well as downregulation of genes in this subband, has been linked to asbestos exposure in lung cancer (Marsit et al., 2004; Nymark et al., 2006). In addition, SCLC have been shown to harbor unbalanced translocations, mainly involving 3q13.2 and chromosome 5 (Ashman et al., 2002). SCLC, as well as LCNEC, often exhibit loss of *RB1* (13q14.2) expression in up to 90% of the cases, mainly attributable to deletions, whereas only 25%

of NSCLC show loss of this gene (Wikman and Kettunen, 2006; Peifer et al., 2012).

Lung cancer patients have higher amounts of free circulating DNA in both sputum and serum (Xue et al., 2006). Single circulating tumor cells (CTC) may be useful in identifying tumors and possibly even for establishing the subtype. Ni et al. (2013) found highly reproducible patterns of CNA in CTC, patterns that were similar among patients with the same subtype; 8q (*MYC*), 5p (*TERT*), 3q29, 17p22, 17q25.3, and 20p13 gains were associated with AdC, while 6p gains were associated with both SCLC and AdC.

Therapeutic importance of acquired genomic aberrations in lung cancer

A novel classification of lung cancer into molecular subtypes, based on the molecular tests and drugs that may be used for treatment, was recently proposed (West et al., 2012). Some of these subtypes are based on cytogenetic changes, such as the *EML4–ALK* fusion (inversion 2p21p23), *PIK3CA* amplification (3q26.3), *PTEN* deletion (10q23.3), or translocations involving *ROS1* (6q22) (see Table 13.1 for the complete list). EGFR was long the only kinase for which FDA-approved TKI had been developed (e.g., erlotinib and gefitinib), but in later years, also crizotinib has been approved and is used in patients whose tumors carry the *EML4–ALK* fusion gene (Soda et al., 2007). Crizotinib also inhibits ROS1 (6q22), indicating that patients whose tumors have acquired aberrations of this gene may also benefit from the drug (Cagle et al., 2013). Other TKIs are being developed such as sunitinib, sorafenib, and vandetanib for lung cancers with *KIF5B–RET* fusion as well as tivantinib and onartuzumab for patients with tumors carrying *MET* (7q31) amplification (Stella et al., 2013). In general, these targetable alterations are largely associated with younger patients, nonsmokers, and AdC histology, and so only these patients respond favorably when treated with TKI. But even in this most favorable subgroup, resistance, either primary or acquired, is not an uncommon phenomenon and is associated with further alterations occurring in the tumor genomes. For example, *HER2* (17q12) and *MET* (7q31) amplifications may cause acquired resistance (Engelman et al., 2007; Stella et al., 2013). Therefore, the so-called irreversible pan-TKIs (e.g., afatinib and XL647) targeting several kinases simultaneously are being explored and developed (Cagle et al., 2013; Stella et al., 2013). Bevacizumab, a monoclonal antibody against the product of *VEGF* (6p21), is another approved treatment for advanced NSCLC and targets angiogenesis (Das and Wakelee, 2012). Several other possibilities for targeted therapy are also being exploited, such as miRNAs and the interaction between *CDK4* (12q14), amplified in a subset of lung cancers, and *KRAS* mutations (Wikman et al., 2005; Puyol et al., 2010; Vannini et al., 2013).

Pleura

Primary pleural tumors are extremely rare (reviewed in Granville et al., 2005). DNA CNA in solitary fibrous tumors (SFT) of the pleura (reviewed in Bertucci et al., 2013) have shown gain of 8p11.23–11.22 in 20% of cases, whereas losses of 8p23.3 and 1p34.2 were seen in 15% (Rodriguez-Gonzalez et al., 2014). Some of the primary pleural tumors are not typical of this tissue and organ; for example, a synovial sarcoma of the pleura has been described, which displayed the specific translocation t(X;18)(p11;q11) causing a *SYT–SSX* fusion gene (Bégueret et al., 2005).

The principal tumor type of the pleura is *malignant pleural mesothelioma* (MPM). Most of these tumors (~80%) are believed to develop as a consequence of previous asbestos exposure but with a very long latency period. Early karyotype and CGH studies indicated a chaotic nature of chromosomal aberrations in MPM (Tiainen et al., 1988, 1989; Björkqvist et al., 1998). Similar to what is the case for lung carcinomas, a detailed view with molecular karyotyping data on the complex acquired genomic imbalances of almost 350 MPM and other pleural tumors is provided in publicly available databases (Scheinin et al., 2008; Cai et al., 2014; Mitelman et al., 2014). The gains in MPM primarily involve chromosome arms 1p, 5p, 7p, 7q, 8q, 9p, 12q, and 17q, whereas losses affect nearly all chromosomes (Figure 13.1B). The epithelial MPM subtype has been associated with gain of 7q and losses at 3p14–21 and 17p12-pter, whereas sarcomatoid MPM typically display gains at 5p, 8q, and 17q and losses at 7q and 15q (Krismann et al., 2002). Losses of chromosomes 1, 4, and 9 and a

breakpoint at 1p11–22 have been related to a high asbestos fiber content in the tumors (Tammilehto et al., 1992).

The overall DNA gain/loss pattern of MPM may be useful in differentiating these tumors from pleural sarcomas and lung carcinomas. CGH profiling has shown that losses at 4p, 4q, 6q, 14q, and 9p and gains at 15q are common in MPM, whereas gains at 8q, 1q, 7p, and 6p dominate in lung carcinomas (Björkqvist et al., 1998; Knuuttila et al., 2006). Other means to discriminate MPM from lung AdC and normal pleura are provided by epigenetic deregulation, that is, miRNA expression (see the following text) and DNA methylation patterns of cancer-associated genes such as *APC* and *CDH1* or global profiles (reviewed by Kettunen and Knuutila, 2014). DNA methylation profiles may also be used as predictors of MPM patient survival (Christensen et al., 2009).

The most common aberration in MPM (>80%) is a homozygous deletion of 9p21.3 affecting *CDKN2A/p16* and occasionally adjacent genes as well (Simon et al., 2005; Musti et al., 2006; Pei et al., 2006; Taniguchi et al., 2007). While *CDKN2A* methylation and mutations (~15%) in MPM did not prove a significant clinical association (Kettunen and Knuutila, 2014), homozygous deletion of *CDKN2A* is of potential diagnostic significance. FISH analysis of *CDKN2A* copy numbers, in adjunction to cytology or karyotyping, improved the sensitivity up to 79% for the detection of MPM in effusions (Factor et al., 2009; Husain et al., 2009). Loss of *CDKN2A* is associated with a bleak prognosis in MPM (Lopez-Rios et al., 2006).

3p21, harboring the TSG *BAP1*, is frequently deleted in MPM. Forty-two percent of MPM show either *BAP1* loss, somatic mutation, or both (Bott et al., 2011). In spite of this, MPM patients with somatic *BAP1* mutations do not display any distinct clinical phenotype (Zauderer et al., 2013). Interestingly, germline *BAP1* mutations were found in a new cancer syndrome that predisposes to MPM in addition to various melanocytic neoplasms, renal cell carcinoma, and potentially also other tumors (Bott et al., 2011; Testa et al., 2011; Wiesner et al., 2011; Carbone et al., 2012; Popova et al., 2013).

The third frequently altered region in MPM is 22q, deleted in 33–70% (Bott et al., 2011; Cai et al., 2014). The region harbors the tumor suppressor neurofibromatosis 2 gene (*NF2*), which is mutated in 35–40% of MPM (Ladanyi et al., 2012). Inactivation of the *NF2* gene product Merlin has been associated with invasiveness in mesothelioma cells (Poulikakos et al., 2006). Merlin may contribute to tumorigenesis through activation of the Hippo signaling pathway. Moreover, MPM may harbor homozygous deletions or inactivating mutations of *LATS2* (13q12), another component of Hippo signaling (Murakami et al., 2011). Loss of Merlin causes activation of the cell survival-promoting mTORC1 signaling in MPM, and Merlin-negative MPM have shown sensitivity to rapamycin, indicating that these tumors could be potential targets for therapeutic options (Lopez-Lago et al., 2009).

Asbestos fibers have been shown to activate EGFR expression. Although mutations only infrequently play a role in the activation of signaling pathways involving receptor tyrosine kinases (RTK) in MPM, the coactivation of overlapping pathways involving RTK such as EGFR, MET, ERBB3, and AXL in MPM cell lines has been demonstrated (Ou et al., 2011). It was therefore suggested that inhibition of multi-RTK signaling (i.e., pan-TKIs) could be a beneficial treatment strategy in MPM, similarly to what is the case in lung cancer (Ou et al., 2011; Favoni et al., 2012).

As for lung carcinomas, insights into the molecular pathology and the introduction of new methodologies have recently enabled analyses providing information on new and potentially therapeutically important genomic aberrations in MPM. Using next-generation RNA sequencing after analysis by banding cytogenetics had hinted at where in the genome the pathogenetically important fusion gene might be, Panagopoulos et al. (2013) described an *EWSR1–YY1* fusion brought about by the translocation t(14;22)(q32;q12) in two MPM. The potential usefulness of long noncoding RNAs (lncRNA) as well as miRNAs for diagnostic and prognostic purposes in MPM has been demonstrated (Wright et al., 2013; Truini et al., 2014). MPM can be distinguished from normal pleura as well as AdC of the lung and metastatic epithelial tumors based on miRNA expression profiles (Guled et al., 2009; Benjamin et al., 2010). Of note, *CDKN2A* and *NF2* are targeted by miR-885-3p, which was shown to be highly expressed in MPM (Guled et al., 2009).

Summary

Benign hamartomas often (60–80% of the tumors) show *HMGA2–LPP* fusion due to a translocation t(3;12)(q27;q14). In bronchial carcinoids, no specific fusions or mutations have been described, but alterations in the TSG *MEN1* have been implicated in tumorigenesis.

The genuine lung cancers show highly distinct patterns of aberrations depending on the histological subtype. Furthermore, the molecular subtypes are based on clinically targetable aberrations. In AdC, *EGFR* (7p12) amplifications and *ALK* (2p23) fusions (e.g., *EML4–ALK*) are currently the most useful clinical cytogenetic markers that can be targeted by molecular drugs (Table 13.1). Guidelines for which patients are eligible for such biological therapies have been published, and one can safely assume that such therapies will increase in importance as well as numbers in the years to come (Cagle et al., 2013). In SCC, several targetable markers at the frequently amplified region in 3q have been identified such as *PIK3CA* and *SOX2* (both at 3q26.3). Also, *FGFR1* (8p11) gains have been exploited for their therapeutic potential. LCLC have recently been shown to exhibit largely the same cytogenetic patterns as either AdC or SCC, and patients with these tumors can be expected to benefit from the same therapies. The research on SCLC has not yet revealed similarly useful targets, although gain of *FGFR1* and loss of *RBM5* may be envisaged in such a role.

In MPM, deletion at 9p21 (*CDKN2A*) is a common and prognostically unfavorable change. Tests for this deletion could help detect MPM in effusions. Somatic and germline mutations of *BAP1* at 3p21 have been found and in the latter setting predispose to a new cancer syndrome. A novel fusion gene, *EWSR1–YY1* resulting from t(14;22)(q32;q12), was recently described in two MPM cases.

References

Anttila S, Raunio H, Hakkola J (2011): Cytochrome P450-mediated pulmonary metabolism of carcinogens: regulation and cross-talk in lung carcinogenesis. *Am J Respir Cell Mol Biol* 44: 583–590.

Ashman JN, Brigham J, Cowen ME, Bahia H, Greenman J, Lind M, et al. (2002): Chromosomal alterations in small cell lung cancer revealed by multicolour fluorescence in situ hybridization. *Int J Cancer* 102: 230–236.

Bégueret H, Galateau-Salle F, Guillou L, Chetaille B, Brambilla E, Vignaud J, et al. (2005): Primary intrathoracic synovial sarcoma: a clinicopathologic study of 40 t(X;18)-positive cases from the French Sarcoma Group and the Mesopath Group. *Am J Surg Pathol* 29: 339–346.

Benjamin H, Lebanony D, Rosenwald S, Cohen L, Gibori H, Barabash N, et al. (2010): A diagnostic assay based on microRNA expression accurately identifies malignant pleural mesothelioma. *J Mol Diagn* 12: 771–779.

Bertucci F, Bouvier-Labit C, Finetti P, Adelaide J, Metellus P, Mokhtari K, et al. (2013): Comprehensive genome characterization of solitary fibrous tumors using high-resolution array-based comparative genomic hybridization. *Genes Chromosomes Cancer* 52: 156–164.

Björkqvist A-M, Tammilehto L, Nordling S, Nurminen M, Anttila S, Mattson K, et al. (1998): Comparison of DNA copy number changes in malignant mesothelioma, adenocarcinoma and large-cell anaplastic carcinoma of the lung. *Br J Cancer* 77: 260–269.

Blank C, Schoenmakers EF, Rogalla P, Huys EH, van Rijk AA, Drieschner N, et al. (2001): Intragenic breakpoint within RAD51L1 in a t(6;14)(p21.3;q24) of a pulmonary chondroid hamartoma. *Cytogenet Cell Genet* 95: 17–19.

Blaukovitsch M, Halbwedl I, Kothmaier H, Gogg-Kammerer M, Popper HH (2006): Sarcomatoid carcinomas of the lung—are these histogenetically heterogeneous tumors? *Virchows Arch* 449: 455–461.

Bott M, Brevet M, Taylor BS, Shimizu S, Ito T, Wang L, et al. (2011): The nuclear deubiquitinase BAP1 is commonly inactivated by somatic mutations and 3p21.1 losses in malignant pleural mesothelioma. *Nat Genet* 43, 668–672.

Brambilla E, Gazzeri S, Moro D, Lantuejoul S, Veyrenc S, Brambilla C (1999): Alterations of Rb pathway (Rb-p16INK4-Cyclin D1) in preinvasive bronchial lesions. *Clin Cancer Res* 5: 243–250.

Cagle PT, Allen TC, Olsen RJ (2013): Lung cancer biomarkers: present status and future developments. *Arch Pathol Lab Med* 137: 1191–1198.

Cai H, Kumar N, Ai N, Gupta S, Rath P, Baudis M (2014): Progenetix: 12 years of oncogenomic data curation. *Nucleic Acids Res* 42: D1055–D1062.

Calio A, Nottegar A, Gilioli E, Bria E, Pilotto S, Peretti U, et al. (2014): ALK/EML4 fusion gene may be found in pure squamous carcinoma of the lung. *J Thorac Oncol* 9: 729–732.

Carbone M, Ferris LK, Baumann F, Napolitano A, Lum CA, Flores EG, et al. (2012): BAP1 cancer syndrome: malignant mesothelioma, uveal and cutaneous melanoma, and MBAITs. *J Transl Med* 10: 179.

Cancer Genome Atlas Research Network (CGARN) (2012): Comprehensive genomic characterization of squamous cell lung cancers. *Nature* 489: 519–525.

Christensen B, Houseman E, Godleski J, Marsit C, Longacker J, Roelofs C, et al. (2009): Epigenetic profiles distinguish pleural mesothelioma from normal pleura and predict lung asbestos burden and clinical outcome. *Cancer Res* 69: 227–234.

The Clinical Lung Cancer Genome Project (CLCGP) and Network Genomic Medicine (NGM) (2013): A genomics-based classification of human lung tumors. *Sci Transl Med* 5: 209ra153.

Cline MS, Craft B, Swatloski T, Goldman M, Ma S, Haussler D, et al. (2013): Exploring TCGA Pan-Cancer data at the UCSC Cancer Genomics Browser. *Sci Rep* 3: 2652.

Dang TP, Gazdar AF, Virmani AK, Sepetavec T, Hande KR, Minna JD, et al. (2000): Chromosome 19 translocation, overexpression of Notch3, and human lung cancer. *J Natl Cancer Inst* 92: 1355–1357.

Das M, Wakelee H (2012): Targeting VEGF in lung cancer. *Expert Opin Ther Targets* 16: 395–406.

Drilon A, Rekhtman N, Ladanyi M, Paik P (2012): Squamous-cell carcinomas of the lung: emerging biology, controversies, and the promise of targeted therapy. *Lancet Oncol* 13: e418–e426.

Engelman JA, Zejnullahu K, Mitsudomi T, Song Y, Hyland C, Park JO, et al. (2007): MET amplification leads to gefitinib resistance in lung cancer by activating ERBB3 signaling. *Science* 316: 1039–1043.

Factor RE, Dal Cin P, Fletcher JA, Cibas ES (2009): Cytogenetics and fluorescence in situ hybridization as adjuncts to cytology in the diagnosis of malignant mesothelioma. *Cancer* 117: 247–253.

Favoni RE, Daga A, Malatesta P, Florio T (2012): Preclinical studies identify novel targeted pharmacological strategies for treatment of human malignant pleural mesothelioma. *Br J Pharmacol* 166: 532–553.

Franklin WA, Veve R, Hirsch FR, Helfrich BA, Bunn PA Jr (2002): Epidermal growth factor receptor family in lung cancer and premalignancy. *Semin Oncol* 29: 3–14.

Garnis C, Lockwood WW, Vucic E, Ge Y, Girard L, Minna JD, et al. (2006): High resolution analysis of non-small cell lung cancer cell lines by whole genome tiling path array CGH. *Int J Cancer* 118: 1556–1564.

Granville L, Laga A, Allen T, Dishop M, Roggli V, Churg A, et al. (2005): Review and update of uncommon primary pleural tumors: a practical approach to diagnosis. *Arch Pathol Lab Med* 129: 1428–1443.

Grepmeier U, Dietmaier W, Merk J, Wild PJ, Obermann EC, Pfeifer M, et al. (2005): Deletions at chromosome 2q and 12p are early and frequent molecular alterations in bronchial epithelium and NSCLC of long-term smokers. *Int J Oncol* 27, 481–488.

Guled M, Lahti L, Lindholm PM, Salmenkivi K, Bagwan I, Nicholson AG, et al. (2009): CDKN2A, NF2, and JUN are dysregulated among other genes by miRNAs in malignant mesothelioma: a miRNA microarray analysis. *Genes Chromosomes Cancer* 48: 615–623.

Hirao T, Nelson HH, Ashok TD, Wain JC, Mark EJ, Christiani DC, et al. (2001): Tobacco smoke-induced DNA damage and an early age of smoking initiation induce chromosome loss at 3p21 in lung cancer. *Cancer Res* 61: 612–615.

Huang YT, Lin X, Liu Y, Chirieac LR, McGovern R, Wain J, et al. (2011): Cigarette smoking increases copy number alterations in nonsmall-cell lung cancer. *Proc Natl Acad Sci USA* 108: 16345–16350.

Husain AN, Colby TV, Ordonez NG, Krausz T, Borczuk A, Cagle PT, et al. (2009): Guidelines for pathologic diagnosis of malignant mesothelioma: a consensus statement from the International Mesothelioma Interest Group. *Arch Pathol Lab Med* 133: 1317–1331.

Jiang F, Yin Z, Caraway NP, Li R, Katz RL (2004): Genomic profiles in stage I primary non small cell lung cancer using comparative genomic hybridization analysis of cDNA microarrays. *Neoplasia* 6: 623–635.

Job B, Bernheim A, Beau-Faller M, Camilleri-Broet S, Girard P, Hofman P, et al. (2010): Genomic aberrations in lung adenocarcinoma in never smokers. *PLoS One* 5: e15145.

Johansson M, Heim S, Mandahl N, Hambraeus G, Johansson L, Mitelman F (1993): Cytogenetic analysis of six bronchial carcinoids. *Cancer Genet Cytogenet* 66: 33–38.

Kawano O, Sasaki H, Endo K, Suzuki E, Haneda H, Yukiue H, et al. (2006): PIK3CA mutation status in Japanese lung cancer patients. *Lung Cancer* 54: 209–215.

Kayser K, Dunnwald D, Kazmierczak B, Bullerdiek J, Kaltner H, Zick Y, et al. (2003): Chromosomal aberrations, profiles of expression of growth-related markers including galectins and environmental hazards in relation to the incidence of chondroid pulmonary hamartomas. *Pathol Res Pract* 199: 589–598.

Kazmierczak B, Meyer-Bolte K, Tran K, Wockel W, Breightman I, Rosigkeit J, et al. (1999): A high frequency of tumors with rearrangements of genes of the HMGI(Y) family in a series of 191 pulmonary chondroid hamartomas. *Genes Chromosomes Cancer* 26: 125–133.

Kettunen E, Knuutila S (2014): Malignant mesothelioma, molecular markers. In: *Occupational Cancers*. (Eds. Anttila SL, Boffetta P). Berlin: Springer.

Kettunen E, El-Rifai W, Björkqvist AM, Wolff H, Karjalainen A, Anttila S, et al. (2000): A broad amplification pattern at 3q in squamous cell lung cancer: a fluorescence in situ hybridization study. *Cancer Genet Cytogenet* 117: 66–70.

Knuuttila A, Jee K, Taskinen E, Wolff H, Knuutila S, Anttila S (2006): Spindle cell tumours of the pleura: a clinical, histological and comparative genomic hybridization analysis of 14 cases. *Virchows Archiv* 448: 135–141.

Krismann M, Müller K, Jaworska M, Johnen G (2002): Molecular cytogenetic differences between histological subtypes of malignant mesotheliomas: DNA cytometry and comparative genomic hybridization of 90 cases. *J Pathol* 197: 363–371.

Ladanyi M, Zauderer MG, Krug LM, Ito T, McMillan R, Bott M, et al. (2012): New strategies in pleural mesothelioma: BAP1 and NF2 as novel targets for therapeutic development and risk assessment. *Clin Cancer Res* 18: 4485–4490.

Li P, Wang K, Zhang J, Zhao L, Liang H, Shao C, et al. (2012): The 3p21.3 tumor suppressor RBM5 resensitizes cisplatin-resistant human non-small cell lung cancer cells to cisplatin. *Cancer Epidemiol* 36: 481–489.

Li N, Ou W, Yang H, Liu QW, Zhang SL, Wang BX, et al. (2014): A randomized phase 2 trial of erlotinib versus pemetrexed as second-line therapy in the treatment of patients with advanced EGFR wild-type and EGFR FISH-positive lung adenocarcinoma. *Cancer* 120: 1379–1386.

Liu Y, Gao W, Siegfried JM, Weissfeld JL, Luketich JD, Keohavong P (2007): Promoter methylation of RASSF1A and DAPK and mutations of K-ras, p53, and EGFR in lung tumors from smokers and never-smokers. *BMC Cancer* 7: 74.

Lopez-Lago MA, Okada T, Murillo MM, Socci N, Giancotti FG (2009): Loss of the tumor suppressor gene NF2, encoding merlin, constitutively activates integrin-dependent mTORC1 signaling. *Mol Cell Biol* 29: 4235–4249.

Lopez-Rios F, Chuai S, Flores R, Shimizu S, Ohno T, Wakahara K, et al. (2006): Global gene expression profiling of pleural mesotheliomas: overexpression of Aurora kinases and P16/CDKN2A deletion as prognostic factors and critical evaluation of microarray-based prognostic prediction. *Cancer Res* 66: 2970–2979.

Marsit C, Hasegawa M, Hirao T, Kim D-H, Aldape K, Hinds P, et al. (2004): Loss of heterozygosity of chromosome 3p21 is associated with mutant TP53 and better patient survival in non-small-cell lung cancer. *Cancer Res* 64: 8702–8707.

Merlo A, Herman JG, Mao L, Lee DJ, Gabrielson E, Burger PC, et al. (1995): 5′ CpG island methylation is associated with transcriptional silencing of the tumour suppressor p16/CDKN2/MTS1 in human cancers. *Nat Med* 1: 686–692.

Mitelman F, Johansson B, Mertens F (Eds) (2014): Mitelman Database of Chromosome Aberrations and Gene Fusions in Cancer. http://cgap.nci.nih.gov/Chromosomes/Mitelman.

Murakami H, Mizuno T, Taniguchi T, Fujii M, Ishiguro F, Fukui T, et al. (2011): LATS2 is a tumor suppressor gene of malignant mesothelioma. *Cancer Res* 71: 873–883.

Musti M, Kettunen E, Dragonieri S, Lindholm P, Cavone D, Serio G, et al. (2006): Cytogenetic and molecular genetic changes in malignant mesothelioma. *Cancer Genet Cytogenet* 170: 9–15.

Mäki-Nevala S, Kaur Sarhadi V, Tuononen K, Lagstrom S, Ellonen P, Ronty M, et al. (2013): Mutated ephrin receptor genes in non-small cell lung carcinoma and their occurrence with driver mutations-targeted resequencing study on formalin-fixed, paraffin-embedded tumor material of 81 patients. *Genes Chromosomes Cancer* 52: 1141–1149.

Mäki-Nevala S, Rönty M, Morel M, Gomez M, Dawson Z, Sarhadi VK, et al. (2014): Epidermal growth factor receptor mutations in 510 Finnish non-small-cell lung cancer patients. *J Thorac Oncol* 9: 886–891.

Ni X, Zhuo M, Su Z, Duan J, Gao Y, Wang Z, et al. (2013): Reproducible copy number variation patterns among single circulating tumor cells of lung cancer patients. *Proc Natl Acad Sci USA* 110: 21083–21088.

Nymark P, Wikman H, Ruosaari S, Hollmén J, Vanhala E, Karjalainen A, et al. (2006): Identification of specific gene copy number changes in asbestos-related lung cancer. *Cancer Res* 16: 5737–5743.

Nymark P, Guled M, Borze I, Faisal A, Lahti L, Salmenkivi K, et al. (2011): Integrative analysis of microRNA, mRNA and aCGH data reveals asbestos- and histology-related changes in lung cancer. *Genes Chromosomes Cancer* 50: 585–597.

Ou WB, Hubert C, Corson JM, Bueno R, Flynn DL, Sugarbaker DJ, et al. (2011): Targeted inhibition of multiple receptor tyrosine kinases in mesothelioma. *Neoplasia* 13: 12–22.

Panagopoulos I, Thorsen J, Gorunova L, Micci F, Haugom L, Davidson B, et al. (2013): RNA sequencing identifies fusion of the EWSR1 and YY1 genes in mesothelioma with t(14;22) (q32;q12). *Genes Chromosomes Cancer* 52: 733–740.

Panani AD, Roussos C (2006): Cytogenetic and molecular aspects of lung cancer. *Cancer Lett* 239: 1–9.

Pei J, Kruger WD, Testa JR (2006): High-resolution analysis of 9p loss in human cancer cells using single nucleotide polymorphism-based mapping arrays. *Cancer Genet Cytogenet* 170: 65–68.

Peifer M, Fernandez-Cuesta L, Sos ML, George J, Seidel D, Kasper LH, et al. (2012): Integrative genome analyses identify key somatic driver mutations of small-cell lung cancer. *Nat Genet* 44: 1104–1110.

Petersen S, Aninat-Meyer M, Schluns K, Gellert K, Dietel M, Petersen I (2000): Chromosomal alterations in the clonal evolution to the metastatic stage of squamous cell carcinomas of the lung. *Br J Cancer* 82: 65–73.

Popova T, Hebert L, Jacquemin V, Gad S, Caux-Moncoutier V, Dubois-d'Enghien C, et al. (2013): Germline BAP1 mutations predispose to renal cell carcinomas. *Am J Hum Genet* 92: 974–980.

Poulikakos PI, Xiao G-H, Gallagher R, Jablonski S, Jhanwar SC, Testa JR (2006): Re-expression of the tumor suppressor NF2//merlin inhibits invasiveness in mesothelioma cells and negatively regulates FAK. *Oncogene* 25: 5960–5968.

Puyol M, Martin A, Dubus P, Mulero F, Pizcueta P, Khan G, et al. (2010): A synthetic lethal interaction between K-Ras oncogenes and Cdk4 unveils a therapeutic strategy for non-small cell lung carcinoma. *Cancer Cell* 18: 63–73.

Rodriguez-Gonzalez M, Novoa NM, Gomez MT, Garcia JL, Ludena D (2014): Factors influencing malignant evolution and long-term survival in solitary fibrous tumours of the pleura. *Histol Histopathol* 29:1445–1454.

Ruosaari ST, Nymark PEH, Aavikko MM, Kettunen E, Knuutila S, Hollmen J, et al. (2008): Aberrations of chromosome 19 in asbestos-associated lung cancer and in asbestos-induced micronuclei of bronchial epithelial cells in vitro. *Carcinogenesis* 29: 913–917.

Sanchez-Cespedes M, Monzo M, Rosell R, Pifarre A, Calvo R, Lopez-Cabrerizo MP, et al. (1998): Detection of chromosome 3p alterations in serum DNA of non-small-cell lung cancer patients. *Ann Oncol* 9: 113–116.

Scheinin I, Myllykangas S, Borze I, Bohling T, Knuutila S, Saharinen J (2008): CanGEM: mining gene copy number changes in cancer. *Nucleic Acids Res* 36: D830–D835.

Shibata T, Uryu S, Kokubu A, Hosoda F, Ohki M, Sakiyama T, et al.2005): Genetic classification of lung adenocarcinoma based on array-based comparative genomic hybridization analysis: its association with clinicopathologic features. *Clin Cancer Res* 11: 6177–6185.

Sholl LM, Yeap BY, Iafrate AJ, Holmes-Tisch AJ, Chou YP, Wu MT, et al. (2009): Lung adenocarcinoma with EGFR amplification has distinct clinicopathologic and molecular features in never-smokers. *Cancer Res* 69: 8341–8348.

Siegel R, Naishadham D, Jemal A (2012): Cancer statistics, 2012. *CA Cancer J Clin* 62: 10–29.

Simon F, Johnen G, Krismann M, Muller K-M (2005): Chromosomal alterations in early stages of malignant mesotheliomas. *Virchows Archiv* 447: 762–767.

Soda M, Choi YL, Enomoto M, Takada S, Yamashita Y, Ishikawa S, et al. (2007): Identification of the transforming EML4-ALK fusion gene in non-small-cell lung cancer. *Nature* 448: 561–566.

Stella GM, Luisetti M, Pozzi E, Comoglio PM (2013): Oncogenes in non-small-cell lung cancer: emerging connections and novel therapeutic dynamics. *Lancet Respir Med* 1: 251–261.

Sutherland LC, Wang K, Robinson AG (2010): RBM5 as a putative tumor suppressor gene for lung cancer. *J Thorac Oncol* 5: 294–298.

Swarts DR, Ramaekers FC, Speel EJ (2012): Molecular and cellular biology of neuroendocrine lung tumors: evidence for separate biological entities. *Biochim Biophys Acta* 1826: 255–271.

Takamochi K, Ogura T, Suzuki K, Kawasaki H, Kurashima Y, Yokose T, et al. (2001): Loss of heterozygosity on chromosomes 9q and 16p in atypical adenomatous hyperplasia concomitant with adenocarcinoma of the lung. *Am J Pathol* 159: 1941–1948.

Takanami I (2005): The prognostic value of overexpression of Skp2 mRNA in non-small cell lung cancer. *Oncol Rep* 13: 727–731.

Tammilehto L, Tuomi T, Tiainen M, Rautonen J, Knuutila S, Pyrhonen S, et al. (1992): Malignant mesothelioma: clinical characteristics, asbestos mineralogy and chromosomal abnormalities of 41 patients. *Eur J Cancer* 28A: 1373–1379.

Taniguchi T, Karnan S, Fukui T, Yokoyama T, Tagawa H, Yokoi K, et al. (2007): Genomic profiling of malignant pleural mesothelioma with array-based comparative genomic hybridization shows frequent non-random chromosomal alteration regions including JUN amplification on 1p32. *Cancer Sci* 98: 438–446.

Testa JR, Cheung M, Pei J, Below JE, Tan Y, Sementino E, et al. (2011): Germline BAP1 mutations predispose to malignant mesothelioma. *Nat Genet* 43: 1022–1025.

Tiainen M, Tammilehto L, Mattson K, Knuutila S (1988): Nonrandom chromosomal abnormalities in malignant pleural mesothelioma. *Cancer Genet Cytogenet* 33: 251–274.

Tiainen M, Tammilehto L, Rautonen J, Tuomi T, Mattson K, Knuutila S (1989): Chromosomal abnormalities and their correlations with asbestos exposure and survival in patients with mesothelioma. *Br J Cancer* 60: 618–626.

Tonon G, Wong KK, Maulik G, Brennan C, Feng B, Zhang Y, et al. (2005a): High-resolution genomic profiles of human lung cancer. *Proc Natl Acad Sci USA* 102: 9625–9630.

Tonon G, Brennan C, Protopopov A, Maulik G, Feng B, Zhang Y, et al. (2005b): Common and contrasting genomic profiles among the major human lung cancer subtypes. *Cold Spring Harb Symp Quant Biol* 70: 11–24.

Torenbeek R, Hermsen MA, Meijer GA, Baak JP, Meijer CJ (1999): Analysis by comparative genomic hybridization of epithelial and spindle cell components in sarcomatoid carcinoma and carcinosarcoma: histogenetic aspects. *J Pathol* 189: 338–343.

Toyooka S, Toyooka K, Maruyama R, Virmani A, Girard L, Miyajima K, et al. (2001): DNA methylation profiles of lung tumors. *Mol Cancer Ther* 1: 61–67.

Truini A, Coco S, Alama A, Genova C, Sini C, Dal Bello MG, et al. (2014): Role of microRNAs in malignant mesothelioma. *Cell Mol Life Sci* 71: 2865–2878.

Tuononen K, Sarhadi VK, Wirtanen A, Ronty M, Salmenkivi K, Knuuttila A, et al. (2013): Targeted resequencing reveals ALK fusions in non-small cell lung carcinomas detected by FISH, immunohistochemistry, and real-time RT-PCR: a comparison of four methods. *Biomed Res Int* 2013: 757490.

Tuononen K, Kero M, Mäki-Nevala S, Sarhadi VK, Tikkanen M, Wirtanen T, et al. (2014): ALK fusion and its association with other driver gene mutations in Finnish non-small cell lung cancer patients. *Genes Chromosomes Cancer* 53: 895–901.

Ullmann R, Schwendel A, Klemen H, Wolf G, Petersen I, Popper HH (1998): Unbalanced chromosomal aberrations in neuroendocrine lung tumors as detected by comparative genomic hybridization. *Hum Pathol* 29: 1145–1149.

Ullmann R, Petzmann S, Sharma A, Cagle PT, Popper HH (2001): Chromosomal aberrations in a series of large-cell neuroendocrine carcinomas: unexpected divergence from small-cell carcinoma of the lung. *Hum Pathol* 32: 1059–1063.

Vaishnavi A, Capelletti M, Le AT, Kako S, Butaney M, Ercan D, et al. (2013): Oncogenic and drug-sensitive NTRK1 rearrangements in lung cancer. *Nat Med* 19: 1469–1472.

Walch AK, Zitzelsberger HF, Aubele MM, Mattis AE, Bauchinger M, Candidus S, et al. (1998): Typical and atypical carcinoid tumors of the lung are characterized by 11q deletions as detected by comparative genomic hybridization. *Am J Pathol* 153: 1089–1098.

van Jaarsveld MT, Helleman J, Boersma AW, van Kuijk PF, van Ijcken WF, Despierre E, et al. (2013): miR-141 regulates KEAP1 and modulates cisplatin sensitivity in ovarian cancer cells. *Oncogene* 32: 4284–4293.

Vannini I, Fanini F, Fabbri M (2013): MicroRNAs as lung cancer biomarkers and key players in lung carcinogenesis. *Clin Biochem* 46: 918–925.

Weir BA, Woo MS, Getz G, Perner S, Ding L, Beroukhim R, et al. (2007): Characterizing the cancer genome in lung adenocarcinoma. *Nature* 450: 893–898.

West L, Vidwans SJ, Campbell NP, Shrager J, Simon GR, Bueno R, et al. (2012): A novel classification of lung cancer into molecular subtypes. *PLoS One* 7: e31906.

Whang-Peng J, Kao-Shan CS, Lee EC, Bunn PA, Carney DN, Gazdar AF, et al. (1982): Specific chromosome defect associated with human small-cell lung cancer; deletion 3p(14–23). *Science* 215: 181–182.

Wiesner T, Obenauf AC, Murali R, Fried I, Griewank KG, Ulz P, et al. (2011): Germline mutations in BAP1 predispose to melanocytic tumors. *Nat Genet* 43: 1018–1021.

Wikman H, Kettunen E (2006): Regulation of the G1/S phase of the cell cycle and alterations in the RB pathway in human lung cancer. *Expert Rev Anticanc* 6: 515–530.

Wikman H, Nymark P, Vayrynen A, Jarmalaite S, Kallioniemi A, Salmenkivi K, et al. (2005): CDK4 is a probable target gene in a novel amplicon at 12q13.3-q14.1 in lung cancer. *Genes Chromosomes Cancer* 42: 193–199.

Wikman H, Ruosaari S, Nymark P, Sarhadi VK, Saharinen J, Vanhala E, et al. (2007): Gene expression and copy number profiling suggests the importance of allelic imbalance in 19p in asbestos-associated lung cancer. *Oncogene* 26: 4730–4737.

Wilkerson MD, Yin X, Hoadley KA, Liu Y, Hayward MC, Cabanski CR, et al. (2010): Lung squamous cell carcinoma mRNA expression subtypes are reproducible, clinically important, and correspond to normal cell types. *Clin Cancer Res* 16: 4864–4875.

Winslow MM, Dayton TL, Verhaak RG, Kim-Kiselak C, Snyder EL, Feldser DM, et al. (2011): Suppression of lung adenocarcinoma progression by Nkx2-1. *Nature* 473: 101–104.

Wright CM, Kirschner MB, Cheng YY, O'Byrne KJ, Gray SG, Schelch K, et al. (2013): Long non coding RNAs (lncRNAs) are dysregulated in malignant pleural mesothelioma (MPM). *PLoS One* 8: e70940.

Xue X, Zhu YM, Woll PJ (2006): Circulating DNA and lung cancer. *Ann N Y Acad Sci* 1075: 154–164.

Yokoi S, Yasui K, Mori M, Iizasa T, Fujisawa T, Inazawa J (2004): Amplification and overexpression of SKP2 are associated with metastasis of non-small-cell lung cancers to lymph nodes. *Am J Pathol* 165: 175–180.

Zauderer MG, Bott M, McMillan R, Sima CS, Rusch V, Krug LM, et al. (2013): Clinical characteristics of patients with malignant pleural mesothelioma harboring somatic BAP1 mutations. *J Thorac Oncol* 8: 1430–1433.

Zhao X, Weir BA, LaFramboise T, Lin M, Beroukhim R, Garraway L, et al. (2005): Homozygous deletions and chromosome amplifications in human lung carcinomas revealed by single nucleotide polymorphism array analysis. *Cancer Res* 65: 5561–5570.

CHAPTER 14

Tumors of the digestive tract

Georgia Bardi[1] and Sverre Heim[2]

[1]BioAnalytica-GenoType SA, Molecular Cytogenetic Research and Applications, Athens, Greece
[2]Section for Cancer Cytogenetics, Institute for Cancer Genetics and Informatics, Oslo University Hospital, Oslo, Norway

Although 40 years have passed since the first chromosome banding analysis of human colonic polyps (Mitelman et al., 1974), our cytogenetic knowledge about digestive tract tumors is still disproportionately limited. These tumors make up no more than 4% of all the cases with abnormal karyotypes included in the database of chromosome aberrations in cancer (Mitelman et al., 2014).

Large intestine

Colorectal cancer, with adenocarcinomas as the dominant tumor type, is one of the most common malignancies in large parts of the world and one whose incidence is rising. Most colorectal adenocarcinomas develop from benign, polyp-like adenomas in what is called the adenoma–carcinoma sequence (Bedenne et al., 1992). The fact that macroscopically recognizable, sometimes symptomatic, premalignant mucosa lesions exist opens up the unique possibility in this organ system to investigate and compare all main stages of carcinogenesis: the benign but malignancy-prone adenomas, the locally infiltrating carcinoma, and the metastatic lesions. In addition, the circumstance that a relatively large proportion of colorectal cancers, perhaps 10–15% (Houlston et al., 1992), is familial makes it possible to compare the pathogenetic events that characterize hereditary and sporadic tumors.

Some increase in survival for patients with colorectal cancer has been registered in recent years (Gao et al., 2013), mostly due to the introduction of novel biological therapies targeting cancer-specific molecules (Ruzzo et al., 2010). However, the extensive new knowledge about the structure, function, and interaction of key genes in large bowel tumorigenesis has not yet brought about corresponding improvements in the clinical handling of patients, especially as regards the sporadic type that constitutes more than 85% of all colorectal cancers. The reasons for this are undoubtedly complex, but one aspect may, in our opinion, be a widespread lack of appreciation of the full extent of the genetic complexity and heterogeneity that characterize colorectal malignant tumors. The vast majority of studies seeking to unravel the acquired genomic changes of large bowel tumor cells were often unnecessarily reductionistic (Heim, 1992), focusing exclusively on gene-level alterations without taking into account the numerous coexisting genomic abnormalities at higher organizational levels, in particular numerical and structural chromosomal abnormalities, and without due recognition of the extensive cell-to-cell variation seen in the neoplastic parenchyma. In only few studies (Brüderlein et al.,

1990; Platzer Upender et al., 2002; Cardoso et al., 2007) were genetic methodologies combined to provide simultaneous, detailed information about changes at the gene level and a global overview of the genomic profile in individual tumors, let alone in individual cells within that tumor. In addition, most series of genetically characterized colorectal cancers are insufficiently accurate when it comes to the clinical and histopathological description of the tumors. Finally, very few attempts have been made to prepare for meta-analysis genetic information about colorectal tumors obtained by different groups of researchers, even when they utilized the same methodological approach.

In total, less than 550 tumors of the large intestine with clonal chromosome aberrations are described in the cytogenetic literature (Mitelman et al., 2014). The main reason for the paucity of data is unquestionably the same as for most solid tumors; it has been very difficult to induce the tumor cells to divide *in vitro*, and often the metaphases have been of poor technical quality, making interpretations unreliable. A particular difficulty with large bowel tumors is the high tendency for infections to develop in the cultures. All these problems notwithstanding, the available data have made it possible to construct a relatively detailed picture of the cytogenetic events of both benign and malignant colorectal tumorigenesis. The cytogenetic investigations have helped (i) to identify early, possibly initiating, genetic events in colorectal tumorigenesis; (ii) to determine the clonal relationship among synchronously growing, macroscopically distinct colorectal adenomas as well as between carcinomas and polyps growing in the same patient; (iii) to describe the cytogenetic makeup of metastatic lesions by comparing karyotypically primary tumors and their local and distal metastases in individual patients; (iv) to demonstrate considerable genetic heterogeneity in colorectal tumors with distinct cytogenetic subgroups corresponding to different oncogenetic pathways in sporadic large bowel cancer, as is known to be the case also in hereditary colorectal tumors; and (v) to reveal a tight correlation of both the overall karyotypic pattern and of specific chromosome alterations with prognosis for colorectal cancer patients. The latter observations are still not widely appreciated, but they do provide valuable and in some instances unique information about the likely clinical outcome and, hence, may come to serve as clues to how colorectal cancer patients should best be treated.

Colorectal tumors are characterized by recurrent chromosome aberrations

Of the more than 500 cytogenetically abnormal colorectal tumors published, less than one-third were classified as adenomas, two-thirds were adenocarcinomas, and the rest were listed as carcinomas not otherwise specified. Clonal chromosome aberrations were detected in nearly 40% of the nonadenomatous polyps, in 80% of the adenomas, in up to 90% of the primary carcinomas, and in all the metastatic cancers reported.

The systematic cytogenetic studies behind these numbers have provided important information that in part corroborates and extends the molecular genetic model of colorectal carcinogenesis proposed by Fearon and Vogelstein (1990). Some discoveries have been unexpected, however, and have yielded novel insights into the processes of initiation and progression of colorectal cancer. The main conclusion reached by karyotyping analysis of colorectal neoplastic cells is that both benign and malignant neoplastic lesions of the large intestine display characteristic patterns of acquired chromosomal abnormalities. No single cytogenetic aberration can be said to distinguish colorectal adenomas from carcinomas with absolute certainty; however, in groupwise comparisons, adenomas come across as karyotypically much simpler than their malignant counterparts.

The development of a wide array of fluorescence *in situ* hybridization (FISH)-based techniques enabled a marriage of banding cytogenetics with molecular genetics, and the resulting molecular cytogenetic techniques have greatly facilitated the genetic analysis of colorectal tumors. In particular, comparative genomic hybridization (CGH) studies on metaphases (chromosomal or cCGH) or utilizing array technology (aCGH) have been performed on several series of colorectal tumors consisting of adenomas, primary carcinomas, and metastases. The DNA copy number pattern revealed by cCGH and aCGH analyses has substantially contributed to our understanding of the cytogenetics of colorectal carcinogenesis, confirming the overall picture arrived at on the basis of karyotyping studies alone and expanding it by detecting also genomic imbalances that are below the detection limit of karyotyping. In the last few years, newly invented sequencing technologies have increasingly been relied on to unravel the molecular acquired genomic changes of colorectal tumors (Fearon, 2011; The Cancer Genome Atlas Research Network, 2012; Nome et al., 2013). A wealth of new information has been obtained, but unfortunately the data thus produced has not been collated with chromosomal tumor features.

Colorectal carcinomas

In all major published series of cytogenetically investigated colorectal carcinomas (Reichman et al., 1981; Muleris et al., 1990; Konstantinova et al., 1991; Bardi et al., 1993a, 1993b, 1995a), clonal aberrations were found in the vast majority of cases. However, a small fraction of tumors, perhaps 10%, do appear to have a normal chromosome complement. Some of these tumors may have only submicroscopic genomic rearrangements or the examined cells may have been of stromal origin; once a cell enters mitosis and is taken through the steps necessary for chromosome analysis, it is no longer possible to determine its phenotype. That stromal or normal epithelial admixture in primary cultures of colorectal carcinomas represents a real problem is evident from the fact that the growth

fraction of tumor parenchyma cells may be as low as 2% (Shroy et al., 1988). At least to some extent, this problem can be overcome, however, as demonstrated by the increased percentage of cytogenetically abnormal cases seen when the culturing techniques are optimized.

The modal chromosome number of colorectal carcinomas displaying clonal chromosome aberrations varies from hypo- or near diploid to near pentaploid. More than half of the cases have had near-diploid or pseudodiploid karyotypes, which is consistent with the finding of diploidy in several DNA flow cytometry studies in as much as 47–54% (Nishida et al., 1995; Tonouchi et al., 1998; Lin et al., 2003). Admittedly, among flow cytometrically normal cases, there may not only be tumors with normal karyotypes or one or few numerical and/or structural changes but also tumors with extensive chromosomal rearrangements leading to no or only small changes in the total DNA content.

When all reported cases with clonal aberrations are pooled, it turns out that although a certain difference in the reported frequencies is apparent, the most common numerical aberrations (Figure 14.1) are monosomy 18 and trisomy 7,

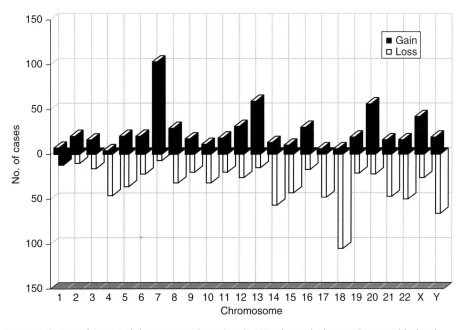

Figure 14.1 Distribution of numerical chromosome aberrations in 338 colorectal adenocarcinomas with clonal chromosome aberrations.

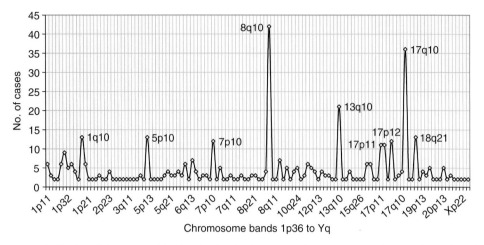

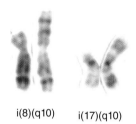

i(8)(q10)   i(17)(q10)

Figure 14.2 Distribution of chromosomal breakpoints involved in structural rearrangements in 338 colorectal adenocarcinomas with clonal chromosome aberrations.

Figure 14.3 i(8)(q10) and i(17)(q10) are the most frequent (10%) structural chromosome aberrations in colorectal adenocarcinomas.

followed in decreasing order of frequency by trisomy 13, monosomy 14, trisomy 20, and monosomy for chromosomes 22, 4, and 21.

With the exception of the Y, all chromosomes have been seen to be involved in structural rearrangements in colorectal carcinomas. The breakpoints recurrently involved in such rearrangements map to no less than 160 chromosome bands, but at variable frequencies in different studies. However, when all data available in the literature are considered, the most marked clustering of breakpoints is seen at 8q10, 17q10, and 13q10, followed by 1q10, 5p10, 7p10, 17p11, 17p12, and 18q21 (Figure 14.2). Several other chromosomal breakpoints are also recurrently involved but in less than 3% of the total number of cytogenetically examined colorectal carcinomas.

The most frequent structural rearrangements in the total material are i(8)(q10) and i(17)(q10) (Figure 14.3) found in about 10%, followed by del(17)(p11 or p12) (8%) and i(13)(q10) and del(18) (q21) (5% each). The net outcome of these rearrangements is loss of 8p and gain of 8q, gain of 13q, loss of 17p, and gain of 17q. Although the aforementioned anomalies were seen repeatedly in all major published series of cytogenetically characterized colorectal carcinomas, the reported frequencies varied considerably. Technical and stochastic factors undoubtedly play a role in bringing about this variability, but systematic differences related to the composition of the series examined could also be important, in particular with regard to possible etiologic and pathogenetic differences, including microsatellite versus chromosomal instability (CIN) status, among different groups of patients.

The consistent losses of genomic material in colorectal cancer presumably exert their pathogenetic influence through loss of tumor suppressor genes (TSG), but the effect of gains remains elusive, even for genomic loci undergoing amplification. Using combined CGH and DNA microarray expression profiling, Platzer Upender et al. (2002) examined the expression of over 2000 genes situated on chromosome arms 7p, 8q, 13q, and 20q, that is, genomic areas that in their study were consistently found amplified in metastatic colorectal cancers. Interestingly, 96.2% of the genes located in areas of chromosome amplification did not show upregulation of expression. On the other hand, Cardoso et al. (2007), who attempted an integration of genomic and expression profiling data of colorectal cancer available in the public domain, found that several aneuploid loci were associated with differential regulation of specific genes. In particular, losses of 4q21–35, 5q31–32, 14q32, 17p12–13, 17q23–25, 18q21, 19p13, and 22q13 and gains of 7p15–22, 7q22–32, 8p11–21, 8q11–24, 13q12–13, 20p12–13, and 20q11–13 identified clusters of genes reported to be, respectively, down- and upregulated by expression analysis. However, in some instances, such as for the *S100P* gene in 4p16, *SPARC* in 5q31–32, and *SOX9* in 17q24–25, the nature of the aneuploidy events and the direction of the corresponding gene expression changes were apparently discordant. That only a proportion of genes undergoing copy number changes because of aneuploidy events that appear to be differentially expressed, can be attributed to a number of mechanisms responsible for normal and abnormal control of gene expression, such as mutation, methylation, and microRNA expression. Nevertheless, recurrent genomic imbalances in colorectal cancer apparently do affect gene expression, albeit in a manner that is not easy to predict, and doubtlessly also the biology of the malignant cells that make up the tumor.

The molecular genetics of colorectal cancer were expertly reviewed by Fearon (2011). A relatively limited number of oncogenes and TSG are mutated in a sizeable fraction of such cancers, most prominently *APC*, *KRAS*, and *TP53*. The molecular data remain largely uncollated with karyotypic tumor features. Even more recently, The Cancer Genome Atlas Research Network (2012) published their genome-scale examination of 276 carcinomas including analyses of exome sequence, DNA copy number, promoter methylation, and messenger RNA and microRNA expression. Of this total, a subset of 97 samples underwent whole-genome sequencing. Twenty-four genes were found to be significantly mutated, and in addition to the expected *APC*, *TP53*, *SMAD4*, *PIK3CA*, and *KRAS* mutations, frequent mutations were also found in *ARID1A*, *SOX9*, and *FAM123B*. Nome et al. (2013) performed RNA sequencing of seven colorectal adenocarcinoma cell lines finding 11 candidate fusion transcripts worthy of further experimental validation (of 3391 fusion candidates altogether), three of which (*AKAP13–PDE8A*, *COMMD10–AP3S1*, and *CTB–35F21.1–PSD2*) were present in most cell lines as well as in a substantial proportion of primary cancer tissues also tested. One can expect more such studies to follow. Again, we emphasize that it would have been advantageous to have also karyotypic data on the tumors subjected to whole-transcriptome sequencing, but so far, this information has been lacking.

Colorectal adenomatous and hyperplastic polyps

Chromosome aberrations have now been reported in nearly 140 such adenomas. The early studies left the impression that gains of whole chromosomes were the only, or at least the predominant, aberrations. As data from new and larger series were added, the consensus picture of the karyotypic characteristics of benign colorectal tumors has undergone considerable refinements. According to Bardi et al. (1993c) and Bomme et al. (1994, 1996a), who karyotyped 82 colorectal polyps, up to 80% of large bowel adenomas carry clonal chromosome aberrations. Other investigators have reported lower percentages of cytogenetically abnormal lesions, from 30% to 50%. In all series, however, most karyotypically abnormal polyps (90%) had only few cytogenetic abnormalities giving rise to pseudo- or near-diploid karyotypes. The remainder are near triploid or near tetraploid with massive chromosome changes, often showing anomalies that are recurrent in colorectal adenocarcinomas as well. At present, therefore, one cannot point to any single karyotypic feature that is capable of distinguishing unequivocally between benign and malignant colorectal tumors. As a group, the adenomas have much simpler karyotypes.

The most frequent chromosome abnormality in colorectal polyps is +7, found in 50% of all reported cases (Figure 14.4) and mostly as the sole anomaly. Although the pathogenetic relevance of +7 in large bowel neoplasms as well as tumors of other tissues has been questioned (Bardi et al., 1991a; Johansson et al., 1993), the finding of this trisomy in the epithelial component of adenomatous polyps (Bardi et al., 1995b; Bomme et al., 1994, 1996a, 1996b, 2001) by chromosome banding analysis of metaphase cells and by interphase FISH analysis with centromere-specific probes supports the early suggestion that it plays a primary role in some colorectal neoplasms. Ly et al. (2011) suggested that the acquisition of +7 precedes loss or truncation of *APC*, a gene-level

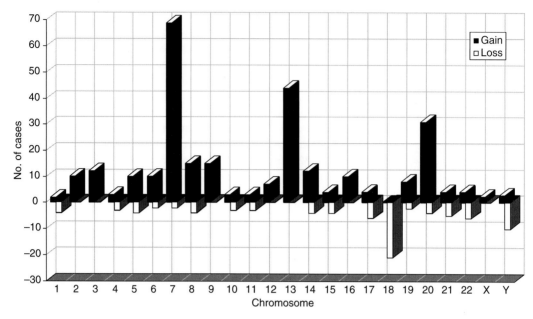

Figure 14.4 Distribution of numerical chromosome aberrations in 139 adenomas of the large intestine with clonal chromosome aberrations.

change that occurs very early in colorectal tumorigenesis. Besides, they found that human colonic epithelial cells with +7 enjoyed a growth advantage over their diploid counterparts and also that such cells exhibited altered migration abilities and aberrant regulation of the *EGFR* gene in 7p. The recent study by Gemoll et al. (2014) showed that trisomy 7, the earliest chromosomal aberration in premalignant stages of colorectal carcinomas, was associated with protein expression changes that affect molecular functions involved in cell growth and proliferation.

Gain of chromosome 13 is the second most common numerical abnormality in large bowel adenomas and has been found in about 30% of the tumors (Figure 14.4). The *GTF3A* and *HMGB1* genes, mapped to 13q12.3–13.1 and 13q12, respectively, have been reported in several independent studies to be differentially expressed (upregulated) in colorectal adenomas (Cardoso et al., 2007). Gain of chromosome 20 has been found in 22% of the cases (Figure 14.4). Frequent gains of at least six distinct genomic loci at both the p and the q arm of chromosome 20 have been identified also by CGH analysis. The *CDC25B* gene at 20p13, involved in protein amino acid phosphorylation, and *AHCY*, localized at 20q10–13.1 and related to 1-carbon

compound metabolism, have both been reported as differentially expressed (upregulated) in colorectal adenomas in more than three independent studies. Other frequent aneusomies in colorectal adenomas are, in decreasing order of frequency, loss of chromosome 18 (15%) and gain of chromosomes 8 and 9, each seen in 10% of the cases (Figure 14.4).

The necessity to culture the tumor cells prior to banding investigation and also the fact that different clones are likely to enter mitosis at different rates reduce the information value of cytogenetic analysis regarding the presence and relative size *in vivo* of clones with numerical changes. To estimate more reliably the clonal composition of colorectal adenomas, Bomme et al. (2001) performed interphase FISH analyses with probes for chromosomes 1, 7, 13, and 20 on a series of previously karyotyped adenomas. Gains of chromosomes 7, 13, and 20 were found in 32–44% of the adenomas, verifying that these trisomies are indeed common and that they occur *in vivo*. Although gain of chromosome 7 usually preceded the other gains in those instances where this could be assessed, this was not always so. Evidently, the end result of the acquired chromosomal imbalances rather than the sequence in which they occur is of the essence in colorectal tumorigenesis.

A deletion of part of the short arm of chromosome 1 (Figure 14.5) is the most common structural rearrangement in intestinal polyps. We have seen it in 30% of all cases with an abnormal karyotype, often as the only anomaly, which led us to suggest that this is an early, possibly primary, genetic change in the development of large bowel tumors (Bardi et al., 1993b). Lips et al. (2007), in a genome-wide single nucleotide polymorphism (SNP) analysis of 78 rectal tumors of different clinical stages, identified loss of 1p36 in 26% of the investigated adenomas; they too concluded that it was an early event as it was not seen more frequently in carcinomas analyzed by the same approach.

The consistency and extent of the 1p loss in colorectal adenomas was also investigated using a combined cytogenetic and molecular genetic approach (Bomme et al., 1998). The deletions were shown to be interstitial with a minimal common deleted region between markers D1S199 and D1S234 in bands 1p35–36 (Figure 14.5), suggesting that this might be the site of the hypothetical TSG presumed to be lost by the deletion. This genomic area contains the human homolog of the tumor modifier gene *Mom1* (1p35–36.1), which, in mice, modifies the number of intestinal tumors in multiple intestinal neoplasia (MIN)-mutated animals. That distal 1p is indeed important in colorectal tumorigenesis was shown functionally by Tanaka et al. (1993), who demonstrated that the introduction of a normal 1p36 segment into a colorectal carcinoma cell line rendered it nontumorigenic. Besides, recent data (Henrich et al., 2012) derived from studies of both human tumors and functional cancer models indicated that the 1p36 genes *CHD5*, *CAMTA1*, *KIF1B*, *CASZ1*, and *miR-34a* contribute to cancer development when reduced in dosage by genomic copy number loss or other mechanisms. The authors suggested potential interactions among these candidate genes and proposed a model whereby heterozygous 1p36 deletion impairs oncosuppressive pathways via simultaneous downregulation of several dosage-dependent TSG.

More than one-third of all investigated hyperplastic large bowel polyps, that is, lesions without any cellular atypia, have been shown to harbor clonal chromosomal abnormalities. Whether these polyps, too, have a tendency to progress toward carcinomas is not yet clear, but the cytogenetic data unequivocally indicate that they are genuine neoplasms with karyotypic features similar to those of small tubular adenomas. Rashid et al. (2000), in a genotype–phenotype retrospective analysis of 129 hyperplastic polyps, identified allelic loss of 1p (1p32–36) as the most frequent genetic alteration. In that series, interestingly, some patients with 1p allelic loss had hyperplastic polyposis (more than 20 hyperplastic polyps), and some of them had family members with colorectal cancer. The authors suggested that 1p loss could be the "starting point" of a hyperplastic polyp–adenocarcinoma sequence.

Deletions of the short arm of chromosome 1 are also seen in large bowel carcinomas although, relatively speaking, not as frequently as in adenomas and often with a larger segment lost. Usually, the del(1p) in carcinomas is accompanied by several other anomalies, but cases also exist in which it was the only karyotypic change. The rest of adenomatous

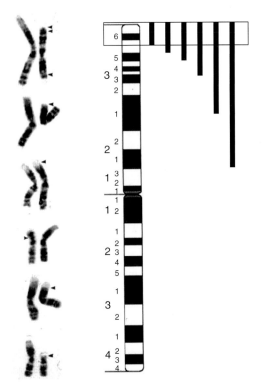

Figure 14.5 Partial karyotypes of chromosome 1 from six benign colon lesions with 1p deletions of various sizes. In the ideogram of chromosome 1 (right), the size of the deleted segment is illustrated for each case. The minimum common deleted region is band 1p36.

tissue were then often found in the tumors, and it has been suggested that the cells showing del(1p) as the only anomaly actually grew from these remnants (Bardi et al., 1995a).

Based on the finding in an allelic imbalance study that colorectal carcinomas lacking 1p deletion in the primary tumor acquired such changes in their metastatic lesions, Thorstensen et al. (2000) suggested that loss of 1p35–36 is of importance both early and late in colorectal tumorigenesis. We share the view expressed by Couturier-Turpin et al. (2001) that one needs to distinguish between loss of 1p occurring in pseudodiploid cells, mostly as the sole cytogenetic change that appears to be of importance in the initiation of carcinogenesis, and the loss of 1p that is often found in massively aneuploid cells, in which case the deletion may have been acquired as a result of complex chromosomal rearrangements occurring during tumor progression.

Clonal relationship among synchronously growing colorectal tumors

Synchronous adenomas

The phenotypic progression of colorectal tumors is driven by their step-by-step acquisition of genomic alterations, which not only signify important changes in carcinogenesis but also constitute highly informative markers of tumor clonality. In a series of 24 adenomas from 11 patients, chromosome banding analysis was used to examine the clonal relationship among synchronously growing, macroscopically distinct colorectal adenomas (Bomme et al., 1996a, 1996b). The main question to be answered was whether these polyps had karyotypic similarities or whether the clonal findings were unrelated, indicating that they arose independently. In six patients, similar clones were found in separate polyps within the same patient, polyps that were always located in the same part of the large bowel. In the remaining two patients, both with one rectal adenoma and one adenoma in the colon, no karyotypic similarity between the lesions was seen. The findings indicate that when macroscopically distinct, synchronous adenomas are growing in the same part of the large bowel, they are karyotypically similar, in contrast to when they grow in different parts (proximal colon, sigmoid, and

rectum). In the former situation, two explanations are possible. Either the same etiologic agent has elicited identical pathogenetic responses from several cells within the same anatomical area (i.e., they have acquired the same chromosomal aberration, probably because that particular etiologic stimulus tends to induce one and the same genomic response), or the morphologically distinct but close adenomas are in fact seemingly separate lesions belonging to the same clone of neoplastically transformed cells. In the latter situation, on the other hand, they are macroscopic manifestations of parallel but pathogenetically independent neoplastic processes. The latter hypothesis can also explain the by and large common loss of heterozygosity (LOH) features identified in 7–13 adenomas from each of seven patients with sporadic colorectal cancer examined in a genome-wide allelotyping analysis by Mao et al. (2006).

Synchronous polyps and carcinomas

Many colorectal carcinomas arise from visible benign precursor lesions, adenomas, in what has been termed the adenoma–carcinoma sequence (Bedenne et al., 1992). Most adenomas do not transform malignantly, however, in spite of the dysplastic changes characterizing their epithelial component. Other carcinomas arise de novo, that is, without a visible precursor lesion. In addition to adenomas, hyperplastic polyps are tumorous yet benign, and in most instances presumably nonneoplastic, lesions frequently seen in the colon and rectum. The identification of genetic similarities and differences between adenomas and carcinomas, and also between polyps that tend to and those that do not tend to transform to malignancy, is likely to shed light on the mechanisms driving tumorigenesis in the large intestine. The developmental relationship among various tumor lesions present at the same time in the same patient is another interesting issue; are they clonally related or not?

To approach these questions, 30 tumor lesions of the large bowel, including carcinomas, adenomas, and nonadenomatous polyps, from seven patients with colorectal cancer were cytogenetically analyzed (Bardi et al., 1997a). Clonal chromosomal abnormalities were found in all adenomas and carcinomas but only in 37.5% of the nonadenomatous polyps. Although the majority of hyperplastic polyps displayed a normal chromosome complement, some

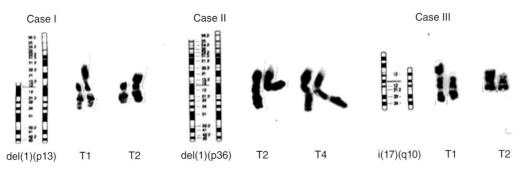

Case I   Case II   Case III

del(1)(p13) T1 T2 del(1)(p36) T2 T4 i(17)(q10) T1 T2

Figure 14.6 Ideograms and partial karyotypes illustrating three structural chromosome aberrations, each detected in two macroscopically distinct colorectal tumors from the same patient: del(1)(p13) was found in a carcinoma (T1) and a hyperplastic polyp (T2) from the same patient (Case I); del(1)(p36) was found in two of several tubulovillous adenomas (T2 and T4) from the same patient (Case II); and i(17)(q10) was found in a carcinoma (T1) and a tubular adenoma (T2) from the same patient (Case III).

showed clonal aberrations that in general seemed to be simpler than those of dysplastic polyps. It is possible that the subset of hyperplastic polyps with cytogenetic aberrations may have had small dysplastic areas that went undetected by conventional histological examination or the chromosome aberrations they carry, which are indistinguishable from those of small tubular adenomas, are not dysplasia specific but rather related to the hyperproliferation in the intestinal mucosa. Finally, the very occurrence of clonal chromosome aberrations in a proportion of hyperplastic polyps, which constitutes strong evidence that these lesions are neoplastic, could be viewed as the genetic corollary of a hyperplastic polyp–carcinoma sequence even in the absence of corresponding histopathological or clinical indications to this effect. Leggett et al. (2001) confirmed our earlier conclusion that some hyperplastic polyps do have acquired genetic changes by finding microsatellite instability (MSI) in three and *KRAS* mutations in eight of 47 hyperplastic polyps examined.

Although some chromosome aberrations have been found in carcinomas but not in adenomas, for example, der(8;17)(q10;q10), indicating that they may be specifically associated with malignant transformation of large bowel mucosa, adenomas and carcinomas occurring simultaneously in the same patient by and large share most of their chromosomal features (Bardi et al., 1997a). This karyotypic similarity between malignant and benign tumors in the same patient, and also sometimes among nonmalignant polyps in the same individual (Figure 14.6), can be interpreted to indicate that the macroscopically distinct lesions arose as part of a single clonal expansion, in spite of the fact that the distance between them was more than 3 cm. The only alternative explanation would be that the same oncogenetic environmental factor(s) induced identical chromosomal rearrangements in more than one cell.

Ried et al. (1996) used CGH to confirm that the frequency and degree of genetic aberrations increase with progression from low-grade adenoma through high-grade adenoma to carcinoma. Only three of their 14 low-grade and five high-grade adenomas showed chromosome abnormalities by CGH, compared with 14 of 16 carcinomas. The most frequently gained chromosome regions were 20q, 13q, 8q, 7p, and 7q, whereas frequent losses were observed from 8p, 18q, 4q, and 17p. Furthermore, the frequency of specific alterations increased with advancing stages of tumor progression. Also, Meijer et al. (1998) found that the average number of chromosomal aberrations increased from adenoma to carcinoma; frequent gains involved 13q, 7p, 7q, 8q, and 20q, and losses most often occurred at 18q, 4q, and 8p. The results of CGH analysis in these studies thus are in almost complete accordance with the pattern of imbalances previously detected in colorectal adenomas and carcinomas by G-banding analysis. Only losses of 4q, which were maybe hidden in unidentified chromosome markers, appeared to be underestimated in G-banding studies compared to the CGH data on colorectal cancer. In spite of the similar findings, however, one should keep in mind while interpreting the combined G-banding and CGH results that CGH can only detect DNA copy number changes that are present in at least 50% of the examined tumor cell population. Karyotypic analysis is in this sense superior because it can also detect balanced changes and very small clones consisting of as little as two abnormal mitoses. Integrating karyotypic and CGH data, Grade et al. (2006) proposed a chromosome aberration-based progression model of colorectal carcinogenesis. In their scheme, the progression from low-grade colorectal adenomas to high-grade adenomas is accompanied by gains of chromosome 7 and chromosome arm 20q, whereas gains of 8q and 13 as well as losses of 4p, 8p, and 18q indicate transition to invasive carcinomas.

Primary and metastatic colorectal carcinomas

The major cause of death in colorectal cancer is metastasis rather than localized disease. It is therefore clear that a better understanding of the metastatic process and the finding of ways to prevent it stand out as prime goals in colorectal cancer research. Given their importance, it is somewhat surprising that so little is known about the genetic profile of metastatic deposits. As a consequence, markers of prognosis or response to therapy are often assessed against the backdrop of data on the primary tumor, with the mostly implicit assumption that they also reflect the situation in the secondary disease loci.

To obtain more information on the karyotypic characteristics of colorectal cancer metastases, Bardi et al. (1997b) examined cytogenetically 18 tumors from 11 patients with metastatic disease. In all cases with matched samples from the primary tumor and lymph node metastases, cytogenetic similarities were found between the primary and the secondary lesions, indicating that many of the chromosomal aberrations were acquired before disease spreading took place. The observed genomic similarities, combined with data showing close transcriptional resemblance between primary tumors and metastases (D'Arrigo et al., 2005), support the notion that larger cell clumps rather than rare sporadic cells from the primary tumor in most instances give rise to the secondaries. The assumed existence of a migrating cancer stem cell (Brabletz et al., 2005) is nevertheless compatible with the genomic and transcriptional similarities

between primary tumors and their matching metastases since cancer stem cell(s) detaching from the primary tumor can form a metastatic lesion with similar genomic and gene expression patterns. Compared with the primaries, the metastases appeared to exhibit less clonal heterogeneity, probably reflecting clonal selection within the primary tumor from which the metastasis was derived, but, concurrently, an increase in the karyotypic complexity of individual clones (Bardi et al., 1997b). In addition to the aberrations del(1)(p34), i(17)(q10), −18, −21, +7, and +20, which were found recurrently in both primary and metastatic lesions, the del(10)(q22) found in metastases has not so far been associated with primary colorectal carcinomas. The finding of loss of 10q24-qter in two more cases in another series of colorectal metastases to the liver (Parada et al., 1999) provides further support for an association between loss of 10q and tumor progression. In a more recent LOH study, Fawole et al. (2002) used a panel of nine highly polymorphic microsatellite markers spanning the long arm of chromosome 10 to examine 114 sporadic colorectal adenocarcinomas. They found the highest LOH frequency at 10q21.1 and suggested that 10q loss is a late event in colorectal tumorigenesis. Using CGH, Paredes-Zaglul et al. (1998) compared the genetic composition of primary colorectal tumors without distant metastases (TNM stages I–III) with liver metastases (TNM stage IV) and found a distinct predominance of genetic losses in the metastatic lesions. Although not all aberrations were the same as those found by us, they too identified two patterns of alterations: (i) changes (+8q, +13q, −4p, −8p, −15q, −17p, −18q, −21q, and −22q) that were more often found in liver metastases than in primary tumors and (ii) changes (−9q, −11q, and −17q) that were unique to the metastatic lesions.

In a comparison between multiple metastatic lesions in the same patient but at different sites (Bardi et al., 1997b), we could demonstrate common karyotypic aberrations in the lesions but not in a single case was the karyotype of one metastatic lesion exactly identical to that of any other metastasis, even when both metastatic samples were from lymph nodes. Such genomic differences between primary and secondary tumors and among separate metastatic lesions have also been reported in several

CGH studies of paired primary colorectal carcinomas and metastases to either lymph nodes or distant organs such as the liver (Al-Mulla et al., 1999; Alcock et al., 2003; Knosel et al., 2004; Grade et al., 2006) and lung (Jiang et al., 2005; Knosel et al., 2005; Mekenkamp et al., 2014). However, the data are not sufficient to distinguish specific genomic patterns, either chromosomal or at the gene level, that could predict or explain the metastatic spreading of colorectal tumor cells to particular organs or tissues.

Correlation between karyotypic and phenotypic features

Cytogenetic pattern and tumor site

Colorectal carcinomas that arise proximal (right) or distal (left) to the splenic flexure exhibit differences in incidence depending on their site and the patient's age and gender. Tumors in the hereditary nonpolyposis colorectal cancer (HNPCC) and familial adenomatous polyposis (FAP) syndromes occur predominantly in the right and left colon, respectively, and the existence of two general categories of colorectal cancer based on the site of origin in the large bowel was proposed many years ago (Bufill, 1990). Differences between normal right- and left-sided colonic segments that could favor progression through different tumorigenic pathways have been recognized (Iacopetta, 2002). Right- and left-sided tumors also exhibit different sensitivities to chemotherapy, possibly related to the genetic characteristics of the tumors, with MSI (MSI[+]) phenotypes being associated predominantly with right-sided tumors and CIN (CIN[+]) with left-sided tumors (Iacopetta, 2002). Chromosomal alterations do not exclusively occur in microsatellite stable colorectal tumors, however. Douglas et al. (2004) investigated 37 primary colorectal carcinomas and 48 cell lines by aCGH and showed that CIN[+] samples had a significantly higher number of aberrations than did MSI[+] samples, particularly gain of chromosome 20 and loss of 18q and 8p. In addition, the target of the 8q gain seemed to differ depending on microsatellite status with 8q24.21 frequently gained in CIN[+] tumors, whereas gain of 8q24.3 occurred more often in MSI[+] tumors. In addition to microsatellite and chromosome instability, the CpG island methylation phenotype (CIMP) distinguished by hypermethylation has been added (Shen et al., 2007) as a third, molecularly distinct pathway. Since the definition of the three pathways is not mutually exclusive, it is possible that tumors can exhibit features of multiple pathways.

Site–karyotype correlations have largely remained unexamined in cytogenetic studies of colorectal cancer. In our series of karyotyped tumors (Bardi et al., 1995b), we found that carcinomas located in the proximal colon and rectum often were near diploid, with simple numerical changes and displaying cytogenetically unrelated clones, whereas carcinomas in the distal colon often had near-triploid to near-tetraploid karyotypes with massive chromosomal aberrations.

Cytogenetic pattern and histology

A statistically significant association was found between the karyotype of colorectal carcinomas and their degree of differentiation when cytogenetically abnormal tumors were divided into those with only numerical changes and those also having structural aberrations (Bardi et al., 1993a, 2004). Carcinomas carrying structural chromosomal rearrangements were more often poorly differentiated, whereas well- and moderately differentiated tumors more often had only numerical aberrations or normal karyotypes.

In large bowel adenomas, an association between cytogenetic pattern and the tumors' degree of dysplasia, histologic type, and size was found (Bomme et al., 1994, 1996a, 1996b). All villous and tubulovillous adenomas, that is, the adenomas most likely to progress to carcinoma, had structural chromosome aberrations. Adenomas with numerical changes only were mildly dysplastic, whereas all but one of the adenomas with structural rearrangements showed either moderate or severe dysplasia. Furthermore, polyps with a normal karyotype had either mild or moderate, but never severe, dysplasia. Polyps with structural chromosomal aberrations were on average larger than polyps with only numerical changes or those with a normal karyotype. The data strongly indicate that the accumulation of chromosomal changes in adenomas correlates with pathologic features: the more malignancy-like the phenotype, the more complex the karyotype. Presumably, this correlation reflects a causal relationship, with the acquired genetic changes enabling the cells to assume an increasingly aggressive growth pattern.

Cytogenetic pattern and prognosis

In spite of our much-improved understanding of the cellular and molecular mechanisms underlying colorectal tumor initiation and progression, little is known about the prognostic impact of particular genomic aberrations or aberration patterns. In a relatively small study 20 years ago, a statistically significant correlation between tumor karyotype and patient survival was demonstrated (Bardi et al., 1993a). Patients with complex tumor karyotypes had shorter survival than did those whose tumors had no or only few and simple chromosome anomalies.

To assess whether the karyotypic pattern provides valuable and independent information about the prognosis of individual patients with colorectal cancer, one decade later we attempted to evaluate simultaneously the prognostic importance of all nonrandom cytogenetic features in 150 patients with colorectal cancer, examined at the time of surgery, taking into account also the impact of classical clinicopathologic parameters (Bardi et al., 2004). In addition to tumor grade and clinical stage, complex structural aberrations as well as rearrangements of chromosomes 8 and 16 were in univariate analysis significantly correlated with shorter overall survival (OS). Karyotypic complexity, rearrangements of chromosomes 8 and 16, and loss of chromosome 4 were significantly correlated with shorter disease-free survival (DFS). In multivariate analysis, in addition to tumor grade, the type of chromosome aberrations (structural or numerical), ploidy, and loss of chromosome 18 came across as independent prognostic factors.

The most striking correlation observed between a specific chromosome aberration and prognosis was the effect of loss of chromosome 18. This loss was, together with tumor grade, found to be an independent predictor of short survival in the entire group of patients. Furthermore, loss of chromosome 18 was shown to be a stronger independent predictor of prognosis than tumor grade in the subset of patients having cancers of the intermediate stages II and III. Also, in a recent genome-scale analysis of 256 primary colorectal carcinomas (The Cancer Genome Atlas Research Network, 2012), deletion of

18q21.2 was picked up as a major marker of aggressive disease. Although several candidate TSG on the long arm of chromosome 18 have been identified, including *DCC*, *DPC4/SMAD4/MADH4*, and *SMAD2/MADH2*, none of them is mutated in most colorectal cancer cases with 18q loss (Woodford-Richens et al., 2001; Zhou et al., 2002). In addition, studies using microsatellite markers to assess allelic imbalances in colorectal carcinomas have shown that larger chromosomal segments were lost significantly more frequently than smaller ones in cases with 18q loss, indicating, as we see it, that the crucial event perhaps is not at the genic but at the genomic level, meaning that, in this case, tumor progression is facilitated by global genomic rearrangements or imbalances rather than by single-gene mutations or losses.

In the subset of patients with stage I and II carcinomas, none of the clinicopathologic variables could independently predict patient survival, whereas the presence of structural chromosomal aberrations was the only independent predictor of poor prognosis (Bardi et al., 2004). In the subset of patients with stage III carcinomas, the presence of structural changes of chromosome 8 was a stronger independent predictor of prognosis than was tumor grade. The correlation of structural rearrangements of chromosome 8 with OS and DFS in univariate analysis, together with the emergence of this chromosomal variable in multivariate analysis as the strongest predictor of poor disease outcome in stage III patients, was also a remarkable finding. It is presently unknown whether, let alone how, the colorectal cancer susceptibility locus identified at 8q24 by SNP genotyping of individuals affected by colorectal cancer and normal controls (Zanke et al., 2007) is in any way linked to the development of the aggressive clinical phenotype we could observe in the clinicocytogenetic correlation analyses.

In a CGH study of 50 colorectal carcinomas with and without lymph node metastases, Ghadimi et al. (2003) found that gain of 8q23–24 was strongly associated with lymph node positivity and therefore suggested that gain of this chromosome region could be used to predict an increased metastatic potential. In another CGH study of 67 sporadic carcinomas (De Angelis et al., 2001), 8p loss was found to be an independent predictor of poor survival, whereas an allelic imbalance study of 508 carcinomas showed that 8p loss was a predictor of dismal outcome in colorectal cancer patients of Astler–Coller stage B2 or C (Halling et al., 1999). Although the above molecular genetic data appear to be at odds with one another, suggesting either amplification of an oncogene at 8q or loss of a TSG at 8p as the pathogenetically important event, they are both explained by the cytogenetic finding of an i(8q), which indeed is the most common structural aberration of chromosome 8 in advanced colorectal cancer (Bardi et al., 1995b). The generation of an i(8q) is therefore associated with the development of lymph node metastases in colorectal cancer, but the molecular mechanisms whereby the simultaneous loss of 8p and gain of 8q exert such an influence remain unknown.

A correlation between the occurrence of structural rearrangements of chromosome 16 in the tumor cells and OS as well as DFS in colorectal cancer patients was for the first time suggested by Bardi et al. (2004). Because such aberrations have been found to be predictors of unfavorable outcome in other advanced malignancies as well (e.g., hepatocellular malignancy and bladder cancer), they might be general markers of tumor aggressiveness whose prognostic information value is not restricted to large bowel cancer. The association of karyotypic loss of chromosome 4 with a shorter DFS, found in the same study, agrees well with previous data by Arribas et al. (1999) indicating that LOH at several chromosome 4 loci was associated with a shorter DFS in colorectal cancer patients, as well as with more recent data by Tzeng et al. (2013) who found a novel candidate TSG, NDST4, at chromosome band 4q26 and suggested that its loss adversely affects prognosis in colorectal cancer.

During the last two decades, several CGH, LOH, and SNP studies have provided evidence that allelic imbalances on several chromosomes correlate with prognosis in colorectal cancer patients (Aragane et al., 2001; De Angelis et al., 2001; Zhou et al., 2002; Knosel et al., 2003; Aust et al., 2004; Diep et al., 2006; Jasmine et al., 2012). The involvement of chromosome regions previously detected by karyotyping alone was also confirmed in a BAC array CGH (aCGH) study of 121 colorectal carcinomas by Nakao et al. (2004).

Multiple pieces of evidence coming from different genome-wide screening studies therefore indicate that cytogenetic tumor features are valuable predictors of prognosis in colorectal cancer patients. Research efforts should, in our opinion, now be focused on the cytogenomic characterization of phenotypically homogeneous subsets of tumors to define more accurate genetic predictors for each distinct phenotypic subset (topography, histopathology, and clinical stage).

Cytogenetic pattern and clinical management of colorectal cancer

The majority of colorectal cancers are not diagnosed in the early stages of disease because the tumors often do not give rise to symptoms or signs until they are quite large, sometimes until they have already metastasized. In spite of this, the development of diagnostic systems based on the early genetic characteristics of colorectal lesions stands out as a prime goal. Such knowledge not only might direct our experimental therapeutic focus toward molecular mechanisms that have gone awry in the recently transformed, neoplastic cells, but also this kind of information might potentially be made use of in high-risk population screening programs or at regular checkup examinations. Multitarget stool DNA tests based on the use of genetic markers for presymptomatic detection or detection of serrated colorectal polyps are examples of how genetic profiling may be used in a clinical setting (Heigh et al., 2014).

The appropriate management of individuals with precursor polyps is of utmost importance; some of these individuals will develop adenomas again, even after endoscopic removal, and a small percentage will go on to have colorectal cancer. The use of appropriately selected panels of genetic markers associated with adenoma recurrence or progression to carcinoma might pave the way for an individualized patient management based on the pathogenetic elements in tumor development. The introduction of molecular cytogenetic techniques, especially the application of FISH probes on interphase cells in histological sections, may serve as a genetic diagnostic system to assess the potential of excised colorectal lesions by detecting chromosome or gene alterations, for example, loss of 17p, that seem to be linked to the carcinoma transition independently of the initiating chromosomal events.

Standard treatment for colorectal cancer includes adjuvant chemotherapy for patients with lymph node metastases, but not for those without metastatic disease. However, 20% of the latter group eventually die from disease spreading. The identification of complex karyotypes and structural rearrangements of specific chromosomes as indicators of poor disease outcome alluded to earlier could assist oncologists in deciding which patients might benefit from adjuvant treatment after surgery. Some possibilities that immediately present themselves but that, we hasten to emphasize, first need to be confirmed in prospective clinicocytogenetic correlation studies and then to be tested out in appropriate trials would be the following: colorectal cancer patients whose tumor profiles differ from the high-risk patterns already mentioned may not require adjuvant treatment even if this would otherwise be recommended on the basis of standard staging. Patients with primary carcinomas having rearrangements of chromosome 8 and/or loss of chromosome 18, even in the absence of apparent lymph node metastases, should be considered to be at high metastatic risk and therefore may be eligible for chemotherapy that would not be warranted for clinically similar patients without aberrations of chromosomes 8 or 18 in their tumor karyotypes. The use of FISH probes specific for loci on chromosome 18 as well as for 8p and 8q could provide information sufficient to perform a preliminary risk grouping of colorectal cancers. Loss of chromosome 18 and i(8q) formation can be detected even in interphase nuclei isolated from histological sections, whereas whole chromosome probes can be used on metaphase cells whenever fresh tumor material is available. A FISH test as part of the routine laboratory evaluation of large bowel cancer is, in some respects, more reliable than analogous DNA tests that have already been proposed for a genetic-based prognostication system, because the cells are examined individually and not as a DNA mixture from normal and malignant cells. It is also much simpler than complete karyotypic analysis of a tumor sample, which requires considerable cytogenetic expertise. Besides, when the independent prognostic value of additional chromosome aberrations (such as that of chromosomes 4 and 16) is definitely proven for a particular clinical subset of colorectal cancer, one might also utilize additional specific FISH probes to assess prognosis more accurately than is possible based on only the standard histopathologic evaluation.

In addition, interindividual genetic differences, such as the mutation status of *KRAS*, *NRAS*, and *BRAF* genes, are already in clinical use to select CRC patients for anti-EGFR therapies. A plethora of other genetic markers are also being considered in the development of new drugs, which may lead to individualized therapies of patients with colorectal cancer. The ultimate goal is to arrive at therapies that are at the same time both rational and individualized: rational because they rely on medications designed to counteract the pathogenetic events that lie at the heart of colorectal carcinogenesis and individualized because they pay proper attention to the genetic peculiarities of both "individuals" locked in combat in cancer diseases, the genetic makeup of the tumor cells as well as that of the host, the patient.

Pancreas

Karyotypic abnormalities of altogether 127 *pancreatic adenocarcinomas* have been reported in six studies (Johansson et al., 1992; Bardi et al., 1993d; Griffin et al., 1994, 1995; Gorunova et al., 1998; Kowalski et al., 2007). The main cytogenetic features revealed by the karyotyping of these carcinomas are the high level of complexity and the extensive intratumor heterogeneity they display. One reason behind this complexity could be that samples for cytogenetic analysis are only made available at very late disease stages. The lack of benign precursor lesions that can be subjected to cytogenetic study diminishes the possibility of distinguishing primary from secondary aberrations in the massively altered genomic picture usually observed in carcinomas of the pancreas. The same holds true also for the possibility of finding genotypic–phenotypic correlations in pancreatic cancer; most tumors are examined at too late stages of disease for this to be feasible.

The available karyotypic information indicates that all chromosomes have been involved in unbalanced structural aberrations as well as gains and losses in pancreatic cancer. Their frequency of involvement differs considerably among the various series, however. Twenty-two carcinomas of the exocrine pancreas with tumor stemlines ranging from hypodiploid to hypotetraploid were described by Johansson et al. (1992) and Bardi et al. (1993d).

The most common numerical aberrations were, in order of falling frequency, −18, −Y, +20, +7, +11, and −12. The karyotypic imbalances brought about by structural rearrangements frequently affected chromosomes 1, 8, and 17. The breakpoints of the structural aberrations clustered to bands 1p32, 1q10, 6q21, 7p22, 8p21, 8q11, 14p11, 15q10–11, and 17q11 (Bardi et al., 1993d). Abnormal karyotypes were more often found in poorly differentiated and anaplastic carcinomas than in moderately and well-differentiated tumors. Patients whose tumors contained complex numerical and structural aberrations had significantly shorter survival than did those with simple tumor karyotypes (Johansson et al., 1994). Griffin et al. (1994, 1995) described another 44 pancreatic carcinomas with karyotypic abnormalities. The most common numerical aberrations were gains of chromosomes 20 and 7 and losses of chromosomes 18, 13, 12, 17, and 6. Two hundred and nine breakpoints were identified as involved in structural rearrangements affecting, in order of decreasing frequency, chromosome arms 1p, 6q, 7q, 17p, 1q, 3p, 11p, and 19q. Extensive intra-tumor cytogenetic heterogeneity (ICH) and a high level of karyotypic complexity were the most impressive cytogenetic features described by Gorunova et al. (1995, 1998) in a series of 25 karyotypically abnormal pancreatic carcinomas. Nineteen of the examined tumors each displayed from 2 to 58 clones. Karyotypically documented clonal evolution in the form of related clones was detected in 16 tumors, whereas seemingly unrelated clones were present in nine tumors. Altogether, 608 breakpoints were involved in structural rearrangements, and a total of 19 recurrent unbalanced structural changes were identified. The main karyotypic imbalances were whole-copy losses of chromosomes 18, Y, and 21; gains of chromosomes 7, 2, and 20; partial or whole-arm losses of 1p, 3p, 6q, 8p, 9p, 15q, 17p, 18q, 19p, and 20p; and partial or whole-arm gains of 1q, 3q, 5p, 6p, 7q, 8q, 11q, 12p, 17q, 19q, and 20q. To explore the mechanisms of ICH, Harada et al. (2002) investigated interglandular variation in 20 primary invasive ductal adenocarcinomas of the pancreas by CGH analysis. The profiles displayed a wide variety of differences between multiple adjacent neoplastic glands within the same tumor in all cases, that is, interglandular cytogenetic heterogeneity as measured also by CGH was pronounced in pancreatic

cancer. Genetic changes detected in all regions of a tumor were classified as "region-independent" alterations, whereas changes seen in at least one but not all regions were designated as "region-dependent" alterations and resulted in ICH. The degree of ICH, which was quantified as the ratio between these two types of alterations, correlated closely with the DNA index, and the authors therefore suggested that DNA index might be a surrogate marker for ICH. The results were interpreted to indicate that tumor progression, ICH, and DNA aneuploidy result from the successive appearance of region-dependent alterations attributable to CIN in tumor cells. Based on their findings, the authors supported the concept of individual cell heterogeneity in pancreatic cancer.

Clonal karyotypic abnormalities in another 36 primary pancreatic carcinomas from patients who had undergone a Whipple resection with curative intent were reported by Kowalski et al. (2007). Most of the tumors were diploid or triploid. Most commonly lost were chromosomes 18, 17, 6, 21, 22, Y, and 4. Chromosome 20 was the most frequently gained. Structural abnormalities were also common, resulting in partial chromosomal gains and losses and with a median number of 7 imbalances per case (range, 1–15). Cytogenetic evidence of gene amplification, double-minute chromosomes and homogeneously staining regions, was seen in 16 carcinomas.

In spite of the different cytogenetic features highlighted in various studies, the pooling of all presently available karyotypic data on pancreatic adenocarcinomas allows us to distinguish some very interesting features (Figure 14.7): monosomy 18, described as a common change in all series, is the most frequent chromosome aberration (60% of all cases). Several other recurrent aneusomies follow, but their frequency is clearly lower than that of −18. Thus, −17, −21, −6, −Y, +7, −4, −X, +20, −12, −22, and −9 are all seen in 25–38% of the cases. Interestingly, none of recurrent breakpoints seen in the plethora of structural rearrangements identified in the six series reach a frequency higher than 13% in the meta-analysis. Chromosome bands 13q10, 19q13, 1q10, 8q10, 14q10, 17p11, and 17q10 are the most common sites of breakpoints (8–13%). Most of them are commonly involved in other gastrointestinal malignancies as well, and with the exception of 19q13, they are all at or close to the centromeres.

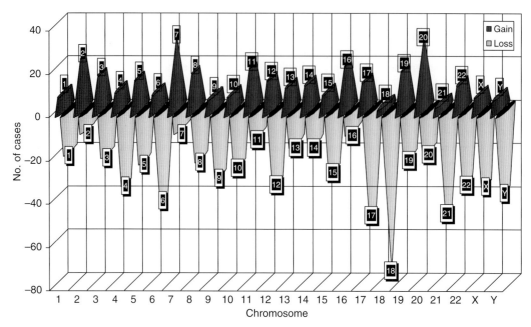

Figure 14.7 Distribution of numerical chromosome aberrations in 127 pancreatic adenocarcinomas with clonal chromosome aberrations.

Additional studies, preferably utilizing multiple investigative technologies, are clearly needed to shed more light on the genetic events underlying pancreatic cancer development and progression. If one is able to integrate all available methodological tools at the genomic, transcriptional, and proteomic level, a more comprehensive assessment of the overall genomic picture of these tumors can surely be arrived at than is possible on the basis of karyotyping alone.

Liver and biliary tract

None of the various types of primary liver tumor have been extensively examined cytogenetically; the available cytogenetic information is restricted to only 173 cases (Mitelman et al., 2014). Regarding *hepatocellular carcinoma*, the most common type of liver cancer and the fourth leading cause of cancer death worldwide, our cytogenetic knowledge is based on only 22 cases with abnormal karyotypes (Simon et al., 1990; Bardi et al., 1992b; Werner et al., 1993; Chen et al., 1996; Lowichik et al., 1996; Hany et al., 1997; Bardi et al., 1998; Parada et al., 1998). The characteristic features that are apparent should therefore be viewed with some caution. The

combined data show that hepatocellular carcinomas are generally highly complex cytogenetically with multiple numerical and structural chromosome aberrations. Although none of the observed chromosome changes appears to be specific for this type of tumors, some abnormalities are frequent (20–35%) and characteristic such as i(8)(q10), deletions of the short arm of chromosome 1, trisomy 7, and monosomy for chromosomes 5, 8, 13, 21, and 22 (Figure 14.8).

Many CGH studies (Wong et al., 1999; Kitay-Cohen et al., 2001; Nishida et al., 2003; Hashimoto et al., 2004; Patil et al., 2005) have not only confirmed the imbalances seen by G-banding analysis but also identified losses and gains of several additional chromosomal regions as nonrandom genomic events in hepatocellular carcinomas. Although the distribution of aberrant chromosomal arms differs among tumors and also among different series, a CGH meta-analysis of 785 human hepatocellular carcinomas and 30 premalignant dysplastic nodules (Moinzadeh et al., 2005) showed that the most prominent amplifications of genomic material took place in 1q (57.1%), 8q (46.6%), 6p (22.3%), and 17q (22.2%), whereas losses were most prevalent in 8p (38%), 16q (35.9%), 4q (34.3%), 17p (32.1%), and 13q

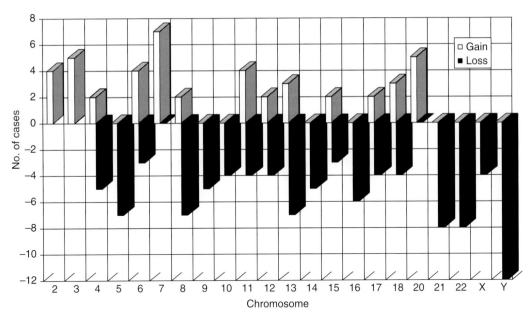

Figure 14.8 Distribution of numerical chromosome aberrations in 22 hepatocellular carcinomas with clonal chromosome aberrations.

(26.2%). In poorly differentiated tumors, 13q and 4q were significantly underrepresented. Moreover, gains of 1q were positively correlated with the occurrence of all other high-frequency alterations. In premalignant dysplastic nodules, amplifications were most frequently present in 1q and 8q, whereas deletions occurred in 8p, 17p, 5p, 13q, 14q, and 16q. The authors concluded that etiology and dedifferentiation correlate with specific genomic alterations in human hepatocellular cancer. That accumulation of genomic imbalances, including the acquisition of specific changes such as gain of 8q, is associated with tumor progression was also found by Patil et al. (2005) in an aCGH study. The identification of other aberrations, such as loss of 1p, not only in well-differentiated hepatocellular carcinomas but also in dysplastic and cirrhotic hepatic nodules suggests that CIN may occur at an early stage during hepatocarcinogenesis, well before the emergence of a malignant phenotype (Nishida et al., 2003).

Molecular genetic studies have revealed a high number of altered genes in hepatocellular cancer, suggesting the existence of at least four different pathogenetic pathways: the TP53 pathway involved in response to DNA damage, the RB1 pathway involved in control of the cell cycle, the TGFB pathway involved in growth inhibition, and the WNT pathway involved in cell–cell adhesion and signal transduction (Saffroy et al., 2006). These main pathways may be alternative to one another, but they could also possibly be complementary. Hiroto et al. (2007) studied 87 hepatocellular carcinomas combining genome-scale chromosome copy number alteration profiles and examination of the mutational status of *TP53* and *CTNNB1*. The results led them to suggest that hepatocellular cancer consists of several genetically homogeneous subclasses, each of which harbors characteristic genetic alterations and even pathognomonic chromosomal amplifications, for example, *MYC*-induced tumors, 6p/1q-amplified tumors, and 17q-amplified tumors. The application of global genomic and proteomic methods to analyze large and clinically well-characterized tumor series should be able to test the proposed hypotheses regarding the cause and functional significance of genomic alterations in human hepatocellular cancer.

In a rare liver cancer subtype affecting adolescents and young adults, fibrolamellar hepatocellular carcinoma, Honeyman et al. (2014) recently identified a chimeric transcript *DNAJB1–PRKACA* brought about by a 400 Kb deletion on chromosome 19. The chimeric RNA is predicted to encode a protein containing the amino-terminal domain of DNAJB1, a homolog of the molecular chaperone DNAJ, fused in frame with PRKACA, the catalytic domain of protein kinase A. The fusion transcript was found in 15 of 15 tumors examined.

The most common liver tumor in childhood is *hepatoblastoma*. At the present time, about 110 cases with abnormal karyotypes are known (Mitelman et al., 2014). The first data came from small studies (Fletcher et al., 1991; Rodriguez et al., 1991; Soukup and Lampkin, 1991; Bardi et al., 1991b, 1992a; Schneider et al., 1997; Sainati et al., 1998; Parada et al., 2000) presenting the karyotypes of single or up to six cases. Only the study by Tomlinson et al. (2005) presented the results of a large series comprising 111 hepatoblastomas karyotyped over a period of 12 years, with abnormal karyotypes being identified in almost half the tumors. Numerical changes were seen in 36% of the total number of cases, whereas only 18% displayed structural rearrangements, which were mostly unbalanced and resulting in gain of 1q. Among the numerical changes, the most frequent were trisomies for chromosomes 2, 8, and 20. Losses of whole chromosomes were less common than gains.

If we merge the data of Tomlinson et al. (2005) with the earlier findings by other groups, we see that the few structural chromosome rearrangements found in hepatoblastomas all are unbalanced and mostly involve chromosomes 1, 4, and 8 at 1q12, 1q10, 4q33–34, and 8q10. The most common numerical abnormality is trisomy 20 (53%), followed by trisomy 2 (39%) and trisomy 8 (34%) (Figure 14.9). None of the chromosome losses reaches a frequency higher than 7% in the total number of reported cases. Also, CGH data indicate that gains of chromosomal material are characteristic imbalances in hepatoblastomas, as they occur almost sevenfold more frequently than losses (Weber et al., 2000). Cytogenetic evidence (Sainati et al., 1998; Parada et al., 2000) suggests that trisomy 20 occurs during clonal evolution as a progression-related change rather than as an early event. As gain of chromosome 2 is also commonly found in embryonal rhabdomyosarcoma, another pediatric neoplasm associated with Beckwith–Wiedemann syndrome, this aberration might constitute a critical step in the development of embryonal tumors. Highly amplified sequences have been identified in some cases mapping to 2q24, 8q11.2–13, and 8q11.2–21.3 (Weber et al., 2000), but the relevant

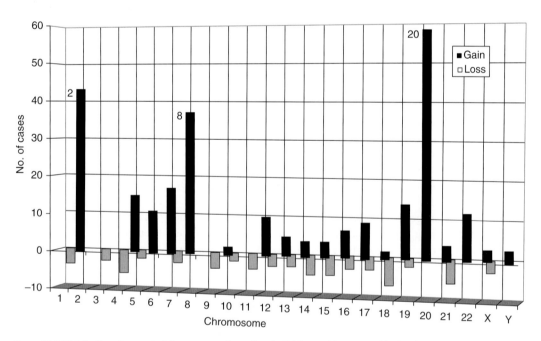

Figure 14.9 Distribution of numerical chromosome aberrations in 110 hepatoblastomas with clonal chromosome aberrations.

target genes of these changes have not yet been found. Of particular clinical interest was the correlation analysis, performed by the same group, between specific genomic alterations and the disease outcome for 34 hepatoblastoma patients; they found that gains of 8q and chromosome 20 were genetic predictors of poor clinical outcome in this disease.

Only isolated reports have described chromosomal aberrations in other types of liver tumors. Mascarello and Krous (1992) were the first to describe the translocation t(11;19)(q13;q13) in mesenchymal liver *hamartoma*. Later reports have confirmed the presence of this translocation in additional cases (Bove et al., 1998; Rakheja et al., 2004; Sharif et al., 2006). More recently, the cloning and DNA sequence analysis of the translocation breakpoints was reported (Rajaram et al., 2007) in an undifferentiated embryonal sarcoma arising in a mesenchymal hamartoma of the liver carrying an identical t(11;19). The breakpoint at 11q13 occurs in the *MALAT1* gene, also known as *ALPHA*. *MALAT1* is also rearranged in renal tumors carrying the t(6;11)(p21;q13) translocation (Chapter 15), and noncoding *MALAT1* transcripts are overexpressed in a number of human carcinomas. The breakpoint at 19q13.4 occurs at a locus referred to as *MHLB1*. Although the *MHLB1* locus does not contain any known gene, several human expressed sequence tags (EST) map to the region, a subset of which show homology to the nuclear RNA export factor (NXF) gene family, and the region is conserved in many mammalian species.

The existing cytogenetic information on biliary tract tumors is restricted to 24 cases, nearly all of them *gallbladder adenocarcinoma*. In the first cytogenetically examined gallbladder carcinomas (Hecht et al., 1983; Bardi et al., 1994), the most prominent feature was the highly complex, abnormal karyotypic pattern, with cytogenetic evidence of gene amplification, aneuploid tumor stemlines, and several recurrent imbalances. Combining G-banding and CGH data on 14 carcinomas, Rijken et al. (1999) found that 11 chromosomal arms were gained entirely or in part, whereas losses occurred from or of nine chromosome arms in at least four tumors each; the lost chromosomal regions were, in decreasing order of frequency, 18q, 6q, 10p, 8p, 12q, 17p, 7q, 12p, and 22q, whereas the most frequently gained regions were 8q, 20q, 12p, 17q, Xp, 2q, 6p, 7p, 11q, 13q, and 19q. On the basis of these data, the

authors suggested that carcinomas of the biliary tract and pancreas share a number of genetic changes. Extensive intratumor heterogeneity, in the form of unrelated clones and altogether 251 breakpoints involved in structural aberrations in seven karyotypically abnormal tumors, was reported by Gorunova et al. (1999). The aberrations del(3) (p13), i(5)(p10), del(6)(q13), del(9)(p13), del(16) (q22), del(17)(p11), i(17)(q10), del(19)(p13), and i(21)(q10), known to occur in other gastrointestinal carcinomas as well, appeared to be recurrent also in gallbladder carcinomas in that study.

Stomach

Clonal chromosome abnormalities have been reported in altogether 133 *gastric carcinomas* (Mitelman et al., 2014). Except for four undifferentiated carcinomas, all were adenocarcinomas, the most common stomach cancers by far. Some were studied as cancerous effusions, and several cases were incompletely karyotyped. Although the evolving picture of gastric cancer karyotypes is still incomplete, several characteristic cytogenetic features are discernible, most of them common to malignancies of the digestive tract in general.

Almost all structural chromosome aberrations reported so far in gastric carcinomas are unbalanced, with the most common (Figure 14.10) being i(8) (q10), found in around 10% of all cases, followed by deletion of 3p21 in about 7%, and rearrangements of 7q22, i(17)(q10), i(13)(q10), deletion of 1p22, and i(5)(p10), all of which are found in roughly 5%.

It is worth emphasizing that all the most frequent numerical chromosomal events in gastric adenocarcinomas represent imbalances repeatedly described also in colorectal cancer: trisomy 8 (22%), trisomy 20 (20%), and trisomies for chromosomes 7 and 13 (10%). Monosomies appear to be more frequent than gains, but this may be a result of incomplete karyotypic description of many complex karyotypes. In any case, the most common losses seem to be monosomy 18, loss of the Y, and monosomies for chromosomes 22, 21, 9, 17, 14, 16, and X, all reported in 20–28% of the cases.

This overall aberration pattern largely corresponds to the gain-and-loss picture that emerged already from early, smaller studies (Ferti-Passantonopoulou et al., 1987; Misawa et al., 1990; Rodriguez et al.,

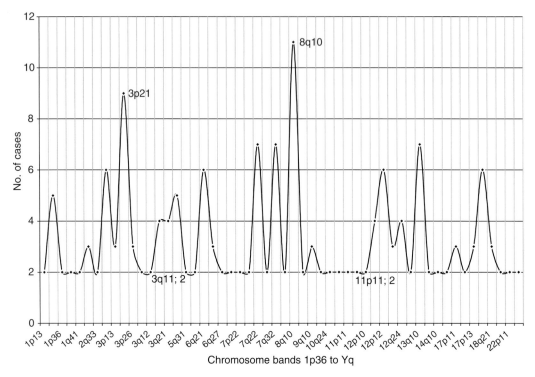

Figure 14.10 Distribution of chromosomal breakpoints involved in structural rearrangements in 129 adenocarcinomas of the stomach with clonal chromosome aberrations.

1990; Xiao et al., 1992; Rao et al., 1993; Seruca et al., 1993). More recently, cytogenetic and FISH studies have highlighted the high incidence of total or partial gain of chromosome 8 material in gastric carcinomas. Xia et al. (1999) suggested that trisomy for chromosomes 8 and 9 and deletion of 7q32-qter are important in the initiation and progression of gastric cancer. Panani et al. (2004), using an alpha-satellite DNA probe for chromosome 8, found trisomy for this chromosome in up to 62% of the cases without apparent preference for any histo-pathologic subtype of tumors. Calcagno et al. (2006) confirmed that chromosome 8 aneuploidy occurs independently of the tumor histological type but observed differences in the amplification and expression status of *MYC* between diffuse and intestinal-type gastric cancer.

Kitayama et al. (2003) investigated 51 formalin-fixed and paraffin-embedded tissue samples of gastric carcinomas with a panel of 18 centromeric probes for chromosomes 1–4, 6–12, 15–18, 20, X, and Y as well as locus-specific probes for *MYC* (8q24) and *TP53* (17p13). Aberrations of chromosomes 1, 8,

17, 20, and X were frequent regardless of histology, although mucocellular-type tumors appeared to have more stable aneusomies than did tubular-type carcinomas. A difference in the clinical outcome of patients whose tumors had aneusomies for chromosomes 3, 10, 11, 12, 17, and Y was suggested; however, the investigators neither screened all chromosomes nor performed multivariate analysis to assess whether the proposed chromosomal predictors could be independent prognostic factors. The prognostic significance of genomic alterations in 74 patients with gastric cancer was also assessed by Suzuki et al. (2003) in a comparative study of paired normal and tumor tissue DNA fingerprints. In a multivariate Cox analysis, they showed that the fraction of genome damage was a prognostic as well as a stage indicator in gastric cancer. Survival was significantly diminished for patients whose tumors showed a genomic damage fraction higher than the cutoff set at 0.22. The degree of genomic damage estimated by arbitrarily primed polymerase chain reaction (AP-PCR) was the only independent factor predicting survival.

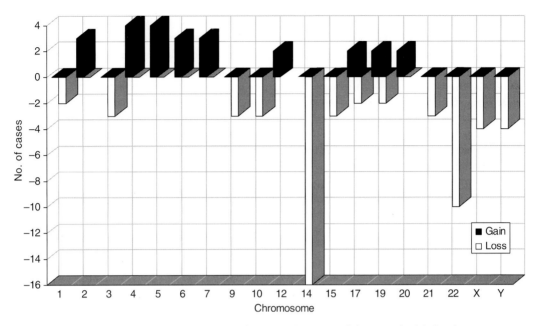

Figure 14.11 Distribution of numerical chromosome aberrations in 31 GIST of the stomach with clonal chromosome aberrations.

Weiss et al. (2003), in a correlation study of tumor genomic profiles and clinicopathologic features of 35 patients with gastric carcinoma, found that chromosomal copy number changes predicted lymph node status and survival. Using a genome-wide scanning array with 2275 BAC and P1 clones giving an average resolution of 1.4 Mb across the genome, they showed that the group of gastric cancers with the lowest mean number of chromosomal events (gains, losses, and amplifications) per case had significantly better survival and lower risk of lymph node metastasis.

Ottini et al. (2006) showed that microsatellite and CIN pathways as well as CpG island methylator phenotype (CIMP) play a role in gastric carcinogenesis. Although the MIS, CIN, and CIMP phenotypes are in general separate, some degree of overlap has been suggested in gastric cancer, as seems to be the case also for other malignancies of the digestive tract (Ottini et al., 2006).

Very little is known about gastric tumors other than carcinomas. There is nothing indicating that leiomyosarcomas of the stomach differ in their karyotypic characteristics from malignant smooth muscle tumors of other locales; the cytogenetics of these tumors is discussed in Chapters 17 and 24.

Similarly, gastric lymphomas such as extranodal marginal zone B-cell lymphomas are discussed in Chapter 11.

Gastrointestinal stromal tumors (GIST) are the most common mesenchymal tumors of the GI tract, arising from the interstitial cells of Cajal, primarily in the stomach and small intestine. Altogether, 31 GIST of the stomach with karyotyped chromosome aberrations have been published. Deletion of 1p11 is the only recurrent structural aberration, identified in two tumors. However, a remarkably high frequency of some numerical chromosome changes (Figure 14.11) has been demonstrated, with monosomy 14 found in 52% and monosomy 22 in 32% of cytogenetically examined GIST. Gunawan et al. (2007), using CGH data from 203 primary GIST, suggested that loss of 14q is mainly detected in tumors with predominantly stable karyotypes and a more favorable clinical course, whereas loss of 1p is associated with increased cytogenetic complexity and more aggressive clinical features. Loss of 22q, more closely associated with loss of 1p than 14q in their study, seemed to mark the transition to an unfavorable cytogenetic subpathway.

The growth of most GIST is driven by oncogenic mutations in either of two tyrosine kinase receptor genes (Hirota et al., 1998), *KIT* (75% of cases) and *PDGFRA* (10%), both residing next to each other on the long arm of chromosome 4, whereas the remaining 15% are negative for mutations in *KIT* and *PDGFRA* (Corless, 2014). In a recent study, Schaefer et al. (2014) analyzed 53 *PDGFRA*-mutated GIST for chromosome imbalances and compared them with a historical series of 122 *KIT*-mutated GIST. They found that *PDGFRA*-mutated GIST displayed the same chromosomal aberrations as did *KIT*-mutated GIST, although they had less CIN in line with their generally favorable outcome.

In an integrated analysis of copy number changes and gene expression in GIST, Astolfi et al. (2010) detected not only frequent involvement of *KIT* and *PDGFRA* but also that the *KIF1B*, *PPM1A*, and *NF2* genes in 1p, 14q, and 22q, respectively, tended to be involved. The genomic segment most frequently found altered in mutated samples was 14q23.1, which contains several potentially important tumor suppressors, including *DAAM1*, *RTN1*, and *DACT1*. In their study, furthermore, the karyotypes of wild-type (WT) GIST displayed fewer genomic alterations than did mutated GIST. The lack of genomic changes in conjunction with overexpression of IGF-1R in WT GIST suggests that the IGF-1 pathway might be a pathogenetic alternative in GIST tumorigenesis.

Treatment with tyrosine kinase inhibitors (TKIs) such as imatinib, sunitinib, and regorafenib is effective in controlling unresectable GIST; however, drug resistance eventually develops in 90% of cases. Adjuvant therapy with imatinib is commonly used to reduce the likelihood of disease recurrence after primary surgery, and for this reason, assessing the prognosis of newly resected tumors remains clinically important (Corless, 2014). The combination of genomic, gene expression, and posttranscriptional profiling may offer a detailed molecular portrait of GIST, providing knowledge necessary to guide the discovery of novel target genes involved in tumor development and progression.

Small intestine

From this relatively neoplasia-free organ, only 34 tumors with clonal chromosome aberrations have been reported (Mitelman et al., 2014). The very limited cytogenetic information consists of case reports or series of only few cases from each of the following mesenchymal tumors: gastrointestinal stromal tumors, leiomyosarcomas, clear cell sarcomas, leiomyomas, as well as a few extranodal marginal zone B-cell lymphomas, carcinoids, and a single case of adenocarcinoma.

The data are much too few to attempt to assess independently the cytogenetic characteristics of these different diagnostic entities that share only the same anatomical location. The reader is referred to other chapters for a general survey of the karyotypic features of mesenchymal tumors and lymphomas.

Summary

Colorectal adenomas are in general karyotypically much simpler than their malignant counterparts, but no single chromosome aberration can distinguish benign from malignant lesions of the large intestine with certainty. Gain of chromosome 7 and deletion of 1p36 appear to be early genetic events in colorectal tumorigenesis. The progression of low-grade to high-grade adenomas and then to colorectal carcinomas, followed by metastasis to lymph nodes and distal organs, is accompanied by the acquisition of additional chromosomal changes, the most common of which are gains of chromosomes 20 and 13, loss of 17p, gain of 17q, monosomy 18, gain of 8q, and losses of 8p and 4p. Metastatic lesions generally show less clonal heterogeneity than do the primary tumors, but instead increased karyotypic complexity of individual clones. Homing of metastasizing colorectal tumor cells to particular organs seems to occur via different patterns of genomic alterations. The overall cytogenetic pattern, the instability status, and the cytogenetic predictors of clinical outcome differ depending on the anatomical site of large bowel tumors. Loss of chromosome 18 and structural rearrangements of chromosome 8, leading to loss of 8p and gain of 8q, are predictors of high metastatic risk, even in the absence of lymph node metastases. Information can therefore be derived from the karyotype about the prognosis of colorectal cancer patients and, hence, could provide clues as to how patients with early- or intermediate-stage tumors should best be treated.

High-level karyotypic complexity and extensive intratumor heterogeneity are the most prominent cytogenetic features of pancreatic adenocarcinomas.

Monosomy 18 is the most frequent aberration present in 60% of all cases. Other frequent aneusomies are −17, −21, −6, −Y, +7, −4, −X, +20, −12, −22, and −9. Recurrent breakpoints mostly are in or near the centromeres: 13q10, 19q13, 1q10, 8q10, 14q10, 17p11, and 17q10. Karyotypic complexity is significantly associated with shorter patient survival.

Several abnormalities, including i(8)(q10), deletions of 1p, trisomy 7, and monosomy for chromosomes 5, 8, 13, 21, and 22, are frequent in hepatocellular carcinomas. Preliminary data indicate that etiology and tumor differentiation correlate with specific genomic alterations. Chromosomal alterations can be found also in dysplastic and cirrhotic hepatic nodules. A chimeric transcript, *DNAJB1-PRKACA*, has been detected in the rare cancer subtype fibrolamellar hepatocellular carcinoma.

Recurrent trisomies, especially +20, +2, and +8, occur frequently in hepatoblastomas. In contrast, monosomies are less common, and the same seems to be the case also for structural aberrations. Structural rearrangements, which always are unbalanced, mostly affect chromosomes 1, 4, and 8 at bands 1q12, 1q10, 4q33–34, and 8q10. Gains of 8q and chromosome 20 may be genetic predictors of poor clinical outcome in hepatoblastoma patients.

A specific balanced translocation, t(11;19)(q13;q13), characterizes liver hamartomas. The gene *MALAT1* (*ALPHA*) is the target in 11q13, whereas the breakpoint in 19q13.4 occurs at a locus referred to as *MHLB1*.

Karyotypic complexity and intratumor heterogeneity as well as several genomic imbalances are the main cytogenetic features of gallbladder carcinomas, a type of tumor that from the cytogenetic point of view seems to have many similarities with pancreatic carcinomas.

Almost all structural aberrations in gastric adenocarcinomas are unbalanced: the most common are i(8)(q10), deletion of 3p21, rearrangements of 7q22, i(17)(q10), i(13)(q10), deletion of 1p22, and i(5)(p10). The numerical chromosome aberrations largely correspond to those known from colorectal cancer: trisomy for chromosomes 8, 20, 7, and 13 and loss of chromosomes 18, Y, 22, 21, 9, 17, 14, 16, and X. A remarkably high frequency of monosomy 14 (52%) and monosomy 22 (32%) is observed in both *KIT*- and *PDGFRA*-mutated gastrointestinal stromal tumors of the stomach. Loss of chromosome 22 is more associated with cytogenetic complexity and unfavorable clinical course than is loss of 14q. The occurrence of submicroscopic mutations of *KIT* and/or *PDGFRA* is important for selecting GIST patients who can benefit from tyrosine kinase inhibitor treatment.

Acknowledgment

Financial support from the Norwegian Cancer Society is gratefully acknowledged.

References

Alcock HE, Stephenson TJ, Royds JA, Hammond DW (2003): Analysis of colorectal tumor progression by microdissection and comparative genomic hybridization. *Genes Chromosomes Cancer* 37:369–380.

Al-Mulla F, Keith WN, Pickford IR, Going JJ, Birnie GD (1999): Comparative genomic hybridisation analysis of primary colorectal carcinomas and their synchronous metastases. *Genes Chromosomes Cancer* 24:306–314.

Aragane H, Sakamura C, Nakanishi M, Yasuoka R, Fujita Y, Tanguchi H, et al. (2001): Chromosomal aberrations in colorectal cancers and liver metastases analyzed by comparative genomic hybridization. *Int J Cancer* 94:623–629.

Arribas R, Ribas M, Risques RA, Masramon L, Tórtola S, Marcuello E, et al. (1999): Prospective assessment of allelic losses at 4p14–16 in colorectal cancer: two mutational patterns and a locus associated with poorer survival. *Clin Cancer Res* 5:3454–3459.

Astolfi A, Nannini M, Pantaleo MA, Di Battista M, Heinrich MC, Santini D, et al. (2010): A molecular portrait of gastrointestinal stromal tumors: an integrative analysis of gene expression profiling and high-resolution genomic copy number. *Lab Invest* 90:1285–1294.

Aust DE, Muders M, Kohler A, Schmidt M, Diebold J, Muller C, et al. (2004): Prognostic relevance of 20q13 gains in sporadic colorectal cancers: a FISH analysis. *Scand J Gastroenterol* 39:766–772.

Bardi G, Johansson B, Pandis N, Heim S, Mandahl N, Andrén-Sandberg Å, et al. (1991a): Trisomy 7 in colorectal adenocarcinomas. *Genes Chromosomes Cancer* 3: 149–152.

Bardi G, Johansson B, Pandis N, Békássy AN, Kullendorff C-M, Hägerstrand I, et al. (1991b): i(8q) as the primary structural chromosome abnormality in a hepatoblastoma. *Cancer Genet Cytogenet* 51:281–283.

Bardi G, Johansson B, Pandis N, Heim S, Mandahl N, Békássy A, et al. (1992a): Trisomy 2 as the sole chromosomal abnormality in a hepatoblastoma. *Genes Chromosomes Cancer* 4:78–80.

Bardi G, Johansson B, Pandis N, Heim S, Mandahl N, Andrén-Sandberg Å, et al. (1992b): Cytogenetic findings in three primary hepatocellular carcinomas. *Cancer Genet Cytogenet* 58:191–195.

Bardi G, Johansson B, Pandis N, Bak-Jensen E, Örndal C, Heim S, et al. (1993a): Cytogenetic aberrations in colorectal adenocarcinomas and their correlation to clinicopathologic features. *Cancer* 71:306–314.

Bardi G, Johansson B, Pandis N, Mandahl N, Bak-Jensen E, Lindström C, et al. (1993b): Cytogenetic analysis of 52 colorectal carcinomas – nonrandom aberration pattern and correlation with pathologic parameters. *Int J Cancer* 55:422–428.

Bardi G, Pandis N, Fenger C, Kronborg O, Bomme L, Heim S (1993c): Deletion of 1p36 as a primary chromosomal aberration in intestinal tumorigenesis. *Cancer Res* 53: 1895–1898.

Bardi G, Johansson B, Pandis N, Mandahl N, Bak-Jensen E, Andrén-Sanberg Å, et al. (1993d): Karyotypic abnormalities in tumors of the pancreas. *Br J Cancer* 67:1106–1112.

Bardi G, Gorunova L, Limon J, Johansson B, Pandis N, Mandahl N, et al. (1994): Cytogenetic findings in three carcinomas of the gallbladder. *Cancer Genet Cytogenet* 76:15–18.

Bardi G, Pandis N, Heim S (1995a): Trisomy 7 as the sole cytogenetic aberration in the epithelial component of a colonic adenoma. *Cancer Genet Cytogenet* 82:82–84.

Bardi G, Sukhikh T, Pandis N, Fenger C, Kronborg O, Heim S (1995b): Karyotypic characterization of colorectal adenocarcinomas. *Genes Chromosomes Cancer* 12:97–109.

Bardi G, Parada LA, Bomme L, Pandis N, Willen R, Johansson B, et al. (1997a): Cytogenetic comparisons of synchronous carcinomas and polyps in patients with colorectal cancer. *Br J Cancer* 76:765–769.

Bardi G, Parada LA, Bomme L, Pandis N, Johansson B, Willen R, et al. (1997b): Cytogenetic findings in metastases from colorectal cancer. *Int J Cancer* 72: 604–607.

Bardi G, Rizou H, Michailakis E, Dietrich C, Pandis N, Heim S (1998): Cytogenetic findings in three primary hepatocellular carcinomas. *Cancer Genet Cytogenet* 104:165–166.

Bardi G, Fenger C, Johansson B, Mitelman F, Heim S (2004): Tumor karyotype predicts clinical outcome in colorectal cancer patients. *J Clin Oncol* 22:2623–2634.

Bedenne L, Faivre JMC, Piard F, Cauvin JM, Hillon P (1992): Adenoma–carcinoma sequence or 'de novo' carcinogenesis? A study of adenomatous remnants in a population-based series of large bowel cancers. *Cancer* 69:883–888.

Bomme L, Bardi G, Pandis N, Fenger C, Kronborg O, Heim S (1994): Clonal karyotypic abnormalities in colorectal adenomas: clues to the early genetic events in the adenoma–carcinoma sequence. *Genes Chromosomes Cancer* 10:190–196.

Bomme L, Bardi G, Fenger C, Kronborg O, Pandis N, Heim S (1996a): Chromosome abnormalities in colorectal adenomas: two cytogenetic subgroups characterized by deletion of 1p and numerical aberrations. *Hum Pathol* 27:1192–1197.

Bomme L, Bardi G, Pandis N, Fenger C, Kronborg O, Heim S (1996b): Cytogenetic analysis of colorectal adenomas: karyotypic comparisons of synchronous tumors. *Cancer Genet Cytogenet* 106:66–71.

Bomme L, Heim S, Bardi G, Fenger C, Kronborg O, Brögger A, et al. (1998): Allelic imbalance and cytogenetic deletion of 1p in colorectal adenomas: a target region identified between D1S199 and D1S234. *Genes Chromosomes Cancer* 21:185–194.

Bomme L, Lothe R, Bardi G, Fenger C, Kronborg O, Heim S (2001): Assessments of clonal composition of colorectal adenomas by FISH analysis of chromosomes 1, 7, 13, and 20. *Int J Cancer* 92:816–823.

Bove KE, Blough RI, Soukup S (1998): Third report of t(19q) (13.4) in mesenchymal hamartoma of liver with comments on link to embryonal sarcoma. *Pediatr Dev Pathol* 1:438–442.

Brabletz T, Jung A, Spaderna S, Hlubek F, Kirchner T (2005): Opinion: migrating cancer stem cells—an integrated concept of malignant tumour progression. *Nat Rev Cancer* 5:744–749.

Brüderlein S, van derBosch K, Schlag P, Schwab M (1990): Cytogenetics and DNA amplification in colorectal cancers. *Genes Chromosomes Cancer* 2:63–70.

Bufill JA (1990): Colorectal cancer: evidence for distinct genetic categories based on proximal or distal tumor location. *Ann Intern Med* 113:779–788.

Calcagno DQ, Leal MF, Seabra AD, Khayat AS, Chen ES, Demachki S, et al. (2006): Interrelationship between chromosome 8 aneuploidy, C-MYC amplification and increased expression in individuals from northern Brazil with gastric adenocarcinoma. *World J Gastroenterol* 12:6207–6211.

Cardoso J, Boer J, Morreau H, Fodde R (2007): Expression and genomic profiling of colorectal cancer. *Biochim Biophys Acta Rev Cancer* 1775:103–137.

Chen HL, Chen YC, Chen DS (1996): Chromosome 1p aberrations are frequent in human primary hepatocellular carcinoma. *Cancer Genet Cytogenet* 86:102–106.

Corless CL (2014) Gastrointestinal stromal tumors: what do we know now? *Mod Pathol* 27:S1–S16.

Couturier-Turpin MH, Bertrand V, Couturier D (2001): Distal deletion of 1p in colorectal tumors: an initial event and/or a step in carcinogenesis? Study by fluorescence *in situ* hybridization interphase cytogenetics. *Cancer Genet Cytogenet* 24:47–55.

D'Arrigo A, Belluco C, Ambrosi A, Digito M, Esposito G, Bertola A, et al. (2005): Metastatic transcriptional pattern revealed by gene expression profiling in primary colorectal carcinoma. *Int J Cancer* 115:256–262.

De Angelis PM, Stokke T, Beigi M, Mjaland O, Clausen OP (2001): Prognostic significance of recurrent chromosomal aberrations detected by comparative genomic hybridization in sporadic colorectal cancer. *Int J Colorectal Dis* 16:38–45.

Diep CB, Kleivi K, Ribeiro FR, Teixeira MR, Lindgjaerde OC, Lothe RA (2006): The order of genetic events associated with colorectal cancer progression inferred from meta analysis of copy number changes. *Genes Chromosomes Cancer* 45:31–41.

Douglas EJ, Fiegler H, Rowan A, Halford S, Bicknell DC, Bodmer W, et al. (2004): Array comparative genomic hybridization analysis of colorectal cancer cell lines and primary carcinomas. *Cancer Res* 64:4817–4825.

Fawole AS, Simpson DJ, Rajagopal R, Elder J, Holland TA, Fryer A, et al. (2002): Loss of heterozygosity on chromosome 10q is associated with earlier onset sporadic colorectal adenocarcinoma. *Int J Cancer* 99:829–833.

Fearon ER (2011): Molecular genetics of colorectal cancer. *Annu Rev Pathol Mech Dis* 6:479–507.

Fearon ER, Vogelstein B (1990): A genetic model for colorectal tumorigenesis. *Cell* 61: 759–767.

Ferti-Passantonopoulou AD, Panani AD, Vlachos JD, Raptis SA (1987): Common cytogenetic findings in gastric cancer. *Cancer Genet Cytogenet* 24:63–73.

Fletcher JA, Kozakewich HP, Pavelka K, Grier HE, Shamberger RC, Korf B, et al. (1991): Consistent cytogenetic aberrations in hepatoblastoma: a common pathway of genetic alterations in embryonal liver and skeletal muscle malignancies? *Genes Chromosomes Cancer* 3:37–43.

Gao P, Song YX, Wang ZN, Xu YY, Tong LL, Sun JX, et al. (2013): Is the prediction of prognosis not improved by the seventh edition of the TNM classification for colorectal cancer? Analysis of the surveillance, epidemiology, and end results (SEER) database. *BMC Cancer* 13:123.

Gemoll T, Habermann JK, Becker S, Szymczak S, Upender MB, Bruch H-P, et al. (2014): Chromosomal aneuploidy affects the global proteome equilibrium of colorectal cancer cells. *Analyt Cell Pathol* 36:149–161.

Ghadimi BM, Grade M, Liersch T, Langer C, Siemer A, Füzesi L, et al. (2003): Gain of chromosome 8q23–24 is a predictive marker for lymph node positivity in colorectal cancer. *Clin Cancer Res* 9:1808–1814.

Gorunova L, Johansson B, Dawiskiba S, Andrén-Sandberg A, Mandahl N, Heim S, et al. (1995): Cytogenetically detected clonal heterogeneity in a duodenal adenocarcinoma. *Cancer Genet Cytogenet* 82:146–150.

Gorunova L, Höglund M, Andrén-Sandberg A, Dawiskiba S, Jin Y, Mitelman F, et al. (1998): Cytogenetic analysis of pancreatic carcinomas: intratumor heterogeneity and nonrandom pattern of chromosome aberrations. *Genes Chromosomes Cancer* 23:81–99.

Gorunova L, Parada LA, Limon J, Jin Y, Hallen M, Hägerstrand I, et al. (1999): Nonrandom chromosomal aberrations and cytogenetic heterogeneity in gallbladder carcinomas. *Genes Chromosomes Cancer* 26:312–321.

Grade M, Becker H, Liersch T, Ried T, Ghadimi BM (2006): Molecular cytogenetics: genomic imbalances in colorectal cancer and their clinical impact. *Cellular Oncol* 28:71–84.

Griffin CA, Hruban RH, Long PP, Morsberger LA, Douna-Issa F, Yeo CJ (1994): Chromosome abnormalities in pancreatic adenocarcinoma. *Genes Chromosomes Cancer* 9:93–100.

Griffin CA, Hruban RH, Morsberger LA, Ellingham T, Long PP, Jaffee EM, et al. (1995): Consistent chromosome abnormalities in adenocarcinoma of the pancreas. *Cancer Res* 55:2394–2399.

Gunawan B, von Heydebreck A, Sander B, Schulten HJ, Haller F, Langer C, et al. (2007): An oncogenetic tree model in gastrointestinal stromal tumours (GISTs) identifies different pathways of cytogenetic evolution with prognostic implications. *J Pathol* 211:463–470.

Halling KC, French AJ, McDonnell SK, Burgart LJ, Schaid DJ, Peterson BJ, et al. (1999): Microsatellite instability and 8p allelic imbalance in stage B2 and C colorectal cancers. *J Natl Cancer Inst* 91:1295–1303.

Hany MA, Betts DR, Schmugge M, Schonle E, Niggli FK, Zachmann M, et al. (1997): A childhood fibrolamellar hepatocellular carcinoma with increased aromatase activity and a near triploid karyotype. *Med Pediatr Oncol* 28:136–138.

Harada T, Okita K, Shiraishi K, Kusano N, Kondoh S, Sasaki K (2002): Interglandular cytogenetic heterogeneity detected by comparative genomic hybridization in pancreatic cancer. *Cancer Res* 62:835–839.

Hashimoto K, Mori N, Tamesa T, Okada T, Kawauchi S, Oga A, et al. (2004): Analysis of DNA copy number aberrations in hepatitis C virus-associated hepatocellular carcinomas by conventional CGH and array CGH. *Mod Pathol* 17:617–622.

Hecht F, Kuban DJ, Berger C, Kaiser-McCaw Hecht B, Sandberg AA (1983): Adenocarcinoma of the gallbladder: chromosome abnormalities in a genetic form of cancer. *Cancer Genet Cytogenet* 8:185–190.

Heigh RI, Yab TC, Taylor WR, Hussain FTN, Smyrk TC, Mahoney DW, et al. (2014): Detection of colorectal serrated polyps by stool DNA testing: comparison with fecal immunochemical testing for occult blood (FIT). *PLoS One* 9:e85659.

Heim S (1992): Is cancer cytogenetics reducible to the molecular genetics of cancer cells? *Genes Chromosomes Cancer* 5:188–196.

Henrich KO, Schwab M, Westermann F (2012): 1p36 tumor suppression – a matter of dosage? *Cancer Res* 72:6079–6088.

Hirota S, Isozaki K, Moriyama Y, Hashimoto K, Nishida T, Ishiguro S, et al. (1998): Gain-of-function mutations of c-kit in human gastrointestinal stromal tumors. *Science* 279:577–580.

Hiroto K, Hidenori O, Akiko K, Shigeru S, Tadashi K, Tomoo K, et al. (2007): Genetically distinct and clinically relevant classification of hepatocellular carcinoma: putative therapeutic targets. *Gastroenterology* 133:1475–1486.

Honeyman JN, Simon EP, Robine N, Chiaroni-Clarke R, Darcy DG, Lim IIP, et al. (2014): Detection of a recurrent DNAJB1-PRKACA chimeric transcript in fibrolamellar hepatocellular carcinoma. *Science* 343:1010–1014.

Houlston RS, Collins A, Slack J, Morton NE (1992): Dominant genes for colorectal cancer are not rare. *Ann Hum Genet* 56:99–103.

Iacopetta B (2002): Are there two sides to colorectal cancer? *Int J Cancer* 101:403–408.

Jasmine F, Rahaman R, Dodsworth C, Roy S, Paul R, Raza M, et al. (2012): A genome-wide study of cytogenetic changes in colorectal cancer using SNP microarrays: opportunities for future personalized treatment. *PLoS One* 7:e31968.

Jiang JK, Chen YJ, Lin CH, Yu IT, Lin JK (2005): Genetic changes and clonality relationship between primary colorectal cancers and their pulmonary metastases – an analysis by comparative genomic hybridisation. *Genes Chromosomes Cancer* 43:25–36.

Johansson B, Bardi G, Heim S, Mandahl N, Mertens F, Bak-Jensen E, et al. (1992): Nonrandom chromosomal abnormalities in pancreatic carcinomas. *Cancer* 69:1674–1681.

Johansson B, Heim S, Mandahl N, Mertens F, Mitelman F (1993): Trisomy 7 in nonneoplastic cells. *Genes Chromosomes Cancer* 6:199–205.

Johansson B, Bardi G, Pandis N, Gorunova L, Bäckman PL, Mandahl N, et al. (1994): Karyotypic pattern of pancreatic adenocarcinomas correlates with survival and tumour grade. *Int J Cancer* 58:8–13.

Kitayama Y, Igarashi H, Watanabe F, Maruyama Y, Kanamori M, Sugimura H (2003): Nonrandom chromosomal numerical abnormality predicting prognosis of gastric cancer: a retrospective study of 51 cases using pathology archives. *Lab Invest* 83:1311–1320.

Kitay-Cohen Y, Amiel A, Ashur Y, Fejgin MD, Herishanu Y Afanasyev F, et al. (2001): Analysis of chromosomal aberrations in large hepatocellular carcinomas by comparative genomic hybridization. *Cancer Genet Cytogenet* 131:60–64.

Knosel T, Schluns K, Stein U, Schwabe H, Schlag PM, Dietel M, et al. (2003): Genetic imbalances with impact on survival in colorectal cancer patients. *Histopathology* 43:323–331.

Knosel T, Schluns K, Stein U, Schwabe H, Schlag PM, Dietel M, et al. (2004): Chromosomal alterations during lymphatic and liver metastasis formation of colorectal cancer. *Neoplasia* 6:23–28.

Knosel T, Schluns K, Dietel M, Petersen I (2005): Chromosomal alterations in lung metastases of colorectal carcinomas: associations with tissue specific tumor dissemination. *Clin Exp Metastasis* 22:533–538.

Konstantinova LN, Fleishman EW, Knisch VI, Perevozchikov AG, Kopnin BP (1991): Karyotypic peculiarities of human colorectal adenocarcinomas. *Hum Genet* 86:491–496.

Kowalski J, Morsberger LA, Blackford A, Hawkins A, Yeo CJ, Hruban RH, et al. (2007): Chromosomal abnormalities of adenocarcinoma of the pancreas: identifying early and late changes. *Cancer Genet Cytogenet* 178:26–35.

Leggett BA, Devereaux B, Biden K, Searle J, Young J, Jass J (2001): Hyperplastic polyposis: association with colorectal cancer. *Am J Surg Pathol* 25:177–184.

Lin JK, Chang SC, Yang YC, Li AF-Y (2003): Loss of heterozygosity and DNA aneuploidy in colorectal adenocarcinoma. *Ann Surg Oncol* 10:1086–1094.

Lips EH, de Graaf EJ, Tollenaar R, van Eijk R, Oosting J, Szuhai K, et al. (2007): Single nucleotide polymorphism array analysis of chromosomal instability patterns discriminates rectal adenomas from carcinomas. *J Pathol* 212:269–277.

Lowichik A, Schneider NR, Tonk V, Ansari MQ, Timmons CF (1996): Report of a complex karyotype in recurrent metastatic fibrolamellar hepatocellular carcinoma and a review of hepatocellular carcinoma cytogenetics. *Cancer Genet Cytogenet* 88:170–174.

Ly P, Eskiocak U, Kim SB, Roig AI, Hight SK, Lulla DR, et al. (2011): Characterization of aneuploid populations with trisomy 7 and 20 derived from diploid human colonic epithelial cells. *Neoplasia* 13:348–357.

Mao X, Hamoudi RA, Talbot IC, Baudis M (2006): Allele-specific loss of heterozygosity in multiple colorectal adenomas: toward an integrated molecular cytogenetic map II. *Cancer Genet Cytogenet* 167:1–14.

Mascarello JT, Krous HF (1992): Second report of a translocation involving 19q13.4 in a mesenchymal hamartoma of the liver. *Cancer Genet Cytogenet* 58:141–142.

Meijer GA, Hermsen MAJA, Baaak JPA, van Diest PJ, Meuwissen SGM, Belien JAM (1998): Progression from colorectal adenoma to carcinoma is associated with nonrandom chromosomal gains as detected by comparative genomic hybridization. *J Clin Pathol* 51:901–909.

Mekenkamp LJM, Haan JC, Israeli D, van Essen HFB, Dijkstra JR, van Cleef P, et al. (2014): Chromosomal copy number aberrations in colorectal metastases resemble their primary counterparts and differences are typically non-recurrent. *PLoS One* 9:e86833.

Misawa S, Horiike S, Taniwaki M, Tsuda S, Okuda T, Kashima K, et al. (1990): Chromosome abnormalities of gastric cancer detected in cancerous effusions. *Jpn J Cancer Res* 81:148–152.

Mitelman F, Mark J, Nilsson PG, Dencker H, Norryd C, Tranberg KG (1974): Chromosome banding pattern in human colonic polyps. *Hereditas* 78:63–68.

Mitelman F, Johansson B, Mertens F, editors (2014): Mitelman Database of Chromosome Aberrations and Gene Fusions in Cancer. http://cgap.nci.nih.gov/Chromosomes/Mitelman.

Moinzadeh P, Breuhahn K, Stützer H, Schirmacher P (2005): Chromosome alterations in human hepatocellular carcinomas correlate with aetiology and histological grade: results of an explorative CGH meta-analysis. *Br J Cancer* 92:935–941.

Muleris M, Salmon R-J, Dutrillaux B (1990): Cytogenetics of colorectal adenocarcinomas. *Cancer Genet Cytogenet* 46:143–156.

Nakao K, Mehta KR, Fridlyand J, Moore DH, Jain AN, Lafuente A, et al. (2004): High-resolution analysis of DNA copy number alterations in colorectal cancer by array-based comparative genomic hybridization. *Carcinogenesis* 25:1345–1357.

Nishida K, Takano H, Yoneda M, Ohtsuki T, Fujii M, Terasawa Y, et al. (1995): Flow cytometric analysis of nuclear DNA content in tissues of colon cancer using endoscopic biopsy specimens. *J Surg Oncol* 59:181–185.

Nishida N, Nishimura T, Ito T, Komeda T, Fukuda Y, Nakao K (2003): Chromosomal instability and human hepatocarcinogenesis. *Histol Histopathol* 18:897–909.

Nome T, Thomassen GOS, Bruun J, Ahlquist T, Bakken AC, Hoff AM, et al. (2013): Common fusion transcripts identified in colorectal cancer cell lines by high-throughput RNA sequencing. *Translat Oncol* 6:546–553.

Ottini L, Falchetti M, Lupi R, Rizzolo P, Agnese V, Colucci G, et al. (2006): Patterns of genomic instability in gastric cancer: clinical implications and perspectives. *Ann Oncol* 17:97–102.

Panani AD, Ferti AD, Avgerinos A, Raptis SA (2004): Numerical aberrations of chromosome 8 in gastric cancer detected by fluorescence in situ hybridization. *Anticancer Res* 24:155–159.

Parada LA, Hallén M, Tranberg KG, Hägerstrand I, Bondeson L, Mitelman F, et al. (1998): Frequent rearrangements of chromosomes 1, 7, and 8 in primary liver cancer. *Genes Chromosomes Cancer* 23:26–35.

Parada LA, Maranon A, Hallen M, Tranberg K-G, Stenram U, Bardi G, et al. (1999): Cytogenetic analyses of secondary liver tumors reveal significant differences in genomic imbalances between primary and metastatic colon carcinomas. *Clin Exp Metastasis* 17:471–479.

Parada LA, Limon J, Iliszko M, Czauderna P, Gisselsson D, Höglund M, et al. (2000): Cytogenetics of hepatoblastoma: further characterization of 1q rearrangements by fluorescence in situ hybridization: an international collaborative study. *Med Pediatr Oncol* 34:165–170.

Paredes-Zaglul A, Kang JJ, Essig YP, Mao WG, Irby R, Wloch M, et al. (1998): Analysis of colorectal cancer by comparative genomic hybridization: evidence for inclusion of the metastatic phenotype by loss of tumor suppressor genes. *Clin Cancer Res* 4:879–886.

Patil MA, Gütgemann I, Zhang J, Ho C, Cheung ST, Ginzinger D, et al. (2005): Array-based comparative genomic hybridization reveals recurrent chromosomal aberrations and Jab1 as a potential target for 8q gain in hepatocellular carcinoma. *Carcinogenesis* 26:2050–2057.

Platzer Upender MB, Wilson K, Willis J, Lutterbaugh J, Norratti A, Willson JKV, et al. (2002): Silence of chromosomal amplifications in colon cancer. *Cancer Res* 62:1134–1138.

Rajaram V, Knezevich S, Bove KE, Perry A, Pfeifer JD (2007): DNA sequence of the translocation breakpoints in undifferentiated embryonal sarcoma arising in mesenchymal hamartoma of the liver harboring the t(11;19)(q11;q13.4) translocation. *Genes Chromosomes Cancer* 46:508–513.

Rakheja D, Margraf LR, Tomlinson GE, Schneider NR (2004): Hepatic mesenchymal hamartoma with translocation involving chromosome band 19q13.4: a recurrent abnormality. *Cancer Genet Cytogenet* 153:60–63.

Rao PH, Mathew S, Lauwers G, Rodriguez E, Kelsen DP, Chaganti RSK (1993): Interphase cytogenetics of gastric and esophageal adenocarcinomas. *Diagn Mol Pathol* 2:264–268.

Rashid A, Houlihan P, Booker S, Petersen G, Giardiello F, Hamilton S (2000): Phenotypic and molecular characteristics of hyperplastic polyposis. *Gastroenterology* 119:323–332.

Reichman A, Levin Martin P, Levin B (1981): Chromosomal banding patterns in human large bowel cancer. *Int J Cancer* 28:431–440.

Ried T, Knutzen R, Steinbeck R, Blegen H, Schrock E, Heselmeyer K, et al. (1996): Comparative genomic hybridization reveals a specific pattern of chromosomal gains and losses during the genesis of colorectal tumors. *Genes Chromosomes Cancer* 15:234–245.

Rijken AM, Hu J, Perlman EJ, Morsberger LA, Long P, Kern SE, et al. (1999): Genomic alterations in distal bile duct carcinoma by comparative genomic hybridization and karyotype analysis. *Genes Chromosomes Cancer* 26:185–191.

Rodriguez E, Rao PH, Ladanyi M, Altorki N, Albino AP, Kelsen DP, et al. (1990): 11p13–15 is a specific region of chromosomal rearrangement in gastric and esophageal adenocarcinomas. *Cancer Res* 50:6410–6416.

Rodriguez E, Reuter VE, Mies C, Bosl GJ, Chaganti RSK (1991): Abnormalities of 2q: a common genetic link between rhabdomyosarcoma and hepatoblastoma? *Genes Chromosomes Cancer* 3:122–127.

Ruzzo A, Graziano F, Canestrari E, Magnani M (2010): Molecular predictors of efficacy to anti-EGFR agents in colorectal cancer patients. *Curr Cancer Drug Targets* 10:68–79.

Saffroy R, Lemoine A, Debuire B (2006): Mechanisms of hepatocarcinogenesis. *Atlas Genet Cytogenet Oncol Haematol.* http://AtlasGeneticsOncology.org/Deep/HepatocarcinogenesisID20055.html (accessed February 3, 2015).

Sainati L, Leszl A, Stella M, Montaldi A, Perilongo G, Rugge M, et al. (1998): Cytogenetic analysis of hepatoblastoma: hypothesis of cytogenetic evolution in such tumors and results of a multicentric study. *Cancer Genet Cytogenet* 104:39–44.

Schaefer I-M, Delfs C, Cameron S, Gunawan B, Agaimy A, Ghadimi M, et al. (2014): Chromosomal aberrations in primary PDGFRA-mutated gastrointestinal stromal tumors. *Hum Pathol* 45:85–97.

Schneider NR, Cooley LD, Finegold MJ, Douglass EC, Tomlinson GE (1997): The first recurring chromosome translocation in hepatoblastoma: der(4)t(1;4)(q12;q34). *Genes Chromosomes Cancer* 19:291–294.

Seruca R, Castedo S, Correia C, Gomes P, Carneiro F, Soares P, et al. (1993): Cytogenetic findings in eleven gastric carcinomas. *Cancer Genet Cytogenet* 68:42–48.

Sharif K, Ramani P, Lochbóhler H, Grundy R, de Ville de Goyet J (2006): Recurrent mesenchymal hamartoma associated with 19q translocation. A call for more radical surgical resection. *Eur J Pediatr Surg* 16:64–67.

Shen L, Toyota M, Kondo Y, Lin E, Zhang L, Guo Y, et al. (2007): Integrated genetic and epigenetic analysis identifies three different subclasses of colon cancer. *Proc Natl Acad Sci USA* 104:18654–18659.

Shroy P, Cohen A, Winawer S, Friedman E (1988): New chemotherapeutic drug sensitivity for colon carcinomas in monolayer culture. *Cancer Res* 48:3236–3244.

Simon D, Munoz SJ, Maddrey WC, Knowles BB (1990): Chromosomal rearrangements in a primary hepatocellular carcinoma. *Cancer Genet Cytogenet* 45:255–260.

Soukup SW, Lampkin BL (1991): Trisomy 2 and 20 in two hepatoblastomas. *Genes Chromosomes Cancer* 3:231–234.

Suzuki K, Ohnami S, Tanabe C, Sasaki H, Yasuda J, Katai H, et al. (2003): The genomic damage estimated by arbitrarily primed PCR DNA fingerprinting is useful for the prognosis of gastric cancer. *Gastroenterology* 25:1330–1340.

Tanaka K, Yanoshita R, Konishi M, Oshimura M, Maede Y, Mori T, et al. (1993): Suppression of tumorigenicity in human colon carcinoma cells by introduction of normal chromosome 1p36 region. *Oncogene* 8:2253–2258.

The Cancer Genome Atlas Research Network (2012): Comprehensive molecular characterization of human colon and rectal cancer. *Nature* 487:330–337.

Thorstensen L, Qvist H, Heim S, Liefers GJ, Nesland JM, Giercksky KE, et al. (2000): Evaluation of 1p losses in primary carcinomas, local recurrences and peripheral metastases from colorectal cancer patients. *Neoplasia* 2:514–522.

Tomlinson GE, Douglass EC, Pollock BH, Finegold MJ, Schneider NR (2005): Cytogenetic evaluation of a large series of hepatoblastomas: numerical abnormalities with recurring aberrations involving 1q12-q21. *Genes Chromosomes Cancer* 44:177–184.

Tonouchi H, Matsumoto K, Kinoshita T, Itoh H, Suzuki H (1998): Prognostic value of DNA ploidy patterns of colorectal adenocarcinoma: univariate and multivariate analysis. *Dig Surg* 15:687–692.

Tzeng ST, Tsai MH, Chen CL, Lee JX, Jao TM, Yu SL, et al. (2013): NDST4 is a novel candidate tumor suppressor gene at chromosome 4q26 and its genetic loss predicts adverse prognosis in colorectal cancer. *PLoS One* 8:e67040.

Weber RG, Pietsch T, von Schweinitz D, Lichter P (2000): Characterization of genomic alterations in hepatoblastomas: a role for gains on chromosomes 8q and 20 as predictors of poor outcome. *Am J Pathol* 157:571–578.

Weiss MM, Kuipers EJ, Postma C, Snijders AM, Siccama I, Pinkel D, et al. (2003): Genomic profiling of gastric cancer predicts lymph node status and survival. *Oncogene* 22:1872–1879.

Werner M, Nolte M, Georgii A, Klempnauer J (1993): Chromosome 1 abnormalities in hepatocellular carcinoma. *Cancer Genet Cytogenet* 66:130.

Wong N, Lai P, Lee SW, Fan S, Pang E, Liew CT, et al. (1999): Assessment of genetic changes in hepatocellular carcinoma by comparative genomic hybridization analysis: relationship to disease stage, tumor size, and cirrhosis. *Am J Pathol* 154:37–43.

Woodford-Richens KL, Rowan AJ, Gorman P, Halford S, Bicknell DC, Wasan HS, et al. (2001): SMAD4 mutations in colorectal cancer probably occur before chromosomal instability, but after divergence of the microsatellite instability pathway. *Proc Natl Acad Sci USA* 98:9719–9723.

Xia J, Xiao S, Zhang J (1999): Direct chromosome analysis and FISH study of primary gastric cancer. *Zhonghua Zhong Liu Za Zhi* 21:345–349.

Xiao S, Geng J-S, Feng X-L, Liu X-Q, Liu Q-Z, Li P (1992): Cytogenetic studies of eight primary gastric cancers. *Cancer Genet Cytogenet* 58:79–84.

Zanke BW, Greenwood CM, Rangrej J, Kustra R, Tenesa A, Farrington SM, et al. (2007): Genome-wide association scan identifies a colorectal cancer susceptibility locus on chromosome 8q24. *Nat Genet* 39:989–994.

Zhou W, Goodman SN, Galizia G, Lieto E, Ferraraccio F, Pignatelli C, et al. (2002): Counting alleles to predict recurrence of early-stage colorectal cancers. *Lancet* 359:219–225.

CHAPTER 15

Tumors of the urinary tract

Paola Dal Cin

Department of Pathology, Brigham and Women's Hospital, Boston, MA, USA

In this organ system, extensive cytogenetic data are available only for the most common tumors, those of the kidney and bladder. Very few ureteral and urethral neoplasms with chromosome abnormalities have been described (Mitelman et al., 2014).

Kidney

The classification of renal tumors has been an evolving process over many years (Weiss et al., 1995; Kovacs et al., 1997; Storkel et al., 1997; Fleming and O'Donnell, 2000). Through international consensus, they were classified by the World Health Organization (WHO) using a scheme that incorporates both morphologic and genetic characteristics (Eble et al., 2004). However, the development did not stop there, and additional tumor entities and morphologic variants of the main tumor categories have subsequently been identified by morphologic, clinical, and molecular means (Cheng et al., 2009; Lopez-Beltran et al., 2009; Srigley and Delahunt, 2009; Crumley et al., 2013; Srigley et al., 2013). Knowledge of these new entities is important for diagnosis, prognostication, and treatment. Unfortunately, the accumulation of cytogenetic and clinicopathologic data for some of these newly described lesions has been slowed by their relative rarity and because not all relevant investigative

techniques were made good use of. A combination of genetic methods should ideally be used to better characterize these entities, so as to overcome the inherent weaknesses of each of them on its own.

Familial predisposition is apparent in less than 4% of renal tumors. Each of these syndromes predisposes to a specific histologic type of renal tumors, and they are therefore mentioned under the relevant tumor subtype.

More than 1,900 cytogenetically abnormal kidney tumors, most of them *renal cell carcinomas* (RCC), have been reported (Mitelman et al., 2014). Systematic cytogenetic analysis with extensive reviews of the field was, in the past, provided by Dal Cin et al. (1988), Walter et al. (1989a), Meloni et al. (1992a), Kovacs (1993), Van Poppel et al. (2000), Weinstein and Dal Cin (2001), Meloni-Ehrig (2002), and Davis et al. (2003).

Benign kidney tumors

Trisomy 7 was observed as the sole abnormality in three of the seven cases of renal *angiomyolipoma* so far reported. However, because cells carrying this abnormality have also been detected in both neoplastic and nonneoplastic renal tissues as well as in other tumors and nonneoplastic lesions (Johansson et al., 1993), it is highly questionable whether +7 should really be viewed as typical of this type of

Cancer Cytogenetics: Chromosomal and Molecular Genetic Aberrations of Tumor Cells, Fourth Edition.
Edited by Sverre Heim and Felix Mitelman.
© 2015 John Wiley & Sons, Ltd. Published 2015 by John Wiley & Sons, Ltd.

(A)

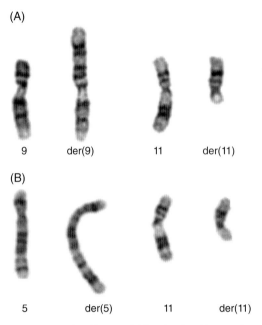

(B)

| 9 | der(9) | 11 | der(11) |
| 5 | der(5) | 11 | der(11) |

Figure 15.1 A t(9;11)(p23;q13) (A) and a t(5;11)(q35;q13) (B) are among the most frequent translocations involving 11q13 in oncocytomas.

benign tumor. Involvement of 12q was observed in two cases, but whether or not 12q rearrangements are unique to a subset of angiomyolipomas remains to be clarified (Debiec-Rychter et al., 1992; Wullich et al., 1997). The presence of bilateral or multifocal angiomyolipomas of the kidneys can also be a feature of tuberous sclerosis, an autosomal dominant, genetically heterogeneous disease featuring multiple benign tumors and caused by mutations in either of the tuberous sclerosis complex genes, *TSC1* (9q34) or *TSC2* (16p13.3) (Crino et al., 2006). Recently, rearrangement of the *TFE3* gene was detected in a few cases of renal epithelioid angiomyolipoma/perivascular epithelioid cell tumor (PEComa) in young patients who did not suffer from tuberous sclerosis (Argani et al., 2010; Ohe et al., 2012).

From a cytogenetic standpoint, *oncocytomas* can be divided into three groups: those with loss of chromosomes 1 and/or 14 and one sex chromosome, most often the Y chromosome (Crotty et al., 1992; Feder et al., 2000; Paner et al., 2007); those with rearrangement of 11q13 (Walter et al., 1989b), with t(9;11) and t(5;11) among the most frequent translocations observed (Figure 15.1); and those with heterogeneous abnormalities, including both numerical and structural aberrations (Jhang et al., 2004). The translocation

t(6;9)(p21;p23) has been observed in three cases of renal oncocytoma (Balzarini et al., 1998; Hudacko et al., 2011). No specific genes involved in oncocytoma development have yet been described.

Multiple oncocytomas can occur in familial form, as the rare *familial renal oncocytoma*. One such family showed a constitutional t(8;9)(q24;q34) in the individuals (Teh et al., 1998).

Hybrid oncocytoma/chromophobe tumor contains a mixture of cells with morphologic features of those seen in renal oncocytoma and chromophobe RCC. It occurs in adult patients sporadically, in association with renal oncocytosis/oncocytomatosis or in patients with *Birt–Hogg–Dube (BHD) syndrome*. The three groups have different genetic features. Sporadic forms are characterized by multiple monosomies and polysomies with monosomy 20 being the most frequent aberration, and the tumors lack mutations in the *VHL, KIT, PDGFRA*, and *FLCN* genes (Petersson et al., 2010). The renal cell neoplasms of oncocytosis exhibit distinct cytogenetic profiles that set them apart from oncocytoma or chromophobic RCC (Gobbo et al., 2010; Kuroda et al., 2012). Germline mutation in the *FLCN* gene at 17p11.2 can be detected in BHD tumors (Klomp et al., 2010).

Only three *metanephric adenomas* (MA) with abnormal karyotypes have been described. A 47, X,−Y, +7,+17 karyotype was reported by Brown et al. (1996). A possible relationship between this tumor type and papillary RCC (see the following text) was suggested because of the finding by FISH of gain of chromosomes 7 and 17 in seven of 11 tumors (Brown et al., 1997). However, Brunelli et al. (2003) did not confirm this link in a study of 70 MA. Lerut et al. (2006) described a 46,XX,t(1;22) (q22;q13),t(15;16)(q21;p13) karyotype in a large MA from a 24-year-old primigravida. A 2p23 deletion was reported as the single abnormality by Stumm et al. (1999), and the possibility of a tumor suppressor gene (TSG) in this interval was suggested by microsatellite analysis (Pesti et al., 2001). Recently, an interstitial deletion of chromosome region 2p14–p26 was detected as the sole chromosome aberration by array CGH (aCGH) analysis. In addition, this case also contained a *BRAF* V600E mutation (Dadone et al., 2013). *BRAF* V600E mutations have been reported in approximately 90% of all MA cases (Choueiri et al., 2012).

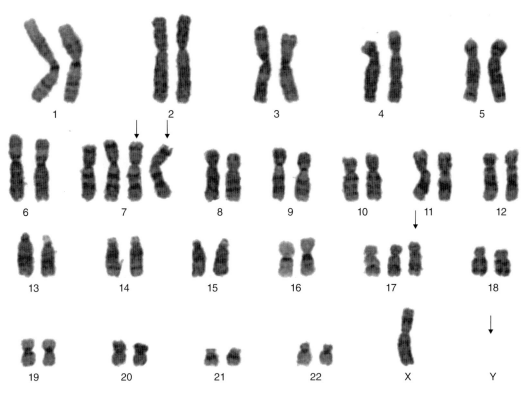

Figure 15.2 A combination of numerical changes (here tetrasomy 7, trisomy 17, and loss of the Y chromosome; arrows indicate gained or missing chromosomes) characterizes papillary adenoma as well as a subgroup of papillary renal cell carcinoma.

Small *cortical epithelial tumors* are common incidental findings at postmortem examinations and in nephrectomy specimens, but distinguishing between benign and malignant tumors is problematic. Small papillary tumors are the most common, and the consensus among pathologists is that the tumors are benign papillary adenomas when they are less than 5 mm in diameter with papillary or tubular architecture of low nuclear grade (Eble et al., 2004). The cytogenetic findings in adenomas are similar to those of papillary RCC and include trisomy for chromosomes 7 and 17 and loss of the Y chromosome (Figure 15.2). The presence of additional karyotypic abnormalities is highly suggestive of malignancy (Dal Cin et al., 1989; Kovacs et al., 1991b; Presti et al., 1991; Van Poppel et al., 2000). Gowrishankar et al. (2014) recently subtyped fine needle aspirates from renal cortical neoplasms based on their FISH signal pattern and pointed out that this added considerable diagnostic power to investigations made by conventional morphological methods used alone.

Malignant kidney tumors

Papillary RCC is the second most common type of RCC, comprising 10–15% of all renal parenchymal epithelial tumors. A combination of trisomy/tetrasomy 7, trisomy 17, and loss of the Y chromosome is the most frequent cytogenetic feature, regardless of tumor size and grade (Figure 15.2). As alluded to in the preceding text, the appearance of additional trisomies, such as those involving chromosomes 12, 16, and 20, as well as +3/+3q (Figure 15.3), is associated with more aggressive behavior. Histologically, two morphologic groups of papillary RCC are now recognized (type 1 and type 2) differing in stage, grade, and prognosis. Cytogenetic analyses suggest that type 2 tumors evolve from type 1 tumors. Both show common chromosomal aberrations, including trisomy for chromosomes 17, 7, 16, 20, 3q, and 12. Hierarchical cluster analysis did not show distinct cytogenetic profiles for the two subgroups (Gunawan et al., 2003).

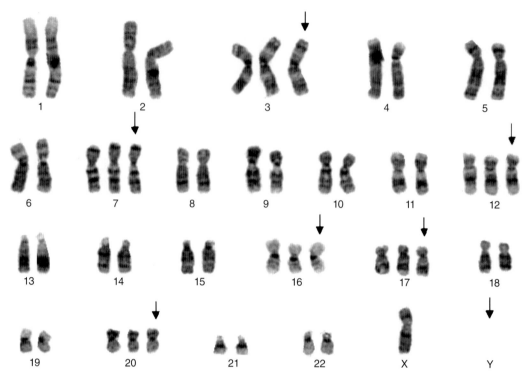

Figure 15.3 Trisomy for chromosomes 3, 7, 12, 16, 17, and 20 and loss of the Y chromosome (arrows indicate gained or lost chromosomes) are observed in clinically aggressive papillary renal cell carcinomas.

Gains of both chromosomes 7 and 17 are more commonly associated with type 1 than type 2 tumors. Papillary type 2 tumors often additionally show aberrations of 1p, 3p, 5q, and monosomy 21 reflecting tumor progression. Loss of 9p correlates with higher stage and tumor grade and poor survival (Klatte et al., 2009b). Loss of 3p can also occur in a subset of papillary tumors (Moch et al., 1998) but is then associated with a more aggressive phenotype and worse survival (Klatte et al., 2009a).

Cytogenetic analyses have not proven useful in determining whether bilateral, multifocal papillary RCC represent single primary tumors with metastases or multiple primary tumors because common numerical anomalies are often detected (Dal Cin et al., 1996).

Two rare morphologic variants of papillary RCC were recently described. Expression profiles of *tubulocystic carcinoma* revealed that this renal lesion is more closely related to papillary RCC than any other renal neoplasms. aCGH analysis showed gain of chromosome 17 but not of chromosome 7 (Yang et al., 2008). However, in another study using FISH, gains of chromosomes 7 and 17 and loss of the Y chromosome were frequent findings (Zhou et al., 2009).

Variable genetic findings have so far been reported for *oncocytic papillary RCC*. Cytogenetic analysis is available on five tumors, none of which showed trisomy for chromosomes 7 and 17. Moreover, a combination of monosomies, including losses of chromosomes 1 and 14 and loss of the Y chromosome, was detected in three cases (Lefevre et al., 2005). In more recent studies, three or more signals for chromosomes 7 and 17 were found by FISH analysis (Hes et al., 2006; Xia et al., 2013).

Hereditary papillary renal cell carcinoma (HPRCC) is a rare, genetically heterogeneous disease featuring relatively late-onset and multiple bilateral papillary RCC (Zbar et al., 1994). HPRCC is associated with mutations in the *MET* proto-oncogene (in 7q31.2), which encodes a tyrosine kinase receptor for hepatocyte growth factor (HGF). Activation mutations of *MET* have been documented both in hereditary forms and in a subset of sporadic papillary RCC (Schmidt et al., 1997).

Furthermore, papillary RCC has been associated with trisomy 7 harboring duplications of mutated *MET* alleles, and the possibility that this event may be a critical step in tumorigenesis was suggested (Zhuang et al., 1998).

Hereditary leiomyomatosis and renal cell carcinoma (HLRCC) is an autosomal dominant disorder predisposing to uterine and cutaneous leiomyomas and papillary RCC type 2. HLRCC results from heterozygous germline mutations in the fumarate hydratase gene (*FH*; in lq43) that encodes an enzyme that catalyzes fumarate to malate in the tricarboxylic acid cycle (Launonen et al., 2001). An estimated 30% of affected individuals develop single renal tumors rather than the multifocal, bilateral tumors seen in other inherited renal cancers (Lehtonen et al., 2004). Recently, *FH* mutations were also detected in rare sporadic papillary RCC type 2 tumors (Gardie et al., 2011).

Most adult malignant kidney tumors (85%) are *clear cell RCC*. Histologically, clear cell RCC is a diverse entity with the three most common architectural patterns being solid, alveolar, and acinar (Eble et al., 2004). Clear cell RCC are the cytogenetically best characterized kidney tumors by far, and several large series have been described (Yoshida et al., 1986; Kovacs et al., 1987; Dal Cin et al., 1988; Kovacs et al., 1989; Meloni et al., 1992a; Dijkhuizen et al., 1996; Iqbal et al., 1996; Verdorfer et al., 1999; Gunawan et al., 2001; Lau et al., 2007). From these analyses, it is obvious that the karyotypic profile of clear cell RCC is markedly different from that of papillary renal cell tumors.

Cytogenetic studies of primary clear cell RCC specimens have identified loss of 3p through a variety of mechanisms: through simple interstitial or terminal deletions; through unbalanced translocation, with a der(3)t(3;5)(p11–22;q13–31) as the most frequent; and through loss of 3pter–3q12 or 3pter–3q21 with a concurrent translocation of the remaining 3q segment to other chromosomes (Figure 15.4) (Balzarini et al., 1998). No specific 3p loss correlates with tumor size, nodal involvement, tumor grade, or metastasis in clear cell RCC. However, patients whose tumors show loss of 3p and gains of 5q31-qter, most often through a der(3)t(3;5), seem to have a better prognosis (Gunawan et al., 2001; Nagao et al., 2005) (Figure 15.5).

Although many deletions involving 3p encompass a relatively large portion of the chromosome arm and identification of a single critical region has proven difficult, three particularly frequently involved target areas have been identified: 3p14, 3p21, and 3p25 (van den Berg and Buys, 1997).

The von Hippel–Lindau (*VHL*) gene at 3p25–26 is known to be frequently mutated in clear cell RCC. *VHL* was identified by positional cloning as the gene responsible for a familial syndrome with renal cancer predisposition, the VHL syndrome (see the following text). Subsequently, *VHL* was found to be biallelically inactivated in approximately 90% of sporadic clear cell RCC. However, VHL inactivation alone does not result in clear cell RCC development, suggesting that involvement of other genes in 3p is required for malignant growth. Specific genes in 3p14 that have been implicated in the pathogenesis of sporadic clear cell RCC include *FHIT* (see the following text) and *FOXOP1* (Toma et al., 2008). Exome-sequencing studies recently identified new candidate TSGs in 3p21, with *SETD2*, *PBRM1*, and *BAP1* being the most frequent (Duns et al., 2012).

Several other nonrandom numerical and structural chromosomal abnormalities can also occur in clear cell RCC. Monosomy is observed for chromosomes 8, 9, 13, and 14, whereas chromosomes 12 and 20 may be gained. Structural abnormalities most commonly involve 5q, 6q, 8p, 9p, 10q, and 14q and may be related to tumor progression. Monosomy 9/9p–, identified either by karyotyping or FISH analysis at the time of surgery, has been correlated with distant metastasis and poor outcome; *INK4a/ARF* and *CAIX* could be the genes behind this clinical consequence (Klatte et al., 2009a; La Rochelle et al., 2010). Also, loss of material from chromosome arm 14q and involvement of the *HIF-1α* gene have been associated with worse outcomes (Kroeger et al., 2013).

Bilateral clear cell RCC mostly occurs as part of inherited cancer syndromes. However, rare cytogenetic studies of bilateral synchronous tumors have shown karyotypic differences, suggesting that independent primary tumors may develop simultaneously (Dal Cin et al., 1996). In contrast, an identical 45,XY,der(3;6)(p10;q10) karyotype was identified in bilateral tumors from a single individual (Hirsch et al., 2002).

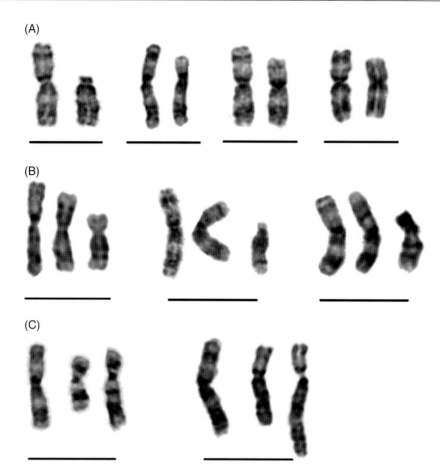

Figure 15.4 Partial karyotypes illustrating three different mechanisms leading to loss of or from 3p in clear cell renal cell carcinoma: (A) terminal or interstitial deletions of 3p (the deleted chromosome 3 is to the right in all four examples); (B) unbalanced transloca-tions involving different 3p regions with 8q (left), 14q (middle), and 9q (right); and (C) loss of 3pter–3q11–12 and 3pter–3q21 through unbalanced translocations between 3q and chromosome 11 (left) or chromosome 6 (right).

Sometimes, simple numerical abnormalities, mostly trisomy for chromosomes 7 and/or 10 or loss of a sex chromosome, are found as the only clonal karyotypic anomaly or as unrelated secondary clones. The neoplastic relevance of these findings is uncertain because nonneoplastic kidney cells may also contain the same numerical aberrations (Kovacs and Brusa, 1989; Kovacs and Frisch, 1989; Elfving et al., 1990; Limon et al., 1990; Emanuel et al., 1992; Johansson et al., 1993). At least in some instances, the cells carrying only trisomy 7 or trisomy 10 seemed to be lymphocytes (Dal Cin et al., 1992). On other occasions, the cells with trisomy 7 seemed to be nonneoplastic epithelial renal cells (Elfving et al., 1995). Trisomy 7 is the most frequently observed trisomy in solid tumors, particularly among epithe-lial neoplasms (Johansson et al., 1993).

VHL syndrome is an autosomal dominant dis-order featuring central nervous system angi-omas, hemangioblastomas, pheochromocytomas, as well as renal cysts and clear cell RCC. The *VHL* gene maps to 3p25–26 and functions as a TSG (Latif et al., 1993). Affected individuals inherit a germline mutation and subsequently suffer a second hit somatically achieved through deletion, mutation, or hypermethylation of the second allele (Knudson's two-hit model) (Gnarra et al., 1994; Herman et al., 1994). The karyotypic profile of autosomal dominant RCC, whether or not it occurs as part of VHL syndrome, does not

(A)

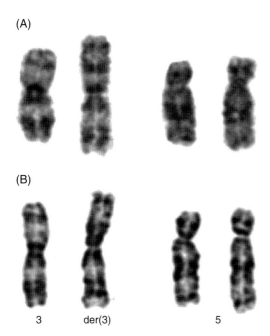

(B)

3   der(3)   5

Figure 15.5 Partial karyotypes (A and B) of a der(3)t(3;5) (p11–22;q13–31), the most frequent structural aberration in clear cell RCC, leading to partial monosomy 3p and partial trisomy 5q.

seem to differ from that of sporadic carcinomas (Kovacs and Kung, 1991; Kovacs et al., 1991a).

Familial clear cell RCC is another cancer syndrome with inherited chromosomal predisposition to renal neoplasms. A constitutional balanced translocation, t(3;8)(p14;q24), was identified in a family with predisposition to both clear cell RCC and thyroid carcinoma (Cohen et al., 1979; Wang and Perkins, 1984). The *FHIT* gene spans the 3p14 breakpoint (Ohta et al., 1996) and, interestingly, is located at the most common aphidicolin-inducible fragile site in the human genome, FRA3B. Affected individuals in the original t(3;8)-positive family showed a *FHIT–TRC8* fusion that joins the 5′ untranslated region of *FHIT* to the coding region of *TRC8* (Gemmill et al., 2002).

Additional constitutional rearrangements cosegregating with RCC have been described in non-VHL families. A significant risk for developing RCC was found among carriers of chromosome 3 translocations, especially those with breakpoints in the pericentromeric regions (Geurts van Kessel et al., 1999). These familial 3p translocations include t(3;6)(p23–24;q23–24), t(3;6)(p13;q25), t(3;11)(p13–14;p15),

t(3;12)(p14;p13), t(3;17)(p25;p13.3), and t(3;21) (p12;q11.2) (Pathak et al., 1982; Kovacs and Hoene, 1988; Kovacs et al., 1989; Gnarra et al., 1995; Motzer et al., 1996). To date, no specific causative genes have been identified that correspond to these 3p breakpoints. In addition, several RCC families with translocation breakpoints in 3p have also been identified, with many of these breakpoints clustering to 3q12 or 3q21 (Geurts van Kessel et al., 1999). Specific examples of translocations involving 3q breakpoints include t(1;3)(q32;q13.3), t(1;3)(q41;q27), t(2;3) (q33;q21), t(2;3)(q35;q21), t(3;6)(q12;q15), t(3;9) (q21;p13), t(3;11)(q29;p15.3), t(3;12)(q13;q24), and t(3;14)(q21;q32) (Kovacs and Hoene, 1988; Meloni et al., 1992a; van den Berg and Buys, 1997; Visser et al., 1997; Bodmer et al., 1998; Koolen et al., 1998; Druck et al., 2001; Eleveld et al., 2001; Kanayama et al., 2001). No specific causative genes have been identified as a result of these rearrangements, with the exception of the t(2;3)(q35;q21), where the 3q21 breakpoint disrupts *DIRC*, although the exact role for this gene in RCC pathogenesis remains unknown (Bodmer et al., 2002a, 2002b; Melendez et al., 2003). It is noteworthy that several sporadic RCC with 3q21 translocations have demonstrated a variety of breakpoints, some of which map up to 1 Mb away from the familial breakpoint and therefore may involve genes other than *DIRC2* (Bodmer et al., 2002a).

Several morphologic variants of clear cell RCC were recently described. *Multilocular cyst RCC* accounts for ~4% of all clear cell RCC and usually presents as solitary lesions affecting mid-age adults. As in clear cell RCC, 3p deletions and VHL mutations have been observed (Halat et al., 2010; Williamson et al., 2012).

Clear cell (tubulo)papillary RCC is composed of clear cells but shows a variable papillary and tubuloacinar architecture. It is mostly a unicentric, unilateral, and small lesion with indolent clinical behavior. The majority of these lesions lack 3p25 deletion, *VHL* mutation, or trisomies for chromosomes 7 and 17 (Gobbo et al., 2008; Aydin et al., 2010).

Cytogenetic studies, CGH, microsatellite, and DNA cytometric analyses have demonstrated that a unique combination of monosomies for chromosomes 1, 2, 6, 10, 13, 17, and 21 characterizes *chromophobe RCC* (Kovacs and Kovacs, 1992; Speicher et al., 1994; Crotty et al., 1995; Bugert et al., 1997) (Figure 15.6). High-resolution DNA

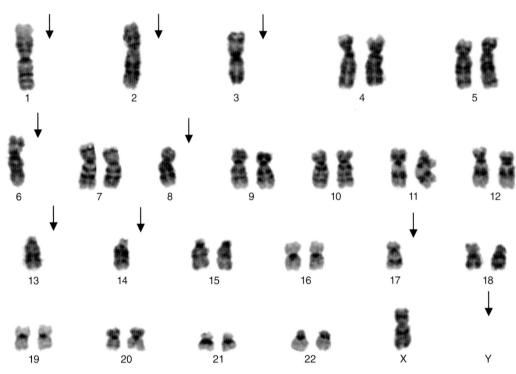

Figure 15.6 A combination of monosomies for chromosomes 1, 2, 3, 6, 8, 13, 14, and 17 and loss of the Y chromosome (arrows indicate missing chromosomes) characterize chromophobe RCC.

microarray analysis did not find smaller, specific alterations indicating that this monosomy pattern is indeed exclusive to the chromophobe subtype of RCC (Yusenko, 2010). The cells from these tumors do not grow well *in vitro*, and the use of complementary molecular techniques may therefore be well advised in order to differentiate this lesion from the eosinophilic variant of clear cell RCC or oncocytoma (Figure 15.7).

The *Xp11.2 translocation renal carcinomas* have been incorporated as a distinct entity in the 2004 WHO classification of renal tumors (Eble et al., 2004). These carcinomas were initially described in pediatric and young adult populations (Argani et al., 2001; Ladanyi et al., 2001) but are now recognized as affecting older individuals as well (Argani et al., 2007; Ross and Argani, 2010). The most common translocations are t(X;1)(p11.2;q21) (Figure 15.8) (de Jong et al., 1986; Meloni et al., 1992b) and t(X;17) (p11.2;q25) (Figure 15.9) (Tomlinson et al., 1991) that result in fusions involving the *TFE3* gene in Xp11.2 with *PRCC* in 1q21.2 (Sidhar et al., 1996; Weterman et al., 1996) or *ASPSCR1 (ASPL)* in 17q25

(Argani et al., 2001; Heimann et al., 2001). Of interest, an unbalanced translocation involving the same chromosome bands and genes, der(X)t(X;17) (p11;q25), has been described in alveolar soft part sarcoma (Ladanyi et al., 2001). Also, other variant Xp11.2 rearrangements have been described, for example, t(X;1)(p11.2;p34), inv(X)(p11.2q12), and t(X;17)(p11.2;q23), in which *TFE3* fuses with *PSF*, *NONO* (Clark et al., 1997), or *CLTC* (Argani et al., 2003), respectively. In those Xp11.2 RCC with t(X;10)(p11;q23) or t(X;3)(p11.2;q23), the identity of the genes fused to *TFE3* remains unknown (Dijkhuizen et al., 1995; Argani et al., 2006). Tumors with different fusion genes may have a slightly different morphology, but common features include a nested to papillary architecture, clear to slightly granular eosinophilic cytoplasm, and psammomatous calcifications (Argani et al., 2001; Altinok et al., 2005; Argani et al., 2007; Ross and Argani, 2010). Several reports initially emphasized the aggressive clinical behavior of some Xp11.2 RCC lesions in adults. However, adults may have a worse prognosis and do poorly because they often present with

(A)   (B)

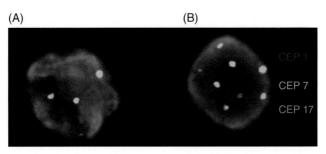

Figure 15.7 FISH evaluation using centromeric probes for chromosomes 1, 7, and 17 performed on interphase nuclei, showing (A) monosomy for chromosomes 1 and 17 and disomy for chromosome 7, consistent with chromophobe type RCC, and (B) trisomy for chromosomes 7 and 17 and disomy for chromosome 1, consistent with papillary type RCC.

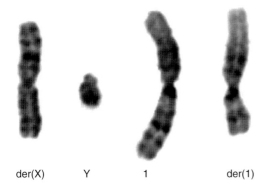

der(X)   Y   1   der(1)

Figure 15.8 t(X;1)(p11.2;q21) is a characteristic translocation in a subgroup of renal carcinomas mostly occurring in children and young adults.

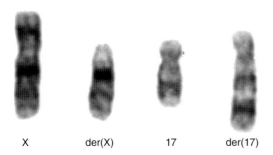

X   der(X)   17   der(17)

Figure 15.9 t(X;17)(p11.2;q25) is a characteristic translocation in a subgroup of renal carcinoma mostly occurring in children and young adults (Courtesy of Dr. Marc Ladanyi).

advanced disease and distant metastasis (Ramphal et al., 2006; Argani et al., 2007; Meyer et al., 2007). Prior exposure to chemotherapy is currently the only known risk factor to development of Xp11.2 translocation RCC (Argani et al., 2006).

Data on the cytogenetic abnormalities of *collecting duct carcinoma* are limited and inconclusive.

Early reports were conflicting with some studies detecting a combination of several monosomies (Fuzesi et al., 1992), while others found more trisomies and structural abnormalities (Cavazzana et al., 1996; Gregori-Romero et al., 1996). Hypodiploid karyotypes with several structural abnormalities, mostly affecting chromosome 1, were described by Antonelli et al. (2003). The most recent CGH analysis revealed recurrent DNA losses (from 8p, 16p, 1p, and 9p); the losses were more common than gains (from 13q and 9q) (Becker et al., 2013).

There is strong evidence that *mucinous tubular and spindle cell carcinoma* (MTSCC) is a distinct RCC entity, characterized by multiple chromosomal losses including losses of 1, 6, 14, 15, and 22, detected by both karyotyping and CGH analyses (Rakozy et al., 2002; Ferlicot et al., 2005; Laury et al., 2011) but lacking the trisomies for chromosomes 7 and 17 that are characteristic of papillary RCC. However, there is some disagreement among the reported studies, probably because the karyotypes often are in the near-triploid range rendering interpretation of CGH data difficult (Brandal et al., 2006; Cossu-Rocca et al., 2006; Dhillon et al., 2009; Kuroda et al., 2011). The use of a combination of FISH probes for chromosomes 7, 15, 17, and 22 has been suggested so as to facilitate the distinction of MTSCC from papillary RCC (Kuroda et al., 2008). However, monosomy for chromosomes 15 and 22 together with disomy for chromosomes 7 and 17 has been described also in a few renal tumors classified as collecting duct carcinoma (Fuzesi et al., 1992). FISH, in combination with morphologic and immunophenotypic findings, can nevertheless aid significantly in the diagnosis of MTSCC, especially when banding cytogenetics for whatever reason cannot be performed.

Tumors that typically arise in soft tissue are being identified with increasing frequency in the kidney. A t(11;22)(q24;q12) has been seen in Ewing sarcoma/primitive neuroectodermal tumor (EWS/PNET) of the kidney (Takeuchi et al., 1997; Vicha et al., 2002; Premalata et al., 2003; Saxena et al., 2006). EWS/PNET can on the basis of morphology alone easily be mistaken for other renal round cell tumors, such as blastema-predominant Wilms' tumors (WTs), and demonstration of the typical t(11;22) or the corresponding *EWSR1–FLI1* fusion gene may clinch the correct diagnosis (Jimenez et al., 2002). A synovial sarcoma with a t(X;18)(p11;q11) has also been reported (Shannon et al., 2005). Synovial sarcoma should be considered in the differential diagnosis of mesenchymal kidney tumors when prominent rhabdoid features are present (Jun et al., 2004). Rubin et al. (1999) reported a t(12;22)(q13;q12) in a clear cell sarcoma of the kidney, and Su et al. (2004) used RT-PCR to identify an *EWSR1–WT1* fusion transcript indicative of a t(11;22)(p13;q12), the characteristic abnormality of desmoplastic round cell tumor. Genetic confirmations by, for example, reverse transcription polymerase chain reaction (RT-PCR) and/or FISH analyses (Argani and Beckwith, 2000; Parham, 2001) will often be relied on for exclusion or confirmation when sarcomas are identified resembling those typically found in soft tissues.

Sarcomatoid transformation may be found in all types of RCC. Therefore, it is not recognized as a single entity but rather as a manifestation of high-grade carcinoma of the cell type from which it arose (Eble et al., 2004). Although the data are sparse, it appears that the genetic aberrations identified in sarcomatoid transformation have little in common with those characterizing each RCC entity (Dal Cin et al., 2002; Brunelli et al., 2007).

The most common renal neoplasm of childhood is *nephroblastoma* or *Wilms' tumor (WT)*, which occurs primarily (95%) as a sporadic unilateral tumor but rarely as an autosomal dominant disease. Most tumors have a favorable histology, but the presence of anaplastic changes generally predicts a poor outcome and calls for more aggressive treatment (Rivera and Haber, 2005).

Approximately 600 WTs with acquired chromosomal abnormalities have now been reported (Soukup et al., 1997; Bown et al., 2002; Gow and

Murphy, 2002; Ehrlich et al., 2003; Kullendorff et al., 2003; Peres et al., 2004; Stewenius et al., 2008; MdZin et al., 2010). WT karyotypes are mostly near diploid or pseudodiploid with only a few polyploid cases. The most common numerical aberrations, in descending order of frequency, are gain of chromosomes 12, 8, and 6, whereas the most common losses arise through structural rearrangements and are 1p−, 11p−, and 16q−. Numerous structural rearrangements have been described involving all chromosomes except the Y. Cytogenetic abnormalities of chromosomes 1, 7, 14, 16, and 17 are observed frequently, and the most common rearrangements are i(1)(q10), der(16)t(1;16)(q10–21;q10–24), and i(7)(q10). Loss of the Y chromosome and trisomy 7 are in rare cases seen as sole aberrations.

WT in the adult population is rare and yet overdiagnosed. Interestingly, i(7)(q10) was observed in a series of adult WT, both by chromosome banding and FISH analysis (Rubin et al., 2000). Two major types of WT have been described. Type I WT is characterized by a stromal-type histology and a high rate of mutations of the *WT1* gene (11p13). Most, or all, *WT1*-mutated cases also carry independent additional somatic mutations of the beta-catenin gene (*CTNNB1*) in 3p21 (Maiti et al., 2000; Royer-Pokora et al., 2008; MdZin et al., 2011).

WTs may occur together with aniridia, genitourinary abnormalities, and mental retardation in the *WAGR syndrome* and *Denys–Drash syndrome* (Little et al., 1993). The majority of these patients have germline *WT1* mutation and a high risk of early onset WT, bilateral tumors, and associated genitourinary abnormalities in males.

Rivera et al. (2007) described the inactivation (via deletion or mutation) of a novel TSG, *WTX*, at Xq11.1 in 30% of sporadic WT. Tumors with *WTX* inactivation lacked *WT1* mutation. Subsequently, the same group reported a microdeletion that included *WTX* in a sporadic WT carrying a t(X;18)(q11;p11) (Han et al., 2007).

Type II WT is associated with epigenetic alteration in the 11p15 region. These tumors have limited nephrogenic differentiation and epithelial-type histology (Breslow et al., 2006). Type II WT can occur in patients with overgrowth syndromes such as *Beckwith–Wiedemann syndrome* and *hemihypertrophy*. Most of these tumors show either loss of imprinting of genes located in 11p15 or chromosome 11 uniparental paternal disomy (Weksberg et al., 2005). A WT2 locus has been postulated at 11p15. Although no gene(s) has been so far identified, the imprinted *HOTS* and *IGF2* genes may be possible candidates (Hu et al., 2011; Onyango and Feinberg, 2011).

In addition to syndromes associated with *WT1* mutations and increased risk for WT, two new emerging risk alleles (FWT1 in 17q12–21 and FWT2 in 19q13.3–4) have recently been proposed (Ruteshouser and Huff, 2004; Royer-Pokora, 2013).

The existence of TSG in 1p, 7p, and 16q has been proposed based on the finding of frequent unbalanced chromosome aberrations with allelic losses. Patients with WT carrying a der(16) t(1;16)(q10–21;q10–24) leading to monosomy 16q and trisomy 1q were found to have a significantly increased risk of relapse and death (Grundy et al., 2005).

Malignant rhabdoid tumors (MRT) were originally described as a "rhabdomyosarcomatous variant" of WT (Beckwith and Palmer, 1978). The majority of MRT have shown a normal karyotype, but in the few cases with chromosomal aberrations, 22q (Biegel et al., 1990; Shashi et al., 1994) and 11p (Hirose et al., 1996; Kaiserling et al., 1996) seem to be nonrandomly involved. LOH studies of primary renal rhabdoid tumors confirmed cytogenetic deletions involving 22q11–12 and 11p15.5 in 80% and 17% of the cases, respectively (Schofield et al., 1996). Concurrent with the aforementioned cytogenetic discoveries, MRT with 22q11.2 rearrangements were described as primary tumors in a variety of extrarenal sites, with the central nervous system as the most common. A TSG, *SMARCB1 (INI1/hSNF5)*, was identified in 22q11.2 through studies of cell lines established from rhabdoid tumors. These lines carried both a rearrangement of 22q11.2 and a homozygous deletion/mutation of *SMARCB1*, changes that were subsequently observed in rhabdoid tumors regardless of their site of origin (Versteege et al., 1998; Biegel et al., 1999).

Differentiating between MRT and WT is critical to prognosis and therapeutic planning because WT is curable, whereas MRT remains one of the most lethal childhood cancers. Loss of *SMARCB1/INI1*

expression as assessed by immunohistochemistry may help distinguish between the two entities.

RCC in children (<18 years) is an uncommon (less than 5%) pediatric renal tumor, and relatively little is known about the cytogenetics of these tumors. Classic "adult-type" RCC may occur also in children, and their clinical and cytogenetic features are identical to those seen in adults. Mainly numerical abnormalities were observed in three pediatric RCC, two with a predominantly papillary pattern and one with a chromophobe pattern (Pedersen et al., 1998; Soller et al., 2007).

Recently, RCC subtypes associated with specific chromosomal rearrangements, namely, translocations involving Xp11.2 and either 1q21 or 17q25, have been recognized in children. These Xp11.2–translocation RCC are recognized by the most recent WHO classification (Eble et al., 2004) and were discussed previously.

Renal carcinoma with t(6;11)(p21;q12) (Figure 15.10) was recently reported as a distinct renal neoplasm showing epithelioid morphology, basement membrane production, and HMB45 immunoreactivity. These rare tumors occur mainly in children and young adults (Argani et al., 2005; Smith et al., 2014a) but have been seen also in adults (Pecciarini et al., 2007). The t(6;11) fuses the *ALPHA* gene at 11q12 and the *TFEB* gene at 6p21. Similar to *TFE3*, which is involved in renal carcinomas with the Xp11.22 translocation, *TFEB* encodes a protein that belongs to the MITF/TFE subfamily of transcription factors (Davis et al., 2003). On the basis of clinical, morphologic, immunohistochemical, and genetic similarities between renal tumors of the Xp11.2

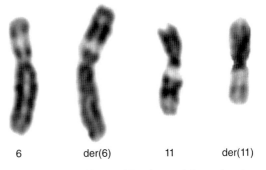

| 6 | der(6) | 11 | der(11) |

Figure 15.10 t(6;11)(p12;q12) is a characteristic translocation in a subgroup of renal carcinomas mostly occurring in children and young adults (Courtesy of Dr. Julia Bridge).

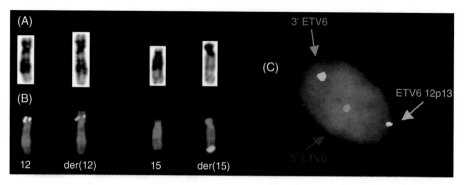

Figure 15.11 This t(12;15)(p13;q26) is a characteristic translocation in congenital mesoblastic nephroma. (A) This is a cryptic translocation; therefore, FISH analysis using the *ETV6* probe at 12p13 is necessary to confirm the translocation either in (B) metaphase chromosomes or in (C) interphase nuclei (Courtesy of Dr. Jonathan Fletcher).

translocation and t(6;11) variety, it has been suggested that they may all be included within the category of *MITF/TFE3 family translocation RCC* (Srigley et al., 2013).

Of interest, a t(6;17)(p21;q24–25) was reported in clear cell RCC (Dal Cin et al., 1991); no specific genes were identified for either breakpoint. Argani et al. (2006) described an association between young patients with a history of cytotoxic chemotherapy and the development of RCC with either an Xp11.2 translocation or a t(6;11)(p21;q12).

Interesting cytogenetic data exist for some children in whom renal neoplasms developed following treatment for neuroblastoma. All four patients in a single series were girls (age 5–13 years), and the tumors were described as oncocytoid RCC. Associated cytogenetic abnormalities were distinct from those typically described in known types of RCC, suggesting a distinct clinicopathologic entity (Medeiros et al., 1999).

Congenital mesoblastic nephromas (CMN) are mostly benign, uncommon renal spindle cell tumors diagnosed in early infancy. Trisomies, often involving chromosome 11 but also chromosomes 8, 10, 17, and 20, were initially believed to be the most consistent karyotypic finding, occurring almost exclusively in the cellular and mixed types of CMN (Dal Cin et al., 1998). However, it was subsequently established that the cellular type of CMN always carries a t(12;15)(p13;q26) (Figure 15.11) resulting in an *ETV6–NTRK3* fusion (Rubin et al., 1998). Considering the cryptic nature of this translocation in the absence of high-resolution banding, the use of a complementary molecular or molecular cytogenetic approach (e.g., RT-PCR or FISH) is highly recommended for such cases. The same pattern of chromosomal trisomies and *ETV6–NTRK3* fusion has been described in infantile fibrosarcoma (Chapter 24) suggesting a link between these two pediatric tumors (Knezevich et al., 1998). An identical *ETV6–NTRK3* fusion has also been detected in secretory breast cancer (Chapter 16) and acute myeloid leukemia (Chapter 6). This illustrates that a single translocation and gene fusion can be involved in multiple tumor types, including those of mesenchymal, hematopoietic, and epithelial origin (Lannon and Sorensen, 2005).

Only a few cases of *clear cell sarcoma of the kidney*, a clinically aggressive and bone metastasizing renal tumor, have been cytogenetically investigated and a recurrent t(10;17)(q22;p13) (Figure 15.12) has been described (Douglass et al., 1985; Punnett et al., 1989; Sheng et al., 1990; Rakheja et al., 2004; Brownlee et al., 2007). The translocation results in fusion of *YWHAE* on chromosome 17 with a member of the *FAM22* gene family on chromosome 10 (Fehr et al., 2012; O'Meara et al., 2012). The same t(10;17)/*YWHAE-FAM22* characterizes also a subset of high-grade endometrial stromal sarcoma (Lee et al., 2012; Chapter 17).

A novel t(2;10)(p22;q22) translocation leading to a *VCL–ALK* fusion gene was recently reported in three renal carcinomas affecting young African American patients with sickle cell trait (Debelenko et al., 2011; Marino-Enriquez et al., 2011; Smith

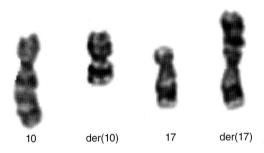

Figure 15.12 t(10;17)(q22;p13) is a characteristic translocation in clear cell sarcoma of the kidney (Courtesy of Dr. Mark Pettenati).

et al., 2014b). Neither *ALK* rearrangement by FISH nor ALK expression by immunohistochemistry could be identified in an additional primary tumor (and lymph node metastasis) carrying an inv(2) (p23q11.2) (Debelenko et al., 2011). Of interest, a diagnosis of *renal medullary carcinoma* was made in two of the renal tumors with t(2;10) (Marino-Enriquez et al., 2011) as well as in a previous renal tumor with inv(2)(p23q11.2) (Swartz et al., 2002). Further investigations of *ALK* rearrangement in large adult RCC series demonstrated four renal tumors with *ALK* rearrangement including two with fusions involving *TPM3* and *ELM4* (Sugawara et al., 2012; Sukov et al., 2012). The affected adults were not afflicted with sickle cell trait, and the morphology of their tumors was nondistinctive. The Mitelman database contains four additional primary kidney tumors with complex karyotype but with one breakpoint at or cytogenetically near the *ALK* locus (Mitelman et al., 2014). It seems that *ALK*-rearranged renal tumors in adults may represent a pathological entity with poor outcome distinct from kidney tumors with *VCL–ALK* fusion in young African American males carrying the sickle cell trait (Hodge et al., 2013). The potential therapeutic implications of *ALK* rearrangement in renal tumors remain to be determined.

Transitional cell carcinoma (TCC) of the kidney is relatively rare, with the earliest cytogenetic description reported more than two decades ago (Berger et al., 1986). The cytogenetic anomalies in renal TCC are often complex and involve chromosomes 3, 5, and 14 (Walter et al., 1989a; Meloni et al., 1992a). The limited karyotypic data suggest that TCC of the kidney are cytogenetically similar to bladder TCC (Fadl-Elmula, 2005).

Epidemiological observations support this notion, as identification of an upper urinary tract tumor predicts an increased likelihood of discovering tumors in the bladder (Kakizoe et al., 1980; Kenworthy et al., 1996). The most commonly observed numerical anomalies include loss of the Y chromosome and trisomy 7, either as the sole aberration or in combination. Indeed, these numerical aberrations are identified frequently in all types of urological tumors.

Bladder

More than 90% of urothelial tumors arise in the bladder, with fewer arising in the renal pelvis, ureter, or urethra. Most of them are classified as TCC. The karyotypes reported to date range from simple to highly complex, and no specific aberrations have been described (Mitelman et al., 2014). Complex karyotypes have been associated with postradiation neoplasias both for ureteral and bladder TCC (Fadl-Elmula et al., 1999). Chromosomal losses or deletions are seen more often than are chromosomal gains. Monosomy 9 or partial 9p/9q deletions are seen particularly frequently (~50%) (Fadl-Elmula, 2005) suggesting that they are early events in TCC development.

Loss of the Y chromosome has been reported as a sole abnormality, but does not appear to correlate with tumor recurrence (Neuhaus et al., 1999). Generally in urological tumors, trisomy 7 and loss of the Y chromosome often occur together (Dal Cin et al., 1999). Interestingly, polysomy Y has been correlated with increasing histological grade of the tumor (Panani and Roussos, 2006). Loss of the X chromosome is rarely seen as the sole abnormality but may occur in complex karyotypes.

Because cells from bladder TCC can be difficult to culture and also hard to karyotype, alternative approaches such as spectral karyotyping (SKY) and, more recently, aCGH have been relied upon for help in the cytogenetic study of these tumors (Fadl-Elmula et al., 2001). *MTSU1* was identified as the most promising deleted gene at 8p21–22 in a CGH analysis of bladder tumors (Rogler et al., 2014). Significant recurrent mutations in 32 genes were found in the comprehensive molecular characterization of urothelial bladder carcinomas recently released by The Cancer Genome Atlas Research Network (2014).

Historically, the difficulty in culturing bladder tumors has adversely impacted the cytogenetic study of these specimens. While no single cytogenetic anomaly is considered diagnostic of bladder TCC, it has been proposed that a combination of chromosomal aberrations be exploited for diagnostic purposes (Sandberg, 2002). Early publications (Meloni et al., 1993; Sandberg, 2002) suggested that the application of molecular cytogenetics to analyze specimens obtained through relatively noninvasive methods (e.g., voided urine and bladder washings) might be a more practical approach. Subsequently, a commercial multitarget FISH assay was developed with several loci interrogated simultaneously (trisomy or tetrasomy for chromosomes 3, 7, and 17 along with loss of 9p), which is now in fairly widespread use (UroVysion; Abbott Molecular) (Figure 15.13). UroVysion is significantly more sensitive than voided urine cytology for detecting bladder cancer in patients evaluated for gross or microscopic hematuria independent of grade and stage in high-risk populations, in particular during follow-up of patients with a history of previous carcinoma *in situ* (Sarosdy et al., 2002, 2006; Skacel et al., 2003; Fritsche et al., 2010).

Relatively few other types of bladder tumors have been investigated cytogenetically. In squamous cell carcinomas, complex karyotypes with many similarities to the profiles obtained in TCC have been found (Hanna et al., 2002). Complex cytogenetic changes have also been seen in a bladder chondrosarcoma (Kingsley et al., 1997), hyperdiploid karyotypes were detected in embryonal rhabdomyosarcoma (Wang-Wuu et al., 1988; Kullendorff et al., 1998; Kapels et al., 2007), a t(10;12)(q24;q13) was seen in an alveolar

rhabdomyosarcoma (Roberts et al., 1992), and, finally, an i(12p) was detected in a choriocarcinoma of the bladder (Hanna et al., 2002). A complex rearrangement involving 2p23 resulting in *ALK–ATIC* fusion was found in an inflammatory myofibroblastic tumor (IMT) (Debiec-Rychter et al., 2003). By FISH analysis, ALK gene alterations were found in as many as 13 of 18 IMT examined (Montgomery et al., 2006).

A malignant PEComa of the urinary bladder with *TFE3* gene rearrangement was recently reported (Williamson et al., 2013).

Ureter

Few tumors arise from the ureter, and cytogenetic findings in only 15 cases have been reported. When the cytogenetics of ureteral cancers could be compared with bladder malignancies from the same patients, largely similar karyotypic features were found (Fadl-Elmula et al., 1999). From these data, it appeared that whereas the presence of a ureteral tumor was associated with an increased likelihood of also discovering tumors in the bladder, the converse association did not hold true (Fadl-Elmula et al., 1999). Epidemiological data support this observation (Kenworthy et al., 1996). Complex karyotypes have been observed in postradiation ureteral tumors (Fadl-Elmula et al., 1999).

Urethra

Cytogenetic analysis of a single urethral cancer, a squamous cell carcinoma, has been published (Fadl-Elmula et al., 1998). A complex, near-diploid

(A)   (B)

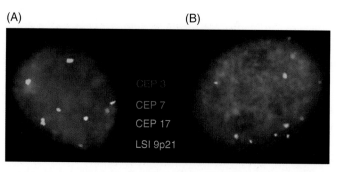

CEP 3
CEP 7
CEP 17
LSI 9p21

Figure 15.13 Interphase FISH analysis of cells from the urinary tract: (A) normal hybridization pattern showing disomy for each probe tested; (B) abnormal hybridization pattern consistent with tetrasomy for chromosomes 3 and 7, trisomy 17, and nullisomy for the 9p21 probe (i.e., homozygous deletion of the corresponding region) (Courtesy of Dr. Stana Weremowicz).

clone and its near-tetraploid duplicate were found. It may be of interest that no rearrangements of chromosomes 9 and 17, both almost ubiquitously involved in TCC of the urinary tract, were seen.

Clinical correlations

Karyotype analysis in uroepithelial tumors is critical because characteristic cytogenetic aberrations are specific for several distinctive neoplastic entities within this organ system and, hence, can be used as highly informative diagnostic markers. In the event that chromosomal analysis cannot be performed, several ancillary methodologies (i.e., flow cytometry, FISH, CGH, LOH, RT-PCR) can be used for diagnostic purposes. Pathologists often rely on immunohistochemistry and in some cases FISH to aid the classification of diagnostically and prognostically challenging renal tumors.

Patients with clear cell RCC have a poor prognosis compared to those with papillary and chromophobe RCC. It is therefore important to distinguish these types of tumors, which sometimes overlap morphologically. For example, the eosinophilic variant of chromophobe RCC mimics clear cell RCC with eosinophilic cytoplasm, as well as oncocytoma. No specific 3p loss correlates with tumor size, nodal involvement, tumor grade, or metastasis in clear cell RCC. However, gains of 5q31-qter, most often through the unbalanced translocation der(3)t(3;5), seem to confer an improved clinical prognosis. On the other hand, losses of 9p and 14q are associated with high-grade tumors, advanced disease, and poor prognosis.

Xp11.2 translocation RCC occur less frequently in adults than in younger patients. However, the incidence in adults could be underestimated because of the morphological overlap with conventional clear cell or papillary RCC. Several reports have indicated more aggressive clinical behavior of some Xp11.2 translocation carcinomas, especially those with a t(X;17). In addition, an interesting association has been reported between RCC in young patients with a history of cytotoxic chemotherapy and either an Xp11.2 translocation or a t(6;11)(p21;q12).

Tumors that typically arise in soft tissues are being identified with increasing frequency in the urinary tract, and they represent special differential diagnostic problems. EWS/PNET can be mistaken for other renal round cell tumors, such as blastema-predominant WT. Similarly, synovial sarcoma should be considered in the differential diagnosis of mesenchymal kidney tumors when prominent rhabdoid features are present. Genetic examinations remain essential for exclusion or confirmation of such diagnostic possibilities. Tumor-specific chromosomal rearrangements can be detected either by FISH or RT-PCR if fresh samples with live cells are not available for karyotyping analysis.

Patients whose WT cells carry a der(16)t(1;16) (q10–21;q10–24) leading to monosomy 16q and trisomy 1q have been found to have a significantly increased risk of relapse and death.

For the purposes of therapeutic selection and prognosis, it is critical to differentiate between WT and MRT because WT is curable, whereas MRT are among the most lethal childhood cancers. The use of karyotyping may be insufficient for this purpose, however, and molecular testing for *SMARCB1/INI1* or immunohistochemical examination is recommended.

Considering the cryptic nature of the t(12;15) (p13;q25) of CMN, even with high-resolution banding, the use of a complementary approach (e.g., RT-PCR or FISH) is highly recommended when this diagnosis is suspected. Importantly, most CMN behave as benign tumors.

ALK rearrangements may in adult patients define a pathological entity with poor outcome different from that of young African American men with sickle cell trait whose kidney tumors have a *VCL–ALK* fusion. The potential therapeutic implications of *ALK* rearrangements in renal tumors remain unexplored.

A multitarget FISH assay has been developed to analyze specimens that may contain TCC cells for aneusomies of chromosomes 3, 7, and 17 as well as for deletions involving 9p. This assay, which can be performed using voided urine cells fixed onto microscope slides, can provide prognostic information when used in conjunction with cystoscopy. The approach may be useful both for initial diagnosis in patients with hematuria and as an adjunct to cystoscopy for monitoring disease recurrence in treated patients.

Summary

RCC are clinically as well as genetically heterogeneous tumors. Specific chromosomal abnormalities have been detected in clear cell RCC (3p deletion), papillary RCC (a combination of trisomies), and chromophobe RCC (a combination of monosomies). In benign renal tumors such as angiomyolipoma, MA, and oncocytoma, these abnormalities are not observed. Cytogenetic analysis cannot distinguish between papillary adenomas and low-grade RCC because of overlapping combinations of numerical changes; therefore, the tumor diameter remains an important diagnostic criterion.

Chromophobe RCC are particularly difficult to culture making karyotyping a challenge. Therefore, complementary diagnostic techniques such as CGH, flow cytometry, and FISH can be used to infer the presence of characteristic cytogenetic aberrations. The most common differential diagnosis includes renal oncocytoma, for which specific chromosomal abnormalities are known (either a combination of −X or −Y, −1/−14, or a translocation involving 11q13).

Familial RCC syndromes, although rare, have provided invaluable models to study the molecular mechanisms of renal carcinogenesis. Fewer than 5% of renal tumors occur as part of hereditary cancer syndromes. The tumors are typically bilateral and multifocal and often occur at an earlier age compared with sporadic forms. The eventual understanding of the molecular pathways for the genes involved promises to have a significant impact on the diagnosis and, especially, treatment of both familial and sporadic RCC. For most of the genes involved, however, we are not there yet.

The recent identification of primary soft tissue tumors arising in the kidney and bladder (e.g., synovial sarcoma, Ewing sarcoma, and IMT, which all have specific translocations and gene fusions) suggests that the use of cytogenetic and/or molecular technologies is essential in confirming or ruling out such diagnoses.

A subset of RCC is characterized by Xp11.2 translocations. This subtype is morphologically heterogeneous and can be misclassified as clear cell or papillary RCC. FISH analysis for *TFE3* rearrangement has proven an effective assay to detect the essential genomic change. Although these tumors were initially described in the pediatric and young adult patient populations, they are now being recognized in older patients as well.

In pediatric renal tumors, some entities correspond to specific diagnostic chromosomal translocations associated with specific gene fusions, including the t(12;15) of CMN, the t(10;17) of clear cell sarcoma of the kidney, and the t(6;11) of renal neoplasms with an epithelioid morphology. In contrast, WT does not feature a single diagnostic chromosomal abnormality. Molecular testing, rather than cytogenetic analysis, is necessary for the diagnosis of MRTs.

It appears that the *ALK*-rearranged renal tumors in adults may represent a pathological entity with poor outcome distinct from kidney tumors with *VCL–ALK* fusion in young African American male with sickle cell trait.

Some newly recognized renal neoplastic tumors are still poorly defined genetically. A combination of investigative methods should be used to better characterize these entities and, hopefully, establish their essential pathogenetic changes.

Complex karyotypes in bladder TCC tend to be associated with a more aggressive clinical course. A multitarget FISH assay (UroVysion) that detects trisomies of chromosomes 3, 7, and 17 as well as deletions of 9p has been introduced in clinical practice. FISH analysis of bladder washings or voided urine specimens can be of considerable value both diagnostically and prognostically, especially when used in an adjunctive role to cystoscopic examination.

Numerical anomalies, such as loss of the Y chromosome, trisomy 7, or a combination of both, are nonspecific findings in a variety of urogenital tumors. Their diagnostic information value is uncertain.

Acknowledgments

The author would like to thank Ms Cynthia McLaughlin for her assistance with figures and Ms Olja Pulluqi for her editorial assistance.

References

Altinok G, Kattar MM, Mohamed A, Poulik J, Grignon D, Rabah R (2005): Pediatric renal carcinoma associated with Xp11.2 translocations/TFE3 gene fusions and clinicopathologic associations. *Pediatr Dev Pathol* 8:168–180.

Antonelli A, Portesi E, Cozzoli A, Zanotelli T, Tardanico R, Balzarini P, et al. (2003): The collecting duct carcinoma of the kidney: a cytogenetical study. *Eur Urol* 43:680–685.

Argani P, Beckwith JB (2000): Metanephric stromal tumor: report of 31 cases of a distinctive pediatric renal neoplasm. *Am J Surg Pathol* 24:917–926.

Argani P, Antonescu CR, Illei PB, Lui MY, Timmons CF, Newbury R, et al. (2001): Primary renal neoplasms with the ASPL-TFE3 gene fusion of alveolar soft part sarcoma: a distinctive tumor entity previously included among renal cell carcinomas of children and adolescents. *Am J Pathol* 159:179–192.

Argani P, Lui MY, Couturier J, Bouvier R, Fournet JC, Ladanyi M (2003): A novel CLTC-TFE3 gene fusion in pediatric renal adenocarcinoma with t(X;17)(p11.2;q23). *Oncogene* 22:5374–5378.

Argani P, Lae M, Hutchinson B, Reuter VE, Collins MH, Perentesis J, et al. (2005): Renal carcinomas with the t(6;11)(p21;q12): clinicopathologic features and demonstration of the specific alpha-TFEB gene fusion by immunohistochemistry, RT-PCR, and DNA PCR. *Am J Surg Pathol* 29:230–240.

Argani P, Lae M, Ballard ET, Amin M, Manivel C, Hutchinson B, et al. (2006): Translocation carcinomas of the kidney after chemotherapy in childhood. *J Clin Oncol* 24:1529–1534.

Argani P, Olgac S, Tickoo SK, Goldfischer M, Moch H, Chan DY, et al. (2007): Xp11 translocation renal cell carcinoma in adults: expanded clinical, pathologic, and genetic spectrum. *Am J Surg Pathol* 31:1149–1160.

Argani P, Aulmann S, Illei PB, Netto GJ, Ro J, Cho HY, et al. (2010): A distinctive subset of PEComas harbors TFE3 gene fusions. *Am J Pathol* 34:1395–1406.

Aydin H, Chen L, Cheng L, Vaziri S, He H, Ganapathi R, et al. (2010): Clear cell tubulopapillary renal cell carcinoma: a study of 36 distinctive low-grade epithelial tumors of the kidney. *Am J Surg Pathol* 34:1608–1621.

Balzarini P, Dal Cin P, Roskams T, Polito P, Van Poppel H, Van Damme B, et al. (1998): Histology may depend on the presence of partial monosomy or partial trisomy 3 in renal cell carcinoma. *Cancer Genet Cytogenet* 105:6–10.

Becker F, Junker K, Parr M, Hartmann A, Fussel S, Toma M, et al. (2013): Collecting duct carcinomas represent a unique tumor entity based on genetic alterations. *PloS One* 8:e78137.

Beckwith JB, Palmer NF (1978): Histopathology and prognosis of Wilms tumors: results from the First National Wilms' Tumor Study. *Cancer* 41:1937–1948.

Berger CS, Sandberg AA, Todd IA, Pennington RD, Haddad FS, Hecht BK, et al. (1986): Chromosomes in kidney, ureter, and bladder cancer. *Cancer Genet Cytogenet* 23:1–24.

Biegel JA, Rorke LB, Packer RJ, Emanuel BS (1990): Monosomy 22 in rhabdoid or atypical tumors of the brain. *J Neurosurg* 73:710–714.

Biegel JA, Zhou JY, Rorke LB, Stenstrom C, Wainwright LM, Fogelgren B (1999): Germ-line and acquired mutations of INI1 in atypical teratoid and rhabdoid tumors. *Cancer Res* 59:74–79.

Bodmer D, Eleveld MJ, Ligtenberg MJ, Weterman MA, Janssen BA, Smeets DF, et al. (1998): An alternative route for multistep tumorigenesis in a novel case of hereditary renal cell cancer and a t(2;3)(q35;q21) chromosome translocation. *Am J Hum Genet* 62:1475–1483.

Bodmer D, Eleveld M, Kater-Baats E, Janssen I, Janssen B, Weterman M, et al. (2002a): Disruption of a novel MFS transporter gene, DIRC2, by a familial renal cell carcinoma-associated t(2;3)(q35;q21). *Hum Mol Genet* 11:641–649.

Bodmer D, Janssen I, Jonkers Y, van den Berg E, Dijkhuizen T, Debiec-Rychter M, et al. (2002b): Molecular cytogenetic analysis of clustered sporadic and familial renal cell carcinoma-associated 3q13 approximately q22 breakpoints. *Cancer Genet Cytogenet* 136:95–100.

Bown N, Cotterill SJ, Roberts P, Griffiths M, Larkins S, Hibbert S, et al. (2002): Cytogenetic abnormalities and clinical outcome in Wilms tumor: a study by the U.K. cancer cytogenetics group and the U.K. Children's Cancer Study Group. *Med Pediatr Oncol* 38:11–21.

Brandal P, Lie AK, Bassarova A, Svindland A, Risberg B, Danielsen H, et al. (2006): Genomic aberrations in mucinous tubular and spindle cell renal cell carcinomas. *Mod Pathol* 19:186–194.

Breslow NE, Beckwith JB, Perlman EJ, Reeve AE (2006): Age distributions, birth weights, nephrogenic rests, and heterogeneity in the pathogenesis of Wilms tumor. *Pediatr Blood Cancer* 47:260–267.

Brown JA, Sebo TJ, Segura JW (1996): Metaphase analysis of metanephric adenoma reveals chromosome Y loss with chromosome 7 and 17 gain. *Urology* 48:473–475.

Brown JA, Anderl KL, Borell TJ, Qian J, Bostwick DG, Jenkins RB (1997): Simultaneous chromosome 7 and 17 gain and sex chromosome loss provide evidence that renal metanephric adenoma is related to papillary renal cell carcinoma. *J Urol* 158:370–374.

Brownlee NA, Perkins LA, Stewart W, Jackle B, Pettenati MJ, Koty PP, et al. (2007): Recurring translocation (10;17) and deletion (14q) in clear cell sarcoma of the kidney. *Arch Pathol Lab Med* 131:446–451.

Brunelli M, Eble JN, Zhang S, Martignoni G, Cheng L (2003): Metanephric adenoma lacks the gains of chromosomes 7 and 17 and loss of Y that are typical of papillary renal cell carcinoma and papillary adenoma. *Mod Pathol* 16:1060–1063.

Brunelli M, Gobbo S, Cossu-Rocca P, Cheng L, Hes O, Delahunt B, et al. (2007): Chromosomal gains in the sarcomatoid transformation of chromophobe renal cell carcinoma. *Mod Pathol* 20:303–309.

Bugert P, Gaul C, Weber K, Herbers J, Akhtar M, Ljungberg B, et al. (1997): Specific genetic changes of diagnostic importance in chromophobe renal cell carcinomas. *Lab Invest* 76:203–208.

Cavazzana AO, Prayer-Galetti T, Tirabosco R, Macciomei MC, Stella M, Lania L, et al. (1996): Bellini duct carcinoma. A clinical and in vitro study): *Eur Urol* 30:340–344.

Cheng L, Zhang S, MacLennan GT, Lopez-Beltran A, Montironi R (2009): Molecular and cytogenetic insights into the pathogenesis, classification, differential diagnosis, and prognosis of renal epithelial neoplasms. *Hum Pathol* 40:10–29.

Choueiri TK, Cheville J, Palescandolo E, Fay AP, Kantoff PW, Atkins MB, et al. (2012): BRAF mutations in metanephric adenoma of the kidney. *Eur Urol* 62:917–922.

Clark J, Lu YJ, Sidhar SK, Parker C, Gill S, Smedley D, et al. (1997): Fusion of splicing factor genes PSF and NonO (p54nrb) to the TFE3 gene in papillary renal cell carcinoma. *Oncogene* 15:2233–2239.

Cohen AJ, Li FP, Berg S, Marchetto DJ, Tsai S, Jacobs SC, et al. (1979): Hereditary renal-cell carcinoma associated with a chromosomal translocation. *N Engl J Med* 301:592–595.

Cossu-Rocca P, Eble JN, Delahunt B, Zhang S, Martignoni G, et al. (2006): Renal mucinous tubular and spindle carcinoma lacks the gains of chromosomes 7 and 17 and losses of chromosome Y that are prevalent in papillary renal cell carcinoma. *Mod Pathol* 19:488–493.

Crino PB, Nathanson KL, Henske EP (2006): The tuberous sclerosis complex. *N Engl J Med* 355:1345–1356.

Crotty TB, Lawrence KM, Moertel CA, Bartelt DH Jr., Batts KP, Dewald GW, et al. (1992): Cytogenetic analysis of six renal oncocytomas and a chromophobe cell renal carcinoma. Evidence that –Y, –1 may be a characteristic anomaly in renal oncocytomas. *Cancer Genet Cytogenet* 61:61–66.

Crotty TB, Farrow GM, Lieber MM (1995): Chromophobe cell renal carcinoma: clinicopathological features of 50 cases. *J Urol* 154:964–967.

Crumley SM, Divatia M, Truong L, Shen S, Ayala AG, Ro JY (2013): Renal cell carcinoma: evolving and emerging subtypes. *World J Clin Cases* 1:262–275.

Dadone B, Ambrosetti D, Carpentier X, Duranton-Tanneur V, Burel-Vandenbos F, Amiel J, et al. (2013): A renal metanephric adenoma showing both a 2p16e24 deletion and BRAF V600E mutation: a synergistic role for a tumor suppressor gene on chromosome 2p and BRAF activation? *Cancer Genet* 206:347–352.

Dal Cin P, Li FP, Prout GR Jr., Huben RP, Limon J, Ferti-Passantonopoulou A, et al. (1988): Involvement of chromosomes 3 and 5 in renal cell carcinoma. *Cancer Genet Cytogenet* 35:41–46.

Dal Cin P, Gaeta J, Huben R, Li FP, Prout GR Jr., Sandberg AA (1989): Renal cortical tumors. Cytogenetic characterization. *Am J Clin Pathol* 92:408–414.

Dal Cin P, van Gool S, Brock P, Proesmans W, Casteels-van Daele M, de Wever I, et al. (1991): Renal cell carcinoma in a child. *Cancer Genet Cytogenet* 57:137–138.

Dal Cin P, Aly MS, Delabie J, Ceuppens JL, Van Gool S, Van Damme B, et al. (1992). Trisomy 7 and trisomy 10 characterize subpopulations of tumor-infiltrating lymphocytes in kidney tumors and in the surrounding kidney tissue. *Proc Natl Acad Sci USA* 89:9744–9748.

Dal Cin P, van Poppel H, van Damme B, Baert L, Van den Berghe H (1996): Cytogenetic investigation of synchronous bilateral renal tumors. *Cancer Genet Cytogenet* 89:57–60.

Dal Cin P, Lipcsei G, Hermand G, Boniver J, Van den Berghe H (1998): Congenital mesoblastic nephroma and trisomy 11. *Cancer Genet Cytogenet* 103:68–70.

Dal Cin P, Roskams T, Van Poppel H, Balzarini P, Van den Berghe H (1999): Cytogenetic investigation of transitional cell carcinomas of the upper urinary tract. *Cancer Genet Cytogenet* 114:117–120.

Dal Cin P, Sciot R, Van Poppel H, Balzarini P, Roskams T, Van den Berghe H (2002): Chromosome changes in sarcomatoid renal carcinomas are different from those in renal cell carcinomas. *Cancer Genet Cytogenet* 134:38–40.

Davis IJ, Hsi BL, Arroyo JD, Vargas SO, Yeh YA, Motyckova G, et al. (2003): Cloning of an Alpha-TFEB fusion in renal tumors harboring the t(6;11)(p21;q13) chromosome translocation. *Proc Natl Acad Sci USA* 100:6051–6056.

de Jong B, Molenaar IM, Leeuw JA, Idenberg VJ, Oosterhuis JW (1986): Cytogenetics of a renal adenocarcinoma in a 2-year-old child. *Cancer Genet Cytogenet* 21:165–169.

Debelenko LV, Raimondi SC, Daw N, Shivakumar BR, Huang D, Nelson M, et al. (2011): Renal cell carcinoma with novel VCL-ALK fusion: new representative of ALK-associated tumor spectrum. *Mod Pathol* 24:430–442.

Debiec-Rychter M, Saryusz-Wolska H, Salagierski M (1992): Cytogenetic analysis of renal angiomyolipoma. *Genes Chromosomes Cancer* 4:101–103.

Debiec-Rychter M, Marynen P, Hagemeijer A, Pauwels P (2003): ALK-ATIC fusion in urinary bladder inflammatory myofibroblastic tumor. *Genes Chromosomes Cancer* 38:187–190.

Dhillon J, Amin MB, Selbs E, Turi GK, Paner GP, Reuter VE (2009): Mucinous tubular and spindle cell carcinoma of the kidney with sarcomatoid change. *Am J Surg Pathol* 33:44–49.

Dijkhuizen T, van den Berg E, Wilbrink M, Weterman M, Geurts van Kessel A, Storkel S, et al. (1995): Distinct Xp11.2 breakpoints in two renal cell carcinomas exhibiting X;autosome translocations. *Genes Chromosomes Cancer* 14:43–50.

Dijkhuizen T, Van den Berg E, Van den Berg A, Storkel S, De Jong B, Seitz G, et al. (1996): Chromosomal findings and p53-mutation analysis in chromophilic renal-cell carcinomas. *Int J Cancer* 68:47–50.

Douglass EC, Wilimas JA, Green AA, Look AT (1985): Abnormalities of chromosomes 1 and 11 in Wilms' tumor. *Cancer Genet Cytogenet* 14:331–338.

Druck T, Podolski J, Byrski T, Wyrwicz L, Zajaczek S, Kata G, et al. (2001): The DIRC1 gene at chromosome 2q33 spans a familial RCC-associated t(2;3)(q33;q21) chromosome translocation. *J Hum Genet* 46:583–589.

Duns G, Hofstra RM, Sietzema JG, Hollema H, van Duivenbode I, Kuik A, et al. (2012): Targeted exome sequencing in clear cell renal cell carcinoma tumors suggests aberrant chromatin regulation as a crucial step in ccRCC development. *Hum Mutat* 33:1059–1062.

Eble JN, Sauter G, Epstein JI, Sesterhenn IA (2004): *World Health Organization Classification of Tumours: Pathology and Genetics of Tumours of the Urinary System and Male Genital Organs*. Lyon: IARC.

Ehrlich M, Hopkins NE, Jiang G, Dome JS, Yu MC, Woods CB, et al. (2003): Satellite DNA hypomethylation in karyotyped Wilms tumors. *Cancer Genet Cytogenet* 141: 97–105.

Eleveld MJ, Bodmer D, Merkx G, Siepman A, Sprenger SH, Weterman MA, et al. (2001): Molecular analysis of a familial case of renal cell cancer and a t(3;6)(q12;q15). *Genes Chromosomes Cancer* 31:23–32.

Elfving P, Cigudosa JC, Lundgren R, Limon J, Mandahl N, Kristoffersson U, et al. (1990): Trisomy 7, trisomy 10, and loss of the Y chromosome in short-term cultures of normal kidney tissue. *Cytogenet Cell Genet* 53:123–125.

Elfving P, Aman P, Mandahl N, Lundgren R, Mitelman F (1995): Trisomy 7 in nonneoplastic epithelial kidney cells. *Cytogenet Cell Genet* 69:90–96.

Emanuel A, Szucs S, Weier HU, Kovacs G (1992): Clonal aberrations of chromosomes X, Y, 7 and 10 in normal kidney tissue of patients with renal cell tumors. *Genes Chromosomes Cancer* 4:75–77.

Fadl-Elmula I (2005): Chromosomal changes in uroepithelial carcinomas. *Cell Chromosome* 4:1.

Fadl-Elmula I, Gorunova L, Mandahl N, Elfving P, Heim S (1998): Chromosome abnormalities in squamous cell carcinoma of the urethra. *Genes Chromosomes Cancer* 23:72–73.

Fadl-Elmula I, Gorunova L, Mandahl N, Elfving P, Lundgren R, Mitelman F, et al. (1999): Cytogenetic monoclonality in multifocal uroepithelial carcinomas: evidence of intraluminal tumour seeding. *Br J Cancer* 81:6–12.

Fadl-Elmula I, Kytola S, Pan Y, Lui WO, Derienzo G, Forsberg L, et al. (2001): Characterization of chromosomal abnormalities in uroepithelial carcinomas by G-banding, spectral karyotyping and FISH analysis. International journal of cancer. *Int J Cancer* 92:824–831.

Feder M, Liu Z, Apostolou S, Greenberg RE, Testa JR (2000): Loss of chromosomes 1 and X in a renal oncocytoma: implications for a possible pseudoautosomal tumor suppressor locus. *Cancer Genet Cytogenet* 123:71–72.

Fehr A, Hansson MC, Kindblom LG, Stenman G (2012): YWHAE-FAM22 gene fusion in clear cell sarcoma of the kidney. *J Pathol* 227:e5–7.

Ferlicot S, Allory Y, Comperat E, Mege-Lechevalier F, Dimet S, Sibony M, et al. (2005): Mucinous tubular and spindle cell carcinoma: a report of 15 cases and a review of the literature. *Virchows Arch* 447:978–983.

Fleming S, O'Donnell M (2000): Surgical pathology of renal epithelial neoplasms: recent advances and current status. *Histopathology* 36:195–202.

Fritsche HM, Burger M, Dietmaier W, Denzinger S, Bach E, Otto W, et al. (2010): Multicolor FISH (UroVysion) facilitates follow-up of patients with high-grade urothelial carcinoma of the bladder. *J Clin Pathol* 134:597–603.

Fuzesi L, Cober M, Mittermayer C (1992): Collecting duct carcinoma: cytogenetic characterization. *Histopathology* 21:155–160.

Gardie B, Remenieras A, Kattygnarath D, Bombled J, Lefevre S, Perrier-Trudova V, et al. (2011): Novel FH mutations in families with hereditary leiomyomatosis and renal cell cancer (HLRCC) and patients with isolated type 2 papillary renal cell carcinoma. *J Med Genet* 48:226–234.

Gemmill RM, Bemis LT, Lee JP, Sozen MA, Baron A, Zeng C, et al. (2002): The TRC8 hereditary kidney cancer gene suppresses growth and functions with VHL in a common pathway. *Oncogene* 21:3507–3516.

Geurts van Kessel AG, Wijnhoven H, Bodmer D, Eleveld M, Kiemeney L, Mulders P, Weterman M, Ligtenberg M, Smeets D, Smits A (1999): Renal cell cancer: chromosome 3 translocations as risk factors. *J Natl Cancer Inst* 91:1159–1160.

Gnarra JR, Tory K, Weng Y, Schmidt L, Wei MH, Li H, et al. (1994): Mutations of the VHL tumour suppressor gene in renal carcinoma. *Nat Genet* 7:85–90.

Gnarra JR, Lerman MI, Zbar B, Linehan WM (1995): Genetics of renal-cell carcinoma and evidence for a critical role for von Hippel-Lindau in renal tumorigenesis. *Semin Oncol* 22:3–8.

Gobbo S, Eble JN, Delahunt B, Grignon DJ, Samaratunga H, Martignoni G, et al. (2010): Renal cell neoplasms of oncocytosis have distinct morphologic, immunohistochemical, and cytogenetic profiles. *Am J Surg Pathol* 34:620–626.

Gobbo S, Eble JN, Grignon DJ, Martignoni G, MacLennan GT, Shah RB, et al. (2008): Clear cell papillary renal cell carcinoma: a distinct histopathologic and molecular genetic entity. *Am J Surg Pathol* 32:1239–1245.

Gow KW, Murphy JJ (2002): Cytogenetic and histologic findings in Wilms' tumor. *J Ped Surg* 37:823–827.

Gowrishankar B, Cahill L, Arndt AE, Al-Ahmadie H, Lin O, Chadalavada K, et al. (2014): Subtyping of renal cortical neoplasms in fine needle aspiration biopsies using a decision tree based on genomic alterations detected by fluorescence in situ hybridization. *BJU Int* 114:881–890.

Gregori-Romero MA, Morell-Quadreny L, Llombart-Bosch A (1996): Cytogenetic analysis of three primary Bellini duct carcinomas. *Genes Chromosomes Cancer* 15: 170–172.

Grundy PE, Breslow NE, Li S, Perlman E, Beckwith JB, Ritchey ML, et al. (2005): Loss of heterozygosity for chromosomes 1p and 16q is an adverse prognostic factor in favorable-histology Wilms tumor: a report from the National Wilms Tumor Study Group. *J Clin Oncol* 23:7312–7321.

Gunawan B, Huber W, Holtrup M, von Heydebreck A, Efferth T, Poustka A, et al. (2001): Prognostic impacts of cytogenetic findings in clear cell renal cell carcinoma: gain of 5q31-qter predicts a distinct clinical phenotype with favorable prognosis. *Cancer Res* 61:7731–7738.

Gunawan B, von Heydebreck A, Fritsch T, Huber W, Ringert RH, Jakse G, et al. (2003): Cytogenetic and morphologic typing of 58 papillary renal cell carcinomas: evidence for a cytogenetic evolution of type 2 from type 1 tumors. *Cancer Res* 63:6200–6205.

Halat S, Eble JN, Grignon DJ, Lopez-Beltran A, Montironi R, Tan PH, et al. (2010): Multilocular cystic renal cell carcinoma is a subtype of clear cell renal cell carcinoma. *Mod Pathol* 23:931–936.

Han M, Rivera MN, Batten JM, Haber DA, Dal Cin P, Iafrate AJ (2007): Wilms' tumor with an apparently balanced translocation t(X;18) resulting in deletion of the WTX gene. *Genes Chromosomes Cancer* 46:909–913.

Hanna NH, Ulbright TM, Einhorn LH (2002): Primary choriocarcinoma of the bladder with the detection of isochromosome 12p. *J Urol* 167:1781.

Heimann P, El Housni H, Ogur G, Weterman MA, Petty EM, Vassart G (2001): Fusion of a novel gene, RCC17, to the TFE3 gene in t(X;17)(p11.2;q25.3)-bearing papillary renal cell carcinomas. *Cancer Res* 61:4130–4135.

Herman JG, Latif F, Weng Y, Lerman MI, Zbar B, Liu S, et al. (1994): Silencing of the VHL tumor-suppressor gene by DNA methylation in renal carcinoma. *Proc Natl Acad Sci USA* 91:9700–9704.

Hes O, Brunelli M, Michal M, Cossu Rocca P, Hora M, Chilosi M, et al. (2006): Oncocytic papillary renal cell carcinoma: a clinicopathologic, immunohistochemical, ultrastructural, and interphase cytogenetic study of 12 cases. *Ann Diagn Pathol* 10:133–139.

Hirose M, Yamada T, Toyosaka A, Hirose T, Kagami S, Abe T, et al. (1996): Rhabdoid tumor of the kidney: a report of two cases with respective tumor markers and a specific chromosomal abnormality, del(11p13). *Med Pediatr Oncol* 27:174–178.

Hirsch MS, Weinstein MH, Thomas A, Dal Cin P (2002): Identical karyotypes in synchronous bilateral clear cell renal cell carcinomas. *Cancer Genet Cytogenet* 139:86–87.

Hodge JC, Pearce KE, Sukov WR (2013): Distinct ALK-rearranged and VCL-negative papillary renal cell carcinoma variant in two adults without sickle cell trait. *Mod Pathol* 26:604–605.

Hu Q, Gao F, Tian W, Ruteshouser EC, Wang Y, Lazar A, et al. (2011): Wt1 ablation and Igf2 upregulation in mice

result in Wilms tumors with elevated ERK1/2 phosphorylation. *J Clin Invest* 121:174–183.

Hudacko R, May M, Aviv H (2011): A new translocation between chromosomes 6 and 9 helps to establish diagnosis of renal oncocytoma. *Ann Diagn Pathol* 15:278–281.

Iqbal MA, Akhtar M, Ali MA (1996): Cytogenetic findings in renal cell carcinoma. *Hum Pathol* 27:949–954.

Jhang JS, Narayan G, Murty VV, Mansukhani MM (2004): Renal oncocytomas with 11q13 rearrangements: cytogenetic, molecular, and immunohistochemical analysis of cyclin D1. *Cancer Genet Cytogenet* 149:114–119.

Jimenez RE, Folpe AL, Lapham RL, Ro JY, O'Shea PA, Weiss SW, et al. (2002): Primary Ewing's sarcoma/primitive neuroectodermal tumor of the kidney: a clinicopathologic and immunohistochemical analysis of 11 cases. *Am J Surg Pathol* 26:320–327.

Johansson B, Heim S, Mandahl N, Mertens F, Mitelman F (1993): Trisomy 7 in nonneoplastic cells. *Genes Chromosomes Cancer* 6:199–205.

Jun SY, Choi J, Kang GH, Park SH, Ayala AG, Ro JY (2004): Synovial sarcoma of the kidney with rhabdoid features: report of three cases. *Am J Surg Pathol* 28:634–637.

Kaiserling E, Ruck P, Handgretinger R, Leipoldt M, Hipfel R (1996): Immunohistochemical and cytogenetic findings in malignant rhabdoid tumor. *Gen Diagn Pathol* 141:327–337.

Kakizoe T, Fujita J, Murase T, Matsumoto K, Kishi K (1980): Transitional cell carcinoma of the bladder in patients with renal pelvic and ureteral cancer. *J Urol* 124:17–19.

Kanayama H, Lui WO, Takahashi M, Naroda T, Kedra D, Wong FK, et al. (2001): Association of a novel constitutional translocation t(1q;3q) with familial renal cell carcinoma. *J Med Genet* 38:165–170.

Kapels KM, Nishio J, Zhou M, Qualman SJ, Bridge JA (2007): Embryonal rhabdomyosarcoma with a der(16)t(1;16) translocation. *Cancer Genet Cytogenet* 174:68–73.

Kenworthy P, Tanguay S, Dinney CP (1996): The risk of upper tract recurrence following cystectomy in patients with transitional cell carcinoma involving the distal ureter. *J Urol* 155:501–503.

Kingsley KL, Peier AM, Meloni-Ehrig AM, Sandberg AA, Klein EA (1997): Cytogenetic findings in a bladder chondrosarcoma. *Cancer Genet Cytogenet* 96:183–184.

Klatte T, Pantuck AJ, Said JW, Seligson DB, Rao NP, LaRochelle JC, et al. (2009a): Cytogenetic and molecular tumor profiling for type 1 and type 2 papillary renal cell carcinoma. *Clin Cancer Res* 15:1162–1169.

Klatte T, Rao PN, de Martino M, LaRochelle J, Shuch B, Zomorodian N, et al. (2009b): Cytogenetic profile predicts prognosis of patients with clear cell renal cell carcinoma. *J Clin Oncol* 27:746–753.

Klomp JA, Petillo D, Niemi NM, Dykema KJ, Chen J, Yang XJ, et al. (2010): Birt-Hogg-Dube renal tumors are genetically distinct from other renal neoplasias and are associated with up-regulation of mitochondrial gene expression. *BMC Med Genom* 3:59.

Knezevich SR, Garnett MJ, Pysher TJ, Beckwith JB, Grundy PE, Sorensen PH (1998): ETV6-NTRK3 gene fusions and trisomy 11 establish a histogenetic link between mesoblastic nephroma and congenital fibrosarcoma. *Cancer Res* 58:5046–5048.

Koolen MI, van der Meyden AP, Bodmer D, Eleveld M, van der Looij E, Brunner H, et al. (1998): A familial case of renal cell carcinoma and a t(2;3) chromosome translocation. *Kidney Int* 53:273–275.

Kovacs G (1993): Molecular cytogenetics of renal cell tumors. *Adv Cancer Res* 62:89–124.

Kovacs G, Hoene E (1988): Loss of der(3) in renal carcinoma cells of a patient with constitutional t(3;12). *Hum Genet* 78:148–150.

Kovacs G, Brusa P (1989): Clonal chromosome aberrations in normal kidney tissue from patients with renal cell carcinoma. *Cancer Genet Cytogenet* 37:289–290.

Kovacs G, Frisch S (1989): Clonal chromosome abnormalities in tumor cells from patients with sporadic renal cell carcinomas. *Cancer Res* 49:651–659.

Kovacs G, Kung HF (1991): Nonhomologous chromatid exchange in hereditary and sporadic renal cell carcinomas. *Proc Natl Acad Sci USA* 88:194–198.

Kovacs A, Kovacs G (1992): Low chromosome number in chromophobe renal cell carcinomas. *Genes Chromosomes Cancer* 4:267–268.

Kovacs G, Szucs S, De Riese W, Baumgartel H (1987): Specific chromosome aberration in human renal cell carcinoma. *Int J Cancer* 40:171–178.

Kovacs G, Brusa P, De Riese W (1989): Tissue-specific expression of a constitutional 3;6 translocation: development of multiple bilateral renal-cell carcinomas. International journal of cancer. *Int J Cancer* 43:422–427.

Kovacs G, Emanuel A, Neumann HP, Kung HF (1991a): Cytogenetics of renal cell carcinomas associated with von Hippel-Lindau disease. *Genes Chromosomes Cancer* 3:256–262.

Kovacs G, Fuzesi L, Emanual A, Kung HF (1991b): Cytogenetics of papillary renal cell tumors. *Genes Chromosomes Cancer* 3:249–255.

Kovacs G, Akhtar M, Beckwith BJ, Bugert P, Cooper CS, Delahunt B, et al. (1997): The Heidelberg classification of renal cell tumours. *J Pathol* 183:131–133.

Kroeger N, Klatte T, Chamie K, Rao PN, Birkhauser FD, Sonn GA, et al. (2013): Deletions of chromosomes 3p and 14q molecularly subclassify clear cell renal cell carcinoma. *Cancer* 119:1547–1554.

Kullendorff CM, Donner M, Mertens F, Mandahl N (1998): Chromosomal aberrations in a consecutive series of childhood rhabdomyosarcoma. *Med Ped Oncol* 30:156–159.

Kullendorff CM, Soller M, Wiebe T, Mertens F (2003): Cytogenetic findings and clinical course in a consecutive series of Wilms tumors. *Cancer Genet Cytogenet* 140:82–87.

Kuroda N, Hes O, Michal M, Nemcova J, Gal V, Yamaguchi T, et al. (2008): Mucinous tubular and spindle cell carcinoma with Fuhrman nuclear grade 3: a histological, immunohistochemical, ultrastructural and FISH study. *Histol Histopathol* 23:1517–1523.

Kuroda N, Naroda T, Tamura M, Taguchi T, Tominaga A, Inoue K, et al. (2011): High-grade mucinous tubular and spindle cell carcinoma: comparative genomic hybridization study. *Ann Diagn Pathol* 15:472–475.

Kuroda N, Tanaka A, Ohe C, Mikami S, Nagashima Y, Sasaki T, et al. (2012): Review of renal oncocytosis (multiple oncocytic lesions) with focus on clinical and pathobiological aspects. *Histol Histopathol* 27:1407–1412.

La Rochelle J, Klatte T, Dastane A, Rao N, Seligson D, Said J, et al. (2010): Chromosome 9p deletions identify an aggressive phenotype of clear cell renal cell carcinoma. *Cancer* 116:4696–4702.

Ladanyi M, Lui MY, Antonescu CR, Krause-Boehm A, Meindl A, Argani P, et al. (2001): The der(17)t(X;17) (p11;q25) of human alveolar soft part sarcoma fuses the TFE3 transcription factor gene to ASPL, a novel gene at 17q25. *Oncogene* 20:48–57.

Lannon CL, Sorensen PH (2005): ETV6-NTRK3: a chimeric protein tyrosine kinase with transformation activity in multiple cell lineages. *Semin Cancer Biol* 15:215–223.

Latif F, Tory K, Gnarra J, Yao M, Duh FM, Orcutt ML, et al (1993): Identification of the von Hippel-Lindau disease tumor suppressor gene. *Science* 260:1317–1320.

Lau LC, Tan PH, Chong TW, Foo KT, Yip S (2007): Cytogenetic alterations in renal tumors: a study of 38 Southeast Asian patients. *Cancer Genet Cytogenet* 175:1–7.

Launonen V, Vierimaa O, Kiuru M, Isola J, Roth S, Pukkala E, et al. (2001): Inherited susceptibility to uterine leiomyomas and renal cell cancer. *Proc Natl Acad Sci USA* 98:3387–3392.

Laury A, Riveros-Angel M, Sabbisetti V, Dal Cin P, Hirsch M (2011): Renal mucinous tubular and spindle cell carcinoma: expanding our knowledge of immunohistochemical and cytogenetic findings. *Mod Pathol* 24:206A.

Lee CH, Marino-Enriquez A, Ou W, Zhu M, Ali RH, Chiang S, et al. (2012): The clinicopathologic features of YWHAE-FAM22 endometrial stromal sarcomas: a histologically high-grade and clinically aggressive tumor. *Am J Surg Pathol* 36:641–653.

Lefevre M, Couturier J, Sibony M, Bazille C, Boyer K, Callard P, et al. (2005): Adult papillary renal tumor with oncocytic cells: clinicopathologic, immunohistochemical, and cytogenetic features of 10 cases. *Am J Surg Pathol* 29:1576–1581.

Lehtonen R, Kiuru M, Vanharanta S, Sjoberg J, Aaltonen LM, Aittomaki K, et al. (2004): Biallelic inactivation of fumarate hydratase (FH) occurs in nonsyndromic uterine leiomyomas but is rare in other tumors. *Am J Pathol* 164:17–22.

Lerut E, Roskams T, Joniau S, Oyen R, Achten R, Van Poppel H, et al. (2006): Metanephric adenoma during pregnancy: clinical presentation, histology, and cytogenetics. *Hum Pathol* 37:1227–1232.

Limon J, Mrozek K, Heim S, Elfving P, Nedoszytko B, Babinska M, et al. (1990): On the significance of trisomy 7 and sex chromosome loss in renal cell carcinoma. *Cancer Genet Cytogenet* 49:259–263.

Little MH, Williamson KA, Mannens M, Kelsey A, Gosden C, Hastie ND, et al. (1993): Evidence that WT1 mutations in Denys-Drash syndrome patients may act in a dominant-negative fashion. *Hum Mol Genet* 2:259–264.

Lopez-Beltran A, Carrasco JC, Cheng L, Scarpelli M, Kirkali Z, Montironi R (2009): 2009 update on the classification of renal epithelial tumors in adults. *Int J Urol* 16:432–443.

Maiti S, Alam R, Amos CI, Huff V (2000): Frequent association of beta-catenin and WT1 mutations in Wilms tumors. *Cancer Res* 60:6288–6292.

Marino-Enriquez A, Ou WB, Weldon CB, Fletcher JA, Perez-Atayde AR (2011): ALK rearrangement in sickle cell trait-associated renal medullary carcinoma. *Genes Chromosomes Cancer* 50:146–153.

MdZin R, Murch A, Charles A (2010): Cytogenetic findings in Wilms' tumour: a single institute study. *Pathology* 42:643–649.

MdZin R, Phillips M, Edwards C, Murch A, Charles A (2011): Perilobar nephrogenic rests and chromosome 22. *Pediatr Dev Pathol* 14:485–492.

Medeiros LJ, Palmedo G, Krigman HR, Kovacs G, Beckwith JB (1999): Oncocytoid renal cell carcinoma after neuroblastoma: a report of four cases of a distinct clinicopathologic entity. *Am J Surg Pathol* 23:772–780.

Melendez B, Rodriguez-Perales S, Martinez-Delgado B, Otero I, Robledo M, Martinez-Ramirez A, et al. (2003): Molecular study of a new family with hereditary renal cell carcinoma and a translocation t(3;8)(p13;q24.1). *Hum Genet* 112:178–185.

Meloni-Ehrig AM (2002): Renal cancer: cytogenetic and molecular genetic aspects. *Am J Med Genet* 115:164–172.

Meloni AM, Bridge J, Sandberg AA (1992a): Reviews on chromosome studies in urological tumors. I. Renal tumors. *J Urol* 148:253–265.

Meloni AM, Sandberg AA, Pontes JE, Dobbs RM Jr. (1992b): Translocation (X;1)(p11.2;q21). A subtype of renal adenocarcinomas. *Cancer Genet Cytogenet* 63:100–101.

Meloni AM, Peier AM, Haddad FS, Powell IJ, Block AW, Huben RP, et al. (1993): A new approach in the diagnosis and follow-up of bladder cancer. FISH analysis of urine, bladder washings, and tumors. *Cancer Genet Cytogenet* 71:105–118.

Meyer PN, Clark JI, Flanigan RC, Picken MM (2007): Xp11.2 translocation renal cell carcinoma with very aggressive course in five adults. *Am J Clin Pathol* 128:70–79.

Mitelman F, Johansson B, Mertens F (2014): Mitelman Database of Chromosome Aberrations and Gene Fusions in Cancer. http://cgap.nci.nih.gov/Chromosomes/Mitelman.

Moch H, Schraml P, Bubendorf L, Richter J, Gasser TC, Mihatsch MJ, et al. (1998): Intratumoral heterogeneity of von Hippel-Lindau gene deletions in renal cell carcinoma detected by fluorescence in situ hybridization. *Cancer Res* 58:2304–2309.

Montgomery EA, Shuster DD, Burkart AL, Esteban JM, Sgrignoli A, Elwood L, et al. (2006): Inflammatory myofibroblastic tumors of the urinary tract: a clinicopathologic study of 46 cases, including a malignant example inflammatory fibrosarcoma and a subset associated with high-grade urothelial carcinoma. *Am J Surg Pathol* 30:1502–1512.

Motzer RJ, Bander NH, Nanus DM (1996): Renal-cell carcinoma. *N Engl J Med* 335:865–875.

Nagao K, Yamaguchi S, Matsuyama H, Korenaga Y, Hirata H, Yoshihiro S, et al. (2005): Allelic loss of 3p25 associated with alterations of 5q22.3 approximately q23.2 may affect the prognosis of conventional renal cell carcinoma. *Cancer Genet Cytogenet* 160:43–48.

Network CGAR (2014): Comprehensive molecular characterization of urothelial bladder carcinoma. *Nature* 507:315–322.

Neuhaus M, Wagner U, Schmid U, Ackermann D, Zellweger T, Maurer R, et al. (1999): Polysomies but not Y chromosome losses have prognostic significance in pTa/pT1 urinary bladder cancer. *Hum Pathol* 30:81–86.

O'Meara E, Stack D, Lee CH, Garvin AJ, Morris T, Argani P, et al. (2012): Characterization of the chromosomal translocation t(10;17)(q22;p13) in clear cell sarcoma of kidney. *J Pathol* 227:72–80.

Ohe C, Kuroda N, Hes O, Michal M, Vanecek T, Grossmann P, et al. (2012): A renal epithelioid angiomyolipoma/perivascular epithelioid cell tumor with TFE3 gene break visualized by FISH. *Med Mol Morphol* 45:234–237.

Ohta M, Inoue H, Cotticelli MG, Kastury K, Baffa R, Palazzo J, et al. (1996): The FHIT gene, spanning the chromosome 3p14.2 fragile site and renal carcinoma-associated t(3;8) breakpoint, is abnormal in digestive tract cancers. *Cell* 84:587–597.

Onyango P, Feinberg AP (2011): A nucleolar protein, H19 opposite tumor suppressor (HOTS), is a tumor growth inhibitor encoded by a human imprinted H19 antisense transcript. *Proc Natl Acad Sci USA* 108:16759–16764.

Panani AD, Roussos C (2006): Sex chromosome abnormalities in bladder cancer: Y polysomies are linked to PT1-grade III transitional cell carcinoma. *Anticancer Res* 26:319–323.

Paner GP, Lindgren V, Jacobson K, Harrison K, Cao Y, Campbell SC, et al. (2007): High incidence of chromosome

1 abnormalities in a series of 27 renal oncocytomas: cytogenetic and fluorescence in situ hybridization studies. *Arch Pathol Lab Med* 131:81–85.

Parham DM (2001): Neuroectodermal and neuroendocrine tumors principally seen in children. *Am J Clin Pathol* 115 Suppl:S113–128.

Pathak S, Strong LC, Ferrell RE, Trindade A (1982): Familial renal cell carcinoma with a 3;11 chromosome translocation limited to tumor cells. *Science* 217:939–941.

Pecciarini L, Cangi MG, Lo Cunsolo C, Macri E, Dal Cin E, Martignoni G, et al. (2007): Characterization of t(6;11) (p21;q12) in a renal-cell carcinoma of an adult patient. *Genes Chromosomes Cancer* 46:419–426.

Pedersen RK, Faurskov B, Hejl M, Kerndrup GB (1998): Chromosome alterations in renal cell carcinoma of childhood may correspond to aberrations in adults. *Cancer Genet Cytogenet* 106:166–169.

Peres EM, Savasan S, Cushing B, Abella S, Mohamed AN (2004): Chromosome analyses of 16 cases of Wilms tumor: different pattern in unfavorable histology. *Cancer Genet Cytogenet* 148:66–70.

Pesti T, Sukosd F, Jones EC, Kovacs G (2001): Mapping a tumor suppressor gene to chromosome 2p13 in metanephric adenoma by microsatellite allelotyping. *Hum Pathol* 32:101–104.

Petersson F, Gatalica Z, Grossmann P, Perez Montiel MD, Alvarado Cabrero I, Bulimbasic S, et al. (2010): Sporadic hybrid oncocytic/chromophobe tumor of the kidney: a clinicopathologic, histomorphologic, immunohistochemical, ultrastructural, and molecular cytogenetic study of 14 cases. *Virchows Arch* 456:355–365.

Premalata CS, Gayathri Devi M, Biswas S, Mukherjee G, Balu S, Sundareshan TS, et al. (2003): Primitive neuroectodermal tumor of the kidney. A report of two cases diagnosed by fine needle aspiration cytology. *Acta Cytol* 47:475–479.

Presti JC Jr., Rao PH, Chen Q, Reuter VE, Li FP, Fair WR, et al. (1991): Histopathological, cytogenetic, and molecular characterization of renal cortical tumors. *Cancer Res* 51:1544–1552.

Punnett HH, Halligan GE, Zaeri N, Karmazin N (1989): Translocation 10;17 in clear cell sarcoma of the kidney. A first report. *Cancer Genet Cytogenet* 41:123–128.

Rakheja D, Weinberg AG, Tomlinson GE, Partridge K, Schneider NR (2004): Translocation (10;17)(q22;p13): a recurring translocation in clear cell sarcoma of kidney. *Cancer Genet Cytogenet* 154:175–179.

Rakozy C, Schmahl GE, Bogner S, Storkel S (2002): Low-grade tubular-mucinous renal neoplasms: morphologic, immunohistochemical, and genetic features. *Mod Pathol* 15:1162–1171.

Ramphal R, Pappo A, Zielenska M, Grant R, Ngan BY (2006): Pediatric renal cell carcinoma: clinical, pathologic,

and molecular abnormalities associated with the members of the mit transcription factor family. *Am J Clin Pathol* 126:349–364.

Rivera MN, Haber DA (2005): Wilms' tumour: connecting tumorigenesis and organ development in the kidney. *Nat Rev Cancer* 5:699–712.

Rivera MN, Kim WJ, Wells J, Driscoll DR, Brannigan BW, Han M, et al. (2007): An X chromosome gene, WTX, is commonly inactivated in Wilms tumor. *Science* 315:642–645.

Roberts P, Browne CF, Lewis IJ, Bailey CC, Spicer RD, Williams J, et al. (1992): 12q13 abnormality in rhabdomyosarcoma. A nonrandom occurrence? *Cancer Genet Cytogenet* 60:135–140.

Rogler A, Hoja S, Giedl J, Ekici AB, Wach S, Taubert H, et al. (2014): Loss of MTUS1/ATIP expression is associated with adverse outcome in advanced bladder carcinomas: data from a retrospective study. *BMC Cancer* 14:214.

Ross H, Argani P (2010): Xp11 translocation renal cell carcinoma. *Pathology* 42:369–373.

Royer-Pokora B (2013): Genetics of pediatric renal tumors. *Pediatr Nephrol* 28:13–23.

Royer-Pokora B, Weirich A, Schumacher V, Uschkereit C, Beier M, Leuschner I, et al. (2008): Clinical relevance of mutations in the Wilms tumor suppressor 1 gene WT1 and the cadherin-associated protein beta1 gene CTNNB1 for patients with Wilms tumors: results of long-term surveillance of 71 patients from International Society of Pediatric Oncology Study 9/Society for Pediatric Oncology. *Cancer* 113:1080–1089.

Rubin BP, Chen CJ, Morgan TW, Xiao S, Grier HE, Kozakewich HP, et al. (1998): Congenital mesoblastic nephroma t(12;15) is associated with ETV6-NTRK3 gene fusion: cytogenetic and molecular relationship to congenital (infantile) fibrosarcoma. *Am J Pathol* 153: 1451–1458.

Rubin BP, Fletcher JA, Renshaw AA (1999): Clear cell sarcoma of soft parts: report of a case primary in the kidney with cytogenetic confirmation. *Am J Surg Pathol* 23:589–594.

Rubin BP, Pins MR, Nielsen GP, Rosen S, Hsi BL, Fletcher JA, et al. (2000): Isochromosome 7q in adult Wilms' tumors: diagnostic and pathogenetic implications. *Am J Surg Pathol* 24:1663–1669.

Ruteshouser EC, Huff V (2004): Familial Wilms tumor. *Am J Med Genet* 129C:29–34.

Sandberg AA (2002): Cytogenetics and molecular genetics of bladder cancer: a personal view. *Am J Med Genet* 115:173–182.

Sarosdy MF, Schellhammer P, Bokinsky G, Kahn P, Chao R, Yore L, et al. (2002): Clinical evaluation of a multi-target fluorescent in situ hybridization assay for detection of bladder cancer. *J Urol* 168:1950–1954.

Sarosdy MF, Kahn PR, Ziffer MD, Love WR, Barkin J, Abara EO, et al. (2006): Use of a multitarget fluorescence in situ hybridization assay to diagnose bladder cancer in patients with hematuria. *J Urol* 176:44–47.

Saxena R, Sait S, Mhawech-Fauceglia P (2006): Ewing sarcoma/primitive neuroectodermal tumor of the kidney: a case report. Diagnosed by immunohistochemistry and molecular analysis. *Ann Diagn Pathol* 10:363–366.

Schmidt L, Duh FM, Chen F, Kishida T, Glenn G, Choyke P, et al. (1997): Germline and somatic mutations in the tyrosine kinase domain of the MET proto-oncogene in papillary renal carcinomas. *Nat Genet* 16:68–73.

Schofield DE, Beckwith JB, Sklar J (1996): Loss of heterozygosity at chromosome regions 22q11–12 and 11p15.5 in renal rhabdoid tumors. *Genes Chromosomes Cancer* 15:10–17.

Shannon BA, Murch A, Cohen RJ (2005): Primary renal synovial sarcoma confirmed by cytogenetic analysis: a lesion distinct from sarcomatoid renal cell carcinoma. *Arch Pathol Lab Med* 129:238–240.

Shashi V, Lovell MA, von Kap-herr C, Waldron P, Golden WL (1994): Malignant rhabdoid tumor of the kidney: involvement of chromosome 22. *Genes Chromosomes Cancer* 10:49–54.

Sheng WW, Soukup S, Bove K, Gotwals B, Lampkin B (1990): Chromosome analysis of 31 Wilms' tumors. *Cancer Res* 50:2786–2793.

Sidhar SK, Clark J, Gill S, Hamoudi R, Crew AJ, Gwilliam R, et al. (1996): The t(X;1)(p11.2;q21.2) translocation in papillary renal cell carcinoma fuses a novel gene PRCC to the TFE3 transcription factor gene. *Hum Mol Genet* 5:1333–1338.

Skacel M, Fahmy M, Brainard JA, Pettay JD, Biscotti CV, Liou LS, et al. (2003): Multitarget fluorescence in situ hybridization assay detects transitional cell carcinoma in the majority of patients with bladder cancer and atypical or negative urine cytology. *J Urol* 169:2101–2105.

Smith NE, Illei PB, Allaf M, Gonzalez N, Morris K, Hicks J, et al. (2014a): t(6;11) Renal cell carcinoma (RCC): expanded immunohistochemical profile emphasizing novel RCC markers and report of 10 new genetically confirmed cases. *Am J Surg Pathol* 38:604–614.

Smith NE, Deyrup AT, Marino-Enriquez A, Fletcher JA, Bridge JA, Illei PB, et al. (2014b): VCL-ALK renal cell carcinoma in children with sickle-cell trait: the eighth sickle-cell nephropathy? Am J Surg Pathol [Epub ahead of print].

Soller MJ, Kullendorff CM, Bekassy AN, Alumets J, Mertens F (2007): Cytogenetic findings in pediatric renal cell carcinoma. *Cancer Genet Cytogenet* 173:75–80.

Soukup S, Gotwals B, Blough R, Lampkin B (1997): Wilms tumor: summary of 54 cytogenetic analyses. *Cancer Genet Cytogenet* 97:169–171.

Speicher MR, Schoell B, du Manoir S, Schrock E, Ried T, Cremer T, et al. (1994): Specific loss of chromosomes 1, 2, 6, 10, 13, 17, and 21 in chromophobe renal cell carcinomas revealed by comparative genomic hybridization. *Am J Pathol* 145:356–364.

Srigley JR, Delahunt B (2009): Uncommon and recently described renal carcinomas. *Mod Pathol* 22 Suppl 2:S2–S23.

Srigley JR, Delahunt B, Eble JN, Egevad L, Epstein JI, Grignon D, et al. (2013): The International Society of Urological Pathology (ISUP) Vancouver Classification of Renal Neoplasia. *Am J Surg Pathol* 37:1469–1489.

Stewenius Y, Jin Y, Ora I, Panagopoulos I, Moller E, Mertens F, et al. (2008): High-resolution molecular cytogenetic analysis of Wilms tumors highlights diagnostic difficulties among small round cell kidney tumors. *Genes Chromosomes Cancer* 47:845–852.

Storkel S, Eble JN, Adlakha K, Amin M, Blute ML, Bostwick DG, et al. (1997): Classification of renal cell carcinoma: workgroup No. 1. Union Internationale Contre le Cancer (UICC) and the American Joint Committee on Cancer (AJCC). *Cancer* 80:987–989.

Stumm M, Koch A, Wieacker PF, Phillip C, Steinbach F, Allhoff EP, et al. (1999): Partial monosomy 2p as the single chromosomal anomaly in a case of renal metanephric adenoma. *Cancer Genet Cytogenet* 115:82–85.

Su MC, Jeng YM, Chu YC (2004): Desmoplastic small round cell tumor of the kidney. *Am J Surg Pathol* 28:1379–1383.

Sugawara E, Togashi Y, Kuroda N, Sakata S, Hatano S, Asaka R, et al. (2012): Identification of anaplastic lymphoma kinase fusions in renal cancer: large-scale immunohistochemical screening by the intercalated antibody-enhanced polymer method. *Cancer* 118:4427–4436.

Sukov WR, Hodge JC, Lohse CM, Akre MK, Leibovich BC, Thompson RH, et al. (2012): ALK alterations in adult renal cell carcinoma: frequency, clinicopathologic features and outcome in a large series of consecutively treated patients. *Mod Pathol* 25:1516–1525.

Swartz MA, Karth J, Schneider DT, Rodriguez R, Beckwith JB, Perlman EJ (2002): Renal medullary carcinoma: clinical, pathologic, immunohistochemical, and genetic analysis with pathogenetic implications. *Urology* 60: 1083–1089.

Takeuchi T, Iwasaki H, Ohjimi Y, Ohshima K, Kaneko Y, Ishiguro M, et al. (1997): Renal primitive neuroectodermal tumor: a morphologic, cytogenetic, and molecular analysis with the establishment of two cultured cell lines. *Diagn Mol Pathol* 6:309–317.

Teh BT, Blennow E, Giraud S, Sahlen S, Hii SI, Brookwell R, et al. (1998): Bilateral multiple renal oncocytomas and cysts associated with a constitutional translocation (8;9) (q24.1;q34.3) and a rare constitutional VHL missense substitution. *Genes Chromosomes Cancer* 21:260–264.

Toma MI, Grosser M, Herr A, Aust DE, Meye A, Hoefling C, et al. (2008): Loss of heterozygosity and copy number abnormality in clear cell renal cell carcinoma discovered by high-density affymetrix 10K single nucleotide polymorphism mapping array. *Neoplasia* 10:634–642.

Tomlinson GE, Nisen PD, Timmons CF, Schneider NR (1991): Cytogenetics of a renal cell carcinoma in a 17-month-old child. Evidence for Xp11.2 as a recurring breakpoint. *Cancer Genet Cytogenet* 57:11–17.

van den Berg A, Buys CH (1997): Involvement of multiple loci on chromosome 3 in renal cell cancer development. *Genes Chromosomes Cancer* 19:59–76.

Van Poppel H, Nilsson S, Algaba F, Bergerheim U, Dal Cin P, Fleming S, et al. (2000): Precancerous lesions in the kidney. *Scand J Urol Nephrol Suppl*:136–165.

Verdorfer I, Hobisch A, Hittmair A, Duba HC, Bartsch G, Utermann G, et al. (1999): Cytogenetic characterization of 22 human renal cell tumors in relation to a histopathological classification. *Cancer Genet Cytogenet* 111:61–70.

Versteege I, Sevenet N, Lange J, Rousseau-Merck MF, Ambros P, Handgretinger R, et al. (1998): Truncating mutations of hSNF5/INI1 in aggressive paediatric cancer. *Nature* 394:203–206.

Vicha A, Stejskalova E, Sumerauer D, Kodet R, Malis J, Kucerova H, et al. (2002): Malignant peripheral primitive neuroectodermal tumor of the kidney. *Cancer Genet Cytogenet* 139:67–70.

Visser O, Coebergh JW, Schouten LJ (1997): *Incidence of Cancer on the Netherlands*. Utrecht: The Netherlands Cancer Registry.

Walter TA, Berger CS, Sandberg AA (1989a): The cytogenetics of renal tumors. Where do we stand, where do we go? *Cancer Genet Cytogenet* 43:15–34.

Walter TA, Pennington RD, Decker HJ, Sandberg AA (1989b): Translocation t(9;11)(p23;q12): a primary chromosomal change in renal oncocytoma. *J Urol* 142:117–119.

Wang-Wuu S, Soukup S, Ballard E, Gotwals B, Lampkin B (1988): Chromosomal analysis of sixteen human rhabdomyosarcomas. *Cancer Res* 48:983–987.

Wang N, Perkins KL (1984): Involvement of band 3p14 in t(3;8) hereditary renal carcinoma. *Cancer Genet Cytogenet* 11:479–481.

Weinstein MH, Dal Cin P (2001): Genetics of epithelial tumors of the renal parenchyma in adults and renal cell carcinoma in children. *Anal Quant Cytol Histol* 23: 362–372.

Weiss LM, Gelb AB, Medeiros LJ (1995): Adult renal epithelial neoplasms. *Am J Clin Pathol* 103:624–635.

Weksberg R, Shuman C, Smith AC (2005): Beckwith-Wiedemann syndrome. *Am J Med Genet C* 137C:12–23.

Weterman MA, Wilbrink M, Janssen I, Janssen HA, van den Berg E, Fisher SE, et al. (1996): Molecular cloning of the papillary renal cell carcinoma-associated translocation (X;1)(p11;q21) breakpoint. *Cytogenet Cell Genet* 75:2–6.

Williamson SR, Halat S, Eble JN, Grignon DJ, Lopez-Beltran A, Montironi R, et al. (2012): Multilocular cystic renal carcinoma: similarities and differences in immunoprofile compared with clear cell renal cell carcinoma. *Am J Surg Pathol* 36:1425–1433.

Williamson SR, Bunde PJ, Montironi R, Lopez-Beltran A, Zhang S, Wang M, et al. (2013): Malignant perivascular epithelioid cell neoplasm (PEComa) of the urinary bladder with TFE3 gene rearrangement: clinicopathologic, immunohistochemical, and molecular features. *Am J Surg Pathol* 37:1619–1626.

Wullich B, Henn W, Siemer S, Seitz G, Freiler A, Zang KD (1997): Clonal chromosome aberrations in three of five sporadic angiomyolipomas of the kidney. *Cancer Genet Cytogenet* 96:42–45.

Xia QY, Rao Q, Shen Q, Shi SS, Li L, Liu B, et al. (2013): Oncocytic papillary renal cell carcinoma: a clinicopathological study emphasizing distinct morphology, extended immunohistochemical profile and cytogenetic features. *Int J Clin Exp Pathol* 6:1392–1399.

Yang XJ, Zhou M, Hes O, Shen S, Li R, Lopez J, et al. (2008): Tubulocystic carcinoma of the kidney: clinicopathologic and molecular characterization. *Am J Surg Pathol* 32: 177–187.

Yoshida MA, Ohyashiki K, Ochi H, Gibas Z, Pontes JE, Prout GR Jr., et al. (1986): Cytogenetic studies of tumor tissue from patients with nonfamilial renal cell carcinoma. *Cancer Res* 46:2139–2147.

Yusenko MV (2010): Molecular pathology of chromophobe renal cell carcinoma: a review. *Int J Urol* 17:592–600.

Zbar B, Tory K, Merino M, Schmidt L, Glenn G, Choyke P, et al. (1994): Hereditary papillary renal cell carcinoma. *J Urol* 151:561–566.

Zhou M, Yang XJ, Lopez JI, Shah RB, Hes O, Shen SS, et al. (2009): Renal tubulocystic carcinoma is closely related to papillary renal cell carcinoma: implications for pathologic classification. *Am J Surg Pathol* 33:1840–1849.

Zhuang Z, Park WS, Pack S, Schmidt L, Vortmeyer AO, Pak E, et al. (1998): Trisomy 7-harbouring non-random duplication of the mutant MET allele in hereditary papillary renal carcinomas. *Nat Genet* 20:66–69.

CHAPTER 16

Tumors of the breast

Manuel R. Teixeira[1]*, Nikos Pandis*[2] *and Sverre Heim*[3]

[1]Department of Genetics, Portugese Oncology Institute, Porto, Portugal
[2]Department of Genetics, Saint Savas Hospital, Athens, Greece
[3]Section for Cancer Cytogenetics, Institute for Cancer Genetics and Informatics,
Osio University Hospital, Oslo, Norway

Breast cancer is the most common malignancy in females in the Western world, with a lifetime risk for a woman in the USA of about one in eight (De Santis et al., 2014). Although most cases are sporadic, as many as 20% occur in familial aggregates, and about 5–10% show a segregation pattern indicative of an autosomal dominant trait (McPherson et al., 2000). A significant proportion of the latter are caused by germline mutations of the *BRCA1* or *BRCA2* genes (Miki et al., 1994; Wooster et al., 1995; Narod and Foulkes, 2004). When, in addition, several environmental breast cancer predisposing factors are known or suspected and also benign breast conditions exist that are associated with an increased risk of carcinoma development (McPherson et al., 2000; Veronesi et al., 2005), it should be obvious that the whole breast neoplasia picture is a complex one indeed.

Benign breast disorders

Hyperproliferative breast disorders of both the epithelial and connective tissues are common; the borderline toward genuinely neoplastic conditions, or perhaps one should rather say clinically significant tumors, may be very vague (Rosen, 1993; Santen and Mansel, 2005). Noguchi et al. (1993) performed clonality analyses on two neoplasias characterized by coproliferation of epithelial and mesenchymal cells: fibroadenomas and phyllodes tumors. They found that whereas the X chromosome inactivation pattern of the fibroadenomas indicated that they were polyclonal, both monoclonal and polyclonal cell components were found in the phyllodes tumors. Closer examination revealed polyclonality of the epithelium in both tumor types and of the connective tissue component in the fibroadenomas, whereas the "stromal" component of the five benign phyllodes tumors was monoclonal. More recent data indicate that although in most cases the stroma of phyllodes tumors is monoclonal and the epithelium polyclonal, sometimes the inverse situation is seen (Kuijper et al., 2002).

Cytogenetic studies, which also are well suited to shed light on clonality issues in neoplastic processes, are sparse in these biphasic breast tumors. Few predominantly epithelial benign hyperproliferations have been karyotypically characterized by chromosome banding analysis. Whereas Bullerdiek et al. (1993) and Lundin et al. (1998a) found numerical chromosome changes (+7 and +16, respectively) to be primary cytogenetic events in breast *papillomas*, Dietrich et al. (1995) detected structural chromosome alterations in four of five such benign tumors, including two with an interstitial 3p deletion and one with several cytogenetically unrelated clones. Rohen et al. (1993) reported two benign epithelial breast lesions showing a clonal chromosomal alteration involving 12q13–15 as the sole cytogenetic change, a t(10;12)(p14–15;q13) in a papilloma with areas of florid epithelial hyperplasia and a t(12;14)(q13–14;q24) in a florid epithelial hyperplasia with adenosis; the latter is cytogenetically similar to the 12;14-translocation that characterizes a large subset of uterine leiomyomas (Chapter 17). On the other hand, a proportion of diffuse *fibrocystic lesions* have shown clonal chromosome aberrations, some of which are known to occur recurrently in breast carcinomas (see following text), such as gain of 1q, interstitial 3p deletion, 6q deletion, and trisomy for chromosomes 7, 18, and 20 (Dietrich et al., 1995; Lundin et al., 1998b; Burbano et al., 2000; Tibiletti et al., 2000; Steinarsdottir et al., 2004). Especially intriguing is the recurrent finding of an interstitial 3p deletion in proliferative lesions from prophylactic mastectomies in women with hereditary predisposition to breast cancer (Petersson et al., 1996; Teixeira et al., 1996a).

Twenty-eight *phyllodes tumors* of the breast with clonal karyotypic changes have been reported (Birdsall et al., 1992, 1995; Dal Cin et al., 1995, 1998; Dietrich et al., 1997, 2004; Polito et al., 1998; Woolley et al., 2000; Ladesich et al., 2002; Barbosa et al., 2004). In general, chromosome banding analysis has revealed relatively simple chromosomal changes in benign phyllodes tumors but complex karyotypes in the malignant ones, indicating that karyotypic complexity is a marker of malignancy in phyllodes tumors (Dietrich et al., 1997). The most recurrent chromosome aberration, found in five tumors, has been i(1)(q10) (Birdsall et al., 1995; Dal Cin et al., 1995; Dietrich et al., 1997, 2004; Polito et al., 1998). The finding of clonal chromosome abnormalities in both the epithelial and connective tissue components of phyllodes tumors, including in the form of cytogenetically unrelated clones, indicates that they are genuinely biphasic, that is, both components are part of the neoplastic parenchyma (Dietrich et al., 1997).

About 80 breast *fibroadenomas* with cytogenetic abnormalities have been published, the most significant series being those of Calabrese et al. (1991), Ozisik et al. (1994), Dietrich et al. (1995), Rohen et al. (1996), Petersson et al. (1997), Tibiletti et al. (2000), and Rizou et al. (2004). Although no clear pattern of nonrandomness has emerged, structural rearrangements of 1p, 6q, 12p, and 12q as well as trisomy for chromosomes 11 and 20 have been seen recurrently. The finding by Calabrese et al. (1991) of an identical t(11;12)(q21;q15) in three fibroadenomas from the same breast indicated that all had their origin in the same transformed cell. Fletcher et al. (1991) attempted to differentiate by immunophenotyping the connective tissue and epithelial tumor components and found that the clonal chromosome aberrations occurred in the former.

Dietrich et al. (1994) used differential culturing of epithelial and mesenchymal cells to study two biphasic breast *adenolipomas*. Both had clonal chromosome anomalies and, in one of them, a rearrangement of 12q13–15, the most typical chromosomal anomaly in sporadic lipomas (Chapter 24), was detected. The cytogenetic changes were found to be present in the mesenchymal but not in the epithelial tissue fractions, indicating that only the former constituted the actual tumor parenchyma. Interestingly, also another breast adenolipoma with a 12q rearrangement (Rohen et al., 1995a) and a breast hamartoma with a 6p21 and *HMGA1* (alias *HMGIY*) rearrangement (Dal Cin et al., 1997) have been reported, pointing to the tumorigenic involvement of the high-mobility group genes in benign mesenchymal tumors of the breast as well as of other tissues and organs (Chapter 24).

Biphasic tumors with high-hyperdiploid karyotypes, particularly common among young children, might constitute a distinct clinicomorphologic subgroup of benign breast tumors (Walther et al., 2013). An adenomyoepithelioma of the breast showed a t(8;16)(p23;q21) (Gatalica et al., 2005), but the molecular consequences of this balanced translocation are unknown. Finally, hidradenoma of the breast is characterized by the recurrent t(11;19)(q21;p13) resulting in the fusion gene *MECT1–MAML2* (Kazakov et al., 2007; Knoedler et al., 2007), genetic changes that are also found in salivary gland mucoepidermoid carcinomas and in clear cell hidradenoma and hidradenocarcinomas of the skin (Chapters 19 and 22, respectively).

Breast carcinoma

Cytogenetic findings

More than 880 carcinomas with clonal karyotypic abnormalities characterized by chromosome banding analysis have been reported (Mitelman et al.,

2014), but a large proportion of the data concern the highly advanced tumor cells of pleural effusions and many karyotypes have been incompletely described. The largest series were reported by Gebhart et al. (1986), Bello and Rey (1989), Dutrillaux et al. (1990), Hainsworth et al. (1991), Lu et al. (1993), Pandis et al. (1993a, 1995a), Thompson et al. (1993), Trent et al. (1993), Rohen et al. (1995b), Steinarsdottir et al. (1995), Cavalli et al. (1997), Bernardino et al. (1998), Adeyinka et al. (1999a), Teixeira et al. (2001), and Wuicik et al. (2007). The field was extensively reviewed by Hainsworth and Garson (1990), Dutrillaux et al. (1993), and Teixeira et al. (2002).

Many of the differences seen among the results reached by various groups, even when the materials examined were similar in the sense that they only included primary tumors, can be put down to differences in investigative techniques (Pandis et al., 1994a). The study of tumor cytogenetics by direct harvesting methods fails to yield information in many cases (those in which the *in vivo* mitotic activity is low) and hence is likely to show only the most malignant tip of the iceberg. Indeed, the proportion of highly abnormal tumor karyotypes of all cases showing aberrations seems to be higher in such studies (Dutrillaux et al., 1990; Hainsworth et al., 1991; Lu et al., 1993) than when short-term cultures are relied upon (Thompson et al., 1993; Trent et al., 1993; Pandis et al., 995a). Examinations using *in vitro* cultures are likely to obtain cytogenetic information—whether the results are always representative of the tumor parenchyma or not is another matter—in a higher percentage of cases; after modification of existing short-term culture protocols to make them better suited for the growth of breast cancer cells (Pandis et al., 1992a), clonal abnormalities were consistently obtained in 80% of the tumors examined (Pandis et al., 1993a, 1995a; Adeyinka et al., 1999a; Teixeira et al., 2001). The fact that in the latter series the number of cases with simple aberrations, sometimes sole anomalies, was markedly higher than when direct or semidirect processing of the tumor tissue was used, perhaps indicates that cells at an earlier stage of neoplastic transformation were being selected for.

Of relevance in the present context is the evidence obtained also by noncytogenetic techniques that far from all malignant breast tumors have complex genomic changes. Investigations of DNA content by flow cytometry have found no aneuploid peak in as many as 40% of breast carcinomas (Levack et al., 1987; Dressler et al., 1988; Wenger et al., 1993). At least one tumorigenic breast carcinoma cell line with a normal karyotype, established from the pleural effusion of a woman with metastatic disease, has been reported (Gioanni et al., 1990). On the other hand, considerable aneuploidy may exist also in certifiably benign proliferative breast disorders (Uccelli et al., 1986; Carpenter et al., 1987; Nielsen and Briand, 1989; Micale et al., 1994). It seems safe to conclude that neither is the demonstration of clonal chromosome anomalies in breast cells sufficient to conclude that the disease is cancerous nor are massive genomic rearrangements a *sine qua non* for even highly malignant tumors. Both these facts need to be kept in mind when assessing the pathogenetic role of the various chromosomal anomalies in breast carcinogenesis.

These caveats should nevertheless not be allowed to confuse the main lesson learned from the many studies that have been performed, namely, that the acquired chromosomal aberrations in breast carcinomas are distinctly nonrandom (Mitelman et al., 2014). The structural chromosome rearrangements most commonly observed are i(1)(q10), der(1;16) (q10;p10), del(3)(p12–13p14–21), del(6)(q21–23), del(1)(p13), del(1)(q11–12), del(1)(p22), i(8)(q10), and del(1)(q42). The most common numerical cytogenetic changes are gain of chromosomes 7, 20, 18, and 8 and loss of chromosomes X, 22, 13, and 17. Of these recurrent karyotypic changes, the best candidates for a primary role in breast carcinogenesis are those that have been detected at least once as the sole change in a clone, and some of these changes will be examined in more detail.

Rearrangements of chromosome 1 are the most common cytogenetic changes in breast carcinomas, in particular unbalanced whole-arm translocation between 1q and 16p (Figure 16.1a) and isochromosome 1q (Figure 16.1b), both of which are frequently present as sole karyotypic anomalies (Pandis et al., 1992b, 1995a; Teixeira et al., 2002). The end result of the unbalanced t(1;16) whole-arm translocation is a karyotype that contains two normal copies of chromosome 1, one normal copy of 16, and a fourth fusion chromosome consisting of 16p and 1q. Probably, the frequency of this

(A)   (B)

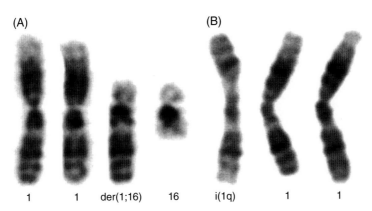

1   1   der(1;16)   16   i(1q)   1   1

Figure 16.1 Chromosomal rearrangements leading to gain of 1q material are common in breast carcinomas. (A) A whole-arm translocation between chromosomes 1 and 16 is found repeatedly both as the sole anomaly and in complex karyotypes, typically leading to 1q gain and 16q loss. (B) Isochromosome 1q is also identified recurrently both as the sole anomaly and together with other chromosome changes in breast carcinomas.

der(1;16)(q10;p10) in breast cancer has been underestimated in the past; Hultén et al. (1993) reinterpreted their early findings (Rodgers et al., 1984) in the light of newer knowledge and now think that what was formerly described by them as del(1p) actually was a der(1;16). It would not be surprising if also some other breast cancer rearrangements described as del(1)(p13) (Mitchell and Santibanez-Koref, 1990) may be similarly reinterpreted. Kokalj-Vokac et al. (1993) used fluorescence *in situ* hybridization (FISH) with probes reacting with alphoid and classic satellite DNA from chromosomes 1 and 16 to demonstrate that the der(1;16) really is a whole-arm translocation. Using the same strategy, these investigators also showed that the breakpoint in the cytogenetically defined i(1q) occurred after breakage in the alpha 1-containing region in six of seven cases, whereas the rearranged chromosome of the last case was dicentric at the molecular cytogenetic level, with breakage in 1p11.2 (Kokalj-Vokac et al., 1993).

The fact that both der(1;16)(q10;p10) and i(1q) have gain of 1q in common suggests that this is the functionally important outcome of the rearrangements (Dutrillaux et al., 1990; Pandis et al., 1992b). The essential result in molecular terms of such an extra 1q copy is unknown, and it is not understood whether the simultaneous loss of 16q associated with the t(1;16) is of any additional pathogenetic importance. Further evidence, albeit still indirect, that der(1;16) really confers on breast epithelial cells a tumorigenic ability was provided by Pandis

et al. (1994b), who found the der(1;16) fusion chromosome as the only cytogenetic abnormality in both a primary breast carcinoma and its axillary metastasis. The same 1;16 whole-arm translocation is by no means restricted to disease processes of the breast, however; it is also a common secondary change in multiple myeloma, several sarcomas, and Wilms' tumor (Chapters 11, 15, and 24). The question of whether the pattern of secondary chromosomal changes in breast carcinomas is also nonrandom and whether it depends on which primary aberration is present has in part been answered for breast carcinomas with der(1;16) and i(1q) as primary abnormalities (Tsarouha et al., 1999). Whereas additional copies of the respective primary change and/or rearrangements leading to loss of material from chromosome arm 11q were equally common in both cytogenetic subsets, the distribution of secondary chromosomal changes otherwise differed, with the frequency of +7 being significantly higher in breast carcinomas carrying a der(1;16) and +20 being more common in breast carcinomas carrying an i(1q).

The conclusion that 1q gain is pathogenetically important in breast carcinogenesis gains further supports from the observation that the variation in exact breakpoint position at the molecular level spans the constitutive heterochromatin in both der(1;16) and i(1q) (Kokalj-Vokac et al., 1993), from the occasional occurrence of der(1;16) as an extra chromosome (leading to gain of 1q and 16p instead of the more common gain of 1q and loss of

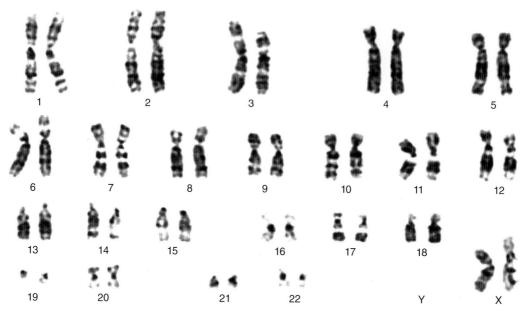

1 2 3 4 5

6 7 8 9 10 11 12

13 14 15 16 17 18

19 20 21 22 Y X

Figure 16.2 Karyogram of a breast carcinoma showing an interstitial 3p deletion (del(3)(p12p14); right homolog) as the sole chromosome abnormality.

16q; Teixeira et al., 2001), and from the observation of occasional gains of 1q through unbalanced translocations between chromosome 1 and other partners than chromosome 16 (Pandis et al., 1995a). It was therefore somewhat surprising when it turned out that also losses of 1q, especially through deletions with breakpoints in the heterochromatic region proximally in the long arm, del(1)(q11–12), are sometimes found in breast carcinomas, either alone or as part of complex karyotypes (Pandis et al., 1995a; Teixeira et al., 2002).

Small *interstitial deletions of the short arm of chromosome 3*, del(3)(p12p14) (Figure 16.2) and del(3)(p13p14), were established as the defining cytogenetic feature of a subset of breast cancers by Pandis et al. (1993b); a del(3)(p13p21) had earlier been described as the sole change also by Zhang et al. (1989). Whereas these interstitial 3p deletions mostly occur as the only visible aberration (Pandis et al., 1993b, 1995a), larger terminal del(3p) are also relatively common and typically occur in complex karyotypes (Teixeira et al., 2002). In parallel with what has been said previously when lung and kidney tumors were discussed, the consistent loss of chromosomal material from proximal 3p raises the suspicion that a tumor suppressor gene important

in breast carcinogenesis might be located here. It is intriguing that, at least at the chromosomal level, the 3p deletions in breast carcinomas seem to cover the same minimal deleted segment in 3p14 that does the group of proximal 3p deletions in renal cancers (Chapter 15). The actual pathogenetic homogeneity or heterogeneity among the various tumors sharing 3p– as a cytogenetic characteristic remains unknown.

Interstitial or terminal *deletions of the long arm of chromosome 6*, often with the proximal breakpoint in 6q21, have also been described both as sole anomalies and together with other aberrations in breast carcinomas (Pandis et al., 1995a; Teixeira et al., 2002). Again, the loss of a tumor suppressor is presumed to be the important DNA-level outcome. The same chromosomal region is recurrently deleted also in several other malignancies, especially lymphatic malignancies, malignant melanomas, and adenocarcinomas of many different organs.

An *isochromosome 8q*, leading to concurrent 8q gain and 8p loss, is the most recurrent structural abnormality of chromosome 8 in breast cancer (Teixeira et al., 2002). However, 8p is also frequently affected at varying breakpoints by different types of aberrations. The nonrandomness of 8p

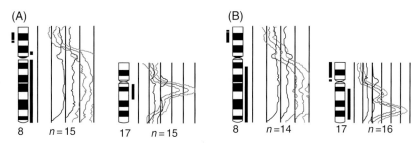

Figure 16.3 Examples of chromosomes 8 and 17 copy number changes identified by chromosome comparative genomic hybridization in breast carcinomas. (A) Breast carcinoma showing loss of 8p21–23 and gains of 8p11–12, 8q, and 17q11–21. (B) Breast carcinoma showing loss of 8p21–23, gain of 8q12–24, and two 17q amplicons centered around 17q12–21 and 17q22–24.

rearrangements in breast carcinomas includes a remarkably high frequency of homogeneously staining regions (hsr) in this chromosome arm (Dutrillaux et al., 1990), whereas the other main cytogenetic manifestation of gene amplification, double minute (dmin) chromosomes, is rare in this tumor type. Using comparative genomic hybridization (CGH) to study carcinomas known to have hsr, Muleris et al. (1994, 1995) found amplifications of 11q13, 9p13, 17q21, 1q21, 16p11, 8q22, 8q24, 10q22, 15q26, 17q23, 20q13, 19q13, and 8p1. The use of chromosome microdissection and *in situ* hybridization to characterize the organization of the amplified sequences demonstrated that hsr are usually formed by amplification of DNA sequences from two to four different chromosomal sites (Guan et al., 1994; Muleris et al., 1995). Bernardino et al. (1998) also presented data indicating that the amplified sequences cannot always be inferred from their genomic sites; although sequences from chromosomes 11 and 17 were mostly found within hsr located on chromosomes 11 and 17, respectively, sequences from chromosome 8 were rarely found within hsr localized on that chromosome. The data at hand therefore show a complex set of 8p rearrangements in breast carcinomas, with a combination of amplification at 8p11–12, break in the 8p12–21 region, and loss of 8p21-pter (Muleris et al., 1995; Teixeira et al., 2002) (Figure 16.3).

Secretory breast carcinoma accounts for less than 1% of all breast cancers and is now known to represent a distinct pathobiologic entity. A t(12;15)(p13;q25) has been found in 92% of secretory breast carcinomas (Tognon et al., 2002; Diallo et al., 2003), that is, the very same chromosome abnormality that characterizes congenital fibrosarcoma (Chapter 24), cellular mesoblastic nephroma (Chapter 15), and salivary mammary analog secretory carcinoma (a recently described entity; Chapter 19), and which is also occasionally seen in acute myeloid leukemia (Chapter 6); this evidently represents a rare example of a cytogenetic aberration causally related to transformation across many cell lineages (molecular consequences discussed in the following text). To assess the frequency of t(12;15)(p13;q25) in breast cancer, Makretsov et al. (2004) used FISH on paraffin-embedded, formalin-fixed tissue sections to detect the presence of this translocation in one secretory breast carcinoma but in none of 201 other cases of breast carcinoma also examined, demonstrating the remarkable consistency of this cytogenetic–pathologic correlation.

Whereas no chromosome losses have been repeatedly found as sole anomalies in breast tumors, trisomies have been described both as the only chromosome-level aberration and as part of complex karyotypes. They would therefore seem to be candidates for a role as pathogenetically important, primary abnormalities. Bullerdiek et al. (1993) suggested that trisomy 8 might constitute such a change; they found +8 as the only or first aberration in two of 15 tumors examined. Pandis et al. (1995a), describing 79 primary breast carcinomas with clonal abnormalities, found trisomy 7 in eight cases, in five of them as the sole change, trisomy 18 likewise in eight cases (in six as the sole change), and trisomy 20 in 10 cases (in two as the sole change). Adeyinka et al. (1997) later identified another subgroup of breast carcinomas cytogenetically characterized by trisomy 12. Some of the same trisomies were also seen in some massively hyperdiploid cases that contained only numerical aberrations, with preferential gain of chromosomes 1, 5, 6, 7, 12, 16, 17, 18, and 19 (Pandis et al., 1993a, 1995a; Adeyinka et al., 1999b; Molist et al., 2005). Whereas well-founded doubts have been expressed as to the neoplasia relevance of a solitary +7 in tumor samples (Johansson et al., 1993), no similar data speak against the importance of the other trisomies mentioned earlier. At least for the time being, they have to be accepted as potential primary chromosome anomalies in breast carcinogenesis. Numerical chromosome changes, including trisomy for chromosomes X, 5, 7, 8, 18, or 20 and monosomy 17, have also been recurrently detected in the about 20 male breast carcinomas with abnormal karyotypes that have been reported (Teixeira et al., 1998a; Mitelman et al., 2014).

One intriguing aspect of many studies of short-term cultured breast carcinomas is the detection of a high frequency of *cytogenetically unrelated clones*, close to 50%, in the tumors (Pandis et al., 1993a, 1995a; Teixeira et al., 2002). In some instances, a highly characteristic aberration such as der(1;16) was present in one clone alongside another showing complex changes but no 1;16-translocation; hence, the circumstantial evidence seems strong that both clones were relevant in carcinogenesis. A detailed cytogenetic study of multiple carcinoma samples (one from each tumor quadrant) as well as normal-looking surrounding breast tissue revealed multiple clones unevenly distributed within the tumor mass in seven of 10 breast carcinomas (Teixeira et al., 1995, 1996b). A similar zonal distribution of cytogenetically distinct cell populations was also demonstrated by CGH (Torres et al., 2007). Furthermore, combined analysis with chromosome banding and CGH (which is not subject to culture bias and detects only those imbalances that are present in a significant proportion of the test sample) has shown that the latter technique can detect changes present in cytogenetically unrelated clones (Persson et al., 1999; Teixeira et al., 2001), providing indirect evidence that the disparate clones are part of the tumor parenchyma. On the contrary, Noguchi et al. (1992, 1994) examined the X chromosome inactivation pattern in breast carcinomas, atypical ductal hyperplasias, and intraductal papillomas and concluded that they always

had predominant inactivation of one particular X chromosome, indicating that these malignancies and precancerous lesions all were of monoclonal origin. The cytogenetic and X chromosome inactivation data need not be mutually exclusive, however, even if it should turn out that the karyotypic abnormalities really are present in cells of the tumor parenchyma and that there is no submicroscopic, unifying mutation common to all of them in every case. The pitfalls of the X chromosome inactivation method are now evident, as it has been shown that the normal breast epithelium is organized in developmentally discrete regions within which all cells have the same inactive X chromosome (Tsai et al., 1996; Diallo et al., 2001), and the method used by Noguchi et al. (1992) recognizes monoclonal cells against a polyclonal background only when the monoclonal cell population is 50% or more (smaller clones may therefore escape detection). Be that as it may, a more recent study of breast cancer clonality using this technique found different X chromosomes inactivated in multiple, morphologically homogeneous tumor samples in four of 12 breast carcinomas (Going et al., 2001), supporting the conclusion that a significant proportion of breast carcinomas are polyclonal (Heim et al., 1997; Going, 2003). Conversely, the only cytogenetic data existing on mammary *carcinosarcomas*, rare malignant biphasic tumors, indicate that both the epithelial and mesenchymal components are part of the neoplastic parenchyma and that they have evolved from a single common stem cell (Teixeira et al., 1998b).

Chromosome banding analysis is ideally suited to evaluate the clonal relationship among multiple breast tumors, be they ipsilateral or bilateral, synchronous or metachronous. The evolutionary relationship among multiple, ipsilateral breast carcinomas was studied by cytogenetic analysis of 37 tumorous lesions from 17 patients (Teixeira et al., 1994, 1997; Pandis et al., 1995b). Nine of 12 patients with at least two karyotypically abnormal, macroscopically distinct carcinoma foci had an evolutionarily related, cytogenetically abnormal clone in the different tumor lesions from the same breast, showing that the dominant mechanism for the origin of multiple ipsilateral breast tumors is intramammary spreading from a single breast cancer. On the other hand, the clonal relationship between bilateral breast carcinomas was analyzed in 20 tumors from 10 patients (Pandis et al., 1995b; Teixeira et al., 1996b; Adeyinka et al., 2000a). The cytogenetic findings in five of the eight cases that were informative with regard to the clonal relationship between the two breast tumors supported the notion that each carcinoma arose independently as a genuinely primary tumor, because the chromosome aberrations they contained were completely disparate. In the remaining three cases, on the other hand, the karyotypic data indicated that spreading of the disease from one breast to the other had taken place, since the same rare chromosome abnormalities were detected from both sides. The conclusion that most ipsilateral breast carcinomas arise through intramammary spreading of a single breast cancer, whereas most patients with bilateral breast carcinomas have two different neoplastic diseases, was also reached by unsupervised hierarchical clustering analysis of chromosomal CGH (Teixeira et al., 2004) and array CGH (Brommesson et al., 2008) data.

Comparison of the karyotypic constitution of breast cancer metastases and their respective primary carcinomas is likely to increase our understanding of the pathogenetic mechanisms underlying the metastatic process in this disease. Of the 17 carcinomas and their corresponding metastatic lesions that have been analyzed by chromosome banding (Pandis et al., 1994b, 1998; Teixeira et al., 1996b; Adeyinka et al., 2000a, 2000b), nine primary tumors and eight metastatic lesions had only simple chromosomal abnormalities, whereas at least one clone with complex aberrations was detected in all the remaining cases. Although metastatic lesions tended to be karyotypically more complex than are unselected primary breast carcinomas, seven out of 17 cases displayed fewer abnormal clones in the metastasis than in the respective primary carcinoma, indicating that the selection pressure facing the neoplastic cells during tumor progression caused a reduction in the number of clones surviving from an initially genotypically heterogeneous tumor cell population. CGH analyses of paired primary-metastatic samples also revealed extensive clonal divergence, indicating that metastases may occur relatively early during breast carcinogenesis (Kuukasjarvi et al., 1997a;

Nishizaki et al., 1997b; Torres et al., 2007). Interestingly, at the other end of the spectrum of tumor progression, the meager existent chromosome banding data on carcinoma *in situ* hinted that this presumed precursor lesion is genetically more advanced than previously anticipated (Nielsen et al., 1989). In fact, subsequent combined tissue microdissection and CGH analyses of lobular or ductal carcinoma *in situ* and adjacent invasive carcinoma areas have shown in most cases an almost identical genetic pattern in the two lesions (Kuukasjarvi et al., 1997b; Buerger et al., 1999, 2000; Aubele et al., 2000a, 2000b, 2000c; Nyante et al., 2004; Shelley Hwang et al., 2004), strongly underlining their role as precursor lesions of invasive breast cancer. Despite the genomic similarities between synchronous DCIS and IDC, Hernandez et al. (2012) provided circumstantial evidence indicating that progression from the former to the latter may be driven by selection of minor clones that harbor a specific repertoire of genetic aberrations.

Molecular genetic findings

Of the many chromosome rearrangements identified in breast carcinomas, the one that is best characterized at the molecular genetic level is the t(12;15)(p13;q25) specific of secretory breast carcinomas. This translocation fuses the dimerization domain of the transcription factor ETS variant gene 6 (*ETV6*, alias *TEL*) with the membrane receptor tyrosine kinase neurotrophin-3 gene (*NTRK3*) (Tognon et al., 2002; Diallo et al., 2003), just as previously described in congenital fibrosarcoma, cellular mesoblastic nephroma, and acute myeloid leukemia and more recently also in salivary mammary analog secretory carcinoma. The resulting *ETV6–NTRK3* fusion oncogene leads to constitutive activation of the RAS–MAPK mitogenic pathway and the PI3K–AKT pathway mediating cell survival, both of which are required for *ETV6–NTRK3* transformation. Retroviral transfer of chimeric *ETV6–NTRK3* into murine mammary epithelial cells results in transformed cells that form tumors in nude mice (Tognon et al., 2002), providing conclusive evidence that this fusion oncogene really is causally related to the development of secretory breast carcinomas. Another example of a pathogenetic relationship between some subtypes of head and neck and breast carcinomas was provided by Persson et al. (2009), who identified a recurrent fusion of the *MYB* and *NFIB* transcription factor genes in adenoid cystic carcinomas arising at both locations. This fusion gene results from a t(6;9)(q21–25;p13–p24) previously observed by chromosome banding analysis in head and neck, mainly salivary gland, adenoid cystic carcinomas (Chapter 19) and subsequently in analogous breast tumors with locus-specific FISH probes. The *MYB–NFIB* chimeric gene consists of *MYB* exon 14 fused to the last coding exons of *NFIB* and results in upregulation of the *MYB* oncogene, presumably by loss of regulatory microRNA target sites at the 3′ end of the gene (Persson et al., 2009).

Other examples of chromosome rearrangements causing gene fusion in breast cancer are scarce. The karyotypic change dic(8;11)(p12;q13) in the breast cancer cell line MDA-MB-175 causes a rearrangement between the neuregulin (*NRL1*) gene at 8p12 and the *ODZ4* (alias *DOC4*) gene at 11q13 (Liu et al., 1999; Wang et al., 1999). Through this cytogenetic rearrangement, *NRG1*, which encodes growth factors that are ligands for tyrosine kinase receptors of the ERBB family, comes under the influence of the *ODZ4* promoter. Although four other breast cancer cell lines (Adelaide et al., 2003) and 4.5–6% of primary breast carcinomas (Huang et al., 2004; Prentice et al., 2005) have been shown to have breakpoints within *NRG1*, no other examples of fusion of this gene could so far be detected. The MCF7 breast cancer cell line has been shown to present coamplification and fusion of the *BCAS3* (17q23) and *BCAS4* (20q13.2) genes (Bärlund et al., 2002) as well as the *TBL1XR1–RGS17* fusion gene resulting from a t(3;6)(q26;q25) (Hahn et al., 2004), but neither fusion transcript has so far been detected in other breast cancer cell lines or primary carcinomas. Finally, a t(3;20)(p14;p11) has been shown to target the *FHIT* gene in the BrCa-MZ-02 cell line but is associated with absence of functional FHIT and does not involve a fusion gene (Popovici et al., 2002). The relevance for breast carcinogenesis of these rare structural gene rearrangements brought about by chromosomal mechanisms and detected in a few cell lines is presently unknown.

Recent technological advances in next-generation sequencing, making use of paired-end transcriptome or whole-genome sequencing, have led to the discovery of a myriad of novel fusion transcripts in breast carcinomas and cancer cell lines, often several per sample (Stephens et al., 2009; Banerji et al., 2012; Robinson et al., 2011). However, these fusion transcripts are rarely found in more than single cases and often the fusion is found only at the mRNA and not at the genomic level, so their role in breast carcinogenesis remains unclear. When genomic rearrangements corresponding to the RNA changes are observed, they are more often intra- than interchromosomal (Stephens et al., 2009), and it has been suggested that many gene fusions in breast cancer in fact represent a by-product of chromosomal amplifications and therefore are passenger rearrangements and not driver oncogenic fusions (Kalyana-Sundaram et al., 2012).

Whereas balanced chromosome rearrangements seem uncommon in primary breast carcinomas, the analysis of more than 6000 tumors by CGH has confirmed the frequent occurrence of genomic imbalances (Cai et al., 2012, 2014). The most common copy number gains and amplifications in breast cancer occur in chromosome arms 1q, 8q, 8p, 11q, 16p, 17q, and 20q (www.progenetix.org; www.arraymap.org). Several of these genomic gains are the result of cytogenetic rearrangements previously identified by chromosome banding analysis (see previous text), whereas others may be masked by the complex karyotypic abnormalities seen in a proportion of breast carcinomas. Array-based CGH has helped pinpoint some of the relevant target genes amplified at these locations (Hyman et al., 2002; Albertson, 2003; Climent et al., 2007; Cai et al., 2012). *ERBB2*, thought to be the driver gene behind the 17q12 amplification found in 15–25% of breast cancers, encodes a tyrosine kinase receptor that is the target of trastuzumab (Slamon et al., 1987, 1989; Borg et al., 1991; Kallioniemi et al., 1992; Vogel et al., 2002). A more distal amplicon at 17q23 is detected in 10–15% of breast carcinomas and results in simultaneous upregulation of several genes (Bärlund et al., 2000; Monni et al., 2001; Pärssinen et al., 2007). On the other hand, the genes *CCND1* and *EMSY* are likely targets of the 11q13 amplification that occurs in 10–20% of breast cancers (Frierson et al., 1996; Hui et al., 1997; Ormandy et al., 2003), often together with amplification also of genes at 8p12 (which may or may not include the *FGFR1* gene; Bautista and

Theillet, 1998; Ugolini et al., 1999; Gelsi-Boyer et al., 2005). The *MYC* oncogene is a likely target of the 8q amplifications that occur in up to 20% of breast carcinomas (Escot et al., 1986; Garcia et al., 1989; Seshadri et al., 1989; Borg et al., 1992), although also other genes in this chromosome arm have been suggested to play a role in breast carcinogenesis (Nupponen et al., 1999; Tsuneizumi et al., 2001). Finally, 20q13 is amplified in 5–15% of breast carcinomas and the genes *AURKA* (alias *STK15*, *BTAK*) and *ZNF217* have been proposed as probable targets for this genomic imbalance (Sen et al., 1997; Collins et al., 1998; Nonet et al., 2001; Hodgson et al., 2003). On the other hand, combined array CGH and expression profiling of breast carcinomas showing 1q copy number gains have identified numerous candidate genes with coordinated overexpression as the result of copy number increase (Orsetti et al., 2006); it is evidently difficult to pinpoint any one single target gene affected by this usually whole-arm imbalance.

The most frequent chromosome losses detected by CGH in breast carcinomas take place at 8p, 11q, 13q, 16q, and 17p (www.progenetix.org; www. arraymap.org). Loss of heterozygosity (LOH) data for the most part corroborate this pattern of genomic loss (Devilee and Cornelisse, 1990; Larsson et al., 1990; Sato et al., 1990, 1991; Andersen et al., 1992), but this approach does not seem to have led to the identification of the target genes in most instances (Devilee et al., 2001). Although recent analyses with array-based CGH have pinpointed loci likely to harbor tumor suppressor genes (Naylor et al., 2005; Chin et al., 2006; van Beers and Nederlof, 2006; Climent et al., 2007; Cai et al., 2012), the relevant target genes of most recurrent genomic losses seen in breast carcinomas remain elusive. A possible exception is the *CDH1* gene in 16q22, which presents inactivating mutations in over 60% of infiltrating lobular carcinomas together with loss of the wild-type allele (Berx et al., 1995, 1996); this gene is also responsible for the association between hereditary diffuse gastric cancer and lobular breast cancer when mutated in the germline (Keller et al., 1999; Kaurah et al., 2007). However, the more common ductal carcinomas also show 16q loss (although less frequently) and do not have inactivating mutations of the second allele, indicating that there is another target gene in

this chromosome arm or that haploinsufficiency is operative in this tumor type (Cleton-Jansen, 2002; Roylance et al., 2003). As to the target of 17p loss, the *TP53* gene at 17p13 is mutated somatically in 20–30% of breast carcinomas (Coles et al., 1992; Olivier and Hainaut, 2001). Germline *TP53* mutations cause the dominantly inherited Li–Fraumeni syndrome that is associated with a markedly increased risk of developing many malignancies but in particular soft tissue sarcomas, brain tumors, osteosarcomas, leukemias, adrenocortical carcinomas, and carcinomas of the breast (Malkin et al., 1990; Srivastava et al., 1990; Olivier et al., 2003). Germline *TP53* mutations are rare in patients with hereditary breast cancer who do not have the Li–Fraumeni syndrome (Børresen et al., 1992; Lidereau and Soussi, 1992).

Contrary to the rare hereditary syndromes mentioned previously, a significant proportion of the hereditary predisposition to breast cancer is caused by germline mutations of the *BRCA1* (17q21) or *BRCA2* (13q12) genes (Miki et al., 1994; Wooster et al., 1995; Narod and Foulkes, 2004). The probability that a *BRCA1/2* mutation will be found in a kindred increases if the family history includes early age at diagnosis, clustering of breast and ovarian cancer (80% *BRCA1*), and male breast cancer (66% *BRCA2*) (Ford et al., 1998; Frank et al., 2002). Data on somatic mutations in hereditary breast carcinomas are sparse, but chromosomal and array CGH analyses indicate that the molecular cytogenetic pathways of *BRCA1* carcinomas are at least partially different from their *BRCA2*-positive and sporadic counterparts (Tirkkonen et al., 1997, 1999; Wessels et al., 2002; Jönsson et al., 2005; van Beers et al., 2005; Joosse et al., 2009, 2012). Other syndromes associated with predisposition to breast cancer are the Cowden syndrome caused by *PTEN* germline mutations, the Peutz–Jeghers syndrome caused by *STK11* germline mutations, and the Reifenstein syndrome caused by androgen receptor gene germline mutations (Wooster et al., 1992; Marsh et al., 1999; Eng, 2000; Narod and Foulkes, 2004; Thull and Vogel, 2004).

Clinicopathologic correlations

With the exception of the t(12;15)(p13;q25) in secretory breast carcinoma, the diagnostic information value of karyotypic data on breast tumors is reduced by the fact that the most common chromosome abnormalities are not exclusively associated with breast carcinoma in general or with a particular histopathologic subgroup. Although the overall pattern of genomic changes is rather characteristic, some of the chromosomal changes consistently found in breast carcinomas are sometimes detected also in other carcinomas and in benign breast proliferations (Lundin and Mertens, 1998; Teixeira et al., 2002). The histopathologic picture, complemented with immunohistochemistry analyses of estrogen and progesterone receptors and a combination of immunohistochemistry and FISH analyses to assess HER2 status, remains the main criterion for the diagnosis and classification of breast cancer, but genetic parameters are expected to provide us with better tools to predict the clinical course of this heterogeneous disease. Pandis et al. (1996) compared karyotypic and histopathologic parameters in a well-characterized series of 125 breast carcinomas. The modal number and the number of chromosome changes were significantly correlated with tumor grade, mitotic activity, and the patients' age. Near-triploid karyotypes were found only in ductal carcinomas and more often in grade III carcinomas, in tumors with high mitotic activity, and in the tumors of patients younger than 40 years. All lobular carcinomas were near-diploid and also papillary, tubular, and mucinous carcinomas tended to have relatively simple karyotypic changes (Pandis et al., 1996; Adeyinka et al., 1998). Medullary carcinomas, on the other hand, appeared to have karyotypes as complex as those found in the more common ductal carcinomas. Unbalanced structural chromosomal changes were positively associated with ductal type carcinomas, with high mitotic activity, and with an infiltrating growth pattern. Cytogenetic polyclonality was more common in infiltrating than in situ carcinomas and in grade II and III than in grade I tumors. Finally, the correlation between modal chromosome number and mitotic activity in vivo and between cytogenetic polyclonality and tumor grade turned out to be statistically significant even in multivariate models (Pandis et al., 1996). Subsequently, Steinarsdottir et al. (2011) showed that polyclonality was significantly associated with poor breast cancer-specific survival independently of tumor size, lymph node metastases, and hormone receptor status.

Informative cytogenetic–pathologic correlations have also been obtained in CGH-based studies. For instance, the higher the mitotic index in vivo, the higher the number of genetic imbalances detected in breast carcinomas (Teixeira et al., 2001; Kleivi et al., 2002), and a nonrandom association between genetic complexity and histologic tumor type is also apparent (Nishizaki et al., 1997a; Tirkkonen et al., 1998; Roylance et al., 1999; Günther et al., 2001). An example of the possible clinical relevance of karyotype complexity is phyllodes tumors of the breast. Benign phyllodes tumors are karyotypically simple whereas malignant phyllodes tumors have complex chromosome abnormalities (Dietrich et al., 1997). As grading individual phyllodes tumors based on their histopathologic features alone can be difficult, the cytogenetic pattern of these tumors may be used to classify them correctly. For breast carcinomas, both chromosome banding (Steinarsdottir et al., 1995) and CGH (Isola et al., 1995; Dellas et al., 2002) data show that patients whose tumors have a higher number of karyotypic abnormalities have significantly lower recurrence-free and overall survival rates.

Preliminary findings indicate that informative correlations may exist also for particular genomic changes. Chromosome banding studies show that different patterns of chromosomal imbalances characterize metastasizing and nonmetastasizing primary breast carcinomas (Adeyinka et al., 1999a), with loss of chromosome 18 being significantly more common in the former and loss of 6q10–21 and 16q in the latter. Patients considered to have a poor prognosis by conventional parameters (e.g., young age, high histologic tumor grade, metastatic disease, and loss of hormonal receptors) more often have hsr in their tumor karyotype (Zafrani et al., 1992), and this cytogenetic feature was also shown to be associated with shorter overall survival (Bernardino et al., 1998). Chromosomal CGH analyses of unselected series of breast carcinomas also indicate that loss of 16q is associated with good prognosis, whereas gains of 11q, 17q, and 20q are associated with poor clinical outcome (Aubele et al., 2002; Hislop et al., 2002; Zudaire et al., 2002). In the particular group of node-negative breast cancer, in addition to gains of 11q, 17q, and 20q, also gain of 3q and 8q and loss of 18q are associated with aggressive clinical behavior (Isola et al., 1995; Hermsen et al., 1998; Dellas et al., 2002; Janssen et al., 2003). Finally, Rennstam et al. (2003) identified three distinct patterns of copy number changes with independent prognostic value: one group characterized by 1q and 16p gains and 16q loss with good prognosis; a second group showing 11q, 20q, and 17q gains and 13q loss with intermediate prognosis; and a third group defined by 8p loss and 8q gain having the worst prognosis. The five-year survival rates varied from 96% in the first group to 56% in the last group, and the prognostic value of the genomic data was independent of node status and tumor size in multivariate analysis.

The genetic heterogeneity underlying the clinical variability of breast cancer has been recognized also at the transcriptional level, with the subclassification into luminal (A and B), basal-like, HER2-positive, and normal-like tumor subtypes (Perou et al., 2000; Sørlie et al., 2001; van de Vijver et al., 2002; van't Veer et al., 2002). Array-based CGH analysis demonstrated that distinct spectra of copy number changes underlie the different subtypes of breast cancer defined by expression profiling (Pollack et al., 2002; Bergamaschi et al., 2006). Whereas the basal-like subtype was associated with higher numbers of genomic gains/losses, the luminal B subset often presented high-level DNA amplification, further indicating that distinct genetic pathways and genomic instability mechanisms are pathogenetically central features (Bergamaschi et al., 2006). Recent exome sequencing data showed that the rate of point mutations in the six most commonly mutated genes in breast cancer (*TP53*, *PIK3CA*, *GATA3*, *MAP3K1*, *MLL3*, and *CDH1*) also differs among the various molecular subtypes: whereas *TP53* mutations are much more common in the basal-like and HER2-positive subgroups, *GATA3* mutations are more common in luminal A and B tumors, *MAP3K1* and *CDH1* mutations in luminal A tumors, and *PIK3CA* mutations in luminal A and B and HER2-positive but not in basal-like tumors (Banerji et al., 2012; Cancer Genome Atlas Network, 2012; Curtis et al., 2012; Ellis et al., 2012; Shah et al., 2012; Stephens et al., 2012; Baird and Caldas, 2013). A new genomic classification of breast cancer into 10 subgroups has been proposed based on integrative genome and transcriptome landscapes, each showing distinct clinical outcomes (Curtis et al., 2012;

Dawson et al., 2013). Besides allowing a molecular subtyping of breast cancer in unprecedented detail, next-generation sequencing analyses of multiple tumor samples and single cells confirm earlier data (discussed previously) as to striking intratumor genetic heterogeneity with clonal divergence between primary and metastatic lesions (Shah et al., 2009, 2012; Ding et al., 2010; Navin et al., 2011; Nik-Zainal et al., 2012a, 2012b).

Summary

Both complex and simple karyotypic changes have been found in carcinomas of the breast. With the exception of the t(12;15)(p13;q25) leading to the *ETV6–NTRK3* fusion gene that characterizes secretory carcinomas and the t(6;9)(q21–25;p13–p24) associated with the *MYB–NFIB* chimeric gene associated with adenoid cystic carcinomas, the recurrent chromosome abnormalities most commonly seen in other breast carcinomas are unbalanced. The most common structural cytogenetic changes are der(1;16)(q10;p10) and i(1)(q10), both of which result in gain of 1q material, and del(3)(p12–13p14–21). Other less frequent structural karyotypic changes are deletions of 1q and 6q, as well as chromosome 8 rearrangements that often combine gain/amplification of 8q, amplification at 8p11–12, a break in 8p12–21, and loss of 8p21-pter. The most common numerical aberrations have been trisomy for chromosomes 7, 8, 12, 18, and 20. The frequent finding of cytogenetically unrelated clones has raised the question whether some carcinomas of the breast have a polyclonal origin. CGH investigations have shown that the most common copy number gains and amplifications in breast cancer occur in chromosome arms 1q, 8q, 8p, 11q, 16p, 17q, and 20q, whereas the most recurrent losses take place at 8p, 11q, 13q, 16q, and 17p. Some of these chromosome rearrangements have also been detected in a few benign or premalignant breast lesions, indicating that they are early events in breast tumorigenesis.

Although many of the relevant target genes of the recurrent genomic imbalances remain elusive, the oncogenes *ERBB2*, *CCND1*, *EMSY*, *FGFR1*, *MYC*, *AURKA*, and *ZNF217* have been shown to be overexpressed as a result of copy number gains in breast carcinomas. Exome sequencing showed that the genes with most frequent point mutations are *TP53, PIK3CA, GATA3, MAP3K1, MLL3,* and *CDH1*, the first and the last playing a role in breast carcinogenesis both somatically and when inherited in the germline. Recent high-throughput, integrated genomic and transcriptomic analyses allow detailed molecular subtyping of breast cancer, promising to improve prediction of the clinical course of this heterogeneous disease as well as detecting keys to personalized, biologically targeted therapies.

Acknowledgment

Financial support from the Norwegian Cancer Society, the Portuguese Cancer Society (LPCC), and the Portuguese Science and Technology Foundation (FCT) is gratefully acknowledged.

References

Adelaide J, Huang HE, Murati A, Alsop AE, Orsetti B, Mozziconacci MJ, et al. (2003): A recurrent chromosome translocation breakpoint in breast and pancreatic cancer cell lines targets the neuregulin/NRG1 gene. *Genes Chromosomes Cancer* 37:333–345.

Adeyinka A, Pandis N, Bardi G, Bonaldi L, Mertens F, Mitelman F, et al. (1997): A subgroup of breast carcinomas is cytogenetically characterized by trisomy 12. *Cancer Genet Cytogenet* 97:119–121.

Adeyinka A, Mertens F, Idvall I, Bondeson L, Ingvar C, Heim S, et al. (1998): Cytogenetic findings in invasive breast carcinomas with prognostically favourable histology: a less complex karyotypic pattern? *Int J Cancer* 79:361–364.

Adeyinka A, Mertens F, Idvall I, Bondeson L, Ingvar C, Mitelman F, et al. (1999a): Different patterns of chromosomal imbalances in metastasising and non-metastasising primary breast carcinomas. *Int J Cancer* 84:370–375.

Adeyinka A, Mertens F, Idvall I, Bondeson L, Pandis N (1999b): Multiple polysomies in breast carcinomas: preferential gain of chromosomes 1, 5, 6, 7, 12, 16, 17, 18, and 19.*Cancer Genet Cytogenet* 111:144–148.

Adeyinka A, Mertens F, Bondeson L, Garne JP, Borg A, Baldetorp B, et al. (2000a): Cytogenetic heterogeneity and clonal evolution in synchronous bilateral breast carcinomas and their lymph node metastases from a male patient without any detectable BRCA2 germline mutation. *Cancer Genet Cytogenet* 118:42–47.

Adeyinka A, Kytola S, Mertens F, Pandis N, Larsson C (2000b): Spectral karyotyping and chromosome banding studies of primary breast carcinomas and their lymph node metastases. *Int J Mol Med* 5:235–240.

Albertson DG (2003): Profiling breast cancer by array CGH. *Breast Cancer Res Treat* 78:289–298.

Andersen TI, Gaustad A, Ottestad L, Farrants GW, Nesland JM, Tveit KM, et al. (1992): Genetic alterations of the tumour suppressor gene regions 3p, 11p, 13q, 17p, and 17q in human breast carcinomas. *Genes Chromosomes Cancer* 4:113–121.

Aubele M, Cummings M, Walsch A, Zitzelsberger H, Nährig J, Höfler H, et al. (2000a): Heterogeneous chromosomal aberrations in intraductal breast lesions adjacent to invasive carcinoma. *Anal Cell Pathol* 20:17–24.

Aubele MM, Cummings MC, Mattis AE, Zitzelsberger HF, Walch AK, Kremer M, et al. (2000b): Accumulation of chromosomal imbalances from intraductal proliferative lesions to adjacent in situ and invasive ductal breast cancer. *Diagn Mol Pathol* 9:14–19.

Aubele M, Mattis A, Zitzelsberger H, Walch A, Kremer M, Welzl G, et al. (2000c): Extensive ductal carcinoma in situ with small foci of invasive ductal carcinoma: evidence of genetic resemblance by CGH. *Int J Cancer* 85:82–86.

Aubele M, Auer G, Braselmann H, Nährig J, Zitzelsberger H, Quintanilla-Martinez L, et al. (2002): Chromosomal imbalances are associated with metastasis-free survival in breast cancer patients. *Anal Cell Pathol* 24:77–87.

Baird RD, Caldas C (2013): Genetic heterogeneity in breast cancer: the road to personalized medicine? *BMC Med* 11:151.

Banerji S, Cibulskis K, Rangel-Escareno C, Brown KK, Carter SL, Frederick AM, et al. (2012): Sequence analysis of mutations and translocations across breast cancer subtypes. *Nature* 486: 405–409.

Barbosa ML, Ribeiro EM, Silva GF, Maciel ME, Lima RS, Cavalli LR, et al. (2004): Cytogenetic findings in phyllodes tumor and fibroadenomas of the breast. *Cancer Genet Cytogenet* 154:156–159.

Bärlund M, Monni O, Kononen J, Cornelison R, Torhorst J, Sauter G, et al. (2000): Multiple genes at 17q23 undergo amplification and overexpression in breast cancer. *Cancer Res* 60:5340–5344.

Bärlund M, Monni O, Weaver JD, Kauraniemi P, Sauter G, Heiskanen M, et al. (2002): Cloning of BCAS3 (17q23) and BCAS4 (20q13) genes that undergo amplification, overexpression, and fusion in breast cancer. *Genes Chromosomes Cancer* 35:311–317.

Bautista S, Theillet C (1998): CCND1 and FGFR1 coamplification results in the colocalization of 11q13 and 8p12 sequences in breast tumor nuclei. *Genes Chromosomes Cancer* 22:268–277.

Bello MJ, Rey JA (1989): Cytogenetic analysis of metastatic effusions from breast tumors. *Neoplasma* 35:71–81.

Bergamaschi A, Kim YH, Wang P, Sørlie T, Hernandez-Boussard T, Lonning PE, et al. (2006): Distinct patterns of DNA copy number alteration are associated with different clinicopathological features and gene-expression subtypes of breast cancer. *Genes Chromosomes Cancer* 45: 1033–1040.

Bernardino J, Apiou F, Gerbault-Seureau M, Malfoy B, Dutrillaux B (1998): Characterization of recurrent homogeneously staining regions in 72 breast carcinomas. *Genes Chromosomes Cancer* 23:100–108.

Berx G, Cleton-Jansen AM, Nollet F, de Leeuw WJ, van de Vijver M, Cornelisse C, et al. (1995): E-cadherin is a tumour/invasion suppressor gene mutated in human lobular breast cancers. *EMBO J* 14:6107–6115.

Berx G, Cleton-Jansen AM, Strumane K, de Leeuw WJ, Nollet F, van Roy F, et al. (1996): E-cadherin is inactivated in a majority of invasive human lobular breast cancers by truncation mutations throughout its extracellular domain. *Oncogene* 13:1919–1925.

Birdsall SH, MacLennan KA, Gusterson BA (1992): t(6;12)(q23;q13) and t(10;16)(q22;p11) in a phyllodes tumor of breast. *Cancer Genet Cytogenet* 60: 74–77.

Birdsall SH, Summersgill BM, Egan M, Fentiman IS, Gusterson BA, et al. (1995): Additional copies of 1q in sequential samples from a phyllodes tumor of the breast. *Cancer Genet Cytogenet* 83:111–114.

Borg Å, Baldetorp B, Fernö M, Killander D, Olsson H, Sigurdsson H (1991): ERBB2 amplification in breast cancer with a high rate of proliferation. *Oncogene* 6:137–143.

Borg Å, Baldetorp B, Fernö M, Olsson H, Sigurdsson H (1992): c-myc Amplification is an independent prognostic factor in postmenopausal breast cancer. *Int J Cancer* 51:687–691.

Børresen A-L, Ikdahl Andersen T, Garber J, Barbier-Piraux N, Thorlacius S, Eyfjord J, et al. (1992): Screening for germ line p53 mutations in breast cancer patients. *Cancer Res* 52:3234–3236.

Brommesson S, Jonsson G, Strand C, Grabau D, Malmstrom P, Ringner M, et al. (2008): Tiling array-CGH for the assessment of genomic similarities among synchronous unilateral and bilateral invasive breast cancer tumor pairs. *BMC Clin Pathol* 8: 6.

Buerger H, Otterbach F, Simon R, Poremba C, Diallo R, Decker T, et al. (1999): Comparative genomic hybridization of ductal carcinoma *in situ* of the breast-evidence of multiple genetic pathways. *J Pathol* 187:396–402.

Buerger H, Simon R, Schäfer KL, Diallo R, Littmann R, Poremba C, et al. (2000): Genetic relation of lobular carcinoma in situ, ductal carcinoma in situ, and associated invasive carcinoma of the breast. *Mol Pathol* 53:118–121.

Bullerdiek J, Leuschner E, Taquia E, Bonk U, Bartnizke S (1993): Trisomy 8 as a recurrent clonal abnormality in breast cancer? *Cancer Genet Cytogenet* 65:64–67.

Burbano RR, Medeiros A, de Amorim MI, Lima EM, Mello A, Neto JB, et al. (2000): Cytogenetics of epithelial hyperplasias of the human breast. *Cancer Genet Cytogenet* 119:62–66.

Cai H, Kumar N, Baudis M (2012): ArrayMap: a reference resource for genomic copy number imbalances in human malignancies. *PLoS One* 7: e36944.

Cai H, Kumar N, Ai N, Gupta S, Rath P, Baudis M (2014): Progenetix: 12 years of oncogenomic data curation. *Nucl Acids Res* 42: D1055–1062.

Calabrese G, Di Virgilio C, Cianchetti E, Guanciali FP, Stuppia L, Parruti G, et al. (1991): Chromosome abnormalities in breast fibroadenomas. *Genes Chromosomes Cancer* 3:202–204.

Cancer Genome Atlas Network (2012): Comprehensive molecular portraits of human breast tumours. *Nature* 490: 61–70.

Carpenter R, Gibbs N, Matthews J, Cooke T (1987): Importance of cellular DNA content in premalignant breast disease and pre-invasive carcinoma of the female breast. *Br J Surg* 74:905–906.

Cavalli LR, Cavalieri LM, Ribeiro LA, Cavalli IJ, Silveira R, Rogatto SR (1997): Cytogenetic evaluation of 20 primary breast carcinomas. *Hereditas* 126:261–268.

Chin K, De Vries S, Fridlyand J, Spellman PT, Roydasgupta R, Kuo WL, et al. (2006): Genomic and transcriptional aberrations linked to breast cancer pathophysiologies. *Cancer Cell* 10:529–541.

Cleton-Jansen AM (2002): E-cadherin and loss of heterozygosity at chromosome 16 in breast carcinogenesis: different genetic pathways in ductal and lobular breast cancer? *Breast Cancer Res* 4:5–8.

Climent J, Garcia JL, Mao JH, Arsuaga J, Perez-Losada J (2007): Characterization of breast cancer by array comparative genomic hybridization. *Biochem Cell Biol* 85: 497–508.

Coles C, Condie A, Chetty U, Steel CM, Evans J, Prosser J (1992): p53 mutations in breast cancer. *Cancer Res* 52:5291–5298.

Collins C, Rommens JM, Kowbel D, Godfrey T, Tanner M, Hwang SI, et al. (1998): Positional cloning of ZNF217 and NABC1: genes amplified at 20q13.2 and overexpressed in breast carcinoma. *Proc Natl Acad Sci USA* 95:8703–8708.

Curtis C, Shah SP, Chin SF, Turashvili G, Rueda OM, Dunning MJ, et al. (2012): The genomic and transcriptomic architecture of 2,000 breast tumours reveals novel subgroups. *Nature* 486: 346–352.

Dal Cin P, Moreman P, De Wever I, Van den Berghe H (1995): Is i(1)(q10) a chromosome marker in phyllodes tumor of the breast? *Cancer Genet Cytogenet* 83:174–175.

Dal Cin P, Wanschura S, Christiaens MR, Van den Berghe I, Moerman P, Polito P, et al. (1997): Hamartoma of the breast with involvement of 6p21 and rearrangement of HMGIY. *Genes Chromosomes Cancer* 20:90–92.

Dal Cin P, Pauwels P, Moerman P, Qi H, Van den Berghe H (1998): Hyperdiploidy in benign breast lesions. *Cancer Genet Cytogenet* 101:162–163.

Dawson SJ, Rueda OM, Aparicio S, Caldas C (2013): A new genome-driven integrated classification of breast cancer and its implications. *EMBO J* 32: 617–628.

De Santis C, Ma J, Bryan L, Jemal A (2014): Breast cancer statistics, 2013. *CA: Cancer J Clin* 64: 52–62.

Dellas A, Torhorst J, Schultheiss E, Mihatsch MJ, Moch H (2002): DNA sequence losses on chromosomes 11p and 18q are associated with clinical outcome in lymph node-negative ductal breast cancer. *Clin Cancer Res* 8:1210–1216.

Devilee P, Cornelisse CJ (1990): Genetics of human breast cancer. *Cancer Surv* 9: 605–630.

Devilee P, Cleton-Jansen AM, Cornelisse CJ (2001): Ever since Knudson. *Trends Genet* 17: 569–573.

Diallo R, Schaefer KL, Poremba C, Shivazi N, Willmann V, Buerger H, et al. (2001): Monoclonality in normal epithelium and in hyperplastic and neoplastic lesions of the breast. *J Pathol* 193:27–32.

Diallo R, Tognon C, Knezevich SR, Sorensen P, Poremba C (2003): Secretory carcinoma of the breast: a genetically defined carcinoma entity. *Verh Dtsch Ges Pathol* 87: 193–203.

Dietrich CU, Pandis N, Andersen JA, Heim S (1994): Chromosome abnormalities in adenolipomas of the breast: karyotypic evidence that the mesenchymal component constitutes the neoplastic parenchyma. *Cancer Genet Cytogenet* 72: 146–150.

Dietrich CU, Pandis N, Teixeira MR, Bardi G, Gerdes AM, Andersen JA, et al. (1995): Chromosome abnormalities in benign hyperproliferative disorders of epithelial and stromal breast tissue. *Int J Cancer* 60:49–53.

Dietrich CU, Pandis N, Rizou H, Petersson C, Bardi G, Qvist H, et al. (1997): Cytogenetic findings in phyllodes tumors of the breast: karyotypic complexity differentiates between malignant and benign tumors. *Hum Pathol* 28:1379–1382.

Dietrich CU, Pandis N, Bardi G, Teixeira MR, Soukhikh T, Petersson C, et al. (2004): Karyotypic changes in phyllodes tumors of the breast. *Cancer Genet Cytogenet* 78:200–206.

Ding L, Ellis MJ, Li S, Larson DE, Chen K, Wallis JW, et al. (2010): Genome remodelling in a basal-like breast cancer metastasis and xenograft. *Nature* 464: 999–1005.

Dressler LG, Seamer LC, Owens MA, Clark GM, McGuire WL (1988): DNA flow cytometry and prognostic factors in 1331 frozen breast cancer specimens. *Cancer* 61:420–427.

Dutrillaux B, Gerbault-Seureau M, Zafrani B (1990): Characterization of chromosomal anomalies in human breast cancer. A comparison of 30 paradiploid cases with few chromosome changes. *Cancer Genet Cytogenet* 49:203–217.

Dutrillaux B, Gerbault-Seureau M, Saint-Ruf C, Prieur M, Muleris M, Bardot V (1993): Cytogenetic characterization of colorectal and breast carcinomas. In: Kirsch IR, editor. *The Causes and Consequences of Chromosomal Aberrations.* Boca Raton, FL: CRC Press, Inc., pp. 447–467.

Ellis MJ, Ding L, Shen D, Luo J, Suman VJ, Wallis JW, et al. (2012): Whole-genome analysis informs breast cancer response to aromatase inhibition. *Nature* 486: 353–360.

Eng C (2000): Will the real Cowden syndrome please stand up: revised diagnostic criteria. *J Med Genet* 37:828–830.

Escot C, Theillet C, Lidereau R, Spyratos F, Champeme M-H, Gest J, et al. (1986): Genetic alteration of the c-myc proto-oncogene (MYC) in human primary breast carcinomas. *Proc Natl Acad Sci USA* 83:4834–4838.

Fletcher JA, Pinkus GS, Weidner N, Morton CC (1991): Lineage-restricted clonality in biphasic solid tumors. *Am J Pathol* 138:1199–1207.

Ford D, Easton DF, Stratton M, Narod S, Goldgar D, Devilee P, et al. (1998): Genetic heterogeneity and penetrance analysis of the BRCA1 and BRCA2 genes in breast cancer families. *Am J Hum Genet* 62:676–689.

Frank TS, Deffenbaugh AM, Reid JE, Hulick M, Ward BE, Lingenfelter B, et al. (2002): Clinical characteristics of individuals with germline mutations in BRCA1 and BRCA2: analysis of 10, 000 individuals. *J Clin Oncol* 20:1480–1490.

Frierson HF Jr, Gaffey MJ, Zukerberg LR, Arnold A, Williams ME (1996): Immunohistochemical detection and gene amplification of cyclin D1 in mammary infiltrating ductal carcinoma. *Mod Pathol* 9:725–730.

Garcia I, Dietrich P-Y, Aapro M, Vauthier G, Vadas L, Engel E (1989): Genetic alterations of c-myc, c-erbB-2, and c-Ha-ras protooncogenes and clinical associations in human breast carcinomas. *Cancer Res* 49:6675–6679.

Gatalica Z, Velagaleti G, Kuivaniemi H, Tromp G, Palazzo J, Graves KM, et al. (2005): Gene expression profile of an adenomyoepithelioma of the breast with a reciprocal translocation involving chromosomes 8 and 16. *Cancer Genet Cytogenet* 156: 14–22.

Gebhart E, Brüderlein S, Augustus M, Siebert E, Feldner J, Schmidt W (1986): Cytogenetic studies on human breast carcinomas. *Breast Cancer Res Treat* 8: 125–138.

Gelsi-Boyer V, Orsetti B, Cervera N, Finetti P, Sircoulomb F, Rougé C, et al. (2005): Comprehensive profiling of 8p11-12 amplification in breast cancer. *Mol Cancer Res* 3:655–667.

Gioanni J, Le Francois D, Zanghellini E, Mazeau C, Ettore F, Lambert J-C, et al. (1990): Establishment and characterization of a new tumorigenic cell line with a normal karyotype derived from a human breast adenocarcinoma. *Br J Cancer* 62:8–13.

Going JJ (2003): Epithelial carcinogenesis: challenging monoclonality. *J Pathol* 200: 1–3.

Going JJ, Abd El-Monem HM, Craft JA (2001): Clonal origins of human breast cancer. *J Pathol* 194:406–412.

Guan XY, Meltzer PS, Dalton WS, Trent JM (1994): Identification of cryptic sites of DNA sequence amplification in human breast cancer by chromosome microdissection. *Nat Genet* 8:155–161.

Günther K, Merkelbach-Bruse S, Amo-Takyi BK, Handt S, Schröder W, Tietze L (2001): Differences in genetic alterations between primary lobular and ductal breast cancers detected by comparative genomic hybridization. *J Pathol* 193:40–47.

Hahn Y, Bera TK, Gehlhaus K, Kirsch IR, Pastan IH, Lee B (2004): Finding fusion genes resulting from chromosome rearrangement by analyzing the expressed sequence databases. *Proc Natl Acad Sci USA* 101:13257–13261.

Hainsworth PJ, Garson OM (1990): Breast cancer cytogenetics and beyond. *Aust NZ J Surg* 60:327–336.

Hainsworth PJ, Raphael KL, Stillwell RG, Bennett RC, Garson OM (1991): Cytogenetic features of twenty-six primary breast cancers. *Cancer Genet Cytogenet* 52:205–218.

Heim S, Teixeira MR, Dietrich CU, Pandis N (1997): Cytogenetic polyclonality in tumors of the breast. *Cancer Genet Cytogenet* 95:16–19.

Hermsen MA, Baak JP, Meijer GA, Weiss JM, Walboomers JW, Snijders PJ, et al. (1998): Genetic analysis of 53 lymph node-negative breast carcinomas by CGH and relation to clinical, pathological, morphometric, and DNA cytometric prognostic factors. *J Pathol* 186:356–362.

Hernandez L, Wilkerson PM, Lambros MB, Campion-Flora A, Rodrigues DN, Gauthier A, et al. (2012): Genomic and mutational profiling of ductal carcinomas in situ and matched adjacent invasive breast cancers reveals intra-tumour genetic heterogeneity and clonal selection. *J Pathol* 227: 42–52.

Hislop RG, Pratt N, Stocks SC, Steel CM, Sales M, Goudie D, et al. (2002): Karyotypic aberrations of chromosomes 16 and 17 are related to survival in patients with breast cancer. *Br J Surg* 89:1581–1586.

Hodgson JG, Chin K, Collins C, Gray JW (2003): Genome amplification of chromosome 20 in breast cancer. *Breast Cancer Res Treat* 78:337–345.

Huang HE, Chin SF, Ginestier C, Bardou VJ, Adelaide J, Iyer NG, et al. (2004): A recurrent chromosome breakpoint in breast cancer at the NRG1/neuregulin 1/heregulin gene. *Cancer Res* 64:6840–6844.

Hui R, Campbell DH, Lee CS, McCaul K, Horsfall DJ, Musgrove EA, et al. (1997): EMS1 amplification can occur independently of CCND1 or INT-2 amplification at 11q13 and may identify different phenotypes in primary breast cancer. *Oncogene* 15:1617–1623.

Hultén MA, Hill SM, Rodgers CS (1993): Chromosomes 1 and 16 in sporadic breast cancer. *Genes Chromosomes Cancer* 8:204.

Hyman E, Kauraniemi P, Hautaniemi S, Wolf M, Mousses S, Rozenblum E, et al. (2002): Impact of DNA amplification on gene expression patterns in breast cancer. *Cancer Res* 62:6240–6245.

Isola JJ, Kallioniemi OP, Chu LW, Fuqua SA, Hilsenbeck SG, Osborne CK, et al. (1995): Genetic aberrations detected by comparative genomic hybridization predict outcome in node-negative breast cancer. *Am J Pathol* 147:905–911.

Janssen EA, Baak JP, Guervós MA, van Diest PJ, Jiwa M, Hermsen MA (2003): In lymph node-negative invasive breast carcinomas, specific chromosomal aberrations are strongly associated with high mitotic activity and predict outcome more accurately than grade, tumour diameter, and oestrogen receptor. *J Pathol* 201: 555–561.

Johansson B, Heim S, Mandahl N, Mertens F, Mitelman F (1993): Trisomy 7 in nonneoplastic cells. *Genes Chromosomes Cancer* 6:199–205.

Jönsson G, Naylor TL, Vallon-Christersson J, Staaf J, Huang J, Ward MR, et al. (2005): Distinct genomic profiles in hereditary breast tumors identified by array-based comparative genomic hybridization. *Cancer Res* 65:7612–7621.

Joosse SA, van Beers EH, Tielen IH, Horlings H, Peterse JL, Hoogerbrugge N, et al. (2009): Prediction of BRCA1-association in hereditary non-BRCA1/2 breast carcinomas with array-CGH. *Breast Cancer Res Treat* 116: 479–489.

Joosse SA, Brandwijk KI, Devilee P, Wesseling J, Hogervorst FB, Verhoef S, et al. (2012): Prediction of BRCA2-association in hereditary breast carcinomas using array-CGH. *Breast Cancer Res Treat* 132: 379–389.

Kallioniemi OP, Kallioniemi A, Kurisu W, Thor A, Chen LC, Smith HS, et al. (1992): ERBB2 amplification in breast cancer analyzed by fluorescence *in situ* hybridization. *Proc Natl Acad Sci USA* 89:5321–5325.

Kalyana-Sundaram S, Shankar S, Deroo S, Iyer MK, Palanisamy N, Chinnaiyan AM, et al. (2012): Gene fusions associated with recurrent amplicons represent a class of passenger aberrations in breast cancer. *Neoplasia* 14: 702–708.

Kaurah P, MacMillan A, Boyd N, Senz J, DeLuca A, Chun N, et al. (2007): Founder and recurrent CDH1 mutations in families with hereditary diffuse gastric cancer. *JAMA* 297:2360–2372.

Kazakov DV, Vanecek T, Belousova IE, Mukensnabl P, Kollertova D, Michal M (2007): Skin-type hidradenoma of the breast parenchyma with t(11;19) translocation: hidradenoma of the breast. *Am J Dermatopathol* 29: 457–461.

Keller G, Vogelsang H, Becker I, Hutter J, Ott K, Candidus S, et al. (1999): Diffuse type gastric and lobular breast carcinoma in a familial gastric cancer patient with an E-cadherin germline mutation. *Am J Pathol* 155:337–342.

Kleivi K, Lothe RA, Heim S, Tsarouha H, Kraggerud SM, Pandis N, et al. (2002): Genome profiling of breast cancer cells selected against in vitro shows copy number changes. *Genes Chromosomes Cancer* 33:304–309.

Knoedler D, Susnik B, Gonyo MB, Osipov V (2007): Giant apocrine hidradenoma of the breast. *Breast J* 13: 91–93.

Kokalj-Vokac N, Alemeida A, Gerbault-Seureau M, Malfoy B, Dutrillaux B (1993): Two-color FISH characterization of i(1q) and der(1;16) in human breast cancer cells. *Genes Chromosomes Cancer* 7:8–14.

Kuijper A, Buerger H, Simon R, Schaefer KL, Croonen A, Boecker W, et al. (2002): Analysis of the progression of fibroepithelial tumours of the breast by PCR-based clonality assay. *J Pathol* 197: 575–581.

Kuukasjarvi T, Karhu R, Tanner M, Kahkonen M, Schaffer A, Nupponen N, et al. (1997a): Genetic heterogeneity and clonal evolution underlying development of asynchronous metastasis in human breast cancer. *Cancer Res* 57:1597–1604.

Kuukasjarvi T, Tanner M, Pennanen S, Karhu R, Kallioniemi OP, Isola J (1997b): Genetic changes in intraductal breast cancer detected by comparative genomic hybridization. *Am J Pathol* 150:1465–1471.

Ladesich J, Damjanov I, Persons D, Jewell W, Arthur T, Rogana J, et al. (2002): Complex karyotype in a low grade phyllodes tumor of the breast. *Cancer Genet Cytogenet* 132:149–151.

Larsson C, Byström C, Skoog L, Rotstein S, Nordenskjöld M (1990): Genomic alterations in human breast carcinomas. *Genes Chromosomes Cancer* 2:191–197.

Levack PA, Mullen P, Anderson TJ, Miller WR, Forrest APM (1987): DNA analysis of breast tumour fine needle aspirates using flow cytometry. *Br J Cancer* 56:643–646.

Lidereau R, Soussi T (1992): Absence of p53 germ-line mutations in bilateral breast cancer patients. *Hum Genet* 89:250–252.

Liu X, Baker E, Eyre HJ, Sutherland GR, Zhou M (1999): Gamma-heregulin: a fusion gene of DOC-4 and neuregulin-1 derived from a chromosome translocation. *Oncogene* 18:7110–7114.

Lu Y-J, Xiao S, Yan Y-S, Fu S-B, Liu Q-Z, Li P (1993): Direct chromosome analysis of 50 primary breast carcinomas. *Cancer Genet Cytogenet* 69:91–99.

Lundin C, Mertens F (1998): Cytogenetics of benign breast lesions. *Breast Cancer Res Treat* 51:1–15.

Lundin CP, Mertens F, Ingvar C, Idvall I, Pandis N (1998a): Trisomy 16 as the primary chromosome aberration in a papilloma of the breast. *Cancer Genet Cytogenet* 106:90–91.

Lundin CP, Mertens F, Rizou H, Idvall I, Georgiou G, Ingvar C, et al. (1998b): Cytogenetic changes in benign proliferative and nonproliferative lesions of the breast. *Cancer Genet Cytogenet* 107:118–120.

Makretsov N, He M, Hayes M, Chia S, Horsman DE, et al. (2004): A fluorescence in situ hybridization study of ETV6-NTRK3 fusion gene in secretory breast carcinoma. *Genes Chromosomes Cancer* 40:152–157.

Malkin D, Li FP, Strong LC, Fraumeni JF Jr, Nelson CE, Kim DH, et al. (1990): Germ line p53 mutations in a familial syndrome of breast cancer, sarcomas, and other neoplasms. *Science* 250: 1233–1238.

Marsh DJ, Kum JB, Lunetta KL, Bennett MJ, Gorlin RJ, Ahmed SF, et al. (1999): TEN mutation spectrum and genotype-phenotype correlations in Bannayan–Riley–Ruvalcaba syndrome suggest a single entity with Cowden syndrome. *Hum Mol Genet* 8: 1461–1472.

McPherson K, Steel CM, Dixon JM (2000): ABC of breast diseases. Breast cancer-epidemiology, risk factors, and genetics. *BMJ* 321:624–628.

Micale MA, Visscher DW, Gulino SE, Wolman SR (1994): Chromosomal aneuploidy in proliferative breast disease. *Hum Pathol* 25:29–35.

Miki Y, Swensen J, Shattuck-Eidens D, Futreal PA, Harshman K, Tavtigian S, et al. (1994): A strong candidate for the breast and ovarian cancer susceptibility gene BRCA1. *Science* 266:66–71.

Mitchell ELD, Santibanez-Koref MF (1990): 1p13 is the most frequently involved band in structural chromosomal rearrangements in human breast cancer. *Genes Chromosomes Cancer* 2:278–289.

Mitelman F, Johansson B, Mertens F, editors (2014): Mitelman Database of Chromosome Aberrations and Gene Fusions in Cancer, http://cgap.nci.nih.gov/Chromosomes/Mitelman (accessed February 3, 2015).

Molist R, Gerbault-Seureau M, Sastre-Garau X, Sigal-Zafrani B, Dutrillaux B, Muleris M (2005): Ductal breast carcinoma develops through different patterns of chromosomal evolution. *Genes Chromosomes Cancer* 43:147–154.

Monni O, Barlund M, Mousses S, Kononen J, Sauter G, Heiskanen M, et al. (2001): Comprehensive copy number and gene expression profiling of the 17q23 amplicon in human breast cancer. *Proc Natl Acad Sci USA* 98:5711–5716.

Muleris M, Almeida A, Gerbault-Seureau M, Malfoy B, Dutrillaux B (1994): Detection of DNA amplification in 17 primary breast carcinomas with homogeneously staining regions by a modified comparative genomic hybridization technique. *Genes Chromosomes Cancer* 10:160–170.

Muleris M, Almeida A, Gerbault-Seureau M, Malfoy B, Dutrillaux B (1995): Identification of amplified DNA sequences in breast cancer and their organization within homogeneously staining regions. *Genes Chromosomes Cancer* 14:155–163.

Narod SA, Foulkes WD (2004): BRCA1 and BRCA 2: 1994 and beyond. *Nat Rev Cancer* 4:665–676.

Navin N, Kendall J, Troge J, Andrews P, Rodgers L, McIndoo J, et al. (2011): Tumour evolution inferred by single-cell sequencing. *Nature* 472: 90–94.

Naylor TL, Greshock J, Wang Y, Colligon T, Yu QC, Clemmer V, et al. (2005): High resolution genomic analysis of sporadic breast cancer using array-based comparative genomic hybridization. *Breast Cancer Res* 7:R1186–R1198.

Nielsen KV, Briand R (1989): Cytogenetic analysis of *in vitro* karyotype evolution in a cell line established from non-malignant human mammary epithelium. *Cancer Genet Cytogenet* 39:103–118.

Nielsen KV, Blichert-Toft M, Andersen J (1989): Chromosome analysis of *in situ* breast cancer. *Acta Oncol* 28:919–921.

Nik-Zainal S, Alexandrov LB, Wedge DC, Van Loo P, Greenman CD, Raine K, et al. (2012a): Mutational processes molding the genomes of 21 breast cancers. *Cell* 149: 979–993.

Nik-Zainal S, Van Loo P, Wedge DC, Alexandrov LB, Greenman CD, Lau KW, et al. (2012b): The life history of 21 breast cancers. *Cell* 149: 994–1007.

Nishizaki T, Chew K, Chu L, Isola J, Kallioniemi A, Weidner N, et al. (1997a): Genetic alterations in lobular breast cancer by comparative genomic hybridization. *Int J Cancer* 74:513–517.

Nishizaki T, De Vries S, Chew K, Goodson WH III, Ljung BM, Thor A, et al. (1997b): Genetic alterations in primary breast cancers and their metastases: direct comparison using modified comparative genomic hybridization. *Genes Chromosomes Cancer* 19:267–272.

Noguchi S, Motomura K, Inaji H, Imaoka S, Koyama H (1992): Clonal analysis of human breast cancer by means of the polymerase chain reaction. *Cancer Res* 52: 6594–6597.

Noguchi S, Motomura K, Inaji H, Imaoka S, Koyama H (1993): Clonal analysis of fibroadenoma and phyllodes tumor of the breast. *Cancer Res* 53:4071–4074.

Noguchi S, Motomura K, Inaji H, Imaoka S, Koyama H (1994): Clonal analysis of predominantly intraductal carcinoma and pre-cancerous lesions of the breast by means of polymerase chain reaction. *Cancer Res* 54:1849–1853.

Nonet GH, Stampfer MR, Chin K, Gray JW, Collins CC, Yaswen P (2001): The ZNF217 gene amplified in breast cancers promotes immortalization of human mammary epithelial cells. *Cancer Res* 61:1250–1254.

Nupponen NN, Porkka K, Kakkola L, Tanner M, Persson K, Borg A, et al. (1999): Amplification and overexpression of p40 subunit of eukaryotic translation initiation factor 3 in breast and prostate cancer. *Am J Pathol* 154:1777–1783.

Nyante SJ, Devries S, Chen YY, Hwang ES (2004): Array-based comparative genomic hybridization of ductal carcinoma in situ and synchronous invasive lobular cancer. *Hum Pathol* 35:759–763.

Olivier M, Hainaut P (2001): TP53 mutation patterns in breast cancers: searching for clues of environmental carcinogenesis. *Semin Cancer Biol* 11:353–360.

Olivier M, Goldgar DE, Sodha N, Ohgaki H, Kleihues P, Hainaut P, et al. (2003): Li–Fraumeni and related syndromes: correlation between tumor type, family structure, and TP53 genotype. *Cancer Res* 63:6643–6650.

Ormandy CJ, Musgrove EA, Hui R, Daly RJ, Sutherland RL (2003): Cyclin D1.EMS1 and 11q13 amplification in breast cancer. *Breast Cancer Res Treat* 78:323–335.

Orsetti B, Nugoli M, Cervera N, Lasorsa L, Chuchana P, Rougé C, et al. (2006): Genetic profiling of chromosome 1 in breast cancer: mapping of regions of gains and losses and identification of candidate genes on 1q. *Br J Cancer* 95:1439–1447.

Ozisik YY, Meloni AM, Stephenson CF, Peier A, Moore GE, Sandberg AA (1994): Chromosome abnormalities in breast fibroadenomas. *Cancer Genet Cytogenet* 77: 125–128.

Pandis N, Heim S, Bardi G, Limon J, Mandahl N, Mitelman F (1992a): Improved technique for short-term culture and cytogenetic analysis of human breast cancer. *Genes Chromosomes Cancer* 5:14–20.

Pandis N, Heim S, Bardi G, Idvall I, Mandahl N, Mitelman F (1992b): Whole-arm t(1;16) and i(1q) as sole anomalies identify gain of 1q as the primary chromosomal abnormality in breast cancer. *Genes Chromosomes Cancer* 5:235–238.

Pandis N, Heim S, Bardi G, Idvall I, Mandahl N, Mitelman F (1993a): Chromosome analysis of 20 breast carcinomas: cytogenetic multiclonality and karyotypic-pathologic correlations. *Genes Chromosomes Cancer* 6:51–57.

Pandis N, Jin Y, Limon J, Bardi G, Idvall I, Mandahl N, et al. (1993b): Interstitial deletion of the short arm of chromosome 3 as the primary chromosome abnormality in carcinomas of the breast. *Genes Chromosomes Cancer* 6:151–155.

Pandis N, Bardi G, Heim S (1994a): Interrelationship between methodological choices and conceptual models in solid tumor cytogenetics. *Cancer Genet Cytogenet* 76: 77–84.

Pandis N, Bardi G, Jin Y, Dietrich C, Johansson B, Andersen J, et al. (1994b): Unbalanced 1;16-translocation as the sole karyotypic abnormality in a breast carcinoma and its lymph node metastasis. *Cancer Genet Cytogenet* 75:158–159.

Pandis N, Jin Y, Gorunova L, Petersson C, Bardi G, Idvall I, et al. (1995a): Chromosome analysis of 97 primary carcinomas of the breast: identification of eight karyotypic subgroups. *Genes Chromosomes Cancer* 12:173–185.

Pandis N, Teixeira MR, Gerdes AM, Limon J, Bardi G, Andersen JA, et al. (1995b): Chromosome abnormalities in bilateral breast carcinomas. Cytogenetic evaluation of the clonal origin of multiple primary tumors. *Cancer* 76:250–258.

Pandis N, Idvall I, Bardi G, Jin Y, Gorunova L, Mertens F, et al. (1996): Correlation between karyotypic pattern and clinicopathologic features in 125 breast cancer cases. *Int J Cancer* 66:191–196.

Pandis N, Teixeira MR, Adeyinka A, Rizou H, Bardi G, Mertens F, et al. (1998): Cytogenetic comparison of primary tumors and lymph node metastases in breast cancer patients. *Genes Chromosomes Cancer* 22:122–129.

Pärssinen J, Kuukasjärvi T, Karhu R, Kallioniemi A (2007): High-level amplification at 17q23 leads to coordinated overexpression of multiple adjacent genes in breast cancer. *Br J Cancer* 96:1258–1264.

Perou CM, Sørlie T, Eisen MB, van de Rijn M, Jeffrey SS, Rees CA, et al. (2000): Molecular portraits of human breast tumours. *Nature* 406:747–752.

Persson K, Pandis N, Mertens F, Borg A, Baldetorp B, Killander D, et al. (1999): Chromosomal aberrations in breast cancer: a comparison between cytogenetics and comparative genomic hybridization. *Genes Chromosomes Cancer* 25:115–122.

Persson M, Andren Y, Mark J, Horlings HM, Persson F, Stenman G (2009): Recurrent fusion of MYB and NFIB transcription factor genes in carcinomas of the breast and head and neck. *Proc Natl Acad Sci USA* 106: 18740–18744.

Petersson C, Pandis N, Mertens F, Adeyinka A, Ingvar C, Ringberg A, et al. (1996): Chromosome aberrations in prophylactic mastectomies from women belonging to breast cancer families. *Genes Chromosomes Cancer* 16:185–188.

Petersson C, Pandis N, Rizou H, Mertens F, Dietrich CU, Adeyinka A, et al. (1997): Karyotypic abnormalities in fibroadenomas of the breast. *Int J Cancer* 70:282–286.

Polito P, Dal Cin P, Pauwels P, Christiaens M, Van den Berghe I, Moerman P, et al. (1998): An important subgroup of phyllodes tumors of the breast is characterized by rearrangements of chromosomes 1q and 10q. *Oncol Rep* 5: 1099–1102.

Pollack JR, Sørlie T, Perou CM, Rees CA, Jeffrey SS, Lonning PE, et al. (2002): Microarray analysis reveals a major direct role of DNA copy number alteration in the transcriptional program of human breast tumors. *Proc Natl Acad Sci USA* 99:12963–12968.

Popovici C, Basset C, Bertucci F, Orsetti B, Adelaide J, Mozziconacci MJ, et al. (2002): Reciprocal translocations in breast tumor cell lines: cloning of a t(3;20) that targets the FHIT gene. *Genes Chromosomes Cancer* 35:204–218.

Prentice LM, Shadeo A, Lestou VS, Miller MA, de Leeuw RJ, Makretsov N, et al. (2005): NRG1 gene rearrangements in clinical breast cancer: identification of an adjacent novel amplicon associated with poor prognosis. *Oncogene* 24:7281–7289.

Rennstam K, Ahlstedt-Soini M, Baldetorp B, Bendahl PO, Borg A, Karhu R, et al. (2003): Patterns of chromosomal imbalances defines subgroups of breast cancer with distinct clinical features and prognosis. A study of 305 tumors by comparative genomic hybridization. *Cancer Res* 63:8861–8868.

Rizou H, Bardi G, Arnaourti M, Apostolikas N, Sfikas K, Charlaftis A, et al. (2004): Metaphase and interphase cytogenetics in fibroadenomas of the breast. *In Vivo* 18:703–711.

Robinson DR, Kalyana-Sundaram S, Wu YM, Shankar S, Cao X, Ateeq B, et al. (2011): Functionally recurrent rearrangements of the MAST kinase and Notch gene families in breast cancer. *Nature Med* 17: 1646–1651.

Rodgers CS, Hill SM, Hultén MA (1984): Cytogenetic analysis in human breast carcinoma. I. Nine cases in the diploid range investigated using direct preparations. *Cancer Genet Cytogenet* 13:95–119.

Rohen C, Bonk U, Staats B, Bartnitzke S, Bullerdiek J (1993): Two human breast tumors with translocations involving 12q13-15 as the sole cytogenetic abnormality. *Cancer Genet Cytogenet* 69:68–71.

Rohen C, Caselitz J, Stern C, Wanschura S, Schoenmakers EF, Van de Ven WJ, et al. (1995a): A hamartoma of the breast with an aberration of 12q mapped to the MAR region by fluorescence *in situ* hybridization. *Cancer Genet Cytogenet* 84:82–84.

Rohen C, Meyer-Bolte K, Bonk U, Ebel T, Staats B, Leuschner E, et al. (1995b): Trisomy 8 and 18 as frequent clonal and single-cell aberrations in 185 primary breast carcinomas. *Cancer Genet Cytogenet* 80:33–39.

Rohen C, Staats B, Bonk U, Bartnitzke S, Bullerdiek J (1996): Significance of clonal chromosome aberrations in breast fibroadenomas. *Cancer Genet Cytogenet* 87: 152–155.

Rosen PP (1993): Proliferative breast "disease." An unresolved diagnostic dilemma. *Cancer* 71:3798–3807.

Roylance R, Gorman P, Harris W, Liebmann R, Barnes D, Hanby A, et al. (1999): Comparative genomic hybridization of breast tumors stratified by histological grade reveals new insights into the biological progression of breast cancer. *Cancer Res* 59:1433–1436.

Roylance R, Droufakou S, Gorman P, Gillett C, Hart IR, Hanby A, et al. (2003): The role of E-cadherin in low-grade ductal breast tumourigenesis. *J Pathol* 200: 53–58.

Santen RJ, Mansel R (2005): Benign breast disorders. *N Engl J Med* 353:275–285.

Sato T, Tanigami A, Yamakawa K, Akiyama F, Kasumi F, Sakamoto G, et al. (1990): Allelotype of breast cancer: cumulative allele losses promote tumor progression in primary breast cancer. *Cancer Res* 50:7184–7189.

Sato T, Akiyama F, Sakamoto G, Kasumi F, Nakamura Y (1991): Accumulation of genetic alterations and progression of primary breast cancer. *Cancer Res* 51: 5794–5799.

Sen S, Zhou H, White RA (1997): A putative serine/threonine kinase encoding gene BTAK on chromosome 20q13 is amplified and overexpressed in human breast cancer cell lines. *Oncogene* 14:2195–2200.

Seshadri R, Matthews C, Dobrovic A, Horsfall DJ (1989): The significance of oncogene amplification in primary breast cancer. *Int J Cancer* 43:270–272.

Shah SP, Morin RD, Khattra J, Prentice L, Pugh T, Burleigh A, et al. (2009): Mutational evolution in a lobular breast tumour profiled at single nucleotide resolution. *Nature* 461: 809–813.

Shah SP, Roth A, Goya R, Oloumi A, Ha G, Zhao Y, et al. (2012): The clonal and mutational evolution spectrum of primary triple-negative breast cancers. *Nature* 486: 395–399.

Shelley Hwang E, Nyante SJ, Yi Chen Y, Moore D, De Vries S, Korkola JE, et al. (2004): Clonality of lobular carcinoma *in situ* and synchronous invasive lobular carcinoma. *Cancer* 100:2562–2572.

Slamon DJ, Clark GM, Wong SG, Levin WJ, Ullrich A, McGuire WL (1987): Human breast cancer: correlation of relapse and survival with amplification of the HER-2/neu oncogene. *Science* 235:177–182.

Slamon DJ, Godolphin W, Jones LA, Holt JA, Wong SG, Keith DE, et al. (1989): Studies of the HER-2/neu proto-oncogene in human breast and ovarian cancer. *Science* 244:707–712.

Sørlie T, Perou CM, Tibshirani R, Aas T, Geisler S, Johnsen H, et al. (2001): Gene expression patterns of breast carcinomas distinguish tumor subclasses with clinical implications. *Proc Natl Acad Sci USA* 98:10869–10874.

Srivastava S, Zou Z, Pirollo K, Blattner W, Chang EH (1990): Germ-line transmission of a mutated p53 gene in a cancer-prone family with Li–Fraumeni syndrome. *Nature* 348:747–749.

Steinarsdottir M, Petursdottir I, Snorradottir S, Eyfjord JE, Ogmundsdottir HM (1995): Cytogenetic studies of breast carcinomas: different karyotypic profiles detected by direct harvesting and short-term culture. *Genes Chromosomes Cancer* 13: 239–248.

Steinarsdottir M, Jonasson JG, Vidarsson H, Juliusdottir H, Hauksdottir H, Ogmundsdottir HM (2004): Cytogenetic changes in nonmalignant breast tissue. *Genes Chromosomes Cancer* 41:47–55.

Steinarsdottir M, Gudmundsson IH, Jonasson JG, Olafsdottir EJ, Eyfjord JE, Ogmundsdottir HM (2011): Cytogenetic polyclonality of breast carcinomas: association with clinico-pathological characteristics and outcome. *Genes Chromosomes Cancer* 50: 930–939.

Stephens PJ, McBride DJ, Lin ML, Varela I, Pleasance ED, Simpson JT, et al. (2009): Complex landscapes of somatic rearrangement in human breast cancer genomes. *Nature* 462: 1005–1010.

Stephens PJ, Tarpey PS, Davies H, Van Loo P, Greenman C, Wedge DC, et al. (2012): The landscape of cancer genes and mutational processes in breast cancer. *Nature* 486: 400–404.

Teixeira MR, Pandis N, Bardi G, Andersen JA, Mandahl N, Mitelman F, et al. (1994): Cytogenetic analysis of multi-focal breast carcinomas: detection of karyotypically unrelated clones as well as clonal similarities between tumour foci. *Br J Cancer* 70:922–927.

Teixeira MR, Pandis N, Bardi G, Andersen JA, Mitelman F, Heim S (1995): Clonal heterogeneity in breast cancer: karyotypic comparisons of multiple intra- and extra-tumorous samples from 3 patients. *Int J Cancer* 63:63–68.

Teixeira MR, Pandis N, Gerdes AM, Dietrich CU, Bardi G, Andersen JA, et al. (1996a): Cytogenetic abnormalities in an *in situ* ductal carcinoma and five prophylactically removed breasts from members of a family with hereditary breast cancer. *Breast Cancer Res Treat* 38:177–182.

Teixeira MR, Pandis N, Bardi G, Andersen JA, Heim S (1996b): Karyotypic comparisons of multiple tumorous and macroscopically normal surrounding tissue samples from patients with breast cancer. *Cancer Res* 56:855–859.

Teixeira MR, Pandis N, Bardi G, Andersen JA, Bohler PJ, Qvist H, et al. (1997): Discrimination between multicentric and multifocal breast carcinoma by cytogenetic investigation of macroscopically distinct ipsilateral lesions. *Genes Chromosomes Cancer* 18:170–174.

Teixeira MR, Pandis N, Dietrich CU, Reed W, Andersen J, Qvist H, et al. (1998a): Chromosome banding analysis of gynecomastias and breast carcinomas in men. *Genes Chromosomes Cancer* 23:16–20.

Teixeira MR, Qvist H, Bohler PJ, Pandis N, Heim S (1998b): Cytogenetic analysis shows that carcinosarcomas of the breast are of monoclonal origin. *Genes Chromosomes Cancer* 22:145–151.

Teixeira MR, Tsarouha H, Kraggerud SM, Pandis N, Dimitriadis E, Andersen JA, et al. (2001): Evaluation of breast cancer polyclonality by combined chromosome banding and comparative genomic hybridization analysis. *Neoplasia* 3:204–214.

Teixeira MR, Pandis N, Heim S (2002): Cytogenetic clues to breast carcinogenesis. *Genes Chromosomes Cancer* 33:1–16.

Teixeira MR, Ribeiro FR, Torres L, Pandis N, Andersen JA, Lothe RA, et al. (2004): Assessment of clonal relationships in ipsilateral and bilateral multiple breast carcinomas by comparative genomic hybridisation and hierarchical clustering analysis. *Br J Cancer* 91:775–782.

Thompson F, Emerson J, Dalton W, Yang J-M, McGee D, Villar H, et al. (1993): Clonal chromosome abnormalities in human breast carcinomas I. Twenty-eight cases with primary disease. *Genes Chromosomes Cancer* 7:185–193.

Thull DL, Vogel VG (2004): Recognition and management of hereditary breast cancer syndromes. *Oncologist* 9:13–24.

Tibiletti MG, Sessa F, Bernasconi B, Cerutti R, Broggi B, Furlan D, et al. (2000): A large 6q deletion is a common cytogenetic alteration in fibroadenomas, pre-malignant lesions, and carcinomas of the breast. *Clin Cancer Res* 6:1422–1431.

Tirkkonen M, Johannsson O, Agnarsson BA, Olsson H, Ingvarsson S, Karhu R, et al. (1997): Distinct somatic genetic changes associated with tumor progression in carriers of BRCA1 and BRCA2 germ-line mutations. *Cancer Res* 57:1222–1227.

Tirkkonen M, Tanner M, Karhu R, Kallioniemi A, Isola J, Kallioniemi OP (1998): Molecular cytogenetics of primary breast cancer by CGH. *Genes Chromosomes Cancer* 21:177–184.

Tirkkonen M, Kainu T, Loman N, Jóhannsson OT, Olsson H, Barkardóttir RB, et al. (1999): Somatic genetic alterations in BRCA2-associated and sporadic male breast cancer. *Genes Chromosomes Cancer* 24:56–61.

Tognon C, Knezevich SR, Huntsman D, Roskelley CD, Melnyk N, Mathers JA, et al. (2002): Expression of the ETV6-NTRK3 gene fusion as a primary event in human secretory breast carcinoma. *Cancer Cell* 2:367–376.

Torres L, Ribeiro FR, Pandis N, Andersen JA, Heim S, Teixeira MR (2007): Intratumor genomic heterogeneity in breast cancer with clonal divergence between primary carcinomas and lymph node metastases. *Breast Cancer Res Treat* 102:143–155.

Trent J, Yang J-M, Emerson J, Dalton W, McGee D, Massey K, et al. (1993): Clonal chromosome abnormalities in human breast carcinomas II. Thirty-four cases with metastatic disease. *Genes Chromosomes Cancer* 7:194–203.

Tsai YC, Lu Y, Nichols PW, Zlotnikov G, Jones PA, Smith HS (1996): Contiguous patches of normal human mammary epithelium derived from a single stem cell: implications for breast carcinogenesis. *Cancer Res* 56:402–404.

Tsarouha H, Pandis N, Bardi G, Teixeira MR, Andersen JA, Heim S (1999): Karyotypic evolution in breast carcinomas with i(1)(q10) and der(1;16)(q10;p10) as the primary chromosome abnormality. *Cancer Genet Cytogenet* 113:156–161.

Tsuneizumi M, Emi M, Nagai H, Harada H, Sakamoto G, Kasumi F, et al. (2001): Overrepresentation of the EBAG9 gene at 8q23 associated with early-stage breast cancers. *Clin Cancer Res* 7:3526–3532.

Uccelli R, Calugi A, Forte D, Mauro F, Polonio-Balbi P, Vecchione A, et al. (1986): Flow cytometrically determined DNA content of breast carcinoma and benign lesions; correlations with histopathological parameters. *Tumori* 72: 171–177.

Ugolini F, Adélaïde J, Charafe-Jauffret E, Nguyen C, Jacquemier J, Jordan B, et al. (1999): Differential expression assay of chromosome arm 8p genes identifies frizzled-related (FRP1/FRZB) and fibroblast growth factor receptor 1 (FGFR1) as candidate breast cancer genes. *Oncogene* 18:1903–1910.

Van Beers EH, Nederlof PM (2006): Array-CGH and breast cancer. *Breast Cancer Res* 8: 210.

Van Beers EH, van Welsem T, Wessels LF, Li Y, Oldenburg RA, Devilee P, et al. (2005): Comparative genomic hybridization profiles in human BRCA1 and BRCA2 breast tumors highlight differential sets of genomic aberrations. *Cancer Res* 65: 822–827.

van't Veer LJ, Dai H, van de Vijver MJ, He YD, Hart AA, Mao M, et al. (2002): Gene expression profiling predicts clinical outcome of breast cancer. *Nature* 415: 530–536.

Veronesi U, Boyle P, Goldhirsch A, Orecchia R, Viale G (2005): Breast cancer. *Lancet* 365: 1727–1741.

van de Vijver MJ, He YD, van't Veer LJ, Dai H, Hart AA, Voskuil DW, et al. (2002):A gene-expression signature as a predictor of survival in breast cancer. *N Engl J Med* 347: 1999–2009.

Vogel CL, Cobleigh MA, Tripathy D, Gutheil JC, Harris LN, Fehrenbacher L, et al. (2002): Efficacy and safety of trastuzumab as a single agent in first-line treatment of HER2-overexpressing metastatic breast cancer. *J Clin Oncol* 20: 719–726.

Walther C, Gisselsson D, Magnusson L, Nilsson J, Grabau D, Kullendorff CM, et al. (2013): Biphasic, hyperdiploid breast tumors in children: a distinct entity? *J Pediatr Hematol Oncol* 35: 64–68.

Wang XZ, Jolicoeur EM, Conte N, Chaffanet M, Zhang Y, Mozziconacci MJ, et al. (1999): gamma-heregulin is the product of a chromosomal translocation fusing the DOC4 and HGL/NRG1 genes in the MDA-MB-175 breast cancer cell line. *Oncogene* 18: 5718–5721.

Wenger CR, Beardslee S, Owens MA, Pounds G, Oldaker T, Vendely P, et al. (1993): DNA ploidy, S-phase, and steroid receptors in more than 127.000 breast cancer patients. *Breast Cancer Res Treat* 28: 9–20.

Wessels LF, van Welsem T, Hart AA, van't Veer LJ, Reinders MJ, Nederlof PM (2002): Molecular classification of breast carcinomas by comparative genomic hybridization: a specific somatic genetic profile for BRCA1 tumors. *Cancer Res* 62: 7110–7117.

Woolley PV, Gollin SM, Riskalla W, Finkelstein S, Stefanik DF, Riskalla L, et al. (2000): Cytogenetics, immunostaining for fibroblast growth factors, p53 sequencing, and clinical features of two cases of cystosarcoma phyllodes. *Mol Diagn* 5: 179–190.

Wooster R, Mangion J, Eeles R, Smith S, Dowsett M, Averill D, et al. (1992): A germline mutation in the androgen receptor gene in two brothers with breast cancer and Reifenstein syndrome. *Nature Genet* 2: 132–134.

Wooster R, Bignell G, Lancaster J, Swift S, Seal S, Mangion J, et al. (1995): Identification of the breast cancer susceptibility gene BRCA2. *Nature* 378: 789–792.

Wuicik L, Cavalli LR, Cornelio DA, Schmid Braz AT, Barbosa ML, Lima RS, et al. (2007): Chromosome alterations associated with positive and negative lymph node involvement in breast cancer. *Cancer Genet Cytogenet* 173: 114–121.

Zafrani B, Gerbault-Seureau M, Mosseri V, Dutrillaux B (1992): Cytogenetic study of breast cancer: clinicopathologic significance of homogeneously staining regions in 84 patients. *Hum Pathol* 23: 542–547.

Zhang R, Wiley J, Howard SP, Meisner LF, Gould MN (1989): Rare clonal karyotypic variants in primary cultures of human breast carcinoma cells. *Cancer Res* 49: 444–449.

Zudaire I, Odero MD, Caballero C, Valenti C, Martínez-Penuela JM, Isola J, et al. (2002): Genomic imbalances detected by comparative genomic hybridization are prognostic markers in invasive ductal breast carcinomas. *Histopathology* 40: 547–555.

CHAPTER 17

Tumors of the female genital organs

Francesca Micci and Sverre Heim

Section for Cancer Cytogenetics, Institute for Cancer Genetics and Informatics,
Oslo University Hospital, Oslo, Norway

The dominating gynecologic malignancies are cancers of the ovaries and uterine cervix. Although more is known cytogenetically about the former than about the latter, the information cannot be said to be extensive or even satisfactory for any of them or, for that matter, for any other malignant tumor of the female reproductive tract. The most complete data exist for the common but clinically benign leiomyomas of the uterine wall. The chromosomal characteristics of these and some of the less common benign and malignant tumors of the female genital organs will be discussed under their respective anatomical subheadings.

Ovary

Less than 50 ovarian *adenomas* showing chromosome abnormalities have been karyotyped. The largest series was reported by Tibiletti et al. (2003), who found a deletion in 6q in almost all tumors, with a possible common deleted region between 6q27 and 6qter. When comparing ovarian tumors of different types, Tibiletti et al. (2003) interpreted their data to indicate that whereas deletions from 6q24 to 6qter were frequently observed in benign and borderline ovarian tumors, the larger deletions

from 6q16 to 6qter were found exclusively in invasive carcinomas. Other aberrations reported at lower frequencies in ovarian adenomas have been trisomy for chromosomes 10 and 12 and monosomy 20 (Pejovic et al., 1990a; Yang-Feng et al., 1991; Tibiletti et al., 2003). Whereas both +10 and +12 were often seen as the sole abnormality in the karyotype, monosomy 20 occurred together with other abnormalities and very often together with del(6q), indicating that it is a secondary aberration.

Only six ovarian adenomas with imbalances detected by comparative genomic hybridization (CGH) have been reported (Hauptmann et al., 2002; Helou et al., 2006). The most frequent gains were from 6p and chromosome 12, whereas losses were seen from 1p, 2q, 4q, 5q, and 6q.

Some 40 ovarian *borderline carcinomas* with chromosomal abnormalities detected by chromosome banding have been reported. Karyotypic simplicity with few or no structural rearrangements seems to be a characteristic of these tumors. Trisomies for chromosomes 7 and 12 have been the most common abnormalities (Yang-Feng et al., 1991; Jenkins et al., 1993; Thompson et al., 1994b; Pejovic et al., 1996b; Grygalewicz et al., 2009; Micci et al., 2010b). Molecular cytogenetic studies are

Cancer Cytogenetics: Chromosomal and Molecular Genetic Aberrations of Tumor Cells, Fourth Edition.
Edited by Sverre Heim and Felix Mitelman.
© 2015 John Wiley & Sons, Ltd. Published 2015 by John Wiley & Sons, Ltd.

also limited but have shown consistent loss of 6q material (Tibiletti et al., 1996; Helou et al., 2006). Tibiletti et al. (1996, 2003), using a combination of YAC probes and microsatellite markers, identified a 300 kb deletion in 6q, which they found was the smallest common deleted region in borderline tumors; however, others did not find this deletion (Micci et al., 2010b). CGH analyses of borderline tumors have been performed by many investigators, the largest series being reported by Wolf et al. (1999), Blegen et al. (2000), Hu et al. (2002), and Osterberg et al. (2006). Of the over 100 tumors analyzed, more than half have shown genomic imbalances. The most frequent abnormalities have been gains of or from chromosomes 5, 8, and 12 and losses from 1p (Wolf et al., 1999; Blegen et al., 2000; Hauptmann et al., 2002; Hu et al., 2002; Staebler et al., 2002; Helou et al., 2006; Micci et al., 2010b). In a few studies, the issue of whether borderline tumors are precursors of invasive carcinomas or a distinct clinical entity was addressed. Blegen et al. (2000), Hauptmann et al. (2002), and Staebler et al. (2002) compared the imbalance pattern of borderline tumors and invasive carcinomas finding that the average number of genetic alterations was significantly higher in the latter. Osterberg et al. (2006) found that whereas the genetic alterations identified in borderline tumors were seen equally often in invasive carcinomas, the latter tumors typically also had additional changes. Micci et al. (2010b) found that specific gains of chromosomal band 8q23 as well as losses of 19p13 and 19q13 were present in both borderline tumors and overt carcinomas and hypothesized that borderline tumors with these aberrations were at particular risk of undergoing further evolutionary changes giving rise to a more malignant phenotype. Grygalewicz et al. (2009) cytogenetically analyzed six primary and five relapsed borderline tumors of the ovary; admittedly, the relapses were not from the same patients as the primary tumors. They found structural aberrations of chromosomes and/or chromosomal arms 1, 6q, 7q, and 10q in relapsed tumors in addition to the gains of chromosomes 7, 8, and 12 found in primary tumors.

Adenocarcinomas make up 75% of all tumors of the ovary and 95% of ovarian malignancies. Many of the known ovarian carcinomas with karyotypically characterized chromosomal aberrations (http://cgap.nci.nih.gov/Chromosomes/Mitelman) were examined as abdominal effusions, that is, at a very late stage in tumor progression, and many were incompletely karyotyped. Knowledge about the chromosomal characteristics of this type of cancer is therefore still far from satisfactory.

Reasonably large series (>10 cases) of karyotypically abnormal ovarian adenocarcinomas were reported by Wake et al. (1980), Whang-Peng et al. (1984), Bello and Rey (1990), Pejovic et al. (1992a), Jenkins et al. (1993), Thompson et al. (1994a), Tibiletti et al. (1996, 2003), Deger et al. (1997), Panani and Roussos (2006), and Micci et al. (2009, 2010a). Based on the findings in 52 ovarian carcinomas with clonal chromosome aberrations, Pejovic et al. (1989, 1990c, 1991, 1992a) concluded that most tumors (46 of the 52) had complex karyotypes, often with a stemline chromosome number that was near triploid or hypodiploid. The most common numerical changes (compared with the nearest euploid level) were losses of chromosomes X, 22, 17, 13, 14, and 8 (each lost in at least 20 tumors). Gains were less common; the most frequent, +20, was seen in 10 tumors. Deletions and unbalanced translocations resulting in loss of chromosomal material were the most common structural abnormalities. These rearrangements preferentially involved (in order of falling frequency) chromosomes 1, 3, 11, 19, 7, 6, and 12. The bands and segments most frequently affected were 19p13 (26 tumors), 19q13 (14 tumors), 1p36 and 11p13 (13 tumors each), 3p12–13 (12 tumors), 1q23 (11 tumors), and 6q21 (10 tumors). Jenkins et al. (1993) examined 36 carcinomas and found abnormal karyotypes in 26. Common chromosomal gains included +1, +2, +3, +6, +7, +9, and +12. The most common losses were –X, –4, –8, –11, –13, –15, –17, and –22. The chromosome arms most often involved in structural changes were 1p, 1q, 3p, 3q, 7p, 9q, 11q, 17q, 19p, and 19q. In the series examined by Thompson et al. (1994a), the breakpoints of structural rearrangements clustered to 1p35, 1p11–q21, 3p11–23, 7p, 11p, 11q, 12p13–q12, and 12q24. The most common numerical changes were loss of one X chromosome and +7. Finally, Tibiletti et al. (1996, 2003) karyotyped a total of 88 ovarian carcinomas with chromosome abnormalities; the most common of

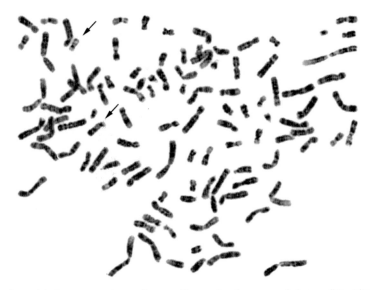

Figure 17.1 Metaphase plate from an ovarian carcinoma with complex chromosomal abnormalities. The arrows point to examples of 19q+, one of the most common rearrangements in this tumor type.

which, irrespective of the tumor's histological grade, was deletion of 6q. The deletions appeared to be terminal but of variable size. The position of the proximal breakpoint varied between bands 6q15 and 6q27 but was mostly mapped to 6q25 and 6q26. All cases with 6q deletion seemed to share a minimal common deleted region between 6q27 and 6qter. The investigators also used locus-specific probes mapping to 6q and found 6q abnormalities in seemingly normal karyotypes. The finding of 6q deletions in borderline, low-grade, intermediate, and high-grade ovarian carcinomas led Tibiletti and coworkers to suggest that this represented an early event in the process of ovarian carcinogenesis. The sometimes simultaneous finding of del(6q) and +12 suggested, in their opinion, that the trisomy was secondary to the deletion. Partial loss of 6q material was detected as the most common imbalance in advanced invasive carcinomas also by Deger et al. (1997), followed in frequency by partial or complete loss of chromosome 1 (frequent breaks in both the p and the q arm were seen). On the other hand, the most commonly rearranged bands in their series were 11p13 and 19p13.

Although the aberration pattern in carcinoma of the ovary thus comes across as distinctly nonrandom, no aberration can be said to be fully specific, let alone pathognomonic, for these malignancies. The early suggestion by Wake et al. (1980) that t(6;14)(q21;q32) is typical of ovarian carcinomas has not been corroborated in later studies. Deletions and unbalanced translocations leading to 6q– are unquestionably common in these tumors, but neither are the rearrangements restricted to any single band, nor is only a single translocation partner involved.

The most common (50%) cytogenetic aberration in ovarian cancer in the experience of Pejovic et al. (1989, 1992a) was a 19p+ marker with unknown material, sometimes looking identical from case to case, added to 19p13. A 19p+ was also described by Tanaka et al. (1989) and Jenkins et al. (1993); otherwise, most investigators have chosen to interpret the rearrangements of chromosome 19 as taking place in 19q13 (Figure 17.1) rather than 19p13 (Whang-Peng et al., 1984; Tanaka et al., 1989; Bello and Rey, 1990). The only other solid tumor in which similar 19p+ rearrangements are consistently registered is malignant fibrous histiocytoma (Chapter 24). The 19p+ has never been seen as the only chromosomal aberration in ovarian carcinoma, and so it seems likely that it is a progressional rather than a primary anomaly. Its molecular consequences are unknown. Åman et al. (1993) mapped the 19p13 breakpoint in one ovarian carcinoma to between the *INSR* and *TCF3* loci. Micci et al. (2009) focused on the rearrangements of chromosome 19 using a combination of chromosomal microdissection and reverse painting to determine the identity of the material present in these markers as well as to determine the breakpoint position on chromosome 19. The analysis showed that particularly common donors to chromosome 19 were chromosome arms 11q, 21q, and 22q. Breakpoint positions were located (in order of decreasing frequency) in the short arm, long arm, pericentromeric region, and centromeric region of chromosome 19 (Micci et al., 2009).

The second most common (one-third of all tumors) structural chromosomal aberration in ovarian carcinoma seen by Pejovic et al. (1989, 1992a) was rearrangement of the short arm of chromosome 11, leading to loss of distal 11p material. A similar involvement of 11p was noted also by Bello and Rey (1990), Jenkins et al. (1993), and Thompson et al. (1994a).

The frequent rearrangements of chromosome 1 in the series examined by Pejovic et al. (1989, 1992a) included deletions of the distal half of 1q and various abnormalities resulting in loss of 1p34–36. Similar patterns of chromosome 1 involvement were observed also by Trent and Salmon (1981), Whang-Peng et al. (1984), Tanaka et al. (1989), Jenkins et al. (1993), Thompson et al. (1994a), and Deger et al. (1997). The variability of the changes and the frequent occurrence of similar aberrations also in other tumor types suggest that they are of a secondary, nonspecific nature.

Deletions and unbalanced translocations resulting in loss of 3p material were seen in one-fourth of the tumors studied by Pejovic et al. (1989, 1992a). Comparable deletions, particularly of 3p13–21, were described in ovarian carcinoma also by Trent and Salmon (1981), Whang-Peng et al. (1984), Panani and Ferti-Passantonopoulou (1985), Teyssier (1987), Tanaka et al. (1989), Jenkins et al. (1993), Thompson et al. (1994a), and Panani and Roussos (2006). Loss of chromosomal material from roughly the same 3p region is common also in many other tumor types, including carcinomas of the lung, kidney, and breast. This consistent loss pattern strongly suggests that one or more tumor suppressor loci, possibly with very low tissue specificity of the genes, may be located here. Because

3p– is not found as a solitary abnormality in carcinomas of the ovary, in contrast to what is the case in renal cell and breast carcinomas (Chapters 15 and 16), it seems less likely that the putative suppressor gene plays any primary role in ovarian carcinogenesis.

Panani and Roussos (2006) analyzed 12 ovarian adenocarcinomas and found i(5)(p10) in seven of them. The aberration was always found in complex karyotypes, but the authors nevertheless suggested that it might constitute a novel recurrent abnormality in ovarian cancer. In the same series, nonrandom involvement of chromosome 11, as add(11)(p15), was also described. A similar rearrangement was later reported in eight additional tumors studied by the same group (Panani, 2007). Rearrangements of the same band (11p15) have also been described in nearly 30 more ovarian carcinomas according to the Mitelman database (http://cgap.nci.nih.gov/Chromosomes/Mitelman).

Ten karyotypically abnormal *endometrioid ovarian carcinomas* have been reported (Yonescu et al., 1996; Micci et al., 2010a). They showed structural rearrangements that most frequently involved chromosomes 1, 3, 6, and 19. More specifically, eight tumors had a deletion in 1p, four tumors had a deletion in 6q, four tumors showed an add(19)(q13), and four tumors had rearrangements of chromosome 3. The observed aberration pattern therefore seems to correspond to that generally seen in carcinomas of the ovary.

Few *undifferentiated carcinomas* of the ovary have been reported with karyotypic abnormalities (Augustus et al., 1986; Atkin and Baker, 1987a, 1987b; Pejovic et al., 1992a; Thompson et al., 1994a; Tibiletti et al., 1996). All had massive numerical and structural rearrangements, which led to an incomplete description.

The simultaneous finding of cancer in both ovaries is common: 50% of all ovarian carcinomas are bilateral. Pejovic et al. (1991) used cytogenetic analysis to address the old question of whether *bilateral ovarian cancer* is the result of spreading from one side to the other or whether the tumors arise independently. The baseline karyotypes in the two tumorous ovaries were identical in each of the 11 patients in whom informative results were obtained, providing strong evidence that the tumors in both sides were monoclonal and arose from the same transformed cell. Because the clonal evolution of the neoplastic tissues in the two locations was similar, it was impossible to determine which tumor was primary and which was metastatic. Micci et al. (2010a) analyzed a series of 32 bilateral ovarian carcinoma cases by means of karyotyping and high-resolution CGH (HR-CGH). The findings showed that spreading to the contralateral ovary gave rise to bilateral cancer cases and that it was a late event in the clonal evolution of the tumors. This was particularly indicated by the large number of similar changes detected by HR-CGH in the different lesions from the same patient. Chromosomal band 5p14 was the most frequently gained band leading to the hypothesis that oncogene(s) involved in bilateral ovarian carcinogenesis or tumor progression might be located there.

Other studies have compared tumor karyotype with clinicopathologic features. The various histologic subtypes of ovarian carcinoma show no marked cytogenetic differences (the main differentiation patterns result in serous, mucinous, endometrioid, and clear cell carcinomas). The initial impression that 19p+ was found only, or at least predominantly, in serous cystadenocarcinomas (Pejovic et al., 1989) could not be corroborated in a more extended later series (Pejovic et al., 1992a). The only difference seems to be that seropapillary tumors carry chromosomal aberrations more often than do the other carcinoma types (Pejovic et al., 1992b). A relationship between karyotypic complexity and tumor grade exists: Pejovic et al. (1990c, 1992a) found that whereas almost all ovarian carcinomas with simple chromosome abnormalities (numerical changes only or a single structural aberration) were well-differentiated, the poorly differentiated carcinomas generally had complex karyotypes. Similar data were also reported by Thompson et al. (1994a). In a correlation analysis between karyotypic pattern and survival, Pejovic et al. (1992b) found that patients with an abnormal tumor karyotype had the shortest survival; the difference was especially noticeable when the abnormalities were complex. Stage, grade, residual tumor after primary surgery, and performance status also correlated with survival time, but a multivariate analysis identified abnormal karyotype as being independently associated with short survival in advanced clinical disease stages.

Höglund et al. (2003) performed a statistical meta-analysis of 387 published ovarian carcinoma karyotypes. Tumors were classified according to whether imbalances were present or absent and statistically analyzed to assess the order of appearance of the chromosomal imbalances and to identify possible karyotypic pathways and cytogenetic subtypes. The analyses led them to suggest that at least two cytogenetic pathways exist, one characterized by +7, +8q, and +12, another by 6q– and 1q–. They further suggested that ovarian carcinomas develop through at least three phases of karyotypic evolution. In the early stages, in phase I, the karyotypic evolution seems to proceed through a stepwise acquisition of genomic changes. The transition to phase II shows signs of an increased chromosome instability and is linked to the presence of imbalances characteristic for the 6q–/1q– pathway. Finally, according to Höglund et al. (2003), triploidization occurs marking the transition to phase III: this too seems to be linked to the 6q–/1q– pathway.

Many studies have examined oncogene activation or loss of heterozygosity (LOH) in ovarian cancer cells. To the extent that one can compare them, the results of these molecular-level investigations by and large tally with the cytogenetic findings outlined in the preceding text. Amplification of, for example, the *ERBB2* oncogene has been found in about 30% of tumors and seems to correlate with advanced clinical disease and shorter survival (Slamon et al., 1989). This may be of particular interest in the cytogenetic context inasmuch as a chromosomal manifestation of (onco)gene amplification in the form of homogeneously staining regions (hsr) is found in about 10% of ovarian carcinomas (Pejovic et al., 1992a). The hsr do not seem to have any preferred site in the genome, and it is mostly not known which loci they contain. The second cytogenetic sign of gene amplification, double minute chromosomes (dmin), is rare in ovarian cancer.

Of interest is the approach chosen by Guan et al. (1995) who combined chromosome microdissection and fluorescence *in situ* hybridization (FISH) analysis to investigate the composition of seven hsr (from five primary tumors and two ovarian carcinoma cell lines) to find specific amplification of bands 4p16, 11q13, 12p12.1, 15q15, 15q22,

16p11–13.2, 16q21, 16q24, and 19q13.1–13.2. Some of these bands are already known to contain genes amplified in ovarian cancer: *KRAS* in 12p12.1 (Filmus et al., 1986), *FGF3* in 11q13 (Lammie and Peters, 1991; Hruza et al., 1993), and *AKT2* in 19q13 (Cheng et al., 1992). The most frequently amplified region was 19q13.1–13.2. In the study by Micci et al. (2009), three chromosome 19 markers were found with hsr, all containing material from 19p. In a subsequent study by array CGH (aCGH), a commonly gained region on 19p13 was found spanning 50 kb and containing 43 genes of which 31 encoded zinc finger proteins (Micci et al., 2010c). Interestingly, Shih et al. (2011) found amplification of the *NACC1* locus in 19p13.2 leading to NAC1 overexpression and hypothesized that this was one of the molecular alterations contributing to early tumor recurrence in ovarian cancer.

Many CGH studies on ovarian carcinomas have been reported. The most common imbalances have been gains of or from chromosome arms 1q, 3q, 8q, 12p, and 20q and losses of or from 4p, 4q, 8p, 13q, 16q, 18q, and Xp. The smallest most frequently involved regions were mapped to 3q26-qter, 8q23-qter, and 12p12 for gains and 18q22-qter, 13q21, and 16q23-qter for losses (Arnold et al., 1996; Sonoda et al., 1997b). Bayani et al. (2002) demonstrated increased expression of four genes, *HGD*, *CASR*, *TM4SF*, and *SST*, mapping to the 3q13–28 seen as consistently gained in their study. A combined analysis of genomic imbalances in ovarian carcinomas was performed by Schraml et al. (2003) using chromosome-based (mCGH) and array-based CGH (aCGH). mCGH showed frequent gains from chromosome arms 3q, 8q, 11q, 17q, and 20q. The aCGH could identify precisely which genes were involved in these gains, namely, *PIK3CA* at 3q26.3, *PAK1* at 11q13.5–14, *KRAS* at 12p12.1, and *STK15* at 20q13. Gene amplification was detected for *MET* on 7q; *MYC* on 8q; *CCND1*, *FGF4/FGF3*, *EMS1*, *GARP*, and *PAK1* on 11q; *ERBB2* on 17q; and *AIB1*, *PTPN1*, and *ZNF217* on 20q.

Tapper et al. (1997) compared endometrioid, mucinous, and serous ovarian carcinomas by CGH analysis and found that the genomic imbalances were different in the three histologic subtypes. Gain from 10q was seen only in endometrioid tumors, whereas gain from 1q was observed in endometrioid and serous tumors, and gains from 11q occurred mostly in serous tumors. The investigators therefore suggested that different pathogenetic pathways were followed by tumors of the three groups. Dent et al. (2003) analyzed 18 clear cell carcinomas and found frequent losses from 9p, 1p, 11q, 16p, and 16q but gains from chromosomes 3 and 13. They concluded that the pattern of genomic alterations in clear cell carcinomas differed from that of other histologic ovarian carcinoma subtypes; however, no genetic changes unique to the clear cell subtype could be identified. Lately, Sung et al. (2013) analyzed 19 clear cell ovarian carcinomas by aCGH and expression array (microarray). They found common gains in 8q and 17q and losses at 5q, 15q, and 22q. 94 genes showed significant correlation between copy number and gene expression, the majority mapping to 8q and 17q with *PTK2* and *PPM1D* being of particular interest. Hauptmann et al. (2002) compared the imbalances of serous and nonserous malignant ovarian tumors and found that gains from 3q and 6p and losses from 4q were common to both subsets. They therefore suggested that these were early, common events in the development of all these tumors.

Hu et al. (2003) performed a comparative analysis of primary and recurrent tumors, albeit not from the same patients, and found that gains from 2p, 19p, and 20q and loss of 5q were more common in the recurrent carcinomas. On the other hand, Israeli et al. (2004) found that genomic imbalances by and large were similar in primary and metastatic ovarian tumors.

In a few studies, patient survival was shown to correlate with the number of chromosomal alterations found in the tumors; patients whose tumors showed a large number of imbalances by CGH had shorter survival (Iwabuchi et al., 1995; Suzuki et al., 2000; Hu et al., 2003). Partheen et al. (2004) analyzed 98 cases of stage III serous papillary adenocarcinoma and found that losses of 4p, 5q, and 8p were common to patients who had died from their disease. They suggested that absence of these chromosomal imbalances might predict a favorable clinical outcome. Finally, Suehiro et al. (2000a) noticed that 8q gain occurred more frequently in tumors of patients who survived disease-free than in those who died or had recurrences. In the latter group, gains of 17q and 20q were the most frequent imbalances and always occurred together.

Different CGH patterns of genomic imbalances have been found in ovarian carcinomas of different stage and grade. In an analysis of 106 tumors, Kiechle et al. (2001) found that poorly differentiated carcinomas typically showed losses from 11q and 13q as well as gains from 8q and 7p, whereas losses of 12p and 18p were significantly more frequent in well- and moderately differentiated tumors. The number of imbalances paralleled tumor grade with the high-grade cancers having the largest number of alterations (Iwabuchi et al., 1995; Kiechle et al., 2001; Bayani et al., 2002; Chene et al., 2013). Suzuki et al. (2000) found that gains at 3q, 8q, and 20q were frequent in both low- and high-grade tumors suggesting that they are early events in ovarian carcinomas. In their experience, furthermore, loss from 4q occurred more frequently in high-grade tumors, and gain from 2q was the most frequent abnormality in low-grade tumors. Birrer et al. (2007) used aCGH to examine 42 high-grade serous ovarian carcinomas and found amplification of the *FGF1* gene on 5q31. The DNA copy number changes were significantly correlated with mRNA copy numbers and protein expression. Shridhar et al. (2001) and Zaal et al. (2012) analyzed by chromosomal- and array-based CGH early- and late-stage ovarian carcinomas. Both studies found similar patterns of imbalances in the two groups of tumors and concluded that late-/advanced-stage ovarian cancer either progresses from early-stage disease or that the two share a common precursor lesion.

Different CGH studies have compared the genomic imbalances in *hereditary and sporadic ovarian carcinomas*. Extensive similarity between the two groups of tumors was found, with gains from 3q, 8q, and 1q and losses of or from 8p, 16q, 18q, and Xp being the most frequent imbalances (Tapper et al., 1998; Zweemer et al., 2001; Israeli et al., 2003). An overall similarity of imbalances was also scored irrespective of whether the patients had *BRCA1* or *BRCA2* mutations (Tapper et al., 1998; Israeli et al., 2003; Bruchim et al., 2009). Although Tapper et al. (1998) found frequent gain at 2q24–32 in the group of inherited cancers, this was not confirmed by other studies, in which gain of the 2q region was seen to be common in sporadic ovarian carcinomas (Israeli et al., 2003, 2004; Partheen et al., 2004; Fishman et al., 2005; Helou et al., 2006).

Bruchim et al. (2009) showed that gain in 5p was associated with a higher risk of recurrence, whereas gain in 1p as well as loss in 5q was associated with a significant decrease in recurrence.

Three carcinomas arising in ovarian endometriosis were analyzed by Mhawech et al. (2002). They showed an imbalanced genome by CGH; more precisely, a serous cystadenocarcinoma presented gains of 1q and 13q and loss of 10p, an endometrioid carcinoma with squamous differentiation showed gain of 8q, and a squamous cell carcinoma (SCC), a rare malignant tumor of the ovary, presented gains of 1q and 8q. The endometriosis tissue showed a normal genomic profile.

LOH as well as other studies have detected nonrandom loss of genetic information from chromosomes and chromosome arms 3p, 4p, 6p, 6q, 8q, 11p, 12, 16, 17, and 19p (Russell et al., 1990; Foulkes et al., 1991; Sato et al., 1991; Eccles et al., 1992; Skirnisdottir et al., 2012). As usual, this translates into the hypothesis that tumor suppressor gene (TSG) loci exist in the lost segments. Much interest has focused on the loss of genetic information from chromosome 17. In the short arm, losses seem to occur especially at 17p13.1 (Godwin et al., 1994; Saretzki et al., 1997) as well as at a more distal locus in 17p13.3 (Godwin et al., 1994; Phillips et al., 1996). Two possible target TSG have been mapped to 17p13.3, *OVCA1* and *OVCA2* (Schultz et al., 1996), but the more proximal 17 changes have received much more attention. Mutation of the gene *TP53* in 17p13.1 is the most common genetic alteration thus far detected in ovarian cancer, with mutation rates as high as 50% in advanced stage carcinomas (Schuijer and Berns, 2003). The frequency of *TP53* alterations varies depending on whether the tumors are benign, borderline, or malignant as well as on the histological subtype, that is, serous, mucinous, endometrioid, or clear cell ovarian carcinoma. In benign epithelial ovarian tumors, neither *TP53* mutation nor overexpression has been described (Shelling et al., 1995; Skilling et al., 1996). In borderline tumors, *TP53* mutation and overexpression may occur, but are not common (Skomedal et al., 1997; Caduff et al., 1999; Schuyer et al., 1999). In malignant tumors, the prevalence of *TP53* gene mutations increases with increasing stage (Shelling et al, 1995). It also seems that gene mutation and overexpression are more common in serous carcinomas followed, in decreasing order of frequency, by endometrioid, mucinous, and clear cell ovarian tumors (Schuijer and Berns, 2003). Finally, even though *TP53* is one of the best-studied genes in relation to prognosis and prediction of response to (adjuvant) chemotherapy, the information value of its mutation and expression status in this regard remains unclear (Schuijer and Berns, 2003).

In the long arm of chromosome 17, losses at 17q12–21 are frequently observed in ovarian carcinomas (Godwin et al., 1994; Cornelis et al., 1995). The breast and ovarian cancer susceptibility gene *BRCA1* maps to 17q21 and could represent a possible gene target.

Pejovic et al. (1999) determined by CGH the genomic imbalances in a well-differentiated mucinous carcinoma in the left ovary and a Brenner tumor in the right ovary of the same woman. They found the same gain of 12q14–21 in both tumors, admittedly among several disparate other abnormalities, and interpreted this as an indication that the tumors were clonally related and, hence, that one was derived from the other. This interpretation presupposes that the 12q gain is a primary change shared by all cells of the putative common clone and also that it did not arise through the effect of some carcinogenic factor that, for whatever reason, induced the same change in two separate cells in separate ovaries.

The first recurrent fusion transcript in serous ovarian carcinomas was reported by Salzman et al. (2011) who used deep paired-end sequencing to detect the fusion gene *ESRRA–C11orf20* in 10 out of 67 (15%) serous ovarian carcinomas examined. The fusion was brought about by rearrangements in the long arm of chromosome 11, in subband 11q13.1. On the other hand, Micci et al. (2014b) found no such fusion transcript in 230 ovarian carcinomas analyzed by RT-PCR and concluded that the frequency of *ESRRA–C11orf20* in serous ovarian carcinomas must be considerably lower than that reported previously (0/163 in their experience compared with 10/67 in the previous study).

The Cancer Genome Atlas (TCGA) Research Network (TCGA, 2011) has conducted a large study covering several aspects of ovarian cancer genetics inasmuch as they analyzed messenger RNA expression, microRNA (miRNA) expression, promoter methylation, DNA copy number in 489 high-grade serous ovarian adenocarcinomas, and the DNA sequence of exons from coding genes in 316 of these tumors. The analyses delineated four ovarian cancer transcriptional subtypes, three miRNA subtypes, four promoter methylation subtypes, and a transcriptional signature associated with survival duration. No karyotypic information on the tumors was available nor was this aspect paid attention to in the TCGA study.

Ten cytogenetically abnormal *mixed mesodermal tumors* and/or *carcinosarcomas* of the ovary have been reported (Atkin and Pickthall, 1977; Atkin and Baker, 1987a; Tanaka et al., 1989; Pejovic et al., 1990b, 1996a; Fletcher et al., 1991b; Guan et al., 1995). All had massive numerical as well as structural changes. The data are too sparse to say whether the karyotypic characteristics of these tumors in any systematic way set them apart from other ovarian malignancies.

Around 80 ovarian *thecomas–thecofibromas–fibromas* have been cytogenetically characterized using karyotyping and/or molecular cytogenetic techniques. The largest series were reported by Streblow et al. (2007) and Micci et al. (2008). Trisomy and/or tetrasomy 12 is the most common chromosomal aberration (Pejovic et al., 1990a; Fletcher et al., 1991a; Taruscio et al., 1993; Persons et al., 1994; Shashi et al., 1994; Liang et al., 2001; Streblow et al., 2007; Micci et al., 2008); however, other aneuploidies are also seen, including trisomies for chromosomes 4, 9, 10, and 18 (Pejovic et al., 1990a; Mrozek et al., 1992; Smith et al., 2002; Streblow et al., 2007; Micci et al., 2008). Monosomies are observed less often (Streblow et al., 2007; Micci et al., 2008). The strictly nonrandom occurrence of these aneuploidies indicates that they play a major pathogenetic role, but how they contribute to tumorigenesis remains unknown. Gain of chromosome 12 is not, however, specific to tumors of this group even in the ovarian context, as it has also been seen in some benign and borderline epithelial tumors (see the preceding text) as well as in granulosa cell tumors (see the following text). The aberration is by no means organ specific, furthermore, since +12 also occurs nonrandomly, and often as the only cytogenetic change, in chronic lymphocytic leukemia, various nonovarian adenocarcinomas, Wilms' tumor, and LM.

Some chromosome banding and molecular cytogenetic analyses have shown that trisomy 12 is a recurrent aberration also in adult *granulosa cell tumors* (Leung et al., 1990; Fletcher et al., 1991a; Halperin et al., 1995), but other studies could not corroborate this conclusion (Persons et al., 1994; Shashi et al., 1994). Persons et al. (1994) suggested that +12 might be more typical of the juvenile form of this tumor and that, hence, different genetic events were involved in the two forms. The finding of monosomy 22 together with trisomy 14 (Lindgren et al., 1996; Van den Berghe et al., 1999; Namiq et al., 2005) led to the hypothesis that −22 followed by acquisition of an extra chromosome 14 could be tumorigenic events in the adult-type tumors. Later reports based on CGH analyses (Mayr et al., 2002; Lin et al., 2005; Mayr et al., 2008) confirmed the high frequency of monosomy 22 in adult granulosa cell tumors, often in association with trisomy 14. Trisomy 12 occurs at lower frequencies.

Some 40 *ovarian teratomas*, both mature and immature, have been karyotyped and shown to harbor chromosome abnormalities. Most of the tumors had a hyperdiploid karyotype with mostly numerical changes. Trisomy 3 was the most frequent aberration, found either as the sole abnormality (Yang-Feng et al., 1988; Lorenzato et al., 1993; Mertens et al., 1998; Bussey et al., 1999) or together with other aberrations (King et al., 1985, 1990; Hoffner et al., 1992; Rodriguez et al., 1995; Bussey et al., 2001). Brassesco et al. (2009) reported a tumor with a t(3;20)(q27;q13.3) and a del(3)(q27) as the sole abnormality in two unrelated clones. Other whole-chromosome gains, in decreasing order of frequency, have been of chromosomes 8, 14, and 12. An isochromosome for the short arm of chromosome 12, i(12p), was reported in few cases. The finding of this isochromosome in different types of germ cell tumor and in both sexes (Speleman et al., 1990, 1992) suggests a common pathogenetic pathway irrespective of the exact eventual phenotype for several germ cell tumors.

Four *seminomas/dysgerminomas* arising in the ovary and harboring chromosome aberrations have been reported. The karyotypes were in the triploid range with many numerical and structural aberrations. An i(12)(p10) was seen in three tumors (Atkin and Baker, 1987a; Jenkyn and McCartney, 1987; Wehle et al., 2008), whereas the fourth tumor showed an add(12)(q11) among other abnormalities (Dal Cin et al., 1996).

Less than 40 dysgerminomas have been characterized by CGH. The major imbalances were gains of 12p, 21q, and the entire chromosome 8 but loss of 13q (Riopel et al., 1998; Kraggerud et al., 2000; Zahn et al., 2006). Gains of 1p, 6p, 12q, 20q, 22q, and the entire chromosomes 7, 17, and 19 were reported at lower frequencies (Kraggerud et al., 2000). CGH analysis of around ten cases of endodermal sinus tumor (Kraggerud et al., 2000) detected gain of 12p as the most frequent aberration, whereas immature teratomas showed gains of chromosome arms 1p and 16p as well as of chromosomes 19 and 22. Based on these findings and literature data, Kraggerud et al. (2000) suggested that the presence of i(12p) in both male (Chapter 18) and female germ cell tumors and the finding of similar, presumably secondary, changes in both, that is, +7, +8, +12, +21, and −13, indicate that these tumors evolve through largely identical pathogenetic mechanisms in both sexes. On the other hand, immature teratomas appear to develop through a different pathway inasmuch as these tumors typically are diploid and do not have i(12p) or other imbalances of chromosome 12. It has also been pointed out that the gain of 12p occurs equally frequently in adult and pediatric cases (Riopel et al., 1998; Kraggerud et al., 2000). Finally, Riopel et al. (1998) reported a case of bilateral dysgerminoma whose imbalance pattern suggested that the contralateral tumor was a metastasis.

A single case of ovarian *ependymoma* with chromosome abnormalities has been reported. It showed a hyperdiploid karyotype with only numerical aberrations, namely, trisomies for chromosomes 5, 8, 19, 20, and 21 and tetrasomies for chromosomes 7 and 13 (Yang-Feng et al., 1988). Also a karyotypically abnormal *endomyometriosis tumor* of the ovary has been reported (Verhest et al., 1996). The only rearrangement was a deletion of the distal part of 2p with breakpoint in 2p21.

Only one *angiosarcoma* of the ovary has been reported with cytogenetic aberrations (Fletcher et al., 1991b). It showed a single balanced translocation involving 1q11 and 3p11 and trisomies for chromosomes 3 and 12.

A single case of *peripheral primitive neuroecto-dermal tumor* (pPNET), which belongs to the PNET/Ewing sarcoma family (see Chapters 23 and 24), arising in the left ovary has been reported (Kawauchi et al., 1998). The typical translocation t(11;22)(q24;q12) was found.

A *fibrosarcoma* arising in the ovary was analyzed by Dal Cin et al. (1998). The tumor had a hyperdiploid karyotype with trisomies for chromosomes 3, 8, 9, 12, and 13 and a der(16)t(12;16)(q13;q13) as the sole structural rearrangement.

Of the four *Sertoli–Leydig cell tumors* that have been karyotypically reported, three showed only a single aberration, trisomy 12 (Taruscio et al., 1993), trisomy 8 (Manegold et al., 2001), and an isochromosome of the long arm of chromosome 1 (Pejovic et al., 1993). The fourth tumor had a hyperdiploid karyotype with both structural and numerical aberrations; among them, trisomy 12 was noted. Molecular investigation of the tumor showed overexpression of the *BCL2* gene (Truss et al., 2004). A fifth tumor was analyzed by CGH and FISH by Verdorfer et al. (2007); it showed loss of chromosome 8 and gains of chromosomes 19 and 22. Finally, Patael-Karasik et al. (2000) analyzed by CGH a Sertoli cell tumor and found gain of 1q and the entire chromosome 6 but loss of 7q.

A *pseudomyxoma* was studied for imbalances by Patael-Karasik et al. (2000). It showed a normal profile.

Uterus

The main neoplastic conditions in this organ are the carcinomas and their precursor lesions in the uterine cervix and, in the uterine body, the myometrial leiomyomas (LM) and sarcomas and the endometrial polyps (EP) and carcinomas. But cytogenetic information nevertheless exists also on some less common entities, including mixed epithelial and mesenchymal tumors and uterine tumors with trophoblastic differentiation.

Uterine corpus

LM are the most common neoplasms of the female genital tract. Since the first reports of chromosomal aberrations in uterine LM 25 years ago (Gibas et al., 1988; Heim et al., 1988; Turc-Carel et al., 1988), some 450 such tumors with abnormal

karyotypes have been described. Large series were reported by Mark et al. (1988, 1990), Nilbert et al. (1988b, 1990a), Kiechle-Schwarz et al. (1991), Vanni et al. (1991), Pandis et al. (1991), Meloni et al. (1992), Stern et al. (1992), Kataoka et al. (2003), and Quade et al. (2003). The pathogenetic and clinical heterogeneity of LM is reflected in the variable cytogenetic findings in these tumors; however, within that heterogeneity, several chromosomally well-defined groups can still be identified (Nilbert et al., 1990a; Pandis et al., 1991) characterized by the presence of t(12;14)(q15;q23–24); del(7)(q21.2q31.2); rearrangements involving 6p21, 10q, and 1p; trisomy 12; deletions of 3q; and changes of the X chromosome. Although no relationship between patient age or parity and the type of chromosomal aberration is apparent, there might exist a positive correlation between the presence of a cytogenetic abnormality and the anatomical location of uterine LM, that is, intramural and serous tumors may be more likely to have abnormal karyotypes than do those of the submucosal type (Brosens et al., 1996, 1998). Another study showed a relationship between karyotype and tumor size, with the largest tumors more often carrying a t(12;14) (Rein et al., 1998). In contrast, tumors with del(7q) were found to be smaller, whereas those with mosaic karyotypes tended to be intermediate in size.

The most common chromosomal aberration in LM, seen in approximately 20% of karyotypically abnormal tumors, is a *t(12;14)(q14–15;q23–24)* (Figure 17.2; Heim et al., 1988; Turc-Carel et al., 1988; Meloni et al., 1992). Alternative rearrangements of 12q14–15, such as paracentric inversions, have also been observed (Vanni et al., 1989; Wanschura et al., 1997; Bullerdiek and Rommel, 1999), and some LM with apparently normal karyotypes have been shown to have cryptic inversions of 12q (Wanschura et al., 1997; Weremowicz and Morton, 1999). In addition, 12q14–15 can also be found rearranged through translocations with chromosomes 1, 5, 8, and 10 (Quade et al., 2003). Frequent secondary changes in LM carrying a t(12;14) are rearrangements of chromosome 1, including ring formation, del(7q), and monosomy 22 (Nilbert et al., 1988a; Pandis et al., 1990).

An interstitial deletion of 7q, *del(7)(q21.2q31.2)* (Figure 17.3), is seen almost as often as the t(12;14)

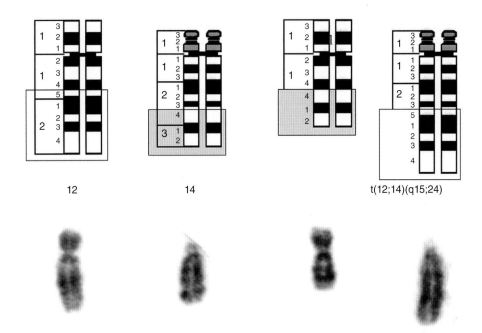

Figure 17.2 A balanced translocation t(12;14)(q14–15;q23–24) is the most characteristic chromosomal rearrangement in uterine leiomyomas.

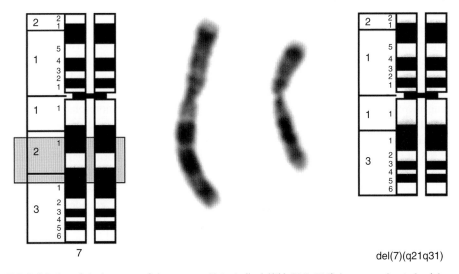

Figure 17.3 A deletion of the long arm of chromosome 7, typically del(7)(q21.2q31.2), is common in uterine leiomyomas. It may occur secondarily during clonal evolution and is also seen as the sole anomaly.

in LM (Boghosian et al., 1988; Nilbert and Heim, 1990; Pandis et al., 1991; Ozisik et al., 1993a; Sargent et al., 1994). The finding of this abnormality as the sole change in some tumors indicates its role as an early, possibly primary, event (Ligon and Morton, 2000). However, del(7q) may also be associated with t(12;14) or t(1;6) (Nilbert et al., 1989), suggesting that its involvement is sometimes secondary.

Rearrangements of 6p21 have been seen in 6% of karyotypically abnormal LM. The most frequent aberrations have been t(1;6)(q32;p21), t(6;14) (p21;q24), and t(6;10)(p21;q22) (Sornberger et al., 1999; Nezhad et al., 2010), but also inversions and translocations with other chromosomal partners were detected (Nilbert et al., 1989; Kiechle-Schwarz et al., 1991; Ozisik et al., 1993b; Sornberger et al., 1999). The 6p21 changes have been seen both as the sole anomaly and together with other abnormalities, including del(7q).

Trisomy 12 is the fourth of the common (frequency around 5%) LM-associated chromosomal aberrations (Nilbert and Heim, 1990; Nilbert et al., 1990b). The nonrandom occurrence of chromosome 12 abnormalities both as a 12q rearrangement and as gain of one entire copy raises the question whether there is any pathogenetic similarity between the two situations. Trisomy 12 is otherwise seen as the sole anomaly particularly in benign and borderline ovarian tumors (see the preceding text) and in B-cell chronic lymphatic leukemia; no biological connection between uterine LM and these two other neoplastic conditions is apparent. Occasionally, clonal evolution is seen in cells carrying +12 as the primary chromosome abnormality. The secondary changes do not then seem to differ from those observed when t(12;14) is the primary aberration (Nilbert et al., 1988a; Pandis et al., 1990); both rearrangements of chromosome 1, including ring formation, del(7q), and monosomy 22 have been seen repeatedly.

Rearrangements of chromosome 10, including monosomy 10 and deletions of 10q (often with breakpoints in 10q22), have also been reported in nearly 5% of uterine LM (Ozisik et al., 1993b, 1994, 1995); they too seem to represent a minor cytogenetic subset of these tumors.

Christacos et al. (2006) reported nine near-diploid uterine LM that showed loss of almost the entire short arm of chromosome 1, described as del(1)(p11p36). The loss of 1p was frequently seen together with other karyotypic aberrations in their study, particularly loss of chromosomes 19 and/or 22. Other rearrangements of both the long and short arms of chromosome 1 have also been described in histologically typical uterine LM, with breakpoints distributed along both arms. Many of these rearrangements give the impression of being random and include deletions, inversions, and various translocations, some of which have been complex (http://cgap.

nci.nih.gov/Chromosomes/Mitelman). The best candidate for a nonrandom chromosome 1 abnormality in uterine LM seems to be rearrangement of 1p36 (Vanni et al., 1990). Finally, a ring chromosome 1 without precise delineation of the breakpoints on either arm has been noted together with other more typical changes, including a t(12;14)(q14–15;q23–24), and represents a route of clonal evolution in these tumors (Nilbert et al., 1988a; Polito et al., 1999; Gross et al., 2004).

A number of rearrangements of chromosome 3 have been observed in uterine LM, both as the sole abnormality and together with other rearrangements. Among them are del(3)(p14), del(3)(q24), del(3)(q13q27, t(3;7)(p11;p11), and ins(2;3)(q31;p12p25) (Nilbert et al., 1990a; Dal Cin et al., 1995a).

Many rearrangements of the X chromosome have also been observed, albeit each aberration only infrequently. These changes include add(X)(q26), del(X)(p11), del(X)(q12), del(X)(q22), der(5)t(X;5)(p11;p15), der(X)t(X;3)(p22;q11), inv(X)(p22q13), t(X;11)(p11;p15), t(X;12)(p22;q15), t(X;22)(p11;p11), t(X;3;14)(q26q27;q22), t(X;5;14)(q2?4;p15;q24), and –X (http://cgap.nci.nih.gov/Chromosomes/Mitelman). The region Xp11–22 has been claimed to be preferentially involved in these abnormalities (Ligon and Morton, 2000).

Locus-specific probes have been utilized in FISH analyses to describe more precisely the chromosomal breakpoints at 12q14–15, 6p21, 7q, 10q, and 14q in LM and to identify the genes involved. At 12q15, the *HMGA2* (formerly *HMG1-C*) gene was found rearranged using YAC probes (Schoenberg Fejzo et al., 1996). This is a highly evolutionarily conserved gene that encodes an architectural factor belonging to the heterogeneous high-mobility group of nonhistone DNA-binding proteins (Ashar et al., 1996; Bustin and Reeves, 1996; Schoenmakers and Van de Ven, 1997). LM with t(12;14) show breaks mapping from as near as 10 kb to more than 100 kb upstream of the coding region of *HMGA2* (Schoenberg Fejzo et al., 1996).

The t(12;14)(q15;q24) has been hypothesized to create pathogenetically significant fusion transcripts derived from *HMGA2* and *RAD51L* in 14q (see also the following text; Ingraham et al., 1999; Schoenmakers et al., 1999; Takahashi et al., 2001). However, the finding of breaks also outside but near *HMGA2* and the results reached by analysis using the rapid amplification of cDNA ends polymerase chain reaction (RACE-PCR) indicate that the formation of a fusion transcript may not be the principal tumorigenic mechanism for uterine LM with this translocation. Instead, dysregulated expression of *HMGA2*, most often achieved by translocation of chromosome 14 sequences to 5′ of this gene (Quade et al., 2003), may be the important outcome. Dysregulated expression of *HMGA2* through a gene dosage mechanism has also been suggested to be the crucial effect of trisomy 12 (Quade et al., 2003; Sandberg, 2005). Enhancement of *HMGA2* after translocation may be a result of altered chromatin structure transmitted from the translocation partner. Klemke et al. (2009) showed that the highest expression level for *HMGA2* was observed in tumors with 12q rearrangements, but although *HMGA2* is expressed at lower levels in LM without such changes or with normal karyotypes, comparison between the expression in myomas and matching myometrial tissue indicates a general upregulation of *HMGA2* regardless of the presence/absence of 12q abnormalities. This suggests a general role of *HMGA2* in the development of fibroids.

The chromosome 14 breakpoint in uterine LM has been mapped within the DNA repair gene *RAD51L1* (also known as *RAD51B*), which spans a large genomic region of ~680 kb (Ingraham et al., 1999; Schoenmakers et al., 1999). RAD51L1 plays a role in DNA repair recombination (Takahashi et al., 2001) and may be essential for cell proliferation (Shu et al., 1999). Chimeric transcripts encoding a *RAD51L1–HMGA2* fusion gene have been detected in some studies (Schoenmakers et al, 1999; Takahashi et al, 2001) but not in others (Quade et al, 2003). Although it is the most common translocation partner, *RAD51L1* clearly is not the only gene recombining with *HMGA2* in uterine LM. Other fusion transcripts for *HMGA2* have been identified in at least five LM: the *COG5* gene at 7q31 (Velagaleti et al., 2010), the *COX6C* gene at 8q22–23 (Kurose et al., 2000), the *ALDH2* gene at 12q24 (Kazmierczak et al., 1995), the *HE110* gene at 14q11 (Mine et al., 2001), and *RTVL-H*-related sequences on chromosome 12 (Kazmierczak et al., 1996).

The *HMGA1* gene in 6p21 belongs to the same family of genes as *HMGA2*. The HMGA1 protein is known to bind to specific AT-rich domains and promoters of a number of genes (Kazmierczak et al., 1995; Kurose et al., 2000; Hauke et al., 2001). The rearrangement of *HMGA1* in LM was demonstrated using locus-specific FISH probes in a tumor with inv(6)(p21q15) (Williams et al., 1997). Nezhad et al. (2010) found that upregulation of *HMGA1* due to 6p21 rearrangements is on average 45-fold up to a maximum of 52.4-fold compared to LM with normal karyotypes. Despite the great extent of sequence and structural similarity between the *HMGA2* and *HMGA1* genes (Tallini and Dal Cin, 1999), their expression patterns are strikingly dissimilar, suggesting the existence of distinct regulatory elements as well as different functional roles (Ram et al., 1993; Tamimi et al., 1993; Chiappetta et al., 1995; Kim et al., 1995; Abe et al., 1999).

The minimal common deleted region on 7q in LM with a del(7q), at the cytogenetic level consistently identified as a del(7)(q21.2q31.2), was narrowed down to less than 500 kb by Sell et al. (2005). Although loss of a TSG seems like an attractive possibility for the crucial pathogenetic outcome of the deletion, this has not yet been proven. *HMGA2* was not found expressed in LM with del(7) as the only abnormality, whereas tumors with both t(12;14) and del(7q) did show HMGA2 expression (Hennig et al., 1997b).

Moore et al. (2004) analyzed four uterine LM with 10q rearrangements and found disruption of the *MORF* gene in 10q22 in all of them. MORF is a member of the MYST family of histone acetylases (histone acetyltransferase). Several acute myeloid leukemias (Chapter 6) have been associated with rearrangements of MYST histone acetyltransferases, one of them a translocation t(10;16)(q22;p13) in a case of childhood leukemia resulting in an in-frame fusion of *MORF* and *CBP* (Panagopoulos et al., 2001). Compared with what happens in the hematopoietic malignancies, the disruption of *MORF* in uterine LM appears to be 5′ in the locus (Moore et al., 2004).

A predisposing gene for *multiple leiomyomatosis*, a condition characterized by the combination of multiple uterine LM and benign tumors arising from the erector pili muscles, has been mapped to 1q42.3–43 (Kiuru et al., 2001; Tomlinson et al., 2002; Dal Cin and Morton, 2002). There is no evidence that this gene plays any role in the development of sporadic LM, and visible involvement of this chromosomal region in such tumors is rare (Dal Cin and Morton, 2002).

Six *plexiform LM* have been cytogenetically characterized, with four of them showing aberrations of chromosome 12. FISH using locus-specific probes demonstrated *HMGA2* alteration confirmed by its overexpression detected both at the mRNA level (247- to 66, 467-fold change compared to matched myometrium) and at the protein level (0- to 5-fold change compared to matched myometrium; Hodge et al., 2008).

Disseminated peritoneal leiomyomatosis (DPL) is a rare condition in females characterized by nodular proliferations of histologically benign smooth muscle throughout the omental and peritoneal surfaces (Quade et al., 1997). Cytogenetic studies have revealed abnormal karyotypes in three of seven DPL lesions (Quade et al., 1997; Ordulu et al., 2010). In one lesion, additional material was present on the long arm of chromosome 12 suggesting that the *HMGA2* gene might be involved. In another lesion, a t(7;18)(q22;p11.3) was seen, that is, an alteration of 7q in the middle of the segment commonly deleted in sporadic LM. In the third lesion, GTG-banding and FISH examinations showed the abnormal karyotype 46,XX,r(1)(p34.3q41),del(3)(q23q26.33),del(9)(q2?2),t(12;14)(q14.3;q24.1) (Ordulu et al., 2010). These similarities with karyotypic features of sporadic smooth muscle tumors suggest that DPL and sporadic LM share pathogenetic mechanisms.

About 15 malignant smooth muscle tumors of the uterine wall, *leiomyosarcomas* (LMS), with chromosomal abnormalities have been described. Only three such tumors have shown a simple rearrangement, a t(10;17)(q22;p13) described by Dal Cin et al. (1988), a t(1;5)(p12;q33) described by Fletcher et al. (1991b), and a t(1;6)(p32;p21) reported by Hennig et al. (1996). Most of the other tumors had massively rearranged karyotypes with numerous structural as well as numerical chromosomal rearrangements. Breakpoints were seen in 1q32 in five cases (Fletcher et al., 1990, 1991b; Nilbert et al., 1990c, 1990d; Iliszko et al., 1998) and in near bands, 1q31, 1q41, and 1q42, in one tumor each (Fletcher et al., 1990; Laxman et al., 1993). Another possibly interesting breakpoint cluster mapped to chromosomal band 10q22, which was seen rearranged in four tumors (Dal Cin et al., 1988; Fletcher et al., 1990; Nilbert et al., 1990d; Iliszko et al., 1998) with the nearest neighboring bands, 10q11 and 10q21, rearranged in an additional case each (Iliszko et al., 1998). Chromosomal band 10q22 has also been found rearranged in LM through a 10;17-translocation (Moore et al., 2004) that involved the *MORF* gene. Interestingly, a t(10;17)(q22;p13) leading to the *YWHAE–FAM22* chimeric fusion was lately found in the so-called high-grade endometrial stromal sarcoma (ESS) (Lee et al., 2012). A t(10;17) with a seemingly identical breakpoint on 10q was also reported in a uterine LMS (Fletcher et al., 1990) as part of an incompletely described karyotype with numerous abnormalities, but whether this reflects actual molecular-level similarity is unknown. To date, only two LMS have been seen to harbor rearrangement of chromosomal bands 12q13–15 (Iliszko et al., 1998) and 14q24 (Nilbert et al., 1990c); the evidence for any pathogenetic similarity between benign and malignant smooth muscle tumors thus seems weak at the moment.

CGH studies have shown that uterine LMS mostly present gains of or from chromosome arms Xp, 1q, 5p, 8q, and 17p and losses of or from 2p, 10q, 11q, 12p, 13q, and 16q (Packenham et al., 1997; Levy et al., 2000; Derre et al., 2001; Hu et al., 2001; Raish et al., 2012). LOH analysis has shown loss of at least one marker on chromosome 10, something that was not noted in benign LM (Quade et al., 1999). The same study also showed that microsatellite instability (MSI) was infrequent in LMS.

About 60 *ESS* with chromosome abnormalities have been karyotyped and scientifically reported (http://cgap.nci.nih.gov/Chromosomes/Mitelman). Although a variety of different aberrations have been described, their pattern of occurrence is nevertheless clearly nonrandom (Figure 17.4). Chromosomes 7 and 17 are recombined in the first genetic hallmark to be discovered in ESS, namely, the translocation t(7;17)(p15;q21), which has been described in altogether 13 tumors, in 12 of them as a balanced rearrangement (Sreekantaiah et al., 1991; Fletcher et al., 1991b; Dal Cin et al., 1992a; Pauwels et al., 1996; Hennig et al., 1997a; Koontz et al., 2001; Satoh et al., 2003; Micci et al., 2003b) and in one as a der(7)t(7;17) (Iliszko et al., 1998). Koontz et al.

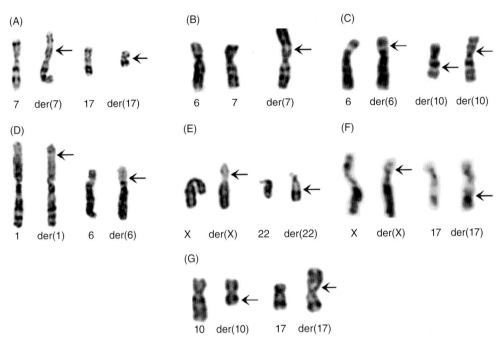

Figure 17.4 Partial karyotypes of different rearrangements found in endometrial stromal sarcomas. Normal chromosomes are presented for comparison. Arrows indicate breakpoints of rearranged chromosomes: (A) t(7;17) (p15;q21), (B) der(7)t(6;7)(p21;p15)del(6)(q21), (C) t(6;10;10)(p21;q22;p11), (D) t(1;6)(p34;p21), (E) t(X;22)(p11;q13), (F) t(X;17)(p11;q23), and (G) t(10;17)(q22;p13).

(2001) demonstrated that two zinc finger genes were recombined by this translocation, the *JAZF1* gene from chromosomal band 7p15 and the *SUZ12* (formerly known as *JJAZ1*) gene from 17q21. In addition to the 7;17-translocation, chromosomal band 7p15–21 was found rearranged in seven ESS with other partners than chromosome 17 (Laxman et al., 1993; Iliszko et al., 1998; Gil-Benso et al., 1999; Micci et al., 2003b, 2006a) suggesting that alternative, pathogenetically equivalent variant translocations exist in this tumor type. Indeed, the first such variant, a t(6;7), was described in two ESS in which a der(7)t(6;7)(p21;p15)del(6)(q21) and a complex derivative chromosome 7 were seen (Micci et al., 2006a). *JAZF1* was found rearranged with the *PHF1* gene from chromosomal band 6p21 in these tumors (Micci et al., 2006a). Band 6p21, which is the third most commonly rearranged band in ESS, was involved in 10 of the reported tumors and with different translocation partners (Fresia et al., 1992; Laxman et al., 1993; Hrynchak et al, 1994; Fuzesi et al., 1995; Gil-Benso et al., 1999; Sonobe et al., 1999; Micci et al., 2003b, 2006a). In four cases, it was

recombined with chromosomal region 7p15–22, and in two of them, the already mentioned *JAZF1–PHF1* fusion gene was identified (Micci et al., 2006a). The consistent involvement of *PHF1* in ESS is further underscored by the demonstration of another seemingly ESS-specific fusion between *PHF1* and the *EPC1* gene from 10p11 in an ESS with a three-way t(6;10;10)(p21;q22;p11) translocation (Micci et al, 2006a). Lately, a new partner mapping to 1p34 was identified, the *MEAF6* gene, recombined through a t(1;6)(p34;p21) (Panagopoulos et al., 2012; Micci et al., 2014a). The involvement of *PHF1* unquestionably defines a pathogenetic subgroup of ESS. Fusion of the *JAZF1*, *SUZ12*, and *PHF1* genes appears to be frequent, although certainly not ubiquitous, in ESS of classic histology but has also been found in other types of endometrial stromal tumors (EST; Chiang et al., 2011).

Chromosomal arm Xp has been found rearranged in seven ESS. Two cases showed an (X;22) (p11;q13) rearrangement, and Panagopoulos et al. (2013) demonstrated the presence of a *ZC3H7B–BCOR* fusion in both. In another two cases with t(X;17)(p11;q23), Dewaele et al. (2014) showed a *MBTD1–Cxorf67* fusion. The last three cases with Xp rearrangement, all reported by Lee et al. (2012), showed complex karyotypes with a del(Xp) and an add(22)(q12–13) among other abnormalities in two cases, whereas the third tumor had an unbalanced X;1-translocation. Since chromosomes X and 22 are rearranged together in two cases, it is likely that these tumors too carry the already mentioned *ZC3H7B–BCOR* fusion.

The cytogenetic literature reports altogether 19 cases with a t(10;17)(q22;p13). The tumors belong to an ESS subtype with more aggressive clinical behavior. Lee et al. (2012) described a *YWHAE–FAM22* chimeric fusion brought about by this rearrangement.

Some ESS show no recurrent chromosomal aberration but carry cryptic rearrangements leading to one of the known fusions characteristic of this tumor type; for example, in one ESS showing an inv(5) as the sole karyotypic rearrangement, an *MEAF6–PHF1*-specific transcript was found (Micci et al., 2014a).

A different approach to the detection of pathogenetic mechanisms operative in EST was taken by Halbwedl et al. (2005) who tested for genomic imbalances nine ESS and three undifferentiated endometrial sarcoma (UES) using CGH. They found a variety of gains and losses that apparently did not correlate with histologic grade. Nor was there any clear-cut increase in copy number changes from ESS to UES, as the average of copy number alterations per case was 3.6 in ESS and 3.0 in UES. The only consistent imbalance seen was loss of chromosomal arm 7p in five cases, with a common overlapping region corresponding to chromosomal band 7p21.

EP (adenomatous) are benign overgrowths of endometrial tissue containing endometrial glands and fibrous stroma. Less than 40 EP have been cytogenetically characterized. As for other benign mesenchymal tumors, the karyotypes are in the diploid range and often present simple chromosomal rearrangements. Different tumor subsets can be distinguished based on whether they have rearrangement of 6p21, 12q13–15, or 7q22. Chromosomal band 6p21 has been found rearranged in 22 tumors (Dal Cin et al., 1991, 1992b, 1995b; Fletcher et al., 1992; Vanni et al., 1995; Kazmierczak et al., 1998). In three

EP, it recombined with chromosomal band 2q35, twice in a balanced two-way translocation (Dal Cin et al, 1995b), in the third case as a t(X;2;6) (Dal Cin et al, 1995b). In another two polyps, 6p21 was recombined with 10q22 in a t(6;10) and a t(6;6;10) (Dal Cin et al., 1995b). Single examples of inversions, duplication, and balanced translocations involving 6p21 with other chromosomal partners have also been reported. Of particular interest may be the finding of two cases with a 2;6;7-translocation (Dal Cin et al., 1995b; Kazmierczak et al., 1998) where the breakpoints involved chromosome bands 2q35, 6p23–25, and 7q22. The nonrandom involvement of chromosomal band 6p21 has been noted in subsets of many benign mesenchymal tumors, including pulmonary chondroid hamartomas, lipomas, and uterine LM (see the preceding text). In all these tumor types, as for EP, the key target gene behind the chromosomal rearrangements appears to be the *HMGA1* (Kazmierczak et al., 1998). Although aberrant *HMGA1* transcripts have been found, most of the breakpoints map outside the gene itself, suggesting that dysregulation of *HMGA1* may be sufficient to induce development of a variety of benign mesenchymal tumors, including EP (Kazmierczak et al., 1998).

Chromosomal region 12q13–15 has been found rearranged in five EP (Vanni et al., 1993, 1995; Dal Cin et al., 1995b; Bol et al., 1996), including a t(12;14)(q15;q24) identical to the translocation seen in uterine LM (Dal Cin et al., 1995b). As in uterine LM, the breakpoint in such rearrangements maps to the *HMGA2* region (Bol et al., 1996).

Chromosomal band 7q22 has been found rearranged in three polyps, in two of them in recombination with 6p, whereas a del(7)(q22q32) was seen in the third (Dal Cin et al., 1995b). Again, the profound karyotypic similarity with LM is obvious (Sreekantaiah and Sandberg, 1991).

More than 100 chromosomally abnormal *endometrial carcinomas* have been reported, the most comprehensive series being those of Milatovich et al. (1990), Sirchia et al. (1997), and Micci et al. (2004). Hyperdiploid karyotypes with simple numerical chromosome aberrations and/or minimal structural rearrangements were seen in two-thirds of the reported tumors, whereas the remainder showed more complex karyotypes with several numerical as well as structural rearrangements.

Chromosome 1 is the most frequently rearranged chromosome in endometrial carcinomas, as indeed in many carcinomas, often with gain of the entire or part of the long arm through an unbalanced translocation and/or isochromosome formation. The most commonly (more than 30%) gained region is 1q21–32. Not only does this 1q change occur frequently in endometrial carcinomas, it sometimes is the only change, which is why Milatovich et al. (1990) and Micci et al. (2004) suggested that it may represent a primary chromosomal abnormality in a subgroup of these tumors.

The second most common aberration is gain of one copy of chromosome 10, found in more than 20% of karyotypically abnormal tumors (Fujita et al., 1985; Dutrillaux and Couturier, 1986; Couturier et al., 1986, 1988; Yoshida et al., 1986; Gibas and Rubin, 1987; Milatovich et al., 1990; Simon et al., 1990; Tharapel et al., 1991; Shah et al., 1994; Bardi et al., 1995; Sirchia et al., 1997; Micci et al., 2004). Although trisomy 10 mostly occurs together with other anomalies, including 1q changes, it has also repeatedly been seen as the sole change (Dutrillaux and Couturier, 1986; Couturier et al., 1986; Milatovich et al., 1990; Simon et al., 1990; Bardi et al., 1995; Sirchia et al., 1997). Also other numerical aberrations are common. Trisomy 7 has been reported in more than 15% of karyotypically abnormal tumors, making it the third most common chromosomal change, and also trisomy 2 and trisomy 12 have been found repeatedly. Again, the aberrations have been seen both alone and together with other abnormalities (Fujita et al., 1985; Dutrillaux and Couturier, 1986; Yoshida et al., 1986; Couturier et al., 1988; Milatovich et al., 1990; Tharapel et al., 1991; Shah et al., 1994; Bardi et al., 1995; Sirchia et al., 1997; Micci et al., 2004). As in other tumor types, the pathogenetic role of trisomies is unknown.

In addition to the breakpoint cluster detected in the centromeric and near-centromeric region of chromosome 1, the centromeres and pericentromeric bands of chromosomes 8, 21, and 22 also seem to be nonrandomly involved. This corresponds to the high frequency of unbalanced whole-arm translocations seen in these carcinomas.

CGH data on nearly 300 endometrial carcinomas have been reported (Sonoda et al., 1997a; Suzuki et al., 1997; Pere et al., 1998b; Suehiro et al., 2000b; Hirasawa et al., 2003; Micci et al., 2004; Muslumanoglu et al., 2005; Levan et al., 2006). The main imbalances are gains of material from 1q and 8q; the different carcinoma subtypes differed with regard to their pattern of copy number changes corresponding to other chromosomal regions. Whereas adenocarcinomas of type I (hormone-dependent tumors) often showed partial losses from 9, 17, and the X chromosome and gains from chromosomes 2 and 10 as additional changes (Sonoda et al., 1997b; Suzuki et al., 1997; Pere et al., 1998b; Suehiro et al., 2000b; Micci et al., 2004), type II adenocarcinomas (i.e., hormone-independent tumors) showed a more complex picture with gains from chromosomes 2, 3, 5, 6, 7, 10, and 20 and losses from chromosomes 5, 17, and the X chromosome (Pere et al., 1998b; Micci et al., 2004). The different histological subtypes, that is, serous papillary and clear cell as well as type I carcinomas of different grade, showed different patterns of genomic imbalances (Sonoda et al., 1997b; Suehiro et al., 2000b; Micci et al., 2004). In general, tumor stage and grade parallel the degree of genomic imbalances, inasmuch as the presence of multiple genomic changes is associated with a less differentiated phenotype. Levan et al. (2006) identified different imbalances in endometrial carcinomas of different stage. Stage I tumors showed gains from 1q, 8q, 19p, and 19q and losses from 4q and 17q. Stage II tumors had gains from 1q, 8p, 10p, and 10q and losses from 5p and 13q. Stage III tumors presented gains from 1q, 7q, 19p, and 19q. Finally, stage IV tumors had gains from 1q, 8p, 8q, 10p, and 10q and losses from 4p, 4q, 5p, and 13q. In the study by Micci et al. (2004), the average number of copy alterations varied between adenocarcinomas of type I, II, and carcinosarcomas, being highest in type II tumors. Of interest is also the study by Suehiro et al. (2000b), in which gains of 8q material were found to correlate with the occurrence of lymph node metastases and losses of or from 9q, 11q, and Xq correlated with an unfavorable prognosis. In the series examined by Levan et al (2006), finally, gains of or from 1q, 18q, 19p, and 20q as well as losses of or from 11q, 13q, and 16q were detected more often in patients who died from their disease.

Also worthy of mention is the CGH study of endometrial hyperplasias by Kiechle et al.

(2000). Genomic imbalances were found in 24 samples out of 47. The most common aberrations were gains from 4q and losses from 1p, 16p, and 20q. The chromosomal imbalances tended to increase in number with the occurrence of cellular atypia.

Carcinosarcomas of the uterus, or malignant mixed Müllerian tumors, are highly malignant tumors composed of a mixture of neoplastic epithelial and mesenchymal elements. Apart from the uterus, such tumors can also arise in the ovaries, fallopian tubes, cervix, vagina, and female peritoneum (Shen et al., 2001; McCluggage, 2002).

Two studies of altogether nearly 40 *carcinosarcomas* have shown that they are chromosomally characterized by overrepresentation of 8q followed in frequency by gains of 1q and losses of 9q (Micci et al., 2004; Schulten et al., 2004). Both reports pointed out that the pattern of genomic imbalances was largely similar to that observed in adenocarcinomas of the uterus, underscoring the central pathogenetic role of the epithelial component in uterine carcinosarcomas. More specifically, Micci et al. (2004) showed that carcinosarcomas whose epithelial component resembled type I endometrial carcinomas exhibited a type I aberration profile, whereas carcinosarcomas with type II carcinoma differentiation had abnormalities similar to those of type II endometrial carcinomas. Finally, homologous carcinosarcomas presented gains from 1p, 1q, 8q, 12q, and 17q as well as losses from 9q and 13q, whereas heterologous tumors showed gains from 1q, 8p, and 8q (Micci et al., 2004). Lately, Chiyoda et al. (2012) compared the gene expression profile of carcinosarcomas, endometrial carcinomas, and uterine sarcomas finding that carcinosarcomas resemble uterine sarcomas more than endometrial carcinomas, with high expression of genes located on chromosome 19. CGH microarray analysis identified amplification of 19p13, 19p12, and 19q13 (Chiyoda et al., 2012). The 19q13 locus includes the *TGFB1* and *AKT2* gene, both of which have been related to epithelial to mesenchymal transition (EMT) in various malignancies (Chaudhury et al., 2010; Ikushima and Miyazono, 2010). Chiyoda et al. (2012) therefore hypothesized that 19q13 amplification, leading to high expression of *TGFB1*, provokes EMT.

Uterine cervix

Cervical carcinoma is the second most common cancer in women worldwide. Chronic infection with human papillomavirus (HPV) is an important predisposing event in the evolution of cervical carcinomas. The incidence of cervical cancer, which is predominantly of the squamous cell type, has markedly declined in many developed countries, mainly due to cytological screening.

Only three cases of *carcinoma in situ* of the uterine cervix have been cytogenetically characterized and reported (Atkin et al., 1983; Sreekantaiah et al., 1987). One had a near-diploid karyotype with some numerical and structural chromosomal aberrations; the other two had massive numerical and structural changes that could only be incompletely described. There were no obvious cytogenetic similarities among the cases beyond the fact that the changes were complex. This is in itself important information; karyotypic complexity alone is evidently not sufficient to explain why some cervical carcinomas invade while others remain *in situ*.

Nearly 100 *invasive cervical carcinomas*, most of them with squamous cell differentiation, have been reported with chromosomal abnormalities, the largest series being reported by Atkin et al. (1990). Most of the cases were incompletely described and often the reports have focused only on the description of a single aberration, usually the presence of an abnormal chromosome 1 (Atkin and Pickthall, 1977; Atkin and Baker, 1979). The cytogenetic knowledge of this tumor type is therefore not only very limited but also biased. Attempts to resolve the complex karyotypes of uterine cervix by multicolor FISH are limited to only a few cases (Brink et al., 2002).

Half of the reported tumors were near diploid, whereas the others had chromosome numbers in the triploid to tetraploid range. Nearly 70% of the tumors showed rearrangement of chromosome 1, mostly as an isochromosome of the long arm, an aberration present also in many other carcinomas. Another frequent aberration was a small metacentric chromosome, possibly an isochromosome for the short arm of chromosome 5 or 4, which was noticed in slightly over 20% of the cases. Chromosome 11 was also found rearranged in 20% of the tumors, mostly by way of unbalanced translocations with different chromosomal partners. Also alterations of chromosome 17 were seen in

20% of the tumors, either as additional material of unknown origin added onto the short arm or as an i(17)(q10). Other chromosomes frequently rearranged (10–15%) were chromosomes 3, 6, 2, and 9.

Chromosomal CGH (cCGH), and increasingly also aCGH, has been utilized to characterize the genomic imbalances of cervical carcinomas more reliably, and data on more than 300 tumors thus analyzed now exist. The largest series were reported by Dellas et al. (1999), Narayan et al. (2003), and Rao et al. (2004). The most common imbalances have been, in decreasing order of frequency, gains of or from chromosome arms 3q, 5p, 1q, 20p, and 20q, whereas losses were scored most frequently of or from chromosome arms 2q, 3p, 4q, 13q, 11q, and 18q. Less frequent imbalances were reported on chromosomes 4, 6, 8, 17, and the X chromosome. High-level amplifications have been found at 3q, 1q, 5p, 20p, and 20q.

Gain of material from 3q seems to be the most frequent aberration detected in these studies. Heselmeyer et al. (1996) found this gain in only one case of severe dysplasia compared with 90% of invasive cervical carcinomas. They therefore proposed that gain of material from chromosome arm 3q occurred at the transition from a premalignant lesion, that is, severe dysplasia/carcinoma *in situ*, to an invasive carcinoma (stage I) and that additional chromosomal aberrations were subsequently acquired during further disease progression to more advanced stages. Kirchhoff et al. (1999), on the other hand, demonstrated 3q gains as well as additional imbalances also in severe dysplasias and opined that this change was more likely to be important for tumor progression. To identify the genes involved in the 3q gains of cervical carcinomas, Ma et al. (2000) combined CGH and molecular techniques. They found that 3q26.3 was a frequently amplified region and that there was a positive correlation between 3q amplification and increased copy number of *PIK3CA*, whose gene product was also excessively expressed. They therefore suggested that *PIK3CA* played an oncogenic role in cervical cancer. Recurrent copy number increases corresponding to genes on chromosome arm 5p have been detected by Heselmeyer et al. (1997); this might correspond to the frequent occurrence of i(5p) alluded to above.

The putative target for these amplifications and lower-level gains remains unknown.

In the study by Dellas et al. (1999), an association between the total number of aberrations and overall survival was found. Furthermore, losses from chromosome arms 18q and 11q were associated with poor prognosis in patients with carcinomas and lymph node metastasis. 9p losses were significantly more frequent in carcinomas with lymph node metastasis than in node-negative tumors.

Narayan et al. (2003) used a combination of CGH and high-resolution LOH deletion mapping of the long arm of chromosome 2 to identify two minimal common deleted regions, at 2q35–36.1 and 2q36.3–37.1, in cervical carcinomas. They also found evidence of downregulated expression of the 2q genes *CFLAR*, *CASP10*, and *PPP1R7*, admittedly in cervical cancer cell lines.

Array-based CGH was used in some studies to delineate more precisely the nature of genomic imbalances observed in cervical cancer. Hidalgo et al. (2005) found that the most common gains in invasive carcinomas included the *RBP1–RBP2* gene at 3q21–22 and the *DAB2* gene at 5p13, whereas losses particularly often involved the *FHIT* gene at 3p14, the *KIT* gene at 4q11q12, *EIF43* at 4q24, and *RBI* at 13q14. Wilting et al. (2006) found that the common SCCs of the uterine cervix showed significantly more gains than did cervical adenocarcinomas; this particularly applied to gains of 3q12–28. However, the limited number of tumors analyzed (nine with squamous cell and seven with adenodifferentiation) makes this result highly tentative. A detailed more recent analysis of copy number increases at 20q showed high-level amplification at 20q11–12, more specifically of the *DNMT3* and *TOP1* genes, in cervical carcinomas (Wilting et al., 2006). Narayan et al. (2007) used a combination of cDNA aCGH, expression arrays, and semiquantitative RT-PCR to identify upregulated expression in cervical cancer relative to normal controls. Particularly high expression was found for *AIM2* mapping on 1q22–23; *RFC4*, *MUC4*, and *HRASLS* on 3q27–29; *SKP2* on 5p12–13; and *UBE2C* on 20q13.1, in addition to other genes in other locations. Wilting et al. (2006) showed that chromosomal gain of 1q, 3q, and 20q resulted in increased expression of genes located at 1q32.1–32.2, 3q13.32–23, 3q26.32–27.3, and 20q11.21–13.33. The 3q gains led to overexpression of *DTX3L*, *PIK3R4*, *ATP2C1*, and *SLC25A36* within 3q21.1–23. The 11q loss was refined as 11q22.3–25.

A single *large cell neuroendocrine carcinoma* of the uterine cervix was reported by Kawauchi et al. (2005). CGH-detected genomic imbalances included gains from 3q and 15q as well as losses from 2q, 18q, and of the entire chromosome 19.

Also, a cytogenetically characterized *alveolar soft part sarcoma* of the uterine cervix has been reported. It showed a simple karyotype with a del(X)(p11) and a der(17)t(X;17)(p11;q25) as the sole abnormalities (Heimann et al., 1998). Ladanyi et al. (2001) demonstrated that in such tumors, admittedly of other sites, the unbalanced X;17-translocation leads to an *ASPL–TFE3* fusion gene (Chapter 24).

Finally, an *embryonal rhabdomyosarcoma* of the uterine cervix with chromosomal abnormalities was reported by Palazzo et al. (1993). It presented a hyperdiploid karyotype with two related clones. The stemline had a deletion of the short arm of chromosome 1 and trisomy for chromosomes 1, 13 and 18. The sideline also showed additional trisomies for chromosomes 2 and 8.

Fallopian tube

Tumors of the fallopian tube are much less common than the corresponding ovarian neoplasms; however, histologically the same surface epithelial–stromal tumor subtypes are recognized. Fallopian tube carcinomas may occur as a component of the hereditary breast–ovarian cancer syndrome caused by *BRCA1* and *BRCA2* germline mutations.

The only *adenocarcinoma* arising in this organ that has been characterized by banding techniques showed a hypodiploid karyotype with several structural as well as numerical aberrations (Bardi et al., 1994). An unusual feature was the presence of triradial and quadriradial figures, something that was noted also in two tumors analyzed before the introduction of banding techniques (Curcio, 1966; Weise and Buttner, 1972).

About 70 primary fallopian tube carcinomas have been analyzed by cCGH and aCGH (Heselmeyer et al., 1998; Pere et al., 1998a; Snijders et al., 2003; Nowee et al., 2007; Chene et al., 2013). The most consistent DNA gains mapped to chromosome arms 1q, 3q, 5p, 7q, 8q, 12p, 19p, 19q, and 20q, whereas losses mapped to 4q, 5q, 8p, 16q, 17p, and 18q. High-level amplifications were scored at 3q with the smallest amplicon in 3q25qter. The aCGH study by Snijders et al. (2003) narrowed down this area to two regions in 3q25–26 and 3q26–27. Heselmeyer et al. (1998) saw a difference between the only carcinoma with endometrioid histology examined by them and the remaining 11 serous papillary carcinomas. The former showed only six aberrations that were either whole-chromosome or whole-chromosome-arm aberrations. Furthermore, it was the only tumor that did not show gain of 3q. The chromosomal imbalances reported by Heselmeyer et al. (1998) are in agreement with the pattern of chromosomal aberrations observed by karyotyping by Bardi et al. (1994), specifically as regards loss of 1p34pter, an iso(8)(q10), and losses of chromosomes 16, 17, 18, and 22. Chene et al. (2013) compared imbalances detected by aCGH in nine tubes with dysplasia and 12 serous tubal intraepithelial carcinomas finding common losses in 6p21 and 11q12. By and large, the pattern of aberrations in this tumor type therefore seems to be similar to that reported for other gynecological cancers, in particular carcinomas of the ovary.

Vagina and vulva

Tumors of the vagina and vulva account for less than 5% of all female genital tract cancer. SCC represents more than 70% of the cases in both locales, followed by melanoma, basal cell carcinoma, Paget's disease, and other carcinoma subtypes.

About 40 *SCCs* of the vulva and vagina have been cytogenetically reported, most of them with complex karyotypes (Worsham et al., 1991; Teixeira et al., 1999; Micci et al., 2003a, 2013). The most common chromosomal imbalances detected have been, in decreasing order of frequency, gains of chromosomal bands 8q11–24, 7p11–12, 7p21–22, 7p13–15, 7q11–36, 5p15, and 5p11–14 and losses of 8p22–23, 8p21, 3p12, 8p11, 3p11, 3p13, 8p12, 3p14, 3p21–26, 18q23, Xp21–22, 5q11–12, 11q23, 11q25, and 18q22. Breakpoint clusters were seen in 11q23, 19p13, 19q13, 9p24, 11p11, 11q13, and

11q21 as well as in the centromeric and pericentro-meric bands of chromosomes 3, 5, 8, and 14. CGH data have been reported on less than 40 vulvar SCCs (Jee et al., 2001; Allen et al., 2002; Micci et al., 2003a), while aCGH data are limited to 13 cases (Micci et al., 2013); the latter study also included microarray analysis of the tumors. The main imbalances were gain of, or from, 3q, 5p, and 8q and loss of, or from, 3p, 4p, 5q, 8p, 9q, qnd 11q. The chromosomal region lost on 3p could be defined more precisely to 3p14.2 by aCGH, that is, the area where the fragile histidine triad (*FHIT*) gene is located (Micci et al., 2013).

Only three cases of *Paget's disease* of the vulva with cytogenetic abnormalities have been described (Teixeira et al., 1999; Micci et al., 2003a). The tumor reported by Teixeira et al. (1999) had three cytogenetically unrelated clones. The other two cases presented two seemingly unrelated clones, one with gain of chromosome 7 as the sole change and the other with loss of the X chromosome either alone or, in one case, together with other and more complex aberrations (Micci et al., 2003a).

A single *adenoid cystic carcinoma of the Bartholin's gland* has been described (Kiechle-Schwarz et al., 1992), showing structural aberrations of chromosomes 1, 4, 6, 11, 14, and 22.

Both simple and complex karyotypes were detected in the five vulvar *malignant melanomas* that have been described (Teixeira et al., 1999; Micci et al., 2003a). Chromosomes 1, 18, and X seemed to be preferentially involved with a breakpoint cluster seen in 1q11–41. Of the two malignant melanomas arising in the vagina that have been cytogenetically characterized, one had an unbalanced 1;8-translocation (Grammatico et al., 1993), while the other presented a near-triploid karyotype with both structural and numerical aberrations (Micci et al., 2003a).

In the five *embryonal rhabdomyosarcomas* of the vagina that have been described cytogenetically (Van den Berg et al., 1992; Kadan-Lottick et al., 2000; Chen et al., 2001; Clawson et al., 2001; Manor et al., 2009), numerical aberrations were more common than structural ones. The most common changes were +8, +13, +2, and +19.

Cytogenetic studies have revealed clonal chromosomal abnormalities in eight *aggressive angiomyxomas* (also termed angioleiomyoma and vascular LM). This is a soft tissue neoplasm with a predilection for the pelvis and peritoneum, and the exact site was not part of the description in all cases. Six tumors had abnormalities involving chromosome 12, including one case with monosomy 12 among other changes (Horsman et al., 1991), and the other five cases showed involvement of 12q13–15 (Betz et al., 1995; Kazmierczak et al., 1998; Nucci et al., 2001; Micci et al., 2006b; Medeiros et al., 2007). The last two tumors showed monosomy of the X chromosome (Kenny-Moynihan et al., 1996) and a t(5;8)(p15;q22) (Tsuji et al., 2007) as the sole karyotypic change. The cases of Kazmierczak et al. (1998), Nucci et al. (2001), Micci et al. (2006b), and Medeiros et al. (2007) of aggressive angiomyxomas with an inv(12)(p11.2q15), t(8;12)(p12;q15), t(11;12)(q23;q15), and t(1;12)(p32;q15), respectively, are of particular interest due to the involvement of 12q15 resulting in aberrant *HMGA2* expression.

The only two cytogenetically characterized vaginal *LM* showed a balanced 7;8-translocation (Horton et al., 2006) and an inv(12)(p12q13–14) (Guardiola et al., 2010) as the only chromosomal change.

Debiec-Rychter et al. (2000) described an *epithelioid sarcoma* in the vagina with multiple structural and numerical chromosomal aberrations.

A single *synovial sarcoma* arising in the vagina has been described with a X;18-translocation (Knight et al., 1992).

Postoperative spindle cell nodule is a localized, nonneoplastic, reparative lesion composed of closely packed proliferating spindle cells and capillaries simulating an LMS. A single *postoperative spindle cell nodule*, arising in the vulva, has been cytogenetically characterized (Micci et al., 2007). Trisomy 7 was the sole karyotypic abnormality.

Summary

Most ovarian carcinomas have complex karyotypes. Chromosomal arms preferentially involved in structural rearrangements include 1p, 1q, 3p, 3q, 6q, 7p, 9q, 11p, 11q, 17q, 19p, and 19q. Unknown material added to 19p and/or 19q may be particularly frequent. Common imbalances detected by CGH have been gains from 1q, 3q, 8q, 12p, and 20q and losses from 4p, 4q, 8p, 13q, 16q, 18q, and Xp.

Well-differentiated carcinomas seem to have simpler karyotypes, even sometimes with +12 as the sole anomaly, although trisomy 12 is more characteristic of benign ovarian tumors. Molecular cytogenetic studies of borderline carcinomas have shown loss of 6q material and sometimes gain of chromosome 12.

The most common abnormalities in uterine LM are t(12;14)(q14–15;q23–24), del(7)(q21.2q31.2), rearrangements of 6p21, and trisomy 12. The molecular events behind these rearrangements are partially known and include the *HMGA2–RAD51L* fusion for the t(12;14) and involvement of *HMGA1* for the 6p21 aberrations. Sometimes, the target genes in 6p and 12q appear to be upregulated rather than involved in fusions. Endometrial stromal sarcomas often show a t(7;17)(p15;q21) leading to a *JAZF1–SUZ12* fusion, but also other specific translocations leading to fusion genes are known. The subgroup of ESS with more aggressive behavior (high-grade ESS) seems to be characterized by a t(10;17)(q22;p13) leading to a *YWHAE–FAM22* fusion transcript. Among EP, different tumor subsets can be distinguished based on whether they have rearrangement of 6p21, 12q13–15, or 7q22. Chromosome 1 is the most commonly rearranged chromosome in endometrial carcinomas, detected both by karyotyping and CGH analysis. The cervical carcinomas that have been cytogenetically characterized showed complex karyotypes. CGH analyses on these tumors have detected gains of or from 1q, 3q, 5p, 20p, and 20q and losses of or from 2q, 3p, 4q, 13q, 11q, and 18q.

Acknowledgment

Financial support from the Norwegian Cancer Society is gratefully acknowledged.

References

Abe N, Watanabe T, Sugiyama M, Uchimura H, Chiappetta G, Fusco A, et al. (1999): Determination of high mobility group I(Y) expression level in colorectal neoplasias: a potential diagnostic marker. *Cancer Res* 59:1169–1174.

Allen DG, Hutchins AM, Hammet F, White DJ, Scurry JP, Tabrizi SN, et al. (2002): Genetic aberrations detected by comparative genomic hybridisation in vulvar cancers. *Br J Cancer* 86:924–928.

Åman P, Pejovic T, Wennborg A, Heim S, Mitelman F (1993): Mapping of the 19p13 breakpoint in an ovarian carcinoma between the INSR and TCF3 loci. *Genes Chromosomes Cancer* 8:134–136.

Arnold N, Hagele L, Walz L, Schempp W, Pfisterer J, Bauknecht T, et al. (1996): Overrepresentation of 3q and 8q material and loss of 18q material are recurrent findings in advanced human ovarian cancer. *Genes Chromosomes Cancer* 16:46–54.

Ashar HR, Cherath L, Przybysz KM, Chada K (1996): Genomic characterization of human HMGIC, a member of the accessory transcription factor family found at translocation breakpoints in lipomas. *Genomics* 31:207–214.

Atkin NB, Baker MC (1979): Chromosome 1 in 26 carcinomas of the cervix uteri: structural and numerical changes. *Cancer* 44:604–613.

Atkin NB, Baker MC (1987a): Abnormal chromosomes including small metacentrics in 14 ovarian cancers. *Cancer Genet Cytogenet* 26:355–361.

Atkin NB, Baker MC (1987b): One or two double minutes in three carcinomas. *Cancer Genet Cytogenet* 25:189–190.

Atkin NB, Pickthall VJ (1977): Chromosomes 1 in 14 ovarian cancers. Heterochromatin variants and structural changes. *Hum Genet* 38:25–33.

Atkin NB, Baker MC, Ferti-Passantonopoulou A (1983): Chromosome changes in early gynecologic malignancies. *Acta Cytol* 27:450–453.

Atkin NB, Baker MC, Fox MF (1990): Chromosome changes in 43 carcinomas of the cervix uteri. *Cancer Genet Cytogenet* 44:229–241.

Augustus M, Bruderlein S, Gebhart E (1986): Cytogenetic and cell cycle studies in metastatic cells from ovarian carcinomas. *Anticancer Res* 6:283–289.

Bardi G, Sukhikh T, Pandis N, Holund B, Heim S (1994): Complex karyotypic abnormalities in a primary carcinoma of the fallopian tube. *Genes Chromosomes Cancer* 10:207–209.

Bardi G, Pandis N, Schousboe K, Holund B, Heim S (1995): Near-diploid karyotypes with recurrent chromosome abnormalities characterize early-stage endometrial cancer. *Cancer Genet Cytogenet* 80:110–114.

Bayani J, Brenton JD, Macgregor PF, Beheshti B, Albert M, Nallainathan D, et al. (2002): Parallel analysis of sporadic primary ovarian carcinomas by spectral karyotyping, comparative genomic hybridization, and expression microarrays. *Cancer Res* 62:3466–3476.

Bello MJ, Rey JA (1990): Chromosome aberrations in metastatic ovarian cancer: relationship with abnormalities in primary tumors. *Int J Cancer* 45:50–54.

Betz JL, Meloni AM, U'Ren LA, Moore GE, Sandberg AA (1995): Cytogenetic findings in a case of aggressive angiomyxoma of the vaginal wall. *Cancer Genet Cytogenet* 84:157.

Birrer MJ, Johnson ME, Hao K, Wong KK, Park DC, Bell A, et al. (2007): Whole genome oligonucleotide-based array comparative genomic hybridization analysis identified fibroblast growth factor 1 as a prognostic marker for advanced-stage serous ovarian adenocarcinomas. *J Clin Oncol* 25:2281–2287.

Blegen H, Einhorn N, Sjovall K, Roschke A, Ghadimi BM, McShane LM, et al. (2000): Prognostic significance of cell cycle proteins and genomic instability in borderline, early and advanced stage ovarian carcinomas. *Int J Gynecol Cancer* 10:477–487.

Boghosian L, Dal CP, Sandberg AA (1988): An interstitial deletion of chromosome 7 may characterize a subgroup of uterine leiomyoma. *Cancer Genet Cytogenet* 34:207–208.

Bol S, Wanschura S, Thode B, Deichert U, Van d, V, Bartnitzke S, et al. (1996): An endometrial polyp with a rearrangement of HMGI-C underlying a complex cytogenetic rearrangement involving chromosomes 2 and 12. *Cancer Genet Cytogenet* 90:88–90.

Brassesco MS, Castro-Gamero AM, Valera ET, Neder L, Elias J Jr., Tone LG (2009): 3q27 aberrations in a childhood ovary teratoma with associated malignant germ cell component. *Pediatr Blood Cancer* 52:398–401.

Brink AA, Wiegant JC, Szuhai K, Tanke HJ, Kenter GG, Fleuren GJ, et al. (2002): Simultaneous mapping of human papillomavirus integration sites and molecular karyotyping in short-term cultures of cervical carcinomas by using 49-color combined binary ratio labeling fluorescence in situ hybridization. *Cancer Genet Cytogenet* 134:145–150.

Brosens I, Johannisson E, Dal Cin P, Deprest J, Van den Berghe H (1996): Analysis of the karyotype and desoxyribonucleic acid content of uterine myomas in premenopausal, menopausal, and gonadotropin-releasing hormone agonist-treated females. *Fertil Steril* 66:376–379.

Brosens I, Deprest J, Dal Cin P, Van den Benghe H (1998): Clinical significance of cytogenetic abnormalities in uterine myomas. *Fertil Steril* 69:232–235.

Bruchim I, Israeli O, Mahmud SM, Aviram-Goldring A, Rienstein S, Friedman E, et al. (2009): Genetic alterations detected by comparative genomic hybridization and recurrence rate in epithelial ovarian carcinoma. *Cancer Genet Cytogenet* 190:66–70.

Bullerdiek J, Rommel B (1999): Diagnostic and molecular implications of specific chromosomal translocations in mesenchymal tumors. *Histol Histopathol* 14:1165–1173.

Bussey KJ, Lawce HJ, Olson SB, Arthur DC, Kalousek DK, Krailo M, et al. (1999): Chromosome abnormalities of eighty-one pediatric germ cell tumors: sex-, age-, site-, and histopathology-related differences – a Children's Cancer Group study. *Genes Chromosomes Cancer* 25:134–146.

Bussey KJ, Lawce HJ, Himoe E, Shu XO, Suijkerbuijk RF, Olson SB, et al. (2001): Chromosomes 1 and 12 abnormalities in pediatric germ cell tumors by interphase fluorescence in situ hybridization. *Cancer Genet Cytogenet* 125:112–118.

Bustin M, Reeves R (1996): High-mobility-group chromosomal proteins: architectural components that facilitate chromatin function. *Prog Nucleic Acid Res Mol Biol* 54:35–100.

Caduff RF, Svoboda-Newman SM, Ferguson AW, Johnston CM, Frank TS (1999): Comparison of mutations of Ki-RAS and p53 immunoreactivity in borderline and malignant epithelial ovarian tumors. *Am J Surg Pathol* 23:323–328.

Chaudhury A, Hussey GS, Ray PS, Jin G, Fox PL, Howe PH (2010): TGF-beta-mediated phosphorylation of hnRNP E1 induces EMT via transcript-selective translational induction of Dab2 and ILEI. *Nat Cell Biol* 12:286–293.

Chen Z, Coffin CM, Smith LM, Issa B, Arndt S, Shepard R, et al. (2001): Cytogenetic-clinicopathologic correlations in rhabdomyosarcoma: a report of five cases. *Cancer Genet Cytogenet* 131:31–36.

Chene G, Tchirkov A, Pierre-Eymard E, Dauplat J, Raoelfils I, Cayre A, et al. (2013): Early telomere shortening and genomic instability in tubo-ovarian preneoplastic lesions. *Clin Cancer Res* 19:2873–2882.

Cheng JQ, Godwin AK, Bellacosa A, Taguchi T, Franke TF, Hamilton TC, et al. (1992): AKT2, a putative oncogene encoding a member of a subfamily of protein-serine/threonine kinases, is amplified in human ovarian carcinomas. *Proc Natl Acad Sci USA* 89:9267–9271.

Chiang S, Ali R, Melnyk N, McAlpine JN, Huntsman DG, Gilks CB, et al. (2011): Frequency of known gene rearrangements in endometrial stromal tumors. *Am J Surg Pathol* 35:1364–1372.

Chiappetta G, Bandiera A, Berlingieri MT, Visconti R, Manfioletti G, Battista S, et al. (1995): The expression of the high mobility group HMGI (Y) proteins correlates with the malignant phenotype of human thyroid neoplasias. *Oncogene* 10:1307–1314.

Chiyoda T, Tsuda H, Tanaka H, Kataoka F, Nomura H, Nishimura S, et al. (2012): Expression profiles of carcinosarcoma of the uterine corpus-are these similar to carcinoma or sarcoma? *Genes Chromosomes Cancer* 51:229–239.

Christacos NC, Quade BJ, Dal Cin P, Morton CC (2006): Uterine leiomyomata with deletions of Ip represent a distinct cytogenetic subgroup associated with unusual histologic features. *Genes Chromosomes Cancer* 45:304–312.

Clawson K, Donner LR, Dobin SM (2001): Isochromosome (17)(q10) as the sole structural chromosomal rearrangement in a case of botryoid rhabdomyosarcoma. *Cancer Genet Cytogenet* 128:11–13.

Cornelis RS, Neuhausen SL, Johansson O, Arason A, Kelsell D, Ponder BA, et al. (1995): High allele loss rates at 17q12-q21 in breast and ovarian tumors from BRCAl-linked families. The Breast Cancer Linkage Consortium. *Genes Chromosomes Cancer* 13:203–210.

Couturier J, Vielh P, Salmon R, Dutrillaux B (1986): Trisomy and tetrasomy for long arm of chromosome 1 in near-diploid human endometrial adenocarcinomas. *Int J Cancer* 38:17–19.

Couturier J, Vielh P, Salmon RJ, Lombard M, Dutrillaux B (1988): Chromosome imbalance in endometrial adeno-carcinoma. *Cancer Genet Cytogenet* 33:67–76.

Curcio S (1966): Cytogenetic study of a primary carcinoma of the fallopian tube. *Arch Ostet Ginecol* 71:450–456.

Dal Cin P, Morton CC (2002): 1q42 approximately q44 is rarely cytogenetically involved in sporadic uterine leiomyomata. *Cancer Genet Cytogenet* 138:92–93.

Dal Cin P, Boghosian L, Crickard K, Sandberg AA (1988): t(10;17) as the sole chromosome change in a uterine leiomyosarcoma. *Cancer Genet Cytogenet* 32:263–266.

Dal Cin P, Van den Berghe H, Brosens I (1991): Involvement of 6p in an endometrial polyp. *Cancer Genet Cytogenet* 51:279–280.

Dal Cin P, Aly MS, De Wever I, Moerman P, Van den Berghe H (1992a): Endometrial stromal sarcoma t(7;17) (p15-21;q12-21) is a nonrandom chromosome change. *Cancer Genet Cytogenet* 63:43–46.

Dal Cin P, De Wolf F, Klerckx P, Van den Berghe H (1992b): The 6p21 chromosome region is nonrandomly involved in endometrial polyps. *Gynecol Oncol* 46:393–396.

Dal Cin P, Moerman P, Deprest J, Brosens I, Van den Berghe H (1995a): A new cytogenetic subgroup in uterine leio-myoma is characterized by a deletion of the long arm of chromosome 3. *Genes Chromosomes Cancer* 13:219–220.

Dal Cin P, Vanni R, Marras S, Moerman P, Kools P, Andria M, et al. (1995b): Four cytogenetic subgroups can be iden-tified in endometrial polyps. *Cancer Res* 55:1565–1568.

Dal Cin P, Marynen P, Moerman P, Vergot I, Van den Berghe H (1996): Ovarian germ cell tumor with chromosome 12 anomaly but without i(12p). *Cancer Genet Cytogenet* 91:61–64.

Dal Cin P, Pauwels P, Van den Berghe H (1998): Fibrosarcoma versus cellular fibroma of the ovary. *Am J Surg Pathol* 22:508–510.

Debiec-Rychter M, Sciot R, Hagemeijer A (2000): Common chromosome aberrations in the proximal type of epithe-lioid sarcoma. *Cancer Genet Cytogenet* 123:133–136.

Deger RB, Faruqi SA, Noumoff JS (1997): Karyotypic anal-ysis of 32 malignant epithelial ovarian tumors. *Cancer Genet Cytogenet* 96:166–173.

Dellas A, Torhorst J, Jiang F, Proffitt J, Schultheiss E, Holzgreve W, et al. (1999): Prognostic value of genomic alterations in invasive cervical squamous cell carcinoma of clinical stage IB detected by comparative genomic hybrid-ization. *Cancer Res* 59:3475–3479.

Dent J, Hall GD, Wilkinson N, Perren TJ, Richmond I, Markham AF, et al. (2003): Cytogenetic alterations in ovarian clear cell carcinoma detected by comparative genomic hybridisation. *Br J Cancer* 88:1578–1583.

Derre J, Lagace R, Nicolas A, Mairal A, Chibon F, Coindre JM, et al. (2001): Leiomyosarcomas and most malignant fibrous histiocytomas share very similar comparative genomic hybridization imbalances: an analysis of a series of 27 leiomyosarcomas. *Lab Invest* 81:211–215.

Dewaele B, Przybyl J, Quattrone A, Finalet FJ, Vanspauwen V, Geerdens E, et al. (2014): Identification of a novel, recurrent MBTD1-CXorf67 fusion in low-grade endome-trial stromal sarcoma. *Int J Cancer* 134:1112–1122.

Dutrillaux B, Couturier J (1986): Chromosome imbalances in endometrial adenocarcinomas: a possible adaptation to abnormal metabolic pathways. *Ann Genet* 29:76–81.

Eccles DM, Russell SE, Haites NE, Atkinson R, Bell DW, Gruber L, et al. (1992): Early loss of heterozygosity on 17q in ovarian cancer. The Abe Ovarian Cancer Genetics Group. *Oncogene* 7:2069–2072.

Filmus J, Trent JM, Pullano R, Buick RN (1986): A cell line from a human ovarian carcinoma with amplification of the K-ras gene. *Cancer Res* 46:5179–5182.

Fishman A, Shalom-Paz E, Fejgin M, Gaber E, Altaras M, Amiel A (2005): Comparing the genetic changes detected in the primary and secondary tumor sites of ovarian can-cer using comparative genomic hybridization. *Int J Gynecol Cancer* 15:261–266.

Fletcher JA, Morton CC, Pavelka K, Lage JM (1990): Chromosome aberrations in uterine smooth muscle tumors: potential diagnostic relevance of cytogenetic instability. *Cancer Res* 50:4092–4097.

Fletcher JA, Gibas Z, Donovan K, Perez-Atayde A, Genest D, Morton CC, et al. (1991a): Ovarian granulosa-stromal cell tumors are characterized by trisomy 12. *Am J Pathol* 138:515–520.

Fletcher JA, Kozakewich HP, Hoffer FA, Lage JM, Weidner N, Tepper R, et al. (1991b): Diagnostic relevance of clonal cytogenetic aberrations in malignant soft-tissue tumors. *N Engl J Med* 324:436–442.

Fletcher JA, Pinkus JL, Lage JM, Morton CC, Pinkus GS (1992): Clonal 6p21 rearrangement is restricted to the mesenchymal component of an endometrial polyp. *Genes Chromosomes Cancer* 5:260–263.

Foulkes W, Black D, Solomon E, Trowsdale J (1991): Allele loss on chromosome 17q in sporadic ovarian cancer. *Lancet* 338:444–445.

Fresia AE, Currie JL, Farrington JE, Laxman R, Griffin CA (1992): Uterine stromal sarcoma cell line. A cytogenetic and electron microscopic study. *Cancer Genet Cytogenet* 60:60–66.

Fujita H, Wake N, Kutsuzawa T, Ichinoe K, Hreshchyshyn MM, Sandberg AA (1985): Marker chromosomes of the long arm of chromosome 1 in endometrial carcinoma. *Cancer Genet Cytogenet* 18:283–293.

Fuzesi L, Gunawan B, Braun S, Karl MC (1995): Endometrial stromal sarcoma with clonal chromosomal aberrations and mixed phenotype. *Cancer Genet Cytogenet* 84:85–88.

Gibas Z, Rubin SC (1987): Well-differentiated adenocarcinoma of endometrium with simple karyotypic changes: a case report. *Cancer Genet Cytogenet* 25:21–26.

Gibas Z, Griffin CA, Emanuel BS (1988): Clonal chromosome rearrangements in a uterine myoma. *Cancer Genet Cytogenet* 32:19–24.

Gil-Benso R, Lopez-Gines C, Navarro S, Carda C, Llombart-Bosch A (1999): Endometrial stromal sarcomas: immunohistochemical, electron microscopical and cytogenetic findings in two cases. *Virchows Arch* 434:307–314.

Godwin AK, Vanderveer L, Schultz DC (1994): A common region of deletion on chromosome 17q in both sporadic and familial epithelial ovarian tumors distal to BRCA1. *Am J Hum Genet* 55:666–677.

Grammatico P, Catricala C, Potenza C, Amantea A, Roccella M, Roccella F, et al. (1993): Cytogenetic findings in 20 melanomas. *Melanoma Res* 3:169–172.

Gross KL, Panhuysen CI, Kleinman MS, Goldhammer H, Jones ES, Nassery N, et al. (2004): Involvement of fumarate hydratase in nonsyndromic uterine leiomyomas: genetic linkage analysis and FISH studies. *Genes Chromosomes Cancer* 41:183–190.

Grygalewicz B, Sobiczewski P, Krawczyk P, Woroniecka R, Rygier J, Pastwinska A, et al. (2009): Comparison of cytogenetic changes between primary and relapsed patients with borderline tumors of the ovary. *Cancer Genet Cytogenet* 195:157–163.

Guan XY, Cargile CB, Anzick SL, Thompson FH, Meltzer PS, Bittner ML, et al. (1995): Chromosome microdissection identifies cryptic sites of DNA sequence amplification in human ovarian carcinoma. *Cancer Res* 55:3380–3385.

Guardiola MT, Dobin SM, Dal CP, Donner LR (2010): Pericentric inversion (12)(p12q13-14) as the sole chromosomal abnormality in a leiomyoma of the vulva. *Cancer Genet Cytogenet* 199:21–23.

Halbwedl I, Ullmann R, Kremser ML, Man YG, Isadi-Moud N, Lax S, et al. (2005): Chromosomal alterations in low-grade endometrial stromal sarcoma and undifferentiated endometrial sarcoma as detected by comparative genomic hybridization. *Gynecol Oncol* 97:582–587.

Halperin D, Visscher DW, Wallis T, Lawrence WD (1995): Evaluation of chromosome 12 copy number in ovarian granulosa cell tumors using interphase cytogenetics. *Int J Gynecol Pathol* 14:319–323.

Hauke S, Rippe V, Bullerdiek J (2001): Chromosomal rearrangements leading to abnormal splicing within intron 4 of HMGIC? *Genes Chromosomes Cancer* 30:302–304.

Hauptmann S, Denkert C, Koch I, Petersen S, Schluns K, Reles A, et al. (2002): Genetic alterations in epithelial ovarian tumors analyzed by comparative genomic hybridization. *Hum Pathol* 33:632–641.

Heim S, Nilbert M, Vanni R, Floderus UM, Mandahl N, Liedgren S, et al. (1988): A specific translocation, t(12;14)(q14-15;q23-24), characterizes a subgroup of uterine leiomyomas. *Cancer Genet Cytogenet* 32:13–17.

Heimann P, Devalck C, Debusscher C, Sariban E, Vamos E (1998): Alveolar soft-part sarcoma: further evidence by FISH for the involvement of chromosome band 17q25. *Genes Chromosomes Cancer* 23:194–197.

Helou K, Padilla-Nash H, Wangsa D, Karlsson E, Osterberg L, Karlsson P, et al. (2006): Comparative genome hybridization reveals specific genomic imbalances during the genesis from benign through borderline to malignant ovarian tumors. *Cancer Genet Cytogenet* 170:1–8.

Hennig Y, Deichert U, Stern C, Ghassemi A, Thode B, Bonk U, et al. (1996): Structural aberrations of chromosome 6 in three uterine smooth muscle tumors. *Cancer Genet Cytogenet* 87:148–151.

Hennig Y, Caselitz J, Bartnitzke S, Bullerdiek J (1997a): A third case of a low-grade endometrial stromal sarcoma with a t(7;17)(p14 approximately 21;q11.2 approximately 21). *Cancer Genet Cytogenet* 98:84–86.

Hennig Y, Rogalla P, Wanschura S, Frey G, Deichert U, Bartnitzke S, et al. (1997b): HMGIC expressed in a uterine leiomyoma with a deletion of the long arm of chromosome 7 along with a 12q14-15 rearrangement but not in tumors showing del(7) as the sole cytogenetic abnormality. *Cancer Genet Cytogenet* 96:129–133.

Heselmeyer K, Schrock E, du Manoir S, Blegen H, Shah K, Steinbeck R, et al. (1996): Gain of chromosome 3q defines the transition from severe dysplasia to invasive carcinoma of the uterine cervix. *Proc Natl Acad Sci USA* 93:479–484.

Heselmeyer K, Macville M, Schrock E, Blegen H, Hellstrom AC, Shah K, et al. (1997): Advanced-stage cervical carcinomas are defined by a recurrent pattern of chromosomal aberrations revealing high genetic instability and a consistent gain of chromosome arm 3q. *Genes Chromosomes Cancer* 19:233–240.

Heselmeyer K, Hellstrom AC, Blegen H, Schrock E, Silfversward C, Shah K, et al. (1998): Primary carcinoma of the fallopian tube: comparative genomic hybridization reveals high genetic instability and a specific, recurring pattern of chromosomal aberrations. *Int J Gynecol Pathol* 17:245–254.

Hidalgo A, Baudis M, Petersen I, Arreola H, Pina P, Vazquez-Ortiz G, et al. (2005): Microarray comparative genomic hybridization detection of chromosomal imbalances in uterine cervix carcinoma. *BMC Cancer* 5:77.

Hirasawa A, Aoki D, Inoue J, Imoto I, Susumu N, Sugano K, et al. (2003): Unfavorable prognostic factors associated with high frequency of microsatellite instability and comparative genomic hybridization analysis in endometrial cancer. *Clin Cancer Res* 9:5675–5682.

Hodge JC, Quade BJ, Rubin MA, Stewart EA, Dal CP, Morton CC (2008): Molecular and cytogenetic characterization of plexiform leiomyomata provide further evidence for genetic heterogeneity underlying uterine fibroids. *Am J Pathol* 172:1403–1410.

Hoffner L, Shen-Schwarz S, Deka R, Chakravarti A, Surti U (1992): Genetics and biology of human ovarian teratomas. III. Cytogenetics and origins of malignant ovarian germ cell tumors. *Cancer Genet Cytogenet* 62:58–65.

Höglund M, Gisselsson D, Hansen GB, Sall T, Mitelman F (2003): Ovarian carcinoma develops through multiple modes of chromosomal evolution. *Cancer Res* 63:3378–3385.

Horsman DE, Berean KW, Salski CB, Clement PB (1991): Aggressive angiomyxoma of the pelvis: cytogenetics findings in a single case. *Cancer Genet Cytogenet* 56:130–131.

Horton E, Dobin SM, biec-Rychter M, Donner LR (2006): A clonal translocation (7;8)(p13;q11.2) in a leiomyoma of the vulva. *Cancer Genet Cytogenet* 170:58–60.

Hruza C, Dobianer K, Beck A, Czerwenka K, Hanak H, Klein M, et al. (1993): HER-2 and INT-2 amplification estimated by quantitative PCR in paraffin-embedded ovarian cancer tissue samples. *Eur J Cancer* 29A:1593–1597.

Hrynchak M, Horsman D, Salski C, Berean K, Benedet JL (1994): Complex karyotypic alterations in an endometrial stromal sarcoma. *Cancer Genet Cytogenet* 77:45–49.

Hu J, Khanna V, Jones M, Surti U (2001): Genomic alterations in uterine leiomyosarcomas: potential markers for clinical diagnosis and prognosis. *Genes Chromosomes Cancer* 31:117–124.

Hu J, Khanna V, Jones MM, Surti U (2002): Genomic imbalances in ovarian borderline serous and mucinous tumors. *Cancer Genet Cytogenet* 139:18–23.

Hu J, Khanna V, Jones MW, Surti U (2003): Comparative study of primary and recurrent ovarian serous carcinomas: comparative genomic hybridization analysis with a potential application for prognosis. *Gynecol Oncol* 89:369–375.

Ikushima H, Miyazono K (2010): TGFbeta signalling: a complex web in cancer progression. *Nat Rev Cancer* 10:415–424.

Iliszko M, Mandahl N, Mrozek K, Denis A, Pandis N, Pejovic T, et al. (1998): Cytogenetics of uterine sarcomas: presentation of eight new cases and review of the literature. *Gynecol Oncol* 71:172–176.

Ingraham SE, Lynch RA, Kathiresan S, Buckler AJ, Menon AG (1999): hREC2, a RAD51-like gene, is disrupted by t(12;14)(q15;q24.1) in a uterine leiomyoma. *Cancer Genet Cytogenet* 115:56–61.

Israeli O, Gotlieb WH, Friedman E, Goldman B, Ben-Baruch G, viram-Goldring A, et al. (2003): Familial vs sporadic ovarian tumors: characteristic genomic alterations analyzed by CGH. *Gynecol Oncol* 90:629–636.

Israeli O, Gotlieb WH, Friedman E, Korach J, Friedman E, Goldman B, et al. (2004): Genomic analyses of primary and metastatic serous epithelial ovarian cancer. *Cancer Genet Cytogenet* 154:16–21.

Iwabuchi H, Sakamoto M, Sakunaga H, Ma YY, Carcangiu ML, Pinkel D, et al. (1995): Genetic analysis of benign, low-grade, and high-grade ovarian tumors. *Cancer Res* 55:6172–6180.

Jee KJ, Kim YT, Kim KR, Kim HS, Yan A, Knuutila S (2001): Loss in 3p and 4p and gain of 3q are concomitant aberrations in squamous cell carcinoma of the vulva. *Mod Pathol* 14:377–381.

Jenkins RB, Bartelt D, Stalboerger P, Persons D, Dahl RJ, Podratz K, et al. (1993): Cytogenetic studies of epithelial ovarian carcinoma. *Cancer Genet Cytogenet* 71:76–86.

Jenkyn DJ, McCartney AJ (1987): A chromosome study of three ovarian tumors. *Cancer Genet Cytogenet* 26:327–337.

Kadan-Lottick NS, Stork L, Ruyle SZ, Koyle M, Hunger SP, McGavran L (2000): Cytogenetic abnormalities in a case of botryoid rhabdomyosarcoma. *Med Pediatr Oncol* 34:293–295.

Kataoka S, Yamada H, Hoshi N, Kudo M, Hareyama H, Sakuragi N, et al. (2003): Cytogenetic analysis of uterine leiomyoma: the size, histopathology and GnRHa-response in relation to chromosome karyotype. *Eur J Obstet Gynecol Reprod Biol* 110:58–62.

Kawauchi S, Fukuda T, Miyamoto S, Yoshioka J, Shirahama S, Saito T, et al. (1998): Peripheral primitive neuroectodermal tumor of the ovary confirmed by CD99 immunostaining, karyotypic analysis, and RT-PCR for EWS/FLI-1 chimeric mRNA. *Am J Surg Pathol* 22:1417–1422.

Kawauchi S, Okuda S, Morioka H, Iwasaki F, Fukuma F, Chochi Y, et al. (2005): Large cell neuroendocrine carcinoma of the uterine cervix with cytogenetic analysis by comparative genomic hybridization: a case study. *Hum Pathol* 36:1096–1100.

Kazmierczak B, Hennig Y, Wanschura S, Rogalla P, Bartnitzke S, Van de Ven, et al. (1995): Description of a novel fusion transcript between HMGI-C, a gene encoding for a member of the high mobility group proteins, and the mitochondrial aldehyde dehydrogenase gene. *Cancer Res* 55:6038–6039.

Kazmierczak B, Pohnke Y, Bullerdiek J (1996): Fusion transcripts between the HMGIC gene and RTVL-H-related sequences in mesenchymal tumors without cytogenetic aberrations. *Genomics* 38:223–226.

Kazmierczak B, Dal Cin P, Wanschura S, Borrmann L, Fusco A, Van den Berghe H, et al. (1998): HMGIY is the target of 6p21.3 rearrangements in various benign mesenchymal tumors. *Genes Chromosomes Cancer* 23:279–285.

Kenny-Moynihan MB, Hagen J, Richman B, McIntosh DG, Bridge JA (1996): Loss of an X chromosome in aggressive angiomyxoma of female soft parts: a case report. *Cancer Genet Cytogenet* 89:61–64.

Kiechle M, Hinrichs M, Jacobsen A, Luttges J, Pfisterer J, Kommoss F, et al. (2000): Genetic imbalances in precursor lesions of endometrial cancer detected by comparative genomic hybridization. *Am J Pathol* 156:1827–1833.

Kiechle M, Jacobsen A, Schwarz-Boeger U, Hedderich J, Pfisterer J, Arnold N (2001): Comparative genomic hybridization detects genetic imbalances in primary ovarian carcinomas as correlated with grade of differentiation. *Cancer* 91:534–540.

Kiechle-Schwarz M, Sreekantaiah C, Berger CS, Pedron S, Medchill MT, Surti U, et al. (1991): Nonrandom cytogenetic changes in leiomyomas of the female genitourinary tract. A report of 35 cases. *Cancer Genet Cytogenet* 53:125–136.

Kiechle-Schwarz M, Kommoss F, Schmidt J, Lukovic L, Walz L, Bauknecht T, et al. (1992): Cytogenetic analysis of an adenoid cystic carcinoma of the Bartholin's gland. A rare, semimalignant tumor of the female genitourinary tract. *Cancer Genet Cytogenet* 61:26–30.

Kim J, Reeves R, Rothman P, Boothby M (1995): The non-histone chromosomal protein HMG-I(Y) contributes to repression of the immunoglobulin heavy chain germ-line epsilon RNA promoter. *Eur J Immunol* 25:798–808.

King ME, Micha JP, Allen SL, Mouradian JA, Chaganti RS (1985): Immature teratoma of the ovary with predominant malignant retinal anlage component. A parthenogenically derived tumor. *Am J Surg Pathol* 9:221–231.

King ME, DiGiovanni LM, Yung JF, Clarke-Pearson DL (1990): Immature teratoma of the ovary grade 3, with karyotype analysis. *Int J Gynecol Pathol* 9:178–184.

Kirchhoff M, Rose H, Petersen BL, Maahr J, Gerdes T, Lundsteen C, et al. 1999): Comparative genomic hybridization reveals a recurrent pattern of chromosomal aberrations in severe dysplasia/carcinoma in situ of the cervix and in advanced-stage cervical carcinoma. *Genes Chromosomes Cancer* 24:144–150.

Kiuru M, Launonen V, Hietala M, Aittomaki K, Vierimaa O, Salovaara R, et al. (2001): Familial cutaneous leiomyomatosis is a two-hit condition associated with renal cell cancer of characteristic histopathology. *Am J Pathol* 159:825–829.

Klemke M, Meyer A, Nezhad MH, Bartnitzke S, Drieschner N, Frantzen C, et al. (2009): Overexpression of HMGA2 in uterine leiomyomas points to its general role for the pathogenesis of the disease. *Genes Chromosomes Cancer* 48:171–178.

Knight J, Reeves B, Smith S, Clark J, Fisher C, Fletcher C, et al. (1992): Cytogenetic and molecular analysis of synovial sarcoma. *Int J Oncol* 1:747–752.

Koontz JI, Soreng AL, Nucci M, Kuo FC, Pauwels P, Van den BH, et al. (2001): Frequent fusion of the JAZF1 and JJAZ1 genes in endometrial stromal tumors. *Proc Natl Acad Sci USA* 98:6348–6353.

Kraggerud SM, Szymanska J, Abeler VM, Kaern J, Eknaes M, Heim S, et al. (2000): DNA copy number changes in malignant ovarian germ cell tumors. *Cancer Res* 60:3025–3030.

Kurose K, Mine N, Doi D, Ota Y, Yoneyama K, Konishi H, et al. (2000): Novel gene fusion of COX6C at 8q22-23 to

HMGIC at 12q15 in a uterine leiomyoma. *Genes Chromosomes Cancer* 27:303–307.

Ladanyi M, Lui MY, Antonescu CR, Krause-Boehm A, Meindl A, Argani P, et al. (2001): The der(17)t(X;17) (p11;q25) of human alveolar soft part sarcoma fuses the TFE3 transcription factor gene to ASPL, a novel gene at 17q25. *Oncogene* 20:48–57.

Lammie GA, Peters G (1991): Chromosome 11q13 abnormalities in human cancer. *Cancer Cells* 3:413–420.

Laxman R, Currie JL, Kurman RJ, Dudzinski M, Griffin CA (1993): Cytogenetic profile of uterine sarcomas. *Cancer* 71:1283–1288.

Lee CH, Ou WB, Marino-Enriquez A, Zhu M, Mayeda M, Wang Y, et al. (2012): 14–3–3 fusion oncogenes in high-grade endometrial stromal sarcoma. *Proc Natl Acad Sci USA* 109:929–934.

Leung WY, Schwartz PE, Ng HT, Yang-Feng TL (1990): Trisomy 12 in benign fibroma and granulosa cell tumor of the ovary. *Gynecol Oncol* 38:28–31.

Levan K, Partheen K, Osterberg L, Helou K, Horvath G. (2006). Chromosomal alterations in 98 endometrioid adenocarcinomas analyzed with comparative genomic hybridization. *Cytogenet Genome Res* 115:16–22.

Levy B, Mukherjee T, Hirschhorn K (2000): Molecular cytogenetic analysis of uterine leiomyoma and leiomyosarcoma by comparative genomic hybridization. *Cancer Genet Cytogenet* 121:1–8.

Liang SB, Sonobe H, Taguchi T, Takeuchi T, Furihata M, Yuri K, et al. (2001): Tetrasomy 12 in ovarian tumors of thecoma-fibroma group: a fluorescence in situ hybridization analysis using paraffin sections. *Pathol Int* 51:37–42.

Ligon AH, Morton CC (2000): Genetics of uterine leiomyomata. *Genes Chromosomes Cancer* 28:235–245.

Lin YS, Eng HL, Jan YJ, Lee HS, Ho WL, Liou CP, et al. (2005): Molecular cytogenetics of ovarian granulosa cell tumors by comparative genomic hybridization. *Gynecol Oncol* 97:68–73.

Lindgren V, Waggoner S, Rotmensch J (1996): Monosomy 22 in two ovarian granulosa cell tumors. *Cancer Genet Cytogenet* 89:93–97.

Lorenzato M, Doco M, Visseaux-Coletto B, Ferre D, Bellaoui H, Evrard G, et al. (1993): Discrepancies of DNA content of various solid tumours before and after culture measured by image analysis. Comparison of cytogenetical data. *Pathol Res Pract* 189:1161–1168.

Ma YY, Wei SJ, Lin YC, Lung JC, Chang TC, Whang-Peng J, et al. (2000): PIK3CA as an oncogene in cervical cancer. *Oncogene* 19:2739–2744.

Manegold E, Tietze L, Gunther K, Fleischer A, mo-Takyi BK, Schroder W, et al. (2001): Trisomy 8 as sole karyotypic aberration in an ovarian metastasizing Sertoli–Leydig cell tumor. *Hum Pathol* 32:559–562.

Manor E, Bodner L, Kachko P, Kapelushnik J (2009): Trisomy 8 as a sole aberration in embryonal rhabdomyosarcoma (sarcoma botryoides) of the vagina. *Cancer Genet Cytogenet* 195:172–174.

Mark J, Havel G, Grepp C, Dahlenfors R, Wedell B (1988): Cytogenetical observations in human benign uterine leiomyomas. *Anticancer Res* 8:621–626.

Mark J, Havel G, Grepp C, Dahlenfors R, Wedell B (1990): Chromosomal patterns in human benign uterine leiomyomas. *Cancer Genet Cytogenet* 44:1–13.

Mayr D, Kaltz-Wittmer C, Arbogast S, Amann G, Aust DE, Diebold J (2002): Characteristic pattern of genetic aberrations in ovarian granulosa cell tumors. *Mod Pathol* 15:951–957.

Mayr D, Hirschmann A, Marlow S, Horvath C, Diebold J (2008): Analysis of selected oncogenes (AKT1, FOS, BCL2L2, TGFbeta) on chromosome 14 in granulosa cell tumors (GCTs): a comprehensive study on 30 GCTs combining comparative genomic hybridization (CGH) and fluorescence-in situ-hybridization (FISH). *Pathol Res Pract* 204:823–830.

McCluggage WG (2002): Uterine carcinosarcomas (malignant mixed Mullerian tumors) are metaplastic carcinomas. *Int J Gynecol Cancer* 12:687–690.

Medeiros F, Erickson-Johnson MR, Keeney GL, Clayton AC, Nascimento AG, Wang X, et al. (2007): Frequency and characterization of HMGA2 and HMGA1 rearrangements in mesenchymal tumors of the lower genital tract. *Genes Chromosomes Cancer* 46:981–990.

Meloni AM, Surti U, Contento AM, Davare J, Sandberg AA (1992): Uterine leiomyomas: cytogenetic and histologic profile. *Obstet Gynecol* 80:209–217.

Mertens F, Kullendorff CM, Hjorth L, Alumets J, Mandahl N (1998): Trisomy 3 as the sole karyotypic change in a pediatric immature teratoma. *Cancer Genet Cytogenet* 102:83–85.

Mhawech P, Kinkel K, Vlastos G, Pelte MF (2002): Ovarian carcinomas in endometriosis: an immunohistochemical and comparative genomic hybridization study. *Int J Gynecol Pathol* 21:401–406.

Micci F, Teixeira MR, Scheistroen M, Abeler VM, Heim S (2003a): Cytogenetic characterization of tumors of the vulva and vagina. *Genes Chromosomes Cancer* 38:137–148.

Micci F, Walter CU, Teixeira MR, Panagopoulos I, Bjerkehagen B, Saeter G, et al. (2003b): Cytogenetic and molecular genetic analyses of endometrial stromal sarcoma: nonrandom involvement of chromosome arms 6p and 7p and confirmation of JAZF1/JJAZ1 gene fusion in t(7;17). *Cancer Genet Cytogenet* 144:119–124.

Micci F, Teixeira MR, Haugom L, Kristensen G, Abeler VM, Heim S (2004): Genomic aberrations in carcinomas of the uterine corpus. *Genes Chromosomes Cancer* 40:229–246.

Micci F, Panagopoulos I, Bjerkehagen B, Heim S (2006a): Consistent rearrangement of chromosomal band 6p21 with generation of fusion genes JAZF1/PHF1 and EPC1/PHF1 in endometrial stromal sarcoma. *Cancer Res* 66:107–112.

Micci F, Panagopoulos I, Bjerkehagen B, Heim S (2006b): Deregulation of HMGA2 in an aggressive angiomyxoma with t(11;12)(q23;q15). *Virchows Arch* 448:838–842.

Micci F, Haugom L, Abeler VM, Bjerkehagen B, Heim S (2007): Trisomy 7 in postoperative spindle cell nodules. *Cancer Genet Cytogenet* 174:147–150.

Micci F, Haugom L, Abeler VM, Trope CG, Danielsen HE, Heim S (2008): Consistent numerical chromosome aberrations in thecofibromas of the ovary. *Virchows Arch* 452:269–276.

Micci F, Weimer J, Haugom L, Skotheim RI, Grunewald R, Abeler VM, et al. (2009): Reverse painting of microdissected chromosome 19 markers in ovarian carcinoma identifies a complex rearrangement map. *Genes Chromosomes Cancer* 48:184–193.

Micci F, Haugom L, Ahlquist T, Abeler VM, Trope CG, et al. (2010a): Tumor spreading to the contralateral ovary in bilateral ovarian carcinoma is a late event in clonal evolution. *J Oncol* 15:646340.

Micci F, Haugom L, Ahlquist T, Andersen HK, Abeler VM, Davidson B, et al. (2010b): Genomic aberrations in borderline ovarian tumors. *J Transl Med* 8–21:21–28.

Micci F, Skotheim RI, Haugom L, Weimer J, Eibak AM, Abeler VM, et al. (2010c): Array-CGH analysis of microdissected chromosome 19 markers in ovarian carcinoma identifies candidate target genes. *Genes Chromosomes Cancer* 49:1046–1053.

Micci F, Panagopoulos I, Haugom L, Dahlback HS, Pretorius ME, Davidson B, et al. (2013): Genomic aberration patterns and expression profiles of squamous cell carcinomas of the vulva. *Genes Chromosomes Cancer* 52:551–563.

Micci F, Gorunova L, Gatius S, Matias-Guiu X, Davidson B, Heim S, et al. (2014a): MEAF6/PHF1 is a recurrent gene fusion in endometrial stromal sarcoma. *Cancer Lett* 347:75–78.

Micci F, Panagopoulos I, Thorsen J, Davidson B, Trope CG, Heim S (2014b): Low frequency of ESRRA-C11orf20 fusion gene in ovarian carcinomas. *PLoS Biol* 12:e1001784.

Milatovich A, Heerema NA, Palmer CG (1990): Cytogenetic studies of endometrial malignancies. *Cancer Genet Cytogenet* 46:41–53.

Mine N, Kurose K, Konishi H, Araki T, Nagai H, Emi M (2001): Fusion of a sequence from HEI10 (14q11) to the HMGIC gene at 12q15 in a uterine leiomyoma. *Jpn J Cancer Res* 92:135–139.

Moore SD, Herrick SR, Ince TA, Kleinman MS, Dal Cin P, Morton CC, et al. (2004): Uterine leiomyomata with t(10;17) disrupt the histone acetyltransferase MORF. *Cancer Res* 64:5570–5577.

Mrozek K, Limon J, Debniak J, Emerich J (1992): Trisomy 12 and 4 in a thecoma of the ovary. *Gynecol Oncol* 45:66–68.

Muslumanoglu HM, Oner U, Ozalp S, Acikalin MF, Yalcin OT, Ozdemir M, et al. (2005): Genetic imbalances in endometrial hyperplasia and endometrioid carcinoma detected by comparative genomic hybridization. *Eur J Obstet Gynecol Reprod Biol* 120:107–114.

Namiq AL, Persons DL, Piehler J, Damjanov I (2005): Monosomy 22 and trisomy 14 in a granulosa tumor metastatic to the lung 20 years after the removal of the primary tumor. *Cancer Genet Cytogenet* 159:192–193.

Narayan G, Pulido HA, Koul S, Lu XY, Harris CP, Yeh YA, et al. (2003): Genetic analysis identifies putative tumor suppressor sites at 2q35-q36.1 and 2q36.3-q37.1 involved in cervical cancer progression. *Oncogene* 22:3489–3499.

Narayan G, Bourdon V, Chaganti S, Arias-Pulido H, Nandula SV, Rao PH, et al. (2007): Gene dosage alterations revealed by cDNA microarray analysis in cervical cancer: identification of candidate amplified and overexpressed genes. *Genes Chromosomes Cancer* 46:373–384.

Nezhad MH, Drieschner N, Helms S, Meyer A, Tadayyon M, Klemke M, et al. (2010): 6p21 rearrangements in uterine leiomyomas targeting HMGA1. *Cancer Genet Cytogenet* 203:247–252.

Nibert M, Heim S (1990): Uterine leiomyoma cytogenetics. *Genes Chromosomes Cancer* 2:3–13.

Nilbert M, Heim S, Mandahl N, Floderus UM, Willen H, Akerman M, et al. (1988a): Ring formation and structural rearrangements of chromosome 1 as secondary changes in uterine leiomyomas with t(12;14)(q14-15;q23-24). *Cancer Genet Cytogenet* 36:183–190.

Nilbert M, Heim S, Mandahl N, Floderus UM, Willen H, Mitelman F (1988b): Karyotypic rearrangements in 20 uterine leiomyomas. *Cytogenet Cell Genet* 49:300–304.

Nilbert M, Heim S, Mandahl N, Floderus UM, Willen H, Mitelman F (1989): Different karyotypic abnormalities, t(1;6) and del(7), in two uterine leiomyomas from the same patient. *Cancer Genet Cytogenet* 42:51–53.

Nilbert M, Heim S, Mandahl N, Floderus UM, Willen H, Mitelman F (1990a): Characteristic chromosome abnormalities, including rearrangements of 6p, del(7q), +12, and t(12;14), in 44 uterine leiomyomas. *Hum Genet* 85:605–611.

Nilbert M, Heim S, Mandahl N, Floderus UM, Willen H, Mitelman F (1990b): Trisomy 12 in uterine leiomyomas. A new cytogenetic subgroup. *Cancer Genet Cytogenet* 45:63–66.

Nilbert M, Jin YS, Heim S, Mandahl N, Floderus UM, Willen H, et al. (1990c): Chromosome rearrangements in two uterine sarcomas. *Cancer Genet Cytogenet* 44:27–35.

Nilbert M, Mandahl N, Heim S, Rydholm A, Helm G, Willen H, et al. (1990d): Complex karyotypic changes, including rearrangements of 12q13 and 14q24, in two leiomyosarcomas. *Cancer Genet Cytogenet* 48:217–223.

Nowee ME, Snijders AM, Rockx DA, de Wit RM, Kosma VM, Hamalainen K, et al. (2007): DNA profiling of primary serous ovarian and fallopian tube carcinomas with array comparative genomic hybridization and multiplex ligation-dependent probe amplification. *J Pathol* 213:46–55.

Nucci MR, Weremowicz S, Neskey DM, Sornberger K, Tallini G, Morton CC, et al. (2001): Chromosomal translocation t(8;12) induces aberrant HMGIC expression in aggressive angiomyxoma of the vulva. *Genes Chromosomes Cancer* 32:172–176.

Ordulu Z, Dal Cin P, Chong WW, Choy KW, Lee C, Muto MG, et al. (2010): Disseminated peritoneal leiomyomatosis after laparoscopic supracervical hysterectomy with characteristic molecular cytogenetic findings of uterine leiomyoma. *Genes Chromosomes Cancer* 49:1152–1160.

Osterberg L, Akeson M, Levan K, Partheen K, Zetterqvist BM, Brannstrom M, et al. (2006): Genetic alterations of serous borderline tumors of the ovary compared to stage I serous ovarian carcinomas. *Cancer Genet Cytogenet* 167:103–108.

Ozisik YY, Meloni AM, Surti U, Sandberg AA (1993a): Deletion 7q22 in uterine leiomyoma. A cytogenetic review. *Cancer Genet Cytogenet* 71:1–6.

Ozisik YY, Meloni AM, Surti U, Sandberg AA (1993b): Involvement of 10q22 in leiomyoma. *Cancer Genet Cytogenet* 69:132–135.

Ozisik YY, Meloni AM, Stone JF, Sandberg AA, Surti U (1994): Spontaneous expression of the chromosome fragile site at 10q23 in leiomyoma. *Cancer Genet Cytogenet* 74:73–75.

Ozisik YY, Meloni AM, Altungoz O, Surti U, Sandberg AA (1995): Translocation (6;10)(p21;q22) in uterine leiomyomas. *Cancer Genet Cytogenet* 79:136–138.

Packenham JP, du Manoir S, Schrock E, Risinger JI, Dixon D, Denz DN, et al. (1997): Analysis of genetic alterations in uterine leiomyomas and leiomyosarcomas by comparative genomic hybridization. *Mol Carcinog* 19:273–279.

Palazzo JP, Gibas Z, Dunton CJ, Talerman A (1993): Cytogenetic study of botryoid rhabdomyosarcoma of the uterine cervix. *Virchows Arch A Pathol Anat Histopathol* 422:87–91.

Panagopoulos I, Fioretos T, Isaksson M, Samuelsson U, Billstrom R, Strombeck B, et al. (2001): Fusion of the MORF and CBP genes in acute myeloid leukemia with the t(10;16)(q22;p13). *Hum Mol Genet* 10:395–404.

Panagopoulos I, Micci F, Thorsen J, Gorunova L, Eibak AM, Bjerkehagen B, et al. (2012): Novel fusion of MYST/Esa1-associated factor 6 and PHF1 in endometrial stromal sarcoma. *PLoS One* 7:e39354.

Panagopoulos I, Thorsen J, Gorunova L, Haugom L, Bjerkehagen B, Davidson B, et al. (2013): Fusion of the ZC3H7B and BCOR genes in endometrial stromal sarcomas carrying an X;22-translocation. *Genes Chromosomes Cancer* 52:610–618.

Panani AD (2007): Preferential involvement of chromosome 11 as add(11)(p15) in ovarian cancer: is it a common cytogenetic abnormality in cancer? *Cancer Lett* 258:262–267.

Panani A, Ferti-Passantonopoulou A (1985): Common marker chromosomes in ovarian cancer. *Cancer Genet Cytogenet* 16:65–71.

Panani AD, Roussos C (2006): Non-random structural chromosomal changes in ovarian cancer: i(5p) a novel recurrent abnormality. *Cancer Lett* 235:130–135

Pandis N, Heim S, Bardi G, Floderus UM, Willen H, Mandahl N, et al. (1990): Parallel karyotypic evolution and tumor progression in uterine leiomyoma. *Genes Chromosomes Cancer* 2:311–317.

Pandis N, Heim S, Bardi G, Floderus UM, Willen H, Mandahl N, et al. (1991): Chromosome analysis of 96 uterine leiomyomas. *Cancer Genet Cytogenet* 55:11–18.

Partheen K, Levan K, Osterberg L, Helou K, Horvath G (2004): Analysis of cytogenetic alterations in stage III serous ovarian adenocarcinoma reveals a heterogeneous group regarding survival, surgical outcome, and substage. *Genes Chromosomes Cancer* 40:342–348.

Patael-Karasik Y, Daniely M, Gotlieb WH, Ben-Baruch G, Schiby J, Barakai G, et al. (2000): Comparative genomic hybridization in inherited and sporadic ovarian tumors in Israel. *Cancer Genet Cytogenet* 121:26–32.

Pauwels P, Dal Cin P, Van de Moosdijk CN, Vrints L, Sciot R, Van den Berghe H (1996): Cytogenetics revealing the diagnosis in a metastatic endometrial stromal sarcoma. *Histopathology* 29:84–87.

Pejovic T, Heim S, Mandahl N, Elmfors B, Floderus UM, Furgyik S, et al. (1989): Consistent occurrence of a 19p+ marker chromosome and loss of 11p material in ovarian seropapillary cystadenocarcinomas. *Genes Chromosomes Cancer* 1:167–171.

Pejovic T, Heim S, Mandahl N, Elmfors B, Floderus UM, Furgyik S, et al. (1990a): Trisomy 12 is a consistent chromosomal aberration in benign ovarian tumors. *Genes Chromosomes Cancer* 2:48–52.

Pejovic T, Heim S, Mandahl N, Floderus UM, Willen H, Mitelman F (1990b): Complex karyotypic anomalies, including an i(5p) marker chromosome, in malignant mixed mesodermal tumor of the ovary. *Cancer Genet Cytogenet* 46:65–69.

Pejovic T, Heim S, Orndal C, Jin YS, Mandahl N, Willen H, et al. (1990c): Simple numerical chromosome aberrations in well-differentiated malignant epithelial tumors. *Cancer Genet Cytogenet* 49:95–101.

Pejovic T, Heim S, Mandahl N, Elmfors B, Furgyik S, Floderus UM, et al. (1991): Bilateral ovarian carcinoma: cytogenetic evidence of unicentric origin. *Int J Cancer* 47:358–361.

Pejovic T, Heim S, Mandahl N, Baldetorp B, Elmfors B, Floderus UM, et al. (1992a): Chromosome aberrations in 35 primary ovarian carcinomas. *Genes Chromosomes Cancer* 4:58–68.

Pejovic T, Himmelmann A, Heim S, Mandahl N, Floderus UM, Furgyik S, et al. (1992b): Prognostic impact of chromosome aberrations in ovarian cancer. *Br J Cancer* 65:282–286.

Pejovic T, Heim S, Alm P, Iosif S, Himmelmann A, Skjaerris J, et al. (1993): Isochromosome 1q as the sole karyotypic abnormality in a Sertoli cell tumor of the ovary. *Cancer Genet Cytogenet* 65:79–80.

Pejovic T, Alm P, Iosif SC, Mitelman F, Heim S (1996a): Cytogenetic findings in four malignant mixed mesodermal tumors of the ovary. *Cancer Genet Cytogenet* 88:53–56.

Pejovic T, Iosif CS, Mitelman F, Heim S (1996b): Karyotypic characteristics of borderline malignant tumors of the ovary: trisomy 12, trisomy 7, and r(1) as nonrandom features. *Cancer Genet Cytogenet* 92:95–98.

Pejovic T, Burki N, Odunsi K, Fiedler P, Achong N, Schwartz PE, et al. (1999): Well-differentiated mucinous carcinoma of the ovary and a coexisting Brenner tumor both exhibit amplification of 12q14-21 by comparative genomic hybridization. *Gynecol Oncol* 74:134–137.

Pere H, Tapper J, Seppala M, Knuutila S, Butzow R (1998a): Genomic alterations in fallopian tube carcinoma: comparison to serous uterine and ovarian carcinomas reveals similarity suggesting likeness in molecular pathogenesis. *Cancer Res* 58:4274–4276.

Pere H, Tapper J, Wahlstrom T, Knuutila S, Butzow R (1998b): Distinct chromosomal imbalances in uterine serous and endometrioid carcinomas. *Cancer Res* 58:892–895.

Persons DL, Hartmann LC, Herath JF, Keeney GL, Jenkins RB (1994): Fluorescence in situ hybridization analysis of trisomy 12 in ovarian tumors. *Am J Clin Pathol* 102:775–779.

Phillips NJ, Zeigler MR, Deaven LL (1996): A cDNA from the ovarian cancer critical region of deletion on chromosome 17p13.3. *Cancer Lett* 102:85–90.

Polito P, Dal Cin P, Kazmierczak B, Rogalla P, Bullerdiek J, Van den Berghe H (1999): Deletion of HMG17 in uterine leiomyomas with ring chromosome 1. *Cancer Genet Cytogenet* 108:107–109.

Quade BJ, McLachlin CM, Soto-Wright V, Zuckerman J, Mutter GL, Morton CC (1997): Disseminated peritoneal leiomyomatosis. Clonality analysis by X chromosome inactivation and cytogenetics of a clinically benign smooth muscle proliferation. *Am J Pathol* 150:2153–2166.

Quade BJ, Pinto AP, Howard DR, Peters WA III, Crum CP (1999): Frequent loss of heterozygosity for chromosome 10 in uterine leiomyosarcoma in contrast to leiomyoma. *Am J Pathol* 154:945–950.

Quade BJ, Weremowicz S, Neskey DM, Vanni R, Ladd C, Dal Cin P, et al. (2003): Fusion transcripts involving HMGA2 are not a common molecular mechanism in uterine leiomyomata with rearrangements in 12q15. *Cancer Res* 63:1351–1358.

Raish M, Khurshid M, Ansari MA, Chaturvedi PK, Bae SM, Kim JH, et al. (2012): Analysis of molecular cytogenetic alterations in uterine leiomyosarcoma by array-based comparative genomic hybridization. *J Cancer Res Clin Oncol* 138:1173–1186.

Ram TG, Reeves R, Hosick HL (1993): Elevated high mobility group-I(Y) gene expression is associated with progressive transformation of mouse mammary epithelial cells. *Cancer Res* 53:2655–2660.

Rao PH, rias-Pulido H, Lu XY, Harris CP, Vargas H, Zhang FF, et al. (2004): Chromosomal amplifications, 3q gain and deletions of 2q33-q37 are the frequent genetic changes in cervical carcinoma. *BMC Cancer* 4:5.

Rein MS, Powell WL, Walters FC, Weremowicz S, Cantor RM, Barbieri RL, et al. (1998): Cytogenetic abnormalities in uterine myomas are associated with myoma size. *Mol Hum Reprod* 4:83–86.

Riopel MA, Spellerberg A, Griffin CA, Perlman EJ (1998): Genetic analysis of ovarian germ cell tumors by comparative genomic hybridization. *Cancer Res* 58:3105–3110.

Rodriguez E, Melamed J, Reuter V, Chaganti RS (1995): Chromosomal abnormalities in choriocarcinomas of the female. *Cancer Genet Cytogenet* 80:9–12.

Russell SE, Hickey GI, Lowry WS, White P, Atkinson RJ (1990): Allele loss from chromosome 17 in ovarian cancer. *Oncogene* 5:1581–1583.

Salzman J, Marinelli RJ, Wang PL, Green AE, Nielsen JS, Nelson BH, et al. (2011): ESRRA-C11orf20 is a recurrent gene fusion in serous ovarian carcinoma. *PLoS Biol* 9:e1001156.

Sandberg AA (2005): Updates on the cytogenetics and molecular genetics of bone and soft tissue tumors: leiomyoma. *Cancer Genet Cytogenet* 158:1–26.

Saretzki G, Hoffmann U, Rohlke P, Psille R, Gaigal T, Keller G, et al. (1997): Identification of allelic losses in benign, borderline, and invasive epithelial ovarian tumors and correlation with clinical outcome. *Cancer* 80:1241–1249.

Sargent MS, Weremowicz S, Rein MS, Morton CC (1994): Translocations in 7q22 define a critical region in uterine leiomyomata. *Cancer Genet Cytogenet* 77:65–68.

Sato T, Saito H, Morita R, Koi S, Lee JH, Nakamura Y (1991): Allelotype of human ovarian cancer. *Cancer Res* 51:5118–5122.

Satoh Y, Ishikawa Y, Miyoshi T, Mukai H, Okumura S, Nakagawa K (2003): Pulmonary metastases from a low-grade endometrial stromal sarcoma confirmed by chromosome aberration and fluorescence in-situ hybridization approaches: a case of recurrence 13 years after hysterectomy. *Virchows Arch* 442:173–178.

Schoenberg Fejzo M, Ashar HR, Krauter KS, Powell WL, Rein MS, Weremowicz S, et al. (1996): Translocation breakpoints upstream of the HMGIC gene in uterine leiomyomata suggest dysregulation of this gene by a mechanism different from that in lipomas. *Genes Chromosomes Cancer* 17:1–6.

Schoenmakers EF, Van de Ven WJ (1997): From chromosome aberrations to the high mobility group protein gene family: evidence for a common genetic denominator in benign solid tumor development. *Cancer Genet Cytogenet* 95:51–58.

Schoenmakers EF, Huysmans C, Van de Ven WJ (1999): Allelic knockout of novel splice variants of human recombination repair gene RAD51B in t(12;14) uterine leiomyomas. *Cancer Res* 59:19–23.

Schraml P, Schwerdtfeger G, Burkhalter F, Raggi A, Schmidt D, Ruffalo T, et al. (2003): Combined array comparative genomic hybridization and tissue microarray analysis suggest PAK1 at 11q13.5-q14 as a critical oncogene target in ovarian carcinoma. *Am J Pathol* 163:985–992.

Schuijer M, Berns EM (2003): TP53 and ovarian cancer. *Hum Mutat* 21:285–291.

Schulten HJ, Gunawan B, Enders C, Donhuijsen K, Emons G, Fuzesi L (2004): Overrepresentation of 8q in carcinosarcomas and endometrial adenocarcinomas. *Am J Clin Pathol* 122:546–551.

Schultz DC, Vanderveer L, Berman DB, Hamilton TC, Wong AJ, Godwin AK (1996): Identification of two candidate tumor suppressor genes on chromosome 17p13.3. *Cancer Res* 56:1997–2002.

Schuyer M, Henzen-Logmans SC, van der Burg ME, Fieret JH, Derksen C, Look MP, et al. (1999): Genetic alterations in ovarian borderline tumours and ovarian carcinomas. *Eur J Obstet Gynecol Reprod Biol* 82:147–150.

Sell SM, Tullis C, Stracner D, Song CY, Gewin J (2005): Minimal interval defined on 7q in uterine leiomyoma. *Cancer Genet Cytogenet* 157:67–69.

Shah NK, Currie JL, Rosenshein N, Campbell J, Long P, Abbas F, et al. (1994): Cytogenetic and FISH analysis of endometrial carcinoma. *Cancer Genet Cytogenet* 73:142–146.

Shashi V, Golden WL, von Kap-Herr C, Andersen WA, Gaffey MJ (1994): Interphase fluorescence in situ hybridization for trisomy 12 on archival ovarian sex cord-stromal tumors. *Gynecol Oncol* 55:349–354.

Shelling AN, Cooke IE, Ganesan TS (1995): The genetic analysis of ovarian cancer. *Br J Cancer* 72:521–527.

Shen DH, Khoo US, Xue WC, Ngan HY, Wang JL, Liu VW, et al. (2001): Primary peritoneal malignant mixed Mullerian tumors. A clinicopathologic, immunohistochemical, and genetic study. *Cancer* 91:1052–1060.

Shih I, Nakayama K, Wu G, Nakayama N, Zhang J, Wang TL (2011): Amplification of the ch19p13.2 NACC1 locus in ovarian high-grade serous carcinoma. *Mod Pathol* 24:638–645.

Shridhar V, Lee J, Pandita A, Iturria S, Avula R, Staub J, et al. (2001): Genetic analysis of early- versus late-stage ovarian tumors. *Cancer Res* 61:5895–5904.

Shu Z, Smith S, Wang L, Rice MC, Kmiec EB (1999): Disruption of muREC2/RAD51L1 in mice results in early embryonic lethality which can Be partially rescued in a p53(–/–) background. *Mol Cell Biol* 19:8686–8693.

Simon D, Heyner S, Satyaswaroop PG, Farber M, Noumoff JS (1990): Is chromosome 10 a primary chromosomal abnormality in endometrial adenocarcinoma? *Cancer Genet Cytogenet* 47:155–162.

Sirchia SM, Pariani S, Rossella F, Garagiola I, De AC, Bulfamante G, et al. (1997): Cytogenetic abnormalities and microsatellite instability in endometrial adenocarcinoma. *Cancer Genet Cytogenet* 94:113–119.

Skilling JS, Sood A, Niemann T, Lager DJ, Buller RE (1996): An abundance of p53 null mutations in ovarian carcinoma. *Oncogene* 13:117–123.

Skirnisdottir I, Mayrhofer M, Rydaker M, Akerud H, Isaksson A (2012): Loss-of-heterozygosity on chromosome 19q in early-stage serous ovarian cancer is associated with recurrent disease. *BMC Cancer* 12:407–412.

Skomedal H, Kristensen GB, Abeler VM, Borresen-Dale AL, Trope C, Holm R (1997): TP53 protein accumulation and gene mutation in relation to overexpression of MDM2 protein in ovarian borderline tumours and stage I carcinomas. *J Pathol* 181:158–165.

Slamon DJ, Godolphin W, Jones LA, Holt JA, Wong SG, Keith DE, et al. (1989): Studies of the HER-2/neu proto-oncogene in human breast and ovarian cancer. *Science* 244:707–712.

Smith LM, Hu P, Meyer LJ, Coffin CM (2002): Complex karyotypic abnormality in ovarian fibroma associated with Gorlin syndrome. *Am J Med Genet* 112:61–64.

Snijders AM, Nowee ME, Fridlyand J, Piek JM, Dorsman JC, Jain AN, et al. (2003): Genome-wide-array-based comparative genomic hybridization reveals genetic homogeneity and frequent copy number increases encompassing CCNE1 in fallopian tube carcinoma. *Oncogene* 22:4281–4286.

Sonobe H, Iwata J, Furihata M, Ohtsuki Y, Taguchi T, Shimizu K (1999): Endometrial stromal sarcoma with clonal complex chromosome abnormalities. Report of a case and review of the literature. *Cancer Genet Cytogenet* 112:34–37.

Sonoda G, du Manoir S, Godwin AK, Bell DW, Liu Z, Hogan M, et al. (1997a): Detection of DNA gains and losses in primary endometrial carcinomas by comparative genomic hybridization. *Genes Chromosomes Cancer* 18:115–125.

Sonoda G, Palazzo J, du Manoir S, Godwin AK, Feder M, Yakushiji M, et al. (1997b): Comparative genomic hybrid-ization detects frequent overrepresentation of chromosomal material from 3q26, 8q24, and 20q13 in human ovarian carcinomas. *Genes Chromosomes Cancer* 20:320–328.

Sornberger KS, Weremowicz S, Williams AJ, Quade BJ, Ligon AH, Pedeutour F, et al. (1999): Expression of HMGIY in three uterine leiomyomata with complex rearrangements of chromosome 6. *Cancer Genet Cytogenet* 114:9–16.

Speleman F, De Potter C, Dal Cin P, Mangelschots K, Ingelaere H, Laureys G, et al. (1990): i(12p) in a malignant ovarian tumor. *Cancer Genet Cytogenet* 45:49–53.

Speleman F, Laureys G, Benoit Y, Cuvelier C, Suijkerbuijk R, de Jong B (1992): i(12p) in a near-diploid mature ovarian teratoma. *Cancer Genet Cytogenet* 60:216–218.

Sreekantaiah C, Sandberg AA (1991): Clustering of aberrations to specific chromosome regions in benign neoplasms. *Int J Cancer* 48:194–198.

Sreekantaiah C, Bhargava MK, Shetty NJ (1987): Cytogenetic findings in two cases of carcinoma in situ of the cervix uterus. *Gynecol Oncol* 28:337–341.

Sreekantaiah C, Li FP, Weidner N, Sandberg AA (1991): An endometrial stromal sarcoma with clonal cytogenetic abnormalities. *Cancer Genet Cytogenet* 55:163–166.

Staebler A, Heselmeyer-Haddad K, Bell K, Riopel M, Perlman E, Ried T, et al. (2002): Micropapillary serous carcinoma of the ovary has distinct patterns of chromosomal imbalances by comparative genomic hybridization compared with atypical proliferative serous tumors and serous carcinomas. *Hum Pathol* 33:47–59.

Stern C, Deichert U, Thode B, Bartnitzke S, Bullerdiek J (1992): Cytogenetic subtyping of 139 uterine leiomyoma. *Geburtshilfe Frauenheilkd* 52:767–772.

Streblow RC, Dafferner AJ, Nelson M, Fletcher M, West WW, Stevens RK, et al. (2007): Imbalances of chromosomes 4, 9, and 12 are recurrent in the thecoma-fibroma group of ovarian stromal tumors. *Cancer Genet Cytogenet* 178:135–140.

Suehiro Y, Sakamoto M, Umayahara K, Iwabuchi H, Sakamoto H, Tanaka N, et al. (2000a): Genetic aberrations detected by comparative genomic hybridization in ovarian clear cell adenocarcinomas. *Oncology* 59:50–56.

Suehiro Y, Umayahara K, Ogata H, Numa F, Yamashita Y, Oga A, et al. (2000b): Genetic aberrations detected by comparative genomic hybridization predict outcome in patients with endometrioid carcinoma. *Genes Chromosomes Cancer* 29:75–82.

Sung CO, Choi CH, Ko YH, Ju H, Choi YL, Kim N, et al. (2013): Integrative analysis of copy number alteration and gene expression profiling in ovarian clear cell adenocarcinoma. *Cancer Genet* 206:145–153.

Suzuki A, Fukushige S, Nagase S, Ohuchi N, Satomi S, Horii A (1997): Frequent gains on chromosome arms 1q and/or 8q in human endometrial cancer. *Hum Genet* 100:629–636.

Suzuki S, Moore DH, Ginzinger DG, Godfrey TE, Barclay J, et al. (2000): An approach to analysis of large-scale correlations between genome changes and clinical endpoints in ovarian cancer. *Cancer Res* 60:5382–5385.

Takahashi T, Nagai N, Oda H, Ohama K, Kamada N, Miyagawa K (2001): Evidence for RAD51L1/HMGIC fusion in the pathogenesis of uterine leiomyoma. *Genes Chromosomes Cancer* 30:196–201.

Tallini G, Dal Cin P (1999): HMGI(Y) and HMGI-C dysregulation: a common occurrence in human tumors. *Adv Anat Pathol* 6:237–246.

Tamimi Y, van der Poel HG, Denyn MM, Umbas R, Karthaus HF, Debruyne FM, et al. (1993): Increased expression of high mobility group protein I(Y) in high grade prostatic cancer determined by in situ hybridization. *Cancer Res* 53:5512–5516.

Tanaka K, Boice CR, Testa JR (1989): Chromosome aberrations in nine patients with ovarian cancer. *Cancer Genet Cytogenet* 43:1–14.

Tapper J, Butzow R, Wahlstrom T, Seppala M, Knuutila S (1997): Evidence for divergence of DNA copy number changes in serous, mucinous and endometrioid ovarian carcinomas. *Br J Cancer* 75:1782–1787.

Tapper J, Sarantaus L, Vahteristo P, Nevanlinna H, Hemmer S, Seppala M, et al. (1998): Genetic changes in inherited and sporadic ovarian carcinomas by comparative genomic hybridization: extensive similarity except for a difference at chromosome 2q24-q32. *Cancer Res* 58:2715–2719.

Taruscio D, Carcangiu ML, Ward DC (1993): Detection of trisomy 12 on ovarian sex cord stromal tumors by fluorescence in situ hybridization. *Diagn Mol Pathol* 2:94–98.

TCGA (2011): Integrated genomic analyses of ovarian carcinoma. *Nature* 474:609–615.

Teixeira MR, Kristensen GB, Abeler VM, Heim S (1999): Karyotypic findings in tumors of the vulva and vagina. *Cancer Genet Cytogenet* 111:87–91.

Teyssier JR (1987): Nonrandom chromosomal changes in human solid tumors: application of an improved culture method. *J Natl Cancer Inst* 79:1189–1198.

Tharapel SA, Qumsiyeh MB, Photopulos G (1991): Numerical chromosome abnormalities associated with early clinical stages of gynecologic tumors. *Cancer Genet Cytogenet* 55:89–96.

Thompson FH, Emerson J, Alberts D, Liu Y, Guan XY, Burgess A, et al. (1994a): Clonal chromosome abnormalities in 54 cases of ovarian carcinoma. *Cancer Genet Cytogenet* 73:33–45.

Thompson FH, Liu Y, Emerson J, Weinstein R, Makar R, Trent JM, et al. (1994b): Simple numeric abnormalities as primary karyotype changes in ovarian carcinoma. *Genes Chromosomes Cancer* 10:262–266.

Tibiletti MG, Bernasconi B, Furlan D, Riva C, Trubia M, Buraggi G, et al. (1996): Early involvement of 6q in surface epithelial ovarian tumors. *Cancer Res* 56:4493–4498.

Tibiletti MG, Bernasconi B, Taborelli M, Facco C, Riva C, Capella C, et al. (2003): Genetic and cytogenetic observations among different types of ovarian tumors are compatible with a progression model underlying ovarian tumorigenesis. *Cancer Genet Cytogenet* 146:145–153.

Tomlinson IP, Alam NA, Rowan AJ, Barclay E, Jaeger EE, Kelsell D, et al. (2002): Germline mutations in FH predispose to dominantly inherited uterine fibroids, skin leiomyomata and papillary renal cell cancer. *Nat Genet* 30:406–410.

Trent JM, Salmon SE (1981): Karyotypic analysis of human ovarian carcinoma cells cloned in short term agar culture. *Cancer Genet Cytogenet* 3:279–291.

Truss L, Dobin SM, Rao A, Donner LR (2004): Overexpression of the BCL2 gene in a Sertoli-Leydig cell tumor of the ovary: a pathologic and cytogenetic study. *Cancer Genet Cytogenet* 148:118–122.

Tsuji T, Yoshinaga M, Inomoto Y, Taguchi S, Douchi T (2007): Aggressive angiomyxoma of the vulva with a sole t(5;8)(p15;q22) chromosome change. *Int J Gynecol Pathol* 26:494–496.

Turc-Carel C, Dal Cin P, Boghosian L, Terk-Zakarian J, Sandberg AA (1988): Consistent breakpoints in region 14q22-q24 in uterine leiomyoma. *Cancer Genet Cytogenet* 32:25–31.

Van den Berg E, Molenaar WM, Hoekstra HJ, Kamps WA, de Jong B (1992): DNA ploidy and karyotype in recurrent and metastatic soft tissue sarcomas. *Mod Pathol* 5:505–514.

Van den Berghe I, Dal Cin P, De Groef K, Michielssen P, Van den Berghe H (1999): Monosomy 22 and trisomy 14 may be early events in the tumorigenesis of adult granulosa cell tumor. *Cancer Genet Cytogenet* 112:46–48.

Vanni R, Nieddu M, Paoli R, Lecca U (1989): Uterine leiomyoma cytogenetics. I. Rearrangements of chromosome 12. *Cancer Genet Cytogenet* 37:49–54.

Vanni R, Dal Cin P, Van den Berghe H (1990): Is the chromosome band 1p36 another hot-spot for rearrangements in uterine leiomyoma? *Genes Chromosomes Cancer* 2:255–256.

Vanni R, Lecca U, Faa G (1991): Uterine leiomyoma cytogenetics. II. Report of forty cases. *Cancer Genet Cytogenet* 53:247–256.

Vanni R, Dal Cin P, Marras S, Moerman P, Andria M, Valdes E, et al. (1993): Endometrial polyp: another benign tumor characterized by 12q13-q15 changes. *Cancer Genet Cytogenet* 68:32–33.

Vanni R, Marras S, Andria M, Faa G (1995): Endometrial polyps with predominant stromal component are characterized by a t(6;14)(p21;q24) translocation. *Cancer Res* 55:31–33.

Velagaleti GV, Tonk VS, Hakim NM, Wang X, Zhang H, Erickson-Johnson MR, et al. (2010): Fusion of HMGA2 to COG5 in uterine leiomyoma. *Cancer Genet Cytogenet* 202:11–16.

Verdorfer I, Horst D, Hollrigl A, Rogatsch H, Mikuz G (2007): Sertoli–Leydig cell tumours of the ovary and testis: a CGH and FISH study. *Virchows Arch* 450:267–271.

Verhest A, Simonart T, Noel JC (1996): A unique clonal chromosome 2 deletion in endomyometriosis. *Cancer Genet Cytogenet* 86:174–176.

Wake N, Hreshchyshyn MM, Piver SM, Matsui S, Sandberg AA (1980): Specific cytogenetic changes in ovarian cancer involving chromosomes 6 and 14. *Cancer Res* 40:4512–4518.

Wanschura S, Dal Cin P, Kazmierczak B, Bartnitzke S, Van den Berghe H, et al. (1997): Hidden paracentric inversions of chromosome arm 12q affecting the HMGIC gene. *Genes Chromosomes Cancer* 18:322–323.

Wehle D, Yonescu R, Long PP, Gala N, Epstein J, Griffin CA (2008): Fluorescence in situ hybridization of 12p in germ cell tumors using a bacterial artificial chromosome clone 12p probe on paraffin-embedded tissue: clinical test validation. *Cancer Genet Cytogenet* 183:99–104.

Weise W, Buttner HH (1972): Analysis of chromosomes in a primary Fallopian tube carcinoma with interpretation of chromosomal peculiarities in uterine corpus carcinoma. *Zentralbl Gynakol* 94:1761–1767.

Weremowicz S, Morton CC (1999): Is HMGIC rearranged due to cryptic paracentric inversion of 12q in karyotypically normal uterine leiomyomas? *Genes Chromosomes Cancer* 24:172–173.

Whang-Peng J, Knutsen T, Douglass EC, Chu E, Ozols RF, Hogan WM, et al. (1984): Cytogenetic studies in ovarian cancer. *Cancer Genet Cytogenet* 11:91–106.

Williams AJ, Powell WL, Collins T, Morton CC (1997): HMGI(Y) expression in human uterine leiomyomata. Involvement of another high-mobility group architectural factor in a benign neoplasm. *Am J Pathol* 150:911–918.

Wilting SM, Snijders PJ, Meijer GA, Ylstra B, van den Ijssel PR, Snijders AM, et al. (2006): Increased gene copy numbers at chromosome 20q are frequent in both squamous cell carcinomas and adenocarcinomas of the cervix. *J Pathol* 209:220–230.

Wolf NG, Abdul-Karim FW, Farver C, Schrock E, du Manoir S, Schwartz S (1999): Analysis of ovarian borderline tumors using comparative genomic hybridization and fluorescence in situ hybridization. *Genes Chromosomes Cancer* 25:307–315.

Worsham MJ, Van Dyke DL, Grenman SE, Grenman R, Hopkins MP, Roberts JA, et al. (1991): Consistent chromosome abnormalities in squamous cell carcinoma of the vulva. *Genes Chromosomes Cancer* 3:420–432.

Yang-Feng TL, Katz SN, Cacangiu ML, Schwartz PE (1988): Cytogenetic analysis of ependymoma and teratoma of the ovary. *Cancer Genet Cytogenet* 35:83–89.

Yang-Feng TL, Li SB, Leung WY, Carcangiu ML, Schwartz PE (1991): Trisomy 12 and K-ras-2 amplification in human ovarian tumors. *Int J Cancer* 48:678–681.

Yonescu R, Currie JL, Hedrick L, Campbell J, Griffin CA (1996): Chromosome abnormalities in primary endometrioid ovarian carcinoma. *Cancer Genet Cytogenet* 87:167–171.

Yoshida MA, Ohyashiki K, Piver SM, Sandberg AA (1986): Recurrent endometrial adenocarcinoma with rearrangement of chromosomes 1 and 11. *Cancer Genet Cytogenet* 20:159–162.

Zaal A, Peyrot WJ, Berns PM, van der Burg ME, Veerbeek JH, Trimbos JB, et al. (2012): Genomic aberrations relate early and advanced stage ovarian cancer. *Cell Oncol* 35:181–188.

Zahn S, Sievers S, Alemazkour K, Orb S, Harms D, Schulz WA, et al. (2006): Imbalances of chromosome arm 1p in pediatric and adult germ cell tumors are caused by true allelic loss: a combined comparative genomic hybridization and microsatellite analysis. *Genes Chromosomes Cancer* 45:995–1006.

Zweemer RP, Ryan A, Snijders AM, Hermsen MA, Meijer GA, Beller U, et al. (2001): Comparative genomic hybridization of microdissected familial ovarian carcinoma: two deleted regions on chromosome 15q not previously identified in sporadic ovarian carcinoma. *Lab Invest* 81:1363–1370.

CHAPTER 18

Tumors of the male genital organs

Manuel R. Teixeira[1] and Sverre Heim[2]

[1]Department of Genetics, Portuguese Oncology Institute, Porto, Portugal
[2]Section for Cancer Cytogenetics, Institute for Cancer Genetics and Informatics, Oslo University Hospital, Oslo, Norway

Tumors of two male genital organs, the testes and, especially, the prostate, are common. Although both benign and malignant prostatic neoplasms almost exclusively affect older or middle-aged men, tumors of the testis typically occur in young adults. Indeed, although prostate cancer is the overall predominant cancer in men in the Western world, germinal neoplasms are the most common form of malignancy in males between 25 and 35 years of age.

Testis

Testicular germ cell tumors (TGCT) are a heterogeneous group of neoplasms that have been classified in various ways. A fundamental dichotomy exists between seminomas and nonseminomatous germ cell tumors (NSGCT), the latter being composed of neoplastic embryonic (embryonal carcinoma, immature and mature teratoma) or extraembryonic tissues (yolk sac tumor and choriocarcinoma). NSGCT sometimes have a seminoma component, and they are then often called combined tumors (CT). About 340 TGCT with clonal chromosome abnormalities have been reported (Mitelman et al., 2014), including 87 seminomas, 174 NSGCT (mostly teratomas), and 72 CT. The largest series were described by Samaniego et al. (1990),

Rodriguez et al. (1992), van Echten et al. (1995a), and Smolarek et al. (1999). The field was extensively reviewed by de Jong et al. (1997), Looijenga et al. (2003b), Frigyesi et al. (2004), Oosterhuis and Looijenga (2005), and Houldsworth et al. (2006). Examination of the data thus accumulated over the years resulted in the recognition of three pathogenetically distinct subgroups of TGCT (Oosterhuis and Looijenga, 2005; Houldsworth et al., 2006), namely, the teratomas and yolk sac tumors of newborns and infants, the seminomatous and nonseminomatous tumors of adolescents and young adults, and the spermatocytic seminomas of older men.

TGCT of adolescents and young adults, by far the most extensively studied of the three TGCT subtypes, have as the only recurrent structural chromosome abnormality an isochromosome for the short arm of chromosome 12, *i(12p)* (Figure 18.1). The isochromosome was first associated with these tumors by Atkin and Baker (1982) and has since been consistently detected in up to 80% of all major TGCT histological subtypes (seminomas, NSGCT, and CT). Although the i(12p) was never the sole anomaly in any of these tumors, the great consistency with which it is found constitutes a strong argument that it is pathogenetically important. The mechanism of origin of the i(12p) was studied by the analysis of restriction

Cancer Cytogenetics: Chromosomal and Molecular Genetic Aberrations of Tumor Cells, Fourth Edition.
Edited by Sverre Heim and Felix Mitelman.

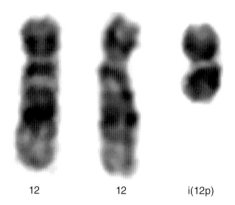

12   12   i(12p)

Figure 18.1 G-banding illustration of an isochromosome 12p occurring together with two normal chromosomes 12. This aberration is typical of testicular germ cell tumors of adolescents and young adults (courtesy of Dr. Paola Dal Cin).

fragment length polymorphisms (RFLP) of 12p markers finding an intensity distribution consistent with a uniparental origin of the two arms of the i(12p) (Sinke et al., 1993). They found no indications that maternal or paternal chromosomes were preferentially involved in the isochromosome formation; hence, there was no sign of genomic imprinting.

i(12p)-negative TGCT do not seem to differ clinically or pathologically from the more numerous i(12p)-positive tumors, and several investigations with FISH have demonstrated that the former contain *alternative chromosomal abnormalities involving 12p*, always resulting in a distinct overrepresentation of short arm sequences (Geurts van Kessel et al., 1993; Rodriguez et al., 1993; Suijkerbuijk et al., 1993; Smolarek et al., 1995). Thus, both i(12p)-positive and i(12p)-negative tumors have a higher than normal number of copies of the entire 12p or of parts of this chromosome arm. Metaphase comparative genomic hybridization (CGH) investigations have confirmed the ubiquitous 12p copy number gain in TGCT of adolescents and young adults and further refined a smallest region of amplification to 12p11.1–12.1 (Korn et al., 1996; Mostert et al., 1998). Zafarana et al. (2002) demonstrated that the *DAD1L* gene (alias *DAD-R*) is amplified and significantly upregulated in seminomas with the restricted 12p amplification compared with seminomas without this amplicon. *DAD1L* is also highly expressed in nonseminomas of various histologies, being associated with inva-

sive growth and decreased apoptosis (Zafarana et al., 2002). On the other hand, triple-color FISH using microdissected probes for the various cytogenetic bands on chromosome arm 12p (12p11.2, p12, and p13) demonstrated independent gain of 12p13 or 12p12–13 in several tumors (Henegariu et al., 1998), indicating that 12p harbors more than one pathogenetically important gene for TGCT oncogenesis and perhaps explaining the reason why i(12p) is the most common mechanism of 12p overrepresentation in this tumor type. Indeed, data obtained by array-based CGH and expression profiling support a mechanistic model in which several 12p genes, including *KRAS* and *CCND2*, cooperate in TGCT pathogenesis (Rodriguez et al., 2003; Zafarana et al., 2003; Korkola et al., 2006; Skotheim et al., 2006; Alagaratnam et al., 2011).

Apart from the 12p gain, the various histological subgroups of TGCT of adolescents and young adults share also other genetic features. Both seminomas and NSGCT are aneuploid and often present additional loss of chromosomes 11, 13, 18, and Y and gain of chromosomes 7, 8, 12, 21, and X, indicating a common pathogenetic origin (van Echten et al., 1995a; de Jong et al., 1997; Oosterhuis and Looijenga, 2005). However, seminomas generally differ from NSGCT by having a higher chromosome number (typically in the triploid to tetraploid range, whereas NSGCT mostly are hypotriploid), more frequent gain of chromosomes 7, 15, 19, and 22, but typically fewer copies of chromosome 17 and i(12p). Clonality analysis of the *CT* by karyotyping and FISH revealed that the seminomatous and nonseminomatous components have a common origin in most cases (Gillis et al., 1994; van Echten et al., 1996; de Jong et al., 1997). All seminomas and NSGCT are supposed to evolve from *carcinoma in situ* (CIS; also called intratubular germ cell neoplasia unclassified lesion) precursors, and in fact, CIS lesions share with adjacent invasive TGCT many of the typical numerical chromosomal changes. However, 12p gain is not consistently detected in the CIS component (Vos et al., 1990; van Echten et al., 1995b; Rosenberg et al., 2000; Summersgill et al., 2001; Ottesen et al., 2003), indicating that overrepresentation of 12p is associated with transition to invasive growth. The cytogenetic data therefore favor a pathogenetic model of TGCT in which seminoma and NSGCT are developmentally related, with the latter being a more advanced tumor that has previously gone through a seminoma stage. Computer simulations indicate that two distinct processes are operative in the karyotypic evolution of these tumors, with whole-chromosome changes originating from a multipolar cell division of a tetraploid cell, whereas structural changes accumulate in a stepwise manner (Frigyesi et al., 2004).

Besides the recurrent chromosome-level aberrations mentioned earlier, activating point mutations have been found in a few genes in a relatively small proportion of TGCT of adolescents and young adults. *KRAS* (located in 12p12.1), besides being amplified in TGCT with 12p rearrangements other than i(12p) (Roelofs et al., 2000), is alternatively found mutated in up to 10% of the cases (Olie et al., 1995; Roelofs et al., 2000; McIntyre et al., 2005a; Sommerer et al., 2005). *NRAS* (Olie et al., 1995; McIntyre et al., 2005a) and *BRAF* (Sommerer et al., 2005) mutations also occur at a similar frequency in a mutually exclusive manner. Some studies have indicated that *KIT* mutations are present in most bilateral TGCT (Looijenga et al., 2003a; Biermann et al., 2007), but analysis of larger series have shown that such mutations are found in only a minority of TGCT (Tian et al., 1999; Sakuma et al., 2003; Kemmer et al., 2004; Willmore-Payne et al., 2006) and that they neither reliably predict bilateral disease (Coffey et al., 2008) nor are involved in familial predisposition (Rapley et al., 2004). *KIT* mutations may take place in primordial germ cells during embryogenesis, since the same somatic mutation is sometimes found in bilateral primary tumors (Looijenga et al., 2003a; Rapley et al., 2004; Biermann et al., 2007). In addition to point mutations, *KIT* copy number gain and overexpression have been recurrently found (McIntyre et al., 2005b). A few case reports have shown striking regression of TGCT overexpressing KIT after treatment with imatinib (Pedersini et al., 2007; Pectasides et al., 2008; Okamura et al., 2010), but this has not been demonstrated in a phase II clinical trial (Einhorn et al., 2006). Although present in only a minority of TGCT overall, *KRAS*, *NRAS*, and *KIT* mutations occur preferentially in seminomas and are only occasionally detected in NSGCT (Olie et al., 1995; Kemmer et al., 2004; McIntyre et al., 2005a, 2005b; Coffey et al., 2008), the opposite being true for *BRAF* mutations (Sommerer et al., 2005; Honecker et al., 2009).

The less common teratomas and yolk sac tumors of newborns and infants and spermatocytic seminomas of the elderly are pathogenetically different from the common TGCT of adolescents and young adults, as illustrated by the absence of i(12p) from these tumor types. Although *immature teratomas* seem to have a normal chromosome complement, *yolk sac tumors* typically have karyotypes characterized by gain of 1q and 20q but loss of 1p, 4q, and 6q (Oosterhuis et al., 1988; Rodriguez et al., 1992; Perlman et al., 1994; Bussey et al., 1999; van Echten et al., 2002), a pattern of genomic copy number changes confirmed by CGH (Mostert et al., 2000; Schneider et al., 2001). A combination of karyotype, CGH, and locus-specific FISH analyses showed that *spermatocytic seminomas* are characterized mainly by numerical chromosomal aberrations, with gain of chromosome 9 present in all and gains of X, 1, and 20 and losses of 7, 16, and 22 also occurring nonrandomly (Rosenberg et al., 1998; Verdorfer et al., 2004). Additional analysis with array-based CGH has confirmed a characteristic pattern of chromosomal imbalances, with gain of chromosome 9 as the only consistent anomaly in spermatocytic seminomas (Looijenga et al., 2006). Based on one case showing amplification of the 9p21.3-pter region and associated RNA expression and immunohistochemistry data on these tumors, Looijenga et al. (2006) proposed *DMRT1* (a male-specific transcriptional regulator) as a likely candidate target gene for 9p involvement in the development of spermatocytic seminomas.

The *clinical value of i(12p)* as a highly informative marker of germ cell neoplasia is undisputed. Since the i(12p) is uncommon in other neoplastic entities, its demonstration can be very helpful in establishing the germ cell origin of metastatic lesions (Kernek et al., 2004). It has been shown that somatic-type malignancies (for instance, carcinomas or sarcomas) that develop in patients with germ cell tumors, more commonly in metastases after chemotherapy than in the primary tumors, are clonally related as they share the i(12p) with the corresponding teratoma lesions (Motzer et al., 1998; Kum et al., 2012). Likewise, cytogenetic analysis has shown that a subset of what seemed to be midline undifferentiated carcinomas have i(12p) and, consequently, that they most probably are extragonadal GCT (Dal Cin et al., 1989; Motzer et al., 1991, 1995; Bosl et al., 1994; Schneider et al., 2006). The fact that these patients respond to cisplatin therapy in a manner indistinguishable from that of patients with TGCT (Greco et al., 1986; Bosl et al., 1994; Motzer et al., 1995) supports the conclusion that the tumors are biologically very similar. Furthermore, extensive cytogenetic evidence exists for a clonal relationship between mediastinal germ cell tumor and acute leukemia present in the same patient (Chaganti et al., 1989; Ladanyi et al., 1990; Orazi et al., 1993; Woodruff et al., 1995), conclusively establishing that the apparent primary bone marrow disease actually resulted from leukemization of the malignant germ cell clone. Finally, resistance to cisplatin treatment, the chemotherapy that is very effective in most TGCT patients, may be predicted by the presence of mismatch repair deficiency or *BRAF* mutation (Honecker et al., 2009) or by a gene expression signature including genes other than those located in 12p (Korkola et al., 2009).

Prostate

Although *prostatic cancer* is the most common malignant disease in men in Western countries, the existing cytogenetic information about these tumors is very limited: only about 200 cases with clonal chromosome abnormalities characterized by banding techniques have been reported (Mitelman et al., 2014). The largest series were described by Lundgren et al. (1992b), Micale et al. (1992), Arps et al. (1993), Breitkreuz et al. (1993), Webb et al. (1996), Teixeira et al. (2000), and Verdorfer et al. (2001). The limited chromosome banding data have subsequently been supplemented by numerous CGH analyses that helped determine the characteristic pattern of chromosome copy number changes of prostate cancer at various disease stages (Visakorpi et al., 1995b; Cher et al., 1996; Alers et al., 2000, 2001; Fu et al., 2000; Mattfeldt et al., 2002; Wolter et al., 2002a, 2002b; Chu et al., 2003; Teixeira et al., 2004; Ribeiro et al., 2006a).

Most prostate carcinomas that have been cytogenetically studied had a normal karyotype. As alluded to repeatedly in several chapters, the fact that no aberrations are detected in a tumor is only scant evidence that none exists. Breitkreuz et al. (1993) found that many prostatic carcinoma

biopsies with an aneuploid DNA content as measured by flow cytometry turned out to be cytogenetically normal. König et al. (1993) used a combination of flow cytometric and FISH techniques to demonstrate that the frequency of aneuploid cells gradually decreased when prostatic carcinoma specimens were cultured *in vitro*. On the other hand, combined analyses by chromosome banding and CGH, a technique not dependent on tissue cell culturing, still showed a smaller but nevertheless significant proportion of prostate carcinomas with no chromosome copy number changes (Verdorfer et al., 2001; Teixeira et al., 2004). The high percentage of normal cases, and as normal must also be considered the tetraploid karyotypes seen in many tumors in some series (Micale et al., 1992; Breitkreuz et al., 1993), may therefore in part be a reflection of inadequate techniques to culture prostate cancer cells and also that some of the genomic aberrations that characterize this tumor type are below the resolution level of chromosome banding (discussed subsequently). The same reasoning may be applied regarding the two most common aberrations that have been detected as sole changes by chromosome banding after *in vitro* culturing, namely, −*Y* and +*7*, as ample evidence exists that these chromosome abnormalities may also be present in nonneoplastic lesions from many tissues (Johansson et al., 1993; see also Chapters 6, 12, and 15).

Despite the methodological considerations and shortcomings mentioned previously, the pattern of cytogenetic changes revealed by chromosome banding and CGH analyses in prostate cancer comes across as clearly nonrandom. *Loss of 8p* through deletions, unbalanced translocations, or i(8q) has been seen in prostate cancer by chromosome banding after *in vitro* culturing (Lundgren et al., 1992b; Webb et al., 1996) and is one of the most common copy number changes detected by metaphase-based CGH (Ribeiro et al., 2006a). Array-based CGH narrowed down the minimal common region of overlap for 8p losses to 12 Mbp between 8p21.2 and 8p22, encompassing more than 50 genes, but no homozygous deletions have been found (Paris et al., 2004; Ribeiro et al., 2006b; Lapointe et al., 2007). *NKX3-1* (a prostate- and testis-specific androgen-regulated homeobox gene at 8p21) has been proposed as the main target,

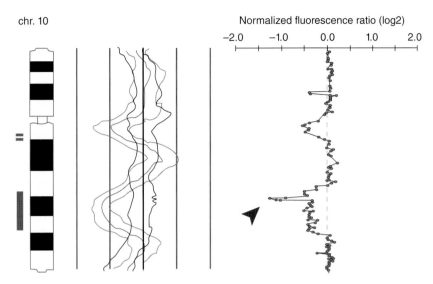

Figure 18.2 Deletions of 10q detected by chromosome comparative genomic hybridization (cCGH) (left) and array CGH (right) in the same prostatic carcinoma. cCGH detected two deletions (in 10q11–21 and 10q22–24), whereas array CGH also identified an additional genomic loss from 10p and a homozygous deletion at 10q23.31 (arrowhead; courtesy of Dr. Franclim R. Ribeiro).

since disruption of *NKX3-1* in mouse models of prostate cancer leads to prostatic epithelial hyperplasia and dysplasia (Abdulkadir et al., 2002) and overexpression of exogenous *NKX3-1* suppresses growth and tumorigenicity in human prostate carcinoma cell lines (Kim et al., 2002a). Importantly, haploinsufficiency of this gene is enough to significantly alter gene expression patterns in the prostate and, therefore, the second inactivating hit expected in a classic tumor suppressor gene may not be necessary (Abdulkadir et al., 2002).

Deletions of 10q were first associated with prostate cancer by Atkin and Baker (1985) and have since been detected repeatedly (Lundgren et al., 1992b; Arps et al., 1993; Webb et al., 1996), sometimes as the sole anomaly. This genomic imbalance is also commonly detected by metaphase-based CGH (Ribeiro et al., 2006a), and array-based CGH studies have further refined the deletion to a 1 Mbp region at 10q23.31 that is often homozygously lost (Paris et al., 2004; Liu et al., 2006; Ribeiro et al., 2006b; Lapointe et al., 2007; Tørring et al., 2007) (Figure 18.2). The likely candidate target gene in this region is *PTEN*, whose expression has been shown to be reduced in most advanced prostate cancers (Halvorsen et al., 2003). Studies of mouse models suggest that the absence of functional

PTEN, even by way of haploinsufficiency (Kwabi-Addo et al., 2001), confers upon proliferating cells the ability to overlook apoptosis even when subjected to apoptotic stimuli and that loss of function of PTEN cooperates with loss of function of NKX3-1 in cancer progression (Kim et al., 2002b). Interestingly, analyses of this multifunctional protein phosphatase generally detect very low mutation frequencies, suggesting that homozygous deletion is in fact the major mechanism of *PTEN* inactivation (Liu et al., 2006; Ribeiro et al., 2006b; Verhagen et al., 2006).

Several other chromosomal regions are recurrently affected by copy number changes in prostate cancer, although the relevant target genes remain uncertain or unknown. Deletions of the long arm of chromosome 7, usually del(7)(q22), have been found by chromosome banding (Atkin and Baker, 1985; Lundgren et al., 1992b; Verdorfer et al., 2001). On the other hand, copy number losses of or from 5q, 6q, 13q, 16q, 17p, and 18q and gains of 8q are commonly detected by CGH (Visakorpi et al., 1995b; Cher et al., 1996; Alers et al., 2000, 2001; Fu et al., 2000; Mattfeldt et al., 2002; Wolter et al., 2002a, 2002b; Chu et al., 2003; Teixeira et al., 2004; Ribeiro et al., 2006a; Lapointe et al., 2007). Even though the entire chromosome arm is usually seen by metaphase-based CGH to be gained in carcinomas with 8q imbalances, array-based CGH has pinpointed several smaller, distinct regions of amplification (van Duin et al., 2005); there is still no conclusive evidence as to which are the most relevant gene targets. After androgen-ablation therapy, extra copies of chromosomal arm Xq encompassing the androgen receptor (AR) locus are also a recurrent finding in prostate cancer (Visakorpi et al., 1995a; Ribeiro et al., 2006a).

Bioinformatic analysis of microarray expression profiling data on prostatic cancer has led to the identification of *fusion oncogenes* involving the androgen-regulated *TMPRSS2* (21q22.3) gene and members of the ETS family of transcription factors *ERG* (21q22.2), *ETV1* (7p21), *ETV4* (17q21), and *ETV5* (3q27) (Tomlins et al., 2005, 2006; Helgeson et al., 2008). More recently, *FLI1* (11q24) has been identified as the fifth *ETS* transcription factor gene involved in fusions in prostate cancer (Paulo et al., 2012a). In addition to *TMPRSS2*, several other less common 5′ fusion partners have also been described (Tomlins et al., 2007; Helgeson et al., 2008; Barros-Silva et al., 2013) (Table 18.1). Although genomic rearrangements of the *ETS* genes *ETV1*, *ETV4*, *ETV5*, and *FLI1* are relatively uncommon (present in 1–10% of primary tumors), the *TMPRSS2–ERG* gene is consistently detected in about 50% of prostate carcinomas (Tomlins et al., 2005; Cerveira et al., 2006; Hermans et al., 2006; Perner et al., 2006; Soller et al., 2006; Wang et al., 2006; Yoshimoto et al., 2006; Mehra et al., 2007b; Rajput et al., 2007; Tu et al., 2007; Paulo et al., 2012a). FISH and array-based CGH analyses have shown that a cytogenetically cryptic deletion between the two genes located in 21q22 is the mechanism giving rise to the fusion gene in 60% of *TMPRSS2–ERG*-positive prostate carcinomas, the remaining being caused by cryptic insertion events (Perner et al., 2006; Yoshimoto et al., 2006; Lapointe et al., 2007; Liu et al., 2007). Contrary to what has been stated by several groups (Hermans et al., 2006; Perner et al., 2007; Tu et al., 2007), and although it is theoretically possible to obtain a *TMPRSS2–ERG* fusion by a reciprocal 21;21-translocation, the split signal pattern detected by the commonly used dual-color, break-apart FISH strategy (flanking *ERG*) identifies an insertion of the genetic material between *ERG* and *TMPRSS2* into another chromosome, not a translocation

(Teixeira, 2008), resulting in fusion of the two genes of the same homolog. In fact, the FISH strategy is not well suited to distinguish a translocation from a deletion as the mechanism of bringing about the *TMPRSS2–ERG* fusion, because the former would lead to the juxtaposition of two green signals that most likely are not spatially distinguishable on tissue sections (Teixeira, 2008). Taking into account the incidence of prostate cancer, the *TMPRSS2–ERG* oncogene may be the most common structural genome aberration in human malignancies, and several potential clinical applications are possible, namely, noninvasive diagnosis of prostate cancer in urine samples (Laxman et al., 2006; Hessels et al., 2007; Tomlins et al., 2011), differential diagnosis in prostate core biopsies in challenging cases (Tomlins et al., 2012), and biologically targeted therapy (Brenner et al., 2011; Han et al., 2013). On the other hand, identification by FISH of the different mechanisms giving rise to *ETS* fusions has shown that multifocal prostate cancer may be a heterogeneous group of diseases arising from multiple, clonally independent expansions (Barry et al., 2007; Mehra et al., 2007a; Paulo et al., 2012a). The 5′ fusion partner most often drives the overexpression of the ETS transcription factor, which affects the expression of ETS target genes and leads to prostate cancer development by altering cell proliferation, differentiation, and/or apoptosis (Tomlins et al., 2005, 2007), although different ETS transcription factors may regulate specific and shared target genes and allow further molecular subtyping of prostate carcinomas (Paulo et al., 2012b). The *TMPRSS2–ERG* fusion oncogene is additionally present in about 20% of high-grade *prostatic intraepithelial neoplasia* (HGPIN) lesions (Cerveira et al., 2006; Perner et al., 2007), the presumed precursor of invasive disease, and may predict subsequent cancer diagnosis (Gao et al., 2012). This indicates that *ETS* gene fusions are initiating events in prostate carcinogenesis (Klezovitch et al., 2008), although existing functional data indicate that other genomic changes might be necessary for a full-blown malignancy (Tomlins et al., 2008; Carver et al., 2009; King et al., 2009). Indeed, earlier CGH data indicate that *ETS* fusions are followed by losses at 8p, then by loss of 13q and 16q and gain of 8q (intermediate events), and then by late secondary events that include losses of 10q, 5q, and 17p (Cerveira et al., 2006; Ribeiro

Table 18.1 Oncogenic gene fusions identified in prostate cancer involving the *ETS* family of transcription factors (*ERG, ETV1, ETV4, ETV5,* and *FLI1*) and various 5′ fusion partners

Translocation partner	Locus	Androgen response	Structure of encoded protein	Gene function
ERG				
TMPRSS2	21q22	Upregulated	NTT; fusion (5aa); WT	Transmembrane serine protease
SLC45A3	1q32	Upregulated	NS	Solute carrier protein
HERPUD1	16q13	Upregulated	Fusion (49aa)	Ubiquitin-like member
NRDG1	8q24.3	Upregulated		Alpha/beta hydrolase
ETV1				
TMPRSS2	21q22	Upregulated	NTT; fusion (5aa)	Transmembrane serine protease
SLC45A3	1q32	Upregulated	NTT	Solute carrier protein
ACSL3	2q36.1	Upregulated	NTT	Acetyl-CoA synthetase
HERV-K22	22q11.23	Upregulated	NTT	Endogenous retrovirus
HERV-K17	17p13.1	Upregulated	NTT	Endogenous retrovirus
FOXP1	3p13	Upregulated	Fusion (19aa)	Forkhead box P1
EST14	14q21.1	Upregulated	NTT; fusion (5aa)	Noncoding RNA
Chr 14	14q13.3–21.1	Upregulated	WT	NA
C15orf21	15q21.1	Downregulated	NTT	Unidentified ORF
HNRPA2B1	7p15	No effect	Fusion (2aa)	Ribonuclear protein
ETV4				
TMPRSS2	21q22	Upregulated	NTT; fusion (5aa)	Transmembrane serine protease
KLK2	19q13.33	Upregulated	NTT	Kallikrein peptidase
CANT1	17q25.3	Upregulated	NTT	Ca-activated nucleotidase
DDX5	17q24.1	No effect	Fusion (102aa)	RNA helicase
ETV5				
TMPRSS2	21q22	Upregulated	WT; fusion (84aa)	Transmembrane serine protease
SLC45A3	1q32	Upregulated	NTT	Solute carrier protein
FLI1				
SLC45A3	1q32	Upregulated	WT	Solute carrier protein

Courtesy of Dr. Joao Barros-Silva.

Ca, calcium; NA, not applicable; NS, not specified; NTT, N-terminal truncated; ORF, open reading frame; WT, wild type.

et al., 2006a, 2006b). More recent data using integrative genomic and transcriptomic profiling have uncovered an association between the *TMPRSS2–ERG* fusion gene and loss of 10q23 (spanning the *PTEN* gene), 17p13 (spanning the *TP53* gene), and 3p14 (spanning the genes *FOXP1, RYBP,* and *SHQ1*) (Taylor et al., 2010). Rarely, fusions involving other genes than those of the *ETS* family have been detected using algorithms applied on paired-end transcriptome next-generation sequencing and aCGH data, namely, *BRAF, RAF1, KRAS,* and *MYC* (Palanisamy et al., 2010; Wang et al., 2011; Wu et al., 2012).

Like for other tumor types, the genetic features of prostate cancer cells are expected to be of *prognostic value* beyond that of standard clinicopathological parameters. Lundgren et al. (1992a) showed that patients whose tumors had an abnormal karyotype had a significantly shorter survival, but they could not demonstrate that the prognostic information contributed by the karyotype was independent of that attributable to other known prognostic factors in this disease. Ribeiro et al. (2006a) reviewed the metaphase CGH findings available on prostate cancers, correlating the data with pertinent clinicopathological information, and identified several genomic features of potential clinical interest: First, both the frequency of cases with copy number changes and the overall genetic complexity were positively associated with pathological grade and clinical stage. Second, several individual genomic copy number changes, like gains of chromosomal arms 7q and 8q and losses of 6q and 10q, were associated in univariate analysis with clinical aggressiveness (development of local and distant metastasis). Finally, 8q gain and 13q loss were associated with extraprostatic disease independent of Gleason score in multivariate analysis, which indicates that genetic features may add significant prognostic information to standard histopathological analyses of prostate cancer specimens. More importantly, Teixeira et al. (2004) showed that it is feasible to consistently obtain whole-genome information from ultrasound-guided sextant needle biopsies by CGH, enabling the acquisition of relevant information about the tumor genome at a time when it can contribute to therapeutic decision making. Ribeiro et al. (2006c) subsequently performed CGH on a large series of prospectively collected biopsies from prostate cancer suspects, which included a wider spectrum of prostate cancer patients than is possible to obtain from a series based on prostatectomy specimens. Patients whose tumors displayed 8q copy number gain were nine times more likely to have a poor outcome, also evidenced by disease-specific survival curves, even when the patients were stratified according to tumor grade or clinical stage (Ribeiro et al., 2006c). This genetic variable seems to be able to identify patients with a worse outcome even in the group of heterogeneous tumors with Gleason score 7, whose clinical behavior is particularly hard to predict (Ribeiro et al., 2006c). The prognostic significance of 8q gain was confirmed using a three-color FISH assay in an independent series of paraffin-embedded diagnostic biopsies with longer follow-up (Ribeiro et al., 2007). The prognostic impact of the *TMPRSS2–ERG* fusion oncogene is controversial regardless of whether biochemical recurrence or disease-specific survival is used as end point. The presence of a *TMPRSS2–ERG* fusion predicted biochemical disease recurrence in multivariate analysis (Nam et al., 2007) both in men with clinically localized prostate cancer treated by prostatectomy and in those conservatively managed (watchful waiting), and lack of this fusion gene was associated with longer disease-specific survival (Demichelis et al., 2007; Attard et al., 2008). However, other studies using FISH analyses (FitzGerald et al., 2008; Gopalan et al., 2009) or immunohistochemistry-based testing of the resulting ERG overexpression (Hoogland et al., 2012; Pettersson et al., 2012) showed no consistent prognostic value for this rearrangement. The relative prognostic value of *TMPRSS2–ERG* and 8q gain in prostate cancer was recently evaluated in a series of diagnostic biopsies from patients with prostate cancer and a long follow-up by Barros-Silva et al. (2011). They showed that whereas *ERG* rearrangements had no impact on disease-specific survival, relative 8q gain was associated with poor prognosis independently of Gleason score, tumor staging, or *ERG* rearrangement status. Reid et al. (2010) found that the poor prognostic influence of 10q deletions was dependent on *ETS* rearrangement status.

Existing cytogenetic information on *benign prostatic hyperplasia* is very scant. The only major study utilizing chromosome banding was reported by Aly et al. (1994), who investigated 28 cases. No structural chromosome rearrangements were detected. Loss of the Y chromosome was the most common change (nine cases), followed by trisomy 7 (five cases). In one case, both anomalies were present in most of the metaphase cells analyzed. The cytogenetic results were confirmed by FISH analysis. The neoplasia relevance of −Y and/or +7 has already been discussed in the previous text. Aly et al. (1994) concluded that trisomy 7 is probably unrelated to the tumor parenchyma cells, which hence might have the rather unspecific −Y as the only chromosomal anomaly. CGH analysis shows no chromosome copy number changes (Ribeiro et al., 2006a) and FISH analysis finds no *TMPRSS2–ERG* rearrangement (Perner et al., 2007) in benign prostatic hyperplasia.

Penis

Carcinoma of the penis is a rare disease and only three squamous cell carcinomas with clonal chromosome abnormalities have been reported. No consistent aberration pattern is apparent.

The tumor examined by Xiao et al. (1992) had a pseudodiploid karyotype with structural rearrangements of chromosomes 2, 4, and 8, a whole-arm translocation between 5 and 15, losses of both chromosomes 13 and one chromosome 15, as well as three unidentified markers. A hypotetraploid karyotype with a rearranged X chromosome, a 1p deletion, an unbalanced translocation between chromosomes 1 and 16, an isochromosome 10q, and several numerical chromosome changes was subsequently reported by Ornellas et al. (1998). Finally, the same group found a hyperdiploid karyotype with a 1q duplication, isochromosomes 1q and 18q, monosomy 3, a rearranged 11q, a 12p deletion, and three markers in the third tumor examined (Ornellas et al., 1999).

Interesting and unexpected cytogenetic findings have been made in *Peyronie's disease*, a localized but progressive fibrosis of unknown cause affecting the tunica albuginea of the penis. Somers et al. (1987) found clonal chromosome abnormalities in seven of 12 lesions examined. The most common karyotypic changes were the numerical aberrations −Y (three cases), +7, and +8, but also nonrecurrent, balanced structural rearrangements were seen in clonal proportions (three cases). No chromosomal abnormalities were found in control cultures from the adjacent tunica, dermis, or blood from the same patients or in other types of penile scars. Guerneri et al. (1991) found clonal chromosome anomalies in nine of 14 Peyronie's disease lesions. Loss of the Y chromosome was again the most common change (six cases), but various other simple numerical aberrations were also seen. In one case, complex structural rearrangements were present in a pseudodiploid karyotype. The authors stressed the fact that four of the nine abnormal cases displayed more than one cytogenetically unrelated clone, which they took to indicate a polyclonal disease origin.

The chromosomal instability discovered by both Somers et al. (1987) and Guerneri et al. (1991) unquestionably gave rise to clonal chromosomal changes, including evidence of clonal evolution, in the examined cell population. But what are the conclusions about the pathogenesis of Peyronie's disease that can be drawn from the cytogenetic data? Of relevance in this context is the finding in another type of fibromatosis, Dupuytren's contracture of

the hand, of similar chromosomal abnormalities (Wurster-Hill et al., 1988). It would be rash to conclude that the karyotypic anomalies necessitate the classification of Peyronie's and Dupuytren's diseases as neoplastic; one now knows that at least some clonal chromosome abnormalities may exist in disease processes that can be called tumorous only if the existing, conventional nomenclature practices are stretched unacceptably (Johansson et al., 1993). Furthermore, it is still unclear whether the karyotypic instability registered by cytogenetic methods represents a primary derangement or if it is a reflection of an even more fundamental defect. In either case, however, it is reasonable to assume that it might contribute significantly to the pathogenetic process.

Summary

Both seminomatous and nonseminomatous TGCT of adolescents and young adults carry an i(12p) as their most common and characteristic chromosomal anomaly; those who have no i(12p) have 12p gain through other mechanisms. Other karyotypic changes that typically are present in these tumors include losses of chromosomes 11, 13, 18, and Y, whereas chromosomes 7, 8, 12, and X are overrepresented. The fact that seminomatous and nonseminomatous TGCT share many karyotypic features strongly indicates that they are pathogenetically related. Compared with their nonseminomatous counterparts, seminomas generally have a higher chromosome number, more frequent gain of chromosomes 7, 15, 19, and 22, but fewer copies of chromosome 17 and i(12p). On the other hand, yolk sac tumors of newborns and infants typically have gain of 1q and 20q and loss of 1p, 4q, and 6q, whereas spermatocytic seminomas of older men are characterized by gain of chromosome 9.

Prostate carcinomas present the *TMPRSS2–ERG* fusion oncogene in about 50% of the cases, as well as rarer variants with alternative 5′ or 3′ fusion partners. The most common chromosome copy number changes are losses of 5q, 6q, 8p, 10q, 13q, 16q, 17p, and 18q and gains of 8q. *TMPRSS2–ERG* is also present in about 20% of HGPIN, the presumed precursor lesion of invasive disease. This indicates that *TMPRSS2–ETS* family gene fusions are early events in prostate carcinogenesis, followed by losses at 8p and then by loss of 13q and 16q and gain of 8q. These alterations seem to be followed by late secondary events that include losses from 10q, 5q, and 17p. No specific karyotypic features have been detected in hyperplasias of the prostate. −Y and +7 have been the most common changes.

Acknowledgment

Financial support from the Norwegian Cancer Society, the Portuguese Cancer Society (LPCC), and the Portuguese Science and Technology Foundation (FCT) is gratefully acknowledged.

References

Abdulkadir SA, Magee JA, Peters TJ, Kaleem Z, Naughton CK, Humphrey PA, et al. (2002): Conditional loss of Nkx3.1 in adult mice induces prostatic intraepithelial neoplasia. *Mol Cell Biol* 22:1495–1503.

Alagaratnam S, Lind GE, Kraggerud SM, Lothe RA, Skotheim RI (2011): The testicular germ cell tumour transcriptome. *Int J Androl* 34:e133–150.

Alers JC, Rochat J, Krijtenburg PJ, Hop WC, Kranse R, Rosenberg C, et al. (2000): Identification of genetic markers for prostatic cancer progression. *Lab Invest* 80:931–942.

Alers JC, Krijtenburg PJ, Vis AN, Hoedemaeker RF, Wildhagen MF, Hop WC, et al. (2001): Molecular cytogenetic analysis of prostatic adenocarcinomas from screening studies: early cancers may contain aggressive genetic features. *Am J Pathol* 158:399–406.

Aly MS, Dal Cin P, Van de Voorde W, van Poppel H, Ameye F, Baert L, et al. (1994): Chromosome abnormalities in benign prostatic hyperplasia. *Genes Chromosomes Cancer* 9:227–233.

Arps S, Rodewald A, Schmalenberger B, Carl P, Bressel M, Kastendieck H (1993): Cytogenetic survey of 32 cancers of the prostate. *Cancer Genet Cytogenet* 66:93–99.

Atkin NB, Baker MC (1982): Specific chromosome change, i(12p), in testicular tumours? *Lancet* 2:1349.

Atkin NB, Baker MC (1985): Chromosome study of five cancers of the prostate. *Hum Genet* 70:359–364.

Attard G, Clark J, Ambroisine L, Fisher G, Kovacs G, Flohr P, et al. (2008): Duplication of the fusion of TMPRSS2 to ERG sequences identifies fatal human prostate cancer. *Oncogene* 27 (3): 253–263.

Barros-Silva JD, Ribeiro FR, Rodrigues A, Cruz R, Martins AT, Jeronimo C, et al. (2011): Relative 8q gain predicts disease-specific survival irrespective of the TMPRSS2-ERG fusion status in diagnostic biopsies of prostate cancer. *Genes Chromosomes Cancer* 50:662–671.

Barros-Silva JD, Paulo P, Bakken AC, Cerveira N, Lovf M, Henrique R, et al. (2013): Novel 5′ fusion partners of ETV1 and ETV4 in prostate cancer. *Neoplasia* 15:720–726.

Barry M, Perner S, Demichelis F, Rubin MA (2007): TMPRSS2–ERG fusion heterogeneity in multifocal prostate cancer: clinical and biologic implications. *Urology* 70:630–633.

Biermann K, Göke F, Nettersheim D, Eckert D, Zhou H, Kahl P, et al. (2007): c-KIT is frequently mutated in bilateral germ cell tumours and down-regulated during progression from intratubular germ cell neoplasia to seminoma. *J Pathol* 213:311–318.

Bosl GJ, Ilson DH, Rodriguez E, Motzer RJ, Reuter VE, Chaganti RSK (1994): Clinical relevance of the i(12p) marker chromosome in germ cell tumors. *J Natl Cancer Inst* 86:349–355.

Breitkreuz T, Romanakis K, Lutz S, Seitz G, Bonkhoff H, Unteregger G, et al. (1993): Genotypic characterization of prostatic carcinomas: a combined cytogenetic, flow cytometry, and in situ DNA hybridization study. *Cancer Res* 53:4035–4040.

Brenner JC, Ateeq B, Li Y, Yocum AK, Cao Q, Asangani IA, et al. (2011): Mechanistic rationale for inhibition of poly(ADP-ribose) polymerase in ETS gene fusion-positive prostate cancer. *Cancer Cell* 19:664–678.

Bussey KJ, Lawce HJ, Olson SB, Arthur DC, Kalousek DK, Krailo M, et al. (1999): Chromosome abnormalities of eighty-one pediatric germ cell tumors: sex-, age-, site-, and histopathology-related differences: a Children's Cancer Group study. *Genes Chromosomes Cancer* 25:134–146.

Carver BS, Tran J, Gopalan A, Chen Z, Shaikh S, Carracedo A, et al. (2009): Aberrant ERG expression cooperates with loss of PTEN to promote cancer progression in the prostate. *Nat Genet* 41:619–624.

Cerveira N, Ribeiro FR, Peixoto A, Costa V, Henrique R, Jerónimo C, et al. (2006): TMPRSS2–ERG gene fusion causing ERG overexpression precedes chromosome copy number changes in prostate carcinomas and paired HGPIN lesions. *Neoplasia* 8:826–832.

Chaganti RS, Ladanyi M, Samaniego F, Offit K, Reuter VE, Jhanwar SC, et al. (1989): Leukemic differentiation of a mediastinal germ cell tumor. *Genes Chromosomes Cancer* 1:83–87.

Cher ML, Bova GS, Moore DH, Small EJ, Carroll PR, Pin SS, et al. (1996): Genetic alterations in untreated metastases and androgen-independent prostate cancer detected by comparative genomic hybridization and allelotyping. *Cancer Res* 56:3091–3102.

Chu LW, Troncoso P, Johnston DA, Liang JC (2003): Genetic markers useful for distinguishing between organ-confined and locally advanced prostate cancer. *Genes Chromosomes Cancer* 36:303–312.

Coffey J, Linger R, Pugh J, Dudakia D, Sokal M, Easton DF, et al. (2008): Somatic KIT mutations occur predominantly in seminoma germ cell tumors and are not predictive of bilateral disease: report of 220 tumors and review of literature. *Genes Chromosomes Cancer* 47:34–42.

Dal Cin P, Drochmans A, Moerman P, Van den Berghe H (1989): Isochromosome 12p in mediastinal germ cell tumor. *Cancer Genet Cytogenet* 42:243–251.

De Jong B, van Echten J, Looijenga LH, Geurts van Kessel A, Oosterhuis JW (1997): Cytogenetics of the progression of adult testicular germ cell tumors. *Cancer Genet Cytogenet* 95:88–95.

Demichelis F, Fall K, Perner S, Andrén O, Schmidt F, Setlur SR, et al. (2007): TMPRSS2–ERG gene fusion associated with lethal prostate cancer in a watchful waiting cohort. *Oncogene* 26:4596–4599.

Einhorn LH, Brames MJ, Heinrich MC, Corless CL, Madani A (2006): Phase II study of imatinib mesylate in chemotherapy refractory germ cell tumors expressing KIT. *Am J Clin Oncol* 29:12–13.

FitzGerald LM, Agalliu I, Johnson K, Miller MA, Kwon EM, Hurtado-Coll A, et al. (2008): Association of TMPRSS2-ERG gene fusion with clinical characteristics and outcomes: results from a population-based study of prostate cancer. *BMC Cancer* 8:230.

Frigyesi A, Gisselsson D, Hansen GB, Soller M, Mitelman F, Höglund M (2004): A model for karyotypic evolution in testicular germ cell tumors. *Genes Chromosomes Cancer* 40:172–178.

Fu W, Bubendorf L, Willi N, Moch H, Mihatsch MJ, Sauter G, et al. (2000): Genetic changes in clinically organ-confined prostate cancer by comparative genomic hybridization. *Urology* 56:880–885.

Gao X, Li LY, Zhou FJ, Xie KJ, Shao CK, Su ZL, et al. (2012): ERG rearrangement for predicting subsequent cancer diagnosis in high-grade prostatic intraepithelial neoplasia and lymph node metastasis. *Clin Cancer Res* 18:4163–4172.

Geurts van Kessel A, Suijkerbuijk RF, Sinke RJ, Looijenga L, Oosterhuis JW, de Jong B (1993): Molecular cytogenetics of human germ cell tumours: I(12p) and related chromosomal anomalies. *Eur Urol* 23:23–29.

Gillis AJ, Looijenga LH, de Jong B, Oosterhuis JW (1994): Clonality of combined testicular germ cell tumors of adults. *Lab Invest* 71:874–878.

Gopalan A, Leversha MA, Satagopan JM, Zhou Q, Al-Ahmadie HA, Fine SW, et al. (2009): TMPRSS2-ERG gene fusion is not associated with outcome in patients treated by prostatectomy. *Cancer Res* 69:1400–1406.

Greco FA, Vaughn WK, Hainsworth JD (1986): Advanced poorly differentiated carcinoma of unknown primary site: recognition of a treatable syndrome. *Ann Intern Med* 104:547–553.

Guerneri S, Stioui S, Mantovani F, Austoni E, Simoni G (1991): Multiple clonal chromosome abnormalities in Peyronie's disease. *Cancer Genet Cytogenet* 52:181–185.

Halvorsen OJ, Haukaas SA, Akslen LA (2003): Combined loss of PTEN and p27 expression is associated with tumor cell proliferation by Ki-67 and increased risk of recurrent disease in localized prostate cancer. *Clin Cancer Res* 9:1474–1479.

Han S, Brenner JC, Sabolch A, Jackson W, Speers C, Wilder-Romans K, et al. (2013): Targeted radiosensitization of ETS fusion-positive prostate cancer through PARP1 inhibition. *Neoplasia* 15:1207–1217.

Helgeson BE, Tomlins SA, Shah N, Laxman B, Cao Q, Prensner JR, et al. (2008): Characterization of TMPRSS2–ETV5 and SLC45A3–ETV5 gene fusions in prostate cancer. *Cancer Res* 68:73–80.

Henegariu O, Vance GH, Heiber D, Pera M, Heerema NA (1998): Triple-color FISH analysis of 12p amplification in testicular germ-cell tumors using 12p band-specific painting probes. *J Mol Med* 76:648–655.

Hermans KG, van Marion R, van Dekken H, Jenster G, van Weerden WM, Trapman J (2006): TMPRSS2–ERG fusion by translocation or interstitial deletion is highly relevant in androgen-dependent prostate cancer, but is bypassed in late-stage androgen receptor-negative prostate cancer. *Cancer Res* 66:10658–10663.

Hessels D, Smit FP, Verhaegh GW, Witjes JA, Cornel EB, Schalken JA (2007): Detection of TMPRSS2–ERG fusion transcripts and prostate cancer antigen 3 in urinary sediments may improve diagnosis of prostate cancer. *Clin Cancer Res* 13:5103–5108.

Honecker F, Wermann H, Mayer F, Gillis AJ, Stoop H, van Gurp RJ, et al. (2009): Microsatellite instability, mismatch repair deficiency, and BRAF mutation in treatment-resistant germ cell tumors. *J Clin Oncol* 27:2129–2136.

Hoogland AM, Jenster G, van Weerden WM, Trapman J, van der Kwast T, Roobol MJ, et al. (2012): ERG immunohistochemistry is not predictive for PSA recurrence, local recurrence or overall survival after radical prostatectomy for prostate cancer. *Mod Pathol* 25:471–479.

Houldsworth J, Korkola JE, Bosl GJ, Chaganti RS (2006): Biology and genetics of adult male germ cell tumors. *J Clin Oncol* 24:5512–5518.

Johansson B, Heim S, Mandahl N, Mertens F, Mitelman F (1993): Trisomy 7 in nonneoplastic cells. *Genes Chromosomes Cancer* 6:199–205.

Kemmer K, Corless CL, Fletcher JA, McGreevey L, Haley A, Griffith D, et al. (2004): KIT mutations are common in testicular seminomas. *Am J Pathol* 164:305–313.

Kernek KM, Brunelli M, Ulbright TM, Eble JN, Martignoni G, Zhang S, et al. (2004): Fluorescence *in situ* hybridization analysis of chromosome 12p in paraffin-embedded tissue is useful for establishing germ cell origin of metastatic tumors. *Mod Pathol* 17:1309–1313.

Kim MJ, Bhatia-Gaur R, Banach-Petrosky WA, Desai N, Wang Y, Hayward SW, et al. (2002a): Nkx3.1 mutant mice recapitulate early stages of prostate carcinogenesis. *Cancer Res* 62:2999–3004.

Kim MJ, Cardiff RD, Desai N, Banach-Petrosky WA, Parsons R, Shen MM, et al. (2002b): Cooperativity of Nkx3.1 and Pten loss of function in a mouse model of prostate carcinogenesis. *Proc Natl Acad Sci USA* 99:2884–2889.

King JC, Xu J, Wongvipat J, Hieronymus H, Carver BS, Leung DH, et al. (2009): Cooperativity of TMPRSS2-ERG with PI3-kinase pathway activation in prostate oncogenesis. *Nat Genet* 41:524–526.

Klezovitch O, Risk M, Coleman I, Lucas JM, Null M, True LD, et al. (2008): A causal role for ERG in neoplastic transformation of prostate epithelium. *Proc Natl Acad Sci USA* 105:2105–2110.

König JJ, Teubel W, van Dongen JW, Hagemeijer A, Romijn JC, Schröder FH (1993): Tissue culture loss of aneuploid cells from carcinomas of the prostate. *Genes Chromosomes Cancer* 8:22–27.

Korkola JE, Houldsworth J, Chadalavada RS, Olshen AB, Dobrzynski D, Reuter VE, et al. (2006): Down-regulation of stem cell genes, including those in a 200-kb gene cluster at 12p13.31, is associated with *in vivo* differentiation of human male germ cell tumors. *Cancer Res* 66:820–827.

Korkola JE, Houldsworth J, Feldman DR, Olshen AB, Qin LX, Patil S, et al. (2009): Identification and validation of a gene expression signature that predicts outcome in adult men with germ cell tumors. *J Clin Oncol* 27:5240–5247.

Korn WM, Oide Weghuis DE, Suijkerbuijk RF, Schmidt U, Otto T, du Manoir S, et al.(1996): Detection of chromosomal DNA gains and losses in testicular germ cell tumors by comparative genomic hybridization. *Genes Chromosomes Cancer* 17:78–87.

Kum JB, Ulbright TM, Williamson SR, Wang M, Zhang S, Foster RS, et al. (2012): Molecular genetic evidence supporting the origin of somatic-type malignancy and teratoma from the same progenitor cell. *Am J Surg Pathol* 36:1849–1856.

Kwabi-Addo B, Giri D, Schmidt K, Podsypanina K, Parsons R, Greenberg N, et al. (2001): Haploinsufficiency of the Pten tumor suppressor gene promotes prostate cancer progression. *Proc Natl Acad Sci USA* 98:11563–11568.

Ladanyi M, Samaniego F, Reuter VE, Motzer RJ, Jhanwar SC, Bosl GJ, et al. (1990): Cytogenetic and immunohistochemical evidence for the germ cell origin of a subset of acute leukemias associated with mediastinal germ cell tumors. *J Natl Cancer Inst* 82:221–227.

Lapointe J, Li C, Giacomini CP, Salari K, Huang S, Wang P, et al. (2007): Genomic profiling reveals alternative genetic pathways of prostate tumorigenesis. *Cancer Res* 67:8504–8510.

Laxman B, Tomlins SA, Mehra R, Morris DS, Wang L, Helgeson BE, et al. (2006): Noninvasive detection of TMPRSS2–ERG fusion transcripts in the urine of men with prostate cancer. *Neoplasia* 8:885–888.

Liu W, Chang B, Sauvageot J, Dimitrov L, Gielzak M, Li T, et al. (2006): Comprehensive assessment of DNA copy number alterations in human prostate cancers using Affymetrix 100 K SNP mapping array. *Genes Chromosomes Cancer* 45:1018–1032.

Liu W, Ewing CM, Chang BL, Li T, Sun J, Turner AR, et al. (2007): Multiple genomic alterations on 21q22 predict various TMPRSS2/ERG fusion transcripts in human prostate cancers. *Genes Chromosomes Cancer* 46:972–980.

Looijenga LH, de Leeuw H, van Oorschot M, van Gurp RJ, Stoop H, Gillis AJ, et al. (2003a): Stem cell factor receptor (c-KIT) codon 816 mutations predict development of bilateral testicular germ-cell tumors. *Cancer Res* 63:7674–7678.

Looijenga LH, Zafarana G, Grygalewicz B, Summersgill B, Debiec-Rychter M, Veltman J, et al. (2003b): Role of gain of 12p in germ cell tumour development. *APMIS* 111:161–171.

Looijenga LH, Hersmus R, Gillis AJ, Pfundt R, Stoop HJ, van Gurp RJ, et al. (2006): Genomic and expression profiling of human spermatocytic seminomas: primary spermatocyte as tumorigenic precursor and DMRT1 as candidate chromosome 9 gene. *Cancer Res* 66:290–302.

Lundgren R, Heim S, Mandahl N, Anderson H, Mitelman F (1992a): Chromosome abnormalities are associated with unfavorable outcome in prostatic cancer patients. *J Urol* 147:784–788.

Lundgren R, Mandahl N, Heim S, Limon J, Henrikson H, Mitelman F (1992b): Cytogenetic analysis of 57 primary prostatic adenocarcinomas. *Genes Chromosomes Cancer* 4:16–24.

Mattfeldt T, Wolter H, Trijic D, Gottfried HW, Kestler HA (2002): Chromosomal regions in prostatic carcinomas studied by comparative genomic hybridization, hierarchical cluster analysis and self-organizing feature maps. *Anal Cell Pathol* 24:167–179.

McIntyre A, Summersgill B, Spendlove HE, Huddart R, Houlston R, Shipley J (2005a): Activating mutations and/or expression levels of tyrosine kinase receptors GRB7, RAS, and BRAF in testicular germ cell tumors. *Neoplasia* 7:1047–1052.

McIntyre A, Summersgill B, Grygalewicz B, Gillis AJ, Stoop J, van Gurp RJ, et al. (2005b): Amplification and overexpression of the KIT gene is associated with progression in the seminoma subtype of testicular germ cell tumors of adolescents and adults. *Cancer Res* 65:8085–8089.

Mehra R, Han B, Tomlins SA, Wang L, Menon A, Wasco MJ, et al. (2007a): Heterogeneity of TMPRSS2 gene rearrangements in multifocal prostate adenocarcinoma: molecular evidence for an independent group of diseases. *Cancer Res* 67:7991–7995.

Mehra R, Tomlins SA, Shen R, Nadeem O, Wang L, Wei JT, et al. (2007b): Comprehensive assessment of TMPRSS2 and ETS family gene aberrations in clinically localized prostate cancer. *Mod Pathol* 20:538–544.

Micale MA, Mohamed A, Sakr W, Powell IJ, Wolman SR (1992): Cytogenetics of primary prostatic adenocarcinoma: clonality and chromosome instability. *Cancer Genet Cytogenet* 61:165–173.

Mitelman F, Johansson B, Mertens F, editors (2014): Mitelman Database of Chromosome Aberrations and Gene Fusions in Cancer. http://cgap.nci.nih.gov/Chromosomes/Mitelman.

Mostert MC, Verkerk AJ, van de Pol M, Heighway J, Marynen P, Rosenberg C, et al. (1998): Identification of the critical region of 12p over-representation in testicular germ cell tumors of adolescents and adults. *Oncogene* 16: 2617–2627.

Mostert M, Rosenberg C, Stoop H, Schuyer M, Timmer A, Oosterhuis W, et al. (2000): Comparative genomic and in situ hybridization of germ cell tumors of the infantile testis. *Lab Invest* 80:1055–1064.

Motzer RJ, Rodriguez E, Reuter VE, Samaniego F, Dmitrovsky E, Bajorin DF, et al. (1991): Genetic analysis as an aid in diagnosis for patients with midline carcinomas of uncertain histologies. *J Natl Cancer Inst* 83:341–346.

Motzer RJ, Rodriguez E, Reuter VE, Bosl GJ, Mazumdar M, Chaganti RS (1995): Molecular and cytogenetic studies in the diagnosis of patients with poorly differentiated carcinomas of unknown primary site. *J Clin Oncol* 13:274–282.

Motzer RJ, Amsterdam A, Prieto V, Sheinfeld J, Murty VV, Mazumdar M, et al. (1998): Teratoma with malignant transformation: diverse malignant histologies arising in men with germ cell tumors. *J Urol* 159:133–138.

Nam RK, Sugar L, Yang W, Srivastava S, Klotz LH, Yang LY, et al. (2007): Expression of the TMPRSS2–ERG fusion gene predicts cancer recurrence after surgery for localised prostate cancer. *Br J Cancer* 97:1690–1695.

Okamura A, Wakahashi K, Ishii S, Katayama Y, Yamamoto K, Matsui T (2010): Possible alternative strategy for stage I imatinib-sensitive testicular seminoma; lessons from a case associated with Philadelphia chromosome-positive acute lymphoblastic leukemia. *Ann Oncol* 21:1129–1130.

Olie RA, Looijenga LH, Boerrigter L, Top B, Rodenhuis S, Langeveld A, et al. (1995): N- and KRAS mutations in primary testicular germ cell tumors: incidence and possible biological implications. *Genes Chromosomes Cancer* 12:110–116.

Oosterhuis JW, Looijenga LH (2005): Testicular germ-cell tumours in a broader perspective. *Nat Rev Cancer* 5:210–222.

Oosterhuis JW, Castedo SM, de Jong B, Seruca R, Buist J, Schraffordt Koops H, et al. (1988): Karyotyping and DNA flow cytometry of an orchidoblastoma. *Cancer Genet Cytogenet* 36:7–11.

Orazi A, Neiman RS, Ulbright TM, Heerema NA, John K, Nichols CR (1993): Hematopoietic precursor cells within the yolk sac tumor component are the source of secondary hematopoietic malignancies in patients with mediastinal germ cell tumors. *Cancer* 71:3873–3881.

Ornellas AA, Ornellas MH, Simoes F, Soares R, Campos MM, Harab RC, et al. (1998): Cytogenetic analysis of an invasive, poorly differentiated squamous cell carcinoma of the penis. *Cancer Genet Cytogenet* 101:78–79.

Ornellas AA, Ornellas MH, Otero L, Simoes F, Campos MM, Harab RC, et al. (1999): Karyotypic finding in two cases of moderately differentiated squamous cell carcinomas of the penis. *Cancer Genet Cytogenet* 115:77–79.

Ottesen AM, Skakkebaek NE, Lundsteen C, Leffers H, Larsen J, Rajpert-De Meyts E (2003): High-resolution comparative genomic hybridization detects extra chromosome arm 12p material in most cases of carcinoma in situ adjacent to overt germ cell tumors, but not before the invasive tumor development. *Genes Chromosomes Cancer* 38:117–125.

Palanisamy N, Ateeq B, Kalyana-Sundaram S, Pflueger D, Ramnarayanan K, Shankar S, et al. (2010): Rearrangements of the RAF kinase pathway in prostate cancer, gastric cancer and melanoma. *Nature Med* 16:793–798.

Paris PL, Andaya A, Fridlyand J, Jain AN, Weinberg V, Kowbel D, et al. (2004): Whole genome scanning identifies genotypes associated with recurrence and metastasis in prostate tumors. *Hum Mol Genet* 13:1303–1313.

Paulo P, Barros-Silva JD, Ribeiro FR, Ramalho-Carvalho J, Jeronimo C, Henrique R, et al. (2012a): FLI1 is a novel ETS transcription factor involved in gene fusions in prostate cancer. *Genes Chromosomes Cancer* 51:240–249.

Paulo P, Ribeiro FR, Santos J, Mesquita D, Almeida M, Barros-Silva JD, et al. (2012b): Molecular subtyping of primary prostate cancer reveals specific and shared target genes of different ETS rearrangements. *Neoplasia* 14:600–611.

Pectasides D, Nikolaou M, Pectasides E, Koumarianou A, Valavanis C, Economopoulos T (2008): Complete response after imatinib mesylate administration in a patient with chemoresistant stage IV seminoma. *Anticancer Res* 28: 2317–2320.

Pedersini R, Vattemi E, Mazzoleni G, Graiff C (2007): Complete response after treatment with imatinib in pre-treated disseminated testicular seminoma with overexpression of c-KIT. *Lancet Oncol* 8:1039–1040.

Perlman EJ, Cushing B, Hawkins E, Griffin CA (1994): Cytogenetic analysis of childhood endodermal sinus tumors: a pediatric oncology group study. *Pediatr Pathol* 14:695–708.

Perner S, Demichelis F, Beroukhim R, Schmidt FH, Mosquera JM, Setlur S, et al. (2006): TMPRSS2–ERG fusion-associated deletions provide insight into the heterogeneity of prostate cancer. *Cancer Res* 66:8337–8341.

Perner S, Mosquera JM, Demichelis F, Hofer MD, Paris PL, Simko J, et al. (2007): TMPRSS2–ERG fusion prostate cancer: an early molecular event associated with invasion. *Am J Surg Pathol* 31:882–888.

Pettersson A, Graff RE, Bauer SR, Pitt MJ, Lis RT, Stack EC, et al. (2012): The TMPRSS2:ERG rearrangement, ERG expression, and prostate cancer outcomes: a cohort study and meta-analysis. *Cancer Epidemiol Biomarkers Prev* 21:1497–1509.

Rajput AB, Miller MA, DeLuca A, Boyd N, Leung S, Hurtado-Coll A, et al. (2007): Frequency of the TMPRSS2–ERG gene fusion is increased in moderate to poorly differentiated prostate cancers. *J Clin Pathol* 60:1238–1243.

Rapley EA, Hockley S, Warren W, Johnson L, Huddart R, Crockford G, et al. (2004): Somatic mutations of KIT in familial testicular germ cell tumours. *Br J Cancer* 90:2397–2401.

Reid AH, Attard G, Ambroisine L, Fisher G, Kovacs G, Brewer D, et al. (2010): Molecular characterisation of ERG, ETV1 and PTEN gene loci identifies patients at low and high risk of death from prostate cancer. *Br J Cancer* 102:678–684.

Ribeiro FR, Diep CB, Jerónimo C, Henrique R, Lopes C, Eknaes M, et al. (2006a): Statistical dissection of genetic pathways involved in prostate carcinogenesis. *Genes Chromosomes Cancer* 45:154–163.

Ribeiro FR, Henrique R, Hektoen M, Berg M, Jerónimo C, Teixeira MR, et al. (2006b): Comparison of chromosomal and array-based comparative genomic hybridization for the detection of genomic imbalances in primary prostate carcinomas. *Mol Cancer* 5:33.

Ribeiro FR, Jerónimo C, Henrique R, Fonseca D, Oliveira J, Lothe RA, et al. (2006c): 8q gain is an independent predictor of poor survival in diagnostic needle biopsies from prostate cancer suspects. *Clin Cancer Res* 12:3961–3970.

Ribeiro FR, Henrique R, Martins AT, Jerónimo C, Teixeira MR (2007): Relative copy number gain of MYC in diagnostic needle biopsies is an independent prognostic factor for prostate cancer patients. *Eur Urol* 52:116–125.

Rodriguez E, Mathew S, Reuter V, Ilson DH, Bosl GJ, Chaganti RSK (1992): Cytogenetic analysis of 124 prospectively ascertained male germ cell tumors. *Cancer Res* 52:2285–2291.

Rodriguez E, Houldsworth J, Reuter VE, Meltzer P, Zhang J, Trent JM, et al. (1993): Molecular cytogenetic analysis of i(12p)-negative human male germ cell tumors. *Genes Chromosomes Cancer* 8:230–236.

Rodriguez S, Jafer O, Goker H, Summersgill BM, Zafarana G, Gillis AJ, et al. (2003): Expression profile of genes from 12p in testicular germ cell tumors of adolescents and adults associated with i(12p) and amplification at 12p11.2–p12.1. *Oncogene* 22:1880–1891.

Roelofs H, Mostert MC, Pompe K, Zafarana G, van Oorschot M, van Gurp RJ, et al. (2000): Restricted 12p amplification and RAS mutation in human germ cell tumors of the adult testis. *Am J Pathol* 157:1155–1166.

Rosenberg C, Mostert MC, Schut TB, van de Pol M, van Echten J, de Jong B, et al. (1998): Chromosomal constitution of human spermatocytic seminomas: comparative genomic hybridization supported by conventional and interphase cytogenetics. *Genes Chromosomes Cancer* 23:286–291.

Rosenberg C, Van Gurp RJ, Geelen E, Oosterhuis JW, Looijenga LH (2000): Overrepresentation of the short arm of chromosome 12 is related to invasive growth of human testicular seminomas and nonseminomas. *Oncogene* 19:5858–5862.

Sakuma Y, Sakurai S, Oguni S, Hironaka M, Saito K (2003): Alterations of the c-kit gene in testicular germ cell tumors. *Cancer Sci* 94:486–491.

Samaniego F, Rodriguez E, Houldsworth J, Murty VVVS, Ladanyi M, Lele KP, et al. (1990): Cytogenetic and molecular genetic analysis of human male germ cell tumors: chromosome 12 abnormalities and gene amplification. *Genes Chromosomes Cancer* 1:289–300.

Schneider DT, Schuster AE, Fritsch MK, Calaminus G, Harms D, Göbel U, et al. (2001): Genetic analysis of childhood germ cell tumors with comparative genomic hybridization. *Klin Padiatr* 213:204–211.

Schneider DT, Zahn S, Sievers S, Alemazkour K, Reifenberger G, Wiestler OD, et al. (2006): Molecular genetic analysis of central nervous system germ cell tumors with comparative genomic hybridization. *Mod Pathol* 19:864–873.

Sinke RJ, Suijkerbuijk RF, de Jong B, Oosterhuis JW, Geurts van Kessel A (1993): Uniparental origin of i(12p) in human germ cell tumors. *Genes Chromosomes Cancer* 6:161–165.

Skotheim RI, Autio R, Lind GE, Kraggerud SM, Andrews PW, Monni O, et al. (2006): Novel genomic aberrations in testicular germ cell tumors by array-CGH, and associated gene expression changes. *Cell Oncol* 28:315–326.

Smolarek TA, Blough RI, Foster RS, Ulbright TM, Palmer CG, Heerema NA (1995): Identification of multiple chromosome 12 abnormalities in human testicular germ cell tumors by two-color fluorescence *in situ* hybridization (FISH). *Genes Chromosomes Cancer* 14:252–258.

Smolarek TA, Blough RI, Foster RS, Ulbright TM, Palmer CG, Heerema NA (1999): Cytogenetic analyses of 85 testicular germ cell tumors: comparison of postchemotherapy and untreated tumors. *Cancer Genet Cytogenet* 108:57–69.

Soller MJ, Isaksson M, Elfving P, Soller W, Lundgren R, Panagopoulos I (2006): Confirmation of the high frequency of the TMPRSS2/ERG fusion gene in prostate cancer. *Genes Chromosomes Cancer* 45:717–719.

Somers KD, Winters BA, Dawson DM, Leffell MS, Wright GL Jr, Devine CJ Jr, et al. (1987): Chromosome abnormalities in Peyronie's disease. *J Urol* 137:672–675.

Sommerer F, Hengge UR, Markwarth A, Vomschloss S, Stolzenburg JU, Wittekind C, et al. (2005): Mutations of BRAF and RAS are rare events in germ cell tumours. *Int J Cancer* 113:329–335.

Suijkerbuijk RF, Sinke RJ, Meloni AM, Parrington JM, van Echten J, de Jong B, et al. (1993): Overrepresentation of chromosome 12p sequences and karyotypic evolution in i(12p)-negative testicular germ-cell tumors revealed by fluorescence *in situ* hybridization. *Cancer Genet Cytogenet* 70:85–93.

Summersgill B, Osin P, Lu YJ, Huddart R, Shipley J (2001): Chromosomal imbalances associated with carcinoma *in situ* and associated testicular germ cell tumours of adolescents and adults. *Br J Cancer* 85:213–220.

Taylor BS, Schultz N, Hieronymus H, Gopalan A, Xiao Y, Carver BS, et al. (2010): Integrative genomic profiling of human prostate cancer. *Cancer Cell* 18:11–22.

Teixeira MR (2008): Chromosome mechanisms giving rise to the TMPRSS2–ERG fusion oncogene in prostate cancer and HGPIN lesions. *Am J Surg Pathol* 32:642–644.

Teixeira MR, Waehre H, Lothe RA, Stenwig AE, Pandis N, Gierchsky KE, et al. (2000): High frequency of clonal chromosome abnormalities in prostatic neoplasms sampled by prostatectomy or ultrasound-guided needle biopsy. *Genes Chromosomes Cancer* 28:211–219.

Teixeira MR, Ribeiro FR, Eknaes M, Waehre H, Stenwig AE, Gierchsky KE, et al. (2004): Genomic analysis of prostate carcinoma specimens obtained via ultrasound-guided needle biopsy may be of use in preoperative decision-making. *Cancer* 101:1786–1793.

Tian Q, Frierson HF Jr, Krystal GW, Moskaluk CA (1999): Activating c-kit gene mutations in human germ cell tumors. *Am J Pathol* 154:1643–1647.

Tomlins SA, Rhodes DR, Perner S, Dhanasekaran SM, Mehra R, Sun XW, et al. (2005): Recurrent fusion of TMPRSS2 and ETS transcription factor genes in prostate cancer. *Science* 310:644–648.

Tomlins SA, Mehra R, Rhodes DR, Smith LR, Roulston D, Helgeson BE, et al. (2006): TMPRSS2–ETV4 gene fusions define a third molecular subtype of prostate cancer. *Cancer Res* 66:3396–3400.

Tomlins SA, Laxman B, Dhanasekaran SM, Helgeson BE, Cao X, Morris DS, et al. (2007): Distinct classes of chromosomal rearrangements create oncogenic ETS gene fusions in prostate cancer. *Nature* 448:595–599.

Tomlins SA, Laxman B, Varambally S, Cao X, Yu J, Helgeson BE, et al. (2008): Role of the TMPRSS2-ERG gene fusion in prostate cancer. *Neoplasia* 10:177–188.

Tomlins SA, Aubin SM, Siddiqui J, Lonigro RJ, Sefton-Miller L, Miick S, et al. (2011): Urine TMPRSS2:ERG fusion transcript stratifies prostate cancer risk in men with elevated serum PSA. *Science Transl Med* 3:94ra72.

Tomlins SA, Palanisamy N, Siddiqui J, Chinnaiyan AM, Kunju LP (2012): Antibody-based detection of ERG rearrangements in prostate core biopsies, including diagnostically challenging cases: ERG staining in prostate core biopsies. *Arch Pathol Lab Med* 136:935–946.

Tørring N, Borre M, Sørensen KD, Andersen CL, Wiuf C, Ørntoft TF (2007): Genome-wide analysis of allelic imbalance in prostate cancer using the Affymetrix 50 K SNP mapping array. *Br J Cancer* 96:499–506.

Tu JJ, Rohan S, Kao J, Kitabayashi N, Mathew S, Chen YT (2007): Gene fusions between TMPRSS2 and ETS family genes in prostate cancer: frequency and transcript variant analysis by RT-PCR and FISH on paraffin-embedded tissues. *Mod Pathol* 20:921–928.

Van Duin M, van Marion R, Vissers K, Watson JE, van Weerden WM, Schröder FH, et al. (2005): High-resolution array comparative genomic hybridization of chromosome arm 8q: evaluation of genetic progression markers for prostate cancer. *Genes Chromosomes Cancer* 44:438–449.

Van Echten J, Oosterhuis JW, Looijenga LH, van de Pol M, Wiersema J, te Meerman GJ, et al. (1995a): No recurrent structural abnormalities apart from i(12p) in primary germ cell tumors of the adult testis. *Genes Chromosomes Cancer* 14:133–144.

Van Echten J, van Gurp RJ, Stoepker M, Looijenga LH, de Jong J, Oosterhuis W (1995b): Cytogenetic evidence that carcinoma *in situ* is the precursor lesion for invasive testicular germ cell tumors. *Cancer Genet Cytogenet* 85:133–137.

Van Echten J, Oosterhuis JW, Looijenga LH, Dam A, Sleijfer DT, Schraffordt Koops H, et al. (1996): Mixed testicular germ cell tumors: monoclonal or polyclonal? *Mod Pathol* 9:371–374.

Van Echten J, Timmer A, van der Veen AY, Molenaar WM, de Jong B (2002): Infantile and adult testicular germ cell tumors. A different pathogenesis? *Cancer Genet Cytogenet* 135:57–62.

Verdorfer I, Hobisch A, Culig Z, Hittmair A, Bartsch G, Erdel M, et al. (2001): Combined study of prostatic carcinoma by classical cytogenetic analysis and comparative genomic hybridization. *Int J Oncol* 19:1263–1270.

Verdorfer I, Rogatsch H, Tzankov A, Steiner H, Mikuz G (2004): Molecular cytogenetic analysis of human spermatocytic seminomas. *J Pathol* 204:277–281.

Verhagen PC, van Duijn PW, Hermans KG, Looijenga LH, van Gurp RJ, Stoop H, et al. (2006): The PTEN gene in locally progressive prostate cancer is preferentially inactivated by bi-allelic gene deletion. *J Pathol* 208:699–707.

Visakorpi T, Hyytinen E, Koivisto P, Tanner M, Keinänen R, Palmberg C, et al. (1995a): *In vivo* amplification of the androgen receptor gene and progression of human prostate cancer. *Nat Genet* 9:401–406.

Visakorpi T, Kallioniemi AH, Syvänen AC, Hyytinen ER, Karhu R, Tammela T, et al. (1995b): Genetic changes in primary and recurrent prostate cancer by comparative genomic hybridization. *Cancer Res* 55:342–347.

Vos AM, Oosterhuis JW, de Jong B, Buist J, Schraffordt Koops H (1990): Cytogenetics of carcinoma *in situ* of the testis. *Cancer Genet Cytogenet* 46:75–81.

Wang J, Cai Y, Ren C, Ittmann M (2006): Expression of variant TMPRSS2/ERG fusion messenger RNAs is associated with aggressive prostate cancer. *Cancer Res* 66:8347–8351.

Wang XS, Shankar S, Dhanasekaran SM, Ateeq B, Sasaki AT, Jing X, et al. (2011): Characterization of KRAS rearrangements in metastatic prostate cancer. *Cancer Discov* 1:35–43.

Webb HD, Hawkins AL, Griffin CA (1996): Cytogenetic abnormalities are frequent in uncultured prostate cancer cells. *Cancer Genet Cytogenet* 88:126–132.

Willmore-Payne C, Holden JA, Chadwick BE, Layfield LJ (2006): Detection of c-kit exons 11- and 17-activating mutations in testicular seminomas by high-resolution melting amplicon analysis. *Mod Pathol* 19:1164–1169.

Wolter H, Gottfried HW, Mattfeldt T (2002a): Genetic changes in stage pT2N0 prostate cancer studied by comparative genomic hybridization. *BJU Int* 89:310–316.

Wolter H, Trijic D, Gottfried HW, Mattfeldt T (2002b): Chromosomal changes in incidental prostatic carcinomas detected by comparative genomic hybridization. *Eur Urol* 41:328–334.

Woodruff K, Wang N, May W, Adrone E, Denny C, Feig SA (1995): The clonal nature of mediastinal germ cell tumors and acute myelogenous leukemia. A case report and review of the literature. *Cancer Genet Cytogenet* 79:25–31.

Wu C, Wyatt AW, Lapuk AV, McPherson A, McConeghy BJ, Bell RH, et al. (2012): Integrated genome and transcriptome sequencing identifies a novel form of hybrid and aggressive prostate cancer. *J Pathol* 227:53–61.

Wurster-Hill DH, Brown F, Park JP, Gibson SH (1988): Cytogenetic studies in Dupuytren contracture. *Am J Hum Genet* 43:285–292.

Xiao S, Feng X-L, Shi Y-H, Liu Q-Z, Li P (1992): Cytogenetic abnormalities in a squamous cell carcinoma of the penis. *Cancer Genet Cytogenet* 64:139–141.

Yoshimoto M, Joshua AM, Chilton-Macneill S, Bayani J, Selvarajah S, Evans AJ, et al. (2006): Three-color FISH analysis of TMPRSS2/ERG fusions in prostate cancer indicates that genomic microdeletion of chromosome 21 is associated with rearrangement. *Neoplasia* 8:465–469.

Zafarana G, Gillis AJ, van Gurp RJ, Olsson PG, Elstrodt F, Stoop H, et al. (2002): Coamplification of DAD-R, SOX5, and EKI1 in human testicular seminomas, with specific overexpression of DAD-R, correlates with reduced levels of apoptosis and earlier clinical manifestation. *Cancer Res* 62:1822–1831.

Zafarana G, Grygalewicz B, Gillis AJ, Vissers LE, van de Vliet W, van Gurp RJ, et al. (2003): 12p-amplicon structure analysis in testicular germ cell tumors of adolescents and adults by array CGH. *Oncogene* 22:7695–7701.

CHAPTER 19

Tumors of endocrine glands

Jörn Bullerdiek[1] and David Gisselsson[2]

[1] Center for Human Genetics, University of Bremen, Bremen, Germany
[2] Department of Clinical Genetics, University of Lund, Lund, Sweden

Cytogenetic information is available (Mitelman et al., 2014) on roughly 600 neoplasms originating from the thyroid, parathyroid, pituitary, and adrenal glands; from the thymus; and from the endocrine pancreas.

Thyroid

Follicular adenomas are frequent benign tumors arising from the thyroid follicular epithelium. About half of them show recurrent structural or numerical chromosome aberrations corresponding to three main cytogenetic subgroups defined by the presence of trisomy 7, translocations involving 19q13, or translocations involving 2p21 (Belge et al., 1998). In addition, recurrent but less common abnormalities such as deletions of the long arm of chromosome 13 have also been described. The rare occurrence of adenoma-like aberrations also in goiters suggests that adenomas can arise as a monoclonal proliferation of cells in preexisting goiters. Apparently, this proliferation can be detected earlier cytogenetically than by histology.

Trisomy 7 is found in 30% of adenomas with clonal cytogenetic aberrations. In the study by Dettori et al. (2003), the cytogenetic changes in oncocytic lesions of the thyroid were examined using karyotyping, fluorescence *in situ* hybridization (FISH), and comparative genomic hybridization (CGH), and the results were compared with *in situ* analysis of mitochondrial accumulation by immunofluorescence. In follicular nodules with oncocytic differentiation, diffuse accumulation of mitochondria within the cell was found to be associated with trisomy 7 and progressive numerical chromosome aberrations. Trisomy 7 is often accompanied by further numerical aberrations such as trisomy for chromosomes 5, 12, 14, 16, and/or 17 (Belge et al., 1994, 1998). More of the same may follow (Belge et al., 1994), occasionally giving rise to adenomas with more than 70 chromosomes per cell, as has also been found by CGH (Perissel et al., 2002; Roque et al., 2003). Interestingly, within that sequence of chromosomal gains starting with trisomy 7, the acquisition of additional whole chromosome copies is associated neither with any structural chromosome instability nor necessarily with transformation to a malignant tumor phenotype.

Translocations involving chromosome band 19q13.4 (Figure 19.1) are the second most frequent cytogenetic aberrations in thyroid adenomas. Given the high prevalence of thyroid adenomas in the population, these translocations may actually represent the most common neoplasia-specific structural chromosome rearrangement in epithelial tumors. The translocation partners are highly variable. By positional cloning, the breakpoints of the

Cancer Cytogenetics: Chromosomal and Molecular Genetic Aberrations of Tumor Cells, Fourth Edition.
Edited by Sverre Heim and Felix Mitelman.
© 2015 John Wiley & Sons, Ltd. Published 2015 by John Wiley & Sons, Ltd.

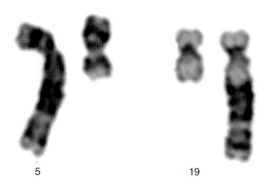

5   19

Figure 19.1 Partial G-banded karyotype of a thyroid adenoma showing the translocation t(5;19)(q13;q13.4). A subset of thyroid adenomas is cytogenetically defined by 19q13 rearrangements.

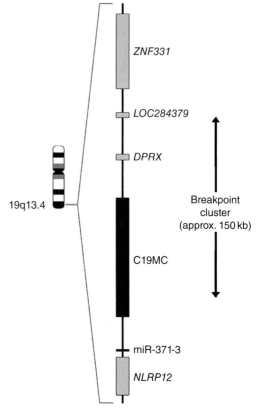

Figure 19.2 Genomic organization of the 19q13.4 breakpoint region. The breakpoint cluster region has a size of approximately 150 kb. Protein-coding genes are represented by light gray and miRNA clusters by dark gray boxes.

translocations have been mapped to a segment of approximately 150 kb within band 19q13.4 (Belge et al., 1997, 2001), but the very high gene density on the long arm of chromosome 19 makes the identification of the target gene difficult. Nevertheless, primary tumors as well as immortalized cell lines of thyroid tumors carrying this translocation show a strong upregulation of two microRNA clusters located within or near the breakpoint cluster region (Figure 19.2) (Rippe et al., 2010). One of these clusters, the so-called chromosome 19 microRNA cluster (C19MC), is the largest known human microRNA cluster, encoding more than 50 mature microRNAs processed from a single Pol II transcript (Bortolin-Cavaillé et al., 2009). The latter gene locus is rearranged, upregulated, or amplified in hamartomas of the liver (Kapur et al., 2014) and aggressive primitive neuroectodermal brain tumors (Li et al., 2009; Nobusawa et al., 2012; Kleinman et al., 2014; Spence et al., 2014). MicroRNAs of C19MC (Flor and Bullerdiek, 2012) as well as of the much smaller miR-371-3 cluster have repeatedly been considered oncomirs, that is, microRNAs with a role in cancer (Esquela-Kerscher and Slack, 2006; Slack and Weidhaas, 2006). On the other hand, there is no evidence that these miRNAs trigger malignant transformation (Rippe et al., 2012) in the case of thyroid tumors. An alternative explanation holds that miRNAs of both clusters could be implicated in immunosurveillance of tumor cells (Bullerdiek and Flor, 2012).

The third main cytogenetic subgroup is defined by *translocations involving chromosomal band 2p21*

(Figure 19.3). As for the 19q13 translocations, the partner chromosomes vary. *THADA* (thyroid adenoma-associated gene) has been identified as the target of the translocations (Rippe et al., 2003).

Follicular carcinomas account for about 15% of malignant thyroid tumors and may be minimally or widely invasive. Minimally invasive carcinomas show limited capsular and/or vascular invasion and are often difficult to distinguish from adenomas. A possible origin of follicular carcinomas from preexisting adenomas has been proposed, something that is supported by the partial similarity of the genetic alterations found in both groups. Studies of follicular carcinomas by chromosome banding with subsequent molecular analyses have revealed a subset of tumors characterized by rearrangements of the peroxisome proliferator-activated

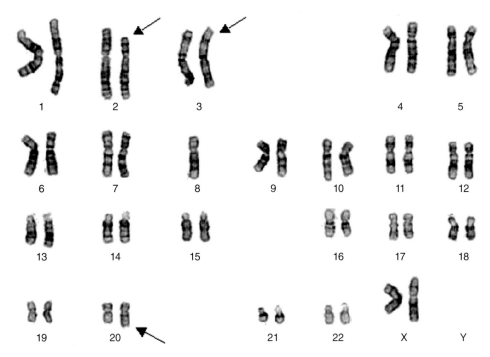

Figure 19.3 Representative G-banded karyotype of a thyroid adenoma with a complex translocation involving 2p21 leading to a *THADA* rearrangement. A subset of thyroid adenomas is cytogenetically defined by 2p21 rearrangements.

receptor gamma (*PPARG*) gene most often due to the translocation t(2;3)(q13;p25) (Figure 19.4) leading to the formation of a chimeric gene of *PAX8* and *PPARG* (Kroll et al., 2000; Giordano et al., 2006). The resulting fusion protein is involved in the WNT signaling pathway (Vu-Phan et al., 2013) and can be detected by RT-PCR as well as by FISH (Chia et al., 2010) on paraffin-embedded samples and even on cytologic smears obtained by fine needle aspiration (Caria et al., 2012, 2014; Ferraz et al., 2012; Klemke et al., 2012; Eszlinger et al., 2014).

Although early RT-PCR studies failed to identify the mRNA of this chimeric gene, Marques et al. (2002) did detect it in five of nine follicular carcinomas and in two of 16 adenomas. More recent data obtained by RT-PCR revealed that, corresponding to cytogenetic data, the fusion is not specific for malignant follicular tumors but occasionally occurs in adenomas as well (Klemke et al., 2011).

Roque et al. (2003) studied by CGH a group of 12 follicular adenomas and 20 follicular carcinomas that had already been characterized by chromosome banding and flow cytometry. In general, considerable similarity was observed between the CGH profiles of

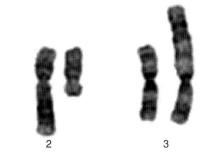

Figure 19.4 Partial G-banded karyotype showing the translocation t(2;3)(q13;p25) that can be found in thyroid adenomas as well as in follicular carcinomas.

the adenomas and the carcinomas. In both the benign and malignant tumors, a combination of gains of or from chromosomes 5, 7, 12, 17, 19, and 20 was observed. Chromosome 7 was the most frequently affected, with three regions of consensus gains: 7p11–12, 7q11.3–21, and 7q31. If an evolutionary continuum between adenomas and follicular carcinomas exists, in particular, minimally invasive carcinomas may represent a mixture of malignant and still nonmalignant cell populations; it is obvious that such a situation may lead to interpretation difficulties with regard to both the genetic profiles and the exact phenotypic classification of such disease lesions.

Papillary carcinomas, too, are believed to originate from cells of the follicular epithelium. The disease outcome for patients with these tumors is usually favorable, but a small group with adverse prognosis exists. The karyotypic abnormalities are usually simple (Bondeson et al., 1989; Jenkins et al., 1990; Teyssier et al., 1990; Herrmann et al., 1991a, 1991b; Antonini et al., 1992; Sozzi et al., 1992). A characteristic intrachromosomal rearrangement, the paracentric inversion inv(10)(q11q21), seems to be specific for this tumor type (Jenkins et al., 1990; Herrmann et al., 1991a, 1991b; Sozzi et al., 1992). Other translocations affecting the two bands 10q11 and 10q21 have also been seen, for example, t(5;10)(p15;q11) (Jenkins et al., 1990) and t(7;10) (q35;q21) (Antonini et al., 1992). The genes in both breakpoints of the inv(10)(q11q21) have been identified. Pierotti et al. (1992) and Sozzi et al. (1992) combined cytogenetic and molecular genetic analyses to show that the inversion generates an oncogenic *RET–PTC* chimeric transcript. So far, one-fourth of all papillary thyroid carcinomas have been demonstrated to carry the transforming *RET–PTC* sequence (Fusco et al., 1987; Bongarzone et al., 1989; Pierotti et al., 1992; de Vries et al., 2012). At least 15 variants of these rearrangements have been described (Chen et al., 2007; Celestino et al., 2012), and generally, rearrangements of 10q11.2 are the most frequent cytogenetic aberrations in tumors of this type (Roque et al., 2001). Some rearrangements, for example, those generating a *RET–PTC3* fusion as the result of a small paracentric inversion, remain undetectable by banding cytogenetics (Minoletti et al., 1994) but can be detected by FISH with appropriate break-apart probes (Chen et al., 2007). For some of the *RET–PTC* rearrangements, an association with previous radiation exposure has been noted. Frau et al. (2007) showed that an isolated trisomy 17 is associated with focal papillary carcinoma changes in follicular-patterned thyroid nodules. This cytogenetic–pathologic association may help to classify these lesions.

Roque et al. (2001) pooled information on breakpoint positions coming from their own study with corresponding published information. In the ensuing meta-analysis, the most commonly affected bands besides 10q11 were 1p32–36, 1p11–13,

1q, 3p25–26, and 7q34–36. It also turned out that some follicular variants of papillary thyroid carcinoma were characterized by chromosomal aberrations commonly found in thyroid follicular adenomas, that is, del(11)(q13q13), t(2;3)(q13;p35), and gains of chromosomes 3, 5, 7, 9, 12, 14, 17, and 20. In the tall-cell papillary thyroid carcinoma variant, an overrepresentation of the long arm of chromosome 2 appeared to occur frequently. Another finding in these studies was an association between complex karyotypes and poorly differentiated tumors. Smit et al. (2001) found the translocation t(3;5)(q12;p15.3) and loss of heterozygosity (LOH) on chromosome 22 in a multifocal follicular variant of papillary thyroid carcinoma presenting with skin metastases. Perissel et al. (2000) suggested that chromosome 22 changes are not part of the karyotypic aberration pattern in pure papillary thyroid tumors but rather could be related to follicular-type histology. In a comparison of follicular and papillary carcinomas, Ward et al. (1998) noted that LOH was much more frequent in the former, suggesting a fundamental difference in genetic stability between these two main types of thyroid cancer.

Poorly differentiated and *undifferentiated (anaplastic) thyroid carcinomas* are highly malignant cancers that are totally or partially composed of undifferentiated cells. Because areas with a higher differentiation are not infrequent, they are thought to originate, at least in part, from preexisting more differentiated carcinomas. Very few chromosome banding studies of this tumor type have been published (Mark et al., 1987; Jenkins et al., 1990; Roque et al., 1998; Bol et al., 2001). No characteristic cytogenetic pattern has emerged. In addition to primary tumors, cell lines are an alternative source to get information on the genetic changes of poorly differentiated and undifferentiated carcinomas. Lee et al. (2007a) analyzed eight cell lines derived from anaplastic thyroid carcinomas by banding cytogenetics, spectral karyotyping (SKY), and CGH. Several nonrandom breakpoints were identified by G-banding and SKY including the novel 1p36 and 17q24–25 as well as 3p21–22 and 15q26 that are also implicated in well-differentiated thyroid cancers. The CGH analyses revealed frequent gains of 20q, indicating that this might be important either in de novo pathogenesis of anaplastic carcinomas or in the progression and dedifferentiation of preexisting thyroid cancers into anaplastic tumors. Several other studies based on CGH and allelotyping have been published as well, often showing inconsistencies with each other and without any characteristic pattern of genomic losses and gains becoming apparent (Hemmer et al., 1999; Komoike et al., 1999; Kitamura et al., 2000; Kleer et al., 2000; Wilkens et al., 2000).

Parathyroid

Very little is known about the cytogenetics of parathyroid neoplasms. No single carcinoma and only two adenomas with an abnormal karyotype have been reported. The case described by Örndal et al. (1990) had a t(1;5)(p22;q32) as the sole clonal anomaly. Of the three parathyroid adenomas studied by Sammarelli et al. (2007), two had a normal karyotype and one showed a clonal t(4;13)(q21;q14). Costa-Guda et al. (2013) performed copy number and LOH analysis on 16 primary parathyroid carcinomas, local recurrences or distant metastases, and matched normal controls from 10 individuals. Overall, recurrent allelic losses were observed from the short arm of chromosome 1, chromosome 3, and 13q, whereas the detection of recurrent gains of or from the long arm of chromosome 1 and chromosome 16 suggested the presence here of genes with tumor suppressive and oncogenic potential, respectively, contributing to the molecular pathology of these tumors (Vaira et al., 2012; Shi et al., 2014). Whole-genome sequencing of a parathyroid carcinoma (Kasaian et al., 2013) also identified loss of the short arm of chromosome 1, along with missense and truncating mutations in CDKN2C and THRAP3 located in 1p, as well as numerous changes in other chromosomes, including two fusion genes—PLD1–AGBL1 and AKAP13–DMXL2—generated by a t(3;15)(q26;q25) and an inv(15)(q21q25), respectively.

Pituitary gland

Almost all pituitary tumors arise from the adenohypophysis and are benign adenomas; carcinomas are very rare. Since the first description of chromosome aberrations in *pituitary adenomas* more than 40 years ago (Mark, 1971), which was based on the examination of unbanded preparations, many cases with abnormal karyotypes identified either by chromosome banding, CGH, FISH, or combinations of these methods have been reported (Rey et al., 1986; Capra et al., 1993; Dietrich et al., 1993; Papi et al., 1993; Rock et al., 1993; Bettio et al., 1997; Hui et al., 1999; Larsen et al., 1999; Finelli et al., 2000; Bello et al., 2001; Trautmann et al., 2001; Wang et al., 2002). Pooling the results obtained by conventional and molecular cytogenetics, roughly one-third of these tumors have revealed chromosomal aberrations with the vast majority showing only numerical changes. Gains repeatedly described in these studies were of chromosomes 5, 7, 8, 9, 12, 19, and 20, whereas losses were noted in more than one study for chromosomes 10, 11, and 13.

As to the frequent occurrence of trisomy 12 in pituitary adenomas, particularly prolactinomas, a key target gene has been suggested based on the fact that transgenic mice overexpressing the wild-type high-mobility group protein gene HMGA2 in 12q14–15 (Schoenmakers et al., 1995) often have prolactinomas (Fedele et al., 2002). Therefore, Finelli et al. (2002) checked prolactinomas for the copy number and the expression of this gene. HMGA2 was found to be amplified in seven of eight prolactinoma samples examined as a result of gain of one or two copies of chromosome 12, der(12) chromosomes, or marker chromosomes bearing amplified 12q14–15 material. Correspondingly, elevated HMGA2 expression occurred in some of these tumors.

Among the cases with structural abnormalities, the most complex was the one reported by Rey et al. (1986), in which the tumor stemline had 58 chromosomes. The most frequently recurring change has been trisomy 9. The only structural rearrangement that has been seen as the sole anomaly is t(1;21)(q32;q22), found by Papi et al. (1993) in a prolactin-producing adenoma in a patient with multiple endocrine neoplasia type 1 (MEN1).

Inherited predisposition to pituitary gland tumors occurs in MEN1, Carney complex, familial acromegaly, and McCune–Albright syndrome. Pack et al. (2000) examined four pituitary gland tumors from patients with a Carney complex, that is, familial multiple neoplasia and lentiginosis syndrome, by means of CGH. The copy number changes included losses of or from 6q, 7q, 11p, and

11q and gains of or from 1p32-pter, 2q35-qter, 9q33-qter, 12q24-qter, 16, 17, 19p, 20p, 20q, 22p, and 22q in the most aggressive tumor, an invasive macroadenoma, whereas no chromosomal changes were seen in the three prospectively diagnosed microadenomas.

Adrenal gland

Neuroblastoma (NB) originates from the sympathicoadrenal lineage of the neural crest. It is the most common extracranial solid tumor in childhood and the most frequently diagnosed malignancy during the first year of life (Maris et al., 2007). The cause of NB is not known. There is some degree of hereditary predisposition (Perri et al., 2002; Zimling et al., 2004; Longo et al., 2007), but only a small minority (<2%) of NB cases are familial. Mutation in the paired-like homeobox 2b (*PHOX2B*) gene was the first specific genetic aberration connected to hereditary NB (Mosse et al., 2004; Trochet et al., 2004). This gene encodes a transcription factor of importance for neuronal differentiation and cell cycle exit, playing a key role in autonomous nervous system development. This is reflected by the fact that the same mutations that cause predisposition to NB are also associated with congenital central hypoventilation syndrome and Hirschsprung's disease (Stovroff et al., 1995; Raabe et al., 2008). The second gene discovered to cause hereditary NB was the anaplastic lymphoma tyrosine kinase (*ALK*) gene (Janoueix-Lerosey et al. 2008; Mosse et al., 2008), which regulates the balance between cellular proliferation and differentiation in the developing sympathicoadrenal lineage. Importantly, also somatic *ALK* mutations are found in 6–8% of sporadic NBs (see following text).

Clinical risk stratification is largely based on age (dichotomized around 18 months), stage before treatment, and absence or presence of amplification of the *MYCN* gene. The histopathological risk classification according to Shimada et al. (1984) classifies tumors as favorable or unfavorable depending on their degree of neuroblast differentiation, Schwannian stroma content, mitotic–karyorrhectic index, and the patient's age at diagnosis. Most NBs occur in the abdomen, and half of them in the adrenal medulla. Approximately 40% of patients present with localized disease,

ranging from a confined adrenal mass to invasive tumors anywhere along the chain of sympathetic ganglia (Brodeur, 2003). About 50% of patients present with metastases to sites such as bone, including the bony orbit, bone marrow, and liver. A specific subtype of metastatic disease, referred to as stage 4S and occurring in 5% of cases, includes infants with a small localized tumor and metastases to the liver, skin, or bone marrow to a minimal extent (Maris et al., 2007). Tumors of this subtype show a high frequency of spontaneous regression. In contrast, widespread disease in older children is still often associated with a very poor outcome despite intensive, multimodal therapy.

The clinical heterogeneity of NB is remarkably well reflected by its cytogenetic and genomic features. Genetic markers are crucial determinants of treatment planning. It is therefore essential to obtain material for genetic analysis at the time of diagnosis. However, chromosome banding analysis of NB is associated with several methodological difficulties, and other analytical approaches have become increasingly important, including flow cytometry for assessment of ploidy, FISH for rapid detection of selected chromosomal aberrations, and genomic arrays for screening the panorama of genomic imbalances.

Brodeur (2003) suggested that NB could be broadly subdivided into two clinicogenetic types. The first is characterized by hyperdiploid to near-triploid modal chromosome numbers with few structural rearrangements. These tumors generally express high levels of the TRKA protein, are prone to differentiation, and occur in patients less than one year of age with low-stage disease and good prognosis. The second type occurs in older children. These tumors are characterized by a near-diploid or tetraploid modal number and structural aberrations that often lead to gain of 17q. Within this class of NB, again, two subtypes can be distinguished. The first is characterized by *MYCN* amplification and loss of 1p sequences. These tumors show high levels of the TRKB protein and its ligand BDNF, which is believed to reflect an autocrine growth-stimulatory pathway. They are highly aggressive, with a rapid clinical course that is often fatal. The second subtype is characterized by 11q deletions and other structural changes. Also, these tumors typically present at an advanced stage but are slowly progressive. The classical genetic classification outlined previously has now been supported by several genome-wide array studies (e.g., George et al., 2007; Mosse et al., 2007; Carén et al., 2010).

Amplification of the MYCN gene in 2p24 occurs in 20–30% of NB (Schwab et al., 1983; Schneiderman et al., 2008). Cytogenetically, the amplicons occur either extrachromosomally as double minutes (dmin) or episomes or intrachromosomally as homoge-

neously staining regions (Figure 19.5). dmin are more commonly found in fresh tumor biopsies, whereas homogeneously staining regions are more common in established NB cell lines. Other genes from 2p24 may be coamplified, but *MYCN* is the only gene that is consistently amplified from this chromosome segment (Reiter and Brodeur, 1996, 1998). *MYCN* amplification is associated with advanced stage and rapid progression, even in infants and patients with low-stage disease at

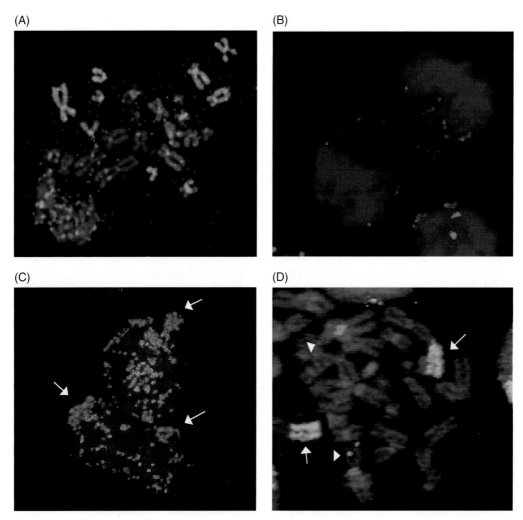

Figure 19.5 Detection of double minutes (dmin) and homogeneously staining regions (hsr) in neuroblastoma by fluorescence *in situ* hybridization, using probes for *MYCN* (red in a, green in b–d). In metaphase spreads, dmin are observed as single or double dots, reflecting their episomal structure (A). The dmin are typically acentric and segregate at anaphase by tethering to centric chromosomes (B). At interphase, dmin occasionally form clusters in nuclear protrusions or micronuclei (arrows), shown here by a three-dimensional reconstruction from a confocal image sequence (C). In contrast, hsr (arrows) contain linear gene amplifications, with a much larger area of *MYCN* signal than the *MYCN* loci in normal homologs of chromosome 2 (arrowheads); red signals correspond to the chromosome 2 centromere (D).

presentation (Schneiderman et al., 2008). Amplification of *MYCN* is strongly associated with overexpression of the corresponding protein (Seeger et al., 1988). The MYCN protein forms a heterodimer with the MAX protein, and the resulting complex functions as a transcriptional activator, ultimately leading to G1 progression (Wenzel and Schwab, 1995). It remains controversial whether overexpression of MYCN protein in the absence of *MYCN* amplification is of any prognostic significance (Chan et al., 1997; Bordow et al., 1998; Cohn et al., 2000).

Loss of material from 1p is a common finding in near-diploid/tetraploid NB, often concurrent with *MYCN* amplification. LOH at 1p has been reported in approximately 35% of near-diploid tumors (Martinsson et al., 1995; White et al., 1995, 2001) and in 23% of all NB (Attiyeh et al., 2005). The independent prognostic value of 1p losses has been debated, but the collected evidence indicates that allelic loss of 1p sequences is clearly associated with disease progression and may also independently predict progression-free survival, at least in tumors without *MYCN* amplification (Gehring et al., 1995; Caron et al., 1996; Maris et al., 2000; Attiyeh et al., 2005). Considerable efforts have been made to define a commonly deleted region in 1p. Several studies have pointed to one or more segments in 1p36, but there is not yet a complete agreement regarding the genomic boundaries (Hogarty et al., 2000; Bauer et al., 2001; Chen et al., 2001; Maris et al., 2001).

Gain of chromosome 17 material has been observed in more than 50% of NB (Caron, 1995; Bown et al., 1999). Hyperdiploid/near-triploid infant tumors often exhibit gain of the entire chromosome. In contrast, near-diploid tumors frequently show unbalanced translocations, most commonly between chromosomes 1 and 17, leading to extra copies of 17q sequences typically spanning 17q22-qter (Lastowska et al., 1998). Such gain of 17q is strongly associated with advanced stage, higher patient age, loss of 1p, and *MYCN* amplification and has been shown to independently predict an adverse outcome in some studies (Bown et al., 1999).

Several studies have shown *loss of 11q*, particularly 11q23 sequences, in NB at frequencies up to 43% (Srivatsan et al., 1993; Guo et al., 1999; Plantaz et al., 2001). Deletion in 11q is strongly associated with 3p and 14q deletions, as well as a wide range of other structural rearrangements, which might be indicative of a chromosomal instability phenotype (George et al., 2007; Carén et al., 2010). Loss of 11q is an adverse prognostic factor in cases with normal *MYCN* copy number (Attiyeh et al., 2005; Carén et al., 2010).

Apart from the previously mentioned abnormalities with clear correlations to clinical features, multiple other recurrent cytogenetic alterations have also been reported in NB. Of the many whole-chromosome gains described in hyperdiploid/near-triploid NB, none has so far been associated specifically with prognostic features. Favorable outcome rather appears to be associated with the ploidy level per se. The most common trisomies described in this type of NB are +17, +12, and +9. Many of these tumors also exhibit losses of a few chromosomes, particularly of chromosome 4 (Gisselsson et al., 2007). The hyperdiploid/near-triploid NBs are typically low-risk with a maturing neuroblastic, Schwannian stroma-rich morphology. It has been demonstrated that the trisomies are confined to the neuroblastic lineage, while the Schwann cells show diploid chromosome numbers, indicating that they are nonneoplastic (Ambros et al., 1996).

Recent next-generation sequencing studies have revealed a relative scarcity of mutations in NB, compared to most common adult cancer types (Molenaar et al., 2012; Cheung et al., 2012; Pugh et al., 2013). Activating mutations of *ALK* are found in 4–12% of sporadic NB (Chen et al., 2008; George et al., 2008; Janoueix-Lerosey et al., 2008; Mosse et al., 2008; Pugh et al., 2013). An additional 3–4% exhibit amplification of this gene, typically in combination with *MYCN*. Also the F1174L *ALK* mutation shows overrepresentation in *MYCN*-amplified cases, and tumors with these two aberrations in combination have a particularly poor prognosis (De Brouwer et al., 2010). Another gene recurrently mutated in sporadic NB is the α-thalassemia/mental retardation syndrome X-linked (*ATRX*) gene (Cheung et al., 2012), although patients with constitutional *ATRX* mutations do not appear to have an increased risk for NB. *ATRX* mutations have primarily been found in the NBs of older children/adolescents with slowly progressing, often lethal, disease. It is a far more common finding than *ALK* mutations, being present in around 17% of children, in 44% of patients over the age of 12, but rarely if ever in infants. Interestingly, *ATRX*-mutated NBs are characterized by elongated telomeres through the ALT pathway, a factor that in itself has been associated with poor outcome in non-*MYCN*-amplified NB (Ohali et al., 2006; Lundberg et al., 2011). Next-generation sequencing also identified chromothripsis, that is, focal dramatic DNA rearrangements, in a subgroup of highly aggressive NB (Molenaar et al., 2012).

Adenomas and carcinomas of the adrenal cortex are rare. In addition to their sporadic occurrence, both types may also be part of inherited tumor syndromes such as the Carney complex and Li–Fraumeni syndrome.

Clonal chromosome abnormalities were reported in adrenocortical adenomas by Gordon et al. (1993). Abnormalities were found in 5/12 cases, all of them male patients. In addition to the loss of the Y chromosome that was a consistent finding in all five tumors, one had loss of chromosome 19 and a second had an unbalanced 6;7-translocation that gave rise to partial trisomy for 7q. A translocation t(7;17)(q22;p13) as a sole karyotypic change in an adrenal adenoma was reported by Bettio et al. (1998). Dohna et al. (2000) analyzed samples from eight adenomas, 14 primary carcinomas, 1 metastasis, and two adrenocortical carcinoma cell lines by CGH. Except for the two smallest adenomas, all tumors showed chromosomal imbalances with a high incidence of gains, most frequently involving chromosomes or chromosome arms 5, 7, 8, 9q, 11q, 12q, 14q, 16, 17q, 19, 20, and 22q. The only significant loss of material was from the distal part of 9p. Recurrent gains and high-level amplifications were identified for chromosomal regions 1p34.3-pter, 1q22–25, 3p24-pter, 3q29, 7p11.2–14, 9q34, 11q12–13, 12q13, 12q24.3, 13q34, 14q11.2–12, 14q32, 16p, 17q24–25, 19p13.3, 19q13.4, and 22q11.2–12. An association between chromosomal imbalances and tumor progression was suggested by the fact that adenomas larger than 4 cm showed gains from regions also overrepresented in carcinomas. The results of another CGH study of 13 malignant, 18 benign, and one adrenocortical tumors of indeterminate malignant potential were reported by Sidhu et al. (2002). Copy number changes were seen in all cancers, in 11 of the 18 adenomas, and in the tumor of indeterminate malignant potential. The most common gains were seen on chromosomes 5 (46%), 12 (38%), 19 (31%), and 4 (31%). Losses were most frequently seen at 1p (62%), 17p (54%), 22 (38%), 2q (31%), and 11q (31%). In the benign adenomas, the most common change was gain of 4q (22%). In part, these results confirmed the earlier data by Zhao et al. (1999) who examined 12 carcinomas, 23 adenomas, and six hyperplasias; genomic imbalances were more frequent in malignant than in benign tumors and were rarely seen in hyperplastic lesions. The most frequent DNA copy number changes in adrenocortical carcinomas included losses of or from 1p21–31, 2q, 3p, 3q, 6q, 9p, and 11q14-qter as well as gains and amplifications of 5q12, 9q32-qter, 12q, and 20q. The imbalances that were most common in adrenocortical adenomas were gains of 17q, 17p, and 9q32-qter. The gains found in two of the six adrenocortical hyperplastic lesions involved chromosome 17 or 17q only. These data indicate that genes determining the early tumorigenesis of adrenocortical tumors may exist on chromosome 17 and that the number of genomic alterations is closely associated with the neoplastic phenotype in adrenocortical tumors. The role of gain of chromosome 17 in the development of adrenocortical tumors was also addressed by Takehara et al. (2005) who studied six adrenal cortical adenomas in patients with Cushing's syndrome, 12 adenomas leading to hyperaldosteronism, three nonfunctioning adenomas, and three adrenal cortical carcinomas by FISH using an alpha-centromeric probe for chromosome 17 on isolated nuclei from frozen samples. Chromosome 17 showed disomy in all adrenocortical adenomas, whereas aberrations were found in two of three carcinomas. Only the latter two cases strongly expressed TP53 protein, indicating that *TP53* may be involved in progression to carcinoma in a subset of patients. In addition, progression from adrenal adenoma to carcinoma may arise from the monoclonal proliferation of cells that have undergone chromosomal duplication at the 11p15.5 locus leading to overexpression of the *IGF2* gene and abrogation of expression of the *CDKN1C* and *H19* genes (for review, see Sidhu et al., 2003).

Shono et al. (2002) reported a FISH study on isolated nuclei from frozen samples using centromere-specific probes for chromosomes 3, 7, 8, 11, and 12. While none of the normal adrenal tissues revealed numerical chromosomal aberrations with these probes, tetrasomy for chromosomes 3, 7, 8, 11, and 12 was detected in 8, 13, 14, 11, and 12, respectively, of the 17 adenomas associated with primary aldosteronism and in 2, 0, 0, 0, and 0, respectively, of the eight cases associated with Cushing's syndrome. One of the two carcinomas also showed aneuploidy.

Also, chromosome banding studies have detected cytogenetic aberrations in adrenocortical carcinomas. Highly complex aberrations were found in two tumors, one with a hypodiploid (Marks et al., 1992) and the other with a hyperdiploid (Limon et al., 1987a) stemline. The karyotypic changes in a third tumor included a t(4;11)(q35; p13) as the primary anomaly and, in addition, some cells with del(1q) as a secondary change (Limon et al., 1987b).

It has been suggested that increased cytogenetic instability may distinguish adrenocortical carcinomas from adenomas, and evidence for increased chromosomal instability with tumor progression was reported by Russell et al. (1999). A significantly increased telomerase activity in adrenocortical carcinomas compared to adenomas was detected by Mannelli et al. (2000) but not by Bamberger et al. (1999). In an adrenocortical carcinoma cell line, telomere maintenance in the absence of telomerase activity was described by Fujiwara et al. (2006). Telomeric associations in an adrenal tumor but not in matching normal adrenal tissue in a patient with Carney complex were reported by Stratakis et al. (1996).

Pheochromocytomas (PCC) originate from the adrenal medulla. In a minority of cases, the tumors occur in patients suffering from MEN2, von Hippel–Lindau syndrome, or von Recklinghausen's disease (neurofibromatosis type 1, NF1). But even in apparently sporadic cases, as many as 25% may actually be due to germline mutations of the *RET*, *VHL*, *SDHB*, or *SDHD* genes (Opocher et al., 2003).

Clonal chromosome changes have been reported in PCC of three patients with von Hippel–Lindau disease. Trisomy 7 was the only anomaly in the two tumors reported by Jordan et al. (1989) and Kiechle-Schwarz et al. (1989). The third case

(Kiechle-Schwarz et al., 1989) had four cytogenetically unrelated clones, each with simple, unbalanced, structural rearrangements.

Gunawan et al. (2004) presented a cytogenetic analysis of five adrenal PCC, including two clinically malignant tumors. The three PCC with benign clinical behavior, including one associated with von Hippel–Lindau syndrome, displayed no clonal chromosomal aberrations. In contrast, both clinically malignant PCC were characterized by hypotriploid chromosome numbers and multiple numerical and structural changes. Generally, the malignant phenotype in PCC is associated with considerable genetic instability leading to highly aneuploid and aberrant karyotypes.

Deletions of the short arm of chromosome 1 seem to play an important role in the development of PCC (Pfragner et al., 1998; Benn et al., 2000). Based on a CGH study, Dannenberg et al. (2000) concluded that the development of PCC is associated with the acquisition of specific genomic aberrations that include losses of 1p, 3q, and 6q and gains of 9q and 17q. Loss of genetic material from 1p and 3q may be involved in early tumorigenesis, while deletions from 6q and 17p contribute to the progression to malignancy. In a comparable CGH study by Edström et al. (2000) of 23 PCC and 11 abdominal paragangliomas, the pattern of copy number changes was found to be similar in these two tumor types, with the most consistent finding being loss of 1cen-p31 (28 of 34 tumors, 82%). Losses were also found of 3q22–25 (41%), 11p (26%), 3p13–14 (24%), 4q (21%), 2q (15%), and 11q22–23 (15%), whereas gains were detected in 19p (26%), 19q (24%), 17q24-qter (21%), 11cen-q13 (15%), and 16p (15%). The progression of genetic events per se did not seem to correspond to any transformation to a malignant phenotype.

To examine more closely the loss of genetic material from the short arm of chromosome 1 in PCC, Opocher et al. (2003) performed a detailed analysis of 1p LOH on 21 sporadic, five MEN2, two NF1, six von Hippel–Lindau, and four nonsyndromatic but familial cases. Complete or partial deletion of 1p was detected in 27/38 (71%) cases, with the most frequently deleted marker mapping to 1p32.1. The data seem to represent strong but indirect evidence that the short arm of chromosome 1 harbors one or more genes responsible for PCC development.

In a CGH study of 36 von Hippel–Lindau-related PCC, loss of chromosomes 3 and 11 was found in 94% and 86%, respectively. The selective loss of chromosome 11 seems to be specific for von Hippel–Lindau-associated tumors (Lui et al., 2002). Finally, a t(12;22)(q13;q12) was found in a primitive small round cell tumor of the adrenal gland by Lam et al. (2001). It seems that these Ewing-type tumors have the same chromosomal characteristics irrespective of their site of origin (Chapter 23).

Thymus

Thymomas and carcinomas of thymic origin are rare and heterogeneous tumors. Clonal chromosome abnormalities have been reported in several *thymomas*, usually as part of near-diploid karyotypes (Kristoffersson et al., 1989; Dal Cin et al., 1993, 1996; Sonobe et al., 1999; Mirza et al., 2000; Goh et al., 2001; Herens et al., 2003) as well as in a few thymic carcinomas (Kubonishi et al., 1991).

Loss of chromosome 6 (Zettl et al., 2000) and deletions of part of the short arm of chromosome 6 due to structural rearrangements are recurrent findings in thymoma, irrespective of tumor subtype. A del(6)(p22p25) was described in a spindle cell thymoma (Mirza et al., 2000) as well as in two thymomas of the AB type (Van den Berghe et al., 2002; Herens et al., 2003). The significance of 6p deletions was also underscored by the findings in the chromosomal CGH study of 28 epithelial tumors of thymic origin by Penzel et al. (2003) and an array CGH study of 39 thymomas of different types by Lee et al. (2007b). Both studies revealed other gains and losses as well and concluded that an association between distinct imbalances and thymoma subtypes existed. A pseudodicentric t(16;12)(q11;p11.2) was described as the sole chromosomal abnormality in a type AB thymoma by Goh et al. (2001), whereas Dal Cin et al. (1996) detected a t(15;22)(p11;q11) in another tumor, again as the only chromosome abnormality.

Based on their own and two other independent observations, Lee et al. (1993) suggested that t(15;19) (q12;p13.1) is a recurrent structural chromosome abnormality in *carcinomas of thymic origin*. Though the breakpoint assignment varied from case to case, with Kubonishi et al. (1991) reporting the translocation as t(15;19)(q15;p13) and Kees et al. (1991) as t(15;19)(p12;q13), this variation may not reflect biological realities.

Lee et al. (2007b) used a microarray approach to investigate 39 thymoma samples from paraffin-embedded tissue. They were able to identify subsets of aberrations correlating with the different thymoma types put forward by the WHO (Marx et al., 2014). Thus, the use of CGH-based techniques may improve thymoma subtyping.

Endocrine pancreas

Little is known about the cytogenetic features of the rare tumors of the endocrine pancreas, at least as far as banding studies are concerned. Scappaticci et al. (1992) karyotyped two pancreatic islet tumors, an insulinoma and a glucagonoma, from two patients with MEN1. The insulinoma had a modal chromosome number of 84 with many complex numerical and structural changes, including dmin in all metaphases, whereas the glucagonoma showed no clonal aberrations. More information comes from studies using mutation analyses, CGH, and the LOH approach (De Lellis et al., 2004; Jonkers et al., 2006). The most frequent genomic imbalances in insulinomas in these studies were losses of or from 11q (11q24, 56%) and 22q (22q13, 67%), as well as gain of 9q (9q32, 63%). The gains of 9q and losses of 22q were interpreted to be early genetic events in insulinoma development.

References

Ambros IM, Zellner A, Roald B, Amann G, Ladenstein R, Printz D, et al. (1996): Role of ploidy, chromosome 1p, and Schwann cells in the maturation of neuroblastoma. *N Engl J Med* 334:1505–1511.

Antonini P, Venuat AM, Caillou B, Berger R, Schlumberger M, Bernheim A, et al. (1992): Cytogenetic studies on 19 papillary thyroid carcinomas. *Genes Chromosomes Cancer* 5:206–211.

Attiyeh EF, London WB, Mosse YP, Wang Q, Winter C, Khazi D, et al. (2005): Chromosome 1p and 11q deletions and outcome in neuroblastoma. *N Engl J Med* 353: 2243–2253.

Bamberger CM, Else T, Bamberger AM, Frilling A, Beil FU, Allolio B, et al. (1999): Telomerase activity in benign and malignant adrenal tumors. *Exp Clin Endocrinol Diabetes* 107:272–275.

Bauer A, Savelyeva L, Claas A, Praml C, Berthold F, Schwab M (2001): Smallest region of overlapping deletion in 1p36 in human neuroblastoma: A 1 Mbp cosmid and PAC contig. *Genes Chromosomes Cancer* 31:228–239.

Belge G, Thode B, Rippe V, Bartnitzke S, Bullerdiek J (1994): A characteristic sequence of trisomies starting with trisomy 7 in benign thyroid tumors. *Hum Genet* 94:198–202.

Belge G, Garcia E, Rippe V, Fusco A, Bartnitzke S, Bullerdiek J (1997): Breakpoints of 19q13 translocations of benign thyroid tumors map within a 400 kilobase region. *Genes Chromosomes Cancer* 20:201–203.

Belge G, Roque L, Soares J, Bruckmann S, Thode B, Fonseca E, et al. (1998): Cytogenetic investigations of 340 thyroid hyperplasias and adenomas revealing correlations between cytogenetic findings and histology. *Cancer Genet Cytogenet* 101:42–48.

Belge G, Rippe V, Meiboom M, Drieschner N, Garcia E, Bullerdiek J (2001): Delineation of a 150-kb breakpoint cluster in benign thyroid tumors with 19q13.4 aberrations. *Cytogenet Cell Genet* 93:48–51.

Bello MJ, deCampos JM, Kusak ME, Vaquero J, Sarasa JL, Rey JA (2001): Chromosomal abnormalities in pituitary adenomas. *Cancer Genet Cytogenet* 124:76–79.

Benn DE, Dwight T, Richardson AL, Delbridge L, Bambach CP, Stowasser M, et al. (2000): Sporadic and familial pheochromocytomas are associated with loss of at least two discrete intervals on chromosome 1p. *Cancer Res* 60:7048–7451.

Bettio D, Rizzi N, Giardino D, Persani L, Pecori-Giraldi F, Losa M, et al. (1997): Cytogenetic study of pituitary adenomas. *Cancer Genet Cytogenet* 98:131–136.

Bettio D, Rizzi N, Giardino D, Virduci T, Loli P, Larizza L (1998): Translocation (7;17)(q22;p13) as a sole karyotypic change in an adrenal adenoma. *Cancer Genet Cytogenet* 103:180–181.

Bol S, Belge G, Thode B, Bonk U, Bartnitzke S, Bullerdiek J (2001): Cytogenetic tetraclonality in a rare spindle cell variant of an anaplastic carcinoma of the thyroid. *Cancer Genet Cytogenet* 125:163–166.

Bondeson AG, Bondeson L, Thompson NW (1989): Hyperparathyroidism after treatment with radioactive iodine: Not only a coincidence? *Surgery* 106:1025–1027.

Bongarzone I, Pierotti MA, Monzini N, Mondellini P, Manenti G, Donghi R, et al. (1989): High frequency of activation of tyrosine kinase oncogenes in human papillary thyroid carcinoma. *Oncogene* 4:1457–1462.

Bordow SB, Norris MD, Haber PS, Marshall GM, Haber M (1998): Prognostic significance of MYCN oncogene expression in childhood neuroblastoma. *J Clin Oncol* 16:3286–3294.

Bortolin-Cavaillé ML, Dance M, Weber M, Cavaillé J (2009): C19MC microRNAs are processed from introns of large Pol-II, non-protein-coding transcripts. *Nucleic Acids Res* 37:3464–3473.

Bown N, Cotterill S, Lastowska M, O'Neill S, Pearson AD, Plantaz D et al. (1999): Gain of chromosome arm 17q and adverse outcome in patients with neuroblastoma. *N Engl J Med* 340:1954–1961.

Brodeur GM (2003): Neuroblastoma: Biological insights into a clinical enigma. *Nat Rev Cancer* 3:203–216.

Bullerdiek J, Flor I (2012): Exosome-delivered microRNAs of "chromosome 19 microRNA cluster" as immunomodulators in pregnancy and tumorigenesis. *Mol Cytogenet* 5:27.

Capra E, Rindi G, Santi G, Spina MP, Scappaticci S (1993): Chromosome abnormalities in a case of pituitary adenoma. *Cancer Genet Cytogenet* 68:140–142.

Carén H, Kryh H, Nethander M, Sjöberg RM, Träger C, Nilsson S, et al. (2010): High-risk neuroblastoma tumors with 11q-deletion display a poor prognostic, chromosome instability phenotype with later onset. *Proc Natl Acad Sci USA* 107:4323–4328.

Caria P, Dettori T, Frau DV, Di Oto E, Morandi L, Parmeggiani A, et al. (2012): Simultaneous occurrence of PAX8-PPARg and RET-PTC3 rearrangements in a follicular variant of papillary thyroid carcinoma. *Am J Surg Pathol* 36:1415–1420.

Caria P, Frau DV, Dettori T, Boi F, Lai ML, Mariotti S, et al. (2014): Optimizing detection of RET and PPARg rearrangements in thyroid neoplastic cells using a home-brew tetracolor probe. *Cancer Cytopathol* 122:377–385.

Caron H (1995): Allelic loss of chromosome 1 and additional chromosome 17 material are both unfavourable prognostic markers in neuroblastoma. *Med Pediatr Oncol* 24:215–221.

Caron H, van Sluis P, de Kraker J, Bokkerink J, Egeler M, Laureys G, et al. (1996): Allelic loss of chromosome 1p as a predictor of unfavorable outcome in patients with neuroblastoma. *N Engl J Med* 334:225–230.

Celestino R, Sigstad E, Løvf M, Thomassen GO, Grøholt KK, Jørgensen LH, et al. (2012): Survey of 548 oncogenic fusion transcripts in thyroid tumors supports the importance of the already established thyroid fusions genes. *Genes Chromosomes Cancer* 51:1154–1164.

Chan HS, Gallie BL, De Boer G, Haddad G, Ikegaki N, Dimitroulakos J, et al. (1997): MYCN protein expression as a predictor of neuroblastoma prognosis. *Clin Cancer Res* 3:1699–1706.

Chen YZ, Soeda E, Yang HW, Takita J, Chai L, Horii A, et al. (2001): Homozygous deletion in a neuroblastoma cell line defined by a high-density STS map spanning human chromosome band 1p36. *Genes Chromosomes Cancer* 31:326–332.

Chen F, Clark DP, Hawkins AL, Morsberger LA, Griffin CA (2007): A break-apart fluorescence in situ hybridization assay for detecting RET translocations in papillary thyroid carcinoma. *Cancer Genet Cytogenet* 178:128–134.

Chen Y, Takita J, Choi YL, Kato M, Ohira M, Sanada M, et al. (2008): Oncogenic mutations of ALK kinase in neuroblastoma. *Nature* 455:971–974.

Cheung NK, Zhang J, Lu C, Parker M, Bahrami A, Tickoo SK, et al. (2012): Association of age at diagnosis and genetic mutations in patients with neuroblastoma. *JAMA* 307: 1062–1071.

Chia WK, Sharifah NA, Reena RM, Zubaidah Z, Clarence-Ko CH, Rohaizak M, et al. (2010): Fluorescence in situ hybridization analysis using PAX8- and PPARG-specific probes reveals the presence of PAX8-PPARG transloca-tion and 3p25 aneusomy in follicular thyroid neoplasms. *Cancer Genet Cytogenet* 196:7–13.

Cohn SL, London WB, Huang D, Katzenstein HM, Salwen HR, Reinhart T, et al. (2000): MYCN expression is not prognostic of adverse outcome in advanced-stage neuroblastoma with nonamplified MYCN. *J Clin Oncol* 18:3604–3613.

Costa-Guda J, Imanishi Y, Palanisamy N, Kawamata N, Phillip Koeffler H, Chaganti RS, et al. (2013): Allelic imbalance in sporadic parathyroid carcinoma and evi-dence for its de novo origins. *Endocrine* 44:489–495.

Dal Cin P, De Wolf-Peeters C, Aly MS, Deneffe G, Van Mieghem W, Van Den Berghe H (1993): Ring chromosome 6 as the only change in a thymoma. *Genes Chromosomes Cancer* 6:243–244.

Dal Cin P, De Wolf-Peeters C, Deneffe G, Fryns JP, Van den Berghe H (1996): Thymoma with a t(15;22)(p11;q11). *Cancer Genet Cytogenet* 89:181–183.

Dannenberg H, Speel EJ, Zhao J, Saremaslani P, van Der Harst E, Roth J, et al. (2000): Losses of chromosomes 1p and 3q are early genetic events in the development of sporadic pheochromocytomas. *Am J Pathol* 157:353–359.

De Brouwer S, De Preter K, Kumps C, Zabrocki P, Porcu M, Westerhout EM, et al. (2010): Meta-analysis of neuroblas-tomas reveals a skewed ALK mutation spectrum in tumors with MYCN amplification. *Clin Cancer Res* 16: 4353–4362.

De Lellis RA, Lloyd RV, Heitz PU, Eng C, editors (2004): *World Health Organization Classification of Tumours. Pathology and Genetics of Tumours of Endocrine Organs.* Lyon: IARC Press.

Dettori T, Frau DV, Lai ML, Mariotti S, Uccheddu A, Daniele GM, et al. (2003): Aneuploidy in oncocytic lesions of the thyroid gland: Diffuse accumulation of mitochondria within the cell is associated with trisomy 7 and progressive numerical chromosomal alterations. *Genes Chromosomes Cancer* 38:22–31.

de Vries MM, Celestino R, Castro P, Eloy C, Máximo V, van der Wal JE, et al. (2012): RET/PTC rearrangement is prev-alent in follicular Hürthle cell carcinomas. *Histopathology* 61:833–843.

Dietrich CU, Pandis N, Bjerre P, Schroder HD, Heim S (1993): Simple numerical chromosome aberrations in two pituitary adenomas. *Cancer Genet Cytogenet* 69:118–121.

Dohna M, Reincke M, Mincheva A, Allolio B, Solinas-Toldo S, Lichter P (2000): Adrenocortical carcinoma is characterized by a high frequency of chromosomal gains and high-level amplifications. *Genes Chromosomes Cancer* 28:145–152.

Edström E, Mahlamäki E, Nord B, Kjellman M, Karhu R, Höög A, et al. (2000): Comparative genomic hybridization reveals frequent losses of chromosomes 1p and 3q in pheo-chromocytomas and abdominal paragangliomas, suggest-ing a common genetic etiology. *Am J Pathol* 156:651–659.

Esquela-Kerscher A, Slack FJ (2006): Oncomirs – MicroRNAs with a role in cancer. *Nat Rev Cancer* 6:259–269.

Eszlinger M, Krogdahl A, Münz S, Rehfeld C, Precht Jensen EM, Ferraz C, et al. (2014): Impact of molecular screening for point mutations and rearrangements in routine air-dried fine-needle aspiration samples of thyroid nodules. *Thyroid* 24:305–313.

Fedele M, Battista S, Kenyon L, Baldassarre G, Fidanza V, Klein-Szanto AJ, et al. (2002): Overexpression of the HMGA2 gene in transgenic mice leads to the onset of pituitary adenomas. *Oncogene* 21:3190–3198.

Ferraz C, Rehfeld C, Krogdahl A, Precht Jensen EM, Bösenberg E, Narz F, et al. (2012): Detection of PAX8/PPARG and RET/PTC rearrangements is feasible in routine air-dried fine needle aspiration smears. *Thyroid* 22:1025–1030.

Flor I, Bullerdiek J (2012): The dark side of a success story: MicroRNAs of the C19MC cluster in human tumours. *J Pathol* 227:270–274.

Finelli P, Giardino D, Rizzi N, Buiatiotis S, Virduci T, Franzin A, et al. (2000): Non-random trisomies of chromosomes 5, 8 and 12 in the prolactinoma sub-type of pituitary ade-nomas: Conventional cytogenetics and interphase FISH study. *Int J Cancer* 86:344–350.

Finelli P, Pierantoni GM, Giardino D, Losa M, Rodeschini O, Fedele M, et al. (2002): The High Mobility Group A2 gene is amplified and overexpressed in human prolactinomas. *Cancer Res* 62:2398–2405.

Frau DV, Lai ML, Caria P, Dettori T, Coni P, Faa G, et al. (2007): Trisomy 17 as a marker for a subset of noninvasive thyroid nodules with focal features of papillary carcinoma: Cytogenetic and molecular analysis of 62 cases and corre-lation with histologic findings. *J Clin Endocrinol Metab* 93:177–181.

Fujiwara M, Kamma H, Wu W, Yano Y, Homma S, Satoh H (2006): Alternative lengthening of telomeres in the human adrenocortical carcinoma cell line H295R. *Int J Oncol* 29:445–451.

Fusco A, Grieco M, Santoro M, Berlingieri MT, Pilotti S, Pierotti MA, et al. (1987): A new oncogene in human thy-roid papillary carcinomas and their lymph-nodal metas-tases. *Nature* 328:170–172.

Gehring M, Berthold F, Edler L, Schwab M, Amler LC (1995): The 1p deletion is not a reliable marker for the prognosis of patients with neuroblastoma. *Cancer Res* 55:5366–5369.

George RE, Attiyeh EF, Li S, Moreau LA, Neuberg D, Li C, et al. (2007): Genome-wide analysis of neuroblastomas using high-density single nucleotide polymorphism arrays. *PLoS ONE* 2: e255.

George RE, Sanda T, Hanna M, Fröhling S, Luther W 2nd, Zhang J, et al. (2008): Activating mutations in ALK provide a therapeutic target in neuroblastoma. *Nature* 455:975–978.

Giordano TJ, Au AY, Kuick R, Thomas DG, Rhodes DR, Wilhelm KG Jr, et al. (2006): Delineation, functional validation, and bioinformatic evaluation of gene expression in thyroid follicular carcinomas with the PAX8-PPARG translocation. *Clin Cancer Res* 12:1983–1993.

Gisselsson D, Lundberg G, Öra I, Höglund M (2007): Distinct evolutionary mechanisms for genomic imbalances in high-risk and low-risk neuroblastomas. *J Carcinog* 6:15.

Goh SG, Lau LC, Sivaswaren C, Chuah KL, Tan PH, Lai D (2001): Pseudodicentric (16;12)(q11;p11.2) in a type AB (mixed) thymoma. *Cancer Genet Cytogenet* 131:42–47.

Gordon RD, Stowasser M, Martin N, Epping A, Conic S, Klemm SA, et al. (1993): Karyotypic abnormalities in benign adrenocortical tumors producing aldosterone. *Cancer Genet Cytogenet* 68:78–81.

Gunawan B, Schlomm T, Schulten HJ, Seseke F, Ringert RH, Fuzesi L (2004): Cytogenetic characterization of 5 pheochromocytomas. *Cancer Genet Cytogenet* 154:163–166.

Guo C, White PS, Weiss MJ, Hogarty MD, Thompson PM, Stram DO, et al. (1999): Allelic deletion at 11q23 is common in MYCN single copy neuroblastomas. *Oncogene* 18:4948–4957.

Hemmer S, Wasenius VM, Knuutila S, Franssila K, Joensuu H (1999): DNA copy number changes in thyroid carcinoma. *Am J Pathol* 154:1539–1547.

Herens C, Radermecker M, Servais A, Quatresooz P, Jardon-Jeghers C, Bours V, et al. (2003): Deletion (6)(p22p25) is a recurrent anomaly of thymoma: Report of a second case and review of the literature. *Cancer Genet Cytogenet* 146:66–69.

Herrmann MA, Hay ID, Bartelt DH Jr, Ritland SR, Dahl RJ, Grant CS, et al. (1991a): Cytogenetic and molecular genetic studies of follicular and papillary thyroid cancers. *J Clin Invest* 88:1596–1604.

Herrmann ME, Mohamed A, Talpos G, Wolman SR (1991b): Cytogenetic study of a papillary thyroid carcinoma with a rearranged chromosome 10. *Cancer Genet Cytogenet* 57:209–217.

Hogarty MD, Liu X, Guo C, Thompson PM, Weiss MJ, White PS, et al. (2000): Identification of a 1-megabase consensus region of deletion at 1p36.3 in primary neuroblastomas. *Med Pediatr Oncol* 35:512–515.

Hui AB, Pang JC, Ko CW, Ng HK (1999): Detection of chromosomal imbalances in growth hormone-secreting pituitary tumors by comparative genomic hybridization. *Hum Pathol* 30:1019–1023.

Janoueix-Lerosey I, Lequin D, Brugières L, Ribeiro A, de Pontual L, Combaret V, et al. (2008): Somatic and germline activating mutations of the ALK kinase receptor in neuroblastoma. *Nature* 455:967–970.

Jenkins RB, Hay ID, Herath JF, Schultz CG, Spurbeck JL, Grant CS, et al. (1990): Frequent occurrence of cytogenetic abnormalities in sporadic nonmedullary thyroid carcinoma. *Cancer* 66:1213–1220.

Jonkers YM, Claessen SM, Feuth T, van Kessel AG, Ramaekers FC, Veltman JA, et al. (2006): Novel candidate tumour suppressor gene loci on chromosomes 11q23–24 and 22q13 involved in human insulinoma tumourigenesis. *J Pathol* 210:450–458.

Jordan DK, Patil SR, Divelbiss JE, Vemuganti S, Headley C, Waziri MH, et al. (1989): Cytogenetic abnormalities in tumors of patients with von Hippel–Lindau disease. *Cancer Genet Cytogenet* 42:227–241.

Kapur RP, Berry JE, Tsuchiya KD, Opheim KE (2014): Activation of the chromosome 19q microRNA cluster in sporadic and androgenetic-biparental mosaicism-associated hepatic mesenchymal hamartoma. *Pediatr Dev Pathol* 17:75–84.

Kasaian K, Wiseman SM, Thiessen N, Mungall KL, Corbett RD, Qian JQ, et al. (2013): Complete genomic landscape of a recurring sporadic parathyroid carcinoma. *J Pathol* 230:249–260.

Kees UR, Mulcahy MT, Willoughby ML (1991): Intrathoracic carcinoma in an 11-year-old girl showing a translocation t(15;19). *Am J Pediatr Hematol Oncol* 13:459–464.

Kiechle-Schwarz M, Neumann HP, Decker HJ, Dietrich C, Wullich B, Schempp W (1989): Cytogenetic studies on three pheochromocytomas derived from patients with von Hippel–Lindau syndrome. *Hum Genet* 82:127–130.

Kitamura Y, Shimizu K, Tanaka S, Ito K, Emi M (2000): Allelotyping of anaplastic thyroid carcinoma: Frequent allelic losses on 1q, 9p, 11, 17, 19p, and 22q. *Genes Chromosomes Cancer* 27:244–251.

Kleer CG, Bryant BR, Giordano TJ, Sobel M, Merino MJ (2000): Genetic changes in chromosomes 1p and 17p in thyroid cancer progression. *Endocr Pathol* 11:137–143.

Kleinman CL, Gerges N, Papillon-Cavanagh S, Sin-Chan P, Pramatarova A, Quang DA, et al. (2014): Fusion of TTYH1 with the C19MC microRNA cluster drives expression of a brain-specific DNMT3B isoform in the embryonal brain tumor ETMR. *Nat Genet* 46:39–44.

Klemke M, Drieschner N, Laabs A, Rippe V, Belge G, Bullerdiek J, et al. (2011): On the prevalence of the PAX8-PPARG fusion resulting from the chromosomal translocation t(2;3)(q13;p25) in adenomas of the thyroid. *Cancer Genet* 204:334–339.

Klemke M, Drieschner N, Belge G, Burchardt K, Junker K (2012): Detection of PAX8-PPARG fusion transcripts in archival thyroid carcinoma samples by conventional RT-PCR. *Genes Chromosomes Cancer* 51:402–408.

Komoike Y, Tamaki Y, Sakita I, Tomita N, Ohue M, Sekimoto M, et al. (1999): Comparative genomic hybridization defines frequent loss on 16p in human anaplastic thyroid carcinoma. *Int J Oncol* 14:1157–1162.

Kristoffersson U, Heim S, Mandahl N, Åkerman M, Mitelman F (1989): Multiple clonal chromosome aberrations in two thymomas. *Cancer Genet Cytogenet* 41:93–98.

Kroll TG, Sarraf P, Pecciarini L, Chen CJ, Mueller E, Spiegelman BM, et al. (2000): PAX8-PPARgamma1 fusion oncogene in human thyroid carcinoma. *Science* 289:1357–1360.

Kubonishi I, Takehara N, Iwata J, Sonobe H, Ohtsuki Y, Abe T, et al. (1991): Novel t(15;19)(q15;p13) chromosome abnormality in a thymic carcinoma. *Cancer Res* 51: 3327–3328.

Lam KY, Lo CY, Shek TW, Ma ES, Au WY, Chan GC (2001): Primitive small round cell tumour of the adrenal gland presenting with fever of unknown origin and t(12;22)(q13;q12) cytogenetic finding. *J Clin Pathol* 54: 966–969.

Larsen JB, Schröder HD, Sörensen AG, Bjerre P, Heim S (1999): Simple numerical chromosome aberrations characterize pituitary adenomas. *Cancer Genet Cytogenet* 114: 144–149.

Lastowska M, Van Roy N, Bown N, Speleman F, Lunec J, Strachan T, et al. (1998): Molecular cytogenetic delineation of 17q translocation breakpoints in neuroblastoma cell lines. *Genes Chromosomes Cancer* 23:116–122.

Lee AC, Kwong YI, Fu KH, Chan GC, Ma L, Lau YL (1993): Disseminated mediastinal carcinoma with chromosomal translocation (15;19). A distinctive clinicopathologic syndrome. *Cancer* 72:2273–2276.

Lee JJ, Foukakis T, Hashemi J, Grimelius L, Heldin NE, Wallin G, et al. (2007a): Molecular cytogenetic profiles of novel and established human anaplastic thyroid carcinoma models. *Thyroid* 17:289–301.

Lee GY, Yang WI, Jeung HC, Kim SC, Seo MY, Park CH, et al. (2007b): Genome-wide genetic aberrations of thymoma using cDNA microarray based comparative genomic hybridization. *BMC Genomics* 8:305.

Li M, Lee KF, Lu Y, Clarke I, Shih D, Eberhart C et al. (2009): Frequent amplification of a chr19q13.41 microRNA polycistron in aggressive primitive neuroectodermal brain tumors. *Cancer Cell* 16:533–546.

Limon J, Dal Cin P, Kakati S, Huben RP, Sandberg AA (1987a): Cytogenetic findings in a primary adrenocortical carcinoma. *Cancer Genet Cytogenet* 26:271–277.

Limon J, Dal Cin P, Gaeta J, Sandberg AA (1987b): Translocation t(4;11)(q35;p13) in an adrenocortical carcinoma. *Cancer Genet Cytogenet* 28:343–348.

Longo L, Panza E, Schena F, Seri M, Devoto M, Romeo G, et al. (2007): Genetic predisposition to familial neuroblastoma: Identification of two novel genomic regions at 2p and 12p. *Hum Hered* 63:205–211.

Lui WO, Chen J, Glasker S, Bender BU, Madura C, Khoo SK, et al. (2002): Selective loss of chromosome 11 in pheochromocytomas associated with the VHL syndrome. *Oncogene* 21:1117–1122.

Lundberg G, Sehic D, Länsberg JK, Øra I, Frigyesi A, Castel V, et al. (2011): Alternative lengthening of telomeres—An enhanced chromosomal instability in aggressive non-*MYCN* amplified and telomere elongated neuroblastomas. *Genes Chromosomes Cancer* 50:250–262.

Mannelli M, Gelmini S, Arnaldi G, Becherini L, Bemporad D, Crescioli C, et al. (2000): Telomerase activity is significantly enhanced in malignant adrenocortical tumors in comparison to benign adrenocortical adenomas. *J Clin Endocrinol Metab* 85:468–470.

Maris JM, Weiss MJ, Guo C, Gerbing RB, Stram DO, White PS, et al. (2000): Loss of heterozygosity at 1p36 independently predicts for disease progression but not decreased overall survival probability in neuroblastoma patients: A Children's Cancer Group study. *J Clin Oncol* 18:1888–1899.

Maris JM, Guo C, Blake D, White PS, Hogarty MD, Thompson PM, et al. (2001): Comprehensive analysis of chromosome 1p deletions in neuroblastoma. *Med Pediatr Oncol* 36:32–36.

Maris JM, Hogarty MD, Bagatell R, Cohn SL (2007): Neuroblastoma. *Lancet* 369:2106–2120.

Mark J (1971): Chromosomal characteristics of human pituitary adenomas. *Acta Neuropathol* 19:99–109.

Mark J, Ekedahl C, Dahlenfors R, Westermark B (1987): Cytogenetical observations in five human anaplastic thyroid carcinomas. *Hereditas* 107:163–174.

Marks JL, Wyandt HE, Beazley RM, Milunsky JM, Sheahan K, Milunsky A (1992): Cytogenetic studies of an adrenal cortical carcinoma. *Cancer Genet Cytogenet* 61:96–98.

Marques AR, Espadinha C, Catarino AL, Moniz S, Pereira T, Sobrinho LG, et al. (2002): Expression of PAX8-PPAR gamma 1 rearrangements in both follicular thyroid carcinomas and adenomas. *J Clin Endocrinol Metab* 87: 3947–3952.

Martinsson T, Sjöberg RM, Hedborg F, Kogner P (1995): Deletion of chromosome 1p loci and microsatellite instability in neuroblastomas analyzed with short-tandem repeat polymorphisms. *Cancer Res* 55:5681–5686.

Marx A, Ströbel P, Badve SS, Chalabreysse L, Chan JK, Chen G, et al. (2014): ITMIG consensus statement on the use of the WHO histological classification of thymoma and thymic carcinoma: Refined definitions, histological criteria, and reporting. *Thorac Oncol* 9:596–611.

Minoletti F, Butti MG, Coronelli S, Miozzo M, Sozzi G, Pilotti S, et al. (1994): The two genes generating RET/

PTC3 are localized in chromosomal band 10q11.2. *Genes Chromosomes Cancer* 11:51–57.

Mitelman F, Johansson B, Mertens F, editors (2014): Mitelman Database of Chromosome Aberrations and Gene Fusions in Cancer. http://cgap.nci.nih.gov/Chromosomes/Mitelman.

Mirza I, Kazimi SN, Ligi R, Burns J, Braza F (2000): Cytogenetic profile of a thymoma. A case report and review of the literature. *Arch Pathol Lab Med* 124:1714–1716.

Molenaar JJ, Koster J, Zwijnenburg DA, van Sluis P, Valentijn LJ, van der Ploeg I, et al. (2012): Sequencing of neuroblastoma identifies chromothripsis and defects in neuritogenesis genes. *Nature* 483:589–593.

Mosse YP, Laudenslager M, Khazi D, Carlisle AJ, Winter CL, Rappaport E, et al. (2004): Germline *PHOX2B* mutation in hereditary neuroblastoma. *Am J Hum Genet* 75:727–730.

Mosse YP, Diskin SJ, Wasserman N, Rinaldi K, Attiyeh EF, Cole K, et al. (2007): Neuroblastomas have distinct genomic DNA profiles that predict clinical phenotype and regional gene expression. *Genes Chromosomes Cancer* 46:936–949.

Mosse YP, Laudenslager M, Longo L, Cole KA, Wood A, Attiyeh EF, et al. (2008): Identification of ALK as a major familial neuroblastoma predisposition gene. *Nature* 455:930–935.

Nobusawa S, Yokoo H, Hirato J, Kakita A, Takahashi H, Sugino T, et al. (2012): Analysis of chromosome 19q13.42 amplification in embryonal brain tumors with ependymoblastic multilayered rosettes. *Brain Pathol* 22:689–697.

Ohali A, Avigad S, Ash S, Goshen Y, Luria D, Feinmesser M, et al. (2006): Telomere length is a prognostic factor in neuroblastoma. *Cancer* 107:1391–1399.

Opocher G, Schiavi F, Vettori A, Pampinella F, Vitiello L, Calderan A, et al. (2003): Fine analysis of the short arm of chromosome 1 in sporadic and familial pheochromocytoma. *Clin Endocrinol* 59:707–715.

Örndal C, Johansson M, Heim S, Mandahl N, Månsson B, Alumets J, et al. (1990): Parathyroid adenoma with t(1;5) (p22;q32) as the sole clonal chromosome abnormality. *Cancer Genet Cytogenet* 48:225–228.

Pack SD, Kirschner LS, Pak E, Zhuang Z, Carney JA, Stratakis CA (2000): Genetic and histologic studies of somatomammotropic pituitary tumors in patients with the "complex of spotty skin pigmentation, myxomas, endocrine overactivity and schwannomas" (Carney complex). *J Clin Endocrinol Metab* 85:3860–3865.

Papi L, Baldassarri G, Montali E, Bigozzi U, Ammannati F, Brandi ML (1993): Cytogenetic studies in sporadic and multiple endocrine neoplasia type 1-associated pituitary adenomas. *Genes Chromosomes Cancer* 7:63–65.

Penzel R, Hoegel J, Schmitz W, Blaeker H, Morresi-Hauf A, Aulmann S, et al. (2003): Clusters of chromosomal imbalances in thymic epithelial tumours are associated with the WHO classification and the staging system according to Masaoka. *Int J Cancer* 105:494–498.

Perri P, Longo L, McConville C, Cusano R, Rees SA, Seri M, et al. (2002): Linkage analysis in families with recurrent neuroblastoma. *Ann N Y Acad Sci* 963:74–84.

Perissel B, Coupier I, DeLatour M, Cardot N, Penault-Llorca F, Jaffray J, et al. (2000): Structural and numerical aberrations of chromosome 22 in a case of follicular variant of papillary thyroid carcinoma revealed by conventional and molecular cytogenetics. *Cancer Genet Cytogenet* 121:33–37.

Perissel B, Bernheim A, Couturier J, Fouilhoux G, Vago P (2002): From the cytogenetics to the cytogenomics of thyroid tumors. *Bull Cancer* 89:588–592.

Pfragner R, Behmel A, Smith DP, Ponder BA, Wirnsberger G, Rinner I, et al. (1998): First continuous human pheochromocytoma cell line: KNA. Biological, cytogenetic and molecular characterization of KNA cells. *J Neurocytol* 27:175–186.

Pierotti MA, Santoro M, Jenkins RB, Sozzi G, Bongarzone I, Grieco M, et al. (1992): Characterization of an inversion on the long arm of chromosome 10 juxtaposing D10S170 and RET and creating the oncogenic sequence RET/PTC. *Proc Natl Acad Sci USA* 89:1616–1620.

Plantaz D, Vandesompele J, Van Roy N, Lastowska M, Bown N, Combaret V, et al. (2001): Comparative genomic hybridization (CGH) analysis of stage 4 neuroblastoma reveals high frequency of 11q deletion in tumors lacking MYCN amplification. *Int J Cancer* 91:680–686.

Pugh TJ, Morozova O, Attiyeh EF, Asgharzadeh S, Wei JS, Auclair D, et al. (2013): The genetic landscape of high-risk neuroblastoma. *Nat Genet* 45:279–284.

Raabe EH, Laudenslager M, Winter C, Wasserman N, Cole K, LaQuaglia M, et al. (2008): Prevalence and functional consequence of PHOX2B mutations in neuroblastoma. *Oncogene* 27:469–476.

Reiter JL, Brodeur GM (1996): High-resolution mapping of a 130-kb core region of the MYCN amplicon in neuroblastomas. *Genomics* 32:97–103.

Reiter JL, Brodeur GM (1998): MYCN is the only highly expressed gene from the core amplified domain in human neuroblastomas. *Genes Chromosomes Cancer* 23:134–140.

Rey JA, Bello MJ, de Campos JM, Kusak ME, Martinez-Castro P, Benitez J (1986): A case of pituitary adenoma with 58 chromosomes. *Cancer Genet Cytogenet* 23:171–174.

Rippe V, Drieschner N, Meiboom M, Murua Escobar H, Bonk U, Belge G, et al. (2003): Identification of a gene rearranged by 2p21 aberrations in thyroid adenomas. *Oncogene* 22:6111–6114.

Rippe V, Dittberner L, Lorenz VN, Drieschner N, Nimzyk R, Sendt W, et al. (2010): The two stem cell microRNA gene clusters C19MC and miR-371-3 are activated by specific chromosomal rearrangements in a subgroup of thyroid adenomas. *PLoS One* 5:e9485.

Rippe V, Flor I, Debler JW, Drieschner N, Rommel B, Krause D, et al. (2012): Activation of the two microRNA clusters C19MC and miR-371-3 does not play prominent role in thyroid cancer. *Mol Cytogenet* 5:40.

Rock JP, Babu VR, Drumheller T, Chason J (1993): Cytogenetic findings in pituitary adenoma: Results of a pilot study. *Surg Neurol* 40:224–229.

Roque L, Soares J, Castedo S (1998): Cytogenetic and fluorescence *in situ* hybridization studies in a case of anaplastic thyroid carcinoma. *Cancer Genet Cytogenet* 103:7–10.

Roque L, Nunes VM, Ribeiro C, Martins C, Soares J (2001): Karyotypic characterization of papillary thyroid carcinomas. *Cancer* 92:2529–2538.

Roque L, Rodrigues R, Pinto A, Moura-Nunes V, Soares J (2003): Chromosome imbalances in thyroid follicular neoplasms: A comparison between follicular adenomas and carcinomas. *Genes Chromosomes Cancer* 36:292–302.

Russell AJ, Sibbald J, Haak H, Keith WN, McNicol AM (1999): Increasing genome instability in adrenocortical carcinoma progression with involvement of chromosomes 3, 9 and X at the adenoma stage. *Br J Cancer* 81:684–689.

Sammarelli G, Zannoni M, Bonomini S, Delsignore R, Rizzoli V, Sianesi M, et al. (2007): A translocation t(4;13) (q21;q14) as single clonal chromosomal abnormality in a parathyroid adenoma. *Tumori* 93:97–99.

Scappaticci S, Arrigoni G, Capra E, Maraschio P, Fraccaro M (1992): Cytogenetics of multiple endocrine neoplasia syndromes. I. Two different, unique clonal chromosome changes in a medullary thyroid carcinoma and in a C-cell thyroid hyperplasia. *Cancer Genet Cytogenet* 59:51–53.

Schneiderman J, London WB, Brodeur GM, Castleberry RP, Look AT, Cohn SL (2008): Clinical significance of MYCN amplification and ploidy in favorable-stage neuroblastoma: A report from the Children's Oncology Group. *J Clin Oncol* 26:913–918.

Schoenmakers EF, Wanschura S, Mols R, Bullerdiek J, Van den Berghe H, Van de Ven WJM (1995): Recurrent rearrangements in the high mobility group protein gene, HMGI-C, in benign mesenchymal tumours. *Nat Genet* 10:436–444.

Schwab M, Alitalo K, Klempnauer KH, Varmus HE, Bishop JM, Gilbert F, et al. (1983): Amplified DNA with limited homology to myc cellular oncogene is shared by human neuroblastoma cell lines and a neuroblastoma tumour. *Nature* 305:245–248.

Seeger RC, Wada R, Brodeur GM, Moss TJ, Bjork RL, Sousa L, et al. (1988): Expression of N-myc by neuroblastomas with one or multiple copies of the oncogene. *Prog Clin Biol Res* 271:41–49.

Shi Y, Hogue J, Dixit D, Koh J, Olson JA Jr (2014): Functional and genetic studies of isolated cells from parathyroid tumors reveal the complex pathogenesis of parathyroid neoplasia. *Proc Natl Acad Sci USA* 111:3092–3097.

Shimada H, Chatten J, NewtonWA Jr, Sachs N, Hamoudi AB, Chiba T, et al. (1984): Histopathologic prognostic factors in neuroblastic tumors: Definition of subtypes of ganglioneuroblastoma and an age-linked classification of neuroblastomas. *J Natl Cancer Inst* 73:405–416.

Shono T, Sakai H, Takehara K, Honda S, Kanetake H (2002): Analysis of numerical chromosomal aberrations in adrenal cortical neoplasms by fluorescence in situ hybridization. *J Urol* 168:1370–1373.

Sidhu S, Marsh DJ, Theodosopoulos G, Philips J, Bambach CP, Campbell P, et al. (2002): Comparative genomic hybridization analysis of adrenocortical tumors. *J Clin Endocrinol Metab* 87:3467–3474.

Sidhu S, Gicquel C, Bambach CP, Campbell P, Magarey C, Robinson BG, et al. (2003): Clinical and molecular aspects of adrenocortical tumourigenesis. *ANZ J Surg* 73:727–738.

Slack FJ, Weidhaas JB (2006): MicroRNAs as a potential magic bullet in cancer. *Future Oncol* 2:73–82.

Smit JW, VanZelderen-Bhola S, Merx R, De Leeuw W, Wessels H, Vink R, et al. (2001): A novel chromosomal translocation t(3;5)(q12;p15.3) and loss of heterozygosity on chromosome 22 in a multifocal follicular variant of papillary thyroid carcinoma presenting with skin metastases. *Clin Endocrinol* 55:543–548.

Sonobe H, Takeuchi T, Ohtsuki Y, Taguchi T, Shimizu K (1999): A thymoma with clonal complex chromosome abnormalities. *Cancer Genet Cytogenet* 110:72–74.

Sozzi G, Bongarzone I, Miozzo M, Cariani CT, Mondellini P, Calderone C, et al. (1992): Cytogenetic and molecular genetic characterization of papillary thyroid carcinomas. *Genes Chromosomes Cancer* 5:212–218.

Spence T, Perotti C, Sin-Chan P, Picard D, Wu W, Singh A, et al. (2014): A novel C19MC amplified cell line links Lin28/let-7 to mTOR signaling in embryonal tumor with multilayered rosettes. *Neuro Oncol* 16:62–71.

Srivatsan ES, Ying KL, Seeger RC (1993): Deletion of chromosome 11 and of 14q sequences in neuroblastoma. *Genes Chromosomes Cancer* 7:32–37.

Stovroff M, Dykes F, Teague WG (1995): The complete spectrum of neurocristopathy in an infant with congenital hypoventilation, Hirschsprung's disease, and neuroblastoma. *J Pediatr Surg* 30:1218–1221.

Stratakis CA, Carney JA, Lin JP, Papanicolaou DA, Karl M, Kastner DL, et al. (1996): Carney complex, a familial multiple neoplasia and lentiginosis syndrome. Analysis of 11 kindreds and linkage to the short arm of chromosome 2. *J Clin Invest* 97:699–705.

Takehara K, Sakai H, Shono T, Irie J, Kanetake H (2005): Proliferative activity and genetic changes in adrenal cortical tumors examined by flow cytometry, fluorescence in situ hybridization and immunohistochemistry. *Int J Urol* 12:121–127.

Teyssier JR, Liautaud-Roger F, Ferre D, Patey M, Dufer J (1990): Chromosomal changes in thyroid tumors. Relation with DNA content, karyotypic features, and clinical data. *Cancer Genet Cytogenet* 50:249–263.

Trautmann K, Thakker RV, Ellison DW, Ibrahim A, Lees PD, Harding B, et al. (2001): Chromosomal aberrations in sporadic pituitary tumors. *Int J Cancer* 91:809–814.

Trochet D, Bourdeaut F, Janoueix-Lerosey I, Deville A, de Pontual L, Schleiermacher G, et al. (2004): Germline mutations of the paired-like homeobox 2B (PHOX2B) gene in neuroblastoma. *Am J Hum Genet* 74:761–764.

Vaira V, Elli F, Forno I, Guarnieri V, Verdelli C, Ferrero S, Scillitani A, et al. (2012): The microRNA cluster C19MC is deregulated in parathyroid tumours. *J Mol Endocrinol* 49:115–124.

Van den Berghe I, Debiec-Rychter M, Proot L, Hagemeijer A, Michielssen P (2002): Ring chromosome 6 may represent a cytogenetic subgroup in benign thymoma. *Cancer Genet Cytogenet* 137:75–77.

Vu-Phan D, Grachtchouk V, Yu J, Colby LA, Wicha MS, Koenig RJ (2013): The thyroid cancer PAX8-PPARG fusion protein activates Wnt/TCF-responsive cells that have a transformed phenotype. *Endocr Relat Cancer* 20:725–739.

Wang Q, Hui GZ, Lin YC, Lu XJ, Yu WH, Wu SR, et al. (2002): Preliminary study of chromosome aberrations in pituitary adenoma. *Ai Zheng* 21:1120–1123.

Ward LS, Brenta G, Medvedovic M, Fagin JA (1998): Studies of allelic loss in thyroid tumors reveal major differences in chromosomal instability between papillary and follicular carcinomas. *J Clin Endocrinol Metab* 83:525–530.

Wenzel A, Schwab M (1995): The mycN/max protein complex in neuroblastoma. Short review. *Eur J Cancer* 31A:516–519.

White PS, Maris JM, Beltinger C, Sulman E, Marshall HN, Fujimori M, et al. (1995): A region of consistent deletion in neuroblastoma maps within human chromosome 1p36.2–36.3. *Proc Natl Acad Sci USA* 92:5520–5524.

White PS, Thompson PM, Seifried BA, Sulman EP, Jensen SJ, Guo C, et al. (2001): Detailed molecular analysis of 1p36 in neuroblastoma. *Med Pediatr Oncol* 36:37–41.

Wilkens L, Benten D, Tchinda J, Brabant G, Potter E, Dralle H, et al. (2000): Aberrations of chromosomes 5 and 8 as recurrent cytogenetic events in anaplastic carcinoma of the thyroid as detected by fluorescence in situ hybridisation and comparative genomic hybridisation. *Virchows Arch* 436:312–318.

Zettl A, Strobel P, Wagner K, Katzenberger T, Ott G, Rosenwald A, et al. (2000): Recurrent genetic aberrations in thymoma and thymic carcinoma. *Am J Pathol* 157:257–266.

Zhao J, Speel EJ, Muletta-Feurer S, Rutimann K, Saremaslani P, Roth J, et al. (1999): Analysis of genomic alterations in sporadic adrenocortical lesions. Gain of chromosome 17 is an early event in adrenocortical tumorigenesis, *Am J Pathol* 155:1039–1045.

Zimling ZG, Rechnitzer C, Rasmussen M, Petersen BL (2004): Familial neuroblastoma: Different histological manifestations in a family with three affected individuals. *APMIS* 112:153–158.

CHAPTER 20

Tumors of the nervous system

Petter Brandal and Sverre Heim

Section for Cancer Cytogenetics, Institute for Cancer Genetics and Informatics, Oslo University Hospital, Oslo, Norway

Tumors of the nervous system are extensively studied cytogenetically; especially, this applies to those within the central nervous system (CNS) that have commanded by far the most scientific attention. Their chromosomal aberrations are the main focus of this chapter. The 2007 WHO classification of CNS tumors recognizes seven different main neoplastic entities (Louis et al., 2007) with metastases from malignant diseases originating outside the CNS as the most common; however, metastases to the brain will not be covered here. Note further that pituitary tumors, most of them adenomas, by the WHO are classified among tumors of endocrine organs (De Lellis et al., 2004) and are covered in Chapter 19. Also, peripheral nervous system (PNS) tumors of the eye and adrenal gland are covered elsewhere in this book (Chapters 21 and 20, respectively), whereas nerve sheath tumors form part of this chapter.

The current WHO classification of CNS tumors (Louis et al., 2007) is almost exclusively based on morphology, and the neoplasms are categorized according to their resemblance to normal cells. Brain tumors are histologically graded from I to IV. Tumors of grades I and II are considered low-grade, whereas grade III and IV tumors are defined as high-grade. An updated version of this classification is expected soon, and given the wealth of cytogenetic and molecular genetic knowledge about several brain tumor entities that has come forth in recent years, it is expected that the new classification will incorporate genetic changes as an integral, important part of its basis.

A total of 2518 karyotypically abnormal CNS tumors are reported in the Mitelman database (Mitelman et al., 2014), a number that includes data on retinoblastoma of the eye. The most extensively studied groups are neuroglial neoplasms ($n = 944$ at the time of writing) and meningiomas ($n = 926$). A pertinent question is, given these high numbers of karyotypically examined tumors, whether the existing cytogenetic information is not now sufficient and, hence, whether further cytogenetic analyses can bring anything of value? Furthermore, in a day when numerous molecular genetic investigative techniques are becoming available, is karyotyping still of value in the brain tumor context, be it for diagnostic or research purposes?

Our answer to these questions is a clear affirmative. One thing is that much of the published data are from an era when the technical quality of G-banding karyotypes was poor compared to what could be obtained in recent years. Most known karyotypes were furthermore published using G-banding as a stand-alone technique, that is, without the use of additional molecular (cyto)genetic methods on the same samples to better characterize the

Cancer Cytogenetics: Chromosomal and Molecular Genetic Aberrations of Tumor Cells, Fourth Edition.
Edited by Sverre Heim and Felix Mitelman.
© 2015 John Wiley & Sons, Ltd. Published 2015 by John Wiley & Sons, Ltd.

aberrations that were detected. Recent understanding of the genetic heterogeneity and complexity of solid neoplasms, including CNS tumors, has underscored the necessity of using several complementary methods to examine neoplasms if a truly informative picture of their pathogenetic changes is to be achieved. The new high-throughput genetic techniques, for example, whole-genome sequencing, have received a lot of attention in this regard, and much faith is put into the targeted therapy that supposedly is going to evolve from a closer study of the high-resolution information they provide. The said present-day techniques generate enormous amounts of data that, although multiple software algorithms exist that help us separate chaff from wheat, are hard to assess in terms of pathogenetic relevance. Karyotyping yields genetic information on individual cells and functions as a nonbiased screening method capable of providing information about both structural and numerical chromosome aberrations. The data thus generated can also serve as starting points for gene-level searches by means of the newer techniques, an approach that has proved fertile also in the brain tumor context (Panagopoulos et al., 2014; Olsen et al., 2015). In line with the title of this book, we shall focus on information provided by studies using karyotyping and other cytogenetic techniques relying on fluorescence *in situ* hybridization such as array and chromosomal comparative genomic hybridization (aCGH and cCGH). Nevertheless, molecular genetic findings of particular interest will also be mentioned, especially if they tie in with acquired genomic changes that are visible at the chromosomal level.

Neuroepithelial tumors

These are the most common primary brain tumors. Multiple subentities exist, including astrocytomas, oligodendrogliomas (ODG), oligoastrocytomas (OA), and ependymomas. It is worthy of note that gliomas differ from other malignant tumors in that they seldom or never give rise to metastases be it inside or outside the CNS. Most of them grow infiltratingly, however, a circumstance that contributes to the well nigh impossibility of achieving complete tumor removal by surgery, and many of them display pronounced cellular as well as clinical aggressiveness. Their malignant potential varies with tumor grade.

Astrocytomas

Astrocytes are cells that provide structural and biochemical support for the neurons. They are important in neurotransmitter turnover and are thought to play a role in maintenance of the blood–brain barrier. The cells are stellate in morphologic appearance (hence their name) and express intermediate filament glial fibrillary acidic protein (GFAP). Genomic changes in astrocytomas will be further discussed for each tumor grade. A study comparing CGH copy number aberrations between astrocytomas of various grades detected grade-specific aberration patterns (Holland et al., 2010).

Grade I astrocytomas (pilocytic astrocytomas, PA): Most WHO grade I astrocytic tumors are classified as PA, which tend to occur in children and young adults. The tumors differ from grade II to IV astrocytomas in that they are circumscribed. Patients with PA can therefore be cured if their tumor is completely resected. PA also, unlike the diffuse astrocytomas (DA), generally do not evolve into more higher-grade tumors with time. As a consequence of these differences, the prognosis for patients with PA is excellent with a 10-year survival rate as high as 90% (Giannini and Scheithauer, 1997).

Intriguingly, many PA occur in patients who suffer from neurofibromatosis type 1 (NF1), a disease associated with mutations in the *NF1* tumor suppressor gene (17q11.2; Listernick et al., 1999). Although PA arising in the setting of neurofibromatosis show inactivation also of the wild-type *NF1* in accordance with Knudson's two-hit hypothesis, inactivation of this gene is not a feature of sporadic PA (Kluwe et al., 2001). Furthermore, gene expression profiling has revealed a distinct molecular signature that separates the neurofibromatosis-associated and sporadic tumors (Sharma et al., 2006). Unlike what is seen in diffusely infiltrating astrocytomas, *TP53* (17p13.1) alterations are uncommon in PA, nor is accumulation of mutant TP53 protein (a hallmark of higher-grade tumors) a feature of PA (Cheng et al., 2000).

Not many PA have been examined by chromosome banding, and only 34 such tumors with an abnormal karyotype, most of them near-diploid, are registered in the Mitelman database. According to Zattara-Cannoni et al. (1998), about half of all

PA are without chromosome aberrations when examined by banding cytogenetics. Some early studies by FISH reported gains of chromosomes 7 and 8, especially the former, as typical of PA (White et al., 1995; Mitelman et al., 2014). Subsequent CGH studies have identified gains of chromosomes 5, 6, 7, and 9 in occasional tumors (Sanoudou et al., 2000). A more recent study using high-resolution aCGH (Jones et al., 2006) found that partial or whole-copy gains of chromosomes 5, 6, 7, 11, 15, and 20 were relatively common in PA; the abnormalities seemed to be more frequent with increasing patient age. The normal karyotype found in many PA suggests that these tumors have genetic alterations too small to be detected at the chromosomal level of genomic organization and also for this reason several higher-resolution platforms have been used to study PA genomes. An aCGH study identified amplification of *HIPK2* at 7q34 in most tumors tested, but found no whole-chromosome losses or gains (Deshmukh et al., 2008), whereas a study by Ward et al. (2010) showed copy number aberrations in 14% of PA. Following the aCGH identification of gains at 7q34 targeting the *BRAF* locus and leading to activation of the MEK and ERK proteins, both downstream of BRAF (Bar et al., 2008; Jones et al., 2008; Pfister et al., 2008), interest in the MAPK pathway in PA pathogenesis rose sharply. A *BRAF–KIAA1549* fusion gene brought about by a tandem duplication of 7q34 was identified (Jones et al., 2008; Sievert et al., 2009) and seems to be present in most PA. Later, also other fusions and other rearrangements involving *BRAF*, including mutations, have been identified (Jones et al., 2009, 2013; Cin et al., 2011). The latter study by Jones and coworkers confirmed that PA harbor few genetic aberrations and that the ones present lead to activation of the MAPK pathway. Not surprisingly, studies investigating targeted therapy based on these findings are underway.

It was initially thought that fusions of the *BRAF* gene were exclusive to PA and never found in other astrocytoma entities (Lawson et al., 2010). This has turned out not to be the case (see Grade II astrocytomas and oligodendrogliomas).

Grade II astrocytomas (DA): Diffuse astrocytomas (DA) are classified as low-grade tumors and are by many regarded as benign. Their incidence is often reported along with grade I astrocytomas, and

taken together, these groups account for about 10% of gliomas in the USA (Zada et al., 2012). DA are, as their name implies, diffusely infiltrating tumors, and they have a tendency to malignant transformation. In principle, they are incurable diseases, but many patients live with their DA for several years and some even for decades (Ohgaki and Kleihues, 2005).

A CGH analysis of grade II astrocytomas conducted by Arslantas et al. (2007) found chromosome copy number abnormalities in over 80% of tumors; however, only zero to five copy number changes were seen per case. Gain of chromosome arm 7q was the most common aberration. Recurrent gain of 7q in diffuse astrocytoma was also seen by Hirose et al. (2003) who pointed out that copy number aberration frequencies in astrocytomas increased with increasing tumor grade. A study combining G-banding and CGH showed that only five of 16 DA had abnormal karyotypes, whereas all 10 analyzed tumors had copy number aberrations (Dahlback et al., 2011a). Most common were 7q gains.

One of the most common genomic changes found in grade II astrocytomas is mutations of the *TP53* tumor suppressor gene in 17p13. This is thought to be an important early step in the malignant progression of DA to higher-grade tumors and, therefore, a parameter indicating poor prognosis (Ohgaki and Kleihues, 2007). In later years, around three-fourths of DA have been shown to carry *IDH1/2* mutations (2q33.3/15q26.1; Gupta et al., 2011; Håvik et al., 2014).

Fusion genes have not been found as often in DA as in PA; however, a *KIAA1549–BRAF* has been reported (Badiali et al., 2012; Ida et al., 2012). In pleomorphic xanthoastrocytoma (PXA), a special subgroup of grade II astrocytoma, the pathogenetic process seems to involve MAPK activation. This activation is primarily mediated via *BRAF* mutations, however, not through fusions of *BRAF* with other genes (Dias-Santagata et al., 2011).

Grade III astrocytomas (anaplastic astrocytomas, AA): AA are high-grade, diffusely infiltrating, intra-axial neoplasms with a more aggressive histopathological pattern than their grade II counterparts; nuclear atypia, increased cellularity, and significant proliferative activity are seen (Louis et al., 2007). AA are often referred to as malignant and represent 8% of gliomas in the USA (Zada et al., 2012). AA carry a dismal prognosis with a relative survival at five years of 24% (Smoll and Hamilton, in press). They also, like DA but even more readily, tend to undergo further malignization and evolve into glioblastoma.

Typical gross cytogenetic abnormalities in AA include loss of 10q, 9p, and 1p as well as gain of 7p. Interestingly, gain of 7p12–13 and loss of 10q tend to occur together (Kunwar et al., 2001; Arslantas et al., 2004), suggesting that two or more genetic loci here may play a synergistic role in the development or progression of these tumors (Arslantas et al., 2007). These genetic regions contain the epidermal growth factor receptor gene (*EGFR* on 7p) and the phosphatase and tensin homolog gene (*PTEN* on 10q). As do grade II astrocytomas, AA frequently carry *TP53* mutations. A recent study of five AA showed a near-diploid karyotype with both numerical and structural chromosome aberrations in all tumors (Holland et al., 2012).

Grade IV astrocytomas (glioblastoma multiforme, GBM): GBM is the most aggressive astrocytoma and accounts for half of all gliomas (Zada et al., 2012). The tumors have a high mitotic index and are usually characterized by pronounced vascular proliferation and necrosis. Some GBM may also contain oligodendroglial features leading to the recognition of a subentity called GBM with an oligodendroglial component (Louis et al., 2007). The prognosis for GBM patients is dismal with a median survival of only 15 months for the youngest and most fit patients (Stupp et al., 2005). GBM are subdivided into primary tumors that arise de novo showing GBM features from the beginning and secondary GBM that develop from a preexisting lower-grade tumor (Louis et al., 2007). Secondary GBM are the less common and carry a (relatively) better prognosis when compared to primary GBM. Genetically, secondary GBM are more similar to lower-grade astrocytomas than to primary GBM (Brennan, 2011).

The vast majority of the 521 high-grade astrocytomas registered in the Mitelman database are GBM. Early cytogenetic studies identified a variety of aberrations in these tumors especially involving chromosomes 1, 6, 7, 9, 11, 13, 16, and 19 (Bigner et al., 1986, 1988; Schrock et al., 1994). Most GBM harbor chromosomal aberrations by G-banding and copy number aberrations by CGH (Dahlback et al., 2009). The karyotypes are typically, but not always, complex. A particularly frequent change is loss of chromosome 10, often occurring together with gain of one copy of chromosome 7 (Figure 20.1). The said combination of monosomy 10 and trisomy 7 is found in 137/521 of all GBM registered in the Mitelman database, but in only 40/1997 other CNS tumors (Mitelman et al., 2014). Putative cytogenetic pathways have been proposed with +7 and –10 as primary changes and losses of 1p, 9p, 13q, and 22q occurring secondarily. No recurrent structural aberrations arousing suspicion of possible fusion genes have been detected. CGH studies have confirmed that +7 and –10 occur together and have discovered also additional nonrandom numerical changes such as –9, +19, +20, and –22 (Dahlback et al., 2009). Similar findings were reported also based on studies using high-throughput techniques aided by statistical algorithms (Beroukhim et al., 2007).

Based on the growing cytogenetic and molecular genetic knowledge about GBM, several key pathogenetic pathways have been suggested (Ohgaki and Kleihues, 2007; Verhaak et al., 2010). Epidermal growth factor (EGF) signaling, which is mediated by several important effector proteins and is vital for cell cycling, seems to play an important role. Aberrant epidermal growth factor receptor gene (*EGFR*) function is often seen in GBM and is usually due to amplification; indeed, 40% of GBM contain *EGFR* amplification resulting in overexpression of the gene (Ekstrand et al., 1991, 1992). Gliomas also acquire aberrant EGFR activity through mutation of the *EGFR* gene, typically together with amplification. The most common variant (*EGFRvIII*) contains a 3′ truncation of the extracellular EGF binding domain (exons 2–7), corresponding to an isoform that is constitutively active also in the absence of a ligand (Moscatello et al., 1996). *EGFR* amplification combined with the presence of *EGFRvIII* variant correlates with the worst prognosis in GBM patients (Shinojima et al., 2003). Whereas *EGFR* maps to chromosome 7 and could constitute a or the target whereby gain of the chromosome acts pathogenetically in GBM, there are several hints that also other genes (including those encoding MET and its ligand HGF) located on this chromosome could play an equally important role (Beroukhim et al., 2007). The best evidence that EGFR is not necessarily the functional target

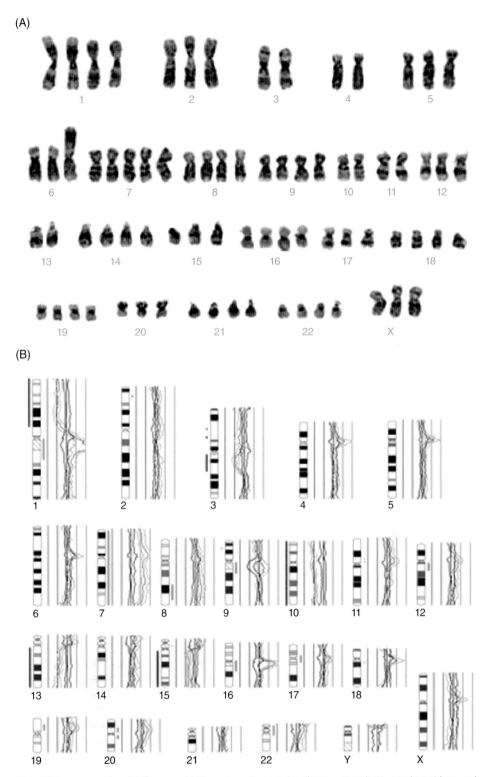

Figure 20.1 (A) Karyogram of a glioblastoma with the commonly occurring changes +7 and –10 together with several other aberrations. (B) CGH profile from the same tumor confirming the relative gain of chromosome 7 and relative loss of chromosome 10 material. Green bars to the right of the chromosome ideograms correspond to areas of gained genomic material; red bars to the left correspond to lost chromosomal areas.

comes from the observation that a large number of GBM have +7 and −10 but no *EGFR* amplification, mutation, or overexpression.

Another genetic alteration that occurs frequently in GBM is inactivation of *PTEN* whose locus in 10q23.3 is deleted in approximately 30% of primary GBM (Dahia, 2000). The primary biological function of PTEN seems to be in cell survival and migration. Briefly, PTEN dephosphorylates the phospholipid phosphatidylinositol 3, 4, 5 triphosphate (PtdIns (3, 4, 5)P3), which directly antagonizes the activity of the phosphatidylinositol 3-kinase (PI3K) (Cantley and Neel, 1999). When fully phosphorylated, PtdIns (3, 4, 5) P3 promotes cell survival and growth by suppressing the activity of AKT (Vanhaesebroeck et al., 1997). In addition, PTEN functions to modulate cell adhesion and migration by antagonizing the activity of FAK (Gu et al., 1999). Although *PTEN* is an important target gene in GBM (and other tumors), there is strong evidence that also other chromosome 10 genes (e.g., *DMBT*) may be altered in high-grade astrocytomas (Somerville et al., 1998). Many GBM have −10 without any sign of *PTEN* inactivation (Fan et al., 2002). Yet again, we witness a situation in which the loss of an entire chromosome cannot be interpreted as functionally equivalent to the loss of one gene locus only.

Other common genetic alterations in GBM include *TP53* mutations (Watanabe et al., 1996) as well as mutation and inactivation of *CDKN2A* and *RB1* (Nakamura et al., 2001a, b). The *CDKN2A* and *RB1* genes, which map to 9p21.3 and 13q14, respectively, are inactivated by deletion or promoter methylation in the majority of GBM. One study found the RB pathway to be functionally inactivated in 86% of the analyzed cases (Ueki et al., 1996). Rollbrocker et al. (1996) suggested that *CDK4* (from 12q14) is amplified in GBM leading to increased CDK4 protein levels. Using a quantitative RT-PCR approach, Zhou et al. (2005) found a statistically significant increase in *CDK4* expression in GBM. This is in agreement with the observation that CDK4/6 inhibition promotes growth arrest of neural progenitor cells and that this arrest is RB dependant (Ferguson et al., 2000).

Another genetic modification commonly associated with GBM is inactivation of the O6-methylguanine-DNA methyltransferase gene

(*MGMT* in 10q26), which encodes a DNA repair protein that removes mutagenic alkyl groups from the O6 position of guanine residues (Gerson, 2004). This gene is silenced in many cancers and is thought to be important in oncogenesis (Esteller, 2002). A common mechanism of *MGMT* silencing is promoter hypermethylation (Esteller et al., 1999). Because MGMT removes alkyl groups from DNA, alkylating compounds such as temozolomide are more effective against tumors that lack normal MGMT activity (Hegi et al., 2005).

Advances in high-throughput techniques have enabled detailed analyses of glioblastoma biology including efforts organized by The Cancer Genome Atlas Research Network (McLendon et al., 2008). In their study from 2008, in which 206 GBM specimens were examined using a multitude of modern techniques, the alterations, including mutations, of many relevant genes such as *EGFR*, *TP53*, *RB1*, *PTEN*, *HER2* (17q12), *PIK3R1* (5q13.1), and *NF1* were assessed. Another focus has been on the elucidation of genetic networks important for the development of GBM, and in a later study, The Cancer Genome Atlas Research Network described a hypermethylator phenotype, G-CIMP, in GBM and lower-grade gliomas (Noushmehr et al., 2010). Verhaak et al. (2010) divided GBM into four different subentities based on genomics and gene expression patterns—classical, proneural, mesenchymal, and neural tumors—with many of the aforementioned genomic aberrations being important for the new classification. In another large-scale genomic sequencing analysis, a specific *IDH1* mutation in the tumors was found to confer on the patients a significantly better prognosis (Parsons et al., 2008).

Several fusion genes have been detected in GBM. According to the Mitelman database, 113 GBM cases with a fusion gene have now been published, 107 of them stemming from two major recent studies (Frattini et al., 2013; Zheng et al., 2013) and the remaining six from five earlier and smaller ones (Charest et al., 2003; Bralten et al., 2010; Badiali et al., 2012; Singh et al., 2012; Brennan et al., 2013). The first fusion gene published originates through a 6q deletion and was called *FIG-ROS* (later changed to *GOPC-ROS1*), where FIG is short for fused in glioblastoma (Charest et al., 2003). *EGFR* was the most frequent fusion gene partner detected in the study by Frattini et al. (2013), whereas Zheng et al. (2013) observed an enrichment of fusion genes in 12q14–15.

Oligodendrogliomas (ODG)

Oligodendrocytes support the neurons and produce the myelin sheath necessary for rapid nerve impulse propagation. The main neoplasms differentiating like oligodendrocytes, ODG, are found either as grade II or grade III tumors with the former being three times more common than the latter. Altogether, ODG account for 10% of gliomas (Zada et al., 2012). Grade III ODG (anaplastic ODG) differ from grade II tumors by their higher mitotic activity, microvascular proliferation, higher cellularity, and nuclear atypia. It has been generally accepted that ODG respond better to chemotherapy than do astrocytic tumors (van den Bent, 2000). In 2013, an updated analysis of two large randomized studies showed that patients with grade III ODG and LOH 1p/19q (see succeeding text) have a better survival when treated with chemotherapy at primary diagnosis (Cairncross et al., 2013; van den Bent et al., 2013). As for astrocytic tumors, patients with low-grade ODG have a better prognosis than those with high-grade ODG with median survival for the former above 10 years and for the latter 4–5 years (van den Bent et al., 2008).

Again in similarity to the situation in astrocytomas, it would have been principally preferable to cover grade II and grade III ODG separately; after all, they were differently graded and named. However, the literature is not always concise on the grading of these brain tumors forcing us to group grades II and III ODG together. The 52 ODG registered in the Mitelman database represent a mixture of grade II and grade III tumors as well as some tumors with oligodendroglial and others with oligoastrocytic features.

The frequency of karyotypic abnormalities in ODG differs considerably among studies (Yamada et al., 1980, 1994; Rey et al., 1987; Jenkins et al., 1989, 2006; Griffin et al., 1992, 2006; Ransom et al., 1992; Thiel et al., 1992; Magnani et al., 1994; Debiec-Rychter et al., 1995; Kim et al., 2009; Dahlback et al., 2011a) but is certainly more than 50%. The most distinguishing genetic feature of these tumors, however, is loss of heterozygosity (LOH) for chromosome arms 1p and 19q (Reifenberger et al., 1994) known

to occur in almost all ODG of both grades II and III as well as in some OA (see succeeding text). The mechanism for the characteristic loss pattern was in 2006 shown to be a centric fusion between chromosomes 1 and 19 with the subsequent loss of the 1p/19q chromosome, whereas the 1q/19p chromosome is retained (Griffin et al., 2006; Jenkins et al., 2006). This translocation is almost never found after short-term culture and G-band analysis, but Jenkins and colleagues tested for it using FISH and found a high concordance between presence of the translocation and FISH-detected 1p/19q loss. It has been known for quite some time that this chromosomal loss pattern correlates with response to chemotherapeutic drugs as well as radiotherapy (Cairncross et al., 1998). The LOH 1p/19q is therefore very important from a diagnostic, prognostic, and therapeutic point of view, as patients whose tumors carry the loss have a better prognosis and, for grade III ODG, also have a better survival when treated with chemotherapy at the time of primary diagnosis.

Apart from LOH 1p/19q, sex chromosome losses and simple aberrations are the most common chromosomal changes in ODG, although more complex abnormalities and aberrations are also occasionally found. Weber et al. (1996) used CGH to identify losses on 4q, 9p, 10q, 11p, and 13q and gains on 1q, 6p, and 20q as the most common imbalances. Other investigators have reported loss of 9p (Bigner et al., 1999) and gain of 8q (Kitange et al., 2005). Reifenberger and Louis (2003) described deletions of 4, 6, 11, 14, and 22. In general, anaplastic ODG have more genomic aberrations than do grade II ODG, with losses of 9p and 10q having been identified as possible progression-related changes. Fusion genes have not been frequently found in ODG, but a *KIAA1549–BRAF* fusion similar to the fusion gene found in astrocytomas (see Grade I and Grade II astrocytomas) was reported by Badiali et al. (2012).

Oligoastrocytomas (OA)

Neoplasms with morphological characteristics reminiscent of both astrocytoma and ODG cells are referred to as OA. OA is a controversial entity as not all neuropathologists recognize it and the morphological borders toward astrocytoma and ODG are not clearly defined. Also, considerable interobserver diagnostic discrepancy exists, and this should be kept in mind when comparing the acquired genomic changes in OA examined at different institutions or at different times from the same institution. In general, some OA have LOH 1p/19q and seem to be more closely related to ODG than to astrocytomas, whereas others have more astrocytoma-like genetic characteristics (Mueller et al., 2002).

More than half of all OA studied by banding techniques had normal karyotypes. In the series of 14 OA of grade II examined by Dahlback et al. (2011a), six were karyotypically abnormal. In five of them, the changes were complex with only –Y and –11 as recurrent aberrations. CGH analysis of the same tumors revealed loss of 19q and 1p as the dominating changes. In a CGH study by Jeuken et al. (2001) of 39 gliomas that had both oligodendroglial and astrocytic elements, 11 low-grade and 28 high-grade tumors, the authors ended up recognizing four genetically different OA subgroups: –1p/–19q, +7/–10, intermediate (both –1p/–19q and +7/–10), and others (neither –1p/–19q nor +7/–10 was seen).

Ependymomas

Ependymomas display differentiation similar to that of the ependymal cells that normally line the cerebral ventricular system and the central canal of the spinal cord. They make up 3% of all gliomas (Zada et al., 2012). Ependymomas are most often found in children and predominantly in the posterior fossa. Adult ependymomas, on the other hand, often occur in the spinal canal. Ependymomas are graded from I to III, but distinguishing between grades II and III is often hard. Grade I tumors are very indolent and slow-growing, grade II tumors are intermediate, and grade III tumors are the most aggressive. If gross total resection is possible, the patient may be cured. Radiotherapy is often used as adjuvant treatment, whereas chemotherapy is of limited value. It has been shown that radial glia, a type of immature neural precursor cell, and stem cells isolated from ependymal tumors share many physical as well as molecular traits, leading to the hypothesis that transformed radial glia may be the source of ependymomas (Taylor et al., 2005). Indeed, tumor stem cells isolated from ependymomas have gene expression patterns similar to those of radial glia from the same anatomical sites (Taylor et al., 2005).

Because of the tumors' relative rarity, little is known about their cytogenetic abnormalities, and only 113 such cases are registered in the Mitelman database. About two-thirds of ependymomas are karyotypically abnormal (Mazewski et al., 1999), and most of these are near-diploid (Griffin et al., 1992; Ransom et al., 1992; Thiel et al., 1992; Vagner-Capodano et al., 1992; Weremowicz et al., 1992). Loss of chromosome 22, the most common aberration, was seen in about a third of the abnormal cases, followed by +7 and +12. Structural abnormalities of chromosome 22 were reported in 11% of the tumors with karyotypic abnormalities. In a large meta-analysis comparing CGH findings in adult and pediatric ependymomas, chromosome 22 was the most common site of genomic loss in both groups (Kilday et al., 2009). 1q gain was significantly more frequent in the pediatric tumors and was indeed the most common aberration overall in this group. Gains of chromosomes 7, 9, and 12 were significantly more common in adult tumors, which also in general had a higher number of genomic imbalances than did pediatric ependymomas. The authors therefore suggested that ependymomas of the two age groups are genetically distinct.

In a CGH study of 23 pediatric ependymomas, Reardon et al. (1999) noted that nearly half displayed no gross copy number variation. It has since been shown that LOH on 22q and 11q is relatively common in ependymomas and that inactivation of genes such as MEN1 in 11q13 and NF2 in 22q12 may play a role in tumorigenesis (Lamszus et al., 2001). A study using a combination of PCR, microarray expression profiling, and CGH discovered a panel of more than a hundred genes that were differentially expressed in ependymomas compared to nonneoplastic brain tissue (Suarez-Merino et al., 2005). In addition to increased WNT5A (3p14) expression, 22q genes such as FBX7, CBX7, and SBF1 were found to be underexpressed. Interestingly, other genes such as CDK2 (12q13), MDM2 (12q), EGFR, and PTEN, which are commonly altered in other CNS tumors, were not found to be differentially expressed in this cohort of ependymal tumors.

It is worthy of note that the cytogenetic abnormalities of ependymomas, as well as their gene expression profiles, seem to vary according to

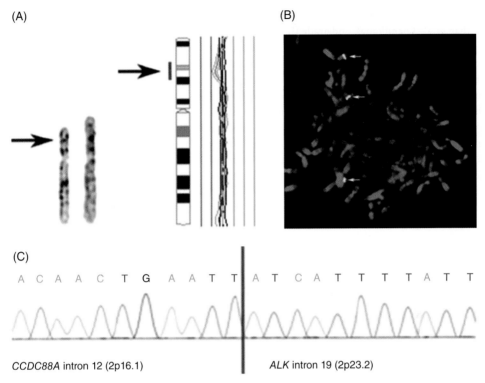

CCDC88A intron 12 (2p16.1)   ALK intron 19 (2p23.2)

Figure 20.2 An ependymal tumor genetically examined at different resolution levels. (A) G-banded chromosomes and corresponding CGH profile. The interstitial 2p deletion from the one aberrant chromosome 2 is marked with an arrow, whereas the normal chromosome 2 is seen to the right. The deletion was confirmed by CGH, which showed breakpoints at 2p16 and 2p23 (marked by arrow and a red bar). (B) FISH analysis using an *ALK* split-apart probe. Three yellow signals (marked with white arrows) indicate nonrearranged *ALK*. Four copies of chromosome 2 are present because this cell was tetraploid. Three normal *ALK* signals are marked by white arrows. The red arrow indicates persisting red signal but loss of green signal (i.e., loss of exons 1–19 of the *ALK* gene) due to the interstitial 2p deletion. (C) The genomic breakpoints of the interstitial 2p deletion leading to the fusion gene *CCDC88A–ALK*.

tumor site. This is true also for histological ependymoma subentities that show clear anatomical predilections. Loss of 22q is more common in spinal cord tumors as well as in tumors of adult patients, whereas gain of 1q is more frequent in intracranial tumors, especially in children (Jeuken et al., 2002). Furthermore, 1q gain may be a marker of more aggressive biological behavior in these tumors (Carter et al., 2002; Dyer et al., 2002). In another study, Rousseau et al. (2007) found an association between trisomy 19 and deletions of 13q21.31–31.2 and chromosome 9, as well as gain of 11q13.3–13.4, and WHO grade III supratentorial tumors in young patients.

Fusion genes in ependymomas have only recently received much attention. *C11orf95–RELA* fusions were reported as common in supratentorial

pediatric ependymomas (Parker et al., 2014). The gene product is thought to drive oncogenic NF-κB signaling in these tumors. In another recent publication (Olsen et al., 2015), two fusion genes, both of them involving *ALK*, were detected in two pediatric supratentorial ependymomas with elements of astrocytic differentiation (Figure 20.2). This is of particular interest because it opens up for the possibility of ALK-targeted therapy and because the tumors may belong to a hitherto unrecognized ependymoma-like entity with both pathogenetic and morphological distinguishing features.

Choroid plexus tumors

Choroid plexus tumors are graded from I to III where grade I is a low-grade and benign choroid plexus papilloma, grade II is an atypical choroid plexus papilloma with a greater likelihood of recurrence than grade I papillomas, and grade III is choroid plexus carcinoma, a microscopically malignant tumor that is also able to metastasize via the cerebrospinal fluid. These rare neoplasms are most often encountered in the pediatric population.

Only 15 choroid plexus tumors with abnormal karyotypes are registered in the Mitelman database, and all except one publication are single-case reports. About half of the cytogenetically abnormal tumors are hyperdiploid as shown by Biegel (1999). In an early FISH study, gains of chromosomes 7 and 12 were the most frequent aberrations (Donovan et al., 1994). This is consistent with karyotypic data showing +7 and +12 as the most common findings among mostly numerical aberrations. By CGH, choroid plexus papillomas were found to have +7q (65%), +5q (62%), +7p (59%), +5p (56%), +9p (50%), and −10q (56%) as the most common aberrations, whereas choroid plexus carcinomas mainly showed +12p, +12q, +20p (60%), +1, +4q, +20q (53%), and −22q (73%) (Rickert et al., 2002). These investigators also compared papillomas and carcinomas, and the former were found to have gains of 5q, 6q, 7q, and 9q as well as loss of 15q significantly more often. On the other hand, carcinomas had gains of 1, 4q, 10, 14q, 20q, and 21q and losses of 5q and 18q more often than did the papillomas. Gain of 9p and loss of 10q were associated with longer survival in the choroid plexus carcinoma group.

Neuronal and mixed neuronal–glial tumors (GNT)

This is a group of diverse neoplasms in which the tumor parenchyma cells show neuronal and/or glial characteristics. The neural and glial components of the tumors have been assumed to originate from a common precursor cell (Zhu et al., 1997). In general, GNT are infrequent and not much is known about their cytogenetic characteristics. In a review looking at the group of GNT as a whole, 31 of 44 tumors were found to be karyotypically normal, whereas 57% were abnormal by CGH. Gains of material most often occurred at chromosomes 7, 12, and X, whereas losses usually were of chromosome 22 material (Coccé et al., 2009).

Gangliogliomas are rare, usually low-grade neoplasms that account for only 1% of all CNS tumors (Johannsson et al., 1981). Although unusual, anaplastic transformation of ganglioglioma does occur. Most gangliogliomas are karyotypically normal. Bhattacharjee et al. (1997) found no chromosomal aberrations in nine of 12 tumors studied. What changes have been detected in banding studies did not give the impression of being specific. CGH studies have indicated that the gain–loss pattern of these tumors may nevertheless be nonrandom. Losses from 9p were seen in some of the tumors examined by Yin et al. (2002). A study comparing the cytogenetic profiles of the benign and malignant components of a ganglioglioma showed losses to be more frequent in the benign parts of the tumor and gains more common in the malignant part (Pandita et al., 2007). A larger CGH study of 61 gangliogliomas showed genomic imbalances in about two-thirds of the tumors: gains were most frequently found for chromosomes 7 (21%) and 5 (16%), whereas losses mostly were of chromosome 22 (Hoischen et al., 2008). The most frequent partial imbalances were loss from 10q25 and gain of 12q13.3–14.1. The authors divided the tumors into two major subgroups based on the imbalance pattern: group I had gain of chromosome 7 and additional gains of 5, 8, or 12, whereas group II had mainly losses of chromosomal material but with no major recurring imbalances.

Neurocytoma is another rare, most often low-grade tumor within this category. They usually arise inside the ventricles, near the foramen of Monro, when they are known as central neurocytomas. The potential for recurrence is considerable if the primary tumor is not completely excised (Bertalanffy et al., 2005). Little information exists on their cytogenetic profile. Gains of chromosome 7 were reported in one study (Taruscio et al., 1997), whereas another found gains of material from chromosomes 2, 10, and 18. The gained region from chromosome 18 included the *BCL2* oncogene (Yin et al., 2000). Although central neurocytomas morphologically resemble ODG, LOH 1p/19q is not found in the former (Leenstra et al., 2007). However, this gain–loss pattern may be present in rare tumors arising in the cerebral hemispheres outside the ventricles, the so-called extraventricular neurocytoma (Perry et al., 2003; Mrak et al., 2004).

Interestingly, a fusion gene has been found in the recently identified GNT entity papillary glioneuronal tumor (Bridge et al., 2013). Three tumors were examined, but for only two of them, a karyotype was established. A t(9;17)(q31;q24) was found as the sole aberration in both. Further analysis using FISH confirmed this finding and showed that the translocation was present also in the third case. Molecular analyses with RT-PCR and DNA sequencing showed that the translocation led to a novel fusion gene, *SLC44A1–PRKCA*. The fusion occurred between *SLC44A1* exon 15 and *PRKCA* exon 9, but the fusion product was smaller in one of the two cases examined because of an additional submicroscopic deletion.

Embryonal tumors

Embryonal CNS tumors are divided in three main groups: medulloblastoma (MB), CNS primitive neuroectodermal tumor (CNS-PNET), and atypical teratoid/rhabdoid tumor (AT/RT). The first two have by many been seen as largely identical except for the fact that MB typically is located in the posterior fossa, whereas CNS-PNET is found in the supratentorial brain.

MB and CNS-PNET: These are the most common high-grade brain tumors in childhood where they account for one-fourth of all brain malignancies. They are only infrequently encountered in adults. MB is thought to occur in approximately one in 200,000 children (Farwell et al., 1984; CBTRUS, 2005). Based on studies of animal models, the cerebellar granular cell layer has been hypothesized to be the source of infratentorial MB (Zindy et al., 2003; Fomchenko and Holland, 2006).

Most MB and CNS-PNET have abnormal karyotypes, and 196 such tumors are registered in the Mitelman database. Aberrations have been found involving chromosomes X, Y, 6, 7, 10, and 22 (Karnes et al., 1992; Mitelman et al., 2014), but the most common abnormality in MB is i(17)(q10) (Bigner et al., 1997). Some studies have identified a 17p gene known as *REN*, which is involved in regulation of the hedgehog-signaling pathway, as implicated in MB development (Di Marcotullio et al., 2004; Argenti et al., 2005).

An interesting specific alteration in MB is loss of function of the patched (*PTCH*) gene. *PTCH* in 9q22 was originally identified in the fruit fly (*Drosophila melanogaster*) based on its mutant phenotype, which involves defects in embryonic

patterning (Hooper and Scott, 1989). Subsequently, mutations in *PTCH* were shown to be associated with the nevoid basal cell carcinoma syndrome (NBCCS) (Hahn et al., 1996). Mice that are homozygous mutants for this gene die during gestation due to perturbed CNS development. Heterozygous mice are carried to term but show an increased incidence of MB (Goodrich et al., 1997).

It has now been established that *PTCH* and members of the sonic hedgehog (Shh) pathway such as smoothened (*Smo*) in 7q32 and *GLI* in 12q13 play key roles in the development of MB as well as many other malignancies (Villavicencio et al., 2000). Based on molecular genetic analysis, subtypes of MB with changes interfering with the WNT/β-catenin pathway have been reported (Thompson et al., 2006), and patients with such tumors have a better prognosis than do other MB patients. Another genetic abnormality associated with MB/CNS-PNET is amplification of the *MYC* oncogene. *MYC* (in 8q24) and *MYCN* (in 2p24) amplification has been reported in 6–8% of MB/CNS-PNET cases, seems to be associated with the large-cell and anaplastic histologic tumor variants, and is an unfavorable prognostic indicator (Lamont et al., 2004).

Building further on the data referenced earlier, Northcott et al. (2011) introduced an interesting classification concept. Based on the transcription profiles and copy number aberrations detected in 103 MB, four distinct, nonoverlapping tumor subgroups could be defined named WNT, SHH, group C, and group D. The two first names reflect the tumors' biological profile (see preceding text), whereas the latter two were without a similarly clear-cut profile. The SHH tumors had 9p gain and often also 9q loss (suggestive of the presence of an isochromosome for 9p) as well as 3q and 21q gain. SHH shared 10q loss with group C, but the tumors of the latter group also had 1q gain, distal 5q loss, and 16q loss. The tumors of groups C and D were somewhat similar genomically but with a higher frequency of 1q gain, distal 5q loss, and 10q loss in group C compared to group D. In contrast, group D tumors more often had i(17)(q10) and X chromosome loss than did group C tumors. Regardless of whether or not the classification suggested by Northcott and coworkers is implemented into clinical trials, increasing knowledge about the tumors' genomic abnormalities has paved the way for a better and more detailed risk stratification scheme of MB (Ellison et al., 2011).

Rhabdoid tumors: AT/RT were in the past often misclassified as CNS-PNET or MB. It is not known from which cell type AT/RT arise, especially because the tumors are polyphenotypic and may express markers of neural, epithelial, and mesenchymal differentiation. This suggests origin from a pluripotent primitive cell. Besides the brain, AT/RT tumors may also be found in the liver, kidney, and soft tissues. Rhabdoid tumors are typically highly aggressive. They have often metastasized at the time of diagnosis and respond poorly to therapy.

The most frequent genomic aberration observed in AT/RT of the CNS is loss of material from 22q, which occurs in 50% of the tumors. It has been shown that mutations in the remaining allele of a gene in 22q called *INI1/hSNF5/SMARCB1* are common in rhabdoid tumors and may play an important role in their formation (Biegel et al., 1999). Absence of the corresponding protein product is a diagnostically useful feature that may be detected by immunohistochemistry.

A rhabdoid tumor predisposition syndrome exists associated with germline mutations in *INI1/ hSNF5/SMARCB1*. This may account for up to one-third of all patients with AT/RT, and rhabdoid tumors outside of the CNS may be particularly common in this situation (Biegel, 2006).

An important differential diagnosis for AT/RT is cribriform neuroepithelial tumor (CRINET), an entity not yet formally established by the WHO but described by Hasselblatt et al. (2009). The genetics of this new and infrequent neoplasm is largely unknown. The first cytogenetic description of a tumor of this type included losses from 1p, 4q, 10p, 10q, and 22q as detected by array CGH (Dahlback et al., 2011b). The karyotype was normal, probably because the cells of the tumor parenchyma could not be induced to divide *in vitro*.

Tumors of the pineal region

Almost all histological tumor types may be found near or within the pineal gland, but only pineocytoma, pineal parenchymal tumor of intermediate differentiation, pineoblastoma, and papillary tumor are by the WHO defined as pineal region tumors (Louis et al., 2007). They are all rare.

Pineoblastomas and pineocytomas are presumed to arise from parenchymal cells of the pineal gland. While the former are poorly differentiated, primitive neuroectodermal tumors that resemble CNS-PNET in other locations, the latter reproduce a lobular growth pattern that is more similar to that of normal pineal gland tissue. In one study of pineoblastoma, all four tumors had aneuploid, complex karyotypes with gain of chromosome arm 17q and rearrangements of chromosome 1 as the most frequent abnormalities (Brown et al., 2006). Mutations in the *RB1* gene have been shown to correlate with a poor prognosis in pineoblastoma patients (Plowman et al., 2004). It is also worthy of note that patients with germline mutation of *RB1* may develop pineoblastomas in addition to retinoblastomas (Chapter 21), a condition sometimes referred to as the "trilateral retinoblastoma syndrome."

A pineocytoma with a karyotype dominated by multiple numerical chromosome abnormalities has been published (Rainho et al., 1992).

Tumors of cranial and paraspinal nerves

Schwannomas

The benign schwannoma emanates from the Schwann cells that surround nerves and nerve roots and the tumors may be intracranial or extracranial. The most typical among the former are the acoustic neuromas or neurinomas that derive from the vestibular branch of the eighth cranial nerve. Bilateral acoustic schwannomas are a hallmark of neurofibromatosis type 2, an autosomal dominant disorder caused by germline mutations in the *NF2* gene.

Chromosomal abnormalities have been reported in close to 90 schwannomas (Mitelman et al., 2014). The two largest series were examined by Bello et al. (1993) and Mertens et al. (2000), the former focusing on intracranial and spinal schwannomas and the latter on soft tissue lesions. Between 45% and 70% of the tumors had chromosome aberrations. Irrespective of site of origin, the most common aberration was monosomy 22 found in two-thirds of karyotypically abnormal cases. It was often the sole change. Most likely, this aberration represents one step in the functional inactivation of the *NF2* gene that maps to 22q12; biallelic inactivating mutations and/or allelic loss has been detected in two-thirds of schwannomas (Jacoby et al., 1996). Other recurrent anomalies, each found in 5–10%, have been losses of chromosomes 12, 15, and X/Y as well as gains of chromosomes 5, 7, and 20. No consistent structural rearrangement has been registered, nor has any fusion gene been described.

In a CGH study of 20 sporadic acoustic schwannomas, loss from 22q was confirmed as the most frequent copy number aberration (Koutsimpelas et al., 2011). Losses were also observed from chromosome arm 9p, whereas gains were seen of 17q, 19p, and 19q.

Neurofibromas

Neurofibromas consist of a mixture of nerve sheath cells, including fibroblasts, Schwann cells, and perineurial-like cells. They may be sporadic or part of von Recklinghausen or type 1 neurofibromatosis, an autosomal dominant disease caused by mutations of the *NF1* gene. Neurofibromas have a tendency to evolve into malignant peripheral nerve sheath tumors (MPNST). It seems that most neurofibromas are karyotypically normal (Mertens et al., 2000). Nonetheless, 12 tumors with an abnormal karyotype characterized by chromosome banding are registered in the Mitelman database. All cases, except one, had a diploid or near-diploid modal chromosome number. Four of the tumors showed rearrangement or loss of 17q where *NF1* maps. The frequent finding of LOH at the *NF1* locus in sporadic and neurofibromatosis-associated cases, as well as the finding of biallelic *NF1* inactivation through chromosomal translocations in one sporadic neurofibroma, provides further evidence for the pathogenetic importance of *NF1* inactivation (Storlazzi et al., 2005). Evidence for such a mechanism was corroborated in a later study by Beert et al. (2012). They found by karyotyping of a sporadic plexiform neurofibroma an insertion of chromosomal bands 1p36–35 at 17q11.2. FISH examinations demonstrated that the insertion disrupted one *NF1* locus, whereas the other *NF1* allele was deleted, a finding that was confirmed by aCGH.

The synovial sarcoma-specific *SS18/SSX* fusion gene has been found in two neurofibromas by RT-PCR (O'Sullivan et al., 2000). However, this study was later criticized, and the generality of these findings remains disputed (Ladanyi et al., 2001).

Perineuriomas

Intraneural perineuriomas are benign, grade I tumors composed of perineurial cells. Soft tissue perineuriomas, on the other hand, may be of grades II and III although most of them are grade I tumors. The Mitelman database contains information on seven perineuriomas with chromosome abnormalities, all displaying a pseudodiploid or near-diploid karyotype. In three of the tumors, loss of material from 22q was found suggesting that *NF2* inactivation is an important pathogenetic mechanism. Also, rearrangement and/or loss of 10q is described in three of these tumors; indeed, it seems that most cytogenetically examined perineuriomas have chromosomal abnormalities (Brock et al., 2005).

Malignant peripheral nerve sheath tumors (MPNST)

MPNST were in the past often referred to as neurofibrosarcoma or malignant schwannoma. They may be sporadic or occur through malignant transformation of large, usually plexiform, neurofibromas in patients with type I neurofibromatosis. Close to 130 MPNST with abnormal karyotypes have been reported, the majority of which had complex changes, often with a modal chromosome number in the near-triploid or near-tetraploid range. Such extreme karyotypic complexity is more common in MPNST than in benign schwannomas (Mertens et al., 2000). The breakpoints of structural rearrangements typically (more than 10% of the cases) involve 1p11, 5p15, 7p22, 9p11, 11q13, 17p11, 17q11, 17q21, 20q13, and 22q11. Frequent (at least 20% of the cases) chromosomal imbalances are loss of 1p21–36, 3p21–23, 5p15, 6q23–27, 7p22, 9p12–24, 10p, 11p, 11q13–25, 12p13, 12q22–24, 13p, 15p, chromosomes 16 and 17, 19p, 20q13, and chromosomes 22 and X but gain of chromosome 7 (Jhanwar et al., 1994; Mertens et al., 2000; Bridge et al., 2004). No recurrent balanced rearrangement has been detected among MPNST nor does there seem to be any clear difference in karyotypic profile between sporadic cases and neurofibromatosis-associated MPNST.

Molecular genetic investigations have revealed that both sporadic and neurofibromatosis-associated

MPNST often display somatic loss or mutation of the *NF1* gene (Bottillo et al., 2009). Other frequent molecular events are amplification of several regions on 17q, inactivation of *TP53*, and disruption of the *RB1* pathway (Berner et al., 1999; Storlazzi et al., 2006; Mantripragada et al., 2008).

Tumors of the meninges

Several neoplastic entities are included in this tumor group, including many rare meningeal sarcomas whose cytogenetic features are unknown. The meningiomas, on the other hand, the most common primary tumors originating from the meningeal coverings of the brain and spinal cord, have been well characterized cytogenetically. Meningiomas are almost exclusively benign grade I tumors, which carry an excellent prognosis; however, some of them grow in surgically inaccessible locations, a few others are grade II with an increased risk of recurrence, and very few are grade III with a malignant cellular picture, a tendency toward locally aggressive growth, and a relatively poor prognosis.

Almost 1000 meningiomas are registered in the Mitelman database. The first report on chromosomal aberrations in meningiomas came as early as 1967 and described the simple loss of a G-group chromosome (Zang and Singer, 1967). When banding methods became available, Mark and coworkers (1972) in Sweden and Zankl and Zang (1972) in Germany demonstrated that the missing chromosome was a 22. By the early 1970s, both groups (Mark, 1977; Zang, 1982) had established the association beyond doubt: the vast majority of meningiomas are cytogenetically characterized by the loss of one chromosome 22.

Since then, also additional abnormalities have been identified, mostly using CGH techniques, indicating that a complex association exists between meningiomas and genomic stability. A study by Arslantas et al. (2002) identified loss of material from chromosomes 1, 9, 10, 14, 15, 18, and 22, whereas gains were seen at 12, 15, and 18.

Patients with neurofibromatosis type 2 have a predisposition to developing meningioma. This led to the discovery that the *NF2* gene in chromosome 22 is mutated in a large proportion of such tumors (Ruttledge et al., 1994).

Much effort has gone into the search for correlations between the genetic characteristics of meningiomas and clinicopathologic features. Tumor site was correlated with karyotype in three large studies (Zang, 1982; Casalone et al., 1990; Doco-Fenzy et al., 1993). All three agreed that abnormal karyotypes were more often seen in meningiomas located at the convexity of the brain hemispheres (50–80%) compared with those found at the base of the skull (20–40%). The highest frequency of chromosomal abnormalities was found in meningiomas of the spinal cord (80–100%); furthermore, these tumors often had monosomy 22 as the sole karyotypic aberration. The latter observation also concurs with the results reported by Al Saadi et al. (1987) who found −22 in all four spinal meningiomas studied, in three of them as the only change.

Female sex hormones seem to play a role in the biology of meningiomas since progesterone receptors are frequently expressed in low-grade tumors but are lost with increasing grade. An interesting study demonstrated that the expression of genes in 22q was affected by progesterone receptor status (Claus et al., 2008).

A recurring theme in the discussion of meningioma biology is that more aggressive tumors evolve from lower-grade precursors and that accumulation of multiple cytogenetic alterations parallels, perhaps brings about, the evolution into more aggressive tumors. Low-grade meningiomas typically harbor only −22, whereas higher-grade tumors show a more diverse genomic profile with alterations that may include losses of or from 1p, 6q, 10, 14q, 17p, and 18q (Rempel et al., 1993; Bello et al., 1994; Lindblom et al., 1994; Menon et al., 1997; Al-Mefty et al., 2004; Perry et al., 2004). In contrast to what is seen in many other tumors, increasing hypodiploidy seems to be characteristic of meningioma progression (Zang, 2001). These findings and conclusions have been confirmed, and alterations on chromosomes 10, 14, and 18 were found to correlate with malignancy (Lopez-Gines et al., 2003). The combination of 1p aberrations and −14 in particular may define a group at increased risk of early relapse, even in histologically benign meningiomas (Maillo et al., 2007; Barbera et al., 2013). A candidate tumor suppressor gene in 14q11.2, *NDRG2*, is consistently altered in anaplastic meningiomas, frequently by promoter hypermethylation

(Lusis et al., 2005). A recently published analysis looked at the prognostic impact of genetic changes and showed that a complex karyotype was one of five parameters with independent predictive value for meningioma recurrence (Domingues et al., 2014). The authors suggested a prognostic score for the risk of meningioma recurrence with complex karyotype as one of the defining variables.

A potential mechanism for the diverse cytogenetic abnormalities in meningiomas is clonal heterogeneity. Performing multicolor FISH examinations of interphase cells, Sayagues et al. (2004) identified what appeared to be multiple independent clones in half of the tumors analyzed.

Fusion genes have been detected in meningiomas. Lekanne Deprez et al. (1995) described a meningioma with a t(4;22) that targeted a gene called *MN1*; its fusion partner remains unknown. Brastianos et al. (2013) used whole-genome and whole-exome sequencing to detect 20 fusion genes in meningiomas. The biological, let alone clinical, relevance of these findings remains unclear.

Summary

Tumors of the CNS vary from benign meningiomas to aggressive glioblastomas with a myriad of different entities existing in between. The next WHO classification update is expected soon and is likely to incorporate (cyto)genetic knowledge in a major way.

Astrocytomas and, in particular, glioblastomas are among the best-studied brain tumors. Common gross genetic abnormalities of glioblastomas include gain of chromosome 7 in combination with loss of chromosome 10. Molecular genetic changes include loss of *MGMT* function via promoter methylation and gain of *EGFR* function (amplification and/or mutationally active variants such as *EGFR VIII*). In PA, *BRAF* changes, including the fusion gene *BRAF–KIAA1549*, have received attention.

Oligodendroglial tumors have codeletion of 1p and 19q as a characteristic cytogenetic abnormality. These deletions are mediated by a centromeric translocation between chromosomes 1 and 19 with subsequent loss of the 1p/19q chromosome. Although the crucial tumor suppressor genes contained within these regions have not been identified, and indeed their existence or at least importance in this context is putative, it is clear that the loss of 1p and 19q correlates with a better prognosis as well as a better response to chemotherapeutic agents and radiotherapy. Oligoastrocytic tumors represent an intermediate form of glioma with both astrocytic and oligodendroglial characteristics, both histologically and genomically.

Ependymomas can display chromosomal deletions of chromosomes 19 and 22 but are relatively normal at the gross karyotypic level. 1q gain is more common in pediatric than in adult ependymomas. Ependymomas appear to arise from immature precursor cells and share phenotypic features with radial glia.

Primitive neuroectodermal tumors, including MB, consist of poorly differentiated cells and typically occur in children. An i(17q) observed in a brain tumor is highly suggestive of MB. A new classification scheme based on transcription profiles and genomic copy number aberrations has been proposed. Rhabdoid tumors are characterized by an increased frequency of deletions and mutations of the *INI1* gene.

The most common aberration in meningiomas is loss of one chromosome 22. Also, deletions of 22q are sometimes seen. Loss of or aberrations affecting chromosome 22 do not help much diagnostically, however, because also several other CNS neoplasms share this characteristic. Secondary anomalies often include rearrangements of chromosomes 1 (typically leading to loss of material from the short arm), 8 (mostly loss of one copy), 14 (usually loss of one copy), and the X or Y (usually loss of one copy).

Fusion genes are being found at increasing frequencies in neoplasms of the CNS. Knowledge about them may pave the way for molecular targeted therapy.

References

Al-Mefty O, Kadri PA, Pravdenkova S, Sawyer JR, Stangeby C, Husain M (2004): Malignant progression in meningioma: documentation of a series and analysis of cytogenetic findings. *J Neurosurg* 101:210–218.

Al Saadi A, Latimer F, Madercic M, Robbins T (1987): Cytogenetic studies of human brain tumors and their clinical significance. II. Meningioma. *Cancer Genet Cytogenet* 26:127–141.

Argenti B, Gallo R, Di Marcotullio L, Ferretti E, Napolitano M, Canterini S, et al. (2005): Hedgehog antagonist REN (KCTD11) regulates proliferation and apoptosis of developing granule cell progenitors. *J Neurosci* 25:8338–8346.

Arslantas A, Artan S, Oner U, Durmaz R, Muslumanoglu H, Atasoy MA, et al. (2002): Comparative genomic hybridization analysis of genomic alterations in benign, atypical and anaplastic meningiomas. *Acta Neurol Belg* 102:53–62.

Arslantas A, Artan S, Oner U, Muslumanoglu H, Durmaz R, Cosan E, et al. (2004): The importance of genomic copy number changes in the prognosis of glioblastoma multiforme. *Neurosurg Rev* 27:58–64.

Arslantas A, Artan S, Oner U, Muslumanoglu MH, Ozdemir M, Durmaz R, et al. (2007): Genomic alterations in low-grade, anaplastic astrocytomas and glioblastomas. *Pathol Oncol Res* 13:39–46.

Badiali M, Gleize V, Paris S, Moi L, Elhouadani S, Arcella A, et al. (2012): KIAA1549-BRAF fusions and IDH mutations can coexist in diffuse gliomas of adults. *Brain Pathol* 22:841–847.

Bar EE, Lin A, Tihan T, Burger PC, Eberhart CG (2008): Frequent gains at chromosome 7q34 involving BRAF in pilocytic astrocytoma. *J Neuropathol Exp Neurol* 67:878–887.

Barbera S, San Miguel T, Gil-Benso R, Muñoz-Hidalgo L, Roldan P, Gonzalez-Darder J, et al. (2013): Genetic changes with prognostic value in histologically benign meningiomas. *Clin Neuropathol* 32:311–317.

Beert E, Brems H, Renard M, Ferreiro JF, Melotte C, Thoelen R, et al. (2012): Biallelic inactivation of NF1 in a sporadic plexiform neurofibroma. *Genes Chromosomes Cancer* 51:852–857.

Bello MJ, de Campos JM, Kusak ME, Vaquero J, Sarasa JL, Pestana A, et al. (1993): Clonal chromosome aberrations in neurinomas. *Genes Chromosomes Cancer* 6:206–211.

Bello MJ, de Campos JM, Kusak ME, Vaquero J, Sarasa JL, Pestana A, et al. (1994): Allelic loss at 1p is associated with tumor progression of meningiomas. *Genes Chromosomes Cancer* 9:296–298.

Berner JM, Sorlie T, Mertens F, Henriksen J, Saeter G, Mandahl N, et al. (1999): Chromosome band 9p21 is frequently altered in malignant peripheral nerve sheath tumors: Studies of CDKN2A and other genes of the pRB pathway. *Genes Chromosomes Cancer* 26:151–160.

Beroukhim R, Getz G, Nghiemphu L, Barretina J, Hsueh T, Linhart D, et al. (2007): Assessing the significance of chromosomal aberrations in cancer: methodology and application to glioma. *Proc Natl Acad Sci USA* 104:20007–20012.

Bertalanffy A, Roessler K, Koperek O, Gelpi E, Prayer D, Knosp E (2005): Recurrent central neurocytomas. *Cancer* 104:135–142.

Bhattacharjee MB, Armstrong DD, Vogel H, Cooley LD (1997): Cytogenetic analysis of 120 primary pediatric brain tumors and literature review. *Cancer Genet Cytogenet* 97:39–53.

Biegel JA (1999): Cytogenetics and molecular genetics of childhood brain tumors. *Neuro Oncol* 1:139–151.

Biegel JA (2006): Molecular genetics of atypical teratoid/rhabdoid tumor. *Neurosurg Focus* 20:E11.

Biegel JA, Zhou JY, Rorke LB, Stenstrom C, Wainwright LM, Fogelgren B (1999): Germ-line and acquired mutations of INI1 in atypical teratoid and rhabdoid tumors. *Cancer Res* 59:74–79.

Bigner SH, Mark J, Bullard DE, Mahaley MS Jr, Bigner DD (1986): Chromosomal evolution in malignant human gliomas starts with specific and usually numerical deviations. *Cancer Genet Cytogenet* 22:121–135.

Bigner SH, Mark J, Burger PC, Mahaley MS Jr, Bullard DE, Muhlbaier LH, et al. (1988): Specific chromosomal abnormalities in malignant human gliomas. *Cancer Res* 48:405–411.

Bigner SH, McLendon RE, Fuchs H, McKeever PE, Friedman HS (1997): Chromosomal characteristics of childhood brain tumors. *Cancer Genet Cytogenet* 97:125–134.

Bigner SH, Matthews MR, Rasheed BK, Wiltshire RN, Friedman HS, Friedman AH, et al. (1999): Molecular genetic aspects of oligodendrogliomas including analysis by comparative genomic hybridization. *Am J Pathol* 155:375–386.

Bottillo I, Ahlquist T, Brekke H, Danielsen SA, van den Berg E, Mertens F, et al. (2009): Germline and somatic NF1 mutations in sporadic and NF1-associated malignant peripheral nerve sheath tumors. *J Pathol* 217:693–701.

Bralten LB, Kloosterhof NK, Gravendeel LA, Sacchetti A, Duijm EJ, Kros JM, et al. (2010): Integrated genomic profiling identifies candidate genes implicated in gliomagenesis and a novel LEO1-SLC12A1 fusion gene. *Genes Chromosomes Cancer* 49:509–517.

Brastianos PK, Horowitz PM, Santagata S, Jones RT, McKenna A, Getz G, et al. (2013): Genomic sequencing of meningiomas identifies oncogenic SMO and AKT1 mutations. *Nat Genet* 45:285–289.

Brennan C (2011): Genomic profiles of glioma. *Curr Neurol Neurosci Rep* 11:291–297.

Brennan CW, Verhaak RG, McKenna A, Campos B, Noushmehr H, Salama SR, et al. (2013): The somatic genomic landscape of glioblastoma. *Cell* 155:462–477.

Bridge RS Jr, Bridge JA, Neff JR, Naumann S, Althof P, Bruch LA (2004): Recurrent chromosomal imbalances and structurally abnormal breakpoints within complex karyotypes of malignant peripheral nerve sheath tumour and malignant triton tumour: A cytogenetic and molecular cytogenetic study. *J Clin Pathol* 57:1172–1178.

Bridge JA, Liu XQ, Sumegi J, Nelson M, Reyes C, Bruch LA, et al. (2013): Identification of a novel, recurrent SLC44A1-PRKCA fusion in papillary glioneuronal tumor. *Brain Pathol* 23:121–128.

Brock JE, Perez-Atayde AR, Kozakewich HPW, Richkind KE, Fletcher JA, Vargas SO (2005): Cytogenetic aberrations in perineurioma: variation with subtype. *Am J Surg Pathol* 29:1164–1169.

Brown AE, Leibundgut K, Niggli FK, Betts DR (2006): Cytogenetics of pineoblastoma: four new cases and a literature review. *Cancer Genet Cytogenet* 170:175–179.

Cairncross JG, Ueki K, Zlatescu MC, Lisle DK, Finkelstein D, Hammond RR, et al. (1998): Specific genetic predictors of chemotherapeutic response and survival in patients with anaplastic oligodendrogliomas. *J Natl Cancer Inst* 90:1473–1479.

Cairncross G, Wang M, Shaw E, Jenkins R, Brachman D, Buckner J, et al. (2013): Phase III trial of chemoradiotherapy for anaplastic oligodendroglioma: long-term results of RTOG 9402. *J Clin Oncol* 31:337–343.

Cantley LC, Neel BG (1999): New insights into tumor suppression: PTEN suppresses tumor formation by restraining the phosphoinositide 3-kinase/AKT pathway. *Proc Natl Acad Sci USA* 96:4240–4245.

Carter M, Nicholson J, Ross F, Crolla J, Allibone R, Balaji V, et al. (2002): Genetic abnormalities detected in ependymomas by comparative genomic hybridisation. *Br J Cancer* 86:929–939.

Casalone R, Simi P, Granata P, Minelli E, Giudici A, Butti G, et al. (1990): Correlation between cytogenetic and histopathological findings in 65 human meningiomas. *Cancer Genet Cytogenet* 45:237–243.

Central Brain Tumor Registry of the United States (CBTRUS) (2005): Statistical Report: Primary Brain Tumors in the United States, 1998–2002. Hinsdale, IL: CBTRUS.

Charest A, Lane K, McMahon K, Park J, Preisinger E, Conroy H, et al. (2003): Fusion of FIG to the receptor tyrosine kinase ROS in a glioblastoma with an interstitial del(6) (q21q21). *Genes Chromosomes Cancer* 37:58–71.

Cheng Y, Pang JC, Ng HK, Ding M, Zhang SF, Zheng J, et al. (2000): Pilocytic astrocytomas do not show most of the genetic changes commonly seen in diffuse astrocytomas. *Histopathology* 37:437–444.

Cin H, Meyer C, Janzarik WG, Lambert S, Jones DT, Jacob K, et al. (2011): Oncogenic FAM131B-BRAF fusion resulting from 7q34 deletion comprises an alternative mechanism of MAPK pathway activation in pilocytic astrocytoma. *Acta Neuropathol* 121:763–774.

Claus EB, Park PJ, Carroll R, Chan J, Black PM (2008): Specific genes expressed in association with progesterone receptors in meningioma. *Cancer Res* 68:314–322.

Coccé MC, Lubieniecki F, Bartuluchi M, Gallego MS (2009): Cytogenetic findings in a rare pediatric mixed glioneuronal tumor and review of the literature. *Childs Nerv Syst* 25):1485–1490.

Dahia PL (2000): PTEN, a unique tumor suppressor gene. *Endocr Relat Cancer* 7:115–129.

Dahlback HS, Brandal P, Meling TR, Gorunova L, Scheie D, Heim S (2009): Genomic aberrations in 80 cases of primary glioblastoma multiforme: pathogenetic heterogeneity and putative cytogenetic pathways. *Genes Chromosomes Cancer* 48:908–924.

Dahlback HS, Gorunova L, Brandal P, Scheie D, Helseth E, Meling TR, et al. (2011a): Genomic aberrations in diffuse low-grade gliomas. *Genes Chromosomes Cancer* 50:409–420.

Dahlback HS, Brandal P, Gorunova L, Widing E, Meling TR, Krossnes BK, et al. (2011b): Genomic aberrations in pediatric gliomas and embryonal tumors. *Genes Chromosomes Cancer* 50:788–799.

Debiec-Rychter M, Alwasiak J, Liberski PP, Nedoszytko B, Babińska M, Mrózek K, et al. (1995): Accumulation of chromosomal changes in human glioma progression. A cytogenetic study of 50 cases. *Cancer Genet Cytogenet* 85:61–67.

De Lellis RA, Lloyd RV, Heitz PU, Eng C, editors (2004): *Pathology and Genetics. Tumours of Endocrine Organs.* Lyon: IARC Press.

Deshmukh H, Yeh TH, Yu J, Sharma MK, Perry A, Leonard JR, et al. (2008): High-resolution, dual-platform aCGH analysis reveals frequent HIPK2 amplification and increased expression in pilocytic astrocytomas. *Oncogene* 27:4745–4751.

Dias-Santagata D, Lam Q, Vernovsky K, Vena N, Lennerz JK, Borger DR, et al. (2011): BRAF V600E mutations are common in pleomorphic xanthoastrocytoma: diagnostic and therapeutic implications. *PLoS One* 6:e17948

Di Marcotullio L, Ferretti E, DeSmaele E, Argenti B, Mincione C, Zazzeroni F, et al. (2004): REN(KCTD11) is a suppressor of Hedgehog signaling and is deleted in human medulloblastoma. *Proc Natl Acad Sci USA* 101:10833–10838.

Doco-Fenzy M, Cornillet P, Scherpereel B, Depernet B, Bisiau-Leconte S, Ferre D, et al. (1993): Cytogenetic changes in 67 cranial and spinal meningiomas: relation to histopathological and clinical pattern. *Anticancer Res* 13:845–850.

Domingues PH, Sousa P, Otero A, Gonçalves JM, Ruiz L, de Oliveira C, et al. (2014): Proposal for a new risk stratification classification for meningioma based on patient age, WHO tumor grade, size, localization, and karyotype. *Neuro Oncol* 16:735–747.

Donovan MJ, Yunis EJ, DeGirolami U, Fletcher JA, Schofield DE (1994): Chromosome aberrations in choroid plexus papillomas. *Genes Chromosomes Cancer* 11:267–270.

Dyer S, Prebble E, Davison V, Davies P, Ramani P, Ellison D, et al. (2002): Genomic imbalances in pediatric intracranial ependymomas define clinically relevant groups. *Am J Pathol* 161:2133–2141.

Ekstrand AJ, James CD, Cavenee WK, Seliger B, Pettersson RF, Collins VP (1991): Genes for epidermal growth factor receptor, transforming growth factor alpha, and epidermal growth factor and their expression in human gliomas *in vivo*. *Cancer Res* 51:2164–2172.

Ekstrand AJ, Sugawa N, James CD, Collins VP (1992): Amplified and rearranged epidermal growth factor receptor genes in human glioblastomas reveal deletions of sequences encoding portions of the N- and/or C-terminal tails. *Proc Natl Acad Sci USA* 89:4309–4313.

Ellison DW, Kocak M, Dalton J, Megahed H, Lusher ME, Ryan SL, et al. (2011): Definition of disease-risk stratification groups in childhood medulloblastoma using combined clinical, pathologic, and molecular variables. *J Clin Oncol* 29:1400–1407.

Esteller M (2002): CpG island hypermethylation and tumor suppressor genes: a booming present, a brighter future. *Oncogene* 21:5427–5440.

Esteller M, Hamilton SR, Burger PC, Baylin SB, Herman JG (1999): Inactivation of the DNA repair gene O6-methylguanine-DNA methyltransferase by promoter hypermethylation is a common event in primary human neoplasia. *Cancer Res* 59:793–797.

Fan X, Munoz J, Sanko SG, Castresana JS (2002): PTEN, DMBT1, and p16 alterations in diffusely infiltrating astrocytomas. *Int J Oncol* 21:667–674.

Farwell JR, Dohrmann GJ, Flannery JT (1984): Medulloblastoma in childhood: an epidemiological study. *J Neurosurg* 61:657–664.

Ferguson KL, Callaghan SM, O'Hare MJ, Park DS, Slack RS (2000): The Rb-CDK4/6 signaling pathway is critical in neural precursor cell cycle regulation. *J Biol Chem* 275:33593–33600.

Fomchenko EI, Holland EC (2006): Mouse models of brain tumors and their applications in preclinical trials. *Clin Cancer Res* 12:5288–5297.

Frattini V, Trifonov V, Chan JM, Castano A, Lia M, Abate F, et al. (2013): The integrated landscape of driver genomic alterations in glioblastoma. *Nat Genet* 45:1141–1149.

Gerson SL (2004): MGMT: Its role in cancer aetiology and cancer therapeutics. *Nat Rev Cancer* 4:296–307.

Giannini C, Scheithauer BW (1997): Classification and grading of low-grade astrocytic tumors in children. *Brain Pathol* 7:785–798.

Goodrich LV, Milenkovic L, Higgins KM, Scott MP (1997): Altered neural cell fates and medulloblastoma in mouse patched mutants. *Science* 277:1109–1113.

Griffin CA, Long PP, Carson BS, Brem H (1992): Chromosome abnormalities in low-grade central nervous system tumors. *Cancer Genet Cytogenet* 60:67–73.

Griffin CA, Burger P, Morsberger L, Yonescu R, Swierczynski S, Weingart JD, et al. (2006): Identification of der(1;19) (q10;p10) in five oligodendrogliomas suggests mechanism of concurrent 1p and 19q loss. *J Neuropathol Exp Neurol* 65:988–994.

Gu J, Tamura M, Pankov R, Danen EH, Takino T, Matsumoto K, et al. (1999): Shc and FAK differentially regulate cell motility and directionality modulated by PTEN. *J Cell Biol* 146:389–403.

Gupta R, Webb-Myers R, Flanagan S, Buckland ME (2011): Isocitrate dehydrogenase mutations in diffuse gliomas: clinical and aetiological implications. *J Clin Pathol* 64:835–844.

Hahn H, Wicking C, Zaphiropoulous PG, Gailani MR, Shanley S, Chidambaram A, et al. (1996): Mutations of the human homolog of Drosophila patched in the nevoid basal cell carcinoma syndrome. *Cell* 85:841–851.

Hasselblatt M, Oyen F, Gesk S, Kordes U, Wrede B, Bergmann M, et al. (2009): Cribriform neuroepithelial tumor (CRINET): a nonrhabdoid ventricular tumor with INI1 loss and relatively favorable prognosis. *J Neuropathol Exp Neurol* 68:1249–1255.

Hegi ME, Diserens AC, Gorlia T, Hamou MF, deTribolet N, Weller M, et al. (2005): MGMT gene silencing and benefit from temozolomide in glioblastoma. *N Engl J Med* 352:997–1003.

Hirose Y, Aldape KD, Chang S, Lamborn K, Berger MS, Feuerstein BG (2003): Grade II astrocytomas are subgrouped by chromosome aberrations. *Cancer Genet Cytogenet* 142:1–7.

Hoischen A, Ehrler M, Fassunke J, Simon M, Baudis M, Landwehr C, et al. (2008): Comprehensive characterization of genomic aberrations in gangliogliomas by CGH, array-based CGH and interphase FISH. *Brain Pathol* 18:326–337.

Holland H, Koschny T, Ahnert P, Meixensberger J, Koschny R (2010): WHO grade-specific comparative genomic hybridization pattern of astrocytoma – a meta-analysis. *Pathol Res Pract* 206:663–668.

Holland H, Ahnert P, Koschny R, Kirsten H, Bauer M, Schober R, et al. (2012): Detection of novel genomic aberrations in anaplastic astrocytomas by GTG-banding, SKY, locus-specific FISH, and high density SNP-array. *Pathol Res Pract* 208:325–330.

Hooper JE, Scott MP (1989): The Drosophila patched gene encodes a putative membrane protein required for segmental patterning. *Cell* 59:751–765.

Håvik AB, Lind GE, Honne H, Meling TR, Scheie D, Hall KS, et al. (2014): Sequencing IDH1/2 glioma mutation hotspots in gliomas and malignant peripheral nerve sheath tumors. *Neuro Oncol* 16:320–322.

Ida CM, Lambert SR, Rodriguez FJ, Voss JS, Mc Cann BE, Seys AR, et al. (2012): BRAF alterations are frequent in cerebellar low-grade astrocytomas with diffuse growth pattern. *J Neuropathol Exp Neurol* 71:631–639.

Jacoby LB, MacCollin M, Barone R, Ramesh V, Gusella JF (1996): Frequency and distribution of *NF2* mutations in schwannomas. *Genes Chromosomes Cancer* 17:45–55.

Jenkins RB, Kimmel DW, Moertel CA, Schultz CG, Scheithauer BW, Kelly PJ, et al. (1989): A cytogenetic study of 53 human gliomas. *Cancer Genet Cytogenet* 39:253–279.

Jenkins RB, Blair H, Ballman KV, Giannini C, Arusell RM, Law M, et al. (2006): A t(1;19)(q10;p10) mediates the combined deletions of 1p and 19q and predicts a better prognosis of patients with oligodendroglioma. *Cancer Res* 66:9852–9861.

Jeuken JW, Sprenger SH, Boerman RH, von Deimling A, Teepen HL, van Overbeeke JJ, et al. (2001): Subtyping of oligo-astrocytic tumours by comparative genomic hybridization. *J Pathol* 194:81–87.

Jeuken JW, Sprenger SH, Gilhuis J, Teepen HL, Grotenhuis AJ, Wesseling P (2002): Correlation between localization, age, and chromosomal imbalances in ependymal tumours as detected by CGH. *J Pathol* 197:238–244.

Jhanwar SC, Chen Q, Li FP, Brennan MF, Woodruff JM (1994): Cytogenetic analysis of soft tissue sarcomas. Recurrent chromosome abnormalities in malignant peripheral nerve sheath tumors (MPNST). *Cancer Genet Cytogenet* 78:138–144.

Johannsson JH, Rekate HL, Roessmann U (1981): Gangliogliomas: pathological and clinical correlation. *J Neurosurg* 54:58–63.

Jones DT, Ichimura K, Liu L, Pearson DM, Plant K, Collins VP (2006): Genomic analysis of pilocytic astrocytomas at 0.97 Mb resolution shows an increasing tendency toward chromosomal copy number change with age. *J Neuropathol Exp Neurol* 65:1049–1058.

Jones DT, Kocialkowski S, Liu L, Pearson DM, Bäcklund LM, Ichimura K, et al. (2008): Tandem duplication producing a novel oncogenic BRAF fusion gene defines the majority of pilocytic astrocytomas. *Cancer Res* 68:8673–8677.

Jones DT, Kocialkowski S, Liu L, Pearsom DM, Ichimura K, Collins VP (2009): Oncogenic RAF1 rearrangement and a novel BRAF mutation as alternatives to KIAA1549:BRAF fusion in activating the MAPK pathway in pilocytic astrocytoma. *Oncogene* 28:2119–2123.

Jones DT, Hutter B, Jäger N, Korshunov A, Kool M, Warnatz HJ, et al. (2013): Recurrent somatic alterations of FGFR1 and NTRK2 in pilocytic astrocytoma. *Nat Genet* 45:927–932.

Karnes PS, Tran TN, Cui MY, Raffel C, Gilles FH, Barranger JA, et al. (1992): Cytogenetic analysis of 39 pediatric central nervous system tumors. *Cancer Genet Cytogenet* 59:12–19.

Kilday JP, Rahman R, Dyer S, Ridley L, Lowe J, Coyle B, et al. (2009): Pediatric ependymoma: biological perspectives. *Mol Cancer Res* 7:765–786.

Kim KE, Kim KU, Kim DC, Park JI, Han JY (2009): Cytogenetic characterizations of central nervous system tumors: the first comprehensive report from a single institution in Korea. *J Korean Med Sci* 24:453–460.

Kitange G, Misra A, Law M, Passe S, Kollmeyer TM, Maurer M, et al. (2005): Chromosomal imbalances detected by array comparative genomic hybridization in human oligodendrogliomas and mixed oligoastrocytomas. *Genes Chromosomes Cancer* 42:68–77.

Kluwe L, Hagel C, Tatagiba M, Thomas S, Stavrou D, Ostertag H, et al. (2001): Loss of NF1 alleles distinguish sporadic from NF1-associated pilocytic astrocytomas. *J Neuropathol Exp Neurol* 60:917–920.

Koutsimpelas D, Felmeden U, Mann WJ, Brieger J (2011): Analysis of cytogenetic aberrations in sporadic vestibular schwannoma by comparative genomic hybridization. *J Neurooncol* 103:437–443.

Kunwar S, Mohapatra G, Bollen A, Lamborn KR, Prados M, Feuerstein BG (2001): Genetic subgroups of anaplastic astrocytomas correlate with patient age and survival. *Cancer Res* 61:7683–7688.

Ladanyi M, Woodruff JM, Scheithauer BW, Bridge JA, Barr FG, Goldblum JR, et al. (2001): Re: O'Sullivan MJ, Kyriakos M, Zhu X, Wick MR, Swanson PE, Dehner LP, Humphrey PA, Pfeifer JD: Malignant peripheral nerve sheath tumors with t(X;18). A pathologic and molecular genetic study. *Mod Pathol* 13:1336–46. Mod Pathol 14:733–73.

Lamont JM, McManamy CS, Pearson AD, Clifford SC, Ellison DW (2004): Combined histopathological and molecular cytogenetic stratification of medulloblastoma patients. *Clin Cancer Res* 10:5482–5493.

Lamszus K, Lachenmayer L, Heinemann U, Kluwe L, Finckh U, Hoppner W, et al. (2001): Molecular genetic alterations on chromosomes 11 and 22 in ependymomas. *Int J Cancer* 91:803–808.

Lawson AR, Tatevossian RG, Phipps KP, Michalski A, Sheer D, Jacques TS, et al. (2010): RAF gene fusions are specific to pilocytic astrocytoma in a broad paediatric brain tumour cohort. *Acta Neuropathol* 120:271–273.

Leenstra JL, Rodriguez FJ, Frechette CM, Giannini C, Stafford SL, Pollock BE, et al. (2007): Central neurocytoma: management recommendations based on a 35-year experience. *Int J Radiat Oncol Biol Phys* 67:1145–1154.

Lekanne Deprez RH, Riegman PH, Groen NA, Warringa UL, van Biezen NA, Molijn AC, et al. (1995): Cloning and characterization of MN1, a gene from chromosome 22q11, which is disrupted by a balanced translocation in a meningioma. *Oncogene* 10:1521–1528.

Lindblom A, Ruttledge M, Collins VP, Nordenskjold M, Dumanski JP (1994): Chromosomal deletions in anaplastic meningiomas suggest multiple regions outside chromosome 22 as important in tumor progression. *Int J Cancer* 56:354–357.

Listernick R, Charrow J, Gutmann DH (1999): Intracranial gliomas in neurofibromatosis type 1. *Am J Med Genet* 89:38–44.

Lopez-Gines C, Gil-Benso R, Collado-Diaz M, Gregori-Romero M, Roldan P, Barbera J, et al. (2003): Meningioma: A model of cytogenetic evolution in tumoral initiation and progression. *Neurocirugia (Astur)*14: 517–525.

Louis DN, Ohgaki H, Wiestler OD, Cavenee WK, editors (2007): *WHO Classification of Tumours of the Central Nervous System.* Lyon: IARC Press.

Lusis EA, Watson MA, Chicoine MR, Lyman M, Roerig P, Reifenberger G, et al. (2005): Integrative genomic analysis identifies NDRG2 as a candidate tumor suppressor gene frequently inactivated in clinically aggressive meningioma. *Cancer Res* 65:7121–7126.

Magnani I, Guerneri S, Pollo B, Cirenei N, Colombo BM, Broggi G, et al. (1994): Increasing complexity of the karyotype in 50 human gliomas. Progressive evolution and de novo occurrence of cytogenetic alterations. *Cancer Genet Cytogenet* 75:77–89.

Maillo A, Orfao A, Espinosa AB, Sayagues JM, Merino M, Sousa P, et al. (2007): Early recurrences in histologically benign/grade I meningiomas are associated with large tumors and coexistence of monosomy 14 and del(1p36) in the ancestral tumor cell clone. *Neuro Oncol* 9:438–446.

Mantripragada KK, Spurlock G, Kluwe L, Chuzhanova N, Ferner RE, Frayling IM, et al. (2008): High-resolution DNA copy number profiling of malignant peripheral nerve sheath tumors using targeted microarray-based comparative genomic hybridization. *Clin Cancer Res* 14:1015–1024.

Mark J (1977): Chromosomal abnormalities and their specificity in human neoplasms: an assessment of recent observations by banding techniques. *Adv Cancer Res* 24:165–222.

Mark J, Levan G, Mitelman F (1972): Identification by fluorescence of the G chromosome lost in human meningomas. *Hereditas* 71:163–168.

Mazewski C, Soukup S, Ballard E, Gotwals B, Lampkin B (1999): Karyotype studies in 18 ependymomas with literature review of 107 cases. *Cancer Genet Cytogenet* 113:1–8.

McLendon R, Friedman A, Bigner D, Van Meir EG, Brat DJ, Mastrogianakis GM, et al. (2008): Comprehensive genomic characterization defines human glioblastoma genes and core pathways. *Nature* 455:1061–1068.

Menon AG, Rutter JL, vonSattel JP, Synder H, Murdoch C, Blumenfeld A, et al. (1997): Frequent loss of chromosome 14 in atypical and malignant meningioma: identification of a putative "tumor progression" locus. *Oncogene* 14:611–616.

Mertens F, Dal Cin P, De Wever I, Fletcher CDM, Mandahl N, Mitelman F, et al. (2000): Cytogenetic characterization of peripheral nerve sheath tumours: a report of the CHAMP study group. *J Pathol* 190:31–38.

Mitelman F, Johansson B, Mertens F, editors (2014): Mitelman Database of Chromosome Aberrations and Gene Fusions in Cancer. http://cgap.nci.nih.gov/Chromosomes/Mitelman.

Moscatello DK, Montgomery RB, Sundareshan P, McDanel H, Wong MY, Wong AJ (1996): Transformational and altered signal transduction by a naturally occurring mutant EGF receptor. *Oncogene* 13:85–96.

Mrak RE, Yasargil MG, Mohapatra G, Earel J Jr, Louis DN (2004): Atypical extraventricular neurocytoma with oligodendroglioma-like spread and an unusual pattern of chromosome 1p and 19q loss. *Hum Pathol* 35:1156–1159.

Mueller W, Hartmann C, Hoffmann A, Lanksch W, Kiwit J, Tonn J, et al. (2002): Genetic signature of oligoastrocytomas correlates with tumor location and denotes distinct molecular subsets. *Am J Pathol* 161:313–319.

Nakamura M, Watanabe T, Klangby U, Asker C, Wiman K, Yonekawa Y, et al. (2001a): p14ARF deletion and methylation in genetic pathways to glioblastomas. *Brain Pathol* 11:159–168.

Nakamura M, Yonekawa Y, Kleihues P, Ohgaki H (2001b): Promoter hypermethylation of the RB1 gene in glioblastomas. *Lab Invest* 81:77–82.

Northcott PA, Korshunov A, Witt H, Hielscher T, Eberhart CG, Mack S, et al. (2011): Medulloblastoma comprises four distinct molecular variants. *J Clin Oncol* 29:1408–1414.

Noushmehr H, Weisenberger DJ, Diefes K, Phillips HS, Pujara K, Berman BP, et al. (2010): Identification of a CpG island methylator phenotype that defines a distinct subgroup of glioma. *Cancer Cell* 17:510–522.

Ohgaki K, Kleihues P (2005). Population-based studies on incidence, survival rates, and genetic alterations in astrocytic and oligodendroglial gliomas. *J Neuropathol Exp Neurol* 64:479–489.

Ohgaki H, Kleihues P (2007): Genetic pathways to primary and secondary glioblastoma. *Am J Pathol* 170:1445–1453.

Olsen TK, Panagopoulos I, Meling TR, Micci F, Gorunova L, Thorsen J, et al. (2015): Fusion genes with ALK as recurrent partner in ependymoma-like gliomas: a new brain tumor entity? *Neuro Oncol* in press.

O'Sullivan MJ, Kyriakos M, Zhu X, Wick MR, Swanson PE, Dehner LP, et al. (2000): Malignant peripheral nerve sheath tumors with t(X;18). A pathologic and molecular genetic study. *Mod Pathol* 13:1336–1346.

Panagopoulos I, Thorsen J, Gorunova L, Micci F, Heim S (2014): Sequential combination of karyotyping and RNA-sequencing in the search for cancer-specific cancer genes. *Int J Biochem Cell Biol.* 53:462–465.

Pandita A, Balasubramaniam A, Perrin R, Shannon P, Guha A (2007): Malignant and benign ganglioglioma: a pathological and molecular study. *Neuro Oncol* 9:124–134.

Parker M, Mohankumar KM, Punchihewa C, Weinlich R, Dalton JD, Li Y, et al. (2014): C11orf95–RELA fusions drive oncogenic NF-κB signalling in ependymoma. *Nature* 506:451–455.

Parsons DW, Jones S, Zhang X, Lin JC, Leary RJ, Angenendt P, et al. (2008): An integrated genomic analysis of human glioblastoma multiforme. *Science* 321:1807–1812.

Perry A, Fuller CE, Banerjee R, Brat DJ, Scheithauer BW (2003): Ancillary FISH analysis for 1p and 19q status: preliminary observations in 287 gliomas and oligodendroglioma mimics. *Front Biosci* 8:a1–9.

Perry A, Gutmann DH, Reifenberger G (2004): Molecular pathogenesis of meningiomas. *J Neurooncol* 70:183–202.

Pfister S, Janzarik WG, Remke M, Ernst A, Werft W, Becker N, et al. (2008): BRAF gene duplication constitutes a mechanism of MAPK pathway activation in low-grade astrocytomas. *J Clin Invest* 118:1739–1749.

Plowman PN, Pizer B, Kingston JE (2004): Pineal parenchymal tumours: II. On the aggressive behaviour of pineoblastoma in patients with an inherited mutation of the RB1 gene. *Clin Oncol* 16:244–247.

Rainho CA, Rogatto SR, de Moraes LC, Barbieri-Neto J (1992): Cytogenetic study of a pineocytoma. *Cancer Genet Cytogenet* 64:127–32.

Ransom DT, Ritland SR, Kimmel DW, Moertel CA, Dahl RJ, Scheithauer BW, et al. (1992): Cytogenetic and loss of heterozygosity studies in ependymomas, pilocytic astrocytomas, and oligodendrogliomas. *Genes Chromosomes Cancer* 5:348–356.

Reardon DA, Entrekin RE, Sublett J, Ragsdale S, Li H, Boyett J, et al. (1999): Chromosome arm 6q loss is the most common recurrent autosomal alteration detected in primary pediatric ependymoma. *Genes Chromosomes Cancer* 24:230–237.

Reifenberger G, Louis DN (2003): Oligodendroglioma: toward molecular definitions in diagnostic neuro-oncology. *J Neuropathol Exp Neurol* 62(2):111–126.

Reifenberger J, Reifenberger G, Liu L, James CD, Wechsler W, Collins VP (1994): Molecular genetic analysis of oligodendroglial tumors shows preferential allelic deletions on 19q and 1p. *Am J Pathol* 145:1175–1190.

Rempel SA, Schwechheimer K, Davis RL, Cavenee WK, Rosenblum ML (1993): Loss of heterozygosity for loci on chromosome 10 is associated with morphologically malignant meningioma progression. *Cancer Res* 53:2386–2392.

Rey JA, Bello MJ, de Campos JM, Kusak ME, Moreno S (1987): Chromosomal composition of a series of 22 human low-grade gliomas. *Cancer Genet Cytogenet* 29:223–37.

Rickert CH, Wiestler OD, Paulus W (2002): Chromosomal imbalances in choroid plexus tumors. *Am J Pathol* 160:1105–1113.

Rollbrocker B, Waha A, Louis DN, Wiestler OD, von Deimling A (1996): Amplification of the cyclin-dependent kinase 4 (CDK4) gene is associated with high cdk4 protein levels in glioblastoma multiforme. *Acta Neuropathol* 92:70–74.

Rousseau E, Palm T, Scaravilli F, Ruchoux MM, Figarella-Branger D, Salmon I, et al. (2007): Trisomy 19 ependymoma, a newly recognized genetico-histological association, including clear cell ependymoma. *Mol Cancer* 6:47.

Ruttledge MH, Xie YG, Han FY, Peyrard M, Collins VP, Nordenskjold M, et al. (1994): Deletions on chromosome 22 in sporadic meningioma. *Genes Chromosomes Cancer* 10:122–130.

Sanoudou D, Tingby O, Ferguson-Smith MA, Collins VP, Coleman N (2000): Analysis of pilocytic astrocytoma by comparative genomic hybridization. *Br J Cancer* 82:1218–1222.

Sayagues JM, Tabernero MD, Maillo A, Espinosa A, Rasillo A, Diaz P, et al. (2004): Intratumoral patterns of clonal evolution in meningiomas as defined by multicolor interphase fluorescence in situ hybridization (FISH): is there a relationship between histopathologically benign and atypical/anaplastic lesions? *J Mol Diagn* 6:316–325.

Schrock E, Thiel G, Lozanova T, du Manoir S, Meffert MC, Jauch A, et al. (1994): Comparative genomic hybridization of human malignant gliomas reveals multiple amplification sites and nonrandom chromosomal gains and losses. *Am J Pathol* 144:1203–1218.

Sharma MK, Watson MA, Lyman M, Perry A, Aldape KD, Deak F, et al. (2006): Matrilin-2 expression distinguishes clinically relevant subsets of pilocytic astrocytoma. *Neurology* 66:127–130.

Shinojima N, Tada K, Shiraishi S, Kamiryo T, Kochi M, Nakamura H, et al. (2003): Prognostic value of epidermal growth factor receptor in patients with glioblastoma multiforme. *Cancer Res* 63:6962–6970.

Sievert AJ, Jackson EM, Gai X, Hakonarson H, Judkins AR, Resnick AC, et al. (2009): Duplication of 7q34 in pediatric low-grade astrocytomas detected by high-density single-nucleotide polymorphism-based genotype arrays results in a novel BRAF fusion gene. *Brain Pathol* 19:449–458.

Singh D, Chan JM, Zoppoli P, Niola F, Sullivan R, Castano A, et al. (2012): Transforming fusions of FGFR and TACC genes in human glioblastoma. *Science* 337:1231–1235.

Smoll NR, Hamilton B (2014): Incidence and relative survival of anaplastic astrocytomas. *Neuro Oncol* 16:1400–1407.

Somerville RP, Shoshan Y, Eng C, Barnett G, Miller D, Cowell JK (1998): Molecular analysis of two putative tumour suppressor genes, PTEN and DMBT, which have been implicated in glioblastoma multiforme disease progression. *Oncogene* 17:1755–1757.

Storlazzi CT, Vult Von Steyern F, Domanski HA, Mandahl N, Mertens F (2005): Biallelic somatic inactivation of the NF1 gene through chromosomal translocations in a sporadic neurofibroma. *Int J Cancer* 117:1055–1057.

Storlazzi CT, Brekke HR, Mandahl N, Brosjö O, Smeland S, Lothe RA, et al. (2006): Identification of a novel amplicon at distal 17q containing the *BIRC5/SURVIVIN* gene in malignant peripheral nerve sheath tumours. *J Pathol* 209:492–500.

Stupp R, Mason WP, van den Bent MJ, Weller M, Fisher B, Taphoorn MJ, et al. (2005): Radiotherapy plus concomitant and adjuvant temozolomide for glioblastoma. *N Engl J Med* 352:987–996.

Suarez-Merino B, Hubank M, Revesz T, Harkness W, Hayward R, Thompson D, et al. (2005): Microarray analysis of pediatric ependymoma identifies a cluster of 112 candidate genes including four transcripts at 22q12.1-q13.3. *Neuro Oncol* 7:20–31.

Taruscio D, Danesi R, Montaldi A, Cerasoli S, Cenacchi G, Giangaspero F (1997): Nonrandom gain of chromosome 7 in central neurocytoma: a chromosomal analysis and fluorescence *in situ* hybridization study. *Virchows Arch* 430:47–51.

Taylor MD, Poppleton H, Fuller C, Su X, Liu Y, Jensen P, et al. (2005): Radial glia cells are candidate stem cells of ependymoma. *Cancer Cell* 8:323–335.

Thiel G, Losanowa T, Kintzel D, Nisch G, Martin H, Vorpahl K, et al. (1992): Karyotypes in 90 human gliomas. *Cancer Genet Cytogenet* 58:109–120.

Thompson MC, Fuller C, Hogg TL, Dalton J, Finkelstein D, Lau CC, et al. (2006): Genomics identifies medulloblastoma subgroups that are enriched for specific genetic alterations. *J Clin Oncol* 24:1924–1931.

Ueki K, Ono Y, Henson JW, Efird JT, von Deimling A, Louis DN (1996): CDKN2/p16 or RB alterations occur in the majority of glioblastomas and are inversely correlated. *Cancer Res* 56:150–153.

Vagner-Capodano AM, Gentet JC, Gambarelli D, Pellissier JF, Gouzien M, Lena G, et al. (1992): Cytogenetic studies in 45 pediatric brain tumors. *Pediatr Hematol Oncol* 9:223–235.

van den Bent MJ (2000): Chemotherapy of oligodendroglial tumours: current developments. *Forum* 10:108–118.

van den Bent MJ, Reni M, Gatta G, Vecht C (2008): Oligodendroglioma. *Crit Rev Oncol Hematol* 66:262–272.

van den Bent MJ, Brandes AA, Taphoorn MJ, Kros JM, Kouwenhoven MC, Delattre JY, et al. (2013): Adjuvant procarbazine, lomustine, and vincristine chemotherapy in newly diagnosed anaplastic oligodendroglioma: long-term follow-up of EORTC brain tumor group study 26951. *J Clin Oncol* 31:344–350.

Vanhaesebroeck B, Leevers SJ, Panayotou G, Waterfield MD (1997): Phosphoinositide 3-kinases: a conserved family of signal transducers. *Trends Biochem Sci* 22:267–272.

Verhaak RG, Hoadley KA, Purdom E, Wang V, Qi Y, Wilkerson MD, et al. (2010): Integrated genomic analysis identifies clinically relevant subtypes of glioblastoma characterized by abnormalities in PDGFRA, IDH1, EGFR, and NF1. *Cancer Cell* 17:98–110.

Villavicencio EH, Walterhouse DO, Iannaccone PM (2000): The sonic hedgehog-patched-gli pathway in human development and disease. *Am J Hum Genet* 67:1047–1054.

Ward SJ, Karakoula K, Phipps KP, Harkness W, Hayward R, Thompson D, et al. (2010): Cytogenetic analysis of paediatric astrocytoma using comparative genomic hybridisation and fluorescence in-situ hybridisation. *J Neurooncol* 98:305–318.

Watanabe K, Tachibana O, Sata K, Yonekawa Y, Kleihues P, Ohgaki H (1996): Overexpression of the EGF receptor and p53 mutations are mutually exclusive in the evolution of primary and secondary glioblastomas. *Brain Pathol* 6:217–223.

Weber RG, Sabel M, Reifenberger J, Sommer C, Oberstrass J, Reifenberger G, et al. (1996): Characterization of genomic alterations associated with glioma progression by comparative genomic hybridization. *Oncogene* 13:983–994.

Weremowicz S, Kupsky WJ, Morton CC, Fletcher JA (1992): Cytogenetic evidence for a chromosome 22 tumor suppressor gene in ependymoma. *Cancer Genet Cytogenet* 61:193–196.

White FV, Anthony DC, Yunis EJ, Tarbell NJ, Scott RM, Schofield DE (1995): Nonrandom chromosomal gains in pilocytic astrocytomas of childhood. *Hum Pathol* 26:979–986.

Yamada K, Kondo T, Yoshioka M, Oami H (1980): Cytogenetic studies in twenty human brain tumors: association of no. 22 chromosome abnormalities with tumors of the brain. *Cancer Genet Cytogenet* 2:293–307.

Yamada K, Kasama, M, Kondo T, Shinoura N, Yoshioka M (1994): Chromosome studies in 70 brain tumors with special attention to sex chromosome loss and single autosomal trisomy. *Cancer Genet Cytogenet* 73:46–52.

Yin XL, Pang JC, Hui AB, Ng HK (2000): Detection of chromosomal imbalances in central neurocytomas by using comparative genomic hybridization. *J Neurosurg* 93:77–81.

Yin XL, Hui AB, Pang JC, Poon WS, Ng HK (2002): Genome-wide survey for chromosomal imbalances in ganglioglioma using comparative genomic hybridization. *Cancer Genet Cytogenet* 134:71–76.

Zada G, Bond AE, Wang YP, Giannotta SL, Deapen D (2012): Incidence trends in the anatomic location of primary malignant brain tumors in the Unites States: 1992–2006. *World Neurosurg* 77:518–524.

Zang KD (1982): Cytological and cytogenetical studies on human meningioma. *Cancer Genet Cytogenet* 6:249–274.

Zang KD (2001): Meningioma: a cytogenetic model of a complex benign human tumor, including data on 394 karyotyped cases. *Cytogenet Cell Genet* 93:207–220.

Zang KD, Singer H (1967): Chromosomal constitution of meningiomas. *Nature* 216:84–85.

Zankl H, Zang KD (1972): Cytological and cytogenetical studies on brain tumors. 4. Identification of the missing G chromosome in human meningiomas as no. 22 by fluorescence technique. *Humangenetik* 14:167–169.

Zattara-Cannoni H, Gambarelli D, Lena G, Dufour H, Choux M, Grisoli F, et al. (1998): Are juvenile pilocytic astrocytomas benign tumors? A cytogenetic study in 24 cases. *Cancer Genet Cytogenet* 104:157–160.

Zheng S, Fu J, Vegesna R, Mao Y, Heathcock LE, Torres-Garcia W, et al. (2013): A survey of intragenic breakpoints in glioblastoma identifies a distinct subset associated with poor survival. *Genes Dev* 27:1462–1472.

Zhou YH, Hess KR, Liu L, Linskey ME, Yung WK (2005): Modeling prognosis for patients with malignant astrocytic gliomas: Quantifying the expression of multiple genetic markers and clinical variables. *Neuro Oncol* 7:485–494.

Zhu JJ, Leon SP, Folkerth RD, Guo SZ, Wu JK, Black PM (1997): Evidence for clonal origin of neoplastic neuronal and glial cells in gangliogliomas. *Am J Pathol* 151:565–571.

Zindy F, Nilsson LM, Nguyen L, Meunier C, Smeyne RJ, Rehg JE, et al. (2003): Hemangiosarcomas, medulloblastomas, and other tumors in Ink4c/p53-null mice. *Cancer Res* 63:5420–5427.

CHAPTER 21

Tumors of the eye

Karen Sisley

Academic Unit of Ophthalmology and Orthoptics, Department of Oncology, The Medical School, University of Sheffield, Sheffield, UK

Eye tumors are classified as intraocular or extraocular. Although primary eye tumors are rare, the eye is the site of a diverse range of both benign and malignant primary neoplasms and is also a common location for metastases from malignancies of the breast, lung, and gastrointestinal tract as well as from cutaneous melanomas. No published cytogenetic analyses of metastases to the eye are available, but in our laboratory, we observed metastatic eye lesions from cutaneous melanoma to have aberrations characteristic of these cutaneous tumors; therefore, it can be assumed that metastases from common primary locations display changes typical of the primary cancer. In children, the most common primary eye malignancy is retinoblastoma (RB), whereas in adults melanomas are the most frequent, mainly affecting the uveal tract of the eye but also involving the conjunctiva. The chromosome changes of both RB and uveal melanoma (UM) have been well documented, less so for conjunctival melanoma, while information on the other forms of primary eye tumors is usually restricted to a few anecdotal cases.

Retinoblastoma (RB)

Tumors affecting the retina are rare in adulthood as the cells of the retina are fully differentiated by the age of three. The presentation of benign retinomas and malignant RB is restricted to childhood as they are thought to develop from the immature retinal cells or retinoblasts, although this is the subject of debate in the light of recent genetic findings (Reis et al., 2012; Kapatai et al., 2013). Hereditary RB (30–40% of cases) is often bilateral and arises early in infancy, sometimes developing in utero and presenting at birth. Sporadic tumors are unilateral and develop later, peaking between 2 and 3 years, but cases have been recorded among late teens and there are reports of benign retinomas transforming into RB in adulthood (Herzog et al., 2001; van der Wal et al., 2003; MacCarthy et al., 2006; Abouzeid et al., 2009). Survivors of RB are at high risk of second cancers later in life (MacCarthy et al., 2013).

The first observations of chromosome changes in RB were made over 50 years ago, but more consistent findings emerged in the 1970s (Hossfeld, 1978; Yunis and Ramsey, 1978). In excess of 130 cases have now been described in detailed reports (Mitelman et al., 2014). Relatively simple pseudodiploid karyotypes with a few, but fairly consistent, alterations are the norm, with less than 5% of cases having higher levels of aneuploidy (Cowell and Hogg, 1992; Horsthemke, 1992; Amare Kadam et al., 2004; Mitelman et al., 2014). The most frequently involved chromosomes are 1, 6, 13, and 16. Alterations of chromosome 6, affecting both

Cancer Cytogenetics: Chromosomal and Molecular Genetic Aberrations of Tumor Cells, Fourth Edition.
Edited by Sverre Heim and Felix Mitelman.
© 2015 John Wiley & Sons, Ltd. Published 2015 by John Wiley & Sons, Ltd.

arms, occur in around 70% of cases, but the most specific cytogenetic change, in approximately 40% of cases, is an isochromosome for the short arm of 6p, i(6p). The best known alteration in RB is a deletion of chromosome 13 and the relevant gene *RB1*, which takes its name from the tumor it gives rise to; it has become the paradigm for the role of tumor suppressor genes (TSG) in cancer development.

Chromosome 13 deletions

Hereditary RB is inherited in an autosomal dominant manner with approximately 90% penetrance, and while studying RB, Knudson theorized how a genetic defect would induce tumorigenesis (Knudson 1971), leading to the now well-known two-hit theory of tumorigenesis. The putative locus for the responsible gene was initially identified through cytogenetic analysis of patients with RB and constitutional deletions of chromosome 13. Although there was speculation as to the locus and deletions varied in size, they always involved loss of band 13q14 (Figure 21.1). Subsequent studies helped refine its location to 13q14.2–13q14.3 (Yunis and Ramsey, 1978; Sparkes et al., 1984; Cowell et al., 1987; Duncan et al., 1987) with the *RB1* gene identified and cloned in the mid-1980s (Friend et al., 1986; Fung et al., 1987; Lee et al., 1987). It is surprising that although sporadic and hereditary cases of RB have deletions, sometimes homozygous, of 13q (Lemieux et al., 1989), cytogenetic analysis only

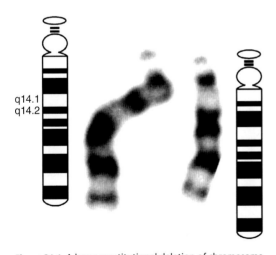

q14.1
q14.2

Figure 21.1 A large constitutional deletion of chromosome 13 affecting band 13q14. Courtesy of Dr D.M. Lillington, St Bartholomew's Hospital.

infrequently provides evidence of 13q abnormalities (Mitelman et al., 2014). The majority of the pathogenetically relevant changes affecting the *RB1* gene are thus submicroscopic, giving rise to both forms of RB, as well as retinomas (Dimaras et al., 2008; Abouzeid et al., 2009). There are, however, around 20% of RB cases without mutations of *RB1* (Lohmann and Horsthemke, 1999; Abouzeid et al., 2007; Rushlow et al., 2013; Thériault et al., 2014). Although it was at first considered that subjugating the action of *RB1* was sufficient to produce RB, this is clearly not the case, and certainly, progression beyond the initial stages of transformation requires the intervention of additional genes. In recent years, there have been a reclassification of the role of *RB1* and also a clearer understanding of the importance that other chromosome changes have, with a realization that different genetic subtypes of RB exist. The genomic background to RB has recently been reviewed comprehensively by Thériault et al. (2014).

Other chromosomes

It is relatively rare to find RBs with complex karyotypes (Mitelman et al., 2014), but as with most cancers, this is thought to signify more advanced aggressive stages, reflecting the acquisition of changes resulting from a later presentation, also because it seems that complex karyotypes are associated with older RB patients (Herzog et al., 2001; Lillington et al., 2003; van der Wal et al., 2003; Gratias et al., 2005; Barros et al., 2012). So if complexity is associated with aggressive/advanced disease, what additional changes are required and is there a sequence of events? Analysis of the clonality of RB has provided clues, but also muddied the waters, with separate tumor foci affecting the left and right eye having different karyotypic profiles (Squire et al., 1985), while a unilateral RB has been reported with two cytogenetically unrelated abnormal clones (Tien et al., 1989). These findings, combined with those of RB with single cytogenetic abnormalities, seem to suggest that the number of additional alterations is random, and there is no favored sequence. It is apparent, however, that even with these discrepancies, certain cytogenetic changes are consistently overrepresented, suggesting that progression of RB is dependent on the involvement of these characteristic chromosome alterations and their underlying genetic drivers.

Among these additional alterations, an isochromosome for the short arm of 6p, i(6p), with a minimal region of gain at 6p22, is the most consistent (Kusnetsova et al., 1982; Mitelman et al., 2014). Cytogenetic observations are likely to be an underestimate, since over 50% of RB cell lines have gain of 6p22 arising from complex translocations (Paderova et al., 2007; Thériault et al., 2014). Of two candidate oncogenes residing within this region, *E2F3* appears to be the most enticing with high gain in primary RB (Thériault et al., 2014). In theory, changes of *E2F3* could potentiate the effects of *RB1* mutations, through promotion of genes for cell cycling, switching from a more quiescent to a proliferative state (Subtil-Rodríguez et al., 2013), an outcome that is maybe further enhanced through coamplification and interaction with the other candidate oncogene in this region, *DEK* (Thériault et al., 2014).

Unbalanced rearrangements of the long arm of chromosome 1 (never in isolation), leading to gain of 1q25–34, are frequent in RB (Mitelman et al., 2014). Refinement of the region to 1q32 (Herzog et al., 2001; Amare Kadam et al., 2004) has led to the hypothesis that both *MDM4* and *KIF14* play important roles in RB progression, as they are amplified in over 50% and have roles in cell cycle regulation (Corson and Gallie, 2007; Sampieri et al., 2008; Thériault et al., 2014). The most common numerical change is monosomy 16, with a minimal deleted region of 16q13–23 reported in tumors, while constitutional analysis has identified a deletion of 16q22 (Amare Kadam et al., 2004). Candidate genes in this region include *CDH11* associated with invasion and *RBL2*, an RB-like gene with a high incidence of allelic loss, that putatively acts synergistically with *RB1*; loss of both genes acts to increase hyperplasia and dysplasia of epithelium in animal models (Haigis et al., 2006; Corson and Gallie, 2007; Dimaras et al., 2008; Sampieri et al., 2008; Priya et al., 2009; Thériault et al., 2014). Lastly, some RBs have homogeneously staining regions (hsr) and/or double minutes (dmin), probably associated with amplification of *MYCN* (Cowell and Hogg, 1992; Amare Kadam et al., 2004; Rushlow et al., 2013; Thériault et al., 2014).

Most aberrations found in RB are also shared by retinomas, the difference being that retinomas are not as genetically unstable and do not individually exhibit as full a range of the critical events, the hypothesis being that when they do, they transform to RB (Corson and Gallie, 2007; Dimaras et al., 2008; Sampieri et al., 2008; Thériault et al., 2014). So can a sequence be defined? It is clear that the sequence starts with deletion/mutation of *RB1* shared by both retinomas and RB (Abouzeid et al., 2009). The other changes are less well characterized, but evidence suggests that changes targeting 1q25–34 (*MDM4*, *KIF14*) are earlier, while 16q abnormalities (*CDH11*) are more likely to occur in advanced RB (Dimaras et al., 2008; Abouzeid et al., 2009; Sampieri et al., 2008; Thériault et al., 2014). It may well be that many of these other changes are interchangeable and compensatory, as it is now deemed likely that there are different genetic subsets of RB. Firstly, there is a small but distinct genetic subgroup without *RB1* mutations, where the transformation is driven by *MYCN* amplification (Rushlow et al., 2013; Thériault et al., 2014). A second group seems to have a defined pathway of instability that features many of the common cytogenetic alterations associated with RB; this is possibly a subset within nonhereditary RB. The third group may be hereditary RB itself, but with these last two groups, the abnormalities are not mutually exclusive and the borders are ill defined at present (Herzog et al., 2001; Lillington et al., 2003; van der Wal et al., 2003; Gratias et al., 2005; Mol et al., 2014). Ultimately, these genetic differences may reflect the cell of origin giving rise to RB (Kapatai et al., 2013), and other factors can also interact to drive the transition from quiescence, such as *CDKN2* and epigenetic regulation (Reis et al., 2012; Thériault et al., 2014).

Other childhood eye tumors

In addition to RB, another eye tumor more common to childhood is orbital rhabdomyosarcoma, which is the most frequent orbital malignancy of children usually presenting within the first decade. Cytogenetic reports are limited but demonstrate the same defining translocations (using fluorescence *in situ* hybridization (FISH)) as those of rhabdomyosarcomas of other locations (Chapter 24). Children are also not immune to the cancers more commonly presenting in adulthood, but cytogenetic investigations under these circumstances are almost nonexistent (Mitelman et al., 2014).

Uveal melanoma (UM)

UM are malignant tumors of neural crest-derived melanocytes that populate the pigmented layer of the eye (uveal tract), which comprises in the anterior segment the iris and in the posterior segment the ciliary body and choroid. They account for approximately 80% of all noncutaneous melanomas and are the most common primary intraocular tumor of adults. Although most frequent among individuals over 55 years, young patients, including some rare instances of preteens, are recorded. The first report of chromosomal changes in UM was of a single tumor metastatic to the brain (Rey et al., 1985), which, unlike the metastases of many solid tumors, was surprisingly devoid of complex karyotypic changes, with alterations of just chromosomes 6 and 8. Changes of these chromosomes are now considered to be among those characteristic of UM. As with RB, the majority of UM are pseudodiploid with comparatively simple karyotypic alterations (Mitelman et al., 2014). It is this simplicity in UM that has allowed clear associations to be drawn between specific cytogenetic changes and their clinical implications. There is, however, a caveat, as the majority of reports come from the aggressive posterior (choroid and ciliary body) tumors. Iris melanomas, because of their rarity and benign nature,

are only infrequently treated by surgery. Iris and conjunctival melanoma will be addressed later.

The first two cytogenetic investigations of more than single cases of posterior UM (in total 20) were almost simultaneous (Prescher et al., 1990; Sisley et al., 1990) and showed great parity of findings, reporting monosomy 3 (M3) as the most frequent alteration, followed by isochromosome for the long arm of chromosome 8, i(8q), and to a lesser degree deletions of 1p and gains of 6p. A number of UM had alterations of chromosomes 3 and 8 occurring together (Figure 21.2), and it was observed that these changes when associated were more likely to be present in melanomas involving the ciliary body (Sisley et al., 1990). To date, in excess of 300 cases have been reported (Mitelman et al., 2014), although duplication of karyotypes among data makes the exact number difficult to establish. There remains a remarkable consistency for cytogenetic changes that mirrors earlier publications from over 20 years ago, confirming that nonrandom involvement of chromosomes 1, 3, 6, and 8 is the most frequent.

Chromosome 3

M3 is the single most consistent cytogenetic change in UM (Figure 21.2), occurring in approximately 50% of cases (Prescher et al., 1990, 1995, 1996;

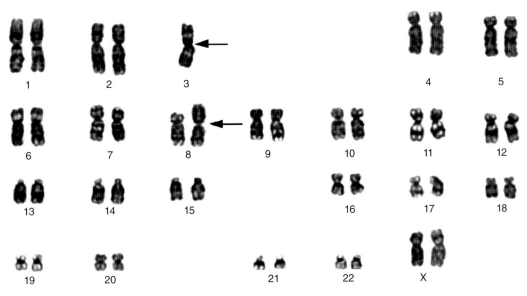

Figure 21.2 Karyotype of a ciliary body uveal melanoma, with characteristic monosomy 3 and i(8q).

Sisley et al., 1990, 2000; Horsman and White, 1993; Wiltshire et al., 1993; Singh et al., 1994; Naus et al., 2001; Kilic et al., 2006). Molecular cytogenetics has suggested that M3 may not actually be the most common change, as both 8q and chromosome 6 are frequently involved in complex rearrangements, leading to their underestimation in earlier cytogenetic investigations (Naus et al., 2001; Sisley et al., 2006; Ehlers et al., 2008; Trolet et al., 2009; Ewens et al., 2013). It is not clear whether this is a true reflection, as M3 is more common among a subset of UM, ciliary body melanomas, the number of which varies between studies (Sisley et al., 1990, 1992, 2006; Dahlenfors et al., 1993; Horsman and White, 1993; Wiltshire et al., 1993; Singh et al., 1994; Prescher et al., 1996; Naus et al., 2001). Cytogenetic investigations imply that M3 is a primary predisposing change since, when present, it is usually found within all abnormal cells analyzed, but FISH analysis suggests that regional heterogeneity for M3 exists among some UM (not necessarily accounting for cytogenetically abnormal cells per se), which has clinical implications when sampling (Maat et al., 2007; Mensink et al., 2009; Bronkhorst et al., 2011; Chang et al., 2013; Aronow et al., 2012).

The preponderance for M3 and paucity of chromosome 3 rearrangements in UM (approximately 5% of cases) suggest that loss of an entire copy is fundamental to UM development, representing the most efficacious way to target multiple genes resident on a single chromosome. Translocations and other rearrangements of both arms identify regional involvement at 3p24–25, 3p13, 3q13–21, and 3q24–26 and correspond to reported molecular deletions in UM (Blasi et al., 1999; Naus et al., 2001; Tschentscher et al., 2001; Parrella et al., 2003; Cross et al., 2006; van Gils et al., 2008; Trolet et al., 2009). The defining events underlying the cytogenetic presentation of M3 remain to be elucidated, but a number of candidate genes, with important regulatory consequences, could act as possible drivers for UM pathogenesis. The clearest association has been made for the BRCA1-associated protein 1 gene (BAP1), residing at 3p21. Mutations of BAP1, thought to occur in approximately 50–80% of UM, correlate with loss of the protein, M3, and poor prognosis as a consequence of metastasis to

the liver (Harbour et al., 2010; Koopmans et al., 2014). The gene interacts with BRCA1, with a potential role in DNA double-strand break repair (Yu et al., 2014) and regulation of genome stability in UM. Its exact role is unclear, as UM generally have low levels of genetic instability (Cross et al., 2006; Hoh et al., 2011; Furney et al., 2013; Mitelman et al., 2014). It seems counterintuitive that a TSG whose loss or mutation should promote genetic instability does not correlate in UM with such an apparent deregulation. Clearly, there is evidence for a biological role important to UM progression, but it remains to be established if mutation of BAP1 is truly a defining event or if other genes on chromosome 3 are equally important or, more so, are drivers of UM pathogenesis.

Chromosome 8

The next most frequent alteration is gain of chromosome arm 8q (approximately 45% of cases), mostly through structural rearrangements and often because an isochromosome for 8q is generated, but covert rearrangements uncovered by molecular cytogenetic studies suggest frequency figures between 55 and 75% may not be unrealistic (Gordon et al., 1994; Speicher et al., 1994; Naus et al., 2001; Sisley et al., 2006; Ehlers et al., 2008; Trolet et al., 2009; Damato et al., 2010; Ewens et al., 2013). There is segregation within UM for 8q gain, as the simplest form of trisomy is found among all posterior UM, while i(8q) is more common in melanomas with ciliary body involvement often with M3 (Figure 21.2), and partial gain of 8q through other rearrangements associates with choroid melanomas (Prescher et al., 1990; Sisley et al., 1990, 2000, 2006; Horsman and White, 1993; Wiltshire et al., 1993; Singh et al., 1994; Prescher et al., 1994, 1995; Naus et al., 2001; Kilic et al., 2006). Gain of 8q is cumulative and the process can best be seen in individual UM, where sublines coexist with either trisomy 8, single i(8q), or multiple i(8q) (Figure 21.3) and variations thereof, while other chromosome abnormalities are maintained at the same level (Horsman and White, 1993; Wiltshire et al., 1993; Prescher et al., 1994; Sisley et al., 2000). Abnormalities of 8q appear to be subsequent to either M3 or 6p gain (Prescher et al.,

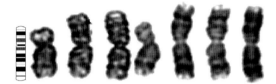

Figure 21.3 Examples of 8q gain from two cases of uveal melanoma. Gain of 8q in the form of an isochromosome, or otherwise, is progressively acquired, and individual karyotypes from the same tumor often show a trend for increasing the copy numbers of the abnormal chromosome 8. Here, in the first example, an i(8q) is duplicated, but in the second case, the abnormal chromosome arises through translocation der(8)t(8;8) (p21;q13), which is subsequently duplicated.

1994; Sisley et al., 1997; Parrella et al., 1999; Ehlers et al., 2008) and are the most consistent aberration of hepatic lesions suggesting that genes targeted by gain of 8q are important to the progression and development of metastases (Parada et al., 1999; Aalto et al., 2001; Taylan et al., 2007; Singh et al., 2009; Trolet et al., 2009; Fang et al., 2012).

As the entire 8q arm is often amplified, defining regional involvement has not been easy with cytogenetic studies initially identifying 8q21-qter as the minimal region (Prescher et al., 1990), whereas later investigations using comparative genomic hybridization (CGH) and spectral karyotyping (SKY) proposed two distinct regions, at 8q21.1–21.2 and again at 8q23–24 (Speicher et al., 1994; Prescher et al., 1995; Naus et al., 2001; Hughes et al., 2005; Trolet et al., 2009). Potential target genes include the *MYC* oncogene (8q24), which is specifically amplified and associated with UM progression (Parrella et al., 2001), *DDEF1*, a gene overexpressed in UM (Ehlers et al., 2005), and *ENPP2*, the gene for autotoxin, which is an independent predictor of UM prognosis (Onken et al., 2004; Singh et al., 2007). It is, however, fair to say that none appear to be strong candidates, particularly as the increased expression of both *MYC* and *ENPP2* is ambiguous, being associated with better outcomes (Chana et al., 1999; Onken et al., 2004; Singh et al., 2007). Furthermore, studies have highlighted deletions of 8p as relevant (Ewens et al., 2013), but as i(8q) is a recurrent cumulative abnormality, it is unclear if genes on 8p are of importance or bystanders in the drive to amplify the long arm.

Chromosome 6

Initially identified in the first cytogenetic studies of these tumors (Rey et al., 1985; Griffin et al., 1988), rearrangements of chromosome 6 affecting both arms have proved to be some of the most consistently observed alterations in UM. Deletions of 6q occur in 22% of UM, while gains of 6p are slightly more frequent (36% of cases); as in RB, they often present as an i(6p) (Prescher et al., 1990, 1995, 1996; Sisley et al., 1990, 2000; Horsman and White, 1993; Wiltshire et al., 1993; Singh et al., 1994; Naus et al., 2001; Kilic et al., 2006). Given that both arms are implicated and the complex nature of some chromosome 6 rearrangements, a more realistic estimate may be as high as 70% of UM, making them the most persistent nonrandom alteration associated with these melanomas (Sisley et al., 2006; Trolet et al., 2009).

A bifurcated tumor pathway was initially proposed, in which gain of 6p and M3 are mutually exclusive early defining events representing two genetic subgroups of UM (Parrella et al., 1999). Cytogenetic studies have clear examples where M3 and 6p gain are present in the same karyotype, however (Prescher et al., 1990; Horsman and White 1993; Sisley et al., 2000; Aalto et al., 2001; Hughes et al., 2005). Gain of 6p does assist in defining genetic subgroups of UM but only in context with both M3 and 8q gain; gain of 6p is twice as likely to arise from unbalanced translocations than as an i(6p), and isochromosome formation, including i(6p) and i(8q), mostly associates with M3 (Prescher et al., 1990; Horsman and White 1993; Sisley et al., 2000; Aalto et al., 2001; Hughes et al., 2005; Damato et al., 2010). These alterations reflect fundamental differences in UM themselves, since i(6p) associates with large melanomas of a mixed cell type and ciliary body involvement, while 6p gain through unbalanced translocations is more frequent among choroid tumors with a spindle cell type (Sisley et al., 2006; van Gils et al., 2008), broadly dividing along the lines of relationship with cell type and tumor location (Figure 21.4).

Although breakpoints in 6p are mainly centromeric, regional involvement of the long arm is poorly defined, with seemingly at least two deleted regions, at 6q24–27 and 6q13–15, and a potential third at 6q21–22 (Prescher et al., 1990; Horsman and White, 1993; Wiltshire et al., 1993; Gordon

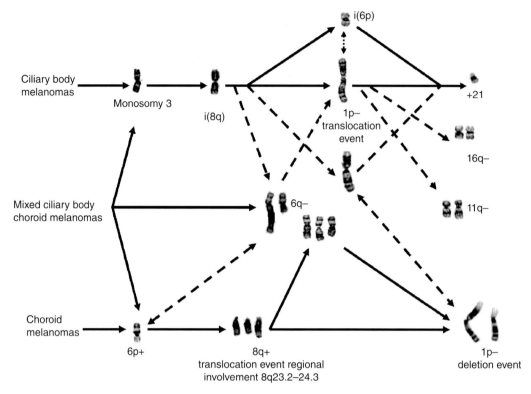

Figure 21.4 Two pathways of sequential chromosome changes are found in uveal melanoma, which correlate essentially with tumor location. There are some shared regions of chromosome involvement, but there are mechanistic differences in how these changes arise. The dashed lines indicate where the sequence is not well established, often where there is possible intersection between the pathways. Tumors with both ciliary body and choroid involvement as a group have features of both pathways, presumably because these melanomas when initially developing would favor the pathway related to their location but are subsequently grouped together.

et al., 1994; Singh et al., 1994; Prescher et al., 1995; Sisley et al., 2000; Kilic et al., 2006; Mitelman et al., 2014). Alterations of chromosome arm 6q appear to be a common feature of all UM and also cutaneous and conjunctival melanomas (White et al., 1995; Sisley et al., 1998; Mudhar et al., 2013; Mitelman et al., 2014). The same genes implicated in cutaneous melanoma are possibly also integral to the development of UM, but although candidate genes have been proposed, their importance has not been clearly established (Abdel-Rahman et al., 2005; Metzelaar-Blok et al., 2005; McCannel et al., 2011).

Chromosome 1

Approximately a quarter of UM have deletion of the short arm, del(1p), either through loss of the distal region or as an unbalanced translocation

(Mitelman et al., 2014). These changes are more frequent among larger UM that have metastasized or are metastases themselves and also correlate with M3, gain of 8q, and ciliary body involvement (Prescher et al., 1990, 1995; Sisley et al., 1990, 2000; Horsman and White 1993; Wiltshire et al., 1993; Singh et al., 1994; Aalto et al., 2001; Naus et al., 2001, 2002; Hausler et al., 2005; Kilic et al., 2005, 2006; Trolet et al., 2009). As a consequence, del(1p) is considered a marker of progressive disease (Aalto et al., 2001; Kilic et al., 2005) occurring after M3 and 8q gain (Figure 21.4). Breakpoints span 1p12–36 but are focused at 1p32–36, and probes mapping to 1p36 are deleted in 35% of UM (Prescher et al., 1990, 1995; Horsman and White, 1993; Sisley et al., 2000; Aalto et al., 2001; Naus et al., 2002; Kilic et al., 2005, 2006). Unbalanced rearrangements usually result in the loss of 1p in its entirety and feature repeated pairings with D group chromosomes and 8q, with breakpoints concentrated in the repetitive sequences of satellites; possibly, their inherent weakness makes them easy targets (Sisley et al., 2000). As similar changes are not a common feature of other cancers, it implies they may have a specific role in UM. Strong candidate genes have not emerged, but since the deletion is large, it would seem reasonable that more than one gene is targeted.

Other chromosome changes

Less is known about the importance of other chromosome changes; certainly, larger UM have greater chromosome instability so many of the less frequent alterations are likely to be unspecific rather than drivers of tumor progression (Sisley et al., 2000; Ehlers et al., 2008). Loss of the Y chromosome may be an early change, as most male patients selectively show it in tumor parenchyma cells but not in cells belonging to the tumor stroma or corresponding lymphocytes, and the change features equally among UM with minimal alterations and those with complex heterogeneous karyotypes (Prescher et al., 1990; Horsman and White, 1993; Wiltshire et al., 1993; Singh et al., 1996; White et al., 1998). Deletion or rearrangement of 9p and alteration of 10q occur in 10–20% of posterior UM, which may be an underestimate (Prescher et al., 1990, 1995; Horsman and White, 1993; Wiltshire et al., 1993; Singh et al., 1994; Gordon et al., 1994; Speicher et al., 1994; Sisley et al., 2000, 2006; Naus et al., 2001; Kilic et al., 2006). The changes are akin to those observed in cutaneous melanoma and potentially target the *P16* and *PTEN* genes, respectively, with possible implications for familial forms of UM (Singh et al., 1996; van der Velden et al., 2001; Abdel-Rahman et al., 2006; Buecher et al., 2010); epigenetic regulation of both genes may be more relevant (Naus et al., 2000; van der Velden et al., 2001). Possibly associated with genetic subtypes of UM are abnormalities of chromosomes 11, 16, and 21. Rearrangements of chromosome 11, affecting 11p15 or as deletion of 11q23–25, are found in 20% of UM, and del(11q) correlates with choroidal melanomas or those of a spindle morphology (Dahlenfors et al., 1993; Horsman and White, 1993; Singh et al., 1994; Speicher et al., 1994; Sisley et al., 2000, 2006). Approximately 10% of UM have deletions of 16q and trisomy 21, both of which occur secondarily to M3, 8q gain, and/or del(1p), indicative of tumor progression (Prescher et al., 1990, 1995; Dahlenfors et al., 1993; Horsman and White, 1993; Wiltshire et al., 1993; Singh et al., 1994; Sisley et al., 2000; Hoglund et al., 2004; Kilic et al., 2006; Trolet et al., 2009).

Specific genes in UM

Surprisingly, a number of mutations have been related to UM in spite of the fact that they occur in genes that are not effectively targeted by the common cytogenetic alterations associated with UM. This does not apply to *BAP1*, which is a potential target for M3 (Harbour et al., 2010). Of the others, the best known is guanine nucleotide binding protein Q polypeptide (*GNAQ*) and its paralog *GNA11* (Van Raamsdonk et al., 2009, 2010; Koopmans et al., 2013), the mutations of which are mutually exclusive affecting around 80% of posterior UM and relating to an upregulation of the mitogen-activated protein kinase (MAPK) pathway. More recently implicated are the splicing factor 3B1 subunit 1 (*SF3B1*) and eukaryotic translation initiation factor 1A, X-linked (*EIF1AX*) genes (Furney et al., 2013; Harbour et al., 2013a; Martin et al., 2013), both of which associate with disomy 3 UM and seem to be correlated with a good prognosis. Whole gene sequencing has confirmed cytogenetic observations suggesting that UM has a relatively uncomplicated genetic basis with a high degree of stability (Furney et al., 2013). These findings suggest that we still have much to learn about the underlying genetic landscape of UM, since the consistency of nonrandom cytogenetic alterations implies specific genes are the target, or at the very least, fundamental deregulatory changes are an issue. It is of interest that UM are singularly unusual by having a lower than normal level of sister chromatid exchanges (SCE), whereas all available evidences in other cancers suggest that genetic instability should lead to an increase in SCE (Hoh et al., 2011). It is possible that loss of the Fanconi anemia group D2 (*FANCD2*) gene is part of the deregulatory changes contributing to the genetic stability of UM (Gravells et al., 2013).

Based on the available cytogenetic information, posterior UM seem to follow either of two genetic pathways (Parrella et al., 1999). Given that they broadly correlate with well-established prognostic criteria and tumor location (Figure 21.4), it is perhaps warranted to consider UM of the choroid and ciliary body as genetically distinct diseases. The alterations of the two pathways are not mutually exclusive, however, and posterior UM with both choroid and ciliary body involvement often have an admixture of chromosome changes; this is not altogether unexpected considering that some of these melanomas would originate within the choroid, while others initiate from the ciliary body. There will always be exception to the rules, and there is undoubtedly crossover whereby potentially the same underlying genetic defects are shared, while other changes may be compensatory but in the end produce the same result. The essential difference is the manner whereby these cytogenetic changes arise, with the M3 ciliary body pathway featuring alterations with a centromeric focus (isochromosome and rearrangements targeting repetitive sequences) and with the implementation of the M3 route providing a drive to metastasis.

Clinical consequences

Even from the early investigations of UM, clear associations between specific chromosome abnormalities and clinical parameters, including patient outcome, were apparent (Sisley et al., 1990, 1997; Prescher et al., 1992, 1996). It is now widely accepted that analysis of the genetic changes in UM is highly and consistently predictive and probably the single most effective predictor of prognosis. The salient genetic changes are those involving chromosomes 3 and 8, with support from rearrangements of 1 and 6. In the first study to demonstrate a clear association, Prescher et al. (1996) found that only 57% of patients with M3 survived for more than 3 years after diagnosis, whereas all patients with disomy 3 were alive. Shortly following, in addition to confirming the importance of M3, 8q gain was also correlated with poor prognosis. A dosage effect was seen whereby the presence of additional copies of 8q was not only found to be predictive but higher amplifications correlated with a reduced disease-free interval

(Sisley et al., 1997). Later associations between del(1p) and a poor prognosis have also been made, specifically when M3 is concurrent with loss of 1p36 (Sisley et al., 2000; Naus et al., 2002; Hausler et al., 2005; Kilic et al., 2005). On the other hand, abnormalities of chromosome 6 seem to indicate a better prognosis (White et al., 1998; Parrella et al., 1999; Onken et al., 2004; Sisley et al., 2006; Damato et al., 2010).

Although M3 was originally considered the most important marker and initially extensively used, predictive reliability is enhanced when more than one change is considered, as seen for M3 in combination with gain of 8q (Sisley et al., 1997; Patel et al., 2001; Trolet et al., 2009; Damato et al., 2010; Onken et al., 2012; van den Bosch et al., 2012). Studies now employ tests that combine the predictive power of changes affecting chromosomes 1, 3, 6, and 8 (Shields et al., 2007; Chang et al., 2013). There are now a plethora of publications demonstrating clear relationships between the essential chromosomal markers and poor prognosis, and genetic testing has become part of the standard clinical assessment of most, but certainly not all, newly presenting UM patients. The relative virtue of testing for these changes has also been the subject of debate, as knowledge of outcome may not essentially alter patient management. Perhaps the most hotly debated area is consideration of which methodology should be advocated, with proponents of array CGH, FISH, mixed ligation-dependent probe amplification, microsatellite analysis, single-nucleotide polymorphisms, and expression arrays differing in their views as to which technology enables the most reliable assessment (Onken et al., 2007, 2012; Damato et al., 2010; McCannel et al., 2011; Aronow et al., 2012; Lake et al., 2012; Thomas et al., 2012; Vaarwater et al., 2012; Ewens et al., 2013; Cassoux et al., 2014). All techniques undoubtedly have their merits, whether it is ease of interpretation, cost, applicability to material (needle biopsies or formalin-fixed sections), and the amount of information they provide. The bottom line is that whatever method is applied, between 5 and 15% of UM will still be assigned incorrectly to risk subgroups. So what are the variables?

Firstly, by considering more reference points on chromosomes 1, 3, 6, and 8, it is hoped that the exact and as yet unknown region of prognostic sensitivity for each chromosome (bearing in mind whole arms are affected) will be included in the test. Certainly, partial deletions or rearrangements of chromosome 3 could be missed in the more simplistic tests, although studies so far suggest UM with structural alterations of chromosome 3 have an intermediate or similar prognosis as disomy 3 UM (Cross et al., 2006; Abdel-Rahman et al., 2011; Thomas et al., 2012). Although deletion of 8p has been linked to the development of metastasis, the majority of studies show stronger evidence for an 8q role (Trolet et al., 2009; Fang et al., 2012; van den Bosch et al., 2012). Since the smallest regional gain of 8q seems less variable and still affects the majority of the arm, selection of probes for 8q should be, but is not necessarily, less of an issue. Gain of 6p is perhaps the least reliable, and when assessing its prognostic power, several points should be considered. Firstly, the observed protective effect could be attributed to either overrepresentation of 6p or loss of 6q. It is likely that gain of 6p is the defining event as 6p gain through unbalanced translocations associates with clinical parameters of a good outcome (spindle morphology) and the nonmetastasizing phenotype, as well as being the first visible alteration of the non-M3 poor prognosis genetic pathway (Parrella et al., 1999; Onken et al., 2004; Sisley et al., 2006). Incorrectly assigning a good prognosis could happen in those UM where the gain is in the form of i(6p) as this change relates ostensibly to tumors with the poor markers of M3 and i(8q) (Figure 21.4).

To improve reliability, techniques that globally assess changes of chromosomes 1, 3, 6, and 8, such as array CGH, whole gene sequencing, or indeed banding cytogenetics itself, should perhaps become the favored option, assuming cost and availability of equipment are not an issue. As always, there is a "but," as there is now increasing evidence that heterogeneity within UM is an issue that can cause sampling problems (Maat et al., 2007; Mensink et al., 2009; Bronkhorst et al., 2011; Aronow et al., 2012; Chang et al., 2013). In addition, it seems that a greater percentage of abnormal cells within a UM population correlates with reduced disease-free interval (van den Bosch et al., 2012) echoing the evidence that increasing dosage of 8q gain shows

the same correlation (Sisley et al., 1997; Patel et al., 2001; van den Bosch et al., 2012). Ultimately, the percentage of burden within UM for certain abnormalities could be the critical factor that relates not only to the inevitability of metastases but the speed at which they present. Tests that consider heterogeneity such as FISH may therefore be preferable, but then we have of course come full circle and are at risk of missing sensitive predictive regions. Finally, most studies have only relatively short periods of follow-up, and in the end, the variations between methodologies may be reduced. Following on from an original study published at the beginning of the millennium (Patel et al., 2001), FISH analysis for copy number changes of chromosomes 3 and 8 has been routinely performed in Sheffield (unpublished data). Considering any combination that gives rise to more copies of chromosome 8 compared to chromosome 3 (termed as a relative genetic imbalance or RGI), in a series of 500 patients studied over 20 years, we found most patients with an RGI died from metastatic disease within 7 years, while at 10 years the majority of patients without an RGI survived, with many still alive at 15 years and above (Figure 21.5).

Assuming cost is not an issue, maybe all UM should be tested by a combination of techniques. The wrong assignments would undoubtedly reduce, as the limitations of individual tests will be compensated for by the others, but there are always going to be UM that are exceptions to the rule. For example, iris melanomas rarely metastasize, yet using expression arrays, they would be misclassified on the basis of their profiles as having a poor prognosis (Harbour et al., 2013b). Until we know exactly why UM get these consistent cytogenetic alterations and what impact they have on melanogenesis, there will always be issues with any test. The general confidence in genetic testing has allowed for the selection of high-risk UM patients to be included into clinical trials, however, although trials use inhibitors that are not specific to the chromosomal markers of high-risk UM patients.

Iris and conjunctival melanoma

As anterior iris melanomas are infrequent (5% of UM) and only rarely removed, there are few cytogenetic reports on such tumors. However, recent

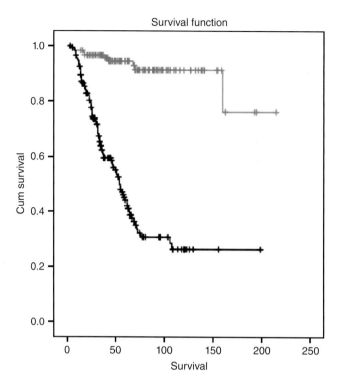

Figure 21.5 Kaplan–Meier survival curve for uveal melanoma patients with a relative genetic imbalance (RGI) for chromosomes 3 and 8. Patients with an RGI have a significantly poorer prognosis (black).

FISH and other studies have provided more background (White et al., 1995; Sisley et al., 1998; Vajdic et al., 2003; Mensink et al., 2011; Shields et al., 2011; Harbour et al., 2013b). Although pseudodiploid, iris melanomas appear more complex than posterior UM in spite of the fact that they share some similarities, such as abnormalities of chromosomes 3, 6, and 8 (White et al., 1995; Sisley et al., 1998; Vajdic et al., 2003). The type of anomaly varies, for example, partial deletions of chromosome 3 are more common in iris tumors (Mensink et al., 2011; Shields et al., 2011), but gain of 8q appears fairly consistent. Alterations of other chromosomes, such as 9p abnormalities, are infrequent in posterior UM but are more of a feature in iris melanomas (Mensink et al., 2011). There are parallels with posterior UM, but iris melanomas share more changes with cutaneous melanoma (e.g., 9p alterations and increased heterogeneity) than with posterior UM. One could perhaps think of iris melanoma as representing a genetic midpoint between posterior UM and cutaneous melanoma, and in this context, it is of interest that reports on the cytogenetic changes found in conjunctival melanoma show a drift toward the genetic characteristics of the cutaneous tumors (Vajdic et al., 2003; Keijser et al., 2007; Griewank et al., 2013; Mudhar et al., 2013). Certainly, conjunctival melanomas share the same mutations of V-RAF murine sarcoma viral oncogene homolog B1 (*BRAF*) that are found in cutaneous but not UM (Griewank et al., 2013). Because of the mutually exclusive nature of *BRAF* (conjunctival and cutaneous melanoma) and *GNAQ/GNA11* (UM), mutational screening can be used to distinguish equivocal cases of eye melanomas.

Other eye tumors

Scant information is available on other forms of primary eye tumors (Mitelman et al., 2014), but where reported, most have pseudodiploid karyotypes that are generally consistent with those observed for the same type of cancer presenting in other locations. Ocular B-cell lymphomas mainly have deletions and rearrangements of chromosome 1, trisomy 3 and deletions of 3p, trisomy 12, and translocations involving chromosome 18, including t(14;18), all characteristic changes of lymphoma (Auer et al., 1997; Cook et al., 2004; Mitelman et al., 2014). A few cases of adenoma and adenoid cystic carcinoma had translocations affecting 8q11–12 (Hrynchak et al., 1994). Sporadic gliomas, peripheral nerve sheath tumors, rhabdomyosarcomas, neurofibrosarcomas, neuroepitheliomas, and medulloepitheliomas mostly had pseudodiploid karyotypes with complex and ill-defined aberrations (Mitelman et al., 2014).

Concluding remarks

With the emergence of high throughput genome sequencing techniques, we can expect over the next decade to gain new and valuable insights into the genetic basis of the rarer forms of eye tumors as well as into the pathogenetic mechanisms of tumors we already know a lot about. Cytogenetic studies have been integral to our growing understanding of how eye tumors occur, with the identification of a deleted 13q in RB providing the foundation upon which an entire branch of cancer genetics has been built. Evidence for a relationship between the secondary changes in both RB and UM has increased. As tumor heterogeneity remains an issue, cytogenetics can still be expected to play an important part in furthering our understanding of how variations in subpopulations affect tumor development and progression.

Acknowledgments

Thank you to Dr D.M. Lillington, St Bartholomew's Hospital Medical College, for the deleted chromosome 13 image. I would like to express my gratitude to the support provided for research by Yorkshire Cancer Research, Trent Regional Health Authority, the Medical Research Council, Weston Park Hospital Cancer Charity, and Yorkshire Eye Research. My thanks go to the contributions made to studies over the past 25 years by David Hammond, David Canovas, Neil Cross, Helen Denney, Kirtikbhai A Patel, Linda Smith Thomas, and Nicola Tattersall and, also, Arran, Bethany, and Finn for their ability to keep you grounded.

References

Aalto Y, Eriksson L, Seregard S, Larsson O, Knuutila S (2001): Concomitant loss of chromosome 3 and whole arm losses and gains of chromosomes 1,6, or 8 in metastasizing primary uveal melanoma. *Invest Ophthalmol Vis Sci* 42:313–317.

Abdel-Rahman MH, Craig EL, Davidorf FH, Eng C (2005): Expression of vascular endothelial growth factor in uveal melanoma is independent of 6p21-region copy number. *Clin Cancer Res* 11:73–78.

Abdel-Rahman MH, Yang Y, Zhou XP, Craig EL, Davidorf FH, Eng C (2006): High frequency of submicroscopic hemizygous deletion is a major mechanism of loss of expression of PTEN in uveal melanoma. *J Clin Oncol* 24:288–295.

Abdel-Rahman MH, Christopher BN, Faramawi MF, Said-Ahmed K, Cole C, McFaddin A, et al. (2011): Frequency, molecular pathology and potential clinical significance of partial chromosome 3 aberrations in uveal melanoma. *Mod Pathol* 24:954–962.

Abouzeid H, Munier FL, Thonney F, Schorderet DF (2007): Ten novel *RB1* gene mutations in patients with retinoblastoma. *Mol Vis* 13:1740–1745.

Abouzeid H, Schorderet DF, Balmer A, Munier FL (2009): Germline mutations in retinoma patients: relevance to low–penetrance and low- expressivity molecular basis. *Mol Vis* 15:771–777.

Amare Kadam PS, Ghule P, Jose J, Bamne M, Kurkure P, Banavali S, et al. (2004): Constitutional genomic instability, chromosome aberrations in tumor cells and retinoblastoma. *Cancer Genet Cytogenet* 150:33–43.

Aronow M, Sun Y, Sauntharararajah Y, Biscotti C, Tubbs R, Triozzi P, et al. (2012): Monosomy 3 by FISH in uveal melanoma: variability in techniques and results. *Surv Ophthalmol* 57:463–473.

Auer IA, Gascoyne RD, Connors JM, Cotter FE, Greiner TC, Sanger WG, et al. (1997): t(11;18)(q21;q21) is the most common translocation in MALT lymphomas. *Ann Oncol* 10:979–985.

Barros JEXS, Soares-Ventura EM, Santos N, Amaral BAS, Oliveira FM, Vera Cruz RS, et al. (2012): New cytogenetic aberrations in a case of aggressive retinoblastoma. *Genet Mol Res* 11:1666–1670.

Blasi MA, Roccella E, Balestrazzi E, Del Porto G, De Felice N, Roccella M, et al. (1999): 3p13 region: a possible location of a tumour suppressor gene involved in uveal melanoma. *Cancer Genet Cytogenet* 108:81–83.

Bronkhorst IHG, Maat W, Jordanova ES, Kroes WGM, Schalij NE, Luyten GPM, et al. (2011): Effect of heterogeneous distribution of monosomy 3 on prognosis in uveal melanoma. *Arch Pathol Lab Med* 135:1042–1047.

Buecher B, Gauthier-Villars M, Desjardins L, Lumbroso-Le Rouic L, Levy C, De Pauw A, et al. (2010): Contribution of CDKN2A/P16INK4A, P14ARF,CDK4 and BRCA1/2 germline mutations in individuals with suspected genetic predisposition to uveal melanoma. *Familial Cancer* 9: 663–667.

Cassoux N, Rodrigues MJ, Plancher C, Asselain B, Lvey-Gabriel C, Lumbroso-Le Rouic L, et al. (2014): Genome-wide profiling is a clinically relevant and affordable prognostic test in posterior uveal melanoma. *Br J Ophthalmol* 98:769–774.

Chana JS, Wilson GD, Cree IA, Alexander RA, Myatt N, Neale M, et al. (1999): C-myc, p53, and Bcl-2 expression and clinical outcome in uveal melanoma. *Br J Ophthalmol* 83:110–114.

Chang MY, Rao NP, Burgess BL, Johnson L, McCannel TA (2013): Heterogeneity of monosomy 3 in fine needle aspiration biopsy of choroidal melanoma. *Mol Vision* 19:1892–1900.

Cook JR, Shekhter-Levin S, Swerdlow SH (2004): Utility of routine classical cytogenetic studies in the evaluation of suspected lymphomas: results of 279 consecutive lymph node/extranodal tissue biopsies. *Am J Clin Pathol* 121:826–835.

Corson TW, Gallie BL (2007): One hit, two hits, three hits, more? Genomic changes in the development of retinoblastoma. *Genes Chromosomes Cancer* 46:617–634.

Cowell JK, Hogg A (1992): Genetics and cytogenetics of retinoblastoma. *Cancer Genet Cytogenet* 64:1–11.

Cowell JK, Hungerford J, Rutland P, Jay M (1987): A chromosomal breakpoint which separates the esterase-D and retinoblastoma predisposition loci in a patient with del(13)(q14-31). *Cancer Genet Cytogenet* 27: 27–31.

Cross NA, Ganesh A, Parpia M, Murray AK, Rennie IG, Sisley K (2006): Multiple locations on chromosome 3 are the targets of specific deletions in uveal melanoma. *Eye* 20:476–481.

Dahlenfors R, Tornqvist G, Wettrell K, Mark J (1993): Cytogenetic observations in nine ocular malignant melanoma. *Anticancer Res* 13:1415–1420.

Damato B, Dopierala JA, Coupland SE (2010): Genotypic profiling of 452 choroidal melanomas with multiplex ligation-dependent probe amplification. *Clin Cancer Res* 16:6083–6092.

Dimaras H, Khetan V, Halliday W, Orlic M, Prigoda NL, Piovesan B, et al. (2008): Loss of RB1 induces non-proliferative retinoma: increasing genomic instability correlates with progression to retinoblastoma. *Hum Mol Genet* 17:1363–1372.

Duncan AMW, Morgan C, Gallie BL, Phillips RA, Squire J (1987): Re-evaluation of the sublocalization of esterase-D and its relation to the retinoblastoma locus by in situ hybridization. *Cytogenet Cell Genet* 44:153–157.

Ehlers JP, Worley L, Onken MD, Harbour JW (2005): DDEF1 is located in an amplified region of chromosome 8q and is overexpressed in uveal melanoma. *Clin Cancer Res* 11: 3609–3613.

Ehlers JP, Worley L, Onken M, Harbour JW (2008): Integrative genomic analysis of aneuploidy in uveal melanoma. *Clin Can Res* 14:115–122.

Ewens KG, Kanetsky PA, Richards-Yutz J, Al-Dahmash S, Carla De Luca M, Bianciotto CG, et al. (2013): Genomic profile of 320 uveal melanoma cases: chromosome 8p-loss and metastatic outcome. *Invest Ophthalmol Vis Sci* 54:5721–5729.

Fang Y, Wang X, Dusza S, Jhanwar S, Abramson D, Busam KJ (2012): Use of fluorescence in situ hybridization to distinguish metastatic uveal melanoma from cutaneous melanoma. *Int J Surg Pathol* 20:246–251.

Friend SH, Bernards R, Rogelj S, Weinberg RA, Rapaport JM, Albert DM, et al. (1986): A human DNA segment with properties of the gene that predisposes to retinoblastoma and osteosarcoma. *Nature* 323:643–646.

Fung YT, Murphree Al, T'ang A, Qian J, Hinrichs SH, Benedict WF (1987): Structural evidence for the authenticity of the human retinoblastoma gene. *Science* 236:1657–1661.

Furney SJ, Pedersen M, Gentien D, Dumont AG, Rapinat A, Desjardins L, et al. (2013): SF3B1 mutations are associated with alternative splicing in uveal melanoma. *Cancer Discov* 3:1122–1129.

Gordon KB, Thompson CT, Char DH, O'Brien JM, Kroll S, Ghazvini S, et al. (1994): Comparative genomic hybridization in the detection of DNA copy number abnormalities in uveal melanoma. *Cancer Res* 54:4764–4768.

Gratias S, Schüler A, Hitpass LK, Stephan H, Rieder H, Schneider S, et al. (2005): Genomic gains on chromosome 1q in retinoblastoma: consequences on gene expression and association with clinical manifestation. *Int J Cancer* 116:555–563.

Gravells P, Hoh L, Solovieva S, Patil A, Dudziec E, Rennie IG, et al. (2013): Reduced FANCD2 influences spontaneous SCE and RAD51 foci formation in uveal melanoma and Fanconi anaemia. *Oncogene* 32:5338–5346.

Griewank K, Westekemper H, Schilling B, Livingstone E, Schimming T, Sucker A, et al. (2013): Conjunctival melanoma harbour BRAF and NRAS mutations-response. *Clin Cancer Res* 19:6331–6332.

Griffin CA, Long PP, Schachat AP (1988): Trisomy 6p in an ocular melanoma. *Cancer Genet Cytogenet* 31:129–132.

Haigis K, Sage J, Glickman J, Shafer S, Jacks T (2006): The related retinoblastoma (pRb) and p130 proteins cooperate to regulate homeostasis in the intestinal epithelium. *J Biol Chem* 281:638–647.

Harbour JW, Onken MD, Roberson ED, Duan S, Cao L, Worley LA, et al. (2010): Frequent mutation of BAP1 in metastasizing uveal melanomas. *Science* 330:1410–1413.

Harbour JW, Roberson EDO, Anbunathan H, Onken MD, Worley LA, Bowcock AM (2013a): Recurrent mutations at codon 625 of the splicing factor SF3B1 in uveal melanoma. *Nat Genet* 45:133–135.

Harbour JW, Wilson D, Finger PT, Worley LA, Onken MD (2013b): Gene expression profiling of iris melanomas. *Ophthalmology* 120:213, 213.e1-3.

Hausler T, Stang A, Anastassiou G, Jockel KH, Mrzyk S, Horsthemke B, et al. (2005): Loss of heterozygosity of 1p in uveal melanomas with monosomy 3. *Int J Cancer* 116: 909–913.

Herzog S, Lohmann DR, Buiting K, Schüler A, Horstheke B, Rehder H, et al. (2001): Marked differences in unilateral isolated retinoblastomas from young and older children studied by comparative genomic hybridization. *Hum Genet* 108:98–104.

Hoglund M, Gisselsson D, Hansen GB, White VA, Sall T, Mitelman F, et al. (2004): Dissecting karyotypic patterns in malignant melanomas: temporal clustering of losses and gains in melanoma karyotypic evolution. *Int J Cancer* 108:57–65.

Hoh L, Gravells P, Canovas D, Ul-Hassan A, Rennie IG, Bryant H, et al. (2011): Atypically low spontaneous sister chromatid exchange formation in uveal melanoma. *Genes Chromosomes Cancer* 50:34–42.

Horsman D E, White V A (1993): Cytogenetic analysis of uveal melanoma. Consistent occurrence of monosomy 3 and trisomy 8q. *Cancer* 71:811–819.

Horsthemke B (1992): Genetics and cytogenetics of retinoblastoma. *Cancer Genet Cytogenet* 63:1–7.

Hossfeld DK (1978): Chromosome 14q + in a retinoblastoma. *Int J Cancer* 21:720–723.

Hughes S, Damato BE, Giddings I, Hiscott PS, Humphreys J, Houlston RS (2005): Microarray comparative genomic hybridisation analysis of intraocular uveal melanomas identifies distinctive imbalances associated with loss of chromosome 3. *Br J Cancer* 93:1191–1196.

Hrynchak M, White V, Berean K, Horsman DE (1994): Cytogenetic findings in seven lacrimal gland neoplasms. *Cancer Genet Cytogenet* 75:133–138.

Kapatai G, Brundler MA, Jenkinson H, Kearns P, Paruleker M, Peet AC, et al. (2013): Gene expression profiling identifies different sub-types of retinoblastoma. *Br J Cancer* 109: 512–525.

Keijser S, Maat W, Missotten GS, de Keizer RJ (2007): A new cell line from a recurrent conjunctival melanoma. *Br J Ophthalmol* 91:1566–1567.

Kiliç E, Naus NC, van Gils W, Klaver CC, Van Til ME, Verbiest MM, et al. (2005): Concurrent loss of chromosome arm 1p and chromosome 3 predicts a decreased disease-free survival in uveal melanoma patients. *Invest Ophthalmol Vis Sci* 46:2253–2257.

Kiliç E, van Gils W, Lodder E, Beverloo HB, van Til ME, Mooy CM, et al. (2006): Clinical and cytogenetic analyses in uveal melanoma. *Invest Ophthalmol Vis Sci* 47:3703–3707.

Knudson AG (1971): Mutation and cancer: statistical study of retinoblastoma. *Proc Natl Acad Sci USA* 68:820–823.

Koopmans AE, Vaarwater J, Paridaens D, Naus NC, Kiliç E, de Klein A, et al. (2013): Patient survival in uveal melanoma is not affected by oncogenic mutations in GNAQ and GNA11. *Br J Cancer* 109:493–496.

Koopmans AE, Verdijsk RM, Brouwer RWW, van den Bosch TPP, van den Berg MMP, Vaarwater J, et al. (2014): Clinical significance of immunohistochemistry for detection of BAP1 mutations in uveal melanoma. *Mod Pathol* 27:1321–1330.

Kusnetsova LE, Prigogina EL, Pogosianz HE, Belkina BM (1982): Similar chromosomal abnormalities in several retinoblastomas. *Hum Genet* 61:201–204.

Lake SL, Kalirai H, Dopieraia J, Damato B, Coupland SE (2012): Comparison of formalin-fixed and snap frozen samples analysed by multiplex ligation-dependent probe amplification for prognostic testing in uveal melanoma. *Invest Ophthalmol Vis Sci* 53:2647–2652.

Lee WH, Bookstein R, Hong F, Young LJ, Shew JY, Lee EYHP (1987): Human retinoblastoma susceptibility gene: cloning, identification, and sequence. *Science* 235:1394–1399.

Lemieux N, Milot J, Barsoum-Homsy M, Michaud J, Leung TK, Richer CL (1989): First cytogenetic evidence of homozygosity for the retinoblastoma deletion in chromosome 13. *Cancer Genet Cytogenet* 43:73–78.

Lillington DM, Kingston JE, Coen PG, Price E, Hungerford J, Domizio P, et al. (2003): Comparative genomic hybridization of 49 retinoblastoma tumors identifies chromosomal regions associated with histopathology, progression and patient outcome. *Genes Chromosom Cancer* 36:121–128.

Lohmann DR, Horsthemke B (1999): No association between the presence of a constitutional RB1 gene mutation and age in 68 patients with isolated unilateral retinoblastoma. *Eur J Cancer* 35:1035–1036.

Maat W, Jordanova ES, van Zelderen-Bhola SL, Barthen ER, Wessels HW, Schalij-Delfos NE, et al. (2007): The heterogeneous distribution of monosomy 3 in uveal melanomas. *Arch Pathol Lab Med* 131:91–96.

MacCarthy A, Draper GJ, Steliarova-Foucher E, Kingston JE (2006): Retinoblastoma incidence and survival in European children (1978–1997): report from the automated childhood cancer information system project. *Eur J Cancer* 42:2092–2102.

MacCarthy A, Bayne AM, Brownbill PA, Bunch KJ, Diggens NL, Draper GJ, et al. (2013): Second and subsequent tumours among 1927 retinoblastoma patients diagnosed in Britain 1951–2004. *Br J Cancer* 108:2455–2463.

Martin M, Masshöfer L, Temming P, Rahmann S, Metz C, Bornfeld N, et al. (2013): Exome sequencing identifies recurrent somatic mutations in EIF1AX and SF3B1 in uveal melanoma with disomy 3. *Nat Genet* 45:933–936.

McCannel TA, Burgess BL, Nelson SF, Eskin A, Straatsma BR (2011): Genomic identification of significant targets in ciliochoroidal melanoma. *Invest Ophthalmol Vis Sci* 52:3018–3022.

Mensink HW, Vaarwater J, Kilic E, Naus NC, Mooy NM, Luyten G, et al. (2009): Chromosome 3 intratumor heterogeneity in uveal melanoma. *Invest Ophthalmol Vis Sci* 50:500–504.

Mensink HW, Vaarwater J, de Keizer RJW, de Wolff-Rouendaal, Mooy CM, de Klein A, et al. (2011): Chromosomal aberrations in iris melanomas. *Br J Ophthalmol* 95:424–428.

Metzelaar-Blok JA, Hurks HM, Naipal A, De Lange P, Keunen JE, Claas FH, et al. (2005): Normal HLA class I, II and MICA gene distribution in uveal melanoma. *Mol Vis* 11:1166–1172.

Mitelman F, Johansson B, Mertens F, editors (2014): Mitelman Database of Chromosome Aberrations and Gene Fusions in Cancer. http://cgap.nci.nih.gov/Chromosomes/Mitelman.

Mol BM, Massink MPG, van der Hout AH, Dommering CJ, Zaman JMA, Bosscha MI, et al. (2014): High resolution SNP array profiling identifies variability in retinoblastoma genome stability. *Genes Chromosomes Cancer* 53:12–14.

Mudhar HS, Smith K, Talley P, Whitworth A, Atkey N Rennie IG (2013): Fluorescence in situ hybridization (FISH) in histologically challenging conjunctival melanocytic lesions. *Br J Ophthalmol* 97:40–46.

Naus NC, Zuidervaart W, Rayman N, Slater R, van Drunen E, Ksander B, et al. (2000): Mutation analysis of the PTEN gene in uveal melanoma cell lines. *Int J Cancer* 87: 151–153.

Naus NC, van Drunen E, De Klein A, Luyten GPM, Paridaens DA, Alers JC, et al. (2001): Characterization of complex chromosomal abnormalities in uveal melanoma by fluorescent in situ hybridization, spectral karyotyping and comparative genomic hybridization. *Genes Chromosomes Cancer* 30:267–273.

Naus NC, Verhoeven AC, van Drunen E, Slater R, Mooy CM, Paridaens DA, et al. (2002): Detection of genetic prognostic markers in uveal melanoma biopsies using fluorescence in situ hybridization. *Clin Cancer Res* 8:534–539.

Onken MD, Worley LA, Ehlers JP, Harbour JW (2004): Gene expression profiling in uveal melanoma reveals two molecular classes and predicts metastatic death. *Cancer Res* 64:7205–7209.

Onken MD, Worley LA, Person E, Char DH, Bowcock AM, Harbour JW (2007): Loss of heterozygosity of chromosome 3 detected with single nucleotide polymorphisms is superior to monosomy 3 for predicting metastasis in uveal melanoma. *Clin Cancer Res* 13:2923–2927.

Onken MD, Worley LA, Char DH, Augsburger JJ, Correa ZM, Nudleman E, et al. (2012): Collaborative ocular oncology group report no. 1: prospective validation of a multi-gene prognostic assay in uveal melanoma. *Ophthalmology* 119:1596–1603.

Paderova J, Orlic-Milacic M, Yoshimoto M, da Cunha Santos G, Gallie B, Squire JA (2007): Novel 6p rearrangements and recurrent translocation breakpoints in retinoblastoma cell lines identified by spectral karyotyping and mBAND analyses. *Cancer Genet Cytogenet* 179:102–111.

Parada LA, Maranon A, Hallen M, Tranberg KG, Stenram U, Bardi G, et al. (1999): Cytogenetic analysis of secondary liver tumours reveal significant differences in genomic imbalances between primary and metastatic colon carcinomas. *Clin Exp Metastasis* 17:471–479.

Parrella P, Sidransky D, Merbs SL (1999): Allelotype of posterior uveal melanoma: implications for a bifurcated tumour progression pathway. *Cancer Res* 59:3032–3037.

Parrella P, Caballero OL, Sidransky D, Merbs SL (2001): Detection of c-myc amplification in uveal melanoma by fluorescent in situ hybridization. *Invest Ophthalmol Vis Sci* 42:1679–1684.

Parrella P, Fazio VM, Gall AP, Sidransky D, Merbs SL (2003): Fine mapping of chromosome 3 in uveal melanoma: identification of a minimal region of deletion on chromosome arm 3p25.1-p25.2. *Cancer Res* 63:8507–8510.

Patel KA, Edmondson ND, Talbot F, Parsons MA, Rennie IG, Sisley K (2001): Prediction of prognosis in patients with uveal melanoma using fluorescence in situ hybridization. *Br J Ophthalmol* 85:1440–1444.

Prescher G, Bornfeld N, Becher R (1990): Non-random chromosomal abnormalities in primary uveal melanoma. *J Natl Cancer Inst* 82:1765–1769.

Prescher G, Bornfeld N, Horsthemke B, Becher R (1992): Chromosomal aberrations defining uveal melanoma of poor prognosis. *Lancet* 339:691–692.

Prescher G, Bornfeld N, Becher R (1994): Two subclones in a case of uveal melanoma. Relevance of monosomy 3 and multiplication of chromosome 8q. *Cancer Genet Cytogenet* 77:144–146.

Prescher G, Bornfeld N, Friedrichs W, Seeber S, Becher R (1995): Cytogenetics of twelve cases of uveal melanoma and patterns of nonrandom anomalies and isochromosome formation. *Cancer Genet Cytogenet* 80:40–46.

Prescher G, Bornfeld N, Hirche H, Horsthemke B, Karl-Heinz Jokel, Becher R (1996): Prognostic implications of monosomy 3 in uveal melanoma. *Lancet* 347: 1222–1225.

Priya K, Jada SR, Quah BL, Quah TC, Lai PS (2009): High incidence of allelic loss at 16q12.2 region spanning RBL2/p130 gene in retinoblastoma. *Cancer Biol Ther* 8:714–7167.

Reis AHO, Vargas FR, Lemos B (2012): More epigenetic hits than meets the eye: microRNAs and genes associated with the tumorigenesis of retinoblastoma. *Frontiers in Genetics* 3: article 284 1–10.

Rey JA, Bello MJ, de Campos JM, Ramos MC, Benitez J (1985): Cytogenetic findings in a human malignant melanoma metastatic to the brain. *Cancer Genet Cytogenet* 16:179–183.

Rushlow DE, Mol BM, Kennett JY, Yee S, Pajovic S, Thériault BL, et al. (2013): Characterization of retinoblastomas without RB1 mutations: genomic, gene expression, and clinical studies. *Lancet Oncology* 14: 327–334.

Sampieri K, Mencarelli MA, Epistolato MC, Toti P, Lazzi S, Bruttini M, et al. (2008): Genomic differences between retinoma and retinoblastoma. *Acta Oncol* 47:1483–1492.

Shields CL, Ganguly A, Materin MA, Teixeira L, Mashayekhi A, Swanson LA, et al. (2007): Chromosome 3 analysis of uveal melanoma using fine-needle aspiration biopsy at the time of plaque radiotherapy in 140 consecutive cases: the Deborah Iverson, MD, Lectureship. *Arch Ophthalmol* 125:1017–1024.

Shields CL, Ramasubramanian A, Ganguly A, Mohan D, Shields JA (2011): Cytogenetic testing of iris melanoma using fine needle aspiration biopsy in 17 patients. *Retina* 31:574–580.

Singh A D, Boghosian-Sell L, Wary KK, Shields CL, De Potter P, Donoso LA, et al. (1994): Cytogenetic findings in primary uveal melanoma. *Cancer Genet Cytogenet* 72: 109–115.

Singh AD, Wang MX, Donoso LA, Shields CL, De Potter P, Shields JA (1996): Genetic aspects of uveal melanoma: a brief review. *Semin Oncol* 23:768–772.

Singh AD, Sisley K, Xu Y, Li J, Faber P, Plummer SJ, et al. (2007): Reduced expression of Autotaxin predicts survival in uveal melanoma. *Br J Ophthalmol* 91:1385–1392.

Singh AD, Tubbs R, Biscotti C, Schoenfield LS, Trizzoi P (2009): Chromosomal 3 and 8 status within hepatic metastasis of uveal melanoma. *Arch Pathol Lab Med* 133: 1223–1227.

Sisley K, Rennie IG, Cottam DW, Potter AM, Potter CW, Rees RC (1990): Cytogenetic findings in six posterior uveal melanomas: involvement of chromosomes 3, 6 and 8. *Genes Chromosomes Cancer* 2:205–209.

Sisley K, Cottam DW, Rennie IG, Parsons MA, Potter AM, Potter CW, et al. (1992): Non-random abnormalities of chromosomes 3, 6, and 8 associated with posterior uveal melanoma. *Genes Chromosomes Cancer* 5:197–200.

Sisley K, Rennie IG, Parsons MA, Jacques R, Hammond DW, Bell SM, et al. (1997): Abnormalities of chromosomes 3 and 8, in posterior uveal melanoma, correlate with prognosis. *Genes Chromosomes Cancer* 19:22–28.

Sisley K, Brand C, Parsons MA, Maltby E, Rees RC, Rennie IG (1998): Cytogenetics of iris melanomas disparity with other uveal melanomas. *Cancer Genet Cytogenet* 101:128–133.

Sisley K, Parsons MA, Garnham J, Potter AM, Curtis DI, Rees RC, et al. (2000): Association of specific chromosome alterations with tumour phenotype in posterior uveal melanoma. *Br J Cancer* 82:330–338.

Sisley K, Tattersall N, Dyson M, Smith K, Mudhar HS, Rennie IG (2006): Multiplex fluorescence in situ hybridization identifies novel rearrangements of chromosomes 6, 15, and 18 in primary uveal melanoma. *Exp Eye Res* 83:554–559.

Sparkes RS, Sparkes MC, Kalina RE, Pagon RA, Salk DJ, Distechne CM (1984): Separation of retinoblastoma and esterase D loci in a patient with sporadic retinoblastoma and del(13)(q14.1q22.3). *Hum Genet* 68:258–259.

Speicher MR, Prescher G, du Manoir S, Jauch A, Horsthemke B, Bornfeld N, et al. (1994): Chromosomal gains and losses in uveal melanoma detected by comparative genomic hybridization. *Cancer Res* 54:3817–3823.

Squire J, Gallie BL, Phillips RA (1985): A detailed analysis of chromosomal changes in heritable and non-heritable retinoblastoma. *Hum Genet* 70:291–301.

Subtil-Rodríguez A, Vázquez-Chávez E, Ceballos-Chávez M, Rodríguez-Paredes M, Martín-Subero JI, Esteller M, et al. (2013): The chromatin remodeller CHD8 is required for E2F-dependent transcription activation of S-phase genes. *Nucleic Acids Res* 42:2185–2196.

Taylan H, Kiratli H, Aktas D (2007): Monosomy 7 mosaicism in metastatic choroidal melanoma. *Cancer Genet Cytogent* 177:70–72.

Thériault BL, Dimaras H, Gallie BL, Corson TW (2014): The genomic landscape of retinoblastoma: a review. *Clin Exp Ophthalmol* 42:33–52.

Thomas S, Pütter C, Weber S, Bornfeld N, Lohmann DR Zeschnigk M (2012): Prognostic significance of chromosome 3 alterations determined by microsatellite analysis in uveal melanoma: a long-term follow up study. *Br J Cancer* 106:1171–1176.

Tien HF, Chuang SM, Chen MS, Lee FY, Hou PK (1989): Cytogenetic evidence of multifocal origin of a unilateral retinoblastoma. A help in genetic counselling. *Cancer Genet Cytogenet* 42:203–208.

Trolet J, Hupe P, Huon I, Lebigot I, Decraene C, Delattre O, et al. (2009): Genomic profiling and identification of high risk uveal melanoma by array CGH analysis of primary tumours and liver metastases. *Invest Ophthalmol Vis Sci* 50:2572–2580.

Tschentscher F, Prescher G, Horsman DE, White VA, Reider H, Anastassiou G, et al. (2001): Partial deletions of the long and short arm of chromosome 3 point to two tumour suppressor genes in uveal melanoma. *Cancer Res* 61:3439–3442.

Vaarwater J, van den Bosch T, Mensink HW, van Kempen C, Verdijk RM, Naus NC, et al. (2012): Multiplex ligation-dependent probe amplification equals fluorescence in situ hybridization for the identification of patients at risk for metastatic disease in uveal melanoma. *Melanoma Res* 22:30–37.

van den Bosch T, van Beek JGM, Vaarwater J, Verdijk RM, Naus NC, Paridaens D, et al. (2012): Higher percentage of FISH-determined monosomy 3 and 8q amplification in uveal melanoma cells relate to poor patient prognosis. *Invest Ophthalmol Vis Sci* 53:2668–2674.

van der Velden PA, Metzelar-Blok JA, Bergman W, Monique H, Hurks H, Frants RR, et al. (2001): Promoter hypomethylation: a common cause of reduced p16(INK4a) expression in uveal melanoma. *Cancer Res* 61:5303–5306.

van der Wal JE, Haremsen MAJA, Gille HJP, Schouten-van Meeteren NYN, Moll AC, Imhof SM, et al. (2003): Comparative genomic hybridisation divides retinoblastomas into high and a low level chromosomal instability group. *J Clin Pathol* 56:26–30.

van Gils W, Lodder EM, Mensink HW, Kileç E, Naus NC, Brüggenwirth HT, et al. (2008): Gene expression profiling in uveal melanoma: two regions on 3p relate to prognosis. *Invest Ophthalmol Vis Sci* 49: 4254–4262.

Van Raamsdonk CD, Bezrookove V, Green G, Bauer J, Gaugler L, O'Brien JM, et al. (2009): Frequent somatic mutations of GNAQ in uveal melanoma and blue naevi. *Nature* 457:599–602.

Van Raamsdonk CD, Griewank KG, Crosby MB, Garrido MC, Vemula S, Wiesner T, et al. (2010): Mutations in GNA11 in uveal melanoma. *N Engl J Med* 363:2191–2199.

Vajdic CM, Hutchins AM, Kricker A, Aitken JF, Armstrong BK, Hayward NK, et al. (2003): Chromosomal gains and losses in ocular melanoma detected by comparative genomic hybridization in an Australian population-based study. *Cancer Genet Cytogenet* 144:12–17.

White V, Horsman DE, Rootman J (1995): Cytogenetic characterization of an iris melanoma. *Cancer Genet Cytogenet* 82:85–87.

White VA, Chambers JD, Courtright PD, Chang W Y, Horsman DE (1998): Correlation of cytogenetic abnormalities with the outcome of patients with uveal melanoma. *Cancer* 83:354–359.

Wiltshire R N, Elner V M, Dennis T, Vine A K, Trent J M (1993): Cytogenetic analysis of posterior uveal melanoma. *Cancer Genet Cytogenet* 66:47–53.

Yu H, Pak H, Hammond-Martel I, Ghram M, Rodrigue A, Daou S, et al. (2014): Tumor suppressor and deubiquitinase BAP1 promotes double-strand break repair. *Proc Natl Acad Sci USA* 111:285–290.

Yunis JJ, Ramsey N (1978): Retinoblastoma and subband deletion of chromosome 13. *Am J Dis Child* 132: 161–163.

CHAPTER 22

Tumors of the skin

Fredrik Mertens¹, Felix Mitelman¹ and Sverre Heim²

¹Department of Clinical Genetics, University of Lund, Lund, Sweden
²Section for Cancer Cytogenetics, Institute for Cancer Genetics and Informatics,
Oslo University Hospital, Oslo, Norway

Skin cancer is the most common malignancy in humans. Behind this simple term hides a plethora of different neoplastic proliferations, however, corresponding to tumors of all the many cell types that normally populate the epidermal and dermal skin layers. Our knowledge about the chromosomal abnormalities of skin cancer is grossly inadequate; in all, only slightly more than 300 cases have been studied, and only for a few of them—basal cell carcinoma (BCC), squamous cell carcinoma (SCC), Merkel cell carcinoma, and malignant melanoma—is cytogenetic information available on more than 25 cases. The diagnostic spectrum of benign neoplasms of the skin is equally complex, but even less is known about the karyotypic abnormalities of these common tumors than about their malignant counterparts. Without any doubt, benign and malignant neoplastic processes of the skin represent one of the most consistently neglected areas of tumor cytogenetics.

In the latest WHO classification (LeBoit et al., 2006), skin tumors are grouped according to their lineage of differentiation, a scheme that will be adhered to also here. Hematolymphoid tumors and soft tissue tumors occurring in the skin are dealt with in other chapters.

Keratinocytic tumors

BCC, also known as basal cell epitheliomas or trichoblastic carcinomas, account for approximately two-thirds of all skin malignancies. They are named after the cells they resemble and from which they presumably originate, the basal cells in the lowermost layer of the epidermis. BCC show malignant behavior in the sense that they infiltrate locally with destruction of the surrounding tissue. They almost never metastasize, however (Weedon et al., 2006). Overwhelming epidemiologic evidence implicates sun exposure, as in most other skin tumors, as the main etiologic factor. BCC are usually sporadic but may also be part of hereditary syndromes, notably the basal cell nevus syndrome, which is caused by mutations in the *PTCH1* gene in chromosome band 9q22.

Clonal chromosome abnormalities have been reported in approximately 100 BCC (Mitelman et al., 2014), the majority of which were part of three large series (Jin et al., 1998, 2001; Casalone et al., 2000). The karyotypes have with few exceptions been pseudo- or near diploid, usually with simple and balanced chromosomal aberrations; less than 5% of the cases have convincingly displayed aneuploid cell populations with <40 or >50

Cancer Cytogenetics: Chromosomal and Molecular Genetic Aberrations of Tumor Cells, Fourth Edition.
Edited by Sverre Heim and Felix Mitelman.
© 2015 John Wiley & Sons, Ltd. Published 2015 by John Wiley & Sons, Ltd.

chromosomes. These results are in contrast with studies of the DNA index of BCC, which show that 80% of the cases have a significant cell population with a DNA index higher than 1.12 or lower than 0.8 (Staibano et al., 2001).

The spectrum of aberrations detected by cytogenetic analysis seems, at least in part, to depend on the culture method used. When assessing the profiles of close to 70 BCC that had been short-term cultured in a medium favoring outgrowth of epithelial cells, Jin et al. (2001) found clonal aberrations at a very high frequency (~90%). Extensive intratumor heterogeneity in the form of cytogenetically unrelated clones was seen in half of the cases, and many had nonclonal aberrations. Two-thirds of the cases harbored structural rearrangements with or without additional numerical changes, whereas the remaining one-third showed one or more numerical changes only. Excluding loss of the Y chromosome in male samples, the most common numerical changes were trisomy or tetrasomy 18, seen in 30% of the cases, followed by gain of chromosomes X, 7, and 9. The most commonly (around 10% of the cases) affected bands in structural rearrangements were 1p36, 1p32, 1p22, 1q11, 1q21, 2q11, 2q37, 3q13, 4q21, 4q31, 7q11, 9q22, 11p15, 16p13, 16q24, 17q21, and 20q13. Recurrent imbalances resulting from structural rearrangements included loss of 1q42-qter, 4q31-qter, 6q23-qter, 8q13-qter, 9p22-pter, and 13q14-qter. The only recurrent balanced change was a t(9;16)(q22;p13), seen in three cases (Jin et al., 1997a, 2001). Also, Casalone et al. (2000) found predominantly near- or pseudodiploid clones in short-term cultured cells, but none of their 73 cases displayed clonal gain of the X chromosome or chromosomes 7, 9, or 18. Furthermore, a much lower frequency of clonal changes (39% vs. 63%) and different aberrations were seen in direct preparations from the same samples. Prompted by the finding of clonal gain of chromosome 6 in two cases, Casalone et al. (2000) also performed interphase FISH on uncultured cells and detected trisomy 6 in one-third of the cases.

The cytogenetic results so far reported for BCC thus differ in at least three respects from what has usually been observed in most other solid tumors and in hematologic malignancies: no one rearrangement has been found to be a common cytogenetic feature, karyotypically unrelated clones are present in a substantial proportion of cases, and the results from different groups of researchers are highly discrepant. Needless to say, these issues will have to be clarified before cytogenetic data can be reliably incorporated into pathogenetic models of BCC tumorigenesis, let alone the clinical management of such skin cancer cases.

The histologic hallmark of *SCC* is the infiltration into the underlying dermis of irregular masses of epidermal cells that may exhibit varying degrees of atypia. In contrast to BCC, SCC set up distant metastases and thus possess all the classic characteristics of malignant tumors.

Less than 30 SCC with clonal chromosome abnormalities have been reported (Mitelman et al., 2014), the largest series comprising 11 cases (Jin et al., 1999). In contrast to BCC, a substantial proportion of the cases display highly complex karyotypes characterized by aneuploidy and multiple numerical as well as structural aberrations. Although no consistent aberration has been detected in these cases, most of them have shown isochromosomes or whole-arm translocations and multiple marker chromosomes, features that are common also in the more extensively analyzed SCC from the upper aerodigestive tract (Chapter 13). In contrast to the latter tumors, however, chromosome band 11q13 has not been reported to be involved in the formation of homogeneously staining regions (hsr) in skin SCC. Recurrent imbalances in cases with complex karyotypes include losses affecting chromosomes and chromosome arms 1p, 4, 8p, 9p, 13, 18, 21, and 22 and gain of 1q, 5p, 8q, 9, and 17q, at least in part corresponding also to sites reported to exhibit loss of heterozygosity (LOH) (Bäckvall et al., 2005).

On the contrary, close to two-thirds of the skin SCC examined have displayed karyotypic features similar to those seen in the majority of BCC, namely, multiple, seemingly unrelated clones with near- or pseudodiploid karyotypes typically displaying structural rearrangements, most of which appear balanced. When numerical changes are present, +7 and +18 predominate.

In contrast to BCC, which has no recognized precursor lesion, SCC of the skin is known to develop through histologic stages, the most important of which are *actinic keratosis* (squamous cell dysplasia) and *carcinoma in situ* (severe dysplasia).

Only two and five such cases, respectively, with clonal changes have been described, and they have invariably displayed near-diploid or near-tetraploid karyotypes with relatively simple numerical and/or structural changes, usually in unrelated clones (Jin et al., 2002). *Keratoacanthoma*, a benign and often spontaneously regressing squamoproliferative tumor with a predilection for hair-bearing skin, is by some regarded as a variant of SCC. Only two cases with abnormal karyotype have been reported, one of which showed a t(2;8)(p13;p23) as the sole change (Kim et al., 2003). The other case had more complex changes, including a der(6)t(2;6)(p13;q23) (Mertens et al., 1989).

Taken at face value, the cytogenetic data on both BCC and squamous cell tumors indicate that a substantial proportion of these skin tumors are of polyclonal origin. Several interpretation difficulties are involved, however, and the most straightforward conclusion may not necessarily be the correct one. As alluded to repeatedly, for example, in Chapter 16 describing the cytogenetics of breast tumors, it is possible to explain the findings in several ways. At the heart of the diagnostic problem lies the realization that, unlike what is the situation in hematologic diseases (with −Y as the only practically important exception), one cannot be certain that a tumorous solid tissue lesion is neoplastic just because it is found to contain clonal karyotypic changes. Chromosomal aberrations, including structural rearrangements, have occasionally been found in what by all classic pathologic criteria are nonneoplastic lesions (Mertens et al., 1992; Rubin et al., 1992; Johansson et al., 1993; Jin et al., 1997b; Broberg et al., 1999). Keeping this in mind, four explanatory possibilities can be envisaged for the importance of the simple clonal chromosome aberrations detected in skin tumors. (i) The clones could be part of the tumor parenchyma, but they are evolutionarily related by a shared, submicroscopic mutation. In this case, the seemingly unrelated clones would actually be subclones and the tumor would be monoclonal. (ii) All the clones could belong to the tumor parenchyma, but there is no unifying mutation. This would mean that the tumor is polyclonal in origin. (iii) At least some of the clones could be descendants of epithelial cells that, although they carry chromosomal mutations, are nevertheless not part of the tumor parenchyma. They represent an admixture of nonneoplastic elements, and the cytogenetic findings are not directly informative about the tumor karyotype. (iv) Finally, the unrelated, aberrant clones could correspond to stromal cells that have somehow acquired cytogenetic abnormalities, perhaps due to the influence of the neighboring tumor parenchyma or the environmental factors that led to neoplastic transformation in the first place. Again, the clones would represent an interesting biological phenomenon, but they would have little information value with regard to the genetic changes that drive the tumorigenic process. At present, the available evidence is not sufficient to confirm or falsify any of these hypotheses, but it is of interest to note that careful molecular analysis of microdissected BCC and SCC has provided support for both a unicellular and a multicellular origin, respectively (Agar et al., 2004; Asplund et al., 2005). It has also been shown that morphologically normal skin keratinocytes may harbor *TP53* mutations and that the incidence of clones with such mutations increases with age and prolonged sun exposure. Undoubtedly, the karyotypic profile of keratinocytic tumors deserves to be better characterized, something that is also likely to improve our understanding at least to some extent of how these tumors arise.

Melanocytic tumors

A wide range of clinically and pathologically different benign and malignant melanocytic tumors are recognized (de Vries et al., 2006). Although more than 100 cases have been cytogenetically examined, the amount of data is nevertheless much too small to offer more than a highly tentative, first glimpse at some of the histologic–cytogenetic correlations that characterize melanocyte tumorigenesis. At the phenotypic level, the process is marked by transitions from nevus to dysplastic nevus and, if the malignant end stage is reached, to the aggressively growing and metastasizing malignant melanoma.

Less than 15 *benign melanocytic tumors* with abnormal karyotypes, all near-diploid or pseudodiploid, have been reported. No recurrent aberration has been identified, but two cases with structural rearrangements both had involvement of the long arm of chromosome 10, as t(9;10)(p24;q24) in a dysplastic nevus (Parmiter and Nowell, 1988) and t(10;15)(q26;q22) in a compound melanocytic nevus (Richmond et al., 1986). A numerical change, trisomy 6 and trisomy 8, respectively, was the only chromosomal abnormality in two nevi (Richmond et al., 1986; Sobey et al., 2007). Patients with dysplastic nevi are at an increased risk of developing melanoma. The limited cytogenetic information available does not indicate that these nevi differ in their pattern of acquired genomic alterations from other types of nevi; all have had near-diploid karyotypes, with one or more structural rearrangements, typically balanced translocations, as the sole changes. No recurrent aberration has been observed. Only two large congenital melanocytic nevi have been analyzed, and both had a translocation of chromosome arm 7q as the sole change (Dessars et al., 2007). Further analysis by molecular (cyto)genetic techniques showed that the case with a t(5;7) (q31;q34) had a fusion of the *FCHSD1* gene in chromosome 5 with the *BRAF* gene in chromosome 7. In the other case, which harbored a t(2;7), no fusion gene was found, but also here, the *BRAF* gene

was disrupted. The authors concluded that the significant outcome of the translocations was removal of the autoinhibitory amino-terminal regulatory domain from the protein kinase domain of BRAF (Dessars et al., 2007). BRAF activation, typically achieved through point mutations, indeed seems to be an early event in melanocytic tumorigenesis and is frequently seen in benign as well as malignant lesions (Indsto et al., 2007).

Although more than 150 *malignant melanomas* with clonal chromosome abnormalities have been reported (Mitelman et al., 2014), the information value with regard to melanoma tumorigenesis is more limited than it may seem, since many of the cases were highly advanced, metastatic tumors. Relatively large series were described by Pedersen et al. (1986), Grammatico et al. (1993), Ozisik et al. (1994), Thompson et al. (1995), and Okamoto et al. (1999), and a review of the field as well as an evaluation of the clinical significance of individual cytogenetic features was provided by Nelson et al. (2000).

Malignant melanoma karyotypes are typically highly aneuploid with multiple numerical as well as structural aberrations (Figure 22.1). Chromosomes

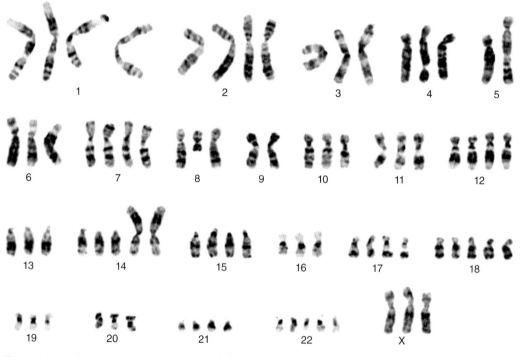

Figure 22.1 Complex karyotype from a cutaneous malignant melanoma illustrating some of the chromosomal rearrangements frequently seen in this tumor type, such as i(1)(q10), loss of chromosome 9, and deletion of distal 10q.

1, 6, 7, 9, 10, and 11 seem to be preferentially involved. The structural rearrangements of chromosome 1, found in 60% of all tumors with abnormal karyotypes, have included isochromosome formation for the long arm as well as various translocations, deletions, and duplications. A certain breakpoint clustering has been seen in the short arm with various terminal deletions, del(1)(p31), del(1)(p22), and del(1)(p13), as recurrent aberrations. In the long arm, the breakpoints of structural rearrangements seem to cluster in or near the centromere and in the constitutive heterochromatic segment. Three translocations, t(1;6)(q11;q11), t(1;19)(q12;p13), and t(1;14)(q21;q32), have been detected in more than one case. Molecular genetic results are in agreement with the cytogenetic data, showing loss of 1p and gain of 1q in more than 20% of the cases (Dracopoli et al., 1989; Böni et al., 1998; Curtin et al., 2005). Studying 47 melanoma cell lines with tiling-resolution array CGH, Jönsson et al. (2007) detected even higher frequencies of 1p loss, with two smallest regions of overlap of losses in 1p22.1 and 1p21.3 and one of gains in 1q23.3–25.3. The putative target genes for deletions in 1p and gains from 1q remain unknown. Finally, Berger et al. (2010) combined RNA sequencing with high-resolution copy number examination identifying 11 novel melanoma gene fusions produced by underlying genomic rearrangements. When they used the data to discover and validate base-pair mutations that had accumulated in the analyzed melanomas, they found a high rate of somatic mutation, lending support to the notion that point mutations constitute the major driver in melanoma development.

Chromosome 6 is rearranged almost as frequently as chromosome 1 in 55–60% of the tumors. Statistical analyses of melanoma karyotypes have suggested that the rearrangements of chromosome 6 occur early in tumorigenesis (Radmacher et al., 2001; Höglund et al., 2004). The most common abnormalities are deletions of the long arm, often with the breakpoints mapping to 6q12–23. The short arm, on the other hand, is more often involved in gains, and an isochromosome for the short arm, i(6)(p10), has been seen repeatedly. Again, these results are in line with molecular data showing frequent loss of 6q, in particular the distal part, and gain of 6p in malignant melanomas

(Millikin et al., 1991; Maitra et al., 2002; Curtin et al., 2005; Namiki et al., 2005; Jönsson et al., 2007). These results suggest that one or more tumor suppressor genes of importance for melanoma development map to 6q. In line with this conclusion, Trent et al. (1990a) presented direct evidence of the tumor suppressor function of chromosome 6 when they introduced a normal copy of the chromosome into melanoma cell lines and showed that the resulting microcell hybrids lost their ability to form tumors in nude mice. When chromosome 6 was lost from the hybrid cells, the cell lines again became tumorigenic. Partly different results, however, were obtained by Welch et al. (1994) and Miele et al. (1996), who found that the transfer of chromosome 6 suppressed metastasis but did not inhibit tumorigenicity in the melanoma cell lines they examined. The *CRSP3* and *UTRN* genes, which map to bands 6q23 and 6q24, respectively, have been put forward as potential targets for the 6q deletions in melanomas (Goldberg et al., 2003; Li et al., 2007).

Structural and/or numerical abnormalities of chromosomes 7 and 10 are each seen in about half of all karyotypically abnormal malignant melanomas. The most common individual aberrations are +7 (38 cases), −7 (five cases), i(7)(q10) (four cases), and −10 (70 cases) and del(10)(q24) (3 cases) (Mitelman et al., 2014). Loss of one chromosome 10 is often accompanied by gain of one or more copies of chromosome 7; this especially occurs during the later stages of melanoma tumorigenesis (Höglund et al., 2004; Jönsson et al., 2007). Although it is unlikely that the cellular outcome of gain of the entire chromosome 7 can be reduced to a copy number increase of a single gene, it is of interest to note that the *BRAF* gene maps to the region of chromosome 7 most commonly gained in melanoma cell lines (Jönsson et al., 2007). Also the *EGFR* gene, which maps to 7p12 and encodes the epidermal growth factor receptor, has been suggested to be a target for trisomy 7; overexpression of *EGFR* correlates with increased copy number of chromosome 7 (Koprowski et al., 1985; Udart et al., 2001; Rákosy et al., 2007) as well as with poor disease outcome (Rákosy et al., 2007). A good candidate tumor suppressor gene on chromosome 10 is *PTEN*, which has been shown to be frequently mutated or heterozygously or homozygously deleted in melanoma cell lines (Pollock et al., 2002; Jönsson et al., 2007). However, such rearrangements and mutations are less common in primary tumors, suggesting that they are late events and that inactivation of or haploinsufficiency for other genes may be at least equally important.

Cytogenetic abnormalities of chromosome 9, too, are found in approximately half of the melanomas with abnormal karyotypes. The most common change is loss of the entire chromosome 9, but structural rearrangements, in particular deletions with breakpoints in 9p11–22, are also recurrent. The high frequency of 9p deletions fits very well with the common finding of allelic imbalance or copy number loss by LOH or CGH analysis (Curtin et al., 2005; Jönsson et al., 2007). Based on the finding that 9p deletions are rare in benign melanocytic nevi but become more frequent with increasing grade of malignancy, as well as on statistical analysis of melanoma karyotypes, it has been suggested that these deletions occur relatively late in melanoma development (Welch et al., 2001; Höglund et al., 2004; Sini et al., 2007). Chromosome arm 9p is frequently deleted in a number of tumor types, strongly suggesting that one or more tumor suppressor genes are located here. Indeed, in 1994, a gene initially named MTS1, now known as CDKN2A, was identified as the target for many of these deletions (Kamb et al., 1994). The CDKN2A gene is unusual in the sense that it encodes two distinct proteins (p16INK4A and p14ARF) that are transcribed from different first exons but share the same second and third exons (Hayward, 2003). Not only is the CDKN2A locus frequently somatically inactivated through deletions visible at the cytogenetic level, but also a number of smaller deletions, point mutations, and epigenetic changes have been reported (Pollock et al., 1996; Hayward, 2003). Constitutional mutations in CDKN2A are associated with an increased risk of melanoma development (Cannon-Albright et al., 1992; Hayward, 2003). Important though CDKN2A may be, several lines of evidence indicate that also other potential tumor suppressor genes exist in 9p, some of which may be involved in melanoma tumorigenesis (Hayward, 2003; Pujana et al., 2007).

The relationship between tumor karyotype and clinical outcome in malignant melanoma has been studied in two patient cohorts by Trent and coworkers (Trent et al., 1990b; Nelson et al., 2000). In the latter series, comprising more than 200 cases, no correlation between the presence of nonrandomly involved chromosomal rearrangements and survival was seen.

Appendageal tumors

Neoplasms showing differentiation toward one or more of the adnexal structures (e.g., sweat glands and hair follicles) of the skin are collectively referred to as appendageal tumors. They are further subdivided into more than 30 benign and malignant subtypes showing apocrine and eccrine differentiation or follicular and sebaceous differentiation (LeBoit, 2006). Little is known about the etiology of these tumors, but some of the entities may be part of the phenotype of inherited tumor syndromes such as tricholemmomas in Cowden disease and sebaceomas in the Muir–Torre syndrome. Apart from the not infrequent finding of acquired TP53 mutations in some malignant subtypes, the somatic cell genetics of appendageal tumors remains virtually unexplored. Although karyotypes are available from only a handful of tumors, including a few hidradenomas and single cases of eccrine spiradenoma, microcystic adnexal carcinoma, and porocarcinoma, these very preliminary results suggest that much could be learned about the biology of appendageal tumors through cytogenetic analysis.

Hidradenoma is a benign neoplasm of apocrine or eccrine origin that is composed of several cell types: clear cells, squamoid cells, mucinous cells, and transitions between them. When the former predominate, the tumor is often referred to as a clear cell hidradenoma (McNiff et al., 2006). Chromosome analysis of a clear cell hidradenoma revealed multiple related and unrelated clones with various structural rearrangements, including a t(11;19)(q21;p13) (Chapter 12, Fig. 12.2) (Gorunova et al., 1994). Molecular genetic analysis showed that the translocation resulted in a fusion of the amino-terminal CREB-binding domain of the cAMP coactivator CRTC1 and the Notch coactivator MAML2 (Behboudi et al., 2005). Further RT-PCR analysis of 20 hidradenomas showed that half of them, all distinguished by the presence of clear cells, harbored the same fusion gene (Winnes et al., 2007). A substantial fraction of hidradenomas with less

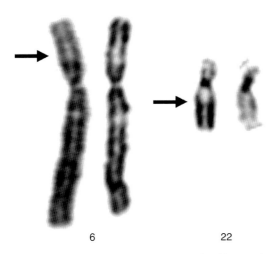

6   22

Figure 22.2 Partial karyotype showing the t(6;22)(p21;q12) in a hidradenoma. The translocation results in fusion of the *EWSR1* gene in band 22q12 with the *POU5F1* gene in 6p21. Arrows indicate breakpoints.

prominent clear cell differentiation seems to be characterized by another balanced translocation, t(6;22)(p21;q12), resulting in fusion of the 5′ part of the *EWSR1* gene with the 3′ part of *POU5F1* (Möller et al., 2008) (Figure 22.2). The former gene is a frequent 5′ partner in a number of sarcoma-associated gene fusions, whereas the latter encodes a key regulator (Oct3/4) of the pluripotent status of germ cells and stem cells (Möller et al., 2008). Both fusion genes so far detected in hidradenomas— *CRTC1–MAML2* and *EWSR1–POU5F1*—have been detected also in other tumor types, raising questions about what roles they play in tumorigenesis. Notably, the *CRTC1–MAML2* chimera is found in approximately 50% of mucoepidermoid carcinomas, the most common malignant salivary gland tumor, with fusion-positive cases being associated with favorable disease outcome (Tonon et al., 2003; Behboudi et al., 2006). Further emphasizing the biological link between mucoepidermoid carcinomas and hidradenomas, also a subset of the former neoplasms harbors the *EWSR1–POU5F1* fusion gene (Möller et al., 2008). In addition, a few cases of Warthin's tumor, a benign salivary gland tumor, with the t(11;19) and/or the *CRTC1–MAML2* chimera have also been reported (Enlund et al., 2004). The *EWSR1–POU5F1* fusion, albeit with different breakpoints at the molecular level, has been described in an undifferentiated malignant bone

tumor, too (Yamaguchi et al., 2005). Thus, it seems unlikely that either of the two fusion genes so far detected in hidradenomas determines the phenotype of the tumor cells.

Cutaneous *hidradenocarcinomas* also exist and may prove their malignant potential by setting up metastases. Kazakov et al. (2009) performed a clinicopathologic, immunohistochemical, and molecular biologic study of 14 such tumors, finding evidence of the aforementioned 11;19-translocation in two of the 11 cases that could be examined for this feature, again illustrating that this translocation can exist in neoplasms of both different differentiation and clinical potential. Whether the finding of a t(11;19) in some tumors signifies malignization of a benign precursor lesion remains unclear.

Another specific translocation leading to a characteristic fusion gene in both a malignant and a benign tumor is the t(6;9)(q22–23;p23–24), leading to a fusion of the two transcription factors genes *MYB* and *NFIB*. Fehr et al. (2011) showed that this acquired genetic event not only is a feature of carcinomas of the breast and head and neck but also of benign dermal *cylindromas*. Their demonstration of the *MYB–NFIB* in eight of 12 cylindromas strengthens the evidence that common molecular pathways exist, providing a pathogenetic link between benign and malignant breast, salivary gland, and adnexal tumors.

Agoston et al. (2010) reported that trisomy 18 is a consistent cytogenetic feature of *pilomatricomas*, also known as calcifying epithelioma of Malherbe, a common adnexal skin tumor that mimics hair growth. They detected the trisomy by G-banding in an index case and by interphase FISH in seven of 11 tumors. The trisomy was only present in a small subset of cells. This, and the fact that trisomy 18 is a frequent finding also in other skin tumors (see preceding text), questions both the specificity of the finding and its role in pilomatricoma tumorigenesis.

Neural tumors

Merkel cell carcinoma is a histologically characteristic tumor that in the past also has been called trabecular or neuroendocrine carcinoma. The tumor cells contain neuroendocrine granules, suggesting a neural crest origin. They share several features with Merkel cells, but a direct histogenetic link remains to be established. Less than 30 Merkel cell carcinomas with abnormal karyotypes have been reported, and apart from three small series (Sozzi et al., 1988; Koduru et al., 1989; Leonard et al., 1993), all were single-case reports. Most cases have had a near-diploid chromosome count, and structural rearrangements seem more common than numerical ones. No consistently recurring abnormality has been identified. The most common changes (about two-thirds of all abnormal cases) have been of chromosome 1, with 12 tumors showing gain of various portions of the long arm and five cases showing rearrangement of 1p35–36. Although both loss of distal 1p and gain of 1q have been seen as the sole aberration in one case each, the generally diverse nature of the chromosome 1 rearrangements—they include deletions of both the long and short arms as well as inversions, balanced and unbalanced translocations, and isochromosome formation—makes it unlikely that they represent primary anomalies. It is of interest to note, however, that also the only reported *granular cell tumor*, another rare neural skin tumor, showed a deletion of 1p (Di Tommaso et al., 2002). The only other recurring cytogenetic aberration also seen as a sole change in Merkel cell carcinoma is trisomy 6, found in four tumors.

Summary

In both BCC and SCC of the skin, multiple cytogenetically unrelated clones have been found repeatedly. Their pathogenetic role is unknown. No consistent chromosomal rearrangement has so far been detected in these tumors, at least not frequently. Benign keratinocytic tumors remain too poorly investigated to allow any meaningful evaluation of their cytogenetic features. Malignant melanomas usually have complex karyotypes with preferential involvement of chromosomes 1, 6, 7, 9, 10, and 11. The most common imbalances are loss of material from 1p, 6q, and 9p; gain of 6p and one copy of chromosome 7; and loss of one copy of chromosomes 9 and 10. Large congenital melanocytic nevi have translocations targeting the *BRAF* gene in band 7q34. Hidradenoma is the only appendageal skin tumor investigated in any greater detail, and most cases seem to be characterized by a t(11;19)(q21;p13) or a t(6;22)(p21;q12), resulting in a *CRTC1–MAML2* or *EWSR1–POU5F1* fusion gene,

respectively. The former translocation may also be found in hidradenocarcinomas. Merkel cell carcinomas have near-diploid karyotypes, often showing rearrangements of chromosome 1. Dermal cylindromas may show similar genetic features to adenoid cystic carcinomas with the occurrence of a t(6;9) (q22-23;p23-24) leading to a *MYB–NFIB* fusion gene.

Acknowledgments

Financial support from the Swedish and Norwegian Cancer Societies is gratefully acknowledged.

References

Agar NS, Halliday GM, Barnetson RSC, Ananthaswamy HN, Wheeler M, Jones AM (2004): The basal layer in human squamous tumors harbors more UVA than UVB fingerprint mutations: a role for UVA in human skin carcinogenesis. *Proc Natl Acad Sci USA* 101:4954–4959.

Agoston AT, Liang C-W, Richkind KE, Fletcher JA, Vargas SO (2010): Trisomy 18 is a consistent cytogenetic feature in pilomatricoma. *Mod Pathol* 23:1147–1150.

Asplund A, Sivertsson A, Bäckvall H, Ahmadian A, Lundeberg J, Pontén F (2005): Genetic mosaicism in basal cell carcinoma. *Exp Dermatol* 14:593–600.

Bäckvall H, Asplund A, Gustafsson A, Sivertsson Å, Lundeberg J, Pontén F (2005): Genetic tumor archeology: microdissection and genetic heterogeneity in squamous and basal cell carcinoma. *Mutat Res* 571:65–79.

Behboudi A, Winnes M, Gorunova L, van denOord JJ, Mertens F, Enlund F, et al. (2005): Clear cell hidradenoma of the skin—a third tumor type with a t(11;19)-associated TORC1-MAML2 gene fusion. *Genes Chromosomes Cancer* 43:202–205.

Behboudi A, Enlund F, Winnes M, Andrén Y, Nordkvist A, Leivo I, et al. (2006): Molecular classification of mucoepidermoid carcinomas—prognostic significance of the MECT1-MAML2 fusion oncogene. *Genes Chromosomes Cancer* 45:470–481.

Berger MF, Levin JZ, Vijayendran K, Sivachenko A, Adiconis X, Maguire J, et al. (2010): Integrative analysis of the melanoma transcriptome. *Genome Res* 20:413–427.

Böni R, Matt D, Voetmeyer A, Burg G, Zhuang Z (1998): Chromosomal allele loss in primary cutaneous melanoma is heterogeneous and correlates with proliferation. *J Invest Dermatol* 110:215–217.

Broberg K, Höglund M, Limon J, Lindstrand A, Toksvig-Larsen S, Mandahl N, et al. (1999): Rearrangement of the neoplasia-associated gene HMGIC in synovia from patients with osteoarthritis. *Genes Chromosomes Cancer* 24:278–282.

Cannon-Albright LA, Goldgar DE, Meyer LJ, Lewis CM, Anderson DE, Fountain JW, et al. (1992): Assignment of a locus for familial melanoma, MLM, to chromosome 9p13-p22. *Science* 258:1148–1152.

Casalone R, Mazzola D, Righi R, Granata P, Minelli E, Salvadore M, et al. (2000): Cytogenetic and interphase FISH analyses of 73 basal cell and three squamous cell carcinomas: different findings in direct preparations and short-term cell cultures. *Cancer Genet Cytogenet* 118:136–143.

Curtin JA, Fridlyand J, Kageshita T, Patel HN, Busam KJ, Kutzner H, et al. (2005): Distinct sets of genetic alterations in melanoma. *N Engl J Med* 353:2135–2147.

Dessars B, DeRaeve LE, ElHousni H, Debouck CJ, Sidon PJ, Morandini R, et al. (2007): Chromosomal translocations as a mechanism of BRAF activation in two cases of large congenital melanocytic nevi. *J Invest Dermatol* 127:1468–1470.

deVries E, Bray F, Coebergh JW, Cerroni L, Ruiter DJ, Elder DE, et al. (2006): Malignant melanoma: introduction. In LeBoit PE, Burg G, Weedon D, Sarasin A (eds.): World Health Organization Classification of Tumours. Pathology and Genetics of Skin Tumours. Lyon: IARC Press, pp. 52–65.

Di Tommaso L, Magrini E, Consales A, Poppi M, Pasquinelli G, Dorji T, et al. (2002): Malignant granular cell tumor of the lateral femoral cutaneous nerve: report of a case with cytogenetic analysis. *Hum Pathol* 33:1237–1240.

Dracopoli NC, Harnett P, Bale SJ, Stanger BZ, Tucker MA, Housman DE, et al. (1989): Loss of alleles from the distal short arm of chromosome 1 occurs late in melanoma tumor progression. *Proc Natl Acad Sci USA* 86:4614–4618.

Enlund F, Behboudi A, Andrén Y, Öberg C, Lendahl U, Mark J, et al. (2004): Altered Notch signaling resulting from expression of a WAMTP1-MAML2 gene fusion in mucoepidermoid carcinomas and benign Warthin's tumors. *Exp Cell Res* 292:21–28.

Fehr A, Kovacs A, Löning T, Frierson Jr HF, van den Oord JJ, Stenman G (2011): The MYB-NFIB gene fusion – a novel genetic link between adenoid cystic carcinoma and dermal cylindroma. *J Pathol* 224:322–327.

Goldberg SF, Miele ME, Hatta N, Takata M, Paquette-Straub C, Freedman LP, et al. (2003): Melanoma metastasis suppression by chromosome 6: evidence for a pathway regulated by CRSP3 and TXNIP. *Cancer Res* 63:432–440.

Gorunova L, Mertens F, Mandahl N, Jonsson N, Persson B, Heim S, et al. (1994): Cytogenetic heterogeneity in a clear cell hidradenoma of the skin. *Cancer Genet Cytogenet* 77:26–32.

Grammatico P, Catricala C, Potenza C, Amantea A, Roccella M, Roccella F, et al. (1993): Cytogenetic findings in 20 melanomas. *Melanoma Res* 3:169–172.

Hayward NK (2003): Genetics of melanoma predisposition. *Oncogene* 22:3053–3062.

Höglund M, Gisselsson D, Hansen GB, White VA, Säll T, Mitelman F, et al. (2004): Dissecting karyotypic patterns in malignant melanomas: temporal clustering of losses and gains in melanoma karyotypic evolution. *Int J Cancer* 108:57–65.

Indsto JO, Kumar S, Wang L, Crotty KA, Arbuckle SM, Mann GJ (2007): Low prevalence of RAS-RAF-activating mutations in Spitz melanocytic nevi compared with other melanocytic lesions. *J Cutan Pathol* 34:448–455.

Jin Y, Mertens F, Persson B, Gullestad HP, Jin C, Warloe T, et al. (1997a): The reciprocal translocation t(9;16) (q22;p13) is a primary chromosome abnormality in basal cell carcinomas. *Cancer Res* 57:404–406.

Jin C, Jin Y, Wennerberg J, Åkervall J, Grenthe B, Mandahl N, et al. (1997b): Clonal chromosome aberrations accumulate with age in upper aerodigestive tract mucosa. *Mutat Res* 374:63–72.

Jin Y, Mertens F, Persson B, Warloe T, Gullestad HP, Salemark L, et al. (1998): Nonrandom numerical chromosome abnormalities in basal cell carcinomas. *Cancer Genet Cytogenet* 103:35–42.

Jin Y, Martins C, Jin C, Salemark L, Jonsson N, Persson B, et al. (1999): Nonrandom karyotypic features in squamous cell carcinomas of the skin. *Genes Chromosomes Cancer* 26:295–303.

Jin Y, Martins C, Salemark L, Persson B, Jin C, Miranda J, et al. (2001): Nonrandom karyotypic features in basal cell carcinomas of the skin. *Cancer Genet Cytogenet* 131:109–119.

Jin Y, Jin C, Salemark L, Wennerberg J, Persson B, Jonsson N (2002): Clonal chromosome abnormalities in premalignant lesions of the skin. *Cancer Genet Cytogenet* 136:48–52.

Johansson B, Heim S, Mandahl N, Mertens F, Mitelman F (1993): Trisomy 7 in nonneoplastic cells. *Genes Chromosomes Cancer* 6:199–206.

Jönsson G, Dahl C, Staaf J, Sandberg T, Bendahl P-O, Ringnér M, et al. (2007): Genomic profiling of malignant melanoma using tiling-resolution array CGH. *Oncogene* 26:4738–4748.

Kamb A, Gruis NA, Weaver-Feldhaus J, Liu Q, Harshman K, Tavtigian SV, et al. (1994): A cell cycle regulator potentially involved in genesis of many tumor types. *Science* 264:436–440.

Kazakov DV, Ivan D, Kutzner H, Spagnolo DV, Grossman P, Vanecek T, et al. (2009): Cutaneous hidradenocarcinoma: a clinicopathological, immunohistochemical, and molecular biologic study of 14 cases, including Her2/neu gene expression/amplification, TP53 gene mutation analysis, and t(11;19) translocation. *Am J Dermatopathol* 31:236–247.

Kim D-K, Kim J-Y, Kim H-T, Han K-H, Shon D-G (2003): A specific chromosome aberration in a keratoacanthoma. *Cancer Genet Cytogenet* 142:70–72.

Koduru PR, Dicostanzo DP, Jhanwar SC (1989): Non random cytogenetic changes characterize Merkel cell carcinoma. *Disease Markers* 7:153–161.

Koprowski H, Herlyn M, Balaban G, Parmiter A, Ross A, Nowell PC (1985): Expression of the receptor for epidermal growth factor correlates with increased dosage of chromosome 7 in malignant melanoma. *Somat Cell Mol Genet* 11:297–302.

LeBoit PE (2006): Appendageal skin tumours: introduction. In *LeBoit PE*, Burg G, Weedon D, Sarasin A (eds.): World Health Organization Classification of Tumours. Pathology and Genetics of Skin Tumours. Lyon: IARC Press, pp. 123–124.

LeBoit PE, Burg G, Weedon D, Sarasin A, editors (2006): *World Health Organization Classification of Tumours. Pathology and Genetics of Skin Tumours.* Lyon: IARC Press.

Leonard JH, Leonard P, Kearsley JH (1993): Chromosomes 1, 11 and 13 are frequently involved in karyotypic abnormalities in metastatic Merkel cell carcinoma. *Cancer Genet Cytogenet* 67:65–70.

Li Y, Huang J, Zhao YL, He J, Wang W, Davies KE, et al. (2007): UTRN on chromosome 6q24 is mutated in multiple tumors. *Oncogene* 26:6220–6228.

Maitra A, Gazdar AF, Moore TO, Moore AY (2002): Loss of heterozygosity analysis of cutaneous melanoma and benign melanocytic nevi: laser capture microdissection demonstrates clonal genetic changes in acquired nevocellular nevi. *Hum Pathol* 33:191–197.

McNiff J, McCalmont TH, Requena L, Sangüeza OP, Vassallo C, Rosso R, et al. (2006): Benign tumours with apocrine and eccrine differentiation. In: *LeBoit PE*, Burg G, Weedon D, Sarasin A (eds.): World Health Organization Classification of Tumours. Pathology and Genetics of Skin Tumours. Lyon: IARC Press, pp. 139–148.

Mertens F, Heim S, Mandahl N, Johansson B, Rydholm A, Biörklund A, et al. (1989): Clonal chromosome aberrations in a keratoacanthoma and a basal cell papilloma. *Cancer Genet Cytogenet* 39:227–232.

Mertens F, Jin Y, Heim S, Mandahl N, Jonsson N, Mertens O, et al. (1992): Clonal structural chromosome aberrations in nonneoplastic cells of the skin and upper aerodigestive tract. *Genes Chromosomes Cancer* 4:235–240.

Miele ME, Robertson G, Lee JH, Coleman A, McGary CT, Fisher PB, et al. (1996): Metastasis suppressed, but tumorigenicity and local invasiveness unaffected, in the human melanoma cell line Me1JuSo after introduction of human chromosomes 1 or 6. *Mol Carcinogenesis* 15:284–299.

Millikin D, Meese E, Vogelstein B, Witkowski C, Trent J (1991): Loss of heterozygosity for loci on the long arm of chromosome 6 in human malignant melanoma. *Cancer Res* 51:5449–5453.

Mitelman F, Johansson B, Mertens F, editors (2014): *Mitelman Database of Chromosome Aberrations and Gene Fusions in Cancer.* http://cgap.nci.nih.gov/Chromosomes/Mitelman.

Möller E, Stenman G, Mandahl N, Hamberg H, Mölne L, van denOord JJ, et al. (2008): POU5F1, encoding a key regulator of stem cell pluripotency, is fused to EWSR1 in hidradenoma and mucoepidermoid carcinoma. *J Pathol* 215:78–86.

Namiki T, Yanagawa S, Izumo T, Ishikawa M, Tachibana M, Kawakami Y, et al. (2005): Genomic alterations in primary cutaneous melanomas detected by metaphase comparative genomic hybridization with laser capture or manual microdissection: 6p gains may predict poor outcome. *Cancer Genet Cytogenet* 157:1–11.

Nelson MA, Radmacher MD, Simon R, Aickin M, Yang J-M, Panda L, et al. (2000): Chromosome abnormalities in malignant melanoma: clinical significance of nonrandom chromosome abnormalities in 206 cases. *Cancer Genet Cytogenet* 122:101–109.

Okamoto I, Pirc-Danoewinata H, Ackermann J, Drach J, Schlagbauer Wadl H, Jansen B, et al. (1999): Deletions of the region 17p11–13 in advanced melanoma revealed by cytogenetic analysis and fluorescence in situ hybridization. *Br J Cancer* 79:131–137.

Ozisik YY, Meloni AM, Altungoz O, Peier A, Karakousis C, Leong SPL, et al. (1994): Cytogenetic findings in 21 malignant melanomas. *Cancer Genet Cytogenet* 77:69–73.

Parmiter AH, Nowell PC (1988): The cytogenetics of human malignant melanoma and premalignant lesions. In Nathanson L (ed.): *Malignant Melanoma: Biology, Diagnosis, and Therapy.* Boston: Kluwer Academic Publishers, pp. 47–61.

Pedersen MI, Bennett JW, Wang N (1986): Nonrandom chromosome structural aberrations and oncogene loci in human malignant melanoma. *Cancer Genet Cytogenet* 20:11–27.

Pollock PM, Pearson JV, Hayward NK (1996): Compilation of somatic mutations of the CDKN2 gene in human cancers: non-random distribution of base substitutions. *Genes Chromosomes Cancer* 15:77–88.

Pollock PM, Walker GJ, Glendening JM, Que Noy T, Bloch NC, Fountain JW, et al. (2002): PTEN inactivation is rare in melanoma tumours but occurs frequently in melanoma cell lines. *Melanoma Res* 12:565–575.

Pujana MA, Ruiz A, Badenas C, Puig-Butille J-A, Nadal M, Stark M, et al. (2007): Molecular characterization of a t(9;12)(p21;q13) balanced chromosome translocation in combination with integrative genomics analysis identifies C9orf14 as a candidate tumor-suppressor. *Genes Chromosomes Cancer* 46:155–162.

Radmacher MD, Simon R, Desper R, Taetle R, Schäffer AA, Nelson MA (2001): Graph models of oncogenesis with an application to melanoma. *J Theor Biol* 212:535–548.

Rákosy Z, Vízkeleti L, Ecsedi S, Vokó Z, Bégány Á, Barok M, et al. (2007): EGFR gene copy number alterations in primary cutaneous malignant melanomas are associated with poor prognosis. *Int J Cancer* 121:1729–1737.

Richmond A, Fine R, Murray D, Lawson DH, Priest JH (1986): Growth factor and cytogenetic abnormalities in cultured nevi and malignant melanomas. *J Invest Dermatol* 86:295–302.

Rubin CM, Nesbit ME Jr, Kim TH, Kersey JH, Arthur DC (1992): Chromosomal abnormalities in skin following total body or total lymphoid irradiation. *Genes Chromosomes Cancer* 4:141–145.

Sini MC, Manca A, Cossu A, Budroni M, Botti G, Ascierto PA, et al. (2007): Molecular alterations at chromosome 9p21 in melanocytic naevi and melanoma. *Br J Dermatol* 158:243–250.

Sobey GJ, Quarrell OW, Williams S, McGrath HM (2007): Mosaic chromosome 6 trisomy in an epidermal nevus. *Pediatr Dermatol* 24:144–146.

Sozzi G, Bertoglio MG, Pilotti S, Rilke F, Pierotti MA, Della Porta G (1988): Cytogenetic studies in primary and metastatic neuroendocrine Merkel cell carcinoma. *Cancer Genet Cytogenet* 30:151–158.

Staibano S, Lo Muzio L, Pannone G, Mezza E, Argenziano G, Vetrani A, et al. (2001): DNA ploidy and cyclin D1 expression in basal cell carcinoma of the head and neck. *Am J Clin Pathol* 115:805–813.

Thompson FH, Emerson J, Olson S, Weinstein R, Leavitt SA, Leong SPL, et al. (1995): Cytogenetics of 158 patients with regional or disseminated melanoma. Subset analysis of near-diploid and simple karyotypes. *Cancer Genet Cytogenet* 83:93–104.

Tonon G, Modi S, Wu L, Kubo A, Coxon AB, Komiya T, et al. (2003): t(11;19)(q21;p13) translocation in mucoepidermoid carcinoma creates a novel fusion product that disrupts a Notch signalling pathway. *Nat Genet* 33:208–213.

Trent JM, Stanbridge EJ, McBride HL, Meese EU, Casey G, Araujo DE, et al. (1990a): Tumorigenicity in human melanoma cell lines controlled by introduction of human chromosome 6. *Science* 247:568–571.

Trent JM, Meyskens FL, Salmon SE, Ryschon K, Leong SPL, Davis JR, et al. (1990b): Relation of cytogenetic abnormalities and clinical outcome in metastatic melanoma. *N Engl J Med* 322:1508–1511.

Udart M, Utikal J, Krähn GM, Peter RU (2001): Chromosome 7 aneusomy. A marker for metastatic melanoma? Expression of the epidermal growth factor receptor gene and chromosome 7 aneusomy in nevi, primary malignant melanomas and metastases. *Neoplasia* 3:245–254.

Weedon D, Marks R, Kao GF, Harwood CA (2006): Keratinocytic tumours: introduction. In: LeBoit PE, Burg G, Weedon D, Sarasin A, editors. *World Health Organization Classification of Tumours. Pathology and Genetics of Skin Tumours.* Lyon: IARC Press, pp 11–12.

Welch DR, Chen P, Miele ME, McGary CT, Bower JM, Stanbridge EJ, et al. (1994): Microcell-mediated transfer of chromosome 6 into metastatic human C8161 melanoma cells suppresses metastasis but does not inhibit tumorigenicity. *Oncogene* 9:255–262.

Welch J, Millar D, Goldman A, Heenan P, Stark M, Eldon M, et al. (2001): Lack of genetic and epigenetic changes in CDKN2A in melanocytic nevi. *J Investi Dermatol* 117:383–384.

Winnes M, Mölne L, Suurküla M, Andrén Y, Persson F, Enlund F, et al. (2007): Frequent fusion of the CRTC1 and MAML2 genes in clear cell variants of cutaneous hidradenomas. *Genes Chromosomes Cancer* 46:559–563.

Yamaguchi S, Yamazaki Y, Ishikawa Y, Kawaguchi N, Mukai H, Nakamura T (2005): EWSR1 is fused to POU5F1 in a bone tumor with translocation t(6;22)(p21;q12). *Genes Chromosomes Cancer* 43:217–222.

CHAPTER 23

Tumors of bone

Fredrik Mertens and Nils Mandahl

Department of Clinical Genetics, University of Lund, Lund, Sweden

Bone tumors constitute a heterogeneous group of neoplasms of skeletal origin. More than 50 distinct subtypes of primary bone tumors have been identified, affecting all age groups and ranging in clinical aggressiveness from totally benign, self-healing lesions to highly malignant tumors associated with a very dismal prognosis. The benign lesions by far outnumber the malignant ones, which when combined constitute only 0.2% of all malignancies. The different diagnostic entities that have been described to date are currently grouped into main categories according to the tumor cells' line of differentiation; it should be emphasized, however, that this does not necessarily reflect the cell of origin, which in most instances remains unknown. In the present review, the current WHO classification of bone tumors (Fletcher et al., 2013) is, in principle, followed. However, since many of the tumors remain poorly characterized at the cytogenetic level, the category with miscellaneous lesions has been expanded. Furthermore, cytogenetic data on plasma cell myeloma are discussed separately in Chapter 11.

Cartilage tumors

Benign cartilage tumors include osteochondroma, subungual exostosis, bizarre parosteal osteochondromatous proliferation (BPOP), chondromas, synovial chondromatosis, chondroblastoma, and chondromyxoid fibroma.

Osteochondroma, also known as osteocartilaginous exostosis, is the most frequent benign bone tumor, representing close to half of the lesions requiring surgical treatment. It arises at the external surface of bones formed by enchondral ossification, typically in the long bones of the limbs. Covered by a fibrous perichondrium that is continuous with the periosteum of the bone, it consists of a cartilage cap covering a sessile or pedunculated bony stalk. Rarely, an osteochondroma may transform into a secondary, peripheral chondrosarcoma, a process heralded by a thickening of the cartilage cap. Such malignant transformation is more common among the approximately 15% of patients who have multiple osteochondromas. Multiple lesions are seen either in the context of microdeletions affecting distal chromosome arm 8q (tricho–rhino–phalangeal syndromes I and II) or, more commonly, in individuals with the autosomal dominant condition multiple osteochondromas. The latter condition is due to an inherited mutation of the *EXT1* gene in band 8q24 or, rarely, the *EXT2* gene in 11p11. It has been established that *EXT1* functions as a classical tumor suppressor gene, that is, both copies are functionally inactivated in osteochondroma cells, with both events

Cancer Cytogenetics: Chromosomal and Molecular Genetic Aberrations of Tumor Cells, Fourth Edition.
Edited by Sverre Heim and Felix Mitelman.
© 2015 John Wiley & Sons, Ltd. Published 2015 by John Wiley & Sons, Ltd.

being somatic in sporadic lesions (Hameetman et al., 2007). It has also been demonstrated that the acquired mutations often are deletions of varying size. In line with this, cytogenetic analysis of osteochondromas has shown a nonrandom involvement of chromosome 8; two-thirds of the close to 30 cases that have been reported showed loss of the entire chromosome 8 or structural rearrangements, most often large deletions, of 8q (Figure 23.1). Cytogenetic evidence for the involvement of the *EXT2* locus is less impressive; only four cases with rearrangements of 11p have been reported. The karyotypes of osteochondromas are, with the single exception of a hereditary osteochondroma, near-diploid (44–47 chromosomes) and of low–moderate complexity (less than 10 rearrangements). Apart from the rearrangements of 8q, no consistent pattern of aberrations has emerged.

Subungual exostosis is a rare tumor that despite its name has nothing to do with ordinary exostoses (osteochondromas). The lesion typically becomes manifest as a slowly growing, painful heterotopic ossification, without continuity with the underlying bone, in the phalanges of the hands and feet. Although it may occur at any age, most patients are between 15 and 25 years old. From the less than 10 cases that have been analyzed, a remarkably homogeneous cytogenetic picture has emerged; all cases share a seemingly balanced t(X;6)(q24–26;q15–25) in half of the tumors as the sole anomaly (Figure 23.2) (Dal Cin et al., 1999; Zambrano et al.,

2004; Storlazzi et al., 2006). Additional changes include other, seemingly random, translocations. Through FISH analysis, the breakpoints have been refined to the regions harboring the collagen genes *COL12A1* and *COL4A5* in chromosome bands 6q13–14 and Xq22, respectively (Storlazzi et al., 2006). Further analysis of gene expression profiles revealed that the *IRS4* gene, located close to *COL4A5* in Xq22, is transcriptionally upregulated in subungual exostoses (Mertens et al., 2011). Presumably, this effect is achieved through regulatory sequences from the translocation partner, *COL12A1*. *IRS4* encodes insulin receptor substrate 4 that mediates signals from growth factors to cytoplasmic proteins containing SH2 domains.

BPOP, also known as Nora lesion, is a rare tumorous lesion with aggressive growth that primarily affects the small tubular bones in the distal extremities and often recurs after excision. Only five cases with clonal chromosome aberrations have been reported, two of which showed an identical t(1;17)(q32;q21) and one a similar t(1;17) (q42;q23) (Nilsson et al., 2004; Endo et al., 2005; Kuruvilla et al., 2011). Using metaphase FISH, Nilsson and coworkers could delineate the breakpoints to regions covered by single BACs in 1q32 and 17q21. Further interphase FISH on paraffin-embedded material from an additional four cases showed that all had a break in the same region in 1q32 and that three of them had a break also in

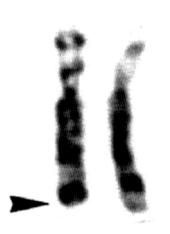

Figure 23.1 Partial karyotype showing a heterozygous del(8)(q24) (arrowhead) in an osteochondroma.

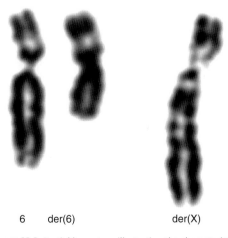

6   der(6)   der(X)

Figure 23.2 Partial karyotype illustrating the characteristic t(X;6)(q24–26;q15–25) in a subungual exostosis.

17q21. The findings strongly indicate that t(1;17) (q32;q21) or variant translocations involving 1q32 are recurrent aberrations in this tumor.

Chondromas account for approximately one-fourth of all benign bone tumors. By far, the most common subtype is *enchondroma*, a benign hyaline cartilage tumor of medullary bone. It may affect all age groups and most commonly occurs in the hands and feet (Lucas and Bridge, 2013). Multiple chondromas—*enchondromatosis*—are seen in the developmental disorders Ollier disease and Maffucci syndrome. Cytogenetic analyses of enchondromas, all of which have been sporadic solitary lesions, have with few exceptions revealed a near-diploid chromosome count. Few recurrent changes have been detected among the close to 20 cases that have been reported, the most common being loss of material from chromosomes 9, 12, and 22 in three cases each. In addition, four cases had a 12q12–13 breakpoint (Tallini et al., 2002; Buddingh et al., 2003a; Sakai Junior et al., 2011). A similar cytogenetic picture is seen in *periosteal chondroma*, which most commonly occurs on the surface of the long bones; however, only five cases have been reported so far. In contrast, *soft tissue chondromas*, two-thirds of which occur in the fingers, show recurrent gain of chromosome 5 and rearrangement of the 12q13–15 region (Tallini et al., 2002; Dahlén et al., 2003). As the *HMGA2* locus in 12q15 is frequently rearranged in other benign mesenchymal tumors, Dahlén et al. (2003) used RT-PCR to investigate the expression of *HMGA2* in six soft tissue chondromas. In four of them, all displaying 12q rearrangements at cytogenetic analysis, a truncated or full-length transcript was found. Furthermore, one case with a t(3;12)(q27;q15) harbored an *HMGA2–LPP* fusion transcript, composed of *HMGA2* exons 1–3 and *LPP* exons 9–11, which is identical to fusion transcripts previously detected in lipoma and pulmonary chondroid hamartoma. Interestingly, single cases of enchondroma and periosteal chondroma with rearrangement of band 12q13 have been reported, which, together with the finding of aberrant expression of *HMGA2* in two cases, suggests that deregulation of this gene may be of pathogenetic importance also in benign chondromatous lesions of skeletal origin (Dahlén et al., 2003). In contrast to the relative lack of recurrent chromosome aberrations, both enchondromas and peripheral chondromas frequently display mutations of the *IDH1* and *IDH2* genes, encoding different forms of isocitrate dehydrogenase (Amary et al., 2011). Mutations of the same two genes during embryogenesis cause enchondromatosis.

Synovial chondromatosis is a rare benign condition characterized by cartilage formation within the synovium. It has been debated whether it is a reactive or a neoplastic disorder. Evidence in favor of the latter interpretation comes from the finding of clonal chromosome aberrations, with involvement of the short arm of chromosome 1 and/or chromosome 6, in particular bands 6p25 and 6q13, in more than half of the cases (Tallini et al., 2002; Buddingh et al., 2003b).

Chondroblastoma is a rare benign, cartilage-producing tumor that typically arises in the epiphyses of the long bones in adolescents and young adults (Kilpatrick and Romeo, 2013). In the largest series examined, six of the seven cases had clonal aberrations (Sjögren et al., 2004). In agreement with previous data, all displayed near-diploid chromosome numbers and only few structural or numerical changes. While no recurrent chromosome aberration has been detected, mutations of the histone H3.3 gene *H3F3B* seem both consistent and specific for chondroblastoma; a mutation—typically, Lys36Met—in this gene was found in 95% of chondroblastomas but only rarely in other cartilaginous tumors (Behjati et al., 2013).

Chondromyxoid fibroma accounts for less than 1% of all bone tumors. It most often presents in the second or third decade of life and is more frequent in males. It can occur in any bone but is most commonly seen in the metaphyseal regions of long bones (Romeo et al., 2013). The cytogenetic information on this lesion is limited, but from the 16 cases that have been reported, a clearly non-random pattern has emerged. All but one have been near-diploid with only one case showing a numerical change. In all but two of the cases, various structural rearrangements of chromosome 6, clustering to 6p23–25, 6q12–13, and 6q23–27, have been present (Figure 23.3). The most common rearrangement is a pericentric inversion, with four cases displaying an apparently identical inv(6)(p25q13) (Granter et al., 1998; Tallini et al., 2002; Sjögren et al., 2004). Transcriptome and exome

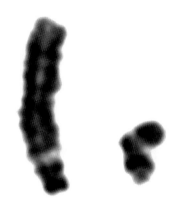

Figure 23.3 Chondromyxoid fibroma with complex rearrangements of both chromosomes 6: der(6)t(6;6)(q15;q27)inv(6)(p25q13) (left) and del(6)(q15) (right).

sequencing revealed that the clustering of breakpoints in chromosome 6 correlates with transcriptional upregulation of the glutamate receptor-encoding gene *GRM1* (Nord et al., 2014). Through inversions, translocations, and/or deletions, the entire *GRM1* gene in 6q24 becomes juxtaposed with a variety of other genes, such as *COL12A1* in 6q13.

Chondrosarcomas, that is, malignant cartilaginous tumors, account for approximately 35% of the primary malignant bone tumors. The incidence increases with age but, apart from a higher risk in patients suffering from multiple osteochondromas or enchondromatosis, predisposing or causative factors are usually unknown. Close to half of the tumors arise in the long bones of the extremities, and also the pelvis and ribs are commonly involved. The tumors are largely insensitive to chemotherapy and radiotherapy, and so the main predictors of poor outcome are inadequate surgical margins and high histologic grade (Bovée et al., 2005; Hogendoorn et al., 2013). The most common subtype is *conventional chondrosarcoma*, which in turn may be subdivided into central and peripheral tumors; the latter, making up less than one-fifth of the cases, originate from the surface of bone, presumably as the result of malignant transformation of a preexisting osteochondroma. With few exceptions, however, no distinction has been made between central and peripheral chondrosarcomas in the cytogenetic literature. In general, the karyotypes seen in conventional chondrosarcoma are much more complex than in benign chondromatous lesions, but among the close to 120 cases that have

been reported, anything from karyotypes with a single numerical or structural rearrangement to highly complex, hyperhexaploid karyotypes have been described (e.g., Bridge et al., 1993; Bovée et al., 2001; Mandahl et al., 2002; Hallor et al., 2009; Niini et al., 2012). Some 15% of the cases are hypodiploid, with a subset displaying remarkably similar hyperhaploid karyotypes, in all cases retaining two copies of chromosomes 5, 7, and 20 (Mandahl et al., 2012; Figure 23.4). Although no specific, diagnostically useful aberration, or in fact any recurrent balanced rearrangement, has been detected, conventional chondrosarcomas have a clearly nonrandom cytogenetic profile dominated by numerical changes. Gains of chromosomes 7, 19, 20, and 21 and losses of the sex chromosomes and chromosomes 1, 4, 6, 9, 10, 11, 13, 14, 17, and 22 are all seen in at least 15% of the cases. Adding imbalances caused by structural rearrangements, minimally gained or lost regions include −1p36, −1p13-22, −5q13-31, −6q22-qter, +7p13-pter, −9p22-pter, −10p, −10q24-qter, −11p13-pter, −11q25, +12q15-qter, −13q21-qter, −14q24-qter, −18p, −18q22-qter, +20pter-q11, and −22q13 (Mandahl et al., 2002). In general, these findings correlate well with results obtained by comparative genomic hybridization (CGH) analyses (Rozeman et al., 2006; Hallor et al., 2009). Approximately half of conventional chondrosarcomas show mutations of *IDH1* or *IDH2*, which are supposed to constitute early events as they are found also in enchondromas (Amary et al., 2011).

Mesenchymal chondrosarcoma is a rare variant of chondrosarcoma that may arise both in bones and in soft tissues (Nakashima et al., 2013). Only 11 cases with cytogenetic data have been reported, typically showing less complex karyotypes than conventional chondrosarcomas. While no specific rearrangement or clustering of breakpoints has been observed among these cases, a tumor-specific *HEY1–NCOA2* fusion was found through global gene expression profiling (Wang et al., 2012). The two genes, located in 8q21 and 8q13, respectively, are fused through an interstitial deletion that is too small to be detectable by chromosome banding. Molecular diagnosis thus requires FISH and/or RT-PCR.

The limited amount of cytogenetic information available on *clear cell* and *dedifferentiated chondrosarcoma* does not indicate the presence of any

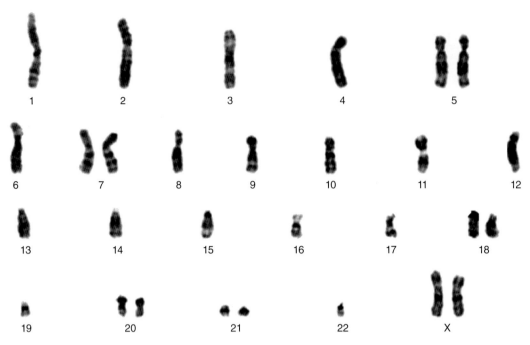

Figure 23.4 Chondrosarcoma with hyperhaploid karyotype. Note retention of two copies of chromosomes 5, 7, and 20.

diagnostic chromosome aberration. In general, the karyotypes seem to resemble those of conventional chondrosarcoma, and no consistent chromosome aberration has emerged. *IDH1* or *IDH2* mutations are found in approximately 50% of dedifferentiated chondrosarcomas but not in clear cell chondrosarcomas (Amary et al., 2011).

Osteogenic tumors

Benign osteogenic tumors are poorly characterized at the cytogenetic level. The few *osteoid osteomas* that have been reported all shared near-diploid karyotypes, with two cases each showing deletion of band 22q13 and loss of parts of or the entire chromosome 17. *Osteoblastomas* seem to have slightly more complex karyotypes, with chromosome numbers ranging from 39 to 52 and, in half the cases, more than 10 structural and/or numerical changes. Still, the level of cytogenetic complexity is far below what is usually seen in osteosarcomas. Loss of material from chromosome 22 is recurrent, but the molecular consequences have not been identified (Nord et al., 2013).

Osteosarcoma is the most common malignant primary bone tumor, with an estimated incidence

of 5 per million inhabitants. The age distribution is bimodal with 60% of osteosarcomas occurring before the age of 25. Based on clinical, roentgenographic, and histopathologic features, several subtypes have been discerned: conventional, telangiectatic, small cell, low-grade central, parosteal, periosteal, and high-grade surface osteosarcomas. In addition, some 15% of osteosarcomas are secondary to a preexisting abnormality, most commonly Paget's disease (Fletcher et al., 2013).

The predominant subtype, *conventional osteosarcoma*, is most common in adolescents, but about one-third occur in patients over 40 years of age. Close to 150 cases have been reported in the cytogenetic literature, and the great majority have shown highly complex karyotypes with gross aneuploidy and a multitude of structural and numerical changes (Figure 23.5). Furthermore, these tumors often display extensive cell-to-cell variation, indicating a high level of genetic instability. It is therefore often difficult or impossible to obtain a complete karyotype using chromosome banding analysis alone (e.g., Mertens et al., 1993; Bridge et al., 1997; Lau et al., 2004). The most common numerical changes are losses of chromosomes 3, 4, 5, 9, 10, 13, 15, 17, 18, 19, and 22, all occurring in

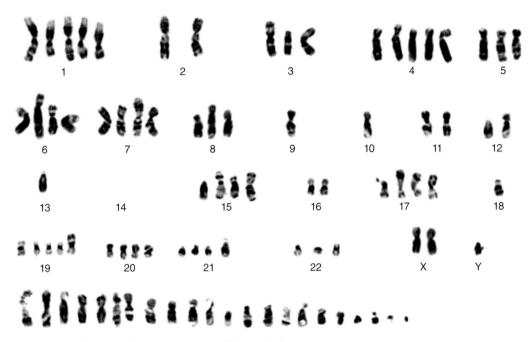

Figure 23.5 High-grade malignant osteosarcoma with complex karyotype.

20–40% of the cases. These findings are in good agreement with results from CGH and loss of heterozygosity (LOH) studies, implicating chromosome arms 3q, 13q, 17p, and 17q as particularly frequent targets for deletions. The *RB1* and *TP53* genes in 13q14 and 17p13, respectively, constitute credible target tumor suppressor genes. Constitutional inactivating mutations in these two genes confer an increased risk of several malignancies, including osteosarcoma. Array-based analyses have, however, also detected several recurrent gene amplifications not found by standard chromosome banding analysis, for example, at 1q21–23, 6p12–21, 8q24, 12q13–15, and 17p. No recurrent balanced aberration has been reported, but breakpoints involved in at least 10% of the cases include 1p11, 1q11, 1q21, 3p11, 11p15, 14p11, 15p11, 17p11, 19p13, 19q13, and 20p11. In spite of their chaotic karyotypes, conventional osteosarcomas have surprisingly few point mutations. Exome sequencing of 13 tumors identified, on average, 15.5 mutations per case, roughly equivalent to the mutation frequency in sarcomas with known gene fusions and few cytogenetic aberrations (Joseph et al., 2014).

Less than five cases each of *telangiectatic*, *small cell*, and *periosteal osteosarcoma* have been reported, precluding any attempt to assess whether they differ cytogenetically from conventional osteosarcomas. However, *parosteal osteosarcoma*, which is a low-grade tumor arising on the surface of bone, has a distinct karyotypic profile. All 10 reported cases have shown one or more supernumerary ring chromosomes, in eight of them as the sole anomaly in at least one clone (Figure 23.6) (Mertens et al., 1993; Heidenblad et al., 2006). FISH and CGH analyses have shown that the ring chromosomes invariably contain material from the long arm of chromosome 12 (Heidenblad et al., 2006; Mejia-Guerrero et al., 2010). The extent and level of the amplicons on 12q vary from case to case, but two regions, each containing a limited set of potential target genes, seem to be involved in all cases: 12q13–14 with *SAS* and *CDK4* and 12q15 with *MDM2*. Thus, both at the cytogenetic level and in terms of distribution of amplicons on chromosome 12, these tumors are highly similar to atypical lipomas/well-differentiated liposarcomas (Heidenblad et al., 2006).

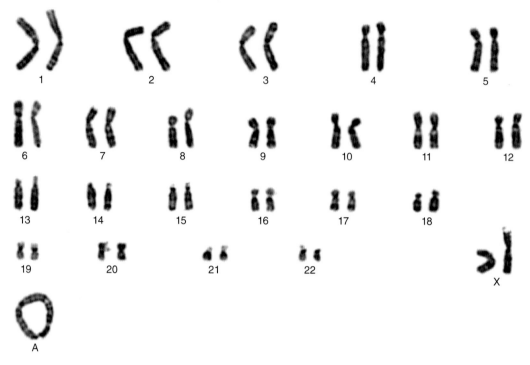

Figure 23.6 Parosteal osteosarcoma with a supernumerary ring chromosome as the sole aberration.

Ewing sarcoma

Ewing sarcomas, also known as *primitive neuroectodermal tumors* (PNET), are highly aggressive small cell round cell sarcomas showing varying degrees of neuroectodermal differentiation. They account for less than 10% of primary malignant bone tumors, with a predilection for the diaphysis of the long bones. However, any bone, as well as the soft tissues and parenchymatous organs, may be affected. Peak age incidence is during the second decade of life, with 80% of the patients being younger than 20 years at diagnosis. Previously, the outcome was invariably fatal, but thanks to the introduction of multimodal treatment, overall survival has increased to almost two-thirds (de Alava et al., 2013).

The cytogenetic hallmark of Ewing sarcoma is a balanced t(11;22)(q24;q12), first described in 1983 by Aurias et al. and Turc-Carel et al. Since then, karyotypes from more than 450 Ewing sarcomas have been reported, with the t(11;22), or variants thereof, being present in close to 75% of the cases (Figure 23.7). In unselected series, the frequency is

even higher, approaching 80–90%, which is in line with figures obtained by FISH and molecular genetic studies (Delattre et al., 1992; Sandberg and Bridge, 2000; Udayakumar et al., 2001; Bridge et al., 2006; Roberts et al., 2008). The importance of the t(11;22) for the origin of Ewing sarcoma is emphasized by the fact that, when present, it is the sole anomaly in close to one-third of the cases. However, most cases display additional changes, and although gross aneuploidy is uncommon in Ewing sarcoma, over 20% have more than 50 chromosomes. The most common secondary anomalies are gain of one or more copies of chromosomes 8 (33%) and 12 (20%), followed by trisomy for chromosomes 2, 14, 18, and 20 and the unbalanced der(16)t(1;16)(q11–21;q11–13), each occurring in approximately 10% of the cases.

The t(11;22)(q24;q12) was the first sarcoma-associated translocation to be characterized at the molecular level (Delattre et al., 1992; Zucman et al., 1992). The translocation fuses the *EWSR1* gene in 22q12 with the *FLI1* gene in 11q24 to generate a novel hybrid gene. *EWSR1* belongs, together with

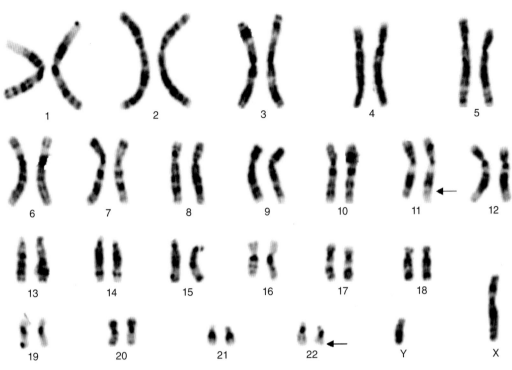

Figure 23.7 Karyotype from a Ewing sarcoma displaying the characteristic t(11;22)(q24;q12) as the sole change. Arrows indicate breakpoints. The translocation results in the creation of an *EWSR1–FLI1* fusion gene.

FUS in 16p11 and *TAF15* in 17q12, two other genes involved in gene fusions in sarcomas, to the so-called *TET* family of genes that share an amino-terminal RNA-binding motif (Riggi et al., 2007). The protein encoded by *FLI1* is a member of the ETS family of transcription factors that target DNA sequences via related structural motifs in their DNA-binding regions, usually located in their carboxy-terminal portions (Riggi et al., 2007). The t(11;22) (q24;q12) joins the 5′ portion of the *EWSR1* gene to the 3′ (DNA-binding) region of *FLI1*, thus resulting in the replacement of its transcription activation domain by *EWSR1* sequences. The breakpoints in the two genes vary, but the most common (~80% of the cases) fusions are between *EWSR1* exon 7 and *FLI1* exon 6 (known as the type 1 transcript) or exon 5 (type 2). It has been shown that expression of the fusion protein causes up- or downregulation of a large number of genes that, consequently, may play a role in the development of Ewing sarcoma (Stoll et al., 2013). Interestingly, the biological effects of the EWSR1–FLI1 chimeric protein seem to be

dependent on the cellular context. Whereas forced expression of the *EWSR1–FLI1* fusion gene is sufficient for transforming mouse primary bone marrow-derived mesenchymal progenitor cells, additional genetic changes are necessary to transform primary mouse embryonic fibroblasts (Deneen and Denny, 2001; Riggi et al., 2005).

Several alternate gene fusions involving the *EWSR1* gene as the 5′-partner and another gene than *FLI1* from the ETS family of transcription factors as the 3′-partner have been described in Ewing sarcomas. The most common of these is the *EWSR1–ERG* fusion, seen in 5–15% of the cases (Zucman et al., 1993). The corresponding t(21;22) (q22;q12) is rarely observed at cytogenetic analysis, probably due to the fact that the two genes are transcribed in opposite directions. Thus, a functional fusion gene cannot arise through a simple balanced translocation. Another 1–5% of Ewing sarcomas harbor a t(7;22)(p21;q12), t(2;22)(q35;q12), or t(17;22)(q21;q12), resulting in fusion of *EWSR1* with *ETV1*, *FEV*, or *ETV4*, respectively (Riggi et al., 2007). In addition, in rare cases of Ewing sarcoma or Ewing-like undifferentiated round cell sarcomas, *EWSR1* becomes fused to *NFATC2* in 20q13, *PATZ1* in 22q12, *POU5F1* in 6p21, *SMARCA5* in 4q31, or *SP3* in 2q31 (Wang et al., 2007; de Alava et al., 2013).

Adding further to the molecular genetic complexity of Ewing sarcoma, EWSR1 may occasionally be exchanged for another member of the TET family of proteins; the t(16;21) (p11;q22) fuses the *FUS* gene in 16p11 with *ERG* and the t(2;16) (q35;p11) results in a *FUS–FEV* chimera (Shing et al., 2003; Ng et al., 2007). The former translocation and fusion gene are recurrently seen also in a subset of acute myeloid leukemias, but it seems as if the transcript types might be different in the sarcoma and the hematologic malignancy (Riggi et al., 2007). With *EWSR1–FLI1* and *EWSR1–ERG* accounting for such an overwhelming majority of the fusion events in Ewing sarcoma, it is difficult to obtain large enough series to evaluate properly the biological and clinical impact of the many rare variants. However, it has been suggested that the less common types of *EWSR1* fusions may be associated with poorly differentiated extraskeletal tumors in children (Wang et al., 2007).

In addition to the many reported permutations on the theme "amino-terminal part of TET family member fusing with carboxy-terminal part of DNA-binding protein," a number of other rare but recurrent fusion events have been described in Ewing-like sarcomas. A subgroup of bone tumors in children and adolescents display a *BCOR–CCNB3* fusion resulting from an inversion in Xp11 (Pierron et al., 2012). Another frequent finding in *EWSR1*-negative cases is the *CIC–DUX4* fusion resulting from a t(4;19)(q35;q13) (Kawamura-Saito et al., 2006; Italiano et al., 2012).

The molecular heterogeneity in Ewing sarcoma notwithstanding, genetic analysis may provide important differential diagnostic information. Ewing sarcomas are phenotypically similar to several other diagnostic entities with the main morphologic feature that they appear as *small cell round cell blue cell tumors*. Although several useful immunohistochemical markers, such as CD99, have been developed during recent years, the differential diagnosis of these usually pediatric malignancies (e.g., rhabdomyosarcoma, small cell osteosarcoma, neuroblastoma, and lymphoma)

may be extremely difficult. The highly consistent occurrence of translocations involving the *EWSR1* gene in Ewing sarcomas, rearrangements not seen in the other tumor types, may thus aid significantly the more traditional, phenotype-based diagnostic efforts. Bearing in mind that the material available for genetic diagnosis is often limited to cells from fine needle or core needle biopsies and that some of the translocations, in particular the t(21;22), are difficult to identify by chromosome banding analysis, directed FISH analysis of the *EWSR1* locus and/or RT-PCR for the most common gene fusions—*EWSR1–FLI1* and *EWSR1–ERG*—come across as the fastest and most reliable methods to verify the suspicion of a Ewing sarcoma.

Several factors negatively influencing the clinical outcome of Ewing sarcoma patients have been identified, including disseminated disease at diagnosis, large tumor size, and axial location. The type of *EWSR1* fusion does not seem to affect outcome (Le Deley et al., 2010; van Doorninck et al., 2010). The same applies to the secondary chromosomal changes frequently seen in Ewing sarcomas. Many individual karyotypic features have been suggested to affect outcome, and in the largest study so far, three overlapping features—complex karyotype (>5 changes), chromosome number greater than 50, and trisomy 20—were all shown to be associated with shorter survival. The authors therefore suggested that karyotypic complexity might constitute a valuable independent prognostic marker (Roberts et al., 2008).

Notochordal tumors

Usually located along the axial skeleton, primarily in the sacrococcygeal and spheno-occipital regions, *chordomas* are believed to be derived from remnants of the embryonal notochord (Vujovic et al., 2006). These tumors are rare accounting for 1–4% of all primary bone sarcomas (Flanagan and Yamaguchi, 2013). Clinically, chordomas manifest as slowly growing, locally destructive lesions with a tendency to infiltrate into adjacent tissues. Metastases are rarely encountered, but because of difficulties in obtaining wide-margin resection of the primary tumor, local recurrences resulting in tissue destruction are common, eventually killing the patient. Most cytogenetically investigated chordomas have displayed near-diploid or moderately hypodiploid karyotypes with several numerical and structural rearrangements (Tallini et al., 2002; Kuzniacka et al., 2004; Brandal et al., 2005; Almefty et al., 2009). Recurrent chromosomal aberrations in chordomas, identified using G-banding, metaphase CGH, and FISH, include loss of the entire or parts of chromosomes 3, 4, 10, 13, and 18, loss or rearrangement of 1p and 9p,

and gain of chromosome 7. An array CGH analysis of 21 cases identified copy number alterations in all samples, and all chromosomes were seen to participate in imbalances (Hallor et al., 2008). The most common imbalance was heterozygous or homozygous loss of a region on 9p encompassing the *CDKN2A* and *CDKN2B* loci (Figure 23.8). Expression of the transcription factor Brachyury in 6q27 is highly specific for chordoma, and copy

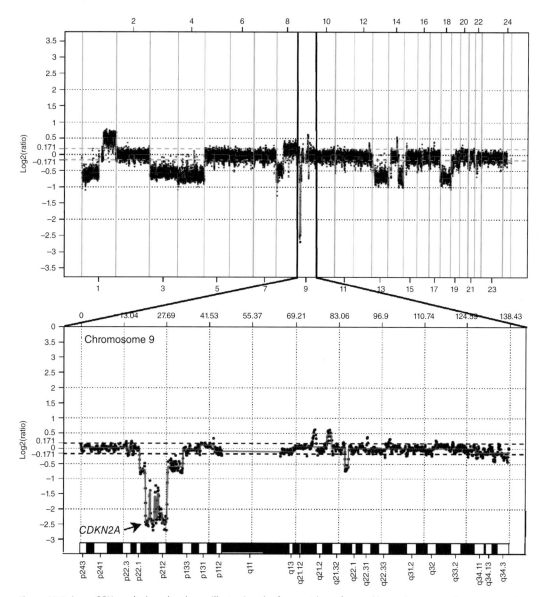

Figure 23.8 Array CGH results in a chordoma, illustrating the frequent loss of several large chromosomal segments and the absence of amplicons in this tumor. The lower part highlights the frequent occurrence of deletions of the 9p21–22 segment harboring the *CDKN2A* tumor suppressor gene.

number gain of the gene encoding this protein is a common finding.

Giant cell tumors

Giant cell tumor of bone is a benign but locally aggressive tumor accounting for approximately 5% of all bone tumors. The peak incidence is in the third to fifth decade of life, and the most common locations are the ends of long bones, in particular the distal femur and radius and the proximal tibia and humerus. The tumor derives its name from the presence of osteoclast-like giant cells, mixed with mononuclear cells. It is generally believed, however, that it is the latter cell type that is neoplastic (Athanasou et al., 2013). This conclusion was further substantiated when it could be shown that driver mutations of the *H3F3A* gene, which are present in more than 90% of the cases, occurred only in nonosteoclastic tumor cells (Behjati et al., 2013). In most cases, short-term culturing does not result in metaphase spreads with clonal chromosome aberrations. A striking feature, however, is the frequent occurrence of telomeric associations (tas), which have been reported to occur in up to 85% of the cases (Bridge et al., 1992; Sciot et al., 2000). Some chromosome ends seem to be more often involved than others. Mandahl et al. (1998) investigated the distribution of 880 clonal and nonclonal breakpoints in telomeric rearrangements and found four chromosome termini that each accounted for more than 5% of the rearrangements: 11p, 15p, 19q, and 21p (Figure 23.9). Whether the increased tendency toward tas formation in giant cell tumors is related to altered H3F3A remains to be investigated.

Close to 40 cases with other changes than tas have been reported in the cytogenetic literature. The great majority of these had a near-diploid chromosome count (45–47 chromosomes), but no consistent aberration has been detected. It could be noted, however, that some of the chromosome arms frequently forming tas, in particular 11p and 19q, are often involved also in other structural rearrangements, such as deletions and ring chromosome formation, suggesting a mechanistic link between these phenomena (Sawyer et al., 2005). Although local recurrences are frequent, metastases are rare, occurring in less than 5% of the

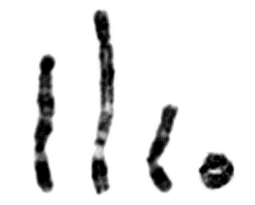

Figure 23.9 Four different rearrangements affecting distal 11p in a giant cell tumor of bone. From left to right: two telomeric associations, one add(11)(p15), and one r(11).

cases. So far, no cytogenetic feature associated with more aggressive behavior has been identified.

Miscellaneous bone tumors

Many tumors that preferentially occur in the soft tissues, such as myoepithelial tumor, epithelioid hemangioendothelioma, and extraskeletal myxoid chondrosarcoma, occasionally also develop as primary lesions in bone. Data on such bone tumors are still very limited, but it seems that they have the same karyotypic and molecular genetic characteristics as their more common soft tissue counterparts. Primary tumors of bone also include a number of entities that remain enigmatic in terms of lineage of differentiation and that have only recently, much thanks to cytogenetic findings, been recognized as true neoplasms.

Aneurysmal bone cyst is a benign, but locally aggressive, osteolytic lesion composed of multiple blood-filled cysts separated by fibrous septae. It usually occurs in the metaphysis of long bones and most commonly affects children or young adults. Rare cases of soft tissue tumors with morphology identical to that of the bone lesions have also been reported. Aneurysmal bone cysts often arise secondarily to other benign or malignant bone tumors, such as giant cell tumor of bone, complicating the differential diagnosis. Aneurysmal bone cyst was long considered a reactive lesion, but in 1999, Panoutsakopoulos and coworkers could firmly establish its neoplastic nature by identifying a recurrent t(16;17)(q22;p13). Since then, karyotypes of close to 40 cases have been reported. All had a pseudo- or near-diploid chromosome count, and one-fourth of the cases harbored an exchange between chromosome arms 16q and 17p (Figure 23.10). The vast majority of the remaining cases display other structural rearrangements, typically translocations, affecting band 17p13, whereas a small number of cases have rearrangements of band 16q22 or other changes (Sciot et al., 2000; Althof et al., 2004; Oliveira et al., 2004a, 2005). In agreement with the cytogenetic data, Oliveira et al. (2004a) demonstrated that the recurrent t(16;17) consistently results in a fusion between the gene for cadherin 11 (*CDH11*) in 16q21 and the gene for ubiquitin-specific protease (*USP6*) in 17p13. More specifically, the translocation puts the entire coding sequence of *USP6* under the control of the promoter region of *CDH11*, which is a gene highly expressed in osteoblasts. Further RT-PCR and interphase FISH analysis of more than 50 aneurysmal bone cysts by Oliveira et al. (2004b) identified the *CDH11–USP6* fusion in 28% of the cases and revealed that the spindle-shaped neoplastic cells were diffusely scattered throughout the tumors. The importance of *USP6* deregulation for the development of aneurysmal bone cysts was later demonstrated by the same group when they showed that four other translocations—t(1;17)(p34;p13), t(3;17)(q21;p13), t(9;17)(q22;p13), and t(17;17)(q12;p13)—all resulted in upregulation of *USP6* transcription through promoter swapping with *THRAP3*, *CNBP*, *OMD*, and *COL1A1*, respectively (Oliveira et al., 2005). Interestingly, not all aneurysmal bone cysts express *USP6*, which, in line with the finding of abnormal karyotypes seemingly without 17p rearrangements, suggests the existence also of alternative molecular pathways.

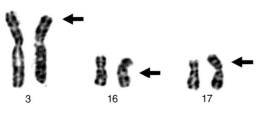

Figure 23.10 Aneurysmal bone cyst with a three-way t(3;16;17)(p2?4;q22;p13) as the sole change. Arrows indicate breakpoints.

The only reported cytogenetically examined soft tissue aneurysmal bone cyst showed a t(11;16)(q13;q22–23) as the sole change (Dal Cin et al., 2000a), suggesting that this unusual variant might be biologically related to the more common bone tumors.

Benign fibro-osseous lesions of bone is a collective term for a number of clinically distinct tumors or tumor-like lesions primarily affecting children and adolescents. Three major morphologic subgroups are currently recognized: *fibrous dysplasia*, *osteofibrous dysplasia*, and *ossifying fibroma*. Whereas no consistent chromosome aberration has been detected in fibrous dysplasias, hyperdiploid karyotypes (47–52 chromosomes) were seen in three of four cases of osteofibrous dysplasia, with gain of chromosomes 7, 8, and 12 as recurrent changes (Bridge et al., 1994; Dal Cin et al., 2000b; Parham et al., 2004). Interestingly, similar karyotypes have been reported also in *adamantinoma*, a low-grade malignant bone tumor that shares clinical and morphologic features with osteofibrous dysplasia. Seven of the nine adamantinomas have had hyperdiploid karyotypes (48–54 chromosomes) with gain of chromosome 7 in six, chromosomes 12 and 19 in five each, and chromosome 8 in four cases (Hazelbag et al., 1997). *Ossifying fibroma*, which is a pediatric tumor showing a marked predilection for the cranial bones and mandible, is still poorly investigated at the cytogenetic level, but from the few cases available, it seems clear that the majority display a t(X;2)(q26;q33) or variants thereof (Sawyer et al., 1995; Parham et al., 2004). Whether this tumor-specific translocation results in a gene fusion remains to be investigated. Skeletal lesions in *Langerhans cell histiocytosis* invariably show normal karyotypes and genomic profiles by array CGH profiling. Half of the cases, however, carry the BRAF V600E mutation, which is also seen in around 50% of *Erdheim–Chester disease* (Badalian-Very et al., 2010; Haroche et al., 2012).

Summary

Cytogenetic analyses of bone tumors have demonstrated that most subtypes carry characteristic, sometimes tumor-specific, chromosomal aberrations that are useful for differential diagnostic purposes (Table 23.1). There is also a general correlation

Table 23.1 Characteristic balanced structural chromosome aberrations and gene fusions in bone tumors

Chromosome rearrangement	Gene fusion	Tumor type
del(X)(p11p11)	BCOR–CCNB3	UDS
t(X;2)(q26;q33)	Unknown	Ossifying fibroma
t(X;6) (q24–26;q15–25)	IRS4 deregulation	Subungual exostosis
t(1;17)(p34;p13)	THRAP3–USP6	Aneurysmal bone cyst
t(1;17) (q32–42;q21–23)	Unknown	BPOP
t(1;22)(q23;q12)	EWSR1–PBX1	Myoepithelial tumor
t(2;16)(q35;p11)	FUS–FEV	Ewing sarcoma
t(2;22)(q35;q12)	EWSR1–FEV	Ewing sarcoma
t(3;17)(q21;p13)	CNBP–USP6	Aneurysmal bone cyst
inv(6)(p25q13), der(6)(q24)	Deregulation of GRM1	Chondromyxoid fibroma
t(6;22)(p21;q12)	EWSR1–POU5F1	UDS
t(7;12)(p22;q13)	ACTB–GLI1	Pericytoma
t(7;19)(q22;q13)	SERPINE1–FOSB	PHA
t(7;22)(p21;q12)	EWSR1–ETV1	Ewing sarcoma
del(8)(q13q21)	HEY1–NCOA2	Mesenchymal CS
t(9;17)(q22;p13)	OMD–USP6	Aneurysmal bone cyst
t(9;22)(q31;q12)	EWSR1–NR4A3	Myxoid chondrosarcoma
t(11;22)(q24;q12)	EWSR1–FLI1	Ewing sarcoma
t(12;22)(q13;q12)	EWSR1–ATF1	UDS
t(16;17)(q22;p13)	CDH11–USP6	Aneurysmal bone cyst
t(16;21)(p11;q22)	FUS–ERG	Ewing sarcoma
t(17;17)(q21;p13)	COL1A1–USP6	Aneurysmal bone cyst
t(17;22)(q21;q12)	EWSR1–ETV4	Ewing sarcoma
t(20;22)(q13;q12)	EWSR1–NFATC2	Ewing sarcoma
t(21;22)(q22;q12)	EWSR1–ERG	Ewing sarcoma
inv(22)(q12q12)	EWSR1–PATZ1	Ewing sarcoma

BPOP, bizarre parosteal osteochondromatous proliferation; mesenchymal CS, mesenchymal chondrosarcoma; PHA, pseudomyogenic hemangioendothelioma; UDS, undifferentiated sarcoma.

between overall level of genomic complexity and the degree of malignancy; benign lesions typically have near-diploid karyotypes with few aberrations, whereas malignant lesions, with the notable exception of Ewing sarcoma, mostly show aneuploidy and multiple structural and numerical changes. Many of the tumor-specific chromosomal rearrangements are balanced translocations, and for the majority of them, the molecular consequences have been clarified, allowing the use of FISH or RT-PCR to verify or exclude their presence preoperatively or before initiating chemotherapy. Most importantly, Ewing sarcomas, which for cure require multimodal treatment, can be readily separated from other malignancies by demonstration of involvement of the *EWSR1* gene, which only rarely is rearranged in tumors posing differential diagnostic problems. For some recurrent balanced rearrangements, such as the t(X;2)(q26;q33) in ossifying fibroma and the t(1;17)(q32–42;q21–23) in BPOP, molecular details are still lacking. Furthermore, many entities, such as fibrogenic and fibrohistiocytic tumors, remain poorly investigated, diminishing the role of cytogenetics in the diagnostic setting.

Much less is known about the prognostic significance of karyotypic variation within tumor entities, but emerging data suggest that the karyotypic pattern is indeed associated with outcome. For instance, it has been suggested that Ewing sarcomas with complex karyotypes and chondrosarcomas with loss of chromosome 13 are more aggressive than the corresponding tumors without these features. In order for such observations to have an impact on the stratification of patients for different treatment protocols, they need to be repeated in larger series and compared with already established prognostic factors.

Acknowledgment

We are grateful to Linda Magnusson for help with the figures.

References

Almefty KK, Pravdenkova S, Sawyer J, Al-Mefty O (2009): Impact of cytogenetic abnormalities on the management of skull base chordomas. *J Neurosurg* 110:715–724.

Althof PA, Ohmori K, Zhou M, Bailey JM, Bridge RS, Nelson M, et al. (2004): Cytogenetic and molecular cytogenetic findings in 43 aneurysmal bone cysts: aberrations of 17p mapped to 17p13.2 by fluorescence in situ hybridization. *Mod Pathol* 17:518–525.

Amary MF, Bacsi K, Maggiani F, Damato S, Halai D, Berisha F, et al. (2011): IDH1 and IDH2 mutations are frequent events in central chondrosarcoma and central and periosteal chondromas but not in other mesenchymal tumours. *J Pathol* 224:334–343.

Athanasou NA, Bansal M, Forsyth R, Reid RP, Sapi Z (2013): Giant cell tumour of bone. In: Fletcher CDM, Bridge JA, Hogendoorn PCW, Mertens F, editors. *WHO Classification of Tumours of Soft Tissue and Bone.* Lyon: IARC Press, pp 321–324.

Aurias A, Rimbaut C, Buffe D, Dubousset J, Mazabraud A (1983): Chromosomal translocations in Ewing's sarcoma. *N Engl J Med* 309:496–497.

Badalian-Very G, Vergilio JA, Degar BA, MacConaill LE, Brandner B, Calicchio ML, et al. (2010): Recurrent BRAF mutations in Langerhans cell histiocytosis. *Blood* 116:1919–1923.

Behjati S, Tarpey PS, Presneau N, Scheipl S, Pillay N, Van Loo P, et al. (2013): Distinct H3F3A and H3F3B driver mutations define chondroblastoma and giant cell tumor of bone. *Nat Genet* 45:1479–1483.

Bovée JVMG, Sciot R, Dal Cin P, Debiec-Rychter M, van Zelderen-Bhola SL, Cornelisse CJ, et al. (2001): Chromosome 9 alterations and trisomy 22 in central chondrosarcoma: a cytogenetic and DNA flow cytometric analysis of chondrosarcoma subtypes. *Diagn Mol Pathol* 10:228–235.

Bovée JVMG, Cleton-Jansen A-M, Taminiau AHM, Hogendoorn PCW (2005): Emerging pathways in the development of chondrosarcoma of bone and implications for targeted therapy. *Lancet Oncol* 6:599–607.

Brandal P, Bjerkehagen B, Danielsen H, Heim S (2005): Chromosome 7 abnormalities are common in chordomas. *Cancer Genet Cytogenet* 160:15–21.

Bridge JA, Neff JR, Mouron BJ (1992): Giant cell tumor of bone. Chromosomal analysis of 48 specimens and review of the literature. *Cancer Genet Cytogenet* 58:2–13.

Bridge JA, Bhatia PS, Anderson JR, Neff JR (1993): Biologic and clinical significance of cytogenetic and molecular cytogenetic abnormalities in benign and malignant cartilaginous lesions. *Cancer Genet Cytogenet* 69:79–90.

Bridge JA, Dembinski A, DeBoer J, Travis J, Neff JR (1994): Clonal chromosomal abnormalities in osteofibrous dysplasia. Implications for histopathogenesis and its relationship with adamantinoma. *Cancer* 73:1746–1752.

Bridge JA, Nelson M, McComb E, McGuire MH, Rosenthal H, Vergara G, et al. (1997): Cytogenetic findings in 73 osteosarcoma specimens and a review of the literature. *Cancer Genet Cytogenet* 95:74–87.

Bridge RS, Rajaram V, Dehner LP, Pfeifer JD, Perry A (2006): Molecular diagnosis of Ewing sarcoma/primitive neuroectodermal tumor in routinely processed tissue: a comparison of two FISH strategies and RT-PCR in malignant round cell tumors. *Mod Pathol* 19:1–8.

Buddingh EP, Naumann S, Nelson M, Neff JR, Birch N, Bridge JA (2003a): Cytogenetic findings in benign cartilaginous neoplasms. *Cancer Genet Cytogenet* 141:164–168.

Buddingh EP, Krallman P, Neff JR, Nelson M, Liu J, Bridge JA (2003b): Chromosome 6 abnormalities are recurrent in synovial chondromatosis. *Cancer Genet Cytogenet* 140:18–22.

Dahlén A, Mertens F, Rydholm A, Brosjö O, Wejde J, Mandahl N, et al. (2003): Fusion, disruption, and expression of HMGA2 in bone and soft tissue chondromas. *Mod Pathol* 16:1132–1140.

Dal Cin P, Pauwels P, Poldermans LJ, Sciot R, Van den Berghe H (1999): Clonal chromosome abnormalities in a so-called Dupuytren's subungual exostosis. *Genes Chromosomes Cancer* 24:162–164.

Dal Cin P, Kozakewich HP, Goumnerova L, Mankin HJ, Rosenberg AE, Fletcher JA (2000a): Variant translocations involving 16q22 and 17p13 in solid variant and extraosseous forms of aneurysmal bone cyst. *Genes Chromosomes Cancer* 28:233–234.

Dal Cin P, Sciot R, Brys P, deWever I, Dorfman H, Fletcher CDM, et al. (2000b): Recurrent chromosome aberrations in fibrous dysplasia of the bone: a report of the CHAMP Study Group. *Cancer Genet Cytogenet* 122:30–32.

de Alava E, Lessnick SL, Sorensen PH (2013): Ewing sarcoma. In: Fletcher CDM, Bridge JA, Hogendoorn PCW, Mertens F, editors. *WHO Classification of Tumours of Soft Tissue and Bone.* Lyon: IARC Press, pp 306–309.

Delattre O, Zucman J, Plougastel B, Desmaze C, Melot T, Peter M, et al. (1992): Gene fusion with an ETS DNA-binding domain caused by chromosome translocation in human tumours. *Nature* 359:162–165.

Deneen B, Denny CT (2001): Loss of p16 pathways stabilizes EWSR/FLI1 expression and complements EWS/FLI1 mediated transformation. *Oncogene* 20:6731–6741.

Endo M, Hasegawa T, Tashiro T, Yamaguchi U, Morimoto Y, Nakatani F, et al. (2005): Bizarre parosteal osteochondromatous proliferation with a t(1;17) translocation. *Virchows Arch* 447:99–102.

Flanagan AM, Yamaguchi T (2013): Chordoma. In: Fletcher CDM, Bridge JA, Hogendoorn PCW, Mertens F, editors. *WHO Classification of Tumours of Soft Tissue and Bone.* Lyon: IARC Press, pp 328–329.

Fletcher CDM, Bridge JA, Hogendoorn PCW, Mertens F, editors (2013): *WHO Classification of Tumours of Soft Tissue and Bone.* Lyon: IARC Press.

Granter SR, Renshaw AA, Kozakewich HP, Fletcher JA (1998): The pericentromeric inversion, inv(6)(p25q13), is a novel diagnostic marker in chondromyxoid fibroma. *Mod Pathol* 11:1071–1074.

Hallor KH, Staaf J, Jönsson G, Heidenblad M, Vult von Steyern F, Bauer HCF, et al. (2008): Frequent deletion of the CDKN2A locus in chordoma: analysis of chromosomal imbalances using array comparative genomic hybridisation. *Br J Cancer* 98:434–442.

Hallor KH, Staaf J, Bovée JVMG, Hogendoorn PCW, Cleton-Jansen A-M, Knuutila S, et al. (2009): Genomic profiling of chondrosarcoma: chromosomal patterns in central and peripheral tumors. *Clin Cancer Res* 15:2685–2694.

Hameetman L, Szuhai K, Yavas A, Knijnenburg J, van Duin M, van Dekken H, et al. (2007): The role of EXT1 in nonhereditary osteochondroma: identification of homozygous deletions. *J Natl Cancer Inst* 99:396–406.

Haroche J, Charlotte F, Arnaud L, von Deimling A, Hélias-Rodzewicz Z, Hervier B, et al.2012): High prevalence of BRAF V600E mutations in Erdheim–Chester disease but not in other non-Langerhans cell histiocytoses. *Blood* 120:2700–2703.

Hazelbag HM, Wessels JW, Mollevangers P, van den Berg E, Molenaar WM, Hogendoorn PCW (1997): Cytogenetic analysis of adamantinoma of long bones: further indications for a common histogenesis with osteofibrous dysplasia. *Cancer Genet Cytogenet* 97:5–11.

Heidenblad M, Hallor KH, Staaf J, Jönsson G, Borg Å, Höglund M, et al. (2006): Genomic profiling of bone and soft tissue tumors with supernumerary ring chromosomes using tiling resolution bacterial artificial chromosome microarrays. *Oncogene* 25:7106–7116.

Hogendoorn PCW, Bovée JVMG, Nielsen GP (2013): Chondrosarcoma (grades I–III), including primary and secondary variants and parosteal chondrosarcoma. In: Fletcher CDM, Bridge JA, Hogendoorn PCW, Mertens F, editors. *WHO Classification of Tumours of Soft Tissue and Bone.* Lyon: IARC Press, pp 264–268.

Italiano A, Sung YS, Zhang L, Singer S, Maki RG, Coindre J-M, et al. (2012): High prevalence of CIC fusion with double-homeobox (DUX4) transcription factors in EWSR1-negative undifferentiated small blue round cell sarcomas. *Genes Chromosomes Cancer* 51:207–218.

Joseph CG, Hwang H, Jiao Y, Wood LD, Kinde I, Wu J, et al. (2014): Exomic analysis of myxoid liposarcomas, synovial sarcomas and osteosarcomas. *Genes Chromosomes Cancer* 53:15–24.

Kawamura-Saito M, Yamazaki Y, Kaneko K, Kawaguchi N, Kanda H, Mukai H, et al. (2006): Fusion between CIC and DUX4 up-regulates PEA3 family genes in Ewing-like sarcomas with t(4;19)(q35;q13) translocation. *Hum Mol Genet* 15:2125–2137.

Kilpatrick SE, Romeo S (2013): Chondroblastoma. In: Fletcher CDM, Bridge JA, Hogendoorn PCW, Mertens F, editors. *WHO Classification of Tumours of Soft Tissue and Bone.* Lyon: IARC Press, pp 262–263.

Kuruvilla S, Marco R, Raymond AK, Al-Ibraheemi A, Tatevian N (2011): Bizarre parosteal osteochondromatous proliferation (Nora's lesion) with translocation t(1;17)

(q32;q21): a case report and role of cytogenetic studies on diagnosis. *Ann Clin Lab Sci* 41:285–287.

Kuzniacka A, Mertens F, Strömbeck B, Wiegant J, Mandahl N (2004): Combined binary ratio labeling fluorescence in situ hybridization analysis of chordoma. *Cancer Genet Cytogenet* 151:178–181.

Lau CC, Harris CP, LuX-Y, Perlaky L, Gogineni S, Chintagumpala M, Hicks J, et al. (2004): Frequent amplification and rearrangement of chromosomal bands 6p12-p21 and 17p11.2 in osteosarcoma. *Genes Chromosomes Cancer* 39:11–21.

Le Deley M-C, Delattre O, Schaefer K-L, Burchill SA, Koehler G, Hogendoorn PCW, et al. (2010): Impact of EWS-ETS fusion type on disease progression in Ewing's sarcoma/peripheral primitive neuroectodermal tumor: prospective results from the cooperative Euro-E.W.I.N.G. 99 trial. *J Clin Oncol* 28:1982–1988.

Lucas DR, Bridge JA (2013): Chondromas: enchondroma, periosteal chondroma. In: Fletcher CDM, Bridge JA, Hogendoorn PCW, Mertens F, editors. World Health Organization Classification of Tumours. Pathology and Genetics of Tumours of Soft Tissue and Bone. Lyon: IARC Press, pp 252–254.

Mandahl N, Mertens F, Willén H, Rydholm A, Kreicbergs A, Mitelman F (1998): Nonrandom pattern of telomeric associations in atypical lipomatous tumors with ring and giant marker chromosomes. *Cancer Genet Cytogenet* 103:25–34.

Mandahl N, Gustafson P, Mertens F, Åkerman M, Baldetorp B, Gisselsson D, et al. (2002): Cytogenetic aberrations and their prognostic impact in chondrosarcoma. *Genes Chromosomes Cancer* 33:188–200.

Mandahl N, Johansson B, Mertens F, Mitelman F (2012): Disease-associated patterns of disomic chromosomes in hyperhaploid neoplasms. *Genes Chromosomes Cancer* 51:536–544.

Mejia-Guerrero S, Quejada M, Gokgoz N, Gill M, Parkes RK, Wunder JS, et al. (2010): Characterization of the 12q15 MDM2 and 12q13-14 CDK4 amplicons and clinical correlations in osteosarcoma. *Genes Chromosomes Cancer* 49:518–525.

Mertens F, Mandahl N, Örndal C, Baldetorp B, Bauer HCF, Rydholm A, et al. (1993): Cytogenetic findings in 33 osteosarcomas. *Int J Cancer* 55:44–50.

Mertens F, Möller E, Mandahl N, Picci P, Perez-Atayde AR, Samson I, et al. (2011): The t(X;6) in subungual exostosis results in transcriptional deregulation of the gene for insulin receptor substrate 4. *Int J Cancer* 128:487–491.

Nakashima Y, de Pinieux G, Ladanyi M (2013): Mesenchymal chondrosarcoma. In: Fletcher CDM, Bridge JA, Hogendoorn PCW, Mertens F, editors. *WHO Classification of Tumours of Soft Tissue and Bone.* Lyon: IARC Press, pp 271–272.

Ng TL, O'Sullivan MJ, Pallen CJ, Hayes M, Clarkson PW, Winstanley M, et al. (2007): Ewing sarcoma with novel translocation t(2;16) producing an in-frame fusion of FUS and FEV. *J Mol Diagn* 9:437–440.

Nilsson M, Domanski HA, Mertens F, Mandahl N (2004): Molecular cytogenetic definition of recurrent translocation breakpoints in bizarre parosteal osteochondromatous proliferation (Nora's lesion). *Hum Pathol* 35:1063–1069.

Niini T, Scheinin I, Lahti L, Savola S, Mertens F, Hollmén J, et al. (2012): Homozygous deletions of cadherin genes in chondrosarcoma – an array comparative genomic hybridization study. *Cancer Genet* 205:588–593.

Nord KH, Nilsson J, Arbajian E, Vult von Steyern F, Brosjö O, Cleton-Jansen AM, et al. (2013): Recurrent chromosome 22 deletions in osteoblastoma affect inhibitors of the wnt/ beta-catenin signaling pathway. *PLoS One* 8:e80725.

Nord KH, Lilljebjörn H, Vezzi F, Nilsson J, Magnusson L, Tayebwa J, et al. (2014): GRM1 is upregulated through gene fusion and promoter swapping in chondromyxoid fibroma. *Nat Genet* 46:474–477.

Oliveira AM, Hsi BL, Weremowicz S, Rosenberg AE, Dal Cin P, Joseph N, et al. (2004a): USP6 (Tre2) fusion oncogenes in aneurysmal bone cyst. *Cancer Res* 64:1920–1923.

Oliveira AM, Perez-Atayde AR, Inwards CY, Medeiros F, Derr V, His B-L, et al. (2004b): USP6 and CDH11 oncogenes identify the neoplastic cell in primary aneurysmal bone cysts and are absent in so-called secondary aneurysmal bone cysts. *Am J Pathol* 165:1773–1780.

Oliveira AM, Perez-Atayde AR, Dal Cin P, Gebhardt MC, Chen CJ, Neff JR, et al. (2005): Aneurysmal bone cyst variant translocations upregulate USP6 transcription by promoter swapping with the ZNF9, COL1A1, TRAP150, and OMD genes. *Oncogene* 24:3419–3426.

Parham DM, Bridge JA, Lukacs JL, Ding Y, Tryka AF, Sawyer JR (2004): Cytogenetic distinction among benign fibro-osseous lesions of bone in children and adolescents: value of karyotypic findings in differential diagnosis. *Pediatr Developmental Pathol* 7:148–158.

Panoutsakopoulos G, Pandis N, Kyriazoglou I, Gustafson P, Mertens F, Mandahl N (1999): Recurrent t(16;17) (q22;p13) in aneurysmal bone cysts. *Genes Chromosomes Cancer* 26:265–266.

Pierron G, Tirode F, Lucchesi C, Reynaud S, Ballet S, Cohen-Gogo S, et al. (2012): A new subtype of bone sarcoma defined by BCOR-CCNB3 gene fusion. *Nat Genet* 44:461–466.

Riggi N, Cironi L, Provero P, Suvà M-L, Kaloulis K, Garcia-Echeverria C, et al. (2005): Development of Ewing's sarcoma from primary bone marrow-derived mesenchymal progenitor cells. *Cancer Res* 65:11459–11468.

Riggi N, Cironi L, Suvà M-L, Stamenkovic I (2007): Sarcomas: genetics, signalling, and cellular origins. Part I: the fellowship of TET. *J Pathol* 213:4–20.

Roberts P, Burchill SA, Brownhill S, Cullinane CJ, Johnston C, Griffiths MJ, et al. (2008): Ploidy and karyotype complexity are powerful prognostic indicators in the Ewing's sarcoma family of tumours: a study by the United Kingdom Cancer Cytogenetics and the Children's Cancer and Leukaemia Group. *Genes Chromosomes Cancer* 47:207–220.

Romeo S, Aigner T, Bridge JA, (2013): Chondromyxoid fibroma. In: Fletcher CDM, Bridge JA, Hogendoorn PCW, Mertens F, editors. *WHO Classification of Tumours of Soft Tissue and Bone.* Lyon: IARC Press, pp 255–256.

Rozeman LB, Szuhai K, Schrage YM, Rosenberg C, Tanke HJ, Taminiau AHM, et al. (2006): Array-comparative genomic hybridization of central chondrosarcoma. Identification of ribosomal protein S6 and cyclin-dependent kinase 4 as candidate target genes for genomic aberrations. *Cancer* 107:380–388.

Sakai Junior N, Abe KT, Formigli LM, Pereira MF, Valverde de Oliveira MD, Cornelio DA, et al. (2011): Cytogenetic findings in 14 benign cartilaginous neoplasms. *Cancer Genet* 204:180–186.

Sandberg AA, Bridge JA (2000): Updates on cytogenetics and molecular genetics of bone and soft tissue tumors: Ewing sarcoma and primitive neuroectodermal tumors. *Cancer Genet Cytogenet* 123:1–26.

Sawyer JR, Tryka AF, Bell JM, Boop FA (1995): Nonrandom chromosome breakpoints at Xq26 and 2q33 characterize cemento-ossifying fibromas of the orbit. *Cancer* 76:1853–1859.

Sawyer JR, Goosen LS, Binz RL, Swanson CM, Nicholas RW (2005): Evidence for telomeric fusions as a mechanism for recurring structural aberrations of chromosome 11 in giant cell tumor of bone. *Cancer Genet Cytogenet* 159:32–36.

Sciot R, Dorfman H, Brys P, Dal Cin P, De Wever I, Fletcher CDM, et al. (2000): Cytogenetic–morphologic correlations in aneurysmal bone cyst, giant cell tumor of bone and combined lesions. A report from the CHAMP Study Group. *Mod Pathol* 13:1206–1210.

Shing DC, McMullan DJ, Roberts P, Smith K, Chin S-F, Nicholson J, et al. (2003): FUS/ERG gene fusions in Ewing's tumors. *Cancer Res* 63:4568–4576.

Sjögren H, Örndal C, Tingby O, Meis-Kindblom JM, Kindblom LG, Stenman G (2004): Cytogenetic and spectral karyotype analyses of benign and malignant cartilage tumours. *Int J Oncol* 24:1385–1391.

Stoll G, Surdez D, Tirode F, Laud K, Barillot E, Zinovyev A, et al. (2013): Systems biology of Ewing sarcoma: a network model of EWS-FLI1 effect on proliferation and apoptosis. *Nucleic Acids Res* 41:8853–8871.

Storlazzi CT, Wozniak A, Panagopoulos I, Sciot R, Mandahl N, Mertens F, et al. (2006): Rearrangement of the COL12A1 and COL4A5 genes in subungual exostosis:

molecular cytogenetic delineation of the tumor-specific translocation t(X;6)(q13–14;q22). *Int J Cancer* 118:1972–1976.

Tallini G, Dorfman H, Brys P, Dal Cin P, De Wever I, Fletcher CDM, et al. (2002): Correlation between clinicopathological features and karyotype in 100 cartilaginous and chordoid tumours. A report from the Chromosomes and Morphology (CHAMP) Collaborative Study Group. *J Pathol* 196:194–203.

Turc-Carel C, Philip I, Berger M-P, Philip T, Lenoir GM (1983): Chromosomal translocations in Ewing's sarcoma. *N Engl J Med* 309:497–498.

Udayakumar AM, Sundareshan TS, Mallana Goud T, Gayathri Devi M, Biswas S, Appaji L, et al. (2001): Cytogenetic characterization of Ewing tumors using fine needle aspiration samples: a 10-year experience and review of the literature. *Cancer Genet Cytogenet* 127:42–48.

van Doorninck JA, Ji L, Schaub B, Shimada H, Wing MR, Krailo MD, et al. (2010): Current treatment protocols have eliminated the prognostic advantage of type 1 fusions in Ewing sarcoma: a report from the Children's Oncology Group. *J Clin Oncol* 28:1989–1994.

Vujovic S, Henderson S, Presneau N, Odell E, Jacques TS, Tirabosco R, et al. (2006): Brachyury, a crucial regulator of notochordal development, is a novel biomarker for chordomas. *J Pathol* 209:157–165.

Wang L, Bhargava R, Zheng T, Wexler L, Collins MH, Roulston D, et al. (2007): Undifferentiated small round cell sarcomas with rare EWS gene fusions. *J Mol Diagn* 9:498–509.

Wang L, Motoi T, Khanin R, Olshen A, Mertens F, Bridge J, et al. (2012): Identification of a novel, recurrent HEY1-NCOA2 fusion in mesenchymal chondrosarcoma based on a genome-wide screen of exon-level expression data. *Genes Chromosomes Cancer* 51:127–139.

Zambrano E, Nosé V, Perez-Atayde AR, Gebhardt M, Hresko MT, Kleinman P, et al. (2004): Distinct chromosomal rearrangements in subungual (Dupuytren) exostosis and bizarre parosteal osteochondromatous proliferation (Nora lesion). *Am J Surg Pathol* 28:1033–1039.

Zucman J, Delattre O, Desmaze C, Plougastel B, Joubert I, Melot T, et al. (1992): Cloning and characterization of the Ewing's sarcoma and peripheral neuroepithelioma t(11;22) translocation breakpoints. *Genes Chromosomes Cancer* 5:271–277.

Zucman J, Melot T, Desmaze C, Ghysdael J, Plougastel B, Peter M, et al. (1993): Combinatorial generation of variable fusion proteins in the Ewing family of tumours. *EMBO J* 12:4481–4487.

CHAPTER 24

Soft tissue tumors

Nils Mandahl and Fredrik Mertens

Department of Clinical Genetics, University of Lund, Lund, Sweden

Soft tissue tumors are highly heterogeneous with more than 100 subtypes. They may occur anywhere in the body but three-fourths are located in the extremities. The large majority are benign; the malignant ones, the sarcomas, are outnumbered by a factor of 100 or more. Soft tissue sarcomas constitute less than 1% of all malignant tumors. Extensive heterogeneity and low incidence mean that most soft tissue sarcoma subtypes are rare. All age groups are affected and males are more often affected than females. However, gender- and age-related incidences vary considerably among the different tumor types. Differential diagnostic dilemmas are frequent and may include difficulties to distinguish benign from malignant lesions, to differentiate between different subtypes of soft tissue tumors, and also to differentiate sarcomas from carcinomas and other neoplasms. In this review, the current WHO classification of soft tissue tumors (Fletcher et al., 2013a) is, in principle, followed. Soft tissue chondro-osseous tumors are dealt with in Chapter 23.

Adipocytic tumors

The cytogenetic database on benign and malignant tumors of adipose tissues is extensive. About 950 cases with clonal chromosome abnormalities, representing more than a dozen morphological subtypes, have been reported. Different subtypes of adipocytic tumors display specific or characteristic patterns of chromosomal changes. An exception to this overall relationship is *angiolipoma*, which most often is found as multiple lesions and for which an increased familial incidence has been recorded. Apart from a single case with a t(X;2), all angiolipomas have revealed a normal karyotype at chromosome banding analysis (Sciot et al., 1997).

By far, the most common adipocytic neoplasm is *lipoma*, a benign tumor composed of mature fat cells, which is also the most common soft tissue neoplasm. Although mitotic figures are rarely seen in histological sections, karyotypes are readily obtained after short-term culturing. About two-thirds of the tumor samples investigated have shown chromosome changes, and close to 500 cases with aberrant karyotypes have been reported (Mitelman et al., 2014). The chromosome number is typically diploid; hyperdiploidy is seen in 10% and polyploidy in 1% of the cases. Cytogenetically detectable clonal evolution is found in 10% of the cases. The spectrum of aberrations is quite diverse and dominated by structural rearrangements. About two-thirds of the karyotypes are seemingly balanced, at least in the stemline. Among the unbalanced karyotypes, loss of chromosome material is more common than gain, and most of the imbalances are partial losses or gains; complete monosomy 13 (see later) and

Cancer Cytogenetics: Chromosomal and Molecular Genetic Aberrations of Tumor Cells, Fourth Edition.
Edited by Sverre Heim and Felix Mitelman.
© 2015 John Wiley & Sons, Ltd. Published 2015 by John Wiley & Sons, Ltd.

trisomy 8 are found in 2 and 1% of the aberrant cases, respectively. Partial losses affect primarily, in decreasing order of frequency, chromosomes 13, 12, 6, and 1. Despite the diversity of aberrations, there is a nonrandom pattern of karyotypic changes that often has been used to categorize lipomas into the following four major cytogenetic subgroups, which are largely mutually exclusive but with an overlap in some 10% of the cases (Sreekantaiah et al., 1991; Mandahl et al., 1994; Bartuma et al., 2007).

1 *Rearrangements of chromosome segment 12q13–15 (two-thirds of abnormal cases).* These changes are primarily translocations involving a large number of bands on all chromosomes. Still, there is a distinct pattern of preferred partner breakpoints with involvement of 3q27–29, seen in more than 20% of the tumors in this subgroup, as the dominating one (Figure 24.1). Other frequent (3–8%) partner breakpoint segments are 1p32–34, 2p22–24, 2q35–37, 5q32–34, 12p11–12, and 12q24. FISH analyses have revealed a higher level of complexity of the genomic reorganization than can be identified by banding (Dahlén et al., 2003; Nilsson et al., 2006). It has been clearly demonstrated that the high-mobility group AT-hook 2 (*HMGA2*) gene, located in 12q14.3, plays a fundamental role in lipoma development. As a consequence of translocations, *HMGA2* may form fusion genes with another gene in the partner breakpoint. The first to be described was the *HMGA2–LPP* gene fusion found in lipomas with the common t(3;12)(q27–28;q13–15) (Ashar et al., 1995; Schoenmakers et al., 1995; Petit et al., 1996). Later, other genes recombining with *HMGA2* were identified, such as *PPAP2B* in 1p32, *CXCR7* in 2q37.3, *EBF1* in 5q33.3, *NFIB* in 9p23, and *LHFP* in 13q13.3 (Petit et al., 1999; Broberg et al., 2002; Nilsson et al., 2005, 2006; Bianchini et al., 2013). These studies have shown that seemingly identical, balanced translocations may result in distinctly different rearrangements at the molecular level, with breakpoints within or flanking *HMGA2*. A common theme is a breakpoint in the large third intron combining the DNA-binding AT-hook domain of *HMGA2* with ectopic sequences replacing the acidic C-terminus. In some cases, a chimeric transcript is formed that may be in frame or out of frame. Frequently, there is a downstream stop codon shortly after the junction, in essence leading to a truncated HMGA2. Involvement

of *HMGA2* has also been demonstrated in lipomas with a normal karyotype and in tumors with cytogenetic aberrations not affecting 12q13–15 (Petit et al., 1996; Bartuma et al., 2007). Both tumors with and without 12q13–15 changes have been shown to express truncated (exons 1–3) and full-length (exons 1–5) HMGA2, a protein that plays a significant role in embryogenesis but is silent in most differentiated adult tissues. These findings, combined with observations in mouse models and human constitutional chromosome rearrangements, strongly indicate that expression of truncated or full-length HMGA2 in a mesenchymal cell has tumorigenic potential and may promote lipoma development (Arlotta et al., 2000; Ligon et al., 2005; Zaidi et al., 2006). The *HMGA2–LPP* fusion gene encodes a protein containing an N-terminal AT-hook domain and C-terminal LIM domains of LPP, constituting a novel transcription factor. The ectopic sequences replacing the HMGA2 C-terminus may affect transcriptional regulation processes, and coexpression of wild-type HMGA2 could act as a stimulating factor (Crombez et al., 2005). *HMGA2* may also be activated through elimination of its 3′ untranslated region containing multiple target sites for the repressing microRNA *let-7* (Lee and Dutta, 2007). Finally, it should be mentioned that the *HMGA2* aberrations described earlier are not unique for lipomas, but have been described also in a variety of other benign solid tumors (Chapters 12, 13, and 17).

2 *Loss of material from 13q (15% of abnormal cases).* This includes monosomy 13, but more often unbalanced translocations and interstitial deletions. Although some tumors have such aberrations as the sole anomaly, it is somewhat questionable to let loss of 13q material define a separate cytogenetic subgroup since partial loss of 13q is seen as an additional aberration in the three other subgroups. The segment deleted in more than half of the tumors runs from 13q12 to 13q32 with a peak incidence at 13q14–22, found in close to 90%. A common minimal deleted region of 13q in lipomas as well as other subtypes of adipose tissue tumors was identified (Dahlén et al., 2003; Bartuma et al., 2011). It was found that some aberrations interpreted as balanced rearrangements of chromosome 13 actually included small deletions, indicating that 13q losses are more common than expected from

banding analyses. The breakpoints were scattered, but the findings indicated that deletion of a segment comprising about 3.5 Mb within 13q14, distal to the *RB1* locus, is of importance in the development of a subset of adipose tissue tumors. The *C13orf1* gene was expressed at significantly lower levels compared with ordinary lipomas without 13q deletion.

3 *Supernumerary ring chromosomes (5–6% of abnormal cases)*. One or more ring chromosomes can be seen in addition to an otherwise normal chromosome complement, but other numerical or structural aberrations may also occur. The ring chromosomes frequently vary in number and size among metaphase cells from the same tumor. Similarly, different cell populations may harbor either ring chromosomes or giant marker rod chromosomes, and in some cells, both structures coexist. The content of the rings and markers in lipomas does not seem to differ from that of atypical lipomatous tumors (ALT) (see following text), which raises the important question of how reliable the histological differentiation between lipoma and ALT/well-differentiated liposarcoma (WDLS) really is. In our opinion, there is a single pathogenetic entity of low-malignant adipocytic tumors characterized by extra chromosomal material usually arranged in supernumerary rings. The less than complete overlap between the genetic and histopathological classification practices for this group of tumors highlights the general issue of which tumor features should be given predominance when diagnoses are reached. With the advent of biological therapies directed specifically against the molecular processes disrupted during tumorigenesis, pathogenetic classifications become increasingly important, but we are not there yet for patients with adipocytic tumors.

4 *Rearrangements of chromosome segment 6p21–23 (5–6% of abnormal cases)*. These are primarily translocations involving a variety of chromosome bands. Less than 30 cases have been reported, and it is uncertain whether there are preferred recombination partners. However, chromosome bands 2q35–36, 3q27–28, 6q21, and 11q13 have been involved in two cases each and 1p35–36 and 12q14–15 in four cases each. The *HMGA2*-related gene *HMGA1* is located in band 6p21. *HMGA1* has been shown to be rearranged in at least a subset of lipomas with breakpoints in 6p (Bartuma et al., 2007). If this is of pathogenetic significance, it remains to be explained why so few lipomas develop along this pathway compared to the *HMGA2* pathway.

The extensive cytogenetic heterogeneity encountered among lipomas shows surprisingly few correlations with clinicopathologic parameters (Bartuma et al., 2007). Apart from the observation that lipomas with ring chromosomes more often are deep seated and larger and occur in older patients compared to lipomas with other aberrations (see above for a discussion of the diagnostic reliability of this tumor subgroup), no correlations with sex, age, tumor size, depth, or location could be detected.

Sixty cases of *lipoblastoma*, a tumor most often presenting in the first three years of life, have been studied by chromosome banding. The karyotypes are, with few exceptions, pseudodiploid, and the vast majority have had aberrations involving chromosome 8, primarily structural rearrangements of 8q with a distinct clustering of breakpoints to 8q11–13. The aberrations include both balanced and unbalanced changes and are frequently seen as the sole anomaly. Many different chromosome bands recombine with 8q11–13. Recurrently involved bands, found in 3–5 cases, are 1p13, 2q23, 3q12–13, 7p22, 7q21–22, 8q24, 14q24, and 16q22. Complete or partial gain of chromosome 8 material, in karyotypes with or without 8q11–13 changes, has been seen in 12% of the cases. Notably, rearrangements of 8q11–13 have been found in 3% of ordinary lipomas.

The target of the 8q11–13 rearrangements is *PLAG1*, a developmentally regulated gene in 8q12.1 encoding a zinc finger transcription factor. So far, it has been found to recombine with the *COL3A1*

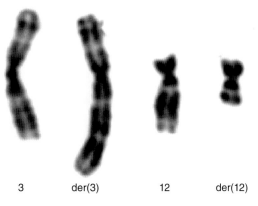

3   der(3)   12   der(12)

Figure 24.1 t(3;12)(q28;q14) in a lipoma.

(in 2q31), *COL1A2* (in 7q21.3), *HAS2* (in 8q24.13), *RAD51L1* (in 14q24), and, in a single case, *RAB2A* (in 8q12) genes (Hibbard et al., 2000; Deen et al., 2013; Yoshida et al., 2014). The promoter regions of at least some of these genes are fused to the entire coding sequence of *PLAG1* that is activated through this promoter-swapping mechanism. It has been suggested that gain of copies of the gene could be an alternative mechanism for tumor development in cases without 8q rearrangement (Gisselsson et al., 2001). However, it remains possible that the extra *PLAG1* copies are not wild type. The same investigators showed that the *PLAG1* changes were present in several types of variably differentiated mesenchymal cells, indicating an origin in a primitive mesenchymal precursor that proliferates and differentiates. Involvement of *PLAG1* has also been implicated in salivary gland tumors (Chapter 12). A single case with rearrangement of *HMGA2* but no *PLAG1* involvement has been described (Pedeutour et al., 2012).

All six reported *chondroid lipomas* have shown a t(11;16)(q13;p13), in four cases as the sole anomaly (Figure 24.2). This resulted in fusion of the *C11orf95* (in 11p) and *MKL2* (in 16p13) genes in 10 of 11 cases investigated by molecular means (Huang et al., 2010; Flucke et al., 2013). *MKL2* is a DNA-binding protein implicated in chromatin remodeling and transcriptional coactivation, whereas *C11orf95* has unknown function.

Angiomyolipomas are poorly characterized cytogenetically. Of the eight cases reported, seven showed unbalanced karyotypes. Three cases had trisomy 7 and one case had trisomy 8 as the sole anomalies, whereas four tumors harbored different structural aberrations.

Spindle cell lipoma and *pleomorphic lipoma* show similar cytogenetic profiles and are therefore lumped together here. The chromosome number ranges from 44 to 46 in the majority of the slightly more than 25 tumors reported (Dahlén et al., 2003; Bartuma et al., 2011). Monosomies or partial chromosome losses due to unbalanced structural rearrangements are the dominating aberrations. The most commonly affected chromosomes are 13 and 16 followed by 10 (most often 10p), 6 (6q), 2 (2q), and 17 (17p). The chromosome region from 13q14 to 13q33 is lost in two-thirds of the cases, whereas 16q13 to 16qter is lost in more than half, and simultaneous losses of 13q and 16q sequences are common. Molecular genetic analyses have revealed two minimal common deleted regions in 13q14 (Bartuma et al., 2011). None of four genes in one of the regions but five genes (*C13orf1, DHRS12, ATP7B, ALG11*, and *VPS36*) in the other region were expressed at significantly lower levels compared with control samples. The expression pattern of *C13orf1* is shared with ordinary lipomas with 13q deletion.

Although less than 20 *hibernomas* with clonal chromosome aberrations have been reported, a clear cytogenetic profile has emerged. The karyotypes are diploid, and 11q13, in a few cases 11q21, is involved in structural aberrations with a variety of chromosome bands, albeit recurrently only with 9q34 and 14q11. FISH analyses have revealed that the rearrangements are much more complex than appreciated by banding analyses, including multiple breakpoints, extensive reorganization, and loss of chromosome segments (Gisselsson et al., 1999; Maire et al., 2003). This affects not only the visibly rearranged chromosome 11 but also its seemingly normal homolog. The deletions cluster to a 3 Mb region in 11q13 covering the tumor suppressor genes *MEN1* and *AIP* (Nord et al., 2010). Among 15 cases, homozygous or heterozygous deletion of *MEN1* was found in ten and five, respectively, and of *AIP* in six and eight cases; both genes were homozygously lost in six cases. Several genes, including *MEN1* and *AIP*, showed low expression, whereas other genes, in particular *UCP1*, were highly expressed.

The intermediate malignant *ALT* and *WDLS* are synonyms for morphologically and karyotypically similar lesions, where ALT denotes tumors located in the limbs and on the trunk and WDLS is used for retroperitoneal and mediastinal lesions.

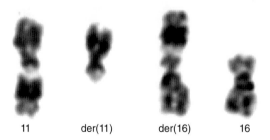

11   der(11)   der(16)   16

Figure 24.2 t(11;16)(q13;p13) in a chondroid lipoma.

These tumors are cytogenetically characterized by one or more supernumerary ring chromosomes and/or giant marker chromosomes in mostly hyperdiploid karyotypes (Figure 24.3). One or both of these aberrations have been present in 90% of the 170 cases reported. Rings occur more frequently than giant rod markers. Both the number and size may vary considerably not only among different tumors but also among cells from the same tumor. More than half of the tumors show r/mar as the sole anomaly; other changes include numerical as well as balanced and unbalanced structural aberrations. Among these, only −13/del(13q) and −22/del(22q) have been found in about 5% of the cases. Most ALT display telomeric associations that may be present in a large fraction of the metaphase cells and show a nonrandom involvement of chromosome termini (Mandahl et al., 1998). The r/mar chromosomes are mitotically unstable structures that undergo breakage–fusion–bridge cycles, which may explain their variable size and composition (Gisselsson et al., 1998); they can transform from r to mar and vice versa.

The origin of the rings and giant rod markers cannot be determined by chromosome banding. By other methods, it has been revealed that their structure is quite complex, invariably including smaller or larger segments from 12q, but frequently also material from other chromosomes, in particular chromosome 1 (Meza-Zepeda et al., 2002; Micci et al., 2002; Italiano et al., 2008). The extension of the 12q and 1q amplicons, which are intermingled with each other in the r/mar, varies and includes both low- and high-level amplification. In chromosome 1, the proximal border of the amplicons seems always to be 1q21, and then they extend down to 1q31 as the most distal border, with a peak incidence in 1q23. In the vast majority of tumors, copy number changes occur within 12q12 down to 12q23, with high-level amplification restricted to 12q13–21 and practically always including 12q14 and 12q15. The amplified 12q sequences are discontinuous, and two distinct amplicons have been identified, one consistently including the target gene *MDM2* in 12q15 and another (absent in some 10% of the cases) including *CDK4* and *TSPAN31* in 12q14, which are most often overexpressed (Berner et al., 1996; Hostein et al., 2004; Singer et al., 2007; Italiano et al., 2008). The more proximal amplicon has, in its centromeric part, a sharp border in the vicinity of *DDIT3*. MDM2 interacts with TP53 and CDK4 with RB1.

The karyotypic profiles of *dedifferentiated liposarcomas* (DDLS) are similar to those of ALT, and most of the 25 cases reported have had one or more ring chromosomes. Three-fourths of the cases have additional chromosome aberrations, and clones with polyploid chromosome numbers occur in half

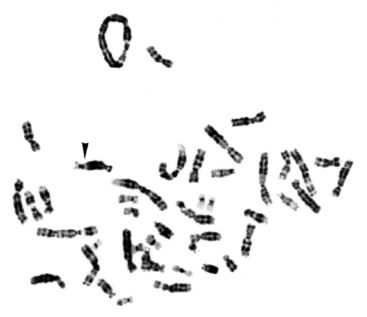

Figure 24.3 Supernumerary ring chromosome in an atypical lipomatous tumor. The arrowhead indicates a telomeric association.

of the cases. The karyotypes may be simple with rings as the sole anomaly or quite complex with multiple numerical and mostly unbalanced structural changes, with no obvious nonrandom pattern. Amplifications of 12q sequences, including *MDM2*, are common, and the extra copies are located in the ring chromosomes (Rieker et al., 2002; Nilsson et al., 2004). Other recurrent copy number changes include the mutually exclusive gains of 1p32 and 6q23 containing the target genes *JUN* and *ASK1*, both involved in the JUN MAP kinase pathway (Coindre et al., 2010; Dei Tos et al., 2013).

The cytogenetic hallmark of *myxoid liposarcoma* (MLS), including tumors with round cell components, is the t(12;16)(q13;p11) (Figure 24.4) (Turc-Carel et al., 1986). Among 100 reported MLS, more than 80% have had recombination between 12q13 and 16p11 as detected by chromosome banding. A variant translocation, t(12;22)(q13;q12), was found in four tumors, and another four showed rearrangement between 12q13 and other bands than 16p11 and 22q12. Thus, more than 90% of these tumors show involvement of 12q13. Various other aberrations have been found in five and 40% of tumors reported as MLS and as round cell liposarcoma, respectively, but in none of the tumors described as mixed liposarcomas. The 12q13 aberrations are present as the sole anomaly in half of the cases, and the chromosome number is typically near diploid or pseudodiploid. The most common secondary aberration is trisomy 8 found in more than 10% of the cases. Other, less common, recurrent imbalances are gains of 1q and 7q and losses of 7p, 6q21–22, and 16q12-qter. Most imbalances of chromosome 7 are caused by an i(7)(q10) or idic(7)(p11).

The molecular genetic consequences of the t(12;16) and t(12;22) are formation of the fusion genes *FUS–DDIT3* and *EWSR1–DDIT3*, respectively (Crozat et al., 1993; Rabbitts et al., 1993; Panagopoulos et al., 1996). *FUS* (in 16p11) and *EWSR1* (in 22q12) show extensive sequence similarities, and both encode nuclear RNA-binding proteins. *DDIT3* (in 12q13) encodes a protein belonging to the C/EBP family of basic leucine zipper transcription factors. At least 11 *FUS–DDIT3* and four *EWSR1–DDIT3* types of chimeric transcripts have been identified, the most common ones fusing exon 5, 7, or 8 of *FUS* with exon 2 of *DDIT3* (Willeke et al., 1998; Panagopoulos et al., 2000; Bode-Lesniewska et al., 2007). The predominance of *FUS–DDIT3* over *EWSR1–DDIT3* (ratio about 20:1) is suggested to depend on the transcriptional orientation of the genes. Whereas *FUS–DDIT3* results in a functional transcript through a reciprocal translocation, additional rearrangements are needed for functioning of the *EWSR1–DDIT3* transcript. The different *FUS–DDIT3* fusion transcript variants do not seem to be associated with histological grade or clinical outcome (Antonescu et al., 2001; Bode-Lesniewska et al., 2007).

Transformation from myxoid to round cell morphology may be associated with activation of the PI3K/Akt pathway through activating mutation of *PIK3CA*, loss of *PTEN*, or high expression of *IGF1R*, all of which are more frequent among round cell tumors than in pure myxoid lesions (Demicco et al., 2012). *TERT* promoter mutations were particularly common in MLS, detected in almost 80% of 24 cases investigated (Killela et al., 2013). Probably, MLS cells maintain telomere lengths through such *TERT* mutations or through alternative lengthening of telomeres.

Chromosome banding analysis of 13 *pleomorphic liposarcomas* has shown that these tumors invariably harbor complex karyotypic changes. Near-diploid karyotypes are seen, but polyploid chromosome numbers are more frequent. Recurrent changes are difficult to discern. The dominance of chromosome losses, involving

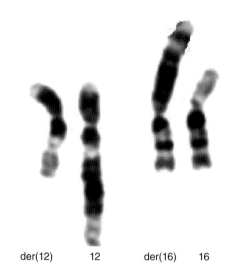

der(12)   12   der(16)   16

Figure 24.4 t(12;16)(q13;p11) in a myxoid liposarcoma.

chromosomes 10, 11, 13, and 22 in half of the cases, may be misleading since all karyotypes are incompletely described by banding. Cytogenetic signs of gene amplification, that is, dmin and ring chromosomes, are present in half of the cases. Metaphase CGH analyses of more than 20 tumors have shown that the imbalances seen in more than half to two-thirds of the cases include gain of sequences from central 1q and 5p, sometimes in the form of high-level amplification, and losses from 2q, 10q, 11q, and 13q (Rieker et al., 2002; Idbaih et al., 2005). Even though no 12q13 aberration has been found cytogenetically, *FUS–DDIT3* chimeric transcripts have been observed in a few cases, including an epithelioid variant (Willeke et al., 1998; De Cecco et al., 2005).

Although different morphologic subtypes of adipose tissue tumors show characteristic karyotypic profiles, some overlapping exists. From a clinical perspective, the precise identification of morphologic subtype is mostly of little importance, since surgery is the dominant treatment for all of them. The overridingly important distinction in the management of patients with lipomatous tumors is whether the tumor is benign or malignant; the former never metastasize and rarely recur locally. Despite some overlapping of genetic features between morphologic subtypes, not least between lipomas and ALT (see preceding text for a discussion of the differential diagnostic information value of the finding of supernumerary rings and marker chromosomes in well-differentiated adipocytic tumors), cytogenetic and molecular genetic analyses do increase the diagnostic precision considerably (Nishio, 2011). In a gene expression profiling study of fat tissue and the major subtypes of adipose tissue tumors, three global clusters could be observed (Singer et al., 2007). The first cluster included normal fat, lipomas, and WDLS only, the second cluster contained all DDLS and pleomorphic liposarcomas as well as a few cases of WDLS, whereas the third cluster comprised MLS and round cell liposarcomas. This is largely in agreement with the genetic findings, although there is a closer cytogenetic similarity between WDLS and DDLS than between DDLS and pleomorphic liposarcomas. Moreover, WDLS, DDLS, and pleomorphic liposarcomas share genetic changes with subsets of undifferentiated pleomorphic sarcomas reported as malignant fibrous histiocytomas (Chibon et al., 2002; Coindre et al., 2004; Idbaih et al., 2005).

Fibroblastic/myofibroblastic tumors

A large number of fibroblastic/myofibroblastic tumor entities have been described. It is debated for several subtypes of low-grade lesions whether they represent true neoplastic lesions or reactive processes. Many investigators have taken the finding of clonal chromosome aberrations as an indication of their neoplastic nature.

Only few cases of *nodular fasciitis* (NF), *proliferative fasciitis*, and *proliferative myositis* with clonal chromosome aberrations have been reported. All karyotypes have been pseudodiploid or near diploid with simple numerical or structural aberrations in the soft tissue lesions, whereas an NF of the breast showed multiple aberrations. Two cases of NF showed different translocations with a breakpoint in 3q21 in common. Molecular studies of 48 cases of NF showed rearrangement of *USP6* in more than 90% of the cases and the presence of a *MYH9–USP6* fusion gene in 60% (Erickson-Johnson et al., 2011). Translocation involving *USP6*, a gene frequently rearranged in aneurysmal bone cysts (Chapter 23), in 17p13 and *MYH9* in 22q12–13 may easily pass undetected at chromosome banding analysis. Fusion of the *MYH9* promoter region to the entire coding region of *USP6* most likely results in transcriptional upregulation of *USP6*. This genetic change is of potential diagnostic relevance since NF may mimic sarcoma.

Chromosome banding analysis has been performed on six cases of *elastofibroma*. All displayed a large fraction of metaphase cells with nonclonal structural aberrations, including many balanced translocations, but only exceptional numerical changes (McComb et al., 2001). In half of the lesions, the aberrant clones were made up of only a few cells. A breakpoint in 3q21 was found in four cases. One-third of 27 elastofibromas analyzed by CGH have shown copy number changes. The only recurrent imbalances were gain of Xq12–22 in six cases and of chromosome 19 in two cases. A clonal origin was demonstrated in two cases using X-inactivation analysis. No recurrent chromosome aberration was identified in three cases of *fibrous hamartoma of infancy*.

Ten out of 11 cases of *desmoplastic fibroblastoma* showed pseudodiploid karyotypes with rearrangement of 11q12 in eight cases and of 11q13 in one. The translocation partner bands were all different, but four breakpoints were located in chromosome 2 (q31–35). In six cases with 11q12 rearrangements, the breakpoints mapped to a 20 Kb region including *FOSL1*, which belongs to a gene family encoding leucine zipper proteins (Macchia et al., 2012). No fusion transcript could be identified. This, combined with the varying translocations, suggests that the functional outcome of the 11q12 aberrations is deregulated expression of *FOSL1*. A similar t(2;11)(q31–32;q12) was reported in a *fibroma of tendon sheath*.

Two cases of *mammary-type myofibroblastoma* displayed partial chromosome losses, in both cases including loss of 13q14–32. Interphase FISH analysis using *RB1* and *FOXO1* probes of a third case revealed loss of 13q14 sequences. A similar FISH study of two *cellular angiofibromas* also showed losses in 13q14. The latter two tumor entities share morphological and immunophenotypic features with spindle cell lipoma, which frequently displays 13q losses (see preceding text). One *giant cell angiofibroma* showed rearrangement of 6q13, whereas another case had a t(12;17)(q15;q23) and del(18)(q21).

A single case of *lipofibromatosis* with a t(4;9;6) (q21;q22;q2?4) as the sole anomaly has been reported. Chromosome banding analyses have revealed clonal, partly nonrandom aberrations in a minor subset of *superficial fibromatoses* (SF) and in a large fraction of *desmoid-type fibromatoses* (DTF) speaking in favor of a neoplastic nature of these lesions (De Wever et al., 2000). SF and DTF display some cytogenetic similarities and some differences. Based on data on 50–60 chromosomally abnormal cases of each type of lesion, including superficial tumors of the foot, hand, and penis and intra- and extra-abdominal tumors, it can be concluded that they generally show near-diploid karyotypes with mostly simple numerical and/or structural aberrations. Trisomy 8 is found in almost one-third of SF and DTF, and loss of the Y chromosome is common. Trisomy 20 has been found in one-fourth of DTF, sometimes together with +8, but never in SF. Similarly, monosomy 5 or deletion of 5q, the only

recurrent structural aberration detected, has been found only in DTF, in about one-sixth of the lesions, with loss of 5q21 common to all cases. Karyotypes with only numerical changes are seen in two-thirds of SF and half of DTF. Complex karyotypes and unbalanced structural aberrations are present in a higher fraction of DTF compared with SF.

In interphase FISH studies of trisomy 8, different investigators have used different cutoff thresholds for accepting the presence of a true trisomic cell population. However, all studies show that +8 is present in only a minority of the cells, 25% or less (Fletcher et al., 1995; Kouho et al., 1997; Brandal et al., 2003). The small clone size is further supported by chromosome CGH studies, which have been unable to detect extra copies of chromosome 8 (Larramendy et al., 1998; Brandal et al., 2003). In contrast, recurrent gain of 1q21 was detected by Larramendy et al. (1998). This is not supported by karyotypic findings and could not be verified by Brandal et al. (2003), who suggested that this might be explained by abdominal and extra-abdominal desmoids developing through different pathogenetic mechanisms. Some observations indicate that DTF with trisomy 8 have a greater tendency to recur locally than do tumors without this aberration (Fletcher et al., 1995; Kouho et al., 1997).

Patients with familial adenomatous polyposis (FAP) coli have an increased risk of developing desmoid tumors. The genetic background of FAP is loss-of-function mutations of the *APC* tumor suppressor gene in 5q22. *APC* mutations have been seen primarily in DTF developing in FAP patients, less often in sporadic tumors. In a series of 42 sporadic DTF, *APC* mutations were found in nine cases, and loss of heterozygosity (LOH) was seen in six of these (Tejpar et al., 1999), which is in good agreement with the cytogenetic findings regarding loss of material from 5q. However, half of the tumors in this study had point mutations in the beta-catenin gene, none of which had *APC* mutation, and all showed increased beta-catenin expression, a feature that seems to distinguish them from various congeners. These genetic events activate the Wnt signaling pathway.

Less than 10 cases with chromosome aberrations have been reported of the recently described fibrovascular neoplasm *soft tissue angiofibroma*.

The majority showed a t(5;8)(p15;q13), most often as the sole anomaly; one case harbored a variant t(7;8;14)(q11;q13;q31). Further analyses revealed two in-frame fusion transcripts, *AHRR–NCOA2* and *NCOA2–AHRR* (Jin et al., 2012). Interphase FISH showed fusion between these two genes in three out of 10 cases. *AHRR* in 5p15 encodes a transcription factor. *NCOA2* in 8q13, encoding a steroid receptor coactivator, is involved in various gene fusions in leukemias (Chapters 6 and 10), rhabdomyosarcomas (see following text), and chondrosarcoma (Chapter 23). The predicted outcome of the fusion is upregulation of AHR/ARNT signaling. In the case with the t(7;8;14), a *GTF2I–NCOA2* fusion gene was identified; the transcription factor gene *GTF2I* maps to 7q11 (Arbajian et al., 2013). This variant fusion indicates that it is *NCOA2* that is essential for soft tissue angiofibroma pathogenesis.

Dermatofibrosarcoma protuberans (DFSP) typically shows hyperdiploid or diploid chromosome numbers. The karyotypes of the vast majority of more than 40 cases reported harbored one or more supernumerary ring chromosomes or marker rod chromosomes that were shown by FISH analyses to contain material from chromosomes 17 and 22 and occasionally also sequences from one or more other chromosomes (Mandahl et al., 1990; Pedeutour et al., 1994; O'Brien et al., 1998). The rod chromosomes were all interpreted as der(22) t(17;22)(q21–23;q13) (Figure 24.5). Other recurrent chromosomal changes include gain of chromosomes 8 and 5, in particular the q arms, seen in 20–25% of the cases.

The molecular consequence of the unbalanced rearrangements involving chromosomes 17 and 22

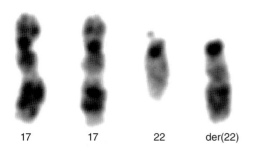

| 17 | 17 | 22 | der(22) |

Figure 24.5 der(22)t(17;22)(q21;q13) together with two normal copies of chromosome 17 in a dermatofibrosarcoma protuberans.

is the fusion of the collagen gene *COL1A1* (in 17q21.33) and the platelet-derived growth factor beta chain gene (*PDGFB*, in 22q13.1) (Simon et al., 1997). In the chimeric transcripts, at least 20 *COL1A1* exons, all within the alpha-helical domain covered by exons 6–49, have been found to fuse to exon 2 of *PDGFB*, whereby the fusion gene comes under control of regulatory sequences of the *COL1A1* gene. The PDGFB receptor is highly expressed indicating stimulation of tumor growth by an autocrine stimulatory loop due to posttranslational processing of the COL1A1–PDGFB protein to yield a fully functional PDGFB. Sequences from 17q and 22q are amplified in ring chromosomes, and the rod der(22)-chromosomes are frequently present in duplicate; CGH analyses have revealed gain of 17q22-qter and 22q13 in almost all tumors investigated and high-level amplification of 17q23-qter in a few cases. The *COL1A1–PDGFB* fusion gene is shared with *giant cell fibroblastoma* (GCF) and *Bednar tumor*, the juvenile and pigmented variant forms of DFSP, as well as superficial adult fibrosarcomas. Only few GCF and Bednar tumors have been investigated by chromosome banding. Seemingly balanced t(17;22) or der(22)t(17;22) were mostly found, whereas ring chromosomes predominate in DFSP. The development of fibrosarcomatous changes in areas of a DFSP has been seen as a sign of tumor progression indicating an increased risk of metastasis. Combined CGH and FISH studies suggest an association between a moderate increase of *COL1A1–PDGFB* copy numbers and fibrosarcomatous changes in a subset of tumors, but this increase does not seem to be a predictor of clinical behavior (Kiuru-Kuhlefelt et al., 2001; Abbott et al., 2006). Probably, other genetic factors contribute to this process. The differential diagnosis of the locally aggressive DFSP may be problematic, but other mimicking tumor entities do not show *COL1A1–PDGFB* fusion or overexpression of PDGFB.

Solitary fibrous tumor (SFT) is a mesenchymal tumor of fibroblastic type, a subset of which was formerly classified as the now obsolete entity hemangiopericytoma (Fletcher et al., 2013b). The cytogenetic profile of SFT is quite disparate. Pseudodiploidy or near diploidy is found in 85% of the more than 60 cases reported. Karyotypes with everything from simple changes to highly complex aberrations have been observed; 25% show a seemingly balanced karyotype. The most conspicuous clustering of breakpoints is to chromosome 12, in particular to 12q13–15 (25% of cases) and 12q24 (10%). Also, 19q13 is involved in 10%, and a recurrent recombination between 12q13 and 19q13 has been found. The most common numerical changes include gain of chromosomes 5, 8, and 21 (5–6%), and partial loss of 13q is frequent.

A pathognomonic *NAB2–STAT6* fusion gene has been identified in 55–100% of almost 150 tumors from various anatomical sites, morphologic subtypes, and malignancy grades (Chmielecki et al., 2013; Mohajeri et al., 2013; Robinson et al., 2013). Complex rearrangements, including inversions and deletions, are needed to obtain a functional chimeric product since the two genes, both located in 12q13, are transcribed in different directions. Several fusion variants have been identified and differ in frequency between different materials; combination of *NAB2* exons 6 or 7 with *STAT6* exons 17 or 18 was found in 75% of the Robinson series compared with 27% in the Mohajeri series, whereas the exon 4–exon 3 combination was found in 6% and 46%, respectively. Most likely, the outcome of the fusion gene formation is disturbed NAB2 function in gene regulation. A *STAT6* and *TRAPPC5* (in 19p13) fusion was detected in a single case with a t(6;12;19). Differential diagnostic problems are considerable regarding SFT. Since cytogenetic analysis is too blunt and because of the need of multiple primer combinations to detect various fusion transcripts by RT-PCR, immunohistochemistry for STAT6 or for deregulated target gene(s) of NAB2–STAT6 could constitute a better diagnostic alternative. Presence of the NAB2–STAT6 chimeric protein was detected in all 17 lesions reported as meningeal hemangiopericytomas (Schweizer et al., 2013).

The cytogenetic findings in more than 20 *inflammatory myofibroblastic tumors* (IMT) are heterogeneous. About half of the IMT have rearrangements of 2p22–24. Structural changes involving this segment are typically found in near-diploid karyotypes with a single or relatively few chromosomal aberrations. Several recombination partner bands have been found. Tumors without a 2p22–24 breakpoint tend to be karyotypically complex. Other frequent aberrations include losses of material from 6q and 22q.

The anaplastic lymphoma kinase gene *ALK* (in 2p23), which encodes a tyrosine kinase receptor, has been shown to fuse with a variety of other genes in IMT, in line with the cytogenetic findings. Thus far, eight fusion partner genes have been identified among IMT that have been proven to be *ALK* fusion positive (referenced in Takeuchi et al., 2011). These include *TPM3* (1q21), *RANBP2* (2q13), *ATIC* (2q35), *SEC31A* (4q21), *CARS* (11p15), *PPFIBP1* (12p11), *CLTC* (17q23), and *TPM4* (19p13). Some of these fusion genes are shared with anaplastic large cell lymphoma (Chapter 11), but the dominating *NPM–ALK* fusion in lymphomas has not yet been detected in IMT. ALK contributes its carboxy-terminus that contains a tyrosine kinase catalytic domain, and the fusion partners encode ubiquitously expressed proteins that promote elevated transcription of the chimera and frequently include amino-terminal oligomerization motifs resulting in autophosphorylation and constitutive activation of the ALK tyrosine kinase. Genomic rearrangement and overexpression of the ALK kinase domain are restricted to the myofibroblastic component. In IMT, there is a strong correlation between *ALK* rearrangements and expression of the kinase domain. As expression of wild-type ALK, through unknown mechanisms, has been reported in smaller or larger fractions of several other soft tissue tumors (Li et al., 2004), detection of the chimeric ALK oncoprotein may be useful to distinguish IMT from its mesenchymal mimics. An *RREB1–TFE3* fusion gene has been reported in a single case of myofibroblastic sarcoma (McPherson et al., 2011). The genes map to 6p24 and Xp11, respectively.

Although less than 30 karyotyped *congenital or infantile fibrosarcomas* have been reported, their cytogenetic characteristics are fairly well mapped. The chromosome number is almost always hyperdiploid due to the presence of 1–5 tri- or tetrasomic chromosomes (Knezevich et al., 1998; Rubin et al., 1998). An extra copy of chromosome 11 is found in 90% of the tumors followed by trisomies for chromosomes 20, 8, and 17, which are present in two-thirds to one-third of the cases (Figure 24.6). Other, more sporadic trisomies occur as well. The other characteristic feature of infantile

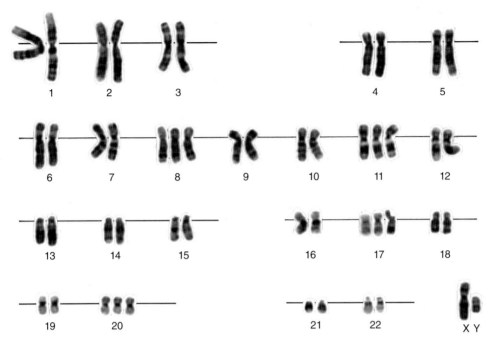

Figure 24.6 Multiple numerical aberrations (+8, +11, +17, and +20) in an infantile fibrosarcoma. Note that the t(12;15) is cytogenetically cryptic.

fibrosarcoma is rearrangement of 12p13 and/or 15q25, which has been found in less than half of the tumors, in one-third of the cases as a balanced or unbalanced t(12;15). The translocation is difficult to detect by chromosome banding and has most likely been missed in earlier studies; molecular genetic investigations show that the aberration is present in a much higher fraction of tumors.

The translocation results in a fusion gene with the pathogenetically important chimeric transcript emanating from the der(15)t(12;15) (Knezevich et al., 1998). The affected genes are *ETV6* (in 12p13) and *NTRK3* (in 15q25). In the *ETV6–NTRK3* fusion, the helix–loop–helix domain of the ETS transcription factor ETV6 is combined with the kinase domain of NTRK3, thus replacing its extracellular ligand-binding and transmembrane domains, resulting in an activation of the NTRK3 kinase. Cytogenetic data do not reveal whether the translocation precedes the numerical changes or vice versa, but molecular findings indicate that the translocation is the earlier event (Rubin et al., 1998). The same fusion gene has been found also in cellular and mixed congenital mesoblastic nephromas, carcinomas, and acute leukemias.

Classic *adult fibrosarcoma* is histologically identical to infantile fibrosarcoma but has a much worse clinical outcome. The genetic aberrations differ from those seen in the infantile counterpart. The majority of a dozen tumors reported show hypodiploid–diploid chromosome numbers and multiple aberrations. The only nonrandom changes that can be discerned are loss of 9p23-pter, with cytogenetic indication of homozygous loss in a few cases, and loss of 10q23-qter. Both have been seen in half of the cases and often together.

The cytogenetic findings in almost 60 *myxofibrosarcomas* reveal a widely scattered spectrum of karyotypic abnormalities. It is possible that diagnostic difficulties may have added to this heterogeneity. In addition, the karyotypic complexity often leads to poor characterization of the chromosome changes; more than half of the karyotypes are designated as incomplete. The chromosome numbers range from 32 to 154 with slightly more than half of the cases being near diploid (Mertens et al., 1998; Willems et al., 2006). Simple karyotypic changes are rare. Cytogenetic evidence of gene amplification, that is, hsr, dmin, and ring chromosomes, are present in one-third of the cases.

Most likely as a consequence of the poor cytogenetic resolution, losses are much more commonly recorded than gains. The only recurrent gain involves chromosome 7, in particular 7q21–35, which is found in almost one-fourth of the cases. Partial losses, found in one-third to one-fourth of the tumors, are from 1p36, 1q23–25, 1q42–44, 3p25, 3q13–29, 5p14–15, 6q21–27, 10p12–15, 12p11–13, 16q23–24, 17p11–13, and 19p13. There is no obvious clustering of breakpoints, with the possible exceptions of 12p11, 19p13, and 19q13.

Although complex karyotypes have been found among all grades, including locally aggressive tumors and lesions with metastatic potential, high-grade tumors showed an overall higher level of cytogenetic complexity, and recurrences showed increase in grade and more complex aberrations than did primary tumors (Willems et al., 2006). An array CGH study of eight myxofibrosarcomas indicated another spectrum of imbalances but was consistent with the cytogenetic findings as regards gain of 7q33–35 and loss of 10p13–14 (Ohguri et al., 2006). The finding of frequent gain of 12q15–21 in this study seems to be at odds with the cytogenetic data, however. In another array CGH study, one case with supernumerary ring chromosomes displayed amplification of 12q sequences (Heidenblad et al., 2006).

More than 10 cases of *myxoinflammatory fibroblastic sarcoma* (MIFS) with chromosome aberrations have been reported. With few exceptions, the chromosome numbers have been near diploid. Some karyotypes showed a single structural aberration, whereas others displayed 5–15, mostly unbalanced, rearrangements. More than half of the cases belonged to the latter category, and all of these tumors had a translocation between chromosomes 1 and 10 (Figure 24.7). The t(1;10)(p22;q24) is often unbalanced and is frequently associated with loss of distal 10q and sometimes also with losses in 1p. Also, chromosome 3 is nonrandomly involved in aberrations, including loss and amplification of sequences from 3p. This amplification seems to be associated with formation of ring chromosomes that may occur separately or together with t(1;10).

Molecular genetic investigations of MIFS with t(1;10) have shown involvement of *TGFBR3* (in 1p22) in a large fraction of cases and that the breakpoint in 10q24 was located in or near the

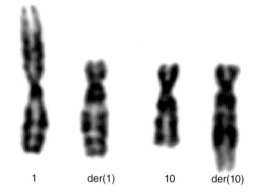

1   der(1)   10   der(10)

Figure 24.7 t(1;10)(p22;q24) in a myxoinflammatory fibroblastic sarcoma.

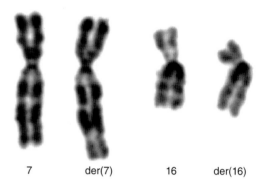

7   der(7)   16   der(16)

Figure 24.8 t(7;16)(q33–34;p11) in a low-grade fibromyxoid sarcoma.

MGEA5 gene, but no fusion transcript or altered expression of these genes (Hallor et al., 2009; Antonescu et al., 2011). On the contrary, *FGF8*, in particular, and also *NPM3*, both close but downstream to *MGEA5*, were expressed at elevated levels. Rearrangements of 3p were associated with amplification and overexpression of genes in 3p11–12, including *VGLL3*. Similar t(1;10) and 3p amplifications have been found also in cases of hemosiderotic fibrolipomatous tumor (see following text) and tumors of mixed morphology.

Two different cytogenetic profiles have been detected in the more than 20 cases of *low-grade fibromyxoid sarcomas* (LGFMS) reported. The most common one, present in two-thirds of the tumors, shows a reciprocal t(7;16)(q33;p11) or more complex variants involving both of these chromosome segments, often as the sole anomaly (Figure 24.8). The majority of the remaining cases are characterized by a single supernumerary ring chromosome. Irrespective of which type of aberration is present, a chimeric *FUS–CREB3L2* gene is found (Panagopoulos et al., 2004). *CREB3L2* (in 7q33–34) encodes a member of the OASIS bZIP family of transcription factors. The bZIP-encoding domain comes under the control of the *FUS* promoter resulting in deregulation of wild-type CREB3L2 target genes. In one case, a related gene fusion, *FUS–CREB3L1*, was detected (Mertens et al., 2005). The *CREB3L1* gene is located in 11p11. An alternative *EWSR1–CREB3L1* fusion gene has been reported in two cases, showing that *EWSR1* can functionally substitute for *FUS* (Lau et al., 2013).

The differential diagnosis of the fairly recently recognized LGFMS may be problematic. Investigation of these fusion genes by RT-PCR in a large series of spindle cell sarcomas representing a variety of diagnoses revealed that the chimeric genes are specific for LGFMS (Panagopoulos et al., 2004; Mertens et al., 2005; Matsuyama et al., 2006). Another large series of LGFMS and non-LGFMS resembling LGFMS obtained from paraffin-embedded tissues were investigated for the presence of fusion genes (Guillou et al., 2007). In more than 80% of the LGFMS group, a chimeric gene was detected, again with a clear predominance (16:1) of the *FUS–CREB3L2* variant. It was detected in less than 10% of non-LGFMS representing various original diagnoses, including *sclerosing epithelioid fibrosarcoma* (SEF). Exons 5, 6, and 7 of *FUS* and exons 5 and 6 of *CREB3L2* were involved in the fusion transcript, with the combination of *FUS* exon 6 and *CREB3L2* exon 5 being found in two-thirds of the fusion-positive tumors followed by the combination exon 7–exon 5 in one-seventh.

All three cases of SEF with chromosome aberrations reported to date have shown near-diploid karyotypes with moderately complex rearrangements. Two of the cases shared several cytogenetic similarities, including monosomy 13, a breakpoint in 10p11, and amplification of sequences from 12q13 and 12q15 in one case and trisomy 12 in the other. In an additional case, immunostaining for MDM2 showed strong nuclear positivity in the majority of tumor cells. Investigations of pure SEF and LGFMS with SEF-like foci, either in the primary tumor or at relapse, have revealed distinct gene fusion patterns (Doyle et al., 2012; Wang et al., 2012; Arbajian et al., 2014). Whereas only

FUS–CREB3L2 has been found in tumors with mixed morphology, the *EWSR1–CREB3L1* fusion gene is clearly dominating among pure SEF, verified or indicated in more than half of 10 cases. Another series showed involvement of *FUS* in two of 22 cases of pure SEF.

So-called fibrohistiocytic tumors

The localized type of *giant cell tumor of tendon sheath* shows pseudodiploid karyotypes with a single or a few structural aberrations (Sciot et al., 1999). In three-fourth of the cases, translocations recombining 1p11–13 with various other bands, in particular 2q35–37, were seen. The only other recurrent translocation partner band identified so far is 5q31. Another recurrently affected breakpoint is 16q24, primarily in tumors without 1p11–13 aberrations. Diffuse-type giant cell tumors have near-diploid karyotypes but are nevertheless cytogenetically heterogeneous (Sciot et al., 1999). A minor subset of tumors show trisomy 5 and/or trisomy 7 as the sole anomalies, and a major subset display simple structural aberrations, with involvement of 1p11–13 in the majority of cases; in a few tumors, these aberrations occur together. Many translocation partners have been found, the only recurrent ones being 2q35–37 and 11q11–12 (Figure 24.9). Thus, gain of chromosomes 5 and 7 is exclusively found in the diffuse type of tumors, whereas translocations with one breakpoint in 1p11–13 are shared by diffuse and localized tumors.

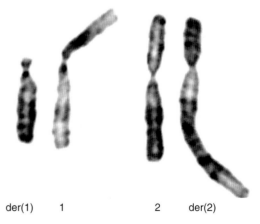

der(1)   1   2   der(2)

Figure 24.9 t(1;2)(p13;q37) in a diffuse-type giant cell tumor.

In the combined data comprising close to 50 cases, t(1;2)(p11–13;q35–37) was present in one-third of tumors with 1p aberrations, followed by t(1;11) (p11–13;q11–12) in 10% of the cases.

Rearrangements of 1p11–13 affect the *CSF1* gene that in some cases recombines with *COL6A3* in 2q37 leading to *CSF1* overexpression (West et al., 2006). It was shown that only a minority of the cells in a tumor express *CSF1*, whereas the majority of cells express its receptor, *CSF1R*. This phenomenon was found both in the localized and diffused forms, and *CSF1* expression was present in tumors with and without rearrangements of the gene, indicating that upregulation of *CSF1* may be caused by some yet unknown alternative mechanism (Cupp et al., 2007; Möller et al., 2008).

About 15 cytogenetically examined cases of *benign fibrous histiocytoma* have been reported. The only recurrent aberrations included t(1;16)(p36;p11) as the sole anomaly in two cases, a breakpoint in 3p21 in three cases, and ring chromosomes in near-tetraploid karyotypes in two cases. Three different fusion genes have been identified in four cases (Plaszczyca et al., 2014). They all included a protein kinase isoform gene, *PRKCB* in 16p11 and *PRKCD* in 3p21, recombined with genes encoding membrane-associated proteins, *PDPN* in 1p36, *CD63* in 12q12–13, and *LAMTOR1* in 11q13. *PDPN–PRKCB* (exons 5–8) was found in the two tumors with t(1;16). The other fusion genes were *LAMTOR1–PRKCD* (exons 1–11) and *CD63–PRKCD* (exons 8–9). The predicted results are chimeric proteins containing membrane-binding parts and the entire catalytic domain of the protein kinase, presumably leading to constitutive kinase activity.

A single case of *aneurysmal fibrous histiocytoma*, which is histologically similar to *angiomatoid fibrous histiocytoma* (AFH), showed a unique t(12;19) (p12;q13). Three cases of *plexiform fibrohistiocytic tumor* showed pseudodiploid karyotypes with no similarities, but one case had a t(4;15)(q21;q15) as the sole anomaly. In a single case of *giant cell tumor of soft tissue*, telomeric associations were found.

Smooth muscle tumors

Less than 10 cases of *leiomyoma* of soft tissues with chromosome aberrations have been reported. The chromosome numbers were invariably near-diploid. The only recurrent aberration, detected in two cases, was one balanced and one unbalanced t(12;14)(q15;q24), the same rearrangement that is the most common cytogenetic change in the extensively studied uterine leiomyomas (Chapter 17).

Roughly 120 *leiomyosarcomas* with chromosome aberrations have been reported, more than half of them soft tissue lesions and the remaining cases primarily gastrointestinal, uterine, and intra-abdominal tumors. No distinct cytogenetic differences can be seen between soft tissue and nonsoft tissue leiomyosarcomas, but the former seem more often to have polyploid chromosome numbers (almost two-thirds vs. more than one-third), and about one-third of them harbor hsr/dmin, which is twice as common as in nonsoft tissue lesions. Some tumors display simple rearrangements, but the majority of cases show highly complex karyotypic changes and extensive intratumor heterogeneity (Mandahl et al., 2000; Wang et al., 2001). No specific structural aberration has been found. Almost 20% of the breakpoints are in chromosome 1, with a clustering to the pericentromeric region (p13 to q21), chromosomes 3 and 7 are also frequently involved, and another breakpoint cluster is seen in 19q13. The most common losses are from 1p32–36; 4q; 9p21–24; 11p; 11q23–25; chromosomes 13, 14, and 18; 19p; 19q13; and 22q. Gains are less common and primarily affect 1q and chromosomes 7 and 20. The rare subtype *inflammatory leiomyosarcoma* seems to display a distinctly different cytogenetic profile. Five of seven karyotyped tumors have shown hyperhaploid stemline karyotypes and one presented with a hyperdiploid karyotype of hyperhaploid origin (Figure 24.10). Molecular genetic analysis has shown that chromosomes 5, 20, and 22 are consistently heterodisomic (Chang et al., 2005; Nord et al., 2012).

Chromosome and array CGH studies of leiomyosarcomas from various sites and representing different malignancy grades have yielded partly different results. The combined data, however, clearly demonstrate the importance of loss of material from 13q and 10q, each found in more than half of the cases (e.g., Larramendy et al., 2006; Meza-Zepeda et al., 2006). Other common (one-third to one-fourth of the cases) imbalances include gain of sequences from 1q, 5p, 8q, 16p, and 17p and losses from 2q, 11q, and 16q. High-level

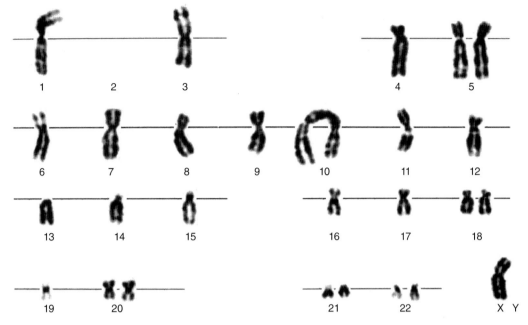

Figure 24.10 Hyperhaploid karyotype in an inflammatory leiomyosarcoma, showing the typical disomies for chromosomes 5, 20, and 21.

amplification is recurrently found in 17p. Discrepancies compared with the cytogenetic findings may be due to tumor heterogeneity and unrepresentative growth of cell populations *in vitro* but possibly also to different diagnostic criteria being used in different studies.

CGH data indicate that loss of 10q sequences and gain of 5p are associated with more aggressive disease. The latter aberration was significantly more common among near-tetraploid tumors compared to near-diploid and near-triploid ones, and loss of 13q13–21 was significantly more frequent among patients surviving less than five years than among those surviving for more than five years (Wang et al., 2003; Hu et al., 2005). Various frequently occurring gene losses and amplifications have been identified in subsets of leiomyosarcomas (Lazar et al., 2013).

Pericytic (perivascular) tumors

No cytogenetic data exists for *glomus tumors* (GT). Molecular genetic analyses of 33 GT revealed rearrangement of either *NOTCH1* (in 9q34), *NOTCH2* (in 1p13), or *NOTCH3* (in 19p13) in 21 cases (Mosquera et al., 2013a). All five malignant GT involved *NOTCH2*. Among 28 benign GT, 12 cases

were positive for *NOTCH2* rearrangement, one for *NOTCH1*, and three for *NOTCH3*, whereas 12 cases showed no involvement of these genes. In one benign and one malignant tumor, a *MIR143–NOTCH2* (exon 1–exon 27) fusion transcript was detected, and in one benign GT, there was a *MIR143–NOTCH3* (exon 1–exon 29). Altogether, *MIR143* (in 5q32) rearrangements were demonstrated by FISH in 12 benign and two malignant GT, indicating the presence of some *MIR143–NOTCH* fusion in a large fraction of GT, regardless of anatomical location and degree of malignancy. The likely outcome is high expression of truncated *NOTCH* through the strong *MIR143* promoter.

A subset of myopericytomas, *pericytoma*, is cytogenetically characterized by a t(7;12)(p22;q13) that was present in all six cases reported, as the sole anomaly in two cases. The karyotypes were pseudo- or hypodiploid. The translocation results in an *ACTB–GLI1* fusion transcript; in a few cases, also, the reciprocal *GLI1–ACTB* transcript has been detected (Dahlén et al., 2004). *ACTB* contributes exon 1, exons 1–2, or exons 1–3 with exons 6–12 or 7–12 coming from *GLI1*. The DNA-binding zinc finger domains of GLI1 are retained, whereas its promoter region is replaced with that of the ubiquitously expressed *ACTB* gene, leading to deregulation of *GLI1* expression. Six *myopericytomas* and nine *myofibromas* investigated for *NOTCH* rearrangement were all negative (Mosquera et al., 2013a).

Only a handful of *angioleiomyomas* have been characterized by chromosome banding. All karyotypes were near diploid with simple aberrations that in half of the cases included monosomies or deletions. No recurrent aberration was identified. In a series of 23 informative angioleiomyomas investigated by CGH, eight revealed copy number changes involving one or two chromosomes in each case (Nishio et al., 2004). Five cases showed losses from chromosome 22, all including 22q11.2, and three cases had gain of Xq sequences, but no high-level amplification was seen. One of 18 tumors investigated was positive for *NOTCH2* (Mosquera et al., 2013a).

Skeletal muscle tumors

About 100 *alveolar rhabdomyosarcomas* (ARMS) have been reported, the vast majority soft tissue lesions. Diploid and polyploid chromosome numbers are equally common (e.g., Gordon et al., 2001). The cytogenetic hallmarks of ARMS are t(2;13)(q36;q14) and, much less frequently, t(1;13)(p36;q14). The translocations, rarely found as the sole anomaly, are often present in duplicate or triplicate, and an extra copy of the der(13)t(2;13) is common. A few tumors without any of these reciprocal translocations showed a breakpoint in either 2q35-37 or 13q14, indicating cryptic or additional variant translocations. Secondary numerical and structural aberrations are common leading to complex karyotypes. A recurrent structural aberration, secondary to t(2;13), is der(16)t(1;16)(q21;q13). Imbalances found in 15-25% of the cases include gain of chromosomes 2, 12, and 20 and of distal 1q and loss of distal 3p and distal 16q. Chromosome-based CGH investigations have yielded partly discrepant results, but gains of 2p, 12q, and 13 have been identified in several studies. A subset of tumors display amplification of sequences from the proximal half of 12q.

The molecular consequences of the translocations are formation of chimeric genes involving *FOXO1* (in 13q14) and either *PAX7* (in 1p36) or *PAX3* (in 2q36), all encoding transcription factors, with breakpoints scattered in intron 7 of the *PAX* genes and intron 1 of *FOXO1* (Xia et al., 2002). The fusion products are composed of the amino-terminal DNA-binding elements of *PAX3* or *PAX7* and the carboxy-terminal transactivation domain of *FOXO1*; the resulting proteins are strong transcriptional activators (Barr, 2001). Roughly 60% of ARMS are *PAX3-FOXO1* positive, 20% are *PAX7-FOXO1* positive, and 20% are negative for both fusions. As expected from the cytogenetic data, variant gene fusions may be present, and in fact, variants have been identified in sporadic cases; *PAX3* fused to *FOXO4* (in Xq13), encoding another forkhead protein, to *NCOA1* (in 2p23) and *NCOA2* (in 8q13), both encoding a nuclear receptor coactivator, as well as a *FOXO1* fused to the growth factor receptor *FGFR1* (in 8p11-12) (Barr et al., 2002; Wachtel et al., 2004; Sumegi et al., 2010; Liu et al., 2011). Most likely, true gene fusion-negative tumors with classical ARMS morphology exist. Genomic amplification of the fusion gene was found in more than 90% of *PAX7-FOXO*-positive tumors but only in less than 10% of *PAX3-FOXO1* cases (Duan et al., 2012). Presence of fusion gene amplification and involvement of *PAX7* were associated with improved outcome. Cytogenetic evidence of gene amplification, dmin and hsr, is found in 20% of the tumors. Apart from amplification of fusion genes and sequences from 12q13-15, about one-fifth of the ARMS display *MYCN* amplification.

RT-PCR is a valuable diagnostic adjunct frequently used in clinical settings, but a FISH assay was reported to carry some advantages, including the ability to identify unusual variant translocations (Nishio et al., 2006). They found that mixed alveolar/embryonal rhabdomyosarcomas (ERMS) were negative for rearrangements of the *PAX* and *FOXO1* genes. Detailed studies of gene expression in 139 rhabdomyosarcomas revealed that ARMS with either of the *PAX-FOXO1A* fusion genes showed a distinctly different expression profile compared to fusion-negative ARMS and other rhabdomyosarcoma subtypes (Davicioni et al., 2006).

Of more than 80 karyotyped ERMS, the majority soft tissue lesions, about two-thirds had hypo- or hyperdiploid chromosome numbers. The karyotypes are frequently complex with multiple numerical changes (e.g., Gordon et al., 2001). Apart from a few cases with t(2;8)(q35–37;q13) as the sole anomaly, no recurrent structural aberration has been found, but the genomic imbalances are nonrandom. Half of the tumors harbor extra copies of chromosomes 2 and 8. Imbalances found in 20–30% of the tumors include gains of distal 1q, distal 7q, distal 11q, and chromosomes 12 and 13 but losses of 9p, distal 15q, and 17p13. Several CGH studies have revealed gains of chromosomes 2, 7, 8, 11, 12, and 13 but losses of distal 1p and 14q. LOH, loss of imprinting, and paternal disomy of loci in 11p15 are recurrent in ERMS. This may lead to an abnormal activation of the normally silent maternal allele of *IGF2*. Combined with the observation in an ERMS of amplification of 15q25–26, encompassing *IGF1R*, a mediator of the biological effect of IGF2, this suggests a role of the IGF pathway in the development of at least a subset of these tumors (Bridge et al., 2002; Slater and Shipley, 2007). Patients with the Beckwith–Wiedemann syndrome, associated with constitutional alterations of 11p15, have an increased risk of developing ERMS. Also, other cancer syndromes predispose to rhabdomyosarcoma (Coffin et al., 2014).

ARMS and ERMS show largely similar patterns of genomic imbalances, although most of them occur at higher frequencies among the latter (Bridge et al., 2002). Based on the cytogenetic findings, the most conspicuous differences are that gains of chromosomes 8 and 13 and of distal 11q are less common, or even rare, among ARMS. This is corroborated by CGH data, in particular as concerns distal 11q. Among the top differentially expressed genes in fusion-positive ARMS compared with ERMS, the only gene showing more than twofold higher expression in ERMS was *APLP2*, which is located in 11q24 (Lae et al., 2007). In one case, the t(2;8) was shown to result in a *PAX3–NCOA2* fusion (Sumegi et al., 2010).

The less than 10 cytogenetically characterized *pleomorphic rhabdomyosarcomas* reported have displayed highly complex karyotypic changes. The *PAX3–FOXO1* fusion gene was found in one case. In a subset of *spindle cell rhabdomyosarcomas*, rearrangements of *NCOA2* were found in children younger than one year (Mosquera et al., 2013b). In one case each, the fusion genes *SRF–NCOA2* and *TEAD1–NCOA2* were identified. *SRF* maps to 6p21 and *TEAD1* to 11p15.

Vascular tumors

Few cytogenetic reports are available on this group of tumors. The karyotypic abnormalities are variable. No recurrent aberrations were detected in four *angiomas*, all displaying near-diploid karyotypes with simple changes. Among more than 10 *angiosarcomas*, half from soft tissues and half from other sites, chromosome numbers ranging from hypodiploidy to hypertriploidy have been found. All from simple to complex karyotypic changes are encountered, and cytogenetically unrelated clones are present in some cases. Recurrent aberrations include gain of 8p12–q24 and 20pter–q13 and loss of 4p14-pter, 4q25–31, 7p15-pter, 13, and 22q13-qter. The combining of these data with data on a handful of nonsoft tissue angiosarcomas investigated by CGH reveals that gains in 8q and 20p and losses in 22q are the most frequent genomic imbalances (Baumhoer et al., 2005). The only recurrent aberration in *Kaposi sarcomas*, with near-diploid karyotypes and mostly simple changes, is a breakpoint in 8q24 in two cases.

In two cases of *pseudomyogenic hemangioendothelioma* (PHE), a t(7;19)(q22;q13) was found as the sole anomaly (Walther et al., 2014). The translocation results in fusion of the *SERPINE1* (in 7q22) and *FOSB* (in 19q13) genes. FISH analyses of sections from eight other cases of PHE identified *SERPINE1–FOSB* fusion in all cases. *SERPINE1* encodes a protein that is a member of the serine protease inhibitor family and is highly expressed in vascular cells, whereas *FOSB* encodes a transcription factor belonging to the FOS family. Probably, the essential outcome is upregulation of *FOSB* through the strong *SERPINE1* promoter.

Among less than 10 cytogenetically investigated *epithelioid hemangioendotheliomas* (EHAE), an identical translocation, t(1;3)(p36;q25), was found in a subset (e.g., Mendlick et al., 2001). Other tumors showed loss of the Y chromosome, supernumerary ring chromosomes, or aberrations involving chromosome 11 in two cases each, but no t(1;3). The translocation has been shown to result in fusion of *WWTR1* (in 3q25), encoding a transcriptional coactivator protein that is highly expressed in endothelial cells, and *CAMTA1* (in 1p36), which encodes a transcriptional regulatory protein that is normally expressed only in the brain (Errani et al., 2011;

Tanas et al., 2011). The *WWTR1–CAMTA1* fusion transcript (exon 2 or 3–exon 9) results in activation of *CAMTA1* expression through a promoter-switch mechanism. The gene fusion is highly specific for EHAE and was detected in 90% of more than 60 tumors tested, whereas some 125 other vascular or potentially mimicking tumors were all negative. A subset of *WWTR1–CAMTA1*-negative EHAE with unusual morphologic features was shown to harbor a *YAP1–TFE3* fusion in eight of 10 cases (Antonescu et al., 2013b). *YAP1* (in 11q22) encodes a transcription factor, and *TFE3* (in Xp11) a transcriptional coactivator sharing functional and sequence homology with *WWTR1*.

Tumors of uncertain differentiation

Less than 10 cases of *ossifying fibromyxoid tumor* (OFMT) of soft tissue with chromosome aberrations have been reported. Most karyotypes were near diploid. Recurrent breakpoints include, in particular, 6p21 followed by 12q24, 12q13, and Xp11. Rearrangements of *PHF1* (in 6p21), encoding a PHD finger protein interacting with polycomb group proteins, were detected in 50–85% of OFMT, including typical, atypical, and malignant variants (Gebre-Medhin et al., 2012; Endo et al., 2013; Graham et al., 2013; Antonescu et al., 2014). The genomic *PHF1* rearrangements are frequently complex. *EP400* (in 12q24), encoding an E1A-binding protein, is the most common fusion partner with *PHF1*; close to 20 cases with *EP400–PHF1* have been reported, representing all three variants of OFMT, although it seems to be less abundant among malignant tumors. Less common, but still recurrent, fusion genes include *MEAF6–PHF1* and *EPC1–PHF1* and *ZC3H7B–BCOR* in a single case. *BCOR* maps to Xp11 and was rearranged in a second case, but not recombined with *ZC3H7B*. A subset of tumors harbor *PHF1* rearrangements, but without involvement of any of the fusion partners mentioned above. *PHF1* has been implicated, as the 3′ fusion partner, also in endometrial stromal sarcomas (Chapter 17). Also, some of the other genes are involved in both tumor entities.

More than 10 *soft tissue myoepitheliomas* (ME) with chromosome changes have been reported. Near-diploid karyotypes predominate. Recurrent aberrations include t(1;22)(q23;q12) in two cases, a breakpoint in Xp11 (three cases), and gain of chromosome 5 in one-third of the cases. Several fusion transcripts have been identified, most of which contain *EWSR1* as the 5′ partner (Brandal et al., 2008, 2009; Hallor et al., 2008; Antonescu et al., 2010, 2013a; Flucke et al., 2012). Rearrangement of *EWSR1* was detected in almost half of soft tissue ME. Recurrent 3′ fusion partners include *PBX1* (in 1q23), *POU5F1* (in 6p21), and less often *ZNF444* (in 19q13), whereas *ATF1* (in 12q13) has only been found in a single case. *EWSR1–POU5F1*-positive tumors occur in children and young adults with deep-seated lesions. *EWSR1*-negative tumors are more often benign and superficial. Studies of such tumors revealed rearrangements of *PLAG1* in more than one-third of the cases, including both skin and soft tissue lesions. In one case, a *LIFR–PLAG1* fusion was found. Thus, ME of soft tissues are genetically heterogeneous, with a subset of tumors sharing *PLAG1* involvement with their salivary gland counterparts.

The few cases of *hemosiderotic fibrolipomatous tumor* with reported chromosome aberrations showed near-diploid karyotypes, balanced or unbalanced t(1;10)(p22–31;q24–25), loss of 3p material, and amplification of genes in 3p11–12, including *VGLL3* (Hallor et al., 2009). The breakpoints map to *TGFBR3* in 1p22 and in or near *MGEA5* in 10q24. These aberrations are shared with MIFS (see preceding text).

The sparse cytogenetic information on AFH has revealed near-diploid karyotypes with simple balanced or moderately complex, unbalanced structural rearrangements. Recurrent breakpoints have been identified in 2q33, 12q13, and 22q12. Based on these findings, RT-PCR analyses of larger series of AFH have revealed three fusion genes, in decreasing order of frequency: *EWSR1–CREB1*, *EWSR1–ATF1*, and *FUS–ATF1*, corresponding to t(2;22)(q33;q12), t(12;22)(q13;q12) (Figure 24.11), and t(12;16)(q13;p11), respectively (Antonescu et al., 2007; Hallor et al., 2007; Rossi et al., 2007). *EWSR1–ATF1* and *EWSR1–CREB1* have also been found in clear cell sarcoma (CCS) (see following text).

Cytogenetic data are available on more than 220 *synovial sarcomas* (SS), including monophasic, biphasic, and poorly differentiated lesions (Limon et al., 1991; Mandahl et al., 1995; Panagopoulos et al.,

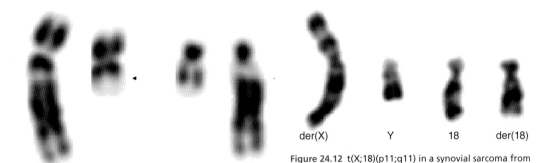

der(X) Y 18 der(18)

Figure 24.12 t(X;18)(p11;q11) in a synovial sarcoma from a man.

12 der(12) 22 der(22)

Figure 24.11 t(12;22)(q13;q12) in an angiomatoid fibrous histiocytoma. Cytogenetically identical translocations are found in clear cell sarcoma of soft tissue and a minor subset of myxoid liposarcomas. In the former two tumor types, an *EWSR1–ATF1* fusion gene is formed, whereas the result in liposarcomas is an *EWSR1–DDIT3* chimera.

2001; Przybyl et al., 2012). Half of the tumors had pseudodiploid karyotypes, hypodiploidy is somewhat more common than hyperdiploidy, and only about 10% had chromosome numbers in the triploid or tetraploid regions. A highly characteristic recombination between chromosome bands Xp11 and 18q11 has been found in more than 90% of the tumors. Mostly a balanced t(X;18)(p11;q11) is seen, in one-third of the cases as the sole anomaly, but also an unbalanced der(X)t(X;18) and insertions and complex translocations involving one to three other chromosomes have been reported (Figure 24.12). A few cases show involvement of Xp11 but not 18q11 or vice versa. With few exceptions, the karyotypic complexity is low or moderate, in particular among primary lesions. Recurrent secondary changes, each seen in 10–15% of the cases, include gain of chromosomes 2 (in particular 2q13–21), 7, 8 (in particular 8q22–24), 12, and 21 and losses of 3p12–26, 11p, and 11q.

The t(X;18) may result in the formation of three different fusion genes involving *SS18* in 18q11 and either of the linked genes *SSX1*, *SSX2*, and *SSX4* in Xp11. A fourth fusion gene variant with involvement of 20q13 and Xp11, *SS18L1–SSX1*, has also been detected. *SS18–SSX1* is found in two-thirds and *SS18–SSX2* in one-third of the cases, whereas *SS18–SSX4* and *SS18L1–SSX1* have been seen only in very occasional tumors. About 15 variant transcripts, with or without inserted sequences in the breakpoint junction, have been reported; in by far the most common one, codon 410 in *SS18* is fused

with codon 111 in *SSX* (Amary et al., 2007; Przybyl et al., 2012). In the resulting chimeric protein, eight amino acids of the C-terminal of SS18 are replaced by 78 amino acids of the SSX C-terminal. This leads to disruption of the QPGY domain of SS18 whereas the Krüppel-associated box of SSX is lost. In biphasic tumors, the chimeric transcript is present in both the spindle cell and epithelial component.

Among patients with *SS18–SSX2*, there is a male to female ratio of 1:2, whereas it is 1:1 among patients with *SS18–SSX1*-positive tumors. *SS18–SSX2*-positive tumors are with few exceptions monophasic, whereas the vast majority of biphasic tumors are *SS18–SSX1* positive. Findings from cytogenetic and chromosome CGH analyses indicate that individual aberrations are not useful for prediction of the clinical outcome in terms of risk of developing metastases. The potential role of the type of gene fusion as an independent prognostic factor has been investigated in about 500 SS (Ladanyi et al., 2002; Guillou et al., 2004; Ren et al., 2013). Still, the results are not conclusive. The finding in one large series that fusion type is the single most significant prognostic factor among patients with localized disease at diagnosis was not corroborated by the results in another large series. Combined cytogenetic and molecular genetic data indicated that patients showing simple karyotypes and *SS18–SSX2* fusion had better clinical outcome than did those with a complex tumor karyotype and *SS18–SSX1* fusion (Panagopoulos et al., 2001). A subset of SS display gain or amplification of 12q sequences, and array CGH analyses indicate that gain of the *SAS* gene is associated with worse overall survival (Nakagawa et al., 2006).

CCS of soft tissue, also known as malignant melanoma of soft parts, show chromosome numbers ranging from hypodiploidy to hypertriploidy and display simple or moderately complex karyotypic changes in most of the less than 40 cases reported (e.g., Panagopoulos et al., 2002a). A characteristic t(12;22)(q13;q12) is present in two-thirds of the tumors, but only rarely as the sole anomaly. A few additional cases have had rearrangement of either 12q13 or 22q12. Polysomy 8 or an isochromosome for 8q is as common as t(12;22). Other aberrations occurring in at least one-fourth of the cases include +7, −1p36, +1q12–41, −9p11, and +17q.

The t(12;22) results in a fusion gene in which the 3′ part of *EWSR1* (in 22q12) is replaced by the 3′ part of the activating transcription factor 1 (*ATF1*) (in 12q13). At least four types of chimeric transcript have been reported. In order of frequency, the following exon fusions of *EWSR1* and *ATF1*, respectively, have been identified: 8–4 (50%), 7–5 (45%), 10–5 (5%), and 7–7 (<1%) (Panagopoulos et al., 2002a; Wang et al., 2009). A variant fusion gene, *EWSR1–CREB1* (exon 7–exon 7), involving an *ATF1*-related *CREB* family member in 2q33, has been found (Wang et al., 2009). *ATF1* is involved in >90% and *CREB1* in >6% of CCS. The chimeric EWSR1–ATF1 protein deregulates promoters harboring an ATF1 binding site. Activating mutations of *BRAF*, which are common in melanomas of the skin, are absent in CCS. The same fusion genes have been identified also in AFH (see preceding text) where *EWSR1–CREB1* is the most common.

Cytogenetic data are available on more than 10 *desmoplastic small round cell tumors* (DSRCT). Most of them were intra-abdominal, but also intra-thoracic and skeletal lesions have been investigated. The karyotypes are usually near diploid with few numerical and/or structural aberrations. Almost always a breakpoint in 22q is found, and most tumors also have a break in 11p13, in about two-thirds of the cases resulting in a t(11;22) (p13;q11–13), sometimes as the sole anomaly (Figure 24.13). Due to the small number of cases investigated by chromosome banding, the pattern of secondary aberrations remains unclear, but +5 and −10 have each been seen in one-fourth of the cases. Much larger series of DSRCT have been investigated by RT-PCR, detecting an *EWSR1–WT1* chimera in 97% of the cases. *EWSR1* contributes its amino-terminal domain, which exhibits strong transactivational properties, and

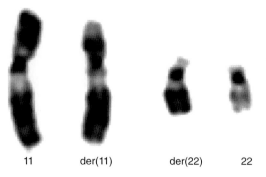

11   der(11)   der(22)   22

Figure 24.13 t(11;22)(p13;q12) in a desmoplastic small round cell tumor.

WT1 with a subset of the DNA-binding zinc fingers to the chimera (Gerald and Haber, 2005). Almost all DSRCT display an in-frame junction of *EWSR1* exon 7 to *WT1* exon 8, but rare variants with other exon combinations have been reported (Murphy et al., 2008). Identification of t(11;22)(p13;q12) or the *EWSR1–WT1* transcript is useful in the differential diagnosis of small cell round cell tumors and may show higher sensitivity than immunohistochemical analyses (Lae et al., 2002). Two pediatric tumors originally diagnosed as leiomyosarcomas showed the cytogenetic and molecular genetic characteristics of DSRCT (Alaggio et al., 2007). These tumors might represent an unusual form of leiomyosarcoma, DSRCT with unusual clinicohistopathologic features, or an unrecognized subgroup of tumors with spindle cell morphology.

Only a few cytogenetically abnormal *soft part myxomas* have been reported. The karyotypes were pseudodiploid or near diploid with few aberrations. Rearrangements affected the 12q13–15 region in four cases, two of which also had a breakpoint in 12p11. Sporadic cases of myxomas from other sites, including larger series of cardiac myxomas, have had rearrangements involving 12p. Five of seven karyotypically aberrant *aggressive angiomyxomas* had breakpoints in 12q13–15 (e.g., Rawlinson et al., 2008). Molecular genetic analyses have revealed fusion of part of *HMGA2* with ectopic sequences or expression of the full-length gene, in similarity with several other benign mesenchymal tumor types.

The karyotypic information available on less than 20 *epithelioid sarcomas* reveals considerable heterogeneity, ranging from a single numerical or structural aberration to more than 20 rearrangements and showing hypodiploid to near-tetraploid chromosome numbers. The only structural change found in two cases is a t(10;22)(q26;q1?); both tumors were proximal-type epithelioid sarcomas (Lualdi et al., 2004). A breakpoint in 22q11–12 has been found in one-third of the cases. Gain of one or more copies of 8q and losses in 22q are present in almost half of the lesions; other frequent imbalances include loss of sequences from 13q and 18p. There may be some differences in the pattern of genomic aberrations between proximal-type and the classic, peripheral epithelioid sarcomas; chromosome 22 aberrations and polyploidy seem to be more frequent among the former. Deletion of the *SMARCB1* gene in 22q11 or inactivation at the protein level was found in most proximal tumors (Modena et al., 2005). Similar changes are also found in malignant rhabdoid tumors.

Of the more than 30 cases of *extraskeletal myxoid chondrosarcoma* (EMC) with chromosome aberrations reported, 90% displayed a pseudo- or near-diploid chromosome number (Panagopoulos et al., 2002b; Sjögren et al., 2003). A breakpoint in 9q22 has been found to be involved in one of three reciprocal translocations—t(9;22)(q22;q12), t(9;17)(q22;q11), and t(9;15)(q22;q21)—one of which occurs as the sole anomaly in more than one-third of the cases (Figure 24.14). The t(9;22), including variant three-way translocations, is present in two-thirds of EMC, the t(9;17) in 20%, while the t(9;15) is represented by a single case. The most common secondary, numerical changes include gains of chromosomes 12, 7, 19, and 8, all of which are present in less than one-fifth of the tumors. Gain of chromosome segment 1q25-qter has been found in one-fourth of EMC.

The three translocations all result in the formation of fusion genes involving *NR4A3* in 9q22–31.1 and *EWSR1* in 22q12, *TAF15* in 17q11 or *TCF12* in 15q21 (Panagopoulos et al., 2002b; Sjögren et al., 2003; Hisaoka and Hashimoto, 2005). A fourth fusion gene, *TFG–NR4A3*, was found in a single case. In the resulting chimeras, the 5′ untranslated portion of *NR4A3* followed by its entire coding sequence is linked to the amino-terminal portion of the partner. A variety of chimeric *EWSR1–NR4A3* transcripts have been identified among about 60 cases investigated, most of which have been found in sporadic cases (Panagopoulos et al., 2002b). In the most common transcript, found in half of the cases, *EWSR1* exon 12 is fused in frame with exon 3 of *NR4A3*, while in the second most common transcript, exons 7 and 2, respectively, are fused. *TAF15* exon 6 is fused to exon 3 of *NR4A3*. Since these fusion genes are pathognomonic, they represent useful diagnostic markers, but the role, if any, of genetic aberrations as prognostic factors remains unknown. The gene expression profile of EMC seems to be quite uniform irrespective of differences in histology and the type of fusion transcript (Sjögren et al., 2003).

Chromosome banding data are available on a dozen *alveolar soft part sarcomas* (ASPS), a rare tumor occurring more often in females (Ladanyi et al., 2001; Folpe and Deyrup, 2006). The karyotypes are near diploid with relatively few aberrations. Almost all tumors have a breakpoint in 17q25 and more than half of the cases another one in Xp11. Recombination between those two chromosome bands is mostly seen as an unbalanced, nonreciprocal translocation, der(17)t(X;17)(p11;q25) (Figure 24.15). As a consequence, there

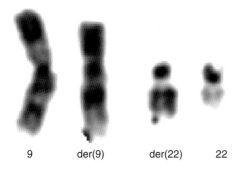

9   der(9)   der(22)   22

Figure 24.14 t(9;22)(q22;q12) in an extraskeletal myxoid chondrosarcoma. The normal chromosome 9 (left) is a constitutional variant with heterochromatin in the short arm.

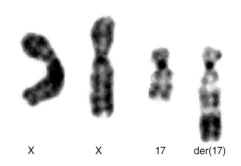

X   X   17   der(17)

Figure 24.15 der(17)t(X;17)(p11;q25) together with two normal copies of the X chromosome in an alveolar soft part sarcoma.

is loss of 17q25-qter in most cases and gain of Xp11-pter in some cases. The combined cytogenetic and molecular data indicate that there is a balanced t(X;17) in 25% of the cases. In the majority of ASPS from men, a normal X chromosome is found, indicating a G_2-phase origin of the rearrangement (Huang et al., 2005); in some women, a der(17)t(X;17) is seen together with two normal X chromosomes. Other recurrent changes include gains of 1q, 5, 12, and 15q.

The ubiquitously expressed *ASPSCR1* gene in 17q25 and the transcription factor gene *TFE3* in Xp11 form an *ASPSCR1–TFE3* fusion gene for which at least two variant transcripts have been identified: exons 1–7 of *ASPSCR1* are fused to exon 6 or exon 5 of *TFE3* (Ladanyi et al., 2001; Aulmann et al., 2007; Hodge et al., 2014), the difference being exclusion or retention of the activating domain of *TFE3*. The chimeric protein acts as a transcription factor causing activation of MET signaling. The same gene fusion has been found also in a subset of pediatric renal cell carcinomas, but in these tumors, the translocation is mostly balanced (Chapter 15).

PEComas have shown rearrangements of *TFE3* (in Xp11), which in one case was fused with *SFPQ* (in 1p34), in a subset of tumors that may have specific clinicomorphologic features (Tanaka et al., 2009; Argani et al., 2010). The few cases investigated cytogenetically have had simple karyotypes with balanced translocations, none of which involved chromosome bands 1p34 or Xp11. A single case of *intimal sarcoma* with a hypertriploid karyotype and multiple numerical and structural chromosome aberrations has been reported (Zhang et al., 2007). FISH analysis of the tumor using probes for six genes in 12q13–15 revealed high-level amplification of *SAS*, *CDK4*, and *MDM2*. In a CGH study of intimal sarcomas, gain or high-level amplification within 12q12–15 was found in six of eight cases (Zhao et al., 2002). Other aberrations seen in three to four cases were losses in 4q, 9p, 11q, 13q, and Xq and gains in 7p and chromosome 17. Additional, less common amplifications were sometimes present. Array CGH revealed frequent amplification of *SAS*, *CDK4*, *MDM2*, and *GLI* and also of *PDGFRA* (in 4q12).

Undifferentiated sarcomas

Undifferentiated small round cell sarcomas represent a heterogeneous group of tumors that are poorly characterized (Fletcher et al., 2013c). Less than 10 cases with chromosome aberrations have been reported. In a subset of these, a t(4;19) (q35;q13) was found in five cases with simple or moderately complex karyotypic changes; in three cases, trisomy 8 was present. The translocation results in the formation of a *CIC–DUX4* fusion gene (e.g., Italiano et al., 2012; Choi et al., 2013; Machado et al., 2013). The mostly aggressive tumors were negative for *EWSR1* rearrangement.

The chromosome numbers of 70 *undifferentiated pleomorphic sarcomas* varied from near haploidy to hyperoctaploidy. More than half of these tumors had complex, incompletely described karyotypes, and more than one-third had cytogenetic signs of gene amplification (Fletcher et al., 2013c; Mitelman et al., 2014). Unbalanced structural aberrations were numerous. A nonrandom distribution of breakpoints could be discerned but may, at least partly, reflect that aberrations of some chromosomes are more readily detected. Bearing these limitations in mind, breakpoint hot spots (≥10% of the cases) seem to be present in 1p36, 1q11, 1q21, 1q32, 4p16, 5p15, 6q15, 12p13, 12q24, 14q11, and 19q13.

Summary

Soft tissue tumors frequently pose differential diagnostic dilemmas, and at times, benign, borderline malignant, and/or malignant tumors may be difficult to distinguish from one another by traditional pathologic methods. Cytogenetic analyses have revealed that practically all soft tissue tumor types harbor acquired chromosome aberrations. The type of aberrations and the level of karyotypic complexity vary considerably from one tumor entity to another. At one end are the pathognomonic translocations that by themselves are extremely useful diagnostic signatures (Table 24.1). Another set of rearrangements are highly characteristic but not unique since they are shared by two or more tumor entities, sometimes including nonsoft tissue tumors. Detection of such aberrations, by cytogenetic or molecular genetic means, is useful in the diagnostic setting

Table 24.1 Characteristic structural chromosome aberrations and corresponding gene fusions in soft tissue tumors

Chromosome aberration	Gene fusion	Tumor type
t(1;2)(p13;q37)	COL6A3–CSF1	Diffuse-type giant cell tumor
t(1;2)(q21;p23)	TPM3–ALK	Inflammatory myofibroblastic tumor
t(1;3)(p36;q25)	WWTR1–CAMTA1	Epithelioid hemangioendothelioma
[t(1;5)(p12;q32)]*	MIR143–NOTCH2	Glomus tumor
t(1;10)(p22;q24)	TGFBR3–FGF8?	Myxoinflammatory fibroblastic sarcoma
		Hemosiderotic fibrolipomatous tumor
t(1;11)(p13;q11–12)	Unknown	Diffuse-type giant cell tumor
t(1;12)(p32;q14)	PPAP2B–HMGA2	Lipoma
t(1;13)(p36;q14)	PAX7–FOXO1	Alveolar rhabdomyosarcoma
[t(1;14)(p12;q31)]*	NOTCH2–CEP128	Glomus tumor
t(1;16)(p36;p11)	PDPN–PRKCB	Benign fibrous histiocytoma
t(1;22)(q23;q12)	EWSR1–PBX1	Soft tissue myoepithelioma
inv(2)(p23q35)	ATIC–ALK	Inflammatory myofibroblastic tumor
t(2;2)(p23;q13)	RANBP2–ALK	Inflammatory myofibroblastic tumor
t(2;2)(p23;q36)	PAX3–NCOA1	Alveolar rhabdomyosarcoma
t(2;4)(p23;q21)	SEC31A–ALK	Inflammatory myofibroblastic tumor
t(2;8)(q36;q13)	PAX3–NCOA2	Alveolar rhabdomyosarcoma
t(2;11)(p23;p15)	CARS–ALK	Inflammatory myofibroblastic tumor
t(2;11)(q31;q12)	FOSL1 deregulation?	Desmoplastic fibroblastoma
		Fibroma of tendon sheath
t(2;12)(p23;p11)	PPFIBP1–ALK	Inflammatory myofibroblastic tumor
t(2;12)(q37;q14)	HMGA2–CXCR7	Lipoma
t(2;13)(q36;q14)	PAX3–FOXO1	Alveolar rhabdomyosarcoma
t(2;17)(p23;q23)	CLTC–ALK	Inflammatory myofibroblastic tumor
t(2;19)(p23;p13)	TPM4–ALK	Inflammatory myofibroblastic tumor
t(2;22)(q33;q12)	EWSR1–CREB1	Angiomatoid fibrous histiocytoma
		Clear cell sarcoma of soft tissue
[t(3;9)(q12;q31)]*	TFG–NR4A3	Extraskeletal myxoid chondrosarcoma
t(3;11)(p21;q13)	LAMTOR1–PRKCD	Benign fibrous histiocytoma
t(3;12)(p21;q12–13)	CD63–PRKCD	Benign fibrous histiocytoma
t(3;12)(q28;q14)	HMGA2–LPP	Lipoma
t(4;19)(q35;q13)	CIC–DUX4	Undifferentiated small round cell sarcoma
[t(5;8)(p13;q12)]*	LIFR–PLAG1	Soft tissue myoepithelioma
t(5;8)(p15;q13)	AHRR–NCOA2	Soft tissue angiofibroma
[t(5;9)(q32;q34)]*	MIR143–NOTCH1	Glomus tumor
t(5;12)(q33;q14)	HMGA2–EBF1	Lipoma
[t(5;19)(q32;p13)]*	MIR143–NOTCH3	Glomus tumor
t(6;12)(p21;q24)	EP400–PHF1	Ossifying fibromyxoid tumor
[t(6;22)(p21;q12)]*	EWSR1–POU5F1	Soft tissue myoepithelioma
t(7;8)(q11;q13)	GTF2I–NCOA2	Soft tissue angiofibroma
t(7;8)(q21;q12)	COL1A2–PLAG1	Lipoblastoma
t(7;12)(p22;q13)	ACTB–GLI1	Pericytoma
t(7;16)(q33;p11)	FUS–CREB3L2	Low-grade fibromyxoid sarcoma
t(7;19)(q22;q13)	SERPINE1–FOSB	Pseudomyogenic hemangioendothelioma
del(8)(q12q24)	HAS2–PLAG1	Lipoblastoma
t(8;13)(p11;q14)	FOXO1–FGFR1	Alveolar rhabdomyosarcoma
t(8;14)(q12;q24)	PLAG1–RAD51L1	Lipoblastoma
t(9;12)(p23;q14)	HMGA2–NFIB	Lipoma
t(9;15)(q22;q21)	TCF12–NR4A3	Extraskeletal myxoid chondrosarcoma

(Continued)

Table 24.1 (*Continued*)

Chromosome aberration	Gene fusion	Tumor type
t(9;17)(q22;q11)	TAF15–NR4A3	Extraskeletal myxoid chondrosarcoma
t(9;22)(q22;q12)	EWSR1–NR4A3	Extraskeletal myxoid chondrosarcoma
t(10;22)(q26;q1?)	Unknown	Epithelioid sarcoma
t(11;16)(p11;p11)	FUS–CREB3L1	Low-grade fibromyxoid sarcoma
t(11;16)(q13;p13)	C11orf95–MKL2	Chondroid lipoma
t(11;22)(p13;q12)	EWSR1–WT1	Desmoplastic small round cell tumor
t(11;22)(p11;q12)	EWSR1–CREB3L1	Low-grade fibromyxoid sarcoma
		Sclerosing epithelioid fibrosarcoma
inv(12)(q13q13)	NAB2–STAT6	Solitary fibrous tumor
t(12;13)(q14;q13)	HMGA2–LHFP	Lipoma
t(12;15)(p13;q25)	ETV6–NTRK3	Infantile fibrosarcoma
t(12;16)(q13;p11)	FUS–ATF1	Angiomatoid fibrous histiocytoma
t(12;16)(q13;p11)	FUS–DDIT3	Myxoid liposarcoma
t(12;22)(q13;q12)	EWSR1–ATF1	Angiomatoid fibrous histiocytoma
		Clear cell sarcoma of soft tissue
[t(12;22)(q13;q12)]*		Soft tissue myoepithelioma
t(12;22)(q13;q12)	EWSR1–DDIT3	Myxoid liposarcoma
t(17;22)(p13;q12–13)	MYH9–USP6	Nodular fasciitis
t(17;22)(q21;q13)	COL1A1–PDGFB	Dermatofibrosarcoma protuberans
		Giant cell fibroblastoma
		Bednar tumor
t(19;22)(q13;q12)	EWSR1–ZNF444	Soft tissue myoepithelioma
[t(X;1)(p11;p34)]*	SFPQ–TFE3	PEComa
t(X;2)(q13;q36)	PAX3–FOXO4	Alveolar rhabdomyosarcoma
t(X;6)(p11;p24)	RREB1–TFE3	Myofibroblastic sarcoma
t(X;11)(p11;q22)	YAP1–TFE3	Epithelioid hemangioendothelioma
t(X;17)(p11;q25)	ASPSCR1–TFE3	Alveolar soft part sarcoma
t(X;18)(p11;q11)	SS18–SSX1	Synovial sarcoma
	SS18–SSX2	
	SS18–SSX4	
t(X;20)(p11;q13)	SS18L1–SSX1	Synovial sarcoma

*Aberration inferred from molecular identification of a fusion gene, but not yet found at cytogenetic analysis.

when combined with clinicopathologic data. For most recurrent translocations, the affected genes in or near the breakpoints have been identified. Tumors studied in larger numbers typically display variant translocations with one gene recombining with two or more partners but most often in one dominating gene combination. Many numerical and partial chromosome imbalances are clearly nonrandom but are frequently shared by several tumor entities. At the other extreme are a set of tumors, primarily pleomorphic tumors, that are characterized by extensive karyotypic complexity and heterogeneity. The results of chromosome banding analysis of such tumors are often highly incomplete. Among all genes involved in fusions, *EWSR1* stands out; it recombines with several other genes in many different tumor entities (Fisher, 2014).

The prognostic impact of the genetic aberrations identified in soft tissue tumors is largely unknown. Although several reports have indicated associations between chromosome aberrations and clinical outcome, these findings are often not corroborated, and chromosome banding is too blunt for such purposes. Variation at the level of gene fusions does not only involve combinations of different genes but also different transcripts from the same gene fusion due to differences in precise breakpoint localization. Several studies have indicated an impact of different transcripts on prognosis, but the data are often contradictory.

Acknowledgment

We are grateful to Linda Magnusson for help with the figures.

References

Abbott JJ, Erickson-Johnson M, Wang X, Nascimento AG, Oliveira AM (2006): Gains of COL1A1-PDGFB genomic copies occur in fibrosarcomatous transformation of dermatofibrosarcoma protuberans. *Mod Pathol* 19:1512–1518.

Alaggio R, Rosolen A, Sartori F, Leszl A, d'Amore ESG, Bisogno G, et al. (2007): Spindle cell tumor with EWS-WT1 transcript and a favorable clinical course: a variant of DSCT, a variant of leiomyosarcoma, or a new entity? Report of 2 pediatric cases. *Am J Surg Pathol* 31:454–459.

Amary MFC, Berisha F, DelCarlo Bernardi F, Herbert A, James M, Reis-Filho JS, et al. (2007): Detection of SS18-SSX fusion transcripts in formalin-fixed paraffin-embedded neoplasms: analysis of conventional RT-PCR, qRT-PCR and dual color FISH as diagnostic tools for synovial sarcoma. *Mod Pathol* 20:482–496.

Antonescu CR, Tschernyavsky SJ, Decuseara R, Leung DH, Woodruff JM, Brennan MF, et al. (2001): Prognostic impact of P53 status, TLS-CHOP fusion transcript structure, and histological grade in myxoid liposarcoma: a molecular and clinicopathologic study of 82 cases. *Clin Cancer Res* 7:3977–3987.

Antonescu CR, Dal Cin P, Nafa K, Teot LA, Surti U, Fletcher CD, et al. (2007): EWSR1-CREB is the predominant gene fusion in angiomatoid fibrous histiocytoma. *Genes Chromosomes Cancer* 46:1051–1060.

Antonescu CR, Zhang L, Chang N-E, Pawel BR, Travis W, Katabi N, et al. (2010): EWSR1-POU5F1 fusion in soft tissue myoepithelial tumors. A molecular analysis of sixty-six cases, including soft tissue, bone, and visceral lesions, showing common involvement of the EWSR1 gene. *Genes Chromosomes Cancer* 49:1114–1124.

Antonescu CR, Zhang L, Nielsen GP, Rosenberg AE, Dal Cin P, Fletcher CDM (2011): Consistent t(1;10) with rearrangements of TGFBR3 and MGEA5 in both myxoinflammatory fibroblastic sarcoma and hemosiderotic fibrolipomatous tumor. *Genes Chromosomes Cancer* 50:757–764.

Antonescu CR, Zhang L, Shao SY, Mosquera J-M, Weinreb I, Katabi N, et al. (2013a): Frequent PLAG1 gene rearrangements in skin and soft tissue myoepithelioma with ductal differentiation. *Genes Chromosomes Cancer* 52:675–682.

Antonescu CR, Le Loarer F, Mosquera J-M, Sboner A, Zhang L, Chen C-L, et al. (2013b): Novel YAP1-TFE3 fusion defines a distinct subset of epithelioid hemangioendothelioma. *Genes Chromosomes Cancer* 52:775–784.

Antonescu CR, Sung Y-S, Chen C-L, Zhang L, Chen H-W, Singer S, et al. (2014): Novel ZC3H7B-BCOR, MEAF6-PHF1, and EPC1-PHF1 fusion in ossifying fibromyxoid tumors – molecular characterization shows genetic overlap with endometrial stromal sarcoma. *Genes Chromosomes Cancer* 53:183–193.

Arbajian E, Magnusson L, Mertens F, Domanski HA, Vult von Steyern F, Nord KH (2013): A novel GTF2I/NCOA2 fusion gene emphasizes the role of NCOA2 in soft tissue angiofibroma development. *Genes Chromosomes Cancer* 52:330–331.

Arbajian E, Puls F, Magnusson L, Thway K, Fisher C, Sumathi PV, et al. (2014): Recurrent EWSR1-CREB3L1 gene fusion in sclerosing epithelioid fibrosarcoma. *Am J Surg Pathol* 38:801–808.

Argani P, Aulmann S, Illei PB, Netto GJ, Ro J, Cho H, et al. (2010): A distinctive subset of PEComas harbors TFE3 gene fusions. *Am J Surg Pathol* 34:1395–1406.

Arlotta P, Tai AK-F Manfioletti G, Clifford C, Jay G, Ono SJ (2000): Transgenic mice expressing a truncated form of the high mobility group I-C protein develop adiposity and an abnormally high prevalence of lipomas. *J Biol Chem* 275:14394–14400.

Ashar HR, Schoenberg Fejzo M, Tkachenko A, Zhou X, Fletcher JA, Weremowicz S, et al. (1995): Disruption of the architectural factor HMGI-C: DNA-binding AT hook motifs fused in lipomas to distinct transcriptional regulatory domains. *Cell* 82:57–65.

Aulmann S, Longerich T, Schirmacher P, Mechtersheimer G, Penzel R (2007): Detection of the ASPSCR1-TFE3 gene fusion in paraffin-embedded alveolar soft part sarcomas. *Histopathology* 50:881–886.

Barr FG (2001): Gene fusions involving PAX and FOX family members in alveolar rhabdomyosarcoma. *Oncogene* 20:5736–5746.

Barr FG, Qualman SJ, Macris MH, Melnyk N, Lawlor ER, Strzelecki DM, et al. (2002): Genetic heterogeneity in the alveolar rhabdomyosarcoma subset without typical gene fusions. *Cancer Res* 62:4704–4710.

Bartuma H, Hallor KH, Panagopoulos I, Collin A, Rydholm A, Gustafson P, et al. (2007): Assessment of the clinical and molecular impact of different cytogenetic subgroups in a series of 272 lipomas with abnormal karyotype. *Genes Chromosomes Cancer* 46:594–606.

Bartuma H, Nord KH, Macchia G, Isaksson M, Nilsson J, Domanski HA, et al. (2011): Gene expression and single nucleotide polymorphism array analyses of spindle cell lipomas and conventional lipomas with 13q14 deletion. *Genes Chromosomes Cancer* 50:619–632.

Baumhoer D, Gunawan B, Becker H, Füzesi L (2005): Comparative genomic hybridization in four angiosarcomas of the breast. *Gynecol Oncol* 97:348–352.

Berner J-M, Forus A, Elkahloun A, Meltzer PS, Fodstad Ö, Myklebost O (1996): Separate amplified regions encompassing CDK4 and MDM2 in human sarcomas. *Genes Chromosomes Cancer* 17:254–259.

Bianchini L, Birtwisle L, Saada E, Bazin A, Long E, Roussel JE, et al. (2013): Identification of PPAP2B as a novel recurrent translocation partner gene of HMGA2 in lipomas. *Genes Chromosomes Cancer* 52:580–590.

Bode-Lesniewska B, Frigerio S, Exner U, Abdou MT, Moch H, Zimmerman DR (2007): Relevance of translocation type in myxoid liposarcoma and identification of a novel EWSR1-DDIT3 fusion. *Genes Chromosomes Cancer* 46:961–971.

Brandal P, Micci F, Bjerkehagen B, Eknäs M, Larramendy M, Lothe RA, et al. (2003): Molecular cytogenetic characterization of desmoid tumors. *Cancer Genet Cytogenet* 146:1–7.

Brandal P, Panagopoulos I, Bjerkehagen B, Gorunova L, Skjeldal S, Micci F, et al. (2008): Detection of a t(1;22) (q23;q12) translocation leading to an EWSR1-PBX1 fusion gene in a myoepithelioma. *Genes Chromosomes Cancer* 47:558–564.

Brandal P, Panagopoulos I, Bjerkehagen B, Heim S (2009): t(19;22)(q13;q12) translocation leading to the novel fusion gene EWSR1-ZNF444 in soft tissue myoepithelial carcinoma. *Genes Chromosomes Cancer* 48:1051–1056.

Bridge JA, Liu J, Qualman SJ, Suijkerbuijk R, Wenger G, Zhang J, et al. (2002): Genomic gains and losses are similar in genetic and histologic subsets of rhabdomyosarcoma, whereas amplification predominates in embryonal with anaplasia and alveolar subtypes. *Genes Chromosomes Cancer* 33:310–321.

Broberg K, Zhang M, Strömbeck B, Isaksson M, Nilsson M, Mertens F, et al. (2002): Fusion of RDC1 with HMGA2 in lipomas as the result of chromosome aberrations involving 2q35–37 and 12q13–15. *Int J Oncol* 21:321–326.

Chang A, Schuetze SM, Conrad EU III, Swisshelm KL, Norwood TH, Rubin BP (2005): So-called "inflammatory leiomyosarcoma": a series of 3 cases providing additional insights into a rare entity. *Int J Surg Pathol* 13:185–195.

Chibon F, Mariani O, Derré J, Malinge S, Coindre J-M, Guillou L, et al. (2002): A subgroup of malignant fibrous histiocytomas is associated with genetic changes similar to those of well-differentiated liposarcomas. *Cancer Genet Cytogenet* 139:24–29.

Chmielecki J, Crago AM, Rosenberg M, O'Connor R, Walker SR, Ambrogio L, et al. (2013): Whole-exome sequencing identifies a recurrent NAB2-STAT6 fusion in solitary fibrous tumors. *Nat Genet* 45:131–132.

Choi EY, Thomas DG, McHugh JB, Patel RM, Roulston D, Schuetze SM, et al. (2013): Undifferentiated small round cell sarcoma with t(4;19)(q35;q13.1) CIC-DUX4 fusion: a novel highly aggressive soft tissue tumor with distinctive histopathology. *Am J Surg Pathol* 37:1379–1386.

Coffin CM, Davis JL, Borinstein SC (2014): Syndrome-associated soft tissue tumours. *Histopathology* 64:68–87.

Coindre J-M, Hostein I, Maire G, Derré J, Guillou L, Leroux A, et al. (2004): Inflammatory malignant fibrous histiocytomas and dedifferentiated liposarcomas: histological review, genomic profile, and MDM2 and CDK4 status favour a single entity. *J Pathol* 203:822–830.

Coindre J-M, Pedeutour F, Aurias A (2010): Well-differentiated and dedifferentiated liposarcomas. *Virchows Arch* 456:167–179.

Crombez KRMO, Vanoirbeek EMR, Van de Ven WJM, Petit MMR (2005): Transactivation functions of the tumor-specific HMGA2/LPP fusion protein are augmented by wild-type HMGA2. *Mol Cancer Res* 3:63–70.

Crozat A, Åman P, Mandahl N, Ron D (1993): Fusion of CHOP to a novel RNA-binding protein in human myxoid liposarcoma. *Nature* 363:640–644.

Cupp JS, Miller MA, Montgomery KD, Nielsen TO, O'Connell JX, Huntsman D, et al. (2007): Translocation and expression of CSF1 in pigmented villonodular synovitis, tenosynovial giant cell tumor, rheumatoid arthritis and other reactive synovitides. *Am J Surg Pathol* 31:970–976.

Dahlén A, Debiec-Rychter M, Pedeutour F, Domanski HA, Höglund M, Bauer HCF, et al. (2003): Clustering of deletions on chromosome 13 in benign and low-malignant lipomatous tumors. *Int J Cancer* 103:616–623.

Dahlén A, Fletcher CDM, Mertens F, Fletcher JA, Perez-Atayde AR, Hicks MJ, et al. (2004): Activation of the GLI oncogene through fusion with the β-actin gene (ACTB) in a group of distinctive pericytic neoplasms. Pericytoma with t(7;12). *Am J Pathol* 164:1645–1653.

Davicioni E, Finckenstein FG, Shahbazian V, Buckley JD, Triche TJ, Anderson MJ (2006): Identification of a PAX-FKHR gene expression signature that defines molecular classes and determines the prognosis of alveolar rhabdomyosarcomas. *Cancer Res* 66:6936–6946.

DeCecco L, Gariboldi M, Reid JF, Lagonigro MS, Tamborini E, Albertini V, et al. (2005): Gene expression profile identifies a rare epithelioid variant case of pleomorphic liposarcoma carrying FUS-CHOP transcript. *Histopathology* 46:334–341.

Deen M, Ebrahim S, Schloff D, Mohamed AN (2013): A novel PLAG1-RAD51L1 gene fusion resulting from a t(8;14)(q12;q24) in a case of lipoblastoma. *Cancer Genet,*206:233–237.

Dei Tos AP, Marino-Enriquez A, Pedeutour F, Rossi S (2013): Dedifferentiated liposarcoma. In: Fletcher CDM, Bridge JA, Hogendoorn PCW, Mertens F, editors. *WHO Classification of Tumours of Soft Tissue and Bone.* IARC: Lyon, pp. 37–38.

Demicco EG, Torres KE, Ghadimi M, Colombo C, Bolshakov S, Hoffman A, et al. (2012): Involvement of the PI3K/Akt pathway in myxoid/round cell liposarcoma. *Mod Pathol* 25:212–221.

De Wever I, Dal Cin P, Fletcher CDM, Mandahl N, Mertens F, Mitelman F, et al. (2000): Cytogenetic, clinical, and morphologic correlations in 78 cases of fibromatosis: a report from the CHAMP study group. *Mod Pathol* 13:1080–1085.

Doyle LA, Wang W, Dal Cin P, Lopez-Terrada D, Mertens F, Lazar AJ, et al. (2012): MUC4 is a sensitive and extremely useful marker for sclerosing epithelioid fibrosarcoma: association with FUS gene rearrangement. *Am J Surg Pathol* 36:1444–1451.

Duan F, Smith LM, Gustafson DM, Zhang C, Dunlevy MJ, Gastier-Foster JM, et al. (2012): Genomic and clinical analysis of fusion gene amplification in rhabdomyosarcoma: a report from the Children's Oncology Group. *Genes Chromosomes Cancer* 51:662–674.

Endo M, Kohashi K, Yamamoto H, Ishii T, Yoshida T, Matsunobu T, et al. (2013): Ossifying fibromyxoid tumor presenting EP400-PHF1 fusion gene. *Hum Pathol* 44:2603–2608.

Erickson-Johnson MR, Chou MM, Evers BR, Roth CW, Seys AR, Jin L, et al. (2011): Nodular fasciitis: a novel model of transient neoplasia induced by MYH9-USP6 gene fusion. *Lab Invest* 91:1427–1433.

Errani C, Zhang L, Sung YS, Hajdu M, Singer S, Maki RG, et al. (2011): A novel WWTR1-CAMTA1 gene fusion is a consistent abnormality in epithelioid hemangioendothelioma of different anatomic sites. *Genes Chromosomes Cancer* 50:644–653.

Fisher C (2014): The diversity of soft tissue tumours with EWSR1 gene rearrangements. *Histopathology* 64:134–150.

Fletcher JA, Naeem R, Xiao S, Corson JM (1995): Chromosome aberrations in desmoid tumors. Trisomy 8 may be a predictor of recurrence. *Cancer Genet Cytogenet* 79:139–143.

Fletcher CDM, Bridge JA, Hogendoorn PCW, Mertens F, editors (2013a): *WHO Classification of Tumours of Soft Tissue and Bone.* IARC: Lyon.

Fletcher CDM, Bridge JA, Lee J-C (2013b): Extrapleural solitary fibrous tumour. In: Fletcher CDM, Bridge JA, Hogendoorn PCW, Mertens F, editors. *WHO Classification of Tumours of Soft Tissue and Bone.* IARC: Lyon, pp. 80–82.

Fletcher CDM, Chibon F, Mertens F (2013c): Undifferentiated/ unclassified sarcomas. In: Fletcher CDM, Bridge JA, Hogendoorn PCW, Mertens F, editors. *WHO Classification of Tumours of Soft Tissue and Bone.* IARC: Lyon, pp. 236–238.

Flucke U, Mentzel T, Verdijk MA, Slootweg PJ, Creytens DH, Suurmeijer AJH, et al. (2012): EWSR1-ATF1 chimeric transcript in a myoepithelial tumor of soft tissue: a case report. *Hum Pathol* 43:764–768.

Flucke U, Tops BB, de Saint Aubin Somerhausen N, Bras J, Creytens DH, Küsters B, et al. (2013): Presence of C11orf95-MKL2 fusion is a consistent finding in chondroid lipomas: a study of eight cases. *Histopathology* 62:925–930.

Folpe AL, Deyrup AT (2006): Alveolar soft-part sarcoma: a review and update. *J Clin Pathol* 59:1127–1132.

Gebre-Medhin S, Nord KH, Möller E, Mandahl N, Magnusson L, Nilsson J, et al. (2012): Recurrent rearrangement of the PHF1 gene in ossifying fibromyxoid tumors. *Am J Pathol* 181:1069–1077.

Gerald WL, Haber DA (2005): The EWS-WT1 gene fusion in desmoplastic small round cell tumor. *Semin Cancer Biol* 15:197–205.

Gisselsson D, Höglund M, Mertens F, Mitelman F, Mandahl N (1998): Chromosomal organization of amplified chromosome 12 sequences in mesenchymal tumors detected by fluorescence in situ hybridization. *Genes Chromosomes Cancer* 23:203–212.

Gisselsson D, Höglund M, Mertens F, Dal Cin P, Mandahl N (1999): Hibernomas are characterized by homozygous deletions in the multiple endocrine neoplasia type I region. Metaphase fluorescence in situ hybridization reveals complex rearrangements not detected by conventional cytogenetics. *Am J Pathol* 155:61–66.

Gisselsson D, Hibbard MK, Dal Cin P, Sciot R, Hsi B-L, Kozakewich HP, et al. (2001): PLAG1 alterations in lipoblastoma. Involvement in varied mesenchymal cell types and evidence for alternative oncogenic mechanisms. *Am J Pathol* 159:955–962.

Gordon T, McManus A, Anderson J, Min T, Swansbury J, Pritchard-Jones K, et al. (2001): Cytogenetic abnormalities in 42 rhabdomyosarcoma: a United Kingdom cancer cytogenetics group study. *Med Pediatr Oncol* 36:259–267.

Graham RP, Weiss SW, Sukov WR, Goldblum JR, Billings SD, Dotlic S, et al. (2013): PHF1 rearrangements in ossifying fibromyxoid tumors of soft parts: a fluorescence in situ hybridization study of 41 cases with emphasis on the malignant variant. *Am J Surg Pathol* 37:1751–1755.

Guillou L, Benhattar J, Binichon F, Gallagher G, Terrier P, Stauffer E, et al. (2004): Histologic grade, but not SYT-SSX fusion type, is an important prognostic factor in patients with synovial sarcoma: a multicenter, retrospective analysis. *J Clin Oncol* 22:4040–4050.

Guillou L, Benhattar J, Gengler C, Gallagher G, Ranchere-Vince D, Collin F, et al. (2007): Translocation-positive low-grade fibromyxoid sarcoma: clinicopathologic and molecular analysis of a series expanding the morphologic spectrum and suggesting potential relationship to sclerosing epithelioid fibrosarcoma. A study from the French sarcoma group. *Am J Surg Pathol* 31:1387–1402.

Hallor KH, Micci F, Meis-Kindblom JM, Kindblom L-G, Bacchini P, Mandahl N, et al. (2007): Fusion genes in angiomatoid fibrous histiocytoma. *Cancer Lett* 251:158–163.

Hallor KH, Teixeira MR, Fletcher CDM, Bizarro S, Staaf J, Domanski HA, et al. (2008): Heterogeneous genetic profiles in soft tissue myoepitheliomas. *Mod Pathol* 21:1311–1319.

Hallor KH, Sciot R, Staaf J, Heidenblad M, Rydholm A, Bauer HCF, et al. (2009): Two genetic pathways, t(1;10) and amplification of 3p11–12, in myxoinflammatory fibroblastic sarcoma, hemosiderotic fibrolipomatous tumor and morphologically similar lesions. *J Pathol* 217:716–727.

Heidenblad M, Hallor KH, Staaf J, Jönsson G, Borg Å, Höglund M, et al. (2006): Genomic profiling of bone and soft tissue tumors with supernumerary ring chromosomes using tiling resolution bacterial artificial chromosome microarrays. *Oncogene* 25:7106–7116.

Hibbard MK, Kozakewich HP, Dal Cin P, Sciot R, Tan X, Xiao S, et al. (2000): PLAG1 fusion oncogenes in lipoblastoma. *Cancer Res* 60:4869–4872.

Hisaoka M, Hashimoto H (2005): Extraskeletal myxoid chondrosarcoma: updated clinicopathological and molecular genetic characteristics. *Pathol Int* 55:453–463.

Hodge JC, Pearce KE, Wang X, Oliveira AM, Greipp PT (2014): Molecular cytogenetic analysis for TFE3 rearrangement in Xp11.2 renal cell carcinoma and alveolar soft part sarcoma: validation and clinical experience with 75 cases. *Mod Pathol* 27:113–127.

Hostein I, Pelmus M, Aurias A, Pedeutour F, Matahoulin-Pélissier S, Coindre JM (2004): Evaluation of MDM2 and CDK4 amplification by real-time PCR on paraffin wax-embedded material: a potential tool for the diagnosis of atypical lipomatous tumours/well-differentiated liposarcomas. *J Pathol* 202:95–102.

Hu J, Rao UNM, Jasani S, Khanna V, Yaw K, Surti U (2005): Loss of DNA copy number of 10q is associated with aggressive behavior of leiomyosarcomas: a comparative genomic hybridization study. *Cancer Genet Cytogenet* 161:20–27.

Huang H-Y, Lui MY, Ladanyi M (2005): Nonrandom cell-cycle timing of a somatic chromosomal translocation: the t(X;17) of alveolar soft part sarcoma occurs in G2. *Genes Chromosomes Cancer* 44:170–176.

Huang D, Sumegi J, Dal Cin P, Reith JD, Yasuda T, Nelson M, et al. (2010): C11orf95-MKL2 is the resulting fusion oncogene of t(11;16)(q13;p13) in chondroid lipoma. *Genes Chromosomes Cancer* 49:810–818.

Idbaih A, Coindre J-M, Derré J, Mariani O, Terrier P, Ranchère D, et al. (2005): Myxoid malignant fibrous histiocytoma and pleomorphic liposarcoma share very similar genomic imbalances. *Lab Invest* 85:176–181.

Italiano A, Bianchini L, Keslair F, Bonnafous S, Cardot-Leccia N, Coindre J-M, et al. (2008): HMGA2 is the partner of MDM2 in well-differentiated liposarcomas whereas CDK4 belongs to a distinct inconsistent amplicon. *Int J Cancer* 122:2233–2241.

Italiano A, Sung YS, Zhang L, Singer S, Maki RG, Coindre J-M, et al. (2012): High prevalence of CIC fusion with double-homeobox (DUX4) transcription factors in EWSR1-negative undifferentiated small blue round cell sarcomas. *Genes Chromosomes Cancer* 51:207–218.

Jin Y, Möller E, Nord KH, Mandahl N, Vult von Steyern F, Domanski HA, et al. (2012): Fusion of the AHRR and NCOA2 genes through a recurrent translocation t(5;8) (p15;q13) in soft tissue angiofibroma results in upregulation of aryl hydrocarbon receptor target genes. *Genes Chromosomes Cancer* 51:510–520.

Killela PJ, Reitman ZJ, Jiao Y, Bettegowda C, Agrawal N, Diaz Jr LA, et al. (2013): TERT promoter mutations occur frequently in gliomas and a subset of tumors derived from cells with low rates of self-renewal. *Proc Natl Acad Sci USA* 110:6021–6026.

Kiuru-Kuhlefelt S, El-Rifai W, Fanburg-Smith J, Kere J, Miettinen M, Knuutila S (2001): Concomitant DNA copy number amplification at 17q and 22q in dermatofibrosarcoma protuberans. *Cytogenet Cell Genet* 92:192–195.

Knezevich SR, McFadden DE, Tao W, Lim JF, Sorensen PHB (1998): A novel ETV6-NTRK3 gene fusion in congenital fibrosarcoma. *Nat Genet* 18:184–187.

Kouho H, Aoki T, Hisaoka M, Hashimoto H (1997): Clinicopathological and interphase cytogenetic analysis of desmoid tumors. *Histopathology* 31:336–341.

Ladanyi M, Lui MY, Antonescu CR, Krause-Boehm A, Meindl A, Argani P, et al. (2001): The der(17)t(X;17) (p11;q25) of human alveolar soft part sarcoma fuses the TFE3 transcription factor gene to ASPL, a novel gene at 17q25. *Oncogene* 20:48–57.

Ladanyi M, Antonescu CR, Leung DH, Woodruff JM, Kawai A, Healey JH, et al. (2002): Impact of SYT-SSX fusion type on the clinical behavior of synovial sarcoma: a multi-institutional retrospective study of 243 patients. *Cancer Res* 62:135–140.

Lae ME, Roche PC, Jin L, Lloyd RV, Nascimento AG (2002): Desmoplastic small round cell tumor. a clinicopathologic, immunohistochemical, and molecular study of 32 tumors. *Am J Surg Pathol* 26:823–835.

Lae M, Ahn EH, Mercado GE, Chuai S, Edgar M, Pawel BR, et al. (2007): Global gene expression profiling of PAX-FKHR fusion-positive alveolar and PAX-FKHR fusion-negative embryonal rhabdomyosarcomas. *J Pathol* 212:143–151.

Larramendy ML, Virolainen M, Tukiainen E, Elomaa I, Knuutila S (1998): Chromosome band 1q21 is recurrently gained in desmoid tumors. *Genes Chromosomes Cancer* 23:183–186.

Larramendy ML, Kaur S, Svarvar C, Böhling T, Knuutila S (2006): Gene copy number profiling of soft-tissue leiomyosarcomas by array-comparative genomic hybridization. *Cancer Genet Cytogenet* 169:94–101.

Lau PPL, Lui PCW, Lau GTC, Yau DTW, Cheung ETY, Chan JKC (2013): EWSR1-CREB3L1 gene fusion: a novel alternative molecular aberration of low-grade fibromyxoid sarcoma. *Am J Surg Pathol* 37:734–738.

Lazar A, Evans HL, Shipley J (2013): Leiomyosarcoma. In: Fletcher CDM, Bridge JA, Hogendoorn PCW, Mertens F, editors. *WHO Classification of Tumours of Soft Tissue and Bone*. IARC: Lyon, pp. 111–113.

Lee YS, Dutta A (2007): The tumor suppressor microRNA let-7 represses the HMGA2 oncogene. *Genes Dev* 21:1025–1030.

Li X-Q, Hisaoka M, Shi D-R, Zhu X-Z, Hashimoto H (2004): Expression of anaplastic lymphoma kinase in soft tissue tumors: an immunohistochemical and molecular study of 249 cases. *Hum Pathol* 35:711–721.

Ligon AH, Moore SDP, Parisi MA, Mealiffe ME, Harris DJ, Ferguson HL, et al. (2005): Constitutional rearrangement of the architectural factor HMGA2: a novel human phenotype including overgrowth and lipomas. *Am J Hum Genet* 76:340–348.

Liu J, Guzman MA, Pezanowski D, Patel D, Hauptman J, Keisling M, et al. (2011): FOXO1-FGFR1 fusion and amplification in a solid variant of alveolar rhabdomyosarcoma. *Mod Pathol* 24:1327–1335.

Limon J, Mrozek K, Mandahl N, Nedoszytko B, Verhest A, Rys J, et al. (1991): Cytogenetics of synovial sarcoma: presentation of ten new cases and review of the literature. *Genes Chromosomes Cancer* 3:338–345.

Lualdi E, Modena P, Debiec-Rychter M, Pedeutour F, Teixeira MT, Facchinetti F, et al. (2004): Molecular cytogenetic characterization of proximal-type epithelioid sarcoma. *Genes Chromosomes Cancer* 41:283–290.

Macchia G, Trombetta D, Möller E, Mertens F, Storlazzi CT, Debiec-Rychter M, et al. (2012): *FOSL1* as a candidate target gene for 11q12 rearrangements in desmoplastic fibroblastoma. *Lab Invest* 92:735–743.

Machado I, Cruz J, Lavernia J, Rubio L, Campos J, Barrios M, et al. (2013): Superficial EWSR1-negative undifferentiated small round cell sarcoma with CIC/DUX4 gene fusion: a new variant of Ewing-like tumors with locoregional lymph node metastasis. *Virchows Arch* 463:837–842.

Maire G, Forus A, Foa C, Bjerkehagen B, Mainguené C, Kresse SH, et al. (2003): 11q13 alterations in two cases of hibernoma: large heterozygous deletions and rearrangement breakpoints near GARP in 11q13.5. *Genes Chromosomes Cancer* 37:389–395.

Mandahl N, Heim S, Willén H, Rydholm A, Mitelman F (1990): Supernumerary ring chromosome as the sole cytogenetic abnormality in a dermatofibrosarcoma protuberans. *Cancer Genet Cytogenet* 49:273–275.

Mandahl N, Höglund M, Mertens F, Rydholm A, Willén H, Brosjö O, et al. (1994): Cytogenetic aberrations in 188 benign and borderline adipose tissue tumors. *Genes Chromosomes Cancer* 9:207–215.

Mandahl N, Limon J, Mertens F, Nedoszytko B, Gibas Z, Denis A, et al. (1995): Nonrandom secondary chromosome aberrations in synovial sarcomas with t(X;18). *Int J Oncol* 7:495–499.

Mandahl N, Mertens F, Willén H, Rydholm A, Kreicbergs A, Mitelman F (1998): Nonrandom pattern of telomeric associations in atypical lipomatous tumors with ring and giant marker chromosomes. *Cancer Genet Cytogenet* 103:25–34.

Mandahl N, Fletcher CDM, Dal Cin P, De Wever I, Mertens F, Mitelman F, et al. (2000): Comparative cytogenetic study of spindle cell and pleomorphic leiomyosarcomas of soft tissues: a report from the CHAMP study group. *Cancer Genet Cytogenet* 116:66–73.

Matsuyama A, Hisaoka M, Shimajiri S, Hayashi T, Imamura T, Ishida T, et al. (2006): Molecular detection of FUS-CREB3L2 fusion transcripts in low-grade fibromyxoid sarcoma using formalin-fixed, paraffin-embedded tissue specimens. *Am J Surg Pathol* 30:1077–1084.

McComb EN, Feely MG, Neff JR, Johansson SL, Nelson M, Bridge JA (2001): Cytogenetic instability, predominantly involving chromosome 1, is characteristic of elastofibroma. *Cancer Genet Cytogenet* 126:68–72.

McPherson A, Hormozdiari F, Zayed A, Giuliany R, Ha G, Sun MGF, et al. (2011): defuse: an algorithm for gene fusion discovery in tumor RNA-seq data. *PLoS Comput Biol* 7:e1001138.

Mendlick MR, Nelson M, Pickering D, Johansson SL, Seemayer TA, Neff JR, et al. (2001): Translocation t(1;3) (p36.3;q25) is a nonrandom aberration in epithelioid hemangioendothelioma. *Am J Surg Pathol* 25:684–687.

Mertens F, Fletcher CDM, Dal Cin P, De Wever I, Mandahl N, Mitelman F, et al. (1998): Cytogenetic analysis of 46 pleomorphic soft tissue sarcomas and correlation with morphologic and clinical features: a report of the CHAMP study group. *Genes Chromosomes Cancer* 22:16–25.

Mertens F, Fletcher CDM, Antonescu CR, Coindre J-M, Colecchia M, Domanski HA, et al. (2005): Clinicopathologic and molecular genetic characterization of low-grade fibromyxoid sarcoma, and cloning of a novel FUS/CREB3L1 fusion gene. *Lab Invest* 85:408–415.

Meza-Zepeda LA, Forus A, Lygren B, Dahlberg AB, Godager LH, South AP, et al. (2002): Positional cloning identifies a novel cyclophilin as a candidate amplified oncogene in 1q21. *Oncogene* 21:2261–2269.

Meza-Zepeda LA, Kresse SH, Barragan-Polania AH, Bjerkehagen B, Ohnstad HO, Namlös HM, et al. (2006): Array comparative genomic hybridization reveals distinct DNA copy number differences between gastrointestinal stromal tumors and leiomyosarcomas. *Cancer Res* 66: 8984–8993.

Micci F, Teixeira MR, Bjerkehagen B, Heim S (2002): Characterization of supernumerary rings and giant marker chromosomes in well-differentiated lipomatous tumors by a combination of G-banding, CGH, M-FISH, and chromosome- and locus-specific FISH. *Cytogenet Genome Res* 97:13–19.

Mitelman F, Johansson B, Mertens F, editors (2014): Mitelman Database of Chromosome Aberrations and Gene Fusions in Cancer. Available at http://cgap.nci.nih.gov/Chromosomes/Mitelman.

Modena P, Lualdi E, Facchinetti F, Galli L, Teixeira MR, Pilotti S, et al. (2005): SMARCB1/INI1 tumor suppressor gene is frequently inactivated in epithelioid sarcomas. *Cancer Res* 65:4012–4019.

Mohajeri A, Tayebwa J, Collin A, Nilsson J, Magnusson L, Vult von Steyern F, et al. (2013): Comprehensive genetic analysis identifies a pathognomonic NAB2/STAT6 fusion gene, nonrandom secondary genomic imbalances, and a characteristic gene expression profile in solitary fibrous tumor. *Genes Chromosomes Cancer* 52:873–886.

Möller E, Mandahl N, Mertens F, Panagopoulos I (2008): Molecular identification of COL6A3-CSF1 fusion transcripts in tenosynovial giant cell tumors. *Genes Chromosomes Cancer* 47:21–25.

Mosquera J-M, Sboner A, Zhang L, Chen C-L, Sung Y-S, Chen H-W, et al. (2013a): Novel MIR143-NOTCH fusions in benign and malignant glomus tumors. *Genes Chromosomes Cancer* 52:1075–1087.

Mosquera JM, Sboner A, Zhang L, Kitabayashi N, Chen C-L, Sung YS, et al. (2013b): Recurrent NCOA2 gene rearrangements in congenital/infantile spindle cell rhabdomyosarcoma. *Genes Chromosomes Cancer* 52:538–550.

Murphy AJ, Bishop K, Pereira C, Chilton-MacNeill S, Ho M, Zielenska M, et al. (2008): A new molecular variant of desmoplastic small round cell tumor: significance of WT1 immunostaining in this entity. *Hum Pathol* 39:1763–1770.

Nakagawa Y, Numoto K, Yoshida A, Kunisada T, Ohata H, Takeda K, et al. (2006): Chromosomal and genetic imbalances in synovial sarcoma detected by conventional and microarray comparative genomic hybridization. *J Cancer Res Clin Oncol* 132:444–450.

Nilsson M, Meza-Zepeda LA, Mertens F, Forus A, Myklebost O, Mandahl N (2004): Amplification of chromosome 1 sequences in lipomatous tumors and other sarcomas. *Int J Cancer* 109:363–369.

Nilsson M, Panagopoulos I, Mertens F, Mandahl N (2005): Fusion of the HMGA2 and NFIB genes in lipoma. *Virchows Arch* 447:855–858.

Nilsson M, Mertens F, Höglund M, Mandahl N, Panagopoulos I (2006): Truncation and fusion of HMGA2 in lipomas with rearrangements of 5q32-q33 and 12q14-q15. *Cytogenet Genome Res* 112:60–66.

Nishio J (2011): Contributions of cytogenetics and molecular cytogenetics to the diagnosis of adipocytic tumors. *J Biomed Biotechnol* 2011:524067.

Nishio J, Iwasaki H, Ohjimi Y, Ishiguro M, Kobayashi K, Nabeshima K, et al. (2004): Chromosomal imbalances in angioleiomyomas by comparative genomic hybridization. *Int J Mol Med* 13:13–16.

Nishio J, Althof PA, Bailey JM, Zhou M, Neff JR, Barr FG, et al. (2006): Use of a novel FISH assay on paraffin-embedded tissues as an adjunct to diagnosis of alveolar rhabdomyosarcoma. *Lab Invest* 86:547–556.

Nord KH, Magnusson L, Isaksson M, Nilsson J, Lilljebjörn H, Domanski HA, et al. (2010): Concomitant deletion of suppressor genes MEN1 and AIP are essential for the pathogenesis of the brown fat tumor hibernoma. *Proc Natl Acad Sci USA* 107:21122–21127.

Nord KH, Paulsson K, Veerla S, Wejde J, Brosjö O, Mandahl N, et al. (2012): Retained heterodisomy is associated with high gene expression in hyperhaploid inflammatory leiomyosarcoma. *Neoplasia* 14:807–812.

O'Brien KP, Seroussi E, Dal Cin P, Sciot R, Mandahl N, Fletcher JA, et al. (1998): Various regions within the alpha-helical domain of the COL1A1 gene are fused to the second exon of the PDGFB gene in dermatofibrosarcomas and giant-cell fibroblastomas. *Genes Chromosomes Cancer* 23:187–193.

Ohguri T, Hisaoka M, Kawauchi S, Sasaki K, Aoki T, Kanemitsu S, et al. (2006): Cytogenetic analysis of myxoid liposarcoma and myxofibrosarcoma by array-based comparative genomic hybridisation. *J Clin Pathol* 59:978–983.

Panagopoulos I, Höglund M, Mertens F, Mandahl N, Mitelman F, Åman P (1996): Fusion of the EWS and CHOP genes in myxoid liposarcoma. *Oncogene* 12:489–494.

Panagopoulos I, Mertens F, Isaksson M, Mandahl N (2000): A novel FUS/CHOP chimera in myxoid liposarcoma. *Biochem Biophys Res Commun* 279:838–845.

Panagopoulos I, Mertens F, Isaksson M, Limon J, Gustafson P, Skytting B, et al. (2001): Clinical impact of molecular and cytogenetic findings in synovial sarcoma. *Genes Chromosomes Cancer* 31:362–372.

Panagopoulos I, Mertens F, Debiec-Rychter M, Isaksson M, Limon J, Kardas I, et al. (2002a): Molecular genetic characterization of the EWS/ATF1 fusion gene in clear cell sarcoma of the tendons and aponeuroses. *Int J Cancer* 99:560–567.

Panagopoulos I, Mertens F, Isaksson M, Domanski HA, Brosjö O, Heim S, et al. (2002b): Molecular genetic characterization of the EWS/CHN and RBP56/CHN fusion genes in extraskeletal myxoid chondrosarcoma. *Genes Chromosomes Cancer* 35:340–352.

Panagopoulos I, Storlazzi CT, Fletcher CDM, Fletcher JA, Nascimento A, Domanski HA, et al. (2004): The chimeric FUS/CREB3L2 gene is specific for low-grade fibromyxoid sarcoma. *Genes Chromosomes Cancer* 40:218–228.

Pedeutour F, Coindre J-M, Sozzi G, Nicolo G, Leroux A, Toma S, et al. (1994): Supernumerary ring chromosomes containing chromosome 17 sequences. A specific feature of dermatofibrosarcoma protuberans? *Cancer Genet Cytogenet* 76:1–9.

Pedeutour F, Deville A, Steyaert H, Ranchere-Vince D, Ambrosetti D, Sirvent N (2012): Rearrangement of HMGA2 in a case of infantile lipoblastomas without Plag1 alteration. *Pediatr Blood Cancer* 58:798–800.

Petit MMR, Mols R, Schoenmakers EFPM, Mandahl N, Van de Ven WJM (1996): LPP, the preferred fusion partner gene of HMGIC in lipomas, is a novel member of the LIM protein gene family. *Genomics* 36:118–129.

Petit MMR, Schoenmakers EFPM, Huysmans C, Geurts JMW, Mandahl N, Van de Ven WJM (1999): LHFP, a novel translocation partner gene of HMGIC in a lipoma, is a member of a new family of LHFP-like genes. *Genomics* 57:438–441.

Plaszczyca A, Nilsson J, Magnusson L, Brosjö O, Larsson O, Vult von Steyern F, et al. (2014): Fusion involving protein kinase C and membrane-associated proteins in benign fibrous histiocytoma. *Int J Biochem Cell Biol* 53:475–81.

Przybyl J, Sciot R, Rutkowski P, Siedlecki JA, Vanspauwen V, Samson I, et al. (2012): Recurrent and novel SS18-SSX fusion transcripts in synovial sarcoma: description of three new cases. *Tumor Biol* 33:2245–2253.

Rabbitts TH, Forster A, Larson R, Nathan P (1993): Fusion of the dominant negative transcription regulator CHOP with a novel gene FUS by translocation t(12;16) in malignant liposarcoma. *Nat Genet* 4:175–180.

Rawlinson NJ, West WW, Nelson M, Bridge JA (2008): Aggressive angiomyxoma with t(12;21) and HMGA2 rearrangement: report of a case and review of the literature. *Cancer Genet Cytogenet* 181:119–124.

Ren T, Lu Q, Guo W, Lou Z, Peng X, Jiao G, et al. (2013): The clinical implication of SS18-SSX fusion gene in synovial sarcoma. *Brit J Cancer* 109:2279–2285.

Rieker RJ, Joos S, Bartsch C, Willeke F, Schwarzbach M, Otano-Joos M, et al. (2002): Distinct chromosomal imbalances in pleomorphic and in high-grade dedifferentiated liposarcomas. *Int J Cancer* 99:68–73.

Robinson DR, Wu Y-M, Kalyana-Sundaram S, Cao X, Lonigro RJ, Sung Y-S, et al. (2013): Identification of recurrent NAB2-STAT6 gene fusion in solitary fibrous tumor by integrative sequencing. *Nat Genet* 45:180–187.

Rossi S, Szuhai K, Ijszenga M, Tanke HJ, Zanatta L, Sciot R, et al. (2007): EWSR1-CREB1 and EWSR1-ATF1 fusion genes in angiomatoid fibrous histiocytoma. *Clin Cancer Res* 13:7322–7328.

Rubin BP, Chen C-J, Morgan TW, Xiao S, Grier HE, Kozakewich HP, et al. (1998): Congenital mesoblastic nephroma t(12;15) is associated with ETV6-NTRK3 gene fusion. Cytogenetic and molecular relationship to congenital (infantile) fibrosarcoma. *Am J Pathol* 153:1451–1458.

Schoenmakers EFPM, Wanschura S, Mols R, Bullerdiek J, Van den Berghe H, Van de Ven WJM (1995): Recurrent rearrangements in the high mobility group protein gene, HMGI-C, in benign mesenchymal tumours. *Nat Genet* 10:436–444.

Schweizer L, Koelsche C, Sahm F, Piro RM, Capper D, Reuss DE, et al. (2013): Meningeal hemangiopericytoma and solitary fibrous tumors carry the NAB2-STAT6 fusion and can be diagnosed by nuclear expression of STAT6 protein. *Acta Neuropathol* 125:651–658.

Sciot R, Akerman M, Dal Cin P, De Wever I, Fletcher CDM, Mandahl N, et al. (1997): Cytogenetic analysis of subcutaneous angiolipoma: further evidence supporting its difference from ordinary pure lipomas. A report of the CHAMP study group. *Am J Surg Pathol* 21:441–444.

Sciot R, Rosai J, Dal Cin P, de Wever I, Fletcher CDM, Mandahl N, et al. (1999): Analysis of 35 cases of localized and diffuse tenosynovial giant cell tumor: a report from the chromosomes and morphology (CHAMP) study group. *Mod Pathol* 12:576–579.

Simon M-P, Pedeutour F, Sirvent N, Grosgeorge J, Minoletti F, Coindre J-M, et al. (1997): Deregulation of the platelet-derived growth factor B-chain gene via fusion with collagen gene COL1A1 in dermatofibrosarcoma protuberans and giant-cell fibroblastoma. *Nat Genet* 15:95–98.

Singer S, Socci ND, Ambrosini G, Sambol E, Decarolis P, Wu Y, et al. (2007): Gene expression profiling of liposarcoma identifies distinct biological types/subtypes and potential therapeutic targets in well-differentiated and dedifferentiated liposarcoma. *Cancer Res* 67:6626–6636.

Sjögren H, Meis-Kindblom JM, Örndal C, Bergh P, Ptaszynski K, Åman P, et al. (2003): Studies on the molecular pathogenesis of extraskeletal myxoid chondrosarcoma—cytogenetic, molecular genetic, and cDNA microarray analyses. *Am J Pathol* 162:781–792.

Slater O, Shipley J (2007): Clinical relevance of molecular genetics to paediatric sarcomas. *J Clin Pathol* 60:1187–1194.

Sreekantaiah C, Leong SPL, Karakousis CP, McGee DL, Rappaport WD, Villar HV, et al. (1991): Cytogenetic profile of 109 lipomas. *Cancer Res* 51:422–433.

Sumegi J, Streblow R, Frayer RW, Dal Cin P, Rosenberg A, Meloni-Ehrig A, et al. (2010): Recurrent t(2;2) and t(2;8) translocations in rhabdomyosarcoma without the canonical PAX-FOXO1 fuse PAX3 to members of the nuclear receptor transcriptional coactivator family. *Genes Chromosomes Cancer* 49:224–236.

Takeuchi K, Soda M, Togashi Y, Sugawara E, Hatano S, Asaka R, et al. (2011): Pulmonary inflammatory myofibroblastic tumor expressing a novel fusion, PPFIBP1-ALK: reappraisal of anti-ALK immunohistochemistry as a tool for novel ALK fusion identification. *Clin Cancer Res* 17:3341–3348.

Tanaka M, Kato K, Gomi K, Matsumoto M, Kudo H, Shinkai M, et al. (2009): Perivascular epithelioid cell tumor with SFPQ/PSF-TFE3 gene fusion in a patient with advanced neuroblastoma. *Am J Surg Pathol* 33:1416–1420.

Tanas MR, Sboner A, Oliveira AM, Erickson-Johnson MR, Hespelt J, Hanwright PJ, et al. (2011): Identification of a disease-defining gene fusion in epithelioid hemangioendothelioma. *Sci Transl Med* 3:98ra82.

Tejpar S, Nollet F, Li C, Wunder JS, Michils G, Dal Cin P, et al. (1999): Predominance of beta-catenin mutations and beta-catenin dysregulation in sporadic aggressive fibromatosis (desmoid tumor). *Oncogene* 18:6615–6620.

Turc-Carel C, Limon J, Dal Cin P, Rao U, Karakousis C, Sandberg AA (1986): Cytogenetic studies of adipose tissue tumors. II. Recurrent reciprocal translocation t(12;16)(q13;p11) in myxoid liposarcomas. *Cancer Genet Cytogenet* 23:291–299.

Wachtel M, Dettling M, Koscielniak E, Stegmaier S, Treuner J, Simon-Klingenstein K, et al. (2004): Gene expression signatures identify rhabdomyosarcoma subtypes and detect a novel t(2;2)(q35;p23) translocation fusing PAX3 to NCOA1. *Cancer Res* 64:5539–5545.

Walther C, Tayebwa J, Lilljebjörn H, Magnusson L, Nilsson J, Vult von Steyern F, et al. (2014): A novel SERPINE1-FOSB fusion gene results in transcriptional upregulation of FOSB in pseudomyogenic hemangioendothelioma. *J Pathol* 232:534–540.

Wang R, Lu Y-J, Fisher C, Bridge JA, Shipley J (2001): Characterization of chromosome aberrations associated with soft-tissue leiomyosarcomas by twenty-four-color karyotyping and comparative genomic hybridization analysis. *Genes Chromosomes Cancer* 31:54–64.

Wang R, Titley JC, Lu Y-J, Summersgill BM, Bridge JA, Fisher C, et al. (2003): Loss of 13q14-q21 and gain of 5p14-pter in the progression of leiomyosarcoma. *Mod Pathol* 16:778–785.

Wang W-L, Mayordomo E, Zhang W, Hernandez VS, Tuvin D, Garcia L, et al. (2009): Detection and characterization of EWSR1/ATF1 and EWSR1/CREB1 chimeric transcripts in clear cell sarcoma (melanoma of soft parts). *Mod Pathol* 22:1201–1209.

Wang W-L, Evans HL, Meis JM, Liegl-Atzwanger B, Bovée JV, Goldblum JR, et al. (2012): FUS rearrangements are rare in "pure" sclerosing epithelioid fibrosarcoma. *Mod Patol* 25:846–853.

West RB, Rubin BP, Miller MA, Subramanian S, Kaygusuz G, Montgomery K, et al. (2006): A landscape effect in tenosynovial giant-cell tumor from activation of CSF1 expression by a translocation in a minority of tumor cells. *Proc Natl Acad Sci USA* 103:690–695.

Willeke F, Ridder R, Mechtersheimer G, Schwarzbach M, Duwe A, Weitz J, et al. (1998): Analysis of FUS-CHOP fusion transcripts in different types of soft tissue liposarcoma and their diagnostic implications. *Clin Cancer Res* 4:1779–1784.

Willems SM, Debiec-Rychter M, Szuhai K, Hogendoorn PCW, Sciot R (2006): Local recurrence of myxofibrosarcoma is associated with increase in tumor grade and cytogenetic aberrations, suggesting a multistep tumour progression model. *Mod Pathol* 19:407–416.

Xia SJ, Pressey JG, Barr FG (2002): Molecular pathogenesis of rhabdomyosarcoma. *Cancer Biol Therapy* 1:97–104.

Yoshida H, Miyachi M, Ouchi K, Kuwahara Y, Tsuchiya K, Iehara T, et al. (2014): Identification of COL3A1 and RAB2A as novel translocation partner genes of PLAG1 in lipoblastomas. Genes Chromosomes Cancer in press.

Zaidi MR, Okada Y, Chada KK (2006): Misexpression of full-length HMGA2 induces benign mesenchymal tumors in mice. *Cancer Res* 66:7453–7459.

Zhang H, MacDonald WD, Erickson-Johnson M, Wang X, Jenkins RB, Oliveira AM (2007): Cytogenetic and molecular cytogenetic findings of intimal sarcoma. *Cancer Genet Cytogenet* 179:146–149.

Zhao J, Roth J, Bode-Lesniewska B, Pfaltz M, Heitz PU, Komminoth P (2002): Combined comparative genomic hybridization and genomic microarray for detection of gene amplifications in pulmonary artery intimal sarcomas and adrenocortical tumors. *Genes Chromosomes Cancer* 34:48–57.

Index

Cancer Cytogenetics: Chromosomal and Molecular Genetic Aberrations of Tumor Cells, Fourth Edition.
Edited by Sverre Heim and Felix Mitelman.
© 2015 John Wiley & Sons, Ltd. Published 2015 by John Wiley & Sons, Ltd.